RHEUMATOID ARTHRITIS

Oxford University Press makes no representation, express or implied, that the drug dosages in this book are correct. Readers must therefore always check the product information and clinical procedures with the most up-to-date published product information and data sheets provided by the manufacturers and the most recent codes of conduct and safety regulations. The authors and the publishers do not accept responsibility or legal liability for any errors in the text or for the misuse or misapplication of material in this work.

RHEUMATOID ARTHRITIS

FRONTIERS IN PATHOGENESIS AND TREATMENT

Edited by

Gary S. Firestein

Professor of Medicine, University of California, San Diego School of Medicine,
La Jolla, USA

Gabriel S. Panayi

Professor of Rheumatology, UMDS Guy's and St Thomas's, London, UK

and

Frank A. Wollheim

Professor of Rheumatology, Lund University Hospital, Lund, Sweden

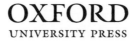
OXFORD
UNIVERSITY PRESS

MT

OXFORD

UNIVERSITY PRESS

Great Clarendon Street, Oxford OX2 6DP
Oxford University Press is a department of the University of Oxford.
It furthers the University's objective of excellence in research, scholarship,
and education by publishing worldwide in

Oxford New York

Athens Auckland Bangkok Bogotá Buenos Aires Calcutta
Cape Town Chennai Dar es Salaam Delhi Florence Hong Kong Istanbul
Karachi Kuala Lumpur Madrid Melbourne Mexico City Mumbai
Nairobi Paris São Paulo Singapore Taipei Tokyo Toronto Warsaw

with associated companies
in Berlin Ibadan

Oxford is a registered trade mark of Oxford University Press
in the UK and in certain other countries

Published in the United States
by Oxford University Press, Inc., New York

© G. S. Firestein, G. S. Panayi, and F. A. Wollheim, 2000

The moral rights of the author have been asserted

Database right Oxford University Press (maker)

First published 2000

A catalogue record for this title is available
from the British Library

Library of Congress Cataloging in Publication Data
Rheumatoid arthritis: frontiers in pathogenesis and treatment/edited by Gary Firestein, Gabriel Panayi, and Frank Wollheim.
Includes bibliographical references.
1. Rheumatoid arthritis. I. Firestein, Gary S. II. Panayi, Gabriel S. (Gabriel Stavros) III. Wollheim, Frank A.
[DNLM: 1. Arthritis, Rheumatoid–therapy 2. Arthritis,
Rheumatoid–physiopathology. WE 346 R47302 2000]
RC933.R4286 2000   616.7'227–dc21   99-059424

1 3 5 7 9 10 8 6 4 2

ISBN 0 19 262972 7 (Hbk)

Typeset by EXPO Holdings, Malaysia

Printed in Great Britain on acid free paper by
Butler & Tanner Ltd,
Frome, Somerset

9/5/0

Preface

In the age of information technology proliferation, do we need another textbook on rheumatoid arthritis? The three editors of this book and the publisher that supported us in planning the chapters and selection of contributors clearly think so. Nevertheless, we have asked ourselves if we did the right thing in accepting such a burden: seeing the results now, however, we are very pleased. In the end, it will be the readers who decide if it has been a worthwhile effort. One of the frustrations in this process is the necessary time lag between conceptualization of the project and completion of the finished product. This two year process has seen many changes in the world of rheumatoid arthritis: the approval and rapid acceptance of anti-cytokine therapy, the discovery of new cytokines and signal transduction pathways, new concepts on the pathogenesis of the disease. Although the final editing process allowed us to include some of this information, there is no way to be completely up to date. Despite this limitation, we hope that the book provides a sound basis for scientists and clinicians to understand and appreciate the nuances of rheumatoid arthritis. Several decades ago George Thorn commented after an impressive meeting on rheumatoid arthritis 'We now know all about the disease, except what causes it and how to treat it.' Perhaps this is still true today. However, a new wave of optimism sweeps this field. Advances in cell biology uncover pathways of inflammation and tissue injury, which lead to better understanding of the pathogenesis. The new knowledge opens possibilities for novel attempts to intervene. The marketing of new pharmaceuticals and biologicals for the therapy of rheumatoid arthritis in 2000 is one tangible example, and experienced rheumatologists are speaking of a paradigm shift. We are approaching a situation where the limited availability of motivated and suitable patients for trials of new treatments may hamper new drug development. This situation calls for the widest possible international co-operation.

TNF inhibition results in impressive symptomatic relief and slowing of structural damage, at least in the short term. One is reminded of the excitement half a century ago, when the early effects of cortisone were presented. It may be good to remember the words of Philip Hench at the famous congress in the Waldorf Astoria: 'this is not the cure for rheumatoid arthritis, but it gives us a new handle to study its nature'. Rheumatoid arthritis is, as all know, a complex disease, and we should not be naïve in hoping for a cause or a cure. More likely, its pathogenesis will turn out to involve both genetic and environmental factors, and effective control will require a combination of treatments. So, returning to the question on the need for a new textbook, we feel that the explosion of new knowledge has a profound impact on the understanding of rheumatoid arthritis and on the management of our patients, and that this motivates a fresh in-depth text. The 44 chapters cover a wide range of topics and bring together current knowledge from the laboratory to the bedside; drug as well as non-drug therapy; psychological and economic impact. The selection of the team of contributors conveys a truly international state-of-the-art picture at the dawn of the new millennium. We are very grateful for the hard work provided by all the contributors. We also want to thank Oxford University Press for their expert help.

La Jolla, London, and Lund
June 2000

Gary S. Firestein
Gabriel S. Panayi
Frank A. Wollheim

Contents

Colour plates are located between pages 272–273

SECTION 6   SURGICAL THERAPY

SECTION 7   FRONTIERS OF THERAPY

Contributors

Alarcón, Graciela S.; Division of Clinical Immunology and Rheumatology, University of Alabama, Birmingham, Alabama, USA.

Arend, William P.; Division of Rheumatology, University of Colorado Health Sciences Center, Denver, Colorado, USA

Badger, Alison M.; Smithkline Beecham Pharmaceuticals, King of Prussia, Pennsylvania, USA

Blake, David; School of Postgraduate Medicine, University of Bath, Bath, UK

Breedveld, Ferdinand C.; Department of Rheumatology, Leiden University Medical Center, Leiden, The Netherlands

Brooks, Peter M.; University of Queensland, Royal Brisbane Hospital, Herston, Australia

Burmester, Gerd-R.; Department of Rheumatology and Clinical Immunology, Charité University Hospital, Humboldt University of Berlin, Germany

Callahan, Leigh F.; Thurston Arthritis Research Center, University of North Carolina, Chapel Hill, North Carolina, USA

Calvo, Franz; Division of Clinical Immunology and Rheumatology, University of Alabama, Birmingham, Alabama, USA

Carson, Dennis A.; Division of Rheumatology, Allergy and Immunology, University of California, San Diego, California, USA

Casey, A.T.H.; Department of Surgical Neurology, The National Hospital for Neurology and Neurosurgery and Royal National Orthopaedic Hospital, London, UK

Chatham, W. Winn; Division of Clinical Immunology and Rheumatology, Department of Medicine, University of Alabama at Birmingham, Birmingham, Alabama, USA

Choy, Ernest H.S.; Academic Rheumatology Unit, Guy's King's Collage and St Thomas' Hospitals Medical and Dental School, London, UK

Coakley, Gerald; Molecular Immunogenetics Unit, Department of Rheumatology, Guy's King's and St Thomas' School of Medicine, London, UK

Conaghan, Philip G.; Rheumatology and Rehabilitation Research Unit, University of Leeds, Leeds, UK

Crockard, H.A.; Department of Surgical Neurology, The National Hospital for Neurology and Neurosurgery, London, UK

Day, Richard; Department of Clinical Pharmacology and Toxicology, St Vincents Hospital, Sydney, Australia

Diallo, S.; Service de Rheumatologie, Groupe Hospitalier Cochin, Paris, France

Dijkmans, Ben A.C.; Free University Hospital, Slotervaart Hospital and Jan van Breemen Institute, Amsterdam, The Netherlands

Doherty, Michael; Academic Rheumatology, City Hospital, Nottingham, UK

Edberg, Jeffrey C.; Division of Clinical Immunology and Rheumatology, Departments of Medicine and Microbiology, University of Alabama at Birmingham, Alabama, USA

Elenkov, Ilia J.; Inflammatory Joint Diseases Section, Arthritis and Rheumatism Branch, National Institute of Arthritis and Musculoskeletal and Skin Diseases, Bethesda, Maryland, USA

Fife, Mark; Molecular Immunogenetics Unit, Department of Rheumatology, Guy's King's and St Thomas' School of Medicine, London, UK

Fox, David A.; Multipurpose Arthritis and Musculoskeletal Disease Center and Division of Rheumatology, University of Michigan Medical Center, Ann Arbor, Michigan, USA

Gabay, Cem; Division of Rheumatology, University of Colorado Health Sciences Center, Denver, Colorado, USA

Gay, Renate E.; Center for Experimental Rheumatology and WHO Collaborating Center for Molecular Biology and Novel Therapeutic Strategies for Rheumatic Diseases, University Hospital, Zürich, Switzerland

Gay, Steffen; Center for Experimental Rheumatology and WHO Collaborating Center for Molecular Biology and Novel Therapeutic Strategies for Rheumatic Diseases, University Hospital, Zürich, Switzerland

Graham, Garry; School of Physiology and Pharmacology and Medicine, University of New South Wales, Australia

Gulko, Pércio S.; Divisions of Rheumatology and Autoimmune and Molecular Diseases, Department of Pediatrics, Columbia University College of Physicians and Surgeons, New York, USA

Hällgren, Roger; Section Rheumatology, Department of Internal Medicine, University Hospital, Uppsala, Sweden

Hamann, Wolfgang; Department of Anaesthetics, King's College, Guy's and Lewisham Hospitals, London, UK

Holmdahl, Rikard; Section for Medical Inflammation Research, Lund University, Lund, Sweden

Huizinga, Tom W.J.; Department of Rheumatology, Leiden University Medical Center, Leiden, The Netherlands

Kalden-Nemeth, Dolores; Department of Internal Medicine III, Friedrich-Alexander University, Erlangen, Germany

Kidd, Bruce; Division of Pharmacology, St Bartholomew's and Royal London School of Medicine, London, UK

Kimberly, Robert P.; Division of Clinical Immunology and Rheumatology, Departments of Medicine and Microbiology, University of Alabama at Birmingham, Alabama, USA

Kingsley, Gabrielle; Guy's King's and St Thomas' School of Medicine, King's College and University Hospital, Lewisham, London, UK

Kinne, Raimund W.; Experimental Rheumatology Unit, Friedrich Schiller University, Jena, Germany

Kroot, Eric-Jan J.A.; University Hospital, Nijmegen, The Netherlands

Kvien, Tore Kristian; Oslo City Department of Rheumatology, Vinderen Diakonhjemmet Hospital, Oslo, Norway

Kyburz, Diego; Division of Rheumatology, Allergy and Immunology, University of California, San Diego, California, USA

Lanchbury, Jerry; Molecular Immunogenetics Unit, Department of Rheumatology, Guy's King's and St Thomas' School of Medicine, London, UK

Lanyon, Peter; Clinical Immunology Unit, University Hospital and Academic Rheumatology City Hospital, Nottingham, UK

Leirisalo-Repo, Marjatta; Department of Rheumatology, University of Lund, Lund, Sweden

Lems, William F.; Free University Hospital, Slotervaart Hospital and Jan van Breemen Institute, Amsterdam, The Netherlands

Lindroth, Ylva; Slottstadens Läkargrupp, Malmö, Sweden

Manger, Bernhard; Department of Internal Medicine III, Friedrich-Alexander University, Erlangen, Germany

Manning, Anthony M.; Signal Pharmaceuticals Inc., San Diego, California, USA

Månsson, Bengt; Department of Cell and Molecular Biology, Lund University, Lund, Sweden

Mapp, Paul; School of Postgraduate Medicine, University of Bath, Bath, UK

March, Lynnette; Department of Rheumatology, Royal North Shore Hospital, Sydney, Australia

Menkes, C.J.; Service de Rheumatologie, Groupe Hospitalier Cochin, Paris, France

Moritz, Ulrich; Department of Physical Therapy, Lund University, Lund, Sweden

Nordenskiöld, Ulla; Department of Occupational Therapy, Sahlgrenska University Hospital, Goteborg, Sweden

O'Gradaigh, Donnchal; Rheumatology Department, Norfolk and Norwich Hospital, Norwich, Norfolk, UK

Palombo-Kinne, Ernesta; Experimental Rheumatology Unit, Friedrich Schiller University, Jena, Germany

Pap, Thomas; Center for Experimental Rheumatology and WHO Collaborating Center for Molecular Biology and Novel Therapeutic Strategies for Rheumatic Diseases, University Hospital, Zürich, Switzerland

Pitzalis, Costantino; Rheumatology Unit, Guy's St Thomas' and King's College, School of Medicine and Dentistry, London, UK

Quinn, David; Department of Medicine, St Vincents Hospital, Sydney, Australia

Rau, Rolf; Department of Rheumatology, Evangelisches Fachkrankenhaus, Ratingen, Germany

Rydholm, Urban; Department of Orthopedics, Lund University, Lund, Sweden

Saxne, Tore; Department of Rheumatology, Lund University, Lund, Sweden

Scott, D.G.I.; Rheumatology Department, Norfolk and Norwich Hospital, Norwich, Norfolk, UK

Scott, David L.; Department of Rheumatology, King's College Hospital, London, UK

Seki, Tetsunori; Division of Autoimmune and Molecular Diseases, Columbia University College of Physicians and Surgeons, New York, New York, USA

Shaw, Tim; Roche Products Ltd. Welwyn Garden City, UK

Sköldstam, Lars; Rheumatology Department, Lasarettet, Kalmar, Sweden

Smedstad, Liv Marit; Oslo City Department of Rheumatology, Vinderen Diakonhjemmet Hospital, Oslo, Norway

Sollerman, Christer; Division E Hand Surgery, Sahlgrenska Hospital, Goteborg, Sweden

Stuhlmüller, Bruno; Department of Rheumatology and Clinical Immunology, Charité University Hospital, Humboldt University of Berlin, Germany

Tak, Paul-Peter; Division of Clinical Immunology and Rheumatology, Academic Medical Center, Amsterdam, The Netherlands

van Riel, Piet L.C.M.; University Hospital, Nijmegen, The Netherlands

Watts, Richards; Rheumatology Department, Norfolk and Norwich Hospital, Norwich, Norfolk, UK

Wilder, Ronald L.; Inflammatory Joint Diseases Section, Arthritis and Rheumatism Branch, National Institute of Arthritis and Musculoskeletal and Skin Diseases, Bethesda, Maryland, USA

Williams, Kenneth; School of Physiology and Pharmacology and Medicine, University of New South Wales, Australia

Winchester, Robert; Divisions of Rheumatology and Autoimmune and Molecular Diseases, Departments of Medicine and Pediatrics, Columbia University College of Physicians and Surgeons, New York, New York, USA

Zvaifler, Nathan J.; Division of Rheumatology, Allergy and Immunology, University of California, San Diego, California, USA

SECTION 1 | *Etiology*

1 | Current perspectives on the genetics of rheumatoid arthritis

Mark Fife, Gerald Coakley, and Jerry Lanchbury

Introduction

The polygenic nature of rheumatoid arthritis (RA) serves as a source of great fascination and frustration for the identification of candidate genes involved in this disease. With the Human Genome Project (HGP) reaching fruition, we now face the prospect that an undefined number of the estimated 60 000–100 000 genes may play a role in disease susceptibility[1,2]. With current and developing methodologies, including the increasingly dense genetic maps generated from the HGP, it is likely that we will soon find ourselves in the auspicious position of clarifying the major genes involved in this complex, immune-mediated disease[3]. To date, the most extensively examined region of the human genome remains the MHC gene cluster on the short arm of chromosome 6 (6p21. 3).

Variation in the human major histocompatibility complex (MHC) has long been associated with autoimmune diseases[4]. More specifically, the HLA region and its contribution to disease susceptibility has been well documented for RA[5,6]. This chapter will focus on HLA and non-HLA genes that predispose individuals to the disease. To appreciate fully the advances made in the dissection of this complex disease it will be important to achieve a basic understanding of the methods and technologies employed for genetic analysis of RA. These concepts will be discussed in the first part of this chapter.

The genetic basis of RA

Traits that show simple dominant or recessive Mendelian inheritance embody a direct relationship between genotype and phenotype. The situation in RA and most other immune-mediated diseases appears to be very different[7,8]. Relatively common complex diseases such as RA are unlikely to be dependent on the inheritance of single disease genes. Rather, it is likely that multiple genes collectively determine susceptibility and/or disease progression, with no individual gene being necessary or sufficient for clinical symptoms of the disease. It is mainly as a result of this incomplete penetrance of polygenic disease genes that progress in the understanding of the genetics of RA has been relatively slow[9]. A consequence of the complexity of the genetic background to RA and the relatively late age of disease onset is that there is unlikely to be strong selection against predisposition genes in a disease-specific context, as is the case for genes causing many monogenic diseases. However, polymorphic loci that contribute to the genetic basis of RA might be under selection in other contexts. HLA is the best discussed example with balancing selection mechanisms, such as heterozygote advantage or frequency-dependent selection, suggested to maintain the high degree of polymorphism[10–12]. For most loci active in maintaining variation in immune system function, infectious disease has been posited as the relevant selective force[13, 14]. Thus in this scenario, the alleles causing RA susceptibility would not be confined to the disease group but found throughout the general population. A further potential level of complexity also exists with susceptibility genes that interact with one another (epistasis) or alternative genes acting independently of one another (genetic heterogeneity) resulting in disease[15,16].

Epidemiologists studying complex diseases like RA employ familial clustering of disease to quantify the genetic component of susceptibility. Familial clustering is classically defined as the ratio of prevalence within families with an affected member to the general population prevalence (expressed as λ_R)[7]. Where affected sib pair families are used for genetic analysis λ_S is used to quantify familial clustering. A λ_S of 1 indicates that there is no risk of disease conferred by genetic (more strictly, familial) factors. Rheumatoid arthritis has a λ_S of between 5 and 7.2[12,17], of which the MHC contribution is estimated to be approximately one-third[5, 18]. Bearing in mind that the total value of λ_S includes any environmental factors contributing to the disease, it is apparent that the remaining non-MHC factors susceptibility components each contribute to a limited extent.

Another epidemiological method of testing familial clustering is the comparison of disease prevalence between monozygotic (MZ) and dizygotic (DZ) twins. In RA the concordance rate, expressed as the fraction of twin pairs that share the disease phenotype (MZ/DZ), is estimated to be 12–15 per cent/ 3.6 per cent[19–21]. Thus, although there is greater concordance in MZ twins compared to DZ twins, generally only one member of an MZ twin pair is affected, despite their identical genetic makeup. In a recent, comparative study of two twin cohorts, the heritability of RA estimated by variance components analysis was 65 per cent in Finland and 53 per cent in the United Kingdom[22]. From these studies it is evident that genetic factors make a significant contribution to RA accounting for approximately 60 per cent of the variance of risk for disease development. However, the 40 per cent residual component shows that both environmental and non-genetic development factors are also likely to play an important role in the development of RA[23].

Despite the challenges encountered by the nature of the genetic predisposition to RA and the problems identifying common environmental triggers, the difficulties in differentiating cause and effect in observational investigation of pathogenesis are also problematical. The genetic approach offers clear theoretical advantages and, given recent technological advances and the development of family-based and population resources for genetic study, we are now in a position to make inroads in understanding the underlying genetic causes of this complex, immune-mediated disease.

Current strategies used in the genetic analysis of RA

Whether one focuses on a single candidate gene, a relatively large chromosomal region, or indeed an extensive genome-wide screen, current methods used for analysis of complex genetic diseases fall into two distinct categories: **association and linkage studies**. Logically, in the absence of prior knowledge of the location of genetic predisposition factors, the current initial strategy is a genome scan. Enthusiasm for this approach, however, has to be tempered by the power limitations of available family collections and the false assignment rate. Well designed candidate gene studies have an important role and ultimately every replicated (and even non-replicated) genome scan should lead to a candidate gene phase. Historically, the first studies on genetic risk loci in RA were carried out in populations using a case-control design since HLA class I and II were suitable *a priori* candidates.

Association studies

The earliest replicated association studies for RA were conducted in the 1970s by Stastny and colleagues in the United States and by Panayi and colleagues in the United Kingdom[24-26] The initial demonstration of an association between a cellular mixed lymphocyte reaction determinant (HLA-Dw4) and RA was followed by a description of significantly raised frequencies of the HLA-DR4 serological determinant. Association studies involve the comparison of affected and unaffected members of a population. An allele of a candidate gene is said to be in association with a phenotypic trait (in this case disease) if the frequency of the allele is shown to be significantly higher in the affected individuals than in the control group. Although this method is an effective statistical tool for genetic analysis, false positive associations can easily be generated if the control group used in the study is not very closely matched to those of the affected group. Consistent with the scientific method, the hypothesis that the gene or gene region of interest is involved in disease susceptibility must be tested by replication studies in case-control populations sharing characteristics with the original study group. Positive associations do not necessarily implicate the tested polymorphisms or locus in disease predisposition due the existence of linkage disequilibrium across the human genome. Linkage disequilibrium is the existence of preferential combinations of alleles across a given genomic region. The consequence is that association with a genetic marker will also be reflected in raised frequencies of those alleles that are in allelic association with the said marker. Independent evidence from biological investigations in addition to the genetic studies is essential to gain a realistic view of the causal relationship between the variation and phenotype. The degree of linkage disequilibrium found across the human genome for a given population depends on a number of factors including current and previous population size, age of polymorphic variants, selection history, and patterns of migration[27-29]. Relatively isolated populations such as the Finns and Icelanders show extensive linkage disequilibrium[30]. Such populations have attracted great interest for disease gene mapping since single disease mutations, contributing to a complex disease, may have undergone only limited meiotic recombination with flanking markers[31-33]. Fine mapping the chromosomal region from the isolated population showing the association may lead to the identification of the genuine disease-causing allele[15,34]. In several diseases with a relatively simple genetic background this strategy has proved effective, though its general utility has yet to be established for complex disease. The relevance of disease-determining polymorphisms from isolated, distantly related populations to the large, outbred continental groups has yet to be evaluated systematically[35].

Whereas true disease association and that seen as a result of linkage disequilibrium of a locus with a disease gene may eventually lead to the identification of the *bona fide* disease susceptibility gene, population stratification or substructure may lead to both false positive and false negative associations, although the parameters for the latter case have not been extensively investigated. The form of population stratification relevant to most common, complex disease studies is that arising in contemporarily large, mixed populations where there has been a significant degree of admixture. In this instance, the case and control samples may at worst be drawn from distinct populations, particularly if the constituent populations differ in the prevalence of the disease in question[15]. Thus when selecting an appropriate case and control population one must ensure ethnic and geographic homogeneity. A number of procedures have now been adopted in an attempt to eliminate the risks brought about by population stratification. The most robust approach currently used is the haplotype relative risk method, where a fictitious individual is generated from the parent alleles not inherited by the affected sibling[15]. This internal control individual eliminates any chance of population stratification because the case and controls now share the same parental chromosomes. Although this method has proved beneficial in a number of association studies, its potential for use in late-onset diseases such as RA, where both parents may not be available, may be overestimated. A further disadvantage is that unusually structured family collections are required and the approach may not be applicable to currently held data sets.

Linkage analysis

Linkage analysis is the archetypal method of examining the segregation of genetic markers with disease within pedigrees. It involves the construction of transmission models to elucidate the inheritance pattern of gene marker loci within families[36]. Initially, it was used to examine the genetics of a number of simple Mendelian traits, but is now being applied to more complex diseases with encouraging results[37–39]. The fundamental aim of linkage analysis is to determine whether there is cosegregation of a general marker and disease within a population. A disease allele will always be inherited with the genetic marker in a family, unless recombination between the two loci occurs. Phenotypic expression, however, may not always occur. Thus the frequency of recombination (θ) is proportional to the distance between the genetic marker of interest and the disease locus. A recombination rate of 10 per cent ($\theta = 0.1$) equates to a genetic distance of 10 centimorgan (cM) or approximately 10 Mb of DNA in physical terms. Where the genetic marker is very close to the gene $\theta = 0$ and the marker will invariably be inherited with the disease.

Before evidence of linkage has been demonstrated for a genetic marker and a disease-causing allele, the distance between them is unknown. The null hypothesis is that the marker and disease genes are unlinked. Since there is at least one recombination event per chromosome in each meiotic division, if the null hypothesis stands then both loci will be inherited together 50 per cent of the time ($\theta = 0.5$). However, if the two loci are in relatively close proximity, or indeed if the genetic marker lies within the disease gene then $\theta = 0$. Having established at what level the marker and disease loci cosegregate within the affected cohort, the probability of observing the segregation pattern can be determined. The ratio of these probabilities is measured as the likelihood ratio: $Z(\theta)$.

$$Z(\theta) = \frac{\text{probability of observing segregation pattern if } \theta = 0}{\text{probability of observing segregation pattern if } \theta = 0.5}$$

The $\log_{10}$ of this ratio is the more conventional method of expressing evidence for linkage, where $\log_{10} Z(\theta)$ is the lod score. In reality, because the distance between the disease allele and the genetic marker is unknown, a best fit value of θ is tested to give the highest lod score for the data. This method is called the maximum likelihood estimation (MLE) method. There is sufficient evidence for linkage when the traditional threshold lod score of 3 is obtained for a set value of θ. This means that for this particular theta value the evidence for linkage is 1000 times greater than for non-linkage.

One of the drawbacks of classical linkage analysis is that an appropriate model must be established to prevent false linkage assignments while not failing to establish genuine linkage. Lander and Kruglyak (1995) proposed a number of guidelines for the interpretation of linkage results for complex traits. These criteria are based on the rate at which one would expect to observe evidence of linkage in a dense genome scan. In this classification there are four levels of observed linkage.

- **Suggestive linkage**: evidence for linkage that would be expected to occur on an average of once in a whole genome scan. Results showing suggestive linkage, although interesting, should be treated with an appropriate level of suspicion. An independent 'extension study' can be used to examine more closely the reported level of linkage.
- **Significant linkage**: evidence for linkage that would be expected to occur no more than 0.05 times in a whole genome scan.

- **Highly significant linkage**: evidence for linkage that would be expected to occur no more than 0.001 times in a whole genome scan.
- **Confirmed linkage**: confirmation of a significant level of linkage in a subsequent independent study. Such a study is specifically referred to as a 'replication study'. As a consequence of the genetic heterogeneity of RA and other complex disease, a replication study may or may not confirm the original study[40,41].

The actual values of the lod scores and significance levels for each of these classes of linkage will vary according to the nature of the statistical method being used for the analysis[42].

Allele-sharing methods

In general the more complex the disease under investigation the more difficult it is to use classical linkage analysis to explore the underlying genetic basis of the disease. Unlike linkage analysis, the allele-sharing method of genetic analysis is a non-parametric method and thus requires no knowledge of the mode of inheritance of a disease. In RA and other complex diseases where penetrance and degree of genetic heterogeneity of the disease is unknown, the allele-sharing method has been accepted as the rational choice for genetic analysis despite its relative insensitivity. Non-parametric linkage analysis can be performed using the sib-pair or the affected-pedigree-member (APM) methods[43]. In a complex multifactorial disease such as RA, where only HLA-linked loci have been implicated in disease susceptibility, single point linkage analysis is seldom used, except in the case of candidate genes. In searching for these additional disease genes, the approach of genome-wide scanning (or screening) has recently been adopted. Unlike single point linkage analysis where the significance level is the likelihood that one would encounter such an extreme deviation at the specific locus by chance, the significance level of a genome screen is the measure of the probability of finding such a deviation across the whole genome. Thus the former involves testing the null hypothesis of no linkage, whereas the latter sifts through a large number of tests in order to find the most significant deviation.

The practicality of genome-wide linkage analysis has been vastly enhanced by identification of large numbers of polymorphic genetic markers. The previous generation of RFLP and variable number tandem repeat (VNTR) DNA markers has been largely superceded by the description and genetic mapping of simple sequence repeat (SSR) markers commonly termed microsatellites[44, 45]. These consist of discrete genetic regions that contain short repetitive elements that vary in length between individuals. The most widely used microsatellite markers are the di-, tri-, and tetranucleotide repeats with a simple repeating unit of two, three, and four nucleotides, respectively. These markers are selected so that the number of repeats is so highly polymorphic within a population that most individuals are heterozygous for any particular microsatellite allele. This extensive heterozygosity allows the inheritance of specific alleles to be traced in families. Current methods of genome screening use approximately 350 markers evenly spread across the entire genome, at an average of one marker per 10 cM[46].

Genetic dissection of RA

At present one extensive genome screen for RA has been completed and published, although several more are ongoing in the academic sector totaling in excess of 1000 affected sibling pairs. The two sets of genome scan data that are available detected the major role of the HLA region while also suggesting novel chromosomal regions that merit further study. Cornelis reported a genome scan performed in 114 European Caucasian RA sib pairs from 97 nuclear families[47]. The group found significant linkage only for HLA ($p < 2.5 \times 10^{-5}$). Nominal linkage was found for 19 markers in 14 other regions ($p < 0.05$). Two of these markers were studied in a second group of families. Support for linkage to chromosome 3 only was extended significantly ($p = 0.002$). This locus accounted for 16 per cent of the genetic component of RA. The relative contributions to the λ_S for RA (assuming $\lambda_S = 5$) for the HLA locus (at TNFα) and that of chromosome 3 marker were estimated to be 1.7 and 1.3, respectively[47]. A previous partial genome scan on 89 affected sib pair families reported linkage to HLA ($p = 0.0003$) and several loci outside HLA[41]. Both these studies reported linkage to the HLA region confirming the capacity of the approach to detect genetic effects already confirmed by association studies at the population level. Interestingly, the region showing linkage to HLA was very extensive, suggesting that strong, genuine positive linkages will be obvious over an extended genomic region. The underlying theoretical basis for this was described by Terwilliger *et al.* (1997) who recognized that true positive peaks are likely to be broader than false positive peaks[48]. However, this does not mean that more limited areas of linkage are necessarily false positives since further loci are unlikely to offer an effect of the magnitude of HLA. None of the data so far available describe additional genomic regions with an effect size equivalent or exceeding that of HLA. Cornelis *et al.* examined the possible interaction between HLA and the genome scan regions by partition of the families in the study according to HLA genotype. The results revealed greater evidence of linkage for the HLA-concordant sib pairs at the chromosome 3 locus than was detected for the remaining sib pairs.

To date the genome scans in RA, and indeed in other simple and complex diseases, have been achieved 'using conventional' microsatellite-based approaches. Microsatellite genotyping is likely to be a short-lived stage in the evolution of genome-wide linkage analysis. It is relatively cumbersome, requires gels (whether slab or capillary), and is not readily fully automatable. Furthermore, the infrequency of microsatellite markers in the human genome and their high mutation rate means that this approach is not indicated for whole genome association linkage disequilibrium mapping of disease-relevant genes. Another class of polymorphic marker is now emerging as the likely future in linkage analysis, specifically for genome-wide screening[3]. Single nucleotide polymorphisms (SNPs), although individually less polymorphic than the microsatellites, are far more abundant (estimated more frequent than 1 SNP per kilobase of DNA). The use of these biallelic genetic markers in linkage and association analysis provides the potential for a substantially higher throughput genotyping technology. Thus, although approximately 2.5 times the number of SNP's will be required to provide the equivalent power of a microsatellite approach, the use of highly automated techniques will greatly enhance our ability to discover new susceptibility loci for RA and other diseases[49].

HLA *as the prototype candidate gene region for RA*

Rheumatoid arthritis is one of the commonest immune-mediated disorders, and is a major cause of morbidity and premature mortality. We have reviewed above several lines of evidence that point to an important genetic contribution to the development of the disease. By far the most extensively studied association in most populations is that with polymorphic human leukocyte antigens alleles (HLA) within the major histocompatibility complex (MHC). RA is both linked to and associated with genetic variation mapping to this locus. Our understanding of disease susceptibility has improved considerably as a consequence. Several original hypotheses of disease causation have arisen from this work, some of which have now been tested. This section will concentrate on recent advances in molecular biology and immunology which have provided a framework for understanding the role of the MHC in the development of rheumatoid arthritis.

Nature of class I and II polymorphisms

The human MHC maps to the short arm of chromosome 6 in the region designated 6p21.3, which represents the most intensively studied area of the human genome. This region occupies approximately four megabases of DNA[50]. Previously, the MHC had been operationally divided into the class I, class II, and class III regions which encode the classical transplantation antigens, the immune response gene products, and a diverse grouping of genes including several complement components, respectively. The location of genes of similar function to particular areas of the MHC is probably a legacy of gene duplication during evolution. Although still useful, this distinction is breaking down as more genes with novel functions are described, such as the peptide transporter genes that map to the HLA class II region but are involved in delivering peptides to HLA class I molecules.

This section is primarily concerned with the HLA class I (A, B, and C) and class II (DR, DQ, and DP) genes. Each of the class II regions DR, DQ, and DP contains at least two genes coding for α and β chains, denoted A and B respectively. The function of MHC molecules is to collect peptide fragments inside the cell and transport them to the cell surface, where the peptide-MHC complex is presented to T cells. The DMA and DMB genes, which map to the class II region, are related structurally to both class I and class II but are apparently involved in the loading of other HLA class II molecules with peptides[51].

Immunological interest in the MHC stems from its role in controlling the specificity of immune responses to protein antigens. Recently, this has been extended to the presentation of non-protein molecules by non-classical HLA and to regulation of natural killer cell activity by classical and non-classical HLA class I. Many HLA class I and class II genes and their products are highly polymorphic, with loci such as HLA-DRB1 currently associated with 221 alleles, and HLA-B with 258[52]. At most of the polymorphic HLA loci, the heterozygosity is about 90 per cent and most of the alleles occur at a frequency below 0.16. The extent of polymorphism has proved useful in uncovering relationships between specific alleles and predisposition to disease, but this process is hampered by extensive linkage disequilibrium. Family studies have shown that recombination in the HLA region is rare, and thus a complete set of alleles is usually inherited as a haplotype. This often leads to difficulties in identifying the precise locus of susceptibility within a linkage group of positively associated alleles. One solution is to examine these disease associations in a variety of ethnic groups where the haplotypes carrying susceptibility alleles may be distinct.

Amino acid polymorphisms in the antigen binding groove

As outlined above, the HLA region is extremely polymorphic, but this polymorphism is not evenly distributed throughout the expressed molecule, and is greatest in the antigen binding groove. The expressed HLA class I molecule comprises a heavy chain encoded by the class I genes of the HLA region, and a light chain encoded by the $\beta 2$ microglobulin gene on chromosome 15. The heavy chain is divided into $\alpha 1$, $\alpha 2$, and $\alpha 3$ domains. The surface of the molecule that binds peptide faces away from the cell, towards the receptor of the incoming 'cytotoxic' T cell. The groove, making up the antigen recognition site, is bordered by two α-helices, and the floor is a β-pleated sheet[53].

The class II molecule is similar in conformation to the class I molecule, although their respective genes are only distantly related. The antigens (DR, DQ, and DP) are composed of an α and a β chain, each of around 200 amino acids, and encoded by A and B genes, respectively. The extracellular part of each chain is divided into two domains, $\alpha 1$, $\alpha 2$ and $\beta 1$, $\beta 2$. These combine to form an $\alpha \beta$ heterodimer, whose antigen recognition site binds and presents antigen to the CD4[+] 'helper' T cell. In a similar manner to class I, the crystal structure of HLA-DR1 has confirmed that the genetic variation of HLA class II alleles is particularly pronounced at the amino acid residues of this antigen recognition site[54]. Presumably this variation has arisen because of the selective advantage gained from the ability to bind a wider range of antigens, and in turn present them to T cells. Mutation analysis supports this view with a strong bias towards replacement amino acid substitutions in the antigen binding site suggesting that natural selection is responsible for the polymorphism observed at class I and class II loci[55,56].

HLA associations with RA

As mentioned earlier, only around two-fifths of the genetic contribution to RA is accounted for by genes in the HLA region. Nevertheless, the region gives rise to by far the strongest and best characterized genetic predisposition to RA. It is clear from serological, cellular, and molecular studies that the greater part of the HLA association is accounted for by molecular polymorphisms that map to the HLA class II region, and to the HLA-DRB1 locus in particular. Positive associations of HLA class I alleles with RA have been reported, but it is likely that the majority (such as B44, B60, and B62) are accounted for by linkage disequilibrium with HLA-DRB1. It remains a possibility that other MHC encoded loci may modify the disease course, and evidence for this will be discussed.

RA in hospital clinics in Northern European, Chinese, New Zealand, Polynesian and most United States population is associated with DRB1*0401, 0404, 0405, and 0408, but is not associated with the closely related subtypes DRB1*0402, 0403, and 0407[57-59]. Of the non-DRB1*04 alleles, DRB1*0101, 1001, and 1402 are associated with RA. Gregersen outlined the 'shared epitope' hypothesis in 1987, proposing that the unit of HLA association with RA was a third hypervariable region (HVR3) pentapeptide motif that would be shared in a conserved form between RA-associated alleles[60]. The DRB*0101 and 1402 alleles share the QRRAA HVR3 motif at positions 70 to 74 with DRB1*0404, 0405, and 0408. DRB1*1001 carries a related sequence RRRAA in its HVR3. Other alleles shown to be negatively associated with RA contain radical substitutions in HVR3 compared to the QRRAA template. The acidic residues that offer protection from RA lie in the wall of the antigen binding cleft, and may prevent the binding of a pathogenic peptide. The implication is that either the QRRAA motif is required to bind and present a putative rheumatoid antigen to class II restricted T cells which then initiate an inflammatory response in the joint, or that the presence of the motif results in a different T cell receptor repertoire due to thymic selection[61]. Another interpretation of the data proffered by Chella David and colleagues suggests that the QRRAA motif is actually presented by HLA-DQB1*03 molecules[62]. This suggestion arose from the observation that HLA-DQB1*0302/0301 transgenic mice can present the 'protective' 65–79 peptide from DRB1*1501 and *0402, but not the shared epitope or 'non-protective' 0101 and *0401, and will discussed in more detail below.

Yet another interpretation of the shared epitope hypothesis was advanced by Auger, who noted that one peptide that binds to the QKRAA (DRB1*0401) and RRRAA (DRB1*1001) motifs can be derived from 70 kD heat shock proteins, either from E. coli or the human constitutive form (HSP73)[63]. Furthermore, HSP73 coprecipitates only with the DRB1*0401 and DRB1*1001 molecules. The function of this HSP is to target selected proteins to lysosomes, and the authors suggest that the association of DR molecules with HSP73 may have a specific effect on the intracellular trafficking of DRB1*0401 and DRB1*1001 molecules and on how they interact with peptide fragments. One problem with this hypothesis is that other HLA-

DRB1 molecules associated with RA do not bind HSP73. In some populations, the association of RA is not with DRB1* 0401 or *1001, and thus cannot be explained by HSP binding.

Although several alleles confer enhanced risk for development of RA, they are not equivalent with important differences between ethnic groups and between subsets of patients. In northern Europe, DRB1*0401 is the most strongly associated allele[57] whereas in Japanese, Jewish, and Greek populations where DRB1*0401 is relatively uncommon, DRB1*0405 is the most common subtype among RA patients[64–66]. Conversely, where the alleles comprising the 'shared epitope' are rare, for example Nigeria, so is RA[67].

Several studies have highlighted limitations of the shared epitope hypothesis. Some studies of mild, early RA in the community have suggested that the presence of the shared epitope is associated with disease severity rather than incidence[68–70]. A case control study has shown the risk of RA in 'compound heterozygote' men who possess two different shared epitope alleles (*0401/*0404) is 90 times that in shared epitope negative individuals, but is more than double this in men under 30 with severe disease[71]. Such an interaction cannot be explained as a dosage effect since the DRB1*0401/0401 genotype is not associated with an equivalent risk.

HLA in clinical subsets of RA: Felty's and large granular lymphocyte syndromes

Felty's syndrome (FS) is a rare complication of RA characterized by neutropenia and splenomegaly. It merits study as a model for investigating the genetic determinants of RA susceptibility. This is because when performing studies to uncover the genetic component of a disease, it is advantageous for the patients studied to be as clinically homogenous as possible. Otherwise, disease heterogeneity will mask all but the strongest genetic effects. FS is far more homogenous than RA, both clinically and genetically.

A number of workers in recent years have identified a related condition known as large granular lymphocyte syndrome, characterized by splenomegaly, neutropenia, and peripheral blood expansion of large granular lymphocytes (LGL)[72]. LGL are thought to be activated cytotoxic T cells, and fall into two subsets. CD3-CD8-CD56+ cells are natural killer cells, and patients with leukemia of this subset follow an aggressive course. The expansion related to Felty's syndrome has the morphology CD3+CD8+CD57+. These cells are thought to be cytotoxic T cells. There is debate about whether this condition is truly a malignancy. Although many patients exhibit clonal genotypes as defined by rearranged T-cell receptor configurations, there is increasing doubt whether such clonality should be equated with malignancy, as it has been in the past. Clinically, the course is chronic, and the majority of patients die with, rather than of, their LGL expansion. For these reasons, many refer to the condition as LGL syndrome rather than leukemia[73].

HLA in FS/LGL

HLA associations studies in FS have shown that, in contrast to RA, FS is genetically homogenous with respect to HLA-DR4. Over 90 per cent of the patients are DR4+, compared with 60–70 per cent of RA patients and approximately 30 per cent of Caucasoid controls[74, 75]. In addition, there is an excess of DR4 homozygotes, particularly *0401/*0404 compound heterozygotes, giving a high relative risk for disease development[76]. Hence, whereas susceptibility to RA is strongly linked to the conserved HLA-DR β epitope QKRAA associated with several DRB1 alleles[61,74], primarily the *0401 allele that is associated with progression to Felty's syndrome or severe RA. Associations have also been identified with the central MHC—notably with complement alleles C4A*3;C4BQ*0[77], in the class I region with HLA-A*02;Cw*0501:B*44[78], and in the class II region with DQB1*0301[74]. However, all these associations appear to be secondary to linkage disequilibrium with HLA-DRB1*0401[78].

HLA in LGL—immunogenetics in disease classification

Immunogenetics can help us understand the relationships between different diseases, and therefore can aid to disease classification. The study of HLA class II in Felty's syndrome and subsets of the LGL syndrome was an example of this[75]. This clinical suspicion was that Felty's and LGL syndrome with arthritis were very similar, if not identical conditions. Support for this hypothesis came from the observation that the same strong (> 90 per cent) association with HLA DRB1*04 seen in Felty's syndrome was also present in LGL with arthritis. LGL without arthritis clearly fell into a different disease group, having the same prevalence of DRB1*04 as the normal population. These findings have recently been confirmed in a North American cohort[79]. A more recent study of HLA class I has shown similar associations with LGL syndrome and arthritis as outlined above for FS[78]. LGL syndrome without arthritis showed no such association.

Hence, immunogenetic studies of FS and LGL syndrome have helped clarify the importance of particular DR4 alleles in progression from simple RA to these severe disease subsets, with implications for disease pathogenesis. Moreover, the HLA studies clarified the relationships between these related but distinct conditions.

Limitations of HLA in disease susceptibility: role of other loci

In RA, a number of groups have looked at regions and candidates within the MHC other than class I and II, and it appears unlikely that transporter associated with antigen processing (TAP) polymorphisms confer susceptibility independent of DRB1[80]. A number of groups have examined the role of TNF polymorphisms. One found that the uncommon allele of tumor necrosis factor α (TNFA*2) was present at three times the frequency of the normal Anglo-Saxon population in patients with RA[81], although this was not accompanied by an increase in production of TNF-α protein. Another group reported a study of five TNF microsatellite markers in 50 multiplex RA families[82]. One of these, TNF a6, b5, c1, d3, e3, was found in 35.3 per cent of affected, but only 20.5 per cent of unaffected, individuals (p < 0.05). Stratification by the presence of the shared epitope showed an independent effect of the TNFc1 allele (p = 0.0003). However, another group reported the same year that the association with TNF a6, b5 microsatellite alleles was secondary to linkage disequilibrium with HLA-DR[83]. Further study will be required before the role of the central MHC in disease susceptibility can be assigned with certainty.

Function of HLA susceptibility loci

As described in the previous section, RA shows significant associations with a number of HLA class II loci. The only known functions of class II molecules are to present self antigens in the thymus in fetal life to allow deletion of self-reactive clones and to shape the T-cell receptor (TCR) repertoire, and to present self or foreign antigens in later life to CD4[+] T cells. The inference is that either subjects with these alleles fail to delete self-reactive T cells efficiently in development, or that they have an enhanced ability to present pathogenic self or foreign antigens to T cells, thus eliciting an inflammatory response. However, amino acids 70–74 primarily face away from the antigen binding site so its role in antigen selection is not clear. A third possibility is that these class II molecules are unable to present pathogenic peptides efficiently to T cells, resulting in a failure of elimination of the pathogen and subsequent disease. Support for the idea that the primary effect is on repertoire selection comes from a study of patients and their mothers. This suggested that patients with RA who were negative for DR4 tended to have DR4[+] mothers, the non-inherited allele therefore apparently affecting fetal TCR repertoire[84]. However, a more recent study of the Arthritis and Rheumatism Council's National Repository of RA families found no such association[85].

Evidence for the alternative, that susceptibility arises from an enhanced ability (or failure) to bind and present pathogenic peptides, has been sought in a number of approaches. One group purified HLA-DR molecules from the spleen of a patient with Felty's syndrome[86]. The endogenous peptides were then isolated and sequenced. A variety of human proteins were found, notably albumin, and a synthesized peptide corresponding to residues 106–120 of albumin bound to HLA-DRB1*0401. Although the findings are interesting, it is difficult to see how this protein could give rise to inflammatory changes seen in RA.

Several groups have carried out site directed mutagenesis on the DRB1*0401 gene. One found that single amino acid substitutions at position 71 resulted in changes in the portion of peptide selected that interacts with the 67–74 area[87]. Another reported that similar changes at position 71 had a critical role in determining T-cell responses to a given peptide, even though binding affinity of the peptide was not significantly altered[88]. Thus, there is some persuasive evidence accumulating that changes in ability to present pathogenic peptide may explain the HLA associations of this disease.

One interesting alternative hypothesis, as mentioned earlier, was recently outlined[62]. Working from mouse models of arthritis, they proposed that HLA-DQ was the arthritogenic peptide-presenting molecule, and that the HLA-DRB1 locus was protective against RA. The proposed mechanism is that DRβ peptides are presented by certain HLA-DQ molecules (DQ4, DQ7, DQ8, and DQ9) in the thymus, positively selecting certain TCR Vβ bearing cells. Shared epitope positive 'non-protective' peptides cannot be presented by HLA-DQ molecules, whereas the 'protective' peptides can[89]. The T cells so selected mature as CD4 cells with T helper 2 (Th2) type characteristics, and remain anergized in the periphery. When the immune system is activated by foreign antigens, specific Th1 cells and eventually DRβ specific anergized Th2 cells are activated. Through antigenic mimicry, the Th1 cells become autoreactive. The Th2 cells then suppress the Th1 cells. Therefore depending on whether the DRB1 locus for that individual is permissive or protective, clinical disease will or will not ensue.

In a subsequent clinical survey comparing the DQ and shared epitope hypotheses in an Early Arthritis Clinic at Leiden, 155 RA patients were studied. Two doses of predisposing DQ alleles strongly predisposed to RA while shared epitope negative DRB1 alleles conferred a dominant protection in DQ5-positive individuals. The group considered this to be evidence in favor of the DQ hypothesis[90]. However, the close linkage between the HLA-DR and DQ loci make these interpretations of data fraught with difficulty, and the model has yet to gain wide acceptance.

Transgenic mouse models and the role of HLA.

The development of mice transgenic for HLA-DR or DQ molecules and human TCR has allowed more extensive testing of the antigen presenting capabilities of these molecules. Mice transgenic for the rearranged Vα1.1 and Vβ8.2 TCR chain genes isolated from a type II collagen (CII)–specific T cell hybridoma do not develop spontaneous arthritis. However, arthritis is seen after immunization with CII in complete Freund's adjuvant[91].

Chimeric (human/mouse) HLA-DR1 mice, when immunized with human type II collagen, develop arthritis with erosions, accompanied by DR1-restricted T and B cell responses to type II collagen[92]. This would suggest that HLA-DR1 is capable of presenting peptides derived from collagen. Arthritis is also induced by human type II collagen in the DRB1*0401 transgenic mouse[93].

Additional studies have shown that mice transgenic for HLA-DQ6, which is not associated with RA, are resistant to collagen arthritis. Those transgenic for HLA-DQ8 are highly susceptible[94], while double transgenics develop moderate collagen arthritis. These studies would support a role for HLA-DQ polymorphism in human RA[95]. The group also found that transgenic with HLA-DQA1*0301/0302 and HLA-DRB1*1502 are less prone to arthritis, suggesting that HLA-DR can modulate disease susceptibility[96]. However, later analysis suggested that the disease seen in the double transgenic mice was more akin to relapsing polychondritis than RA[97]. Zanelli analyzed the immunogenicity of the DRB1*0402 third hypervariablity region peptide in DQ8-transgenic mice. He found that the motif DERAA, seen on shared epitope negative DR molecules, guaranteed DQ8-restricted immunogenicity, and that the main anchor residue for binding of the DRB1*0402 peptide to DQ was R. Moreover, the p1 pocket, which probably controls binding of the R residue, was identical in all four RA-associated DQ molecules. These results imply that the association of RA with some DR subtypes might be explained by their linkage with DQ alleles displaying a binding site for similar 'arthritogenic' peptides[98].

The development of transgenic models has allowed further dissection of the roles of the various susceptibility molecules in arthritis. They do not answer all the questions of interest, particularly since their relationship to human rheumatoid arthritis is not clear, but they do allow crucial *in vivo* interrogation of the role of various components of the HLA/TCR interaction.

Non-HLA genes in RA

At the molecular level, our understanding of the interaction of susceptibility-conferring HLA molecule, putative pathogenic peptide and T-cell receptor has increased to the point where the goal of specific immunotherapies for RA appears more realistic. At the same time, the limitations of HLA in explaining these diseases has been recognized, and the role of genes within and without the MHC has been explored. The focus of most research for non-HLA genes implicated in RA has primarily involved candidate genes central to the control and regulation of the immune response. An initial torrent of putative candidate genes, such as T-cell receptors, cytokines, and cytokine receptors, has later proved disappointingly inconclusive. The explanation for the apparently confused and contradictory nature of these reports lies predominantly with the lack of understanding of the candidate genes and their involvement in the disease. However, another major factor responsible for these inconsistent reports lies in the interpretation of the epidemiological and statistical data for this complex disease[42]. This section will focus primarily on recent advances in the identification of putative candidate genes involved in RA and is, by choice, partial given the huge number of unconfirmed reports of association. Recently, microsatellite markers, which have advantages of convenience to be weighed against relative insensitivity when used in affected sibling allele sharing designs, have been evaluated. Alternatively, nucleotide polymorphisms have been extensively studied on a case-control basis with enhanced sensitivity but with the limitations described earlier. As yet, few family based association studies have been reported.

In one of the most extensive studies, an investigation of candidate susceptibility genes for RA using clinically stratified affected sibling pair families. A total of 200 RA affected sibling pair families were genotyped for microsatellite markers mapping within 3 cM from: IFN–α, IFN–γ, IFN–β, IL–1α, IL–1β, IL–1R, IL–2, IL–6, IL–5R, IL–8R, bcl2, CD40L, NOS3, NRAMP, α_1-antitrypsin, and α-antichymotryspin. Genetic linkage was investigated by defining allele sharing between sibling pairs and assessed using the MLE method. An increase in allele sharing was seen for IL-5R in female sibling pairs (lod 0.91, p = 0.03) and for IFN-γ in sibling pairs with an affected male (lod 0.96, p = 0.03). However, the most significant linkage was observed for IL-2 in sibling pairs where at least one of the pair was rheumatoid factor negative (lod 1.05, p = 0.02). Although these linkages are at best suggestive as previously discussed, this can be attributed to the genetic heterogeneity of the disease [99]. The issue of false positives due to multiple testing is also critical in interpretation of these results.

Interestingly, studies failed to show significant linkage with the gene involved in macrophage activation (NRAMP1), whereas one other study using essentially the same family material has reported evidence for a role of this locus in determining human susceptibility to RA[100]. Multicase rheumatoid arthritis families were used to examine the occurrence of a dinucleotide repeat in the NRAMP1 promoter region with four additional marker genes, TNP1, IL-8R, VIL1, and DES. Identity by descent (IBD) sibling pair analysis using a three locus haplotype NRAMP1-IL-8RB-VIL1, or NRAMP1 alone, provided preliminary evidence (maximum lod score = 1.01, p = 0.024) for a gene in this region contributing to susceptibility for RA. Candidacy for NRAMP1 as the disease susceptibility gene was supported by a significant bias (p = 0.048) towards transmission of the NRAMP1 promoter region of allele 3 in affected offspring.

One hypothesis for the involvement of NRAMP1 in RA states that a functional Z-DNA forming repeat polymorphism in the promoter region of this gene contributes directly to disease susceptibility. Four alleles have been observed: alleles 1 and 4 are rare (gene frequencies approximately equal to 0.001), alleles 2 and 3 occur at gene frequencies approximately 0.25 and 0.75, respectively. Experimental observation demonstrates that alleles 1,2, and 4 are poor promoters of the gene while allele 3 drives high expression. While allele 3 shows allelic association with autoimmune disease susceptibility, allele 2 is associated with susceptibility in infectious disease. Thus it is possible that balancing selection is responsible for maintaining these two alleles in the human population. The association of NRAMP1 with RA susceptibility may be related to one of the multiple pleiotropic effects linked to macrophage activation. Recently however, involvement of NRAMP1 in iron transport has aroused more interesting speculation that regulation of iron transport many contribute directly to the disease phenotype in arthritic disease. Patients suffering from RA show increased deposition of iron in the synovial membrane, which may contribute to free radical generation and local inflammation. Further analysis of NRAMP1 function will continue to be of importance in understanding the molecular basis to immune-mediated disease susceptibility[100].

Possible genetic association between interleukin–1α (IL–1α) gene polymorphism and the severity of chronic polyarthritis has recently been highlighted. The promoter region and fifth exon of the IL–1α gene were analyzed for polymorphism in 51 patients with destructive and 47 with non-destructive RA, as well as in 94 controls. The two biallelic polymorphisms in the promoter region and exon V were found to be 100 per cent linked. The occurence rate of the rare allele (IL–1A2) was 45 per cent in the control population, whereas this rate increased in destructive (54.4 per cent) and decreased in non-destructive RA (26.8 per cent, destructive versus non-destructive, p = 0.007). All indices of joint destruction and disease activity were significantly lower in the patients positive for IL–1A1, and higher in those positive for IL–1A2. These findings suggest that this IL-1A gene polymorphism may contribute to the pathogenesis of chronic polyarthritis [101].

By virtue of its function as the ligand for HLA class I and II, the classical αβ T-cell receptor has been an attractive candidate susceptibility molecule for disease-related genetic variation, either by virtue of structural amino acid polymorphism or in the way that its rearrangement and expression are developmentally regulated. There is weak evidence that TCRA is an RA susceptibility locus[102]. Cornelis *et al.* conducted an extensive RA case-control study involving a total of 1579 northwest Europeans: 766 patients with erosive RF-positive disease and 813 control subjects. Productive genetically encoded amino acid changes in segments TCRAV6S1, TCRAV7S1, TCRAV8S1, TCRAV10S2, and TCRBV6S1, TCRBV6S7 were investigated by single-strand conformation polymorphisms (SSCP). The TCRAV8S1 association was confirmed by restriction fragment length polymorphism (RFLP). In the systematic study (77 patients and 119 controls), an increase in 1 TCRAV8S1 genotype was found in the RA patients (P = 0.0004). This observation was replicated in two further populations; one from France (212 patients and 254 controls) and the other from Britain (477 patients and 440 controls), with a similar odds ratio (OR), which allowed pooling of the data and confirmation of the association (OR 1.3, p = 0.008)[102]. In another smaller study of Swiss patients, an association between TCRAV5S1 and RA after stratification for DR4 status was observed though this did not survive correction for multiple testing[103]. No such association was seen in patient groups from other European centers. Interestingly, there is weak evidence for linkage of RA to TCRA but not to TCRB[104], while in ankylosing spondylitis weak effects map to the TCRB (p = 0.01 lod 1.1) but not the TCRA locus[105]. The authors have been careful to point out that no evidence of major loci has been uncovered although one may speculate that these weak and difficult to replicate effects are to be expected in a genetically heterogeneous disease with a polygenic background. Expectations conditioned on the degree of understanding we have gained by studying the HLA locus in RA are likely to be unhelpful when attempting to unravel the rest of the puzzle.

IL-10 as a candidate gene in RA

In light of the putative importance of interleukin 10 (IL-10) in synovial inflammation, the role of polymorphism variation in the IL-10 gene in RA predisposition has attracted considerable interest. Three polymorphisms within the promoter of the IL-10 gene have been identified; their gene frequencies studied in a healthy population of the cytokine by lymphocytes *in vitro* have been assessed [106]. One of the polymorphisms, at position –1087 from the transcription start site, was associated with varying levels of cytokine production after stimulation with concanavalin A (Con A). This was compatible with an earlier study using a luciferase assay to show that a positive regulatory region resided between –1100 and –900[107]. There are clearly many reasons why IL-10 production might be elevated in RA or FS, but one possibility is that a genetic predisposition to high IL-10 production might be an important contributory factor. Indeed,

recent work has demonstrated a high degree of heritability of IL-10 production from lymphocytes stimulated *in vitro*[108]. For this reason, several groups have studied the frequencies of promoter polymorphisms in RA.

One recent study of RA and Felty's syndrome demonstrated no difference in the frequency of IL-10 promoter polymorphisms between RA and FS patients and controls[109]. A related study also showed no association with RA as a whole, although there was an association between the –1082*A allele and IgA RF positive patients [110]. However, a more recent study, as yet unpublished, showed significant correlation between the –1082*G allele and erosive disease[111] In this study, high IL-10 production *in vitro* was associated with the –1082A allele. This would intuitively make sense, since IL-10 is considered to have anti-inflammatory properties, and so patients with high levels would be expected to have fewer erosions. However, in another study the –1082*A allele was associated with low IL-10 production.[106] The assays were done on different cell populations, and different stimuli were used, so that both results could be valid. However, these contradictory results make it likely that the area will remain controversial in the near future.

Alleles at two microsatellite loci in the 4 kb immediately upstream of the human IL-10 transcription initiation site have been defined[112]. The IL10.G and IL10.R microsatellites are located 1.2 kb and 4.0 kb upstream of the coding region respectively. Hence, the IL10.G allele is close to the minus1082G/A polymorphism discussed above. Lipopolysaccrharide–included IL–10 secretion varies with IL–10 promoter haplotype. Those haplotypes containing the allele IL10.R3 are associated with lower IL–10 secretion than haplotypes containing any other IL10.R allele[112]. A study by Eskdale and collegues showed no association between RA and the IL10.G allele, but there was a weak association with the high IL–10 producing IL10.R2 allele[113]. Hence this study would imply that having the high IL–10 producing haplotype predisposes individuals to RA, which some consider a Th1 type organ-specific immune-mediated disease. Current immunological dogma would predict the opposite, namely that Th2 type disease such as asthma and systemic lupus erythematosus would be more likely in this situation. Further work to replicate these findings will be required before the role of IL–10 promoter polymorphisms in RA pathogenesis becomes clear.

The future of genetic studies in rheumatoid arthritis

Currently investigators are making valiant efforts to map genetic effects of unknown, and in all likelihood, small magnitude with crude genetic markers in family collections of inadequate size and with inevitable limitations due to clinicogenetic heterogeneity. This approach might lead to the discovery and biological verification of allelic polymorphisms accounting for a proportion of the genetic variance in disease risk. What is unavoidable is that despite the massive resources devoted to mapping studies in RA and other disease with a complex basis, there are no examples of the approach yet delivering a causative polymorphism. The key to resolution of this problem is an intersection of the following five resources:

(1)   a high throughput, high resolution mapping platform;

(2)   multiple large, well matched case-control cohorts;

(3)   a comprehensive gene map rich mRNA and protein expression information for candidate tissues relevant to stages of disease development;

(4)   manipulation of biological systems to examine single locus effects;

(5)   relevant biological systems for the introduction and interpretation of variation due to two loci and more.

An extension to such a scheme, which provides a comprehensive pathophysiological database integrated with disease-specific genome variation data, has been proposed[114]. There is little doubt that the mapping platform will be SNP-based for reasons discussed earlier and both public and private initiatives are currently scouring the genome for available variation[3]. The dominant platform for whole genome association mapping though is currently undefined and would seem to be a choice between hybridization chip, mass spectrometric, and fluidic technologies. Despite problems relating to stratification effects on the distribution of marker and disease related allelic variation, the scale of availability of populations of unrelated cases and controls and the inherent sensitivity advantages over linkage-based approaches argues that controlled population association will be the preferred mode of disease locus discovery. A degree of development of robust statistical tools for such analyses that compensate for disease-unrelated human population variation is still necessary. An exciting avenue of research will be the correlation and eventual predictive use of functional SNPs in disease outcome, drug toxicity, and efficacy. Much has been written about so-called genetically tailored therapies and the new field of pharmocogenomics. The challenge for the immediate future is to take on the degree of existing human genetic diversity and to distinguish causal pathways from merely population-associated variation.

References

1. Collins, F.S., *et al*. New goals for the U.S. Human Genome Project: 1998–2003. *Sciene*, 1998;**282**:682–9.
2. Chakravarti, A., Population genetics—making sense out of sequence. *Nat Genet*, 1999;**21**(1 Suppl):56–60.
3. Collins, F.S., L.D. Brooks, and A. Chakravarti, A DNA polymorphism discovery resource for research on human genetic variation.*Genome Res*, 1998;**8**:1229–31.
4. Tiwari, J.L. and P.I., Terasaki, *HLA and Disease Associations*. 1985, New York: Springer-Verlag.
5. Wordsworth, B.P., *et al*., HLA-DR4 subtype frequencies in rheumatoid arthritis indicate that DRB1 is the major susceptibility locus within the HLA class II region. *Proc Natl Acad Sci USA*, 1989;**86**:10049–53.
6. Lanchburg, J.S., L.I. Sakkas, and G.S. Panayi, Genetic factors in rheumatoid arthritis. In *Rheumatoid Arthritis: Recent Research Advances*, (J.S. Smolen, J.Kalden, and R.N. Maini, eds). 1993, Springer-Verlag: Berlin. pp. 17–28.
7. Risch, N., Assessing the role of HLA-linked and unlinked determinants of disease. *Am J Hum Genet,*1987.**40**:1–14.
8. Vyse, T.J. and J.A. Todd, Genetic analysis of autoimmune disease. *Cell*, 1996;**85**:311–18.
9. Ollier, W.E. and A. MacGregor, Genetic epidemiology of rheumatoid disease. *Br Med Bull*, 1995;**51**:267–85.
10. Bodmer, W.F., Evolutionary significance of the HL-A system. *Nature*, 1972;**237**:139–45.
11. Bodmer, W.F., The major histocompatibility gene clusters of man and mouse. *Prog Clin Biol Res*, 1981;**45**:213–29
12. Thomas D.J., *et al*., Evidence for an association between rheumatoid arthritis and autoimmune endocrine disease. *Ann Rheum Dis*, 1983;**42**:297–300.
13. Hill, A.V.S., *et al*., Common West African antigens are associated with protection from severe malaria. *Nature*, 1991;**352**:595–600.
14. Carrington, M., *et al*., HLA and HIV–1: heterozygote advantage and B*35–Cw*04 disadvantage. *Science*, 1999;**283**:1748–52.
15. Lander, E.S. and N.J. Schork, Genetic dissection of complex traits. *Science*, 1994;**265**:2037–48.
16. Frankel, W.N. and N.J. Schork, Who's afraid of epistasis? *Nat Genet*, 1996;**14**:371–3.
17. del Junco, D., *et al*., The familial aggregation of rheumatoid arthritis and its relationship to the HLA-DR4 association. *Am J Epidemiol*, 1984;**119**:813–29.
18. Marlow, A., *et al*., The sensitivity of different analytical methods to detect disease susceptibility genes in rheumatoid arthritis sibling pair families. *J Rheumatol*, 1997;**24**:208–11.
19. Silman, A.J., *et al*., Twin concordance rates for rheumatoid arthritis: results from a nationwide study. *Br J Rheumatol*, 1993;**32**:903–7.
20. Lawrence, J.S., *et al*., Rheumatoid factors in families. *Ann Rheum Dis*, 1970;**29**:269–74.
21. Aho, K., *et al*., Occurrence of rheumatoid arthritis in a nationwide series of twins. *J Rheumatol* 1986;**13**:899–902.
22. MacGregor, A.J., *et al*., Characterising the quantitative genetic contribution to rheumatoid arthritis using data from twins. *Arthritis Rheum*, 1999 (in press)
23. Gregersen, P.K., Discordance for autoimmunity in monozygotic twins. Are 'identical' twins really identical? *Arthritis Rheum*, 1993;**36**:1185–92.
24. Stastny, P., Association of the B-cell alloantigen DRw4 with rheumatoid arthritis. *N Eng J Med*, 1978;**289**:869–71.
25. Panayi, G.S., P. Wooley, and J.R. Batchelor, Genetic basis of rheumatoid disease: HLA antigens, disease manifestations, and toxic reactions to drugs. *Br Med J*, 1978;**2**:1326–8.
26. Stastny, P., Mixed lymphocyte culture typing cells from patients with rheumatoid arthritis. *Tissue Antigens*, 1974;**4**:572–9.
27. Jorde, L.B., Linkage disequilibrium as a gene-mapping tool. *Am J Hum Genet*, 1995;**56**:11–4.
28. Laan, M. and S. Paabo, Demographic history and linkage disequilibrium in human populations *Nat Genet*, 1997;**17**:435–8.
29. Slatkin, M., Linkage disequilibrium in growing and stable populations. *Genetics*, 1995;**137**:331–6.
30. de la Chapelle, A. and F.A. Wright, Linkage disequilibrium mapping in isolated populations: the example of Finland revisited. *Proc Natl Acad Sci USA*, 1998;**95**:12416–23.
31. Laitinen, T., *et al*., Genetic control of serum IgE levels and asthma: linkage and linkage disequilibrium studies in an isolated populations. *Hum Mol Genet*, 1997;**6**:2069–76.
32. Schleutker, J., *et al*., Linkage disequilibrium utilized to establish a refined genetic position of the Salla disease locus on 6q14-q15. *Genomics*, 1995;**27**:286–92.
33. Mannikko, M., *et al*., Fine mapping and haplotype analysis of the locus for congenital nephrotic syndrome on chromosome 19q13.1. *Am J Hum Genet*, 1995;**57**:1377–83.
34. Kruglyak, L. and E.S. Lander, High-resolution genetic mapping of complex traits. *Am J Hum Genet*, 1995;**56**:1212–23.
35. Terwilliger, J.D., *et al*., Mapping genes through the use of linkage disequilibrium generated by genetic drift: 'drift mapping' in small

populations with no demographic expansion. *Hum Hered*, 1998;**48**:138–54.

36. Kruglyak, L., *et al.*, Parametric and nonparametric linkage analysis: a unified multipoint approach. *Am J Hum Genet*, 1996;**58**:1347–63.

37. Davies, J.L., *et al.*, A genome-wide search for human type 1 diabetes susceptibility genes. *Nature*, 1994;**371**:130–6.

38. Saweer, S., *et al.*, A genome screen in multiple sclerosis reveals susceptibility loci on chromosome 6p21 and 17q22. *Nat Gene*, 1996;**13**:464–8.

39. Satsangi, J., *et al.*, Two stage genome-wide search in inflammatory bowel disease provides evidence for susceptibility loci on chromosomes 3, 7 and 12. *Nat Gene*, 1996;**14**:199–202.

40. Bell, J.I. and G.M. Lathrop, Multiple loci for multiple sclerosis. *Nat Gene*, 1996;**13**:377–8.

41. Hardwick, L.J., *et al.*, Genetic mapping of susceptibility loci in the genes involved in rheumatoid arthritis. *J Rheumatol*, 1997;**24**:197–8.

42. Lander, E. and L. Kruglyak, Genetic dissection of complex traits: guidelines for interpreting and reporting linkage results. *Nat Genet*, 1995;**11**:241–7.

43. Weeks, D.E. and K. Lange, The affected-pedigree-member method of linkage analysis. *Am J Hum Genet*, 1988;**42**:315–26.

44. Murray, J.C., *et al.*, A comprehensive human linkage map with centimorgan density. Cooperative Human Linkage Center (CHLC). *Science*, 1994;**265**:2049–54.

45. Dib, C., *et al.*, A comprehensive genetic map of the human genome based on 5,264 microsatellites. *Nature*, 1996. **380**:152–4.

46. Risch, N. and K. Merikangas, The future of genetic studies of complex human disease. *Science*, 1996;**273**:1516–17.

47. Cornelis, F., *et al.*, New susceptibility locus for rheumatoid arthritis suggested by a genome-wide linkage study. *Proc Natl Acad Sci USA*, 1998;**95**:10746–50.

48. Terwilliger, J.D., *et al.*, True and false positive peaks in genomewide scans: applications of length-biased sampling to linkage mapping. *Am J Hum Genet*, 1997;**61**:430–8.

49. Kruglyak, L., The use of genetic map of biallelic markers in linkage studies. *Nat Genet*, 1997;**17**:21–4.

50. Trowsdale, J. and R.D. Campbell, Complexity in the major histocompatibility complex. *Euro J Immunogen*, 1992;**19**:45–55.

51. Sloan, V.S., *et al.*, Mediation by HLA-DM of dissociation of peptides from HLA-DR. *Nature*, 1995;**375**:802–6.

52. Marsh, S.G.E., HLA Informatics Group, in http://www.anthonynolan.com/HIG/index.html. 1999.

53. Bjorkman, P.J., *et al.*, The foreign antigen binding site and T cell recognition regions of class I histocompatibility antigens, *Nature*, 1987;**329**:512–18.

54. Brown, J.H., *et al.*, Three-dimensional structure of the human class II histocompatibility antigen HLA-DR1, *Nature*, 1993;**364**:33–9.

55. Hughes, A.L. and M. Nei, Pattern of nucleotide substitution at major histocompatibility complex class I loci reveals overdominant selection. *Nature*, 1988;**335**:167–70.

56. Hughes, A.L. and M. Nei, Nucleotide substitution at major histocompatibility complex class II loci : evidence for overdominant selection. *Proc Natl Acad Sci USA*, 1989;**86**:958–62.

57. Wordsworth, B.P., *et al.*, HLA-DR4 subtype frequencies in rheumatoid arthritis indicate that DRB1 is the major susceptibility locus within the HLA class II region. *Proc Natl Acad Sci USA*, 1989;**86**:10049–53.

58. Gao, X., *et al.*, HLA-DR alleles with naturally occurring amino acid substitutions and risk for development of rheumatoid arthritis. *Arthritis Rheum*, 1990;**33**:939–46.

59. Tan, P.L., *et al.*, HLA-DR4 subtypes in New Zealand Polynesians. Predominance of Dw13 in the healthy population and association of Dw15 with rheumatoid arthritis. *Arthritis Rheum*, 1993;**36**:15–9.

60. Gregersen, P., J. Silver, and R. Winchester, The shared epitope hypothesis. An approach to understanding the molecular genetics of susceptibility to rheumatoid arthritis. *Arthritis Rheum*, 1987;**30**:1205–13.

61. Gregersen, P.K., HLA associations with rheumatoid arthritis: a piece of the puzzle. *J Rheumatol*, 1992;**32**(suppl):7–11.

62. Zanelli, E., M.A. Gonzalez-Gay, and C.S. David, Could HLA-DRB1 be the protective locus in rheumatoid arthritis? *Immunology Today*, 1995;**16**:274–8.

63. Auger, I., *et al.*, HLA-DR4 and HLA-DR10 motifs that carry susceptibility to rheumatoid arthritis bind 70-kD heat shock proteins. *Nat Med*, 1996;**2**:306–10.

64. Watanabe, Y., *et al.*, Putative amino acid sequence of HLA-DRB chain contributing of rheumatoid arthritis. *J Exp Med*, 1989;**169**:2263–8.

65. Gao, X. and S.W. Serjeantson, Diversity in HLA-DR4-related DR, DQ haplotypes in Australia, Oceania, and China. *Human Immun*, 1991;**32**:269–76.

66. Boki, K.A., *et al.*, HLA class II sequence polymorphisms and susceptibility to rheumatoid arthritis in Greeks. The HLA-DR beta shared-epitope hypothesis accounts for the disease in only a minority of Greek patients. *Arthritis Rheum*, 1992;**35**:749–55.

67. Silman, A.J., *et al.*, Absence of rheumatoid arthritis in rural Nigerian population. *J Rheumatol*, 1993;**20**:618–22.

68. Deighton, C.M., P.J. Kelly, and D.J. Walker, Linkage of rheumatoid arthritis with HLA. *Ann Rheum Dis*, 1993;**52**:638–42.

69. Thomson, W., *et al.*, Absence of an association between HLA-DRB1*04 and rheumatoid arthritis in newly diagnosed cases from the community. *Ann Rheum Dis*, 1993;**52**:539–41.

70. Weyand, C.M., *et al.*, The influence of HLA-DRB1 genes on disease severity in rheumatoid arthritis. *Ann Int Med*, 1992;**117**:801–6.

71. MacGregor, A., *et al.*, HLA-DRB1*0401/0404 genotype and rheumatoid arthritis: increased association in men, young age at onset, and disease severity. *J Rheumatol*, 1995;**22**:1032–6.

72. Loughran, T.P., Jr., Clonal diseases of large granular lymphocytes. *Blood*, 1993;**82**:1–14.

73. Bowman, S.J., *et al.*, T cell receptor alpha-chain and beta-chain junctional region homology in clonal CD3+, CD8+ T lymphocyte expansions in Felty's syndrome. *Arthritis Rheum*, 1997;**40**:615–23.

74. Lanchbury, J.S., *et al.*, Strong primary selection for the Dw4 subtype of DR4 accounts for the HLA-DQw7 association with Felty's syndrome. *Human Immun*, 1991;**32**:56–64.

75. Bowman, S.J., *et al.*, The large granular lymphocyte syndrome with rheumatoid arthritis. Immunogenetic evidence for a broader definition of Felty's syndrome. *Arthritis Rheum*, 1994;**37**:1326–30.

76. Wordsworth, P., *et al.*, HLA heterozygosity contributes to susceptibility to rheumatoid arthritis. *Am J Human Genet*, 1992;**51**:585–91.

77. Hammond, A., W. Ollier, and M.J. Walport, Effects of C4 null alleles and homoduplications on quantitative expression of C4A and C4B. *Clin Exp Immun*, 1992;**88**:163–8.

78. Coakley, G., *et al.*, MHC haplotypic associations in Felty's and Large Granular Lymphocyte Syndromes are secondary to allelic association with HLA-DRB1*0401., 1999 (submitted).

79. Starkebaum, G., *et al.*, Immunogenetic similarities between patients with Felty's syndrome and those with clonal expansions of large granular lymphocytes in rheumatoid arthritis. *Arthritis Rheum*, 1997;**40**:624–6.

80. Marsal, S., *et al.*, Association of TAP2 polymorphism with rheumatoid arthritis is secondary to allelic association with HLA-DRB1. *Arthrit Rheum*, 1994;**37**:504–13.

81. Danis, V.A., *et al.*, Increased frequency of the uncommon allele of a tumour necrosis factor alpha gene polymorphism in rheumatoid arthritis and systemic lupus erythematosus. *Disease Markers*, 1995;**12**:127–33.

82. Mulcahy, B., *et al.*, Genetic variability in the tumour necrosis factor-lymphotoxin region influences susceptibility to rheumatoid arthritis. *Am J Human Genet*, 1996;**59**:676–83.

83. Hajeer, A.H., *et al.*, Association of tumor necrosis factor microsatellite polymorphism with HLA-DRB1*04–bearing haplotypes in rheumatoid arthritis patients. *Arthritis Rheum*, 1996;**39**:1109–14.

84. ten Wolde, S., *et al.*, Influence of non-inherited maternal HLA antigens on occurence of rheumatoid arthritis. *Lancet*, 1993;**341**: 200–2.

85. Silman A.J., *et al.*, Lack of influence of non-inherited maternal HLA-DR alleles on susceptibility to rheumatoid arthritis. *Ann Rheum Dis*, 1995;**54**:311–3.

86. Gordon, R.D., *et al.*, Purification and characterization of endogenous peptides extracted from HLA-DR isolated from the spleen of a patient with rheumatoid arthritis. *Eur J Immun*, 1995;**25**:1473–6.

87. Hammer, J., *et al.*, Peptide binding specificity of HLA-DR4 molecules: correlation with rheumatoid arthritis association. *J Exp Med*, 1995;**181**:1847–55.

88. Signorelli, K.L., L.M. Watts, and L.E. Lambert, The importance of DR4Dw4 beta chain residues 70, 71, and 86 in peptide binding and T cell recognition. *Cell Immun*, 1995;**162**:217–24.

89. Zanelli, E., *et al.*, Immune response of HLA-DQ8 transgenic mice to peptides from the third hypervariable region of HLA-DRB1 correlates with predisposition to rheumatoid arthritis. *Proc Natl Acad Sci USA*, 1996;**93**:1814–9.

90. van der Horst-Bruinsma, I.E., *et al.*, HLA-DQ-associated predisposition to and dominant HLA-DR-associated protection against rheumatoid arthritis. *Human Immunol*, 1999;**60**:152–8.

91. Osman, G.E., *et al.*, Expression of a type II collagen-specific TCR transgene accelerates the onset of arthritis in mice. *Int Immunol*, 1998;**10**:1613–22.

92. Rosloniec, E.F., *et al.*, An HLA-DR1 transgene confers susceptibility to collagen-induced arthritis elicited with human type II collagen. *J Exp Med*, 1997;**185**:1113–22.

93. Rosloniec, E.F., *et al.*, Induction of autoimmune arthritis in HLA-DR4 (DRB1*0401) transgenic mice by immunization with human and bovine type II collagen. *J Immunol*, 1998;**160**:2573–8.

94. Nabozny, G.H., *et al.*, HLA-DQ8 transgenic mice are highly susceptible to collagen-induced arthritis: a novel model for human polyarthritis. *J Exp Med*, 1996;**183**:27–37.

95. Bradley, D.S., *et al.*, HLA-DQB1 polymorphism determines incidence, onset, and severity of collagen-induced arthritis in transgenic mice. Implications in human rheumatoid arthritis. *J Clin Invest*, 1997;**100**:2227–34.

96. Taneja, V., *et al.*, Modulation of HLA-DQ-restricted collagen-induced arthritis by HLA-DRB1 polymorphism. *Int Immunol*, 1998;**10**:1449–57.

97. Bradley, D.S., *et al.*, HLA-DQ6/8 double transgenic mice develop auricular chondritis following type II collagen immunization: a model for human relapsing polychondritis. *J Immunol*, 1998;**161**:5046–53.

98. Zanelli, E., C.J. Krco, and C.S. David, Critical residues on HLA-DRB1*0402 HV3 peptide for HLA-DQ8-restricted immunogenicity: implications for rheumatoid arthritis predisposition. *J Immunol*, 1997;**158**:3545–51.

99. John S., *et al.*, Linkage of cytokine genes to rheumatoid arthritis. Evidence of genetic heterogeneity. *Ann Rheum Dis*, 1998;**57**:361–5.

100. Shaw, M.A., *et al.*, Linkage of rheumatoid arthritis to the candidate gene NRAMP1 on 2q35. *J Exp Genet*, 1996;**33**:672–7.

101. Jouvenne, P., *et al.*, Possible genetic association between interleukin-1 alpha gene polymorphism and the severity of chronic polyarthritis. *Eur Cytokine Netw*, 1999;**10**:33–6.

102. Cornelis, F., *et al.*, Association of rheumatoid arthritis with an amino acid allelic variation of the T cell receptor. *Arthritis Rheum*, 1997;**40**:1387–90.

103. Ibberson, M., *et al.*, Analysis of T cell receptor V alpha polymorphisms in rheumatoid arthritis. *Ann Rheum Dis*, 1998;**57**:49–51.

104. Hall, F.C., *et al.*, A linkage study across the T cell receptor A and T cell receptor B loci in families with rheumatoid arthritis. *Arthritis Rheum*, 1997;**40**:1798–802.

105. Brown, M.A., *et al.*, The role of germline polymorphisms in the T-cell receptor in susceptibility to ankylosing spondylitis. *Br J Rheumatol*, 1998;**37**:454–8

106. Turner, D.M., *et al.*, An investigation of polymorphism in the interleukin-10 gene promoter. *Eur J Immunogen*, 1997;**24**:1–8.

107. Kube, D., *et al.*, Isolation of the human interleukin 10 promoter. Characterization of the promoter activity in Burkitt's lymphoma cell lines. *Cytokine*, 1995;**7**:1–7.

108. Westendorp, R.G., *et al.*, Genetic influence on cytokine production and fatal meningococcal disease. *Lancet*, 1997;**349**:170–3.

109. Coakley, G., *et al.*, Interleukin-10 promoter polymorphisms in rheumatoid arthritis and Felty's syndrome. *Br J Rheumatol*, 1998;**37**:988–91.

110. Hajeer, A.H., *et al.*, IL–10 gene promoter polymorphisms in rheumatoid arthritis.*Scand J Rheumatol*, 1998;27:142–5.

111. Huizinga, T.W.J., *et al.*, Differences in IL–10 production are associated with joint damage. (submitted).

112. Eskdale, J., *et al.*, Interleukin 10 secretion in relation to human IL–10 locus haplotypes. *Proc Natl Acad Sci USA*, 1998;**95**:9465–70.

113. Eskdale, J., *et al.*, Interleukin-10 microsatellite polymorphisms and IL–10 locus alleles in rheumatoid arthritis susceptibility [letter]. *Lancet*, 1998;**352**:1282–3.

114. Schork, N.J. and J.S. Lanchbury, Intergrated phenotyping, disease models, and pathophysiologic databases. (submitted).

2 | *Epidemiology of rheumatoid arthritis*

Franz Calvo and Graciela S. Alarcón

Introduction

The study of the distribution of rheumatoid arthritis (RA) among distinct human groups, at different times, and its impact on the individual affected with it falls within the scope of Descriptive Epidemiology. Analyses of individuals at risk for developing RA of variable severity (by virtue of a given attribute or risk factor), on the other hand, fall within the realm of Analytical Epidemiology. This knowledge may have direct impact in the management of such patients and it has, therefore, not only theoretical but also practical implications. We will limit this section to adult RA.

Descriptive epidemiology

Descriptive studies of diseases still lacking a clear etiology are hampered by the sensitivity, specificity, and positive and negative predictive value of the criteria used to classify cases[1]. In RA, earlier studies (conducted prior to the discovery and widespread utilization of the rheumatoid factor) may have included cases of 'rheumatoid spondylitis', rheumatic fever, gout, and osteoarthritis. If cases are only diagnosed when typical deformities and/or radiographically demonstrable damage has occurred, there will be relatively little misclassification of cases (with diseases other than RA), but patients with early RA might be totally missed[2]. On the other hand, if RA is defined as the presence of characteristic symmetric synovitis with morning stiffness, early cases will be included but non-RA cases are likely to be included as well. Finally, it should be noted that in the criteria for the classification of RA, adopted by the American College of Rheumatology (ACR) in 1987[3], the categories of probable, definite, and classical disease, as defined in 1958[4], are no longer considered (cases diagnosed as having probable RA are unlikely to meet criteria for RA at later times). Thus, it is hard to merge clinical data obtained using the 1958 classification criteria with more recent studies in which these categories are not used at all. The previous criteria also included a long list of exclusions that were hard to meet in either practice-based or population-based studies and thus they were also dropped. Likewise, since in actual practice tissue from either joint cavities or subcutaneous nodules is not obtained, the histopathological criteria were removed. The ACR revised criteria were developed using patients from tertiary care facilities but they, too, have been tested in populations (such as the Pima Indian population of Arizona) and found to perform adequately if present at more than one point in time[5]. Consequently, the revised criteria can be used both in population-based and practice-based studies. These and other methodological considerations need to be kept in mind when the epidemiological literature pertaining to RA is examined.

Prevalence

Although RA is currently described as occurring world-wide in about one per cent of the adult population[6], its regional and temporal prevalence has been variable. The disease is about five times more frequent among indigenous populations of the North American sub-continent than in Caucasian populations from either North America or Europe[7]. Asian and African populations, who presumably came in contact with these indigenous populations later than Europeans, have a much lower prevalence of RA than Caucasians[8]. Moreover, evidence for the existence of RA before the 17th and 20th centuries in Europe and in Africa, respectively, have led investigators to hypothesize that RA originated in North America and was transported to the Old World by returning Spanish conquistadores[9,10]. This contrasted with other rheumatic diseases such as ankylosing spondylitis, osteoarthritis, and some infectious arthritis (tuberculosis) for which there is clear pictorial, graphical, and/or physical (skeletal remains) evidence of their existence in the Old World from ancient times[11–15]. RA might thus be a unique disease among chronic rheumatic disorders. It can be argued, however, that RA is much harder to identify both pictorially and in skeletal remains than diseases that primarily affect larger anatomical structures such as the spine or the weight-bearing joints, and thus we may never be able to affirm categorically that the disease was non-existent in Europe prior to the discovery of the Americas. Another factor that can partially account for the lower prevalence of RA in some developing countries such as Indonesia and Pakistan is its particular demographic distribution: life expectancy is lower than that of Western populations, with women becoming outnumbered by men by the fifth decade of life[16,17] with the consequent decrease in the number of individuals potentially at risk for developing RA. It is intriguing that the risk of developing RA doubles for Pakistanis after living several years in a Western environment such as England[18].

Table 2.1 presents prevalence data for RA in different population groups. These populations have been divided into those

Table 2.1 Prevalence of RA*

Population	Prevalence*
High prevalence	
Yakima Indians, USA	6.0
Chippewa Indians, USA	5.3
Pima Indians, USA	5.3
Intermediate prevalence	
Europe	
Bulgaria	0.9
Denmark	0.9
England	1.1
Greece	0.2
Netherlands	0.9
Sweden	0.9
North America (Caucasians)	
USA	1.0
Sudbury, Massachusetts	0.9
South America and Caribbean	
Brazil	0.6
Colombia	0.1
Jamaica	1.9
Low prevalence	
Asia	
China, a rural island	0.3
China, mainland	0.3
Hong Kong	0.2
Indonesia, rural	0.2
Indonesia, urban	0.3
Japan	0.3
Pakistan	0.1
Philippines	0.2
Taiwan	0.3
Africa	
Lesotho	0.3
Nigeria and Liberia	0
Nigeria	0
South Africa, rural	0
Middle East	
Egypt	0.2
Israel	0.3
Oman	0.4

* Adapted from Abdel-Nasser A.M., Rasker J.J., Valkenburg H.A. Epidemiological and clinical aspects relating to the variability of rheumatoid arthritis. *Semin Arthritis Rheum.* 1997;27:123–40. Figures have been rounded and are shown with only one decimal.

with high, intermediate, and low prevalence rates of the disease which closely agree with the geographic area in which they are located[19–22].

Incidence

The few community-based incidence studies of RA performed in indigenous and non-indigenous populations of North America support the prevalence data just reviewed, with RA occurring at a higher rate in the Pima Indians and other Native American tribes than in Caucasian populations from Europe and North America[20,23–25]. There are no incidence studies from Latin American or African countries. Nevertheless, the existing data support the hypothesis that RA may have originated in North America. Data from available studies are summarized in Table 2.2[19].

Table 2.2 Annual incidence rate (per 100 population) of definite RA in different populations*

Population	Study period	Incidence
Native-American Indians		
Alaskan	1970–84	0.09
Pima	1966–73	0.89
Pima	1974–82	0.62
Pima	1983–90	0.38
USA (Caucasians)		
Rochester, MI	1950–74	0.04
Seattle, WA	1987–89	0.02
Worcester, MA	1987–90	0.03
Europe		
England and Wales	1970–72	0.02
England and Wales	1980–82	0.19
England	1990	0.02
Finland	1974–75	0.04
Finland	1980–90	0.04
France	1980–84	0.01
Netherlands	1947–65	0.05
Norway	1969–84	0.02
Asia		
Japan	1958–64	0.04
Japan	1962–66	0.06
Japan	1965–67	0.09

* Reproduced with permission from Abdel-Nasser A.M., Rasker J.J., Valkenburg H.A. Epidemiological and clinical aspects relating to the variability of rheumatoid arthritis. *Semin Arthritis Rheum.* 1997;27:123–40.

Person-related attributes: age and gender

RA occurs predominantly in women rather than in men (2:1 to 3:1 ration in most studies), which suggests the existence of a higher (genetic) threshold requirement for RA in men. Consistent with this model, several studies have shown that the association between genetic markers and RA is stronger in men than in women[26,27]. The role of hormonal factors in triggering or modulating the onset of the disease and its manifestations will be discussed later.

The influence of gender in the clinical expression of the disease continues to be an interesting topic. RA of comparable severity occurs in both men and women, although some clinical forms such as the 'robust' (or 'robustus') form of the disease is characteristically more common in men who are physical laborers. These patients seem to have only a modest amount of pain and develop little incapacitation over time[28,29]. An alternative explanation is that the robust type of RA is due to the (stoic) personality of some individuals—preferentially men[30].

Weyand and collaborators, based on data from Olmsted County, Minnesota, have recently postulated that gender significantly influences the phenotype of the disease, as more women than men experience structural consequences of the disease (measured as the need for surgery) despite the fact that radiographically men tend to have more erosive disease. A close examination of these data, however, reveals that the differences in surgical rates are primarily due to foot and hand surgery rather than to large joint arthroplasties, suggesting that reasons other than structural damage of the joints may be behind the decision to perform these surgical procedures (footwear, appearance, to cite but a few). In any case, these data substantiate

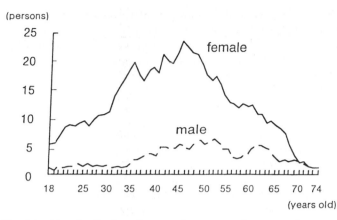

(persons)

(years old)

Fig. 2.1 The distribution of age at disease onset for men and women with RA. The polyarticular form of juvenile rheumatoid arthritis (JRA) can be regarded as the left tail of the distribution. (Reproduced with permission from Yukioka M., Wakitani S., Murata N., Toda Y., Ogawa R., Kaneshige T. *et al.* Elderly on-set rheumatoid arthritis and its association with HLA-DRB1 alleles in Japanese. *Br J Rheumatol*, 1998;37:98–101).

clinical observations made over the years: some extra-articular manifestations, particularly rheumatoid nodules and rheumatoid lung, are more common in men than in women[31]. These phenotypic differences could also result from associated factors such as trauma, smoking, and work-related exposure to toxins rather than to genetic or hormonal differences between the genders[32].

The peak age of onset of RA is in the fifth decade of life[33], but it may occur as early as in the second decade. A seropositive, polyarticular form of juvenile rheumatoid arthritis (JRA) occurs predominantly in adolescent girls. Although it is hard to state whether this JRA subtype is one of the tails of the age distribution for RA as shown in Fig. 2.1[33], common clinic, serologic, radiographic, and immunogenetic characteristics suggest this (Table 2.3)[34,35]. The age of onset of RA appears to be shifting towards later in life, but whether this is a real trend or only an artifact resulting from the aging of the population and/or an increase in access to specialized care among the elderly, has not been sorted out to date[33,36]. In fact, it is not uncommon to see new onset RA in octa- or even nonagenarian individuals, which would have been unheard of a few decades ago[37].

Age also appears to modulate the clinical expression of RA, resulting in some controversy as to the course and final outcome

of the apparently more favorable cases of elderly-onset RA[33,38]. In some of these patients it is unclear whether, in fact, they may have polymyalgia rheumatica, RS₃PE (the syndrome described by McCarty as seronegative symmetric synovitis with pitting edema and characteristic occurrence in elderly men)[39], a transient polyarthritis, or RA *per se*[40].

Other person-related attributes

Some other person-related attributes, particularly formal education[41] and marital status [42] (proxies for socioeconomic status), appear to impact the course and ultimate outcome of the disease rather than the susceptibility to its occurrence. Smoking appears to influence not only the course of the disease in a dose-dependent manner[32,43], but also to increase the risk of developing RA[44-46]. Smoking may exert systemic deleterious effects by altering nitric oxide pathways, perturbing local and systemic immune functions as well as the vascular endothelium[47]. Finally, a diet rich in Ω-3 fatty acids as consumed by Eskimo and some Pacific Islander populations has been found to protect them from the occurrence of RA[48]. These facts prompted the use of dietary supplementation with fish oil to treat RA in the 1980s with very modest results[49-51].

Secular trends in RA prevalence and incidence

For reasons not yet clear, a decline in both the prevalence and incidence of RA, which may have reached an all time high in the 1960s, has been observed in some Native Americans of the United States, Caucasians from North America and Europe, and in Japanese populations (Fig. 2.2)[25,37,52-55]. In contrast, RA appears to be on the rise in African countries, where it has supposedly emerged later[56]. The possibility that the decline in the occurrence of RA relates to the introduction of oral contraceptives in the Western world has been considered, based on large epidemiological studies from North America and Europe[57]. However, the data have not been entirely consistent and thus a final conclusion has not been reached (see below).

The phenotype of the disease also appears to be changing over time. Overall it seems that we are not seeing as many patients with severe articular and extra-articular disease as we saw decades ago[58-61]. This decline in the severity of RA coupled with a decrease in its incidence and prevalence, as already mentioned,

Table 2.3 Comparative features between RA and JRA subtypes

	Rheumatoid arthritis	Polyarticular JRA* (RF+)	Other JRA subtypes
	-	10% of JRA	90% of JRA
Gender (W:M)	3:1	W > M	Variable
Clinical	Symmetric arthritis	Indistinguishable from RA	Variable
Autoantibodies other than RF	Usual	SSA, SSB may appear during the course of the disease	Unusual
Radiological	Erosive arthritis	Erosive arthritis	Usually non-erosive
HLA-DR4 positivity	Usual	≥ 60%	15%

* Juvenile rheumatoid arthritis.

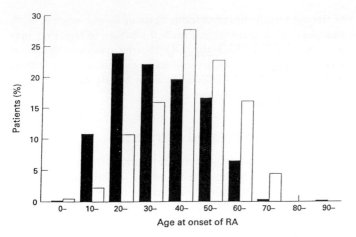

Fig. 2.2   Increase in age at onset of RA in Japan. ■: patients from 1960 to 1965; □: patients from 1985 to 1990. (Reproduced with permission from Imanaka T., Shichikawa K., Inoue K., Shimaoka Y., Takenaka Y., Wakitani S. Increase in age at onset of rheumatoid arthritis in Japan over a 30 year period. *Ann Rheum Dis.*, 1997;56:313–6).

have led some investigators to postulate that RA might eventually disappear as a human malady[62]. Although we would like to share such optimism and enthusiasm, we think caution is in order, as these observations may result from differences in case ascertainment, case selection, access to health care, and other methodological problems rather than from a true decline in the occurrence of the disease or a change in its phenotype.

Impact of RA

According to Fries, the impact of any given disorder should be examined along five defined dimensions: survival, disability, discomfort, iatrogenesis/comorbidities, and economic losses[63]. Some of these dimensions of outcome will be examined in detail in different chapter; thus we will only discuss in this chapter survival and comorbidities directly related to the disease or its treatments.

Survival and causes of death

It is unquestionable that patients with RA die earlier than their peers. Hospital-based studies have shown excess death rates ranging from 30 to 200 per cent[64]. In population-based studies excess mortality rates have been less evident, but still significantly higher than in controls[65,66]. Causes contributing to excess mortality are infectious[67–69], renal[67–69], respiratory[68], and gastrointestinal diseases[67,70]. Malignancies of the reticuloendothelial system have been reported with increased frequency, but, overall, the data on malignancies are controversial[69,71]. The leading cause of death in rheumatoid arthritis is, however, cardiovascular diseases, accounting for almost half of the mortality[66,72]. Hence, the majority of patients with RA die from the same causes as the general population, but at a younger age. In populations where other comorbid conditions account for the main causes of death, these are also the causes among patients with RA. That is the case, for example, of the Pima Indians of

Arizona, where alcohol-related deaths are the leading cause among the general population as well as among RA patients[65].

A greater number of involved joints, older age, fewer number of years of education, significant functional losses, and the presence of comorbid cardiovascular conditions are all significant predictors of mortality in RA[73]. In fact, Pincus *et al.* have suggested that, like patients with malignant disorders or coronary artery disease (CAD), patients with RA could simply be 'staged', based on the number of joints involved to predict correctly their probability of survival at five or 10 years. Patients with RA and a large number of joints involved (or significant functional impairment) may have a five year survival probability of only 40–60 per cent, which is comparable to that of patients with stage IV Hodgkin's lymphoma or three-vessel CAD[74].

An increase in the death rate due to cardiovascular and cerebrovascular diseases as a consequence of the utilization of methotrexate (resulting in elevated levels of homocysteine in the blood) has been proposed but not supported by available data[75]. A possible increment in the occurrence of lung cancer (and deaths due to it) in methotrexate-treated RA patients was reported in a study from Canada[76], but such findings have not been corroborated in studies from other centers[77].

In general, it can be said that RA appears to decrease the expected survival of affected individuals anywhere from three to 10 years. Survival curves for RA patients from North America are shown in Fig. 2.3[78].

Morbidity

RA is capable of inflicting significant structural damage on the affected individual; damage that occurs primarily on the musculoskeletal system. So debilitated may these patients become, that some authors have urged rheumatologists to consider the 'side-effects' of the disease when evaluating the possible 'side-effects' of effective remedies used to treat this condition (and weigh them before making therapeutic decisions)[79]. Patients with RA may become considerably catabolic, even in the absence of exogenous compounds such as corticosteroids, probably due to the systemic effects of proinflammatory cytokines such as IL-1β and TNF-α. They may also experience significant anorexia and their ability to cook may be compromised. Thus, it is not uncommon for RA patients to become markedly malnourished (rheumatoid cachexia)[80,81]. These malnourished patients tend to have a poorer prognosis than patients who are able to maintain their ideal body weight[82]. Sedentarism, coupled with extremely poor eating habits, on the other hand, may lead to obesity with detrimental consequences in already damaged weight-bearing joints and other organ systems[83].

As opposed to SLE, no international consortium of investigators has yet developed a damage index to measure the impact of the disease (or of the drugs used) in RA. This absence may be related to the fact that the 'irreversible' damage produced by the disease, at least in the musculoskeletal system, is quite obvious. In any case, RA is measurable. The disease has been staged radiographically for over five decades using the Steinbrocker Staging System but this system has some deficiencies, including its lack of correlation with other outcome parameters[84,85]. More refined radiographic methods have been developed both in Europe and

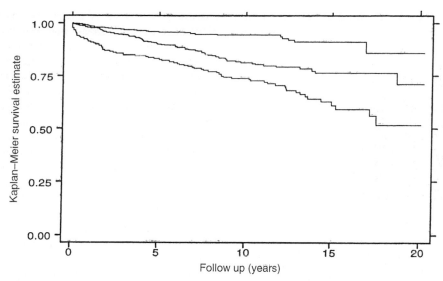

Figure 2.3 Cumulative probability of survival for a cohort of RA patients according with the Health Assessment Questionnaire (HAQ) Disability index scores of 0–1 (top), 1–2 (intermediate), or 2–3 (lower curve). (Reproduced with permission from Wolfe F., Zwillich S.H. The long-term outcomes of rheumatoid arthritis. A 23-year prospective, longitudinal study of total joint replacement and its predictors in 1600 patients with rheumatoid arthritis. *Arthritis Rheum*, 1998;41:1072–82).

North America (the Larsen[86] and Sharp[87,88] methods respectively), and modified subsequently for easier applicability in the clinical setting. Only recently, investigators from both sides of the Atlantic have agreed on establishing guidelines for the use of radiographic methods for the assessment of joint destruction (damage) in patients with RA[89].

From a comprehensive perspective, damage is also caused by the medications used to treat a disease. Efforts have been made to quantify the deleterious effect of some therapeutic agents commonly used in RA (pharmaco epidemiology) such as non-steroidal anti-inflammatory agents (NSAIDs) and disease modifying antirheumatic drugs (DMARDs), particularly methotrexate.

The use of NSAIDs is associated with various gastroduodenal mucosal lesions, collectively referred to as NSAID gastropathy[90]. This is probably one of the most frequent 'rheumatic' disorders at present, and the most frequent adverse effect reported to the United States Food and Drug Administration[91]. Patients who take NSAIDs have a four- to six-fold increased risk of developing peptic ulcers[92,93] (point prevalence of about 20 per cent when all ulcers in these patients are considered NSAID-related), and the annual incidence of serious complications in these patients—hemorrhage or perforation—is about 4 per cent[94]. In the United States alone, direct medical costs attributable to NSAID gastropathy and its complications were estimated to exceed $4 (£2.4) billion a year in 1993[95].

Corticosteroids also have a defined and important toxicity profile[96,97], and although it has recently been reported that daily oral corticosteroids, contrary to popular belief, may protect patients from the occurrence of bone and joint destruction[98], this fact has not been borne out in an early RA cohort[99] and it is certainly not the experience of seasoned clinicians. Nevertheless, corticosteroids are used since they are still the most potent anti-inflammatory drugs available to date and as such are capable of significantly alleviating the symptoms and signs of inflammation which typify this disease[100].

Felson and collaborators have established a comparative safety (and efficacy) profile for the commonly used DMARDs[47], and Morgan *et al.* have empirically developed a toxicity index to quantify the side-effects resulting from the administration of methotrexate, an index that proved to be useful in their folic acid supplementation studies[101].

Finally, the long-term toxicity profile of methotrexate is becoming apparent as we complete the second decade of its use and of its widespread utilization in rheumatology. Whereas some clearly folate deficiency toxicities (abdominal discomfort, alopecia, oral ulcerations) have been curbed with the concomitant administration of folic acid, that is not the case (or it is unclear) with hepatic, pulmonary, and malignant events related to its administration[102–105]. Risk factors for the occurrence of methotrexate-induced clinically significant liver disease include older age and cumulative methotrexate dose (and probably diabetes)[106–108]. For the occurrence of pulmonary toxicity these factors include age older than 60 years, diabetes, hypoalbuminemia, underlying RA pleuropulmonary involvement, and previous use of other DMARD[109,110]. No risk factors have been found, thus far, for EBV-related (or unrelated) B cell lymphomas occurring in methotrexate-treated RA patients[111,112].

Analytical epidemiology

RA as a multifactorial disease

Although the cause (or causes) of what we currently call RA remain elusive, the general consensus is that factors or attributes contributing to its occurrence and course are probably both genetic and environmental, with RA resulting from their interaction. Genetic factors have been suspected for decades based on the clustering of the disease among families and among individuals from highly inbred populations, as well as by the degree of concordance for the disease among monozygotic twins (15–30 per cent). Likewise, environmental triggers have been suspected all along with the number of agents purported as causal agents of RA coming and going over the years (see below).

Genetic factors

RA is a complex, oligogenic disease where genetic factors may account for as much as 60 per cent of disease susceptibility[113]. The study of the genetic factors predisposing to the occurrence of RA is relatively recent. It was only two decades ago that the association between RA and some class II HLA alleles (HLA-Dw4, now HLA-DR4) was reported in Caucasian patients[114]. Since then we have learned that the association is not with HLA-DR4 *per se* but with a sequence motif present in the α helical portion (third hypervariable region) of the β chain of the HLA-DRB1 molecule that forms one side of the peptide binding groove. This sequence motif (QKRAA, QRRAA, OR RRRAA), also called 'rheumatoid epitope', is encoded by HLA-DR4 (*0401, *0404, and *0405 alleles) and some non-DR4 haplotypes, such as HLA-DR1, DR6, and DR10. The initial studies conducted at the Mayo Clinic in 1992 suggested that the rheumatoid epitope (its dose and the alleles carrying it) were important determinants of disease severity as measured by the need for joint surgery, the presence of subcutaneous nodules, and the occurrence of extra-articular manifestations. These studies were, however, conducted in a highly selected sample of Caucasian RA patients with established and advanced disease followed at a tertiary care facility[115]. Based on these data, it was postulated that the course and final outcome of RA could be determined at disease onset based on the genotype of the afflicted person (genotype predicting phenotype) and the patient should be treated accordingly[116,117]. This initial enthusiasm has been followed by caution as the shared epitope appears less relevant to disease severity in some non-Caucasian racial groups, such as North Americans of Hispanic[118] or African descent[119], and Pakistanis[120]. Moreover, in studies of patients with early RA, the frequency of the epitope was comparable among those individuals who evolved to articular destruction and those who completely resolved their articular manifestations, invalidating the value of genotyping to approach more accurately the treatment of patients with early pre-erosive disease. Nevertheless, most studies have shown that there is correlation between disease progression as determined radiographically and the shared epitope[121]. These studies are summarized in Table 2.4[7,26,33,122–132].

In contrast to these 'susceptibility genes', a number of DR specificities have been reported to be protective of RA, as they appear to occur with increased frequency in unaffected individuals. However, the molecular basis for this 'protection' is at the present time unknown. These protective alleles include some DRB1[133,134], HLA-DR1/DR5, DR2, DR2/DR3, DR3/DR7, and DR8[26,135].

The role other MHC genes such as HLA-DQB1 may play in susceptibility to RA or its severity remains unclear to date[136,137]. The associations described may relate only to linkage disequilibrium between some HLA-DR and HLA-DQ alleles. Genes located in chromosome 6, and specifically within the MHC region, have been the subject of intense investigation in patients with RA, as their products appear to play a pivotal role in the inflammatory process which characterizes this condition. One of these is the cytokine TNF-α, currently a strong candidate susceptibility gene for RA. Some studies have found associations between certain TNF-α alleles and susceptibility to RA or disease severity[27,138–141], but others could not detect any independent contribution of the TNF locus to the genetic etiology of RA in Caucasians[142,143].

Environmental factors

As noted above, a possible infectious involvement in the etiology of RA has been a theme of interest in the rheumatology community for decades[144–147]. Different infectious agents have been implicated in the causation of this disease, but even if they can induce a syndrome clinically indistinguishable from RA, they are relatively infrequent and thus can only explain a fraction of the cases (or of the cause) of RA (attributable risk)[148]. That is the case, for example, for *Borrelia burgdorferi* (Lyme disease), Parvovirus B-19 (Fifth disease), or rubella virus, to cite but a few[149,150]. Given the world-wide distribution of RA, more than one microbe must be involved in its causation. It is possible, however, that the infectious agent responsible for RA originated in the Americas and become distributed world-wide after Europeans came in contact with the native populations of the New World[8]. We know that infectious agents may be relatively isolated by geographic barriers, lack of proper ecological requirements to complete their vital cycle, or lack of exposure to humans. In fact syphilis, for example, was unknown to the

Table 2.4   Association of HLA-DR alleles with RA in various ethnic groups

Allele	Assoc. with susceptibility	Assoc. with severity	Ethnic groups
DRB1*0101	✔		Asian Indians, Jews, Caucasians, Greek, Japanese
DRB1*0102	✔		Israeli Jews
DRB1*0401	✔	✔	Koreans, Caucasians, Greek
DRB1*0404	✔	✔	Chinese, Caucasians
DRB1*0405	✔	✔	Koreans, Japanese, Chinese, Spanish, Greek
DRB1*0408		✔	Caucasians
DRB1*0410	✔	✔	Japanese, Chinese
DRB1*1001	✔		Southern Africans, Spanish
DRB1*1402	✔		Yakima Indians, Peruvians

inhabitants of the Old World prior to Columbus, Lyme disease is limited to ecosystems with the capabilities of sustaining the vital cycle of *Borrelia burgdorferi*, and several viral infections which have originated in Africa have only appeared in humans relatively recently (*Ebola* virus, and the human immunodeficiency virus, to cite but a few)[151,152].

It is conceivable that, in the genetically predisposed individual, more than one environmental noxa, infectious or not, triggers the development of RA by initiating an immunopathologic reaction leading to a cascade of events initially characterized by inflammation (predominantly at the articular level) and later by joint destruction. If an infectious agent (not necessarily the entire organism, but a microbial product) is involved in RA, it is likely to be through molecular mimicry of specific microbial peptides with autologous molecules such as the rheumatoid epitope or cartilage-derived epitopes rather than by actual conventional seeding of the joint cavity and its structures[153–155].

Other factors

RA, as many other rheumatic disorders associated with alterations of the immune system/response, occurs more frequently in women (and during their reproductive years) than in men, leading investigators to pursue the role sex hormones may play in disease susceptibility and modulation. In general, estrogens exert an stimulatory effect on the immune system by inhibiting T-cell suppressor function and facilitating T-cell maturation[156].

Pregnancy

The beneficial effect of pregnancy in the clinical manifestations of RA was first reported by Garrrod over a century ago and confirmed by Hench during the 1930s[157]. An improvement in the symptoms occurs in about three-fourths of pregnancies, but, with rare exception, arthritis returns by the third to fourth month after delivery[158,159]. This effect was initially linked to the production of steroids by the placenta. Subsequent studies demonstrated that the placenta produces a pregnancy-associated glycoprotein or PAG[160], an anti-inflammatory/immunomodulatory protein which is present in high concentrations during pregnancy (and declining levels in the post-partum period), in those women with RA experiencing improvement of their symptoms during pregnancy.

Other non-HLA factors that probably contribute to the amelioration and ultimate reactivation of the disease in pregnancy are IgG galactosylation abnormalities[161]. Healthy individuals, with exception of the perinatal period and ages older than 40 years, maintain a low proportion of agalactosyl IgG (IgG-G0), a glycosylation pattern also normally found during pregnancy. RA patients exhibit increased IgG-G0, and animal models suggest that these IgGs may be directly involved in the pathogenesis of the disease[162]. The findings of (i) a correlation between changes in disease activity and changes in IgG-G0 during pregnancy and postpartum[163] and (ii) an elevation in the IgG-G0 level preceding the first clinical symptoms of RA in Pima Indians, support the hypothesis that IgG galactosylation abnormalities may constitute an independent susceptibility factor in RA[164].

Finally, it has been proposed that remissions occurring during pregnancy relate to the maternal immune response to the paternal HLA antigens, as remissions are more likely to occur when there is maternal–paternal HLA disparity (for HLA-DRB1, -DQA, and -DQB) than when there is none[165]. The interplay between the immune system and sex hormones is further supported by the increased occurrence of RA after the first pregnancy in which there was fetal–maternal HLA disparity.

The data reviewed suggest that the remissions observed during pregnancy relate to the transient effect of hormonal and non-hormonal factors. These effects, which revert or normalize in the post-partum period, explain the flares observed in the post-partum period in women experiencing remissions of their disease while pregnant. The net effect of pregnancy in the long-term prognosis of women with RA, however, is not known.

The relationship between parity and RA is also being elucidated. Women that have been pregnant are less likely to develop RA than nulliparous women, independent of family history and the use of oral contraceptives. As shown by Dugowson *et al.*[156], parity has a protective effect, or nulliparity is a risk factor for RA with an odds ratio (OR) of 2.2. In an extension of the prior study, Nelson *et al.* found that in a comparison of parous to nulliparous women the OR for developing RA 1 to 2 years after a term pregnancy was 0.4, for 2 to 3 years 0.3, and for 3 to 4 years 0.2[159].

Oral contraceptives

The possible protective and modulatory effect of oral contraceptives (OC) in RA has been extensively studied. Two independently conducted studies in the United States and England and published in the late 1970s–early 1980s supported the possible protective role of the birth control pill in RA[167]. In the United States study, a secular declining trend (coinciding with the introduction and utilization of the birth control pill) was observed among women but not men[25] while in the English study RA occurred less frequently among users versus non-users of the pill[167]. Studies that have not supported the protective role of the pill have been interpreted as reflecting differences in the populations studied rather than true differences. So far, one of the most plausible explanations for these discrepancies has come from the meta-analysis conducted by Spector and Hochberg, who divided the studies according to whether they were hospital-based or population-based. The pooled OR from the hospital-based studies was 0.49 whereas it was 0.95 for the population-based studies. These differences suggest that OCs protect against severe disease which requires hospital referral rather than protecting against its occurrence[168]. Overall, however, it has not been possible to reach consensus as to the purported protective effect of OCs in RA[57].

Estrogen replacement therapy

The use of estrogen replacement therapy (ERT) during the post-menopausal years has been associated with the occurrence of systemic lupus erythematosus (relative risk of 2.1 for ever-users and 2.5 for current users) and with lupus flares[169]. On the contrary, ERT may have a beneficial effect in RA by ameliorating bone loss without exacerbating the joint disease[170] while at the same time protecting patients from the occurrence of cardio-vascular comorbid conditions. There may even be a modest reduction in the risk of developing RA among progestin users[171].

Androgens

Lower concentrations of androgenic corticosteroids have been found in both men and women with RA[172,173] and it has been proposed that androgens may have a slight disease modifying effect in RA[174].

Conclusions

Significant advances have been made over the last few decades in understanding the events leading to joint destruction in patients with RA. As the factors responsible for disease causation and modulation are better understood and new therapies are developed, it is conceivable that patients can be better categorized at disease onset into subsets with divergent expected outcomes, patients treated accordingly, and the devastating effects of the disease significantly curtailed. Large, multicenter, multinational cohorts of patients with early disease in whom sociodemographic, clinical, radiographic, functional, serologic, cellular, hormonal, genetic, and tissue datasets and repositories are established will certainly be necessary for success to occur.

References

1. Hayse S. Design and conduct collaborative international epidemiological studies of rheumatic disease. *Rheum Dis Clin North Am*, 1990;**16**:763–72.
2. Allander E. Conflict between epidemiological and clinical diagnosis of rheumatoid arthritis in a population sample. *Scand J Rheumatol*, 1973;**2**:109–12.
3. Arnett F.C., Edworthy S.M., Bloch D.A., McShane D.J., Fries J.F., Cooper N.S. *et al*. The American Rheumatism Association 1987 revised criteria for the classification of rheumatoid arthritis. *Arthritis Rheum*, 1988;**31**:315–24.
4. Ropes M.S., Bennett G.A., Cobb S. 1958 revision of diagnostic criteria for rheumatoid arthritis. *Bulletin Rheum Dis*, 1958;**9**:175–6.
5. Jacobsson L.T.H., Knowler W.C., Pillemer S., Hanson R.L., Pettitt D.J., McCance D.R. *et al*. A cross-sectional and longitudinal comparison of the Rome criteria for active rheumatoid arthritis (equivalent to the American College of Rheumatology 1958 criteria) and the American College of Rheumatology 1987 criteria for rheumatoid arthritis. *Arthritis Rheum*, 1994;**37**:1479–86.
6. Lawrence R.C., Hochberg M.C., Kelsey J.L., McDuffie F.C., Medsger T.A., Jr., Felts W.R. *et al*. Estimates of the prevalence of selected arthritic and musculoskeletal diseases in the United States. *J Rheumatol*, 1989;**16**:427–41.
7. Castro F., Angulo J., Acevedo E., Quispe E., Perich R., Ciusani E. *et al*. [Fenotipo clase II del complejo mayor de histocompatibilidad en artritis reumatoide: Primer reporte en pacientes peruanos]. Type II major histocompatibility complex phenotypes in rheumatoid arthritis: First report in Peruvian patients. *Bol Asoc Peruan Rheum*, 1994;**13**:14.
8. Rothschild B.M., Woods R.J., Rothschild C., Sebes J.I. Geographic distribution of rheumatoid arthritis in ancient North America: Implications for pathogenesis. *Semin Arthritis Rheum*, 1992;**22**:181–7.
9. Mijiyawa M. Epidemiology and semiology of rheumatoid arthritis in third world countries. *Rev Rhum Eng Ed*, 1995;**62**:121–6.
10. Halberg P. Rheumatoid arthritis. In: *Rheumatology* (Klippel J.H., Dieppe P.A., eds). London: Mosby-Year Book; 1994:21–4.
11. Arriaza B.T., Salo W., Aufderheide A.C., Holcomb T.A. Pre-Columbian tuberculosis in Northern Chile: molecular and skeletal evidence. *Am J Phys Anthropol*, 1995;**98**:37–45.
12. Horvath R., Horackova L., Benesova L., Bartos M., Votava M. [Detekce DNA specificke pro mycobacterium tuberculosis v archeologickych materialech metodou polymerazove retezove reakce] Detection of DNA specific for mycobaterium tuberculosis in archeological material using the polymerase chain reaction. *Epidemiol Mikrobiol Imunol*, 1997;**46**:9–12.
13. Martinez-Lavin M., Mansilla J., Pineda C., Pijoan C. Ankylosing spondylitis is indigenous to Mesoamerica. *J Rheumatol*, 1995;**22**:2327–30.
14. Palfi G.Y., Panuel M., Gyetvay A., Molnar E., Bende L., Dutour O. [Spondylarthrite ankylosante evoluee chez un sujet du VIIIe siecle] Advanced-stage ankylosing spondylitis in a subject in the 8th century. *J Radiol*, 1996;**77**:283–5.
15. Rothschild B.M. Paleopathology, its character and contribution to understanding and distinguishing among rheumatologic disease: perspectives on rheumatoid arthritis and spondyloarthropathy. *Clin. Exp. Rheumatol*, 1995;**13**:657–62.
16. Darmawan J., Muirden K., Vakenburg H, Wigley R. The epidemiology of rheumatoid arthritis in Indonesia. *Br J Rheumatol*, 1993;**32**:357–40.
17. Hameed K., Gibson T., Kadir M., Sultana S., Fatima Z., Syed A. the prevalence of rheumatoid arthritis in affluent and poor urban communities of Pakistan. *Br J Rheumatol*, 1995;**34**:252–6.
18. Hameed K, Gibson T. A comparison of the prevalence of rheumatoid arthritis and other rheumatic diseases among Pakistanis living in England and Pakistan. *Br J Rheumatol*, 1997;**36**:781–5.
19. Abdel-Nasser A.M., Rasker J.J., Valkenburg H.A. Epidemiological and clinical aspects relating to the variability of rheumatoid arthritis. *Semin Arthritis Rheum*, 1997;**27**:123–40.
20. Willkens R.F., Blandau R.L., Aoyama D.T., Beasley P. Studies of rheumatoid arthritis among a tribe of Northwest Indians. *J Rheumatol*, 1976;**3**:9–14.
21. Harvey J., Lotze M., Arnett F.C., Bias W.B., Billingsley L.M., Harvey E. *et al*. Rheumatoid arthritis in a Chippewa band. II. Field study with clinical, serological, and HLA-D correlations. *J Rheumatol*, 1983;**10**:28–32.
22. Drosos A.A., Alamanos I., Voulgari P.V., Psychos D.N., Katsaraki A., Papadopoulos I. *et al*. Epidemiology of adult rheumatoid arthritis in Northwest Greece 1987–1995. *J Rheumatol*, 1997;**24**:2129–33.
23. Harvey J., Arnett F.C., Bias W.B., Hsu S.H., Stevens M.B. Heterogeneity of HLA-DR4 in the rheumatoid arthritis of a Chippewa band. *J Rheumatol*, 1981;**8**:797–803.
24. Jacobsson L.T.H., Pillemer S.R. What can we learn about rheumatic diseases by studying Pima Indians? *J Rheumatol*, 1994;**21**:1179–80.
25. Linos A., Worthington J.W., O'Fallon W.M., Kurland L.T. The epidemiology of rheumatoid arthritis in Rochester Minnesota: A study of incidence prevalence and mortality. *Am J Epidemiol*, 1980;**111**:87–98.
26. Wakitani S., Murata N., Toda Y., Ogawa R., Kaneshige T., Nishimura Y. *et al*. The relationship between HLA-DRB1 alleles and disease subsets of rheumatoid arthritis in Japanese. *Br J Rheumatol*, 1997;**36**:630–6.
27. Hajeer A., John S., Ollier W.E., Silman A.J., Dawes P., Hassell A. *et al*. Tumor necrosis factor microsatellite haplotypes are different in male and female patients with rheumatoid arthritis. *J Rheumatol*, 1997;**24**:217–9.
28. Chopra A., Raghunath D., Singh A. Chronic inflammatory polyarthritides in a select population of young men. A prospective study. *J Assoc Physicians India*, 1989;**37**:748–51.
29. Dequeker J., Siebrandus S. Evidence of rheumatoid arthritis of the robust reaction type in a seventeeth century Dutch priest. *Ann Rheum Dis*, 1993;**52**:316.
30. Barker J.A., Sebes J.I. Rheumatoid arthritis of the robust-reaction type. *Arthritis Rheum*, 1998;**41**:1131–2.

31. Weyand C.M., Schmidt D., Wager U. Goronzy J.J. The influence of sex on the phenotype of rheumatoid arthritis. *Athritis Rheum* 1998;41:817–22.

32. Saag K.G., Cerhan J.R., Kolluri S., Ohashi K., Hunninghake G.W., Schwartz D.A. Cigarette smoking and rheumatoid arthritis severity. *Ann Rheum Dis*, 1997;56:463–9.

33. Yukioka M., Wakitani S., Murata N., Toda Y., Ogawa R., Kaneshige T. et al. Elderly-onset rheumatoid arthritis and its association with HLA-DRB1 alleles in Japanese. *Br J Rheumatol*, 1998;37:98–101.

34. Cerna M., Vavrincova P., Havelka S., Ivaskova E., Stastny P. Class II alleles in juvenile arthritis in Czech children. *J Rheumatol*, 1994;21:159–64.

35. Thomson W., Pepper L., Payton A., Carthy D., Scott D., Ollier W. et al. Absence of an association between HLA-DRB1*04 and rheumatoid arthritis in newly diagnosed cases from the community. *Ann Rheum Dis*, 1993;52:539–41.

36. Silman A.J. Problems complicating the genetic epidemiology of rheumatoid arthritis. *J Rheumatol*, 1997;24:194–6.

37. Imanaka T., Shichikawa K., Inoue K., Shimaoka Y., Takenaka Y., Wakitani S. Increase in age at onset of rheumatoid arthritis in Japan over a 30 year period. *Ann Rheum Dis*, 1997;56:313–6.

38. Shiozawa K., Tanaka Y., Imura S., Shiozawa S. Elderly-onset rheumatoid arthritis: Ageing as an independent marker for better prognosis. *Arthritis Rheum*, 1997;40:S151.

39. McCarty D.J., O'Duffy J.D., Pearson L., Hunter J.B., Remitting seronegative symmetrical synovitis with pitting edema. RS₃PE Syndrome. *J Am Med Assoc*, 1985:254:2763–7.

40. Olivieri I., Salvarani C., Cantini F. Remitting distal extremity swelling with pitting edema: a distinct syndrome or a clinical feature of different inflammatory rheumatic diseases? *J Rheumatol*, 1997;224:249–52.

41. Pincus T., Callahan L.F. Formal education as a marker for increased morality and morbidity in rheumatoid arthritis. *J Chronic Dis*, 1985;38:973–84.

42. Ward M.M., Leigh J.P. Marital status and the progression of functional disability in patients with rheumatoid arthritis. *Arthritis Rheum*, 1993;36:581–8.

43. McDonagh J.E., Walker D.J. Smoking and rheumatoid arthritis-observations from a multicase family study. *Arthritis Rheum*, 1997;40:594.

44. Masi A.T., Fecht T., Aldag J.C., Malamet R.L., Hazes J.M.W. Smoking and rheumatoid arthritis: comment on the letter by McDonagh and Walker. *Arthritis Rheum*, 1998;41:184.

45. Symmons D.P.M., Bankhead C.R., Harrison B.J., Brennan P., Barrett E.M., Scott D.G.I. et al. Blood transfusion, smoking, and obesity as risk factors for the development of rheumatoid arthritis. Results from a primary care-based incident case-control study in Norfolk, England. *Arthritis Rheum*, 1997;40:1955–61.

46. Wolfe F., Johnston D. Smoking is associated with premature development of rheumatoid arthritis and osteoarthritis. *Arthritis Rheum*, 1997;40:S312.

47. Farrell A.J., Blake D.R. Nitric oxide. *Ann Rheum Dis*, 1996;55: 7–20.

48. Horrobin D.F. Low prevalences of coronary heart disease, psoriasis, asthma, and rheumatoid arthritis in Eskimos: are they caused by high dietary intake of eicosapentaenoic acid (EPA), a genetic variation of essential fatty acid (EFA) metabolism or a combination of both? *Med Hypotheses*, 1987;22:421–8.

49. Kjeldsen-Kragh J., Lund J.A., Riise T., Finnanger B., Haaland K., Finstad R et al. Dietary omega-3 fatty acid supplementation and naproxen treatment in patients with rheumatoid arthritis. *J Rheumatol*, 1992;19:1531–6.

50. Nielsen G.L., Faarvang K.L., Thomsen B.S., Teglbjaerg K.L., Jensen L.T., Hansen T.M. et al. The effects of dietary supplementation with n-3 polyunsaturated fatty acids in patients with rheumatoid arthritis: a randomized, double blind trial. *Eur J Clin Invest*, 1992;22:687–91.

51. Skoldstam L., Borjesson O., Kjallman A., Seiving B., Akesson B. Effect of six months to fish oil supplementation in stable rheuma-

toid arthritis. A double-blind, controlled study. *Scand J Rheumatol*, 1992;21:178–85.

52. Silman A., Bankhead C., Rowlingson B., Brennan P., Symmons D., Gatrell A. Do new cases of rheumatoid arthritis cluster in time or in space? *Int J Epidemiol*, 1997;26:628–34.

53. Hochberg M.C. Changes in the incidence and prevalence of rheumatoid arthritis in England and Wales, 1970–1982. *Semin Arthritis Rheum*, 1990;19:294–302.

54. Dugowson C.E., Koepsell T.D., Voight L.F., Bley L., Nelson J.L., Daling J.R. Rheumatoid arthritis in women. Incidence rates in group health cooperative, Seattle, Washington, 1987–1989. *Arthritis Rheum*, 1991;34:1502–7.

55. Jacobsson L.T.H., Hanson R.L., Knowler W.C., Pillemer S., Pettitt D.J., McCance D.R. et al. Decreasing incidence and prevalence of rheumatoid arthritis in Pima Indians over a twenty-five-year period. *Arthritis Rheum*, 1994;37:1158–65.

56. Adebajo A.O. Rheumatoid arthritis: a twentieth century disease in Africa? *Arthritis Rheum*, 1991;34:248–9.

57. Brennan P., Bankhead C., Silman A., Symmons D., Oral contraceptives and rheumatoid arthritis: Results from a primary care-based incident case-control study. *Semin Arthritis Rheum*, 1997;26:817–23.

58. Heikkila S., Isomaki H. Long-term outcome of rheumatoid arthritis has improved. *Scand J Rheumatol*, 1994;23:13–5.

59. Silman A.J. Recent trends in rheumatoid arthritis (letter). *Br J Rheumatol*, 1992;31:326–30.

60. Silman A.J. Trends in the incidence and severity of rheumatoid arthritis. *J Rheumatol*, 1992;32:(Suppl) 71–3.

61. Laurent R., Robinson R.G., Beller E.M., Buchanan W.W. Incidence and severity of rheumatoid arthritis—the view from Australia. *Br J Rheumatol*, 1989;28:360–1.

62. Buchanan W.W., Murdoch R.M. Hypothesis: that rheumatoid arthritis will disappear. *J Rheumatol*, 1979;6:324–9.

63. Fries J.F., Toward an understanding of patient outcome measurement. *Arthritis Rheum*, 1983;26:697–704.

64. Wolfe F., Mitchell D.M., Sibley J.T., Fires J.F., Bloch D.A., Williams C.A. et al. The mortality of rheumatoid arthritis. *Arthritis Rheum*, 1994;37:481–94.

65. Jacobsson L.T.H., Knowler W.C., Pillemer S., Hanson R.L., Pettitt D.J., Nelson R.G. et al. Rheumatoid arthritis and mortality. A longitudinal study in Pima Indians. *Arthritis Rheum*, 1993;36: 1045–53.

66. Myllykangas-Luosujarvi R., Aho K., Kautiainen H., Isomaki H. Cardiovascular mortality in women with rheumatoid arthritis. *J Rheumatol*, 1995;22:1065–7.

67. Vandenbroucke J.P., Hazevoet H.M., Cats A. Survival and cause of death in rheumatoid arthritis: A 25-year prospective follow-up. *J Rheumatol*, 1984;11:158–61.

68. Prior P., Symmons D.P.M., Scott D.L., Brown R., Hawkins C.F. Cause of death in rheumatoid arthritis. *Br J Rheumatol*, 1984;23:92–9.

69. Mutru O., Laakso M., Isomaki H., Koota K. Ten year mortality and causes of death in patients with rheumatoid arthritis. *Br Med J*, 1985;290:1811–3.

70. Mitchell D.M., Spitz P.W., Young D.Y., Bloch D.A., McShane D.J., Fries J.F. Survival prognosis, and causes of death in rheumatoid arthritis. *Arthritis Rheum*, 1986;29:706–14.

71. Cibere J., Sibley J., Haga M. Rheumatoid arthritis and the risk of malignancy. *Arthritis Rheum*, 1997;40:1580–6.

72. Wallberg-Jonsson S., Ohman M.L., Dahlqvist S.R. Cardiovascular morbidity and mortality in patients with seropositive rheumatoid arthritis in Northern Sweden, *J Rheumatol*, 1997;24:445–51.

73. Callahan L.F., Pincus T., Huston J.W., III., Brooks R.H., Nance E.P., Jr., Kaye J.J. Measures of activity and damage in rheumatoid arthritis: depiction of changes and prediction of morality over five years. *Arthritis Care Res*, 1997;10;381–94.

74. Pincus T., Brooks R.H., Callahan L.F. Prediction of long-term mortality in patients with rheumatoid arthritis according to simple questionnaire and joint count measures. *Ann Intern Med*, 1994;120;26–34.

75. Morgan S.L., Baggott J.E., Jeannette Y.L., Alarcón G.S. Folic acid supplementation prevents deficient blood folate levels and hyperhomocysteinemia during long-term, low dose methotrexate therapy for rheumatoid arthritis: Implications or cardiovascular disease prevention. *J Rheumatol*, 1993;25:441–6.

76. McKendry R.J.R., Dale P. Adverse effects of low dose methotrexate therapy in rheumatoid arthritis. *J Rheumatol*, 1993;20:1850–6.

77. Alarcón G.S., Tracy I.C., Strand G.M., Singh K., Macaluso M. Survival and drug discontinuation analyses in a large cohort of methotrexate-treated rheumatoid arthritis patients. *Ann Rheum Dis*, 1995;54;708–12.

78. Wolfe F., Zwillich S.H. The long-term outcomes of rheumatoid arthritis. A 23-year prospective, longitudinal study of total joint replacement and its predictors in 1600 patients with rheumatoid arthritis. *Arthritis Rheum*, 1998;41:1072–82.

79. Callahan L.F., Pincus T. Reassessment of twelve traditoinal paradigms concerning the diagnosis, prevalence, morbidity and mortality of rheumatoid arthritis. *Scand J Rheumatol*, 1989;79 Suppl: 67–95.

80. Roubenoff R., Roubenoff R.A., Cannon J.G., Kehayias J.J., Zhuang H., Dawson-Hughes B.*et al.* Rheumatoid cachexia: cytokine-driven hypermetabolism accompanying reduced body cell mass in chronic inflammation. *J Clin Invest*, 1994;93:2379–86.

81. Roubenoff R., Robenoff R.A., Selhub J., Nadeau M.R., Cannon J.G., Freeman L.M. *et al.* Abnormal vitamin B6 status in rheumatoid cachexia association with spontaneous tumor necrosis factor alpha production and markers of inflammation. *Arthritis Rheum*, 1995;38:105–9.

82. Collins R., Jr., Dunn T.L., Walthaw J., Harrell P., Alarcón G.S. Malnutrition in rheumatoid arthritis. *Clin Rheumatol*, 1987;6:391–8.

83. Engelhart M., Kondrup J., Hoie L.H., Andersen V., Kristensen J.H., Heitmann B.L. Weight reduction in obese patients with rheumatoid arthritis, with preservation of body cell mass and improvement of physical fitness. *Clin Exp Rheumatol*, 1996;14:289–93.

84. Kaye J.J., Fuchs H.A., Moseley J.W., Nance E.P., Jr., Callahan L.F., Pincus T. Problems with the Steinbrocker Staging System for radiographic assessment of the rheumatoid hand and wrist. *Investig Radiol*, 1993;25:536–44.

85. Regan Smith M.G., O'Connor G.T., Kwoh C.K., Brown L.A., Olmsted E.M., Burnett J.B. Lack of correlation between the Steinbrocker staging of hand radiographs and the functional health status of individuals with rheumatoid arthritis. *Arthritis Rheum*, 1989;32:128–33.

86. Larsen A. Radiological grading of rheumatoid arthritis. An interobserver study. *Scand J Rheumatol*, 1973;2:136–8.

87. Sharp J.T., Lidsky M.D., Collins L.C., Moreland J. Methods of scoring the progression of radiologic changes in rheumatoid arthritis. Correlation of radiologic, clinical and laboratory abnormalities. *Arthritis Rheum*, 1971;14:706–20.

88. Sharp J.T., Young D.Y., Bluhm G.B., Brook A., Brower A.C., Corbett M. *et al.* How many joints in the hands and wrists should be included in a score of radiologic abnormalities used to assess rheumatoid arthritis? *Arthritis Rheum*, 1985;28:1326–35.

89. Molenaar T.H.E., Boers M., van der Heijde D.M.F.M., Alarcón G.S., Bresnihan B., Cardiel M *et al.* Imaging in rheumatoid arthritis: Results of group discussion. *J Rheumatol*, 1999 (in press).

90. Lee M., Feldman M. The aging stomach: implications for NSAID gastropathy. *Gut*, 1997;41:425–6.

91. Ament P.W., Childers R.S. Prophylaxis and treatment of NSAID–induced gastropathy. *Am Fam Phy*, 1998;55:1323–32.

92. Fries J. F., Williams C.A., Bloch D.A., Michel B.A. Nonsteroidal anti-inflammatory drug-associated gastropathy: Incidence and risk factor models *Am J Med*, 1991;91:213–22.

93. Langman M.J., Weil J., Wainwright P., Lawson D.H., Rawlins M.D., Logan R.F. *et al.* Risks of bleeding peptic ulcer associated with individual non-steroidal anti-inflammatory drugs. *Lancet*, 1994;343:1075–8.

94. Hawkey C.J. The gastroenterologist's caseload: contribution of the rheumatologist. *Sem Arthritis Rheum*, 1997;26:11–5.

95. Kendall B.J., Peura D.A. NSAID-associated gastrointestinal damage and the elderly. *Practical Gastroenterol*, 1993;17:13–29.

96. Hansen M., Florescu A., Stoltenberg M., Podenphant J., Pedersen-Zbinden B., Horslev-Petersen K. *et al.* Bone loss in rheumatoid arthritis. Influence of disease activity, duration of the disease, functional capacity, and corticosteroid treatment. *Scand J Rheumatol*, 1996;25:367–76.

97. Verhoeven A.C., Boers M. Limited bon loss due to corticosteroids; a systemic review of prospective studies in rheumatoid arthritis and other diseases. *J Rheumatol*, 1997;24:1495–503.

98. Kirwan J.R. The effect of glucocorticoids on joint destruction in rheumatoid arthritis. The Arthritis and Rheumatism Council Low-Dose Glucocorticoid Study Group. *N. Engl J Med*, 1995;333:142–6.

99. Paulus H., DiPrimeo D., Sanda M., Lynch J., Schwartz B., Sharp J. *et al.* Progression of radiographic joint erosions during low-dose prednisone treatment of rheumatoid arthritis. *Arthritis Rheum*, 1996;39:S320.

100. Saag K.G., Criswell L.A., Sems K.M., Nettleman M.D., Kolluri S. Low-dose corticosteroids in rheumatoid arthritis: A meta-analysis of their moderate-term effectiveness. *Arthritis Rheum*, 1996;39:1818–25.

101. Morgan S.L., Baggott J.E., Vaughn W.H., Austin J.S., Veitch T.A., Lee J.Y. *et al.* Supplementation with folic acid during methotrexate therapy for rheumatoid arthritis. A double-blind, placebocontrolled trial. *Ann Intern Med*, 1994;121:833–41.

102. Ortiz Z., Shea B., Suarez-Almazor M., Moher D., Wells G., Tugwell P. The efficacy of folic acid and folinic acid in reducing methotrexate side effects in rheumatoid arthritis. A meta-analysis of randomized controlled trials. *J Rheumatol*, 1998;25:36–43.

103. Bologna C., Picot M.C., Jorgensen C., Viu P., Verdier R., Sany J. Study of eight cases of cancer in 426 rheumatoid arthritis patients treated with methotrexate. *Ann Rheum Dis*, 1997;56:97–102.

104. Kremer J.M. Safety, efficacy, and mortality in a long-term cohort of patients with rheumatoid arthritis taking methotrexate: followup after a mean of 13.3 years. *Arthritis Rheum*, 1997;40:984–5.

105. McKendry R.J.R. The remarkable spectrum of methotrexate toxicities. *Rheum Dis Clin N Am*, 1997;23:939–55.

106. Walker A.M., Funch D., Dreyer N.A., Tolman K.G., Kremer J.M., Alarcón G.S. *et al.* Determinants of serious liver disease among patients receiving low-dose methotrexate of rheumatoid arthritis. *Arthritis Rheum*, 1993;36:329–35.

107. Erikson A.R., Reddy V., Vogelgesang S.A., West S.G. Usefulness of the American College of Rheumatology recommendations for liver biopsy in methotrexate-treated rheumatoid arthritis patients. *Arthritis Rheum*, 1995;38:1115–9.

108. Beyeler C., Reichen J., Thomann S.R., Lauterburg B.H., Gerber N.J. Quantitative liver function in patients with rheumatoid arthritis treated with low-dose methotrexate: a longitudinal study. *Br J Rheumatol*, 1997;36:338–44.

109. Alarcón G.S., Kremer J.M., Macaluso M., Weinblatt M.E., Cannon G.W., Palmer *et al.* Risk factors for methotrexate-induced lung injury in patients with rheumatoid arthritis. A multicenter, case-control study. Methotrexate-Lung Study Group. *Ann Intern Med*, 1997;127:356–64.

110. Cannon G.W. Methotrexate pulmonary toxicity. *Rheum Dis Clin North Am*, 1997;23:917–37.

111. Salloum E., Cooper D.L., Howe G., Lacy J., Tallini G., Crouch J. *et al.* Spontaneous regression of lymphoproliferative disorders in patients treated with methotrexate for rheumatoid arthritis and other rheumatic disease. *J Clin Oncol*, 1996;14:1943–9.

112. Thomason R.W., Craig F.E., Banks P.M., Sears D.L., Myerson G.E., Gulley M.L. Epstein-Barr virus and lymphoproliferation in methotrexate-treated rheumatoid arthritis. *Mod Pathol*, 1996;9:261–6.

113. Ollier W., MacGregor A. Genetic epidemiology of rheumatoid arthritis. *British Med J*, 1995;51:267–285. [Abstract]

114. Stastny P. Association of the B-cell alloantigen DRw4 with rheumatoid arthritis. *N Engl J Med*, 1978;298:869–71.

115. Weyand C.M., Hicok K.C., Conn D.L., Goronzy J.J. The influence of HLA-DRB1 genes on disease severity in rheumatoid arthritis. *Ann Intern Med*, 1992;117:801–6.

116. Weyand C.M., Xie C., Goronzy J.J. Homozygosity for the HLA-DRB1 allele selects for extraarticular manifestations in rheumatoid arthritis. *J Clin Invest*, 1992;89:2033–9.

117. Weyand C.M., McCarthy T.G., Goronzy J.J. Correlation between disease phenotype and genetic heterogeneity in rheumatoid arthritis. *J Clin Invest*, 1995;95:2120–6.

118. Templin D.W., Boyer G.S., Lanier A.P., Nelson J.L., Barrington R.A., Hasen J.A., *et al.* Rheumatoid arthritis in Tlingit Indians: clinical characterization and HLA associations. *J Rheumatol*, 1994;21:1238–44.

119. McDaniel D.O., Alarcón G.S., Pratt P.W., Reveille J.D. Most African-American patients with rheumatoid arthritis do not have the rheumatoid antigenic determinant (epitope). *Ann Intern Med*, 1995;123:181–7.

120. Hameed K., Bowman S., Kondeatis E., Vaughan R., Gibson T. Association of HLA-DRB genes and the shared epitope with rheumatoid arthritis in Pakistan. *Br J Rheumatol*, 1997;36:1184–8.

121. Toda Y., Minamikawa Y., Akagi S., Sugano H., Mori Y., Nishimura H. *et al.* Rheumatoid susceptible alleles of HLA-DRB1 are genetically recessive to non-susceptible alleles in the progression of bone destruction in the wrists and fingers of patients with R.A. *Ann Rheum Dis*, 1994;53:587–92.

122. Nichol F.E., Woodrow J.C. HLA DR antigens in Indian patients with rheumatoid arthritis. *Lancet*, 1991;1:220–1.

123. Schiff B., Mizrachi Y., Orgad S., Yaron N., Gazit E. Association of HLA-Aw31 and HLA-DR1 with adult rheumatoid arthritis. *Ann Rheumatoid arthritis. Ann Rheum Dis*, 1982;41:403–4.

124. Christiansen F.G., Kelly H., Dawkins R.L. Hystocompatibility Testing. In: *Rheumatoid arthritis*. (Alber E.D., Baur M.P., Mayr W.R., eds). Berlin: Springer-Verlag; 1984:378–83.

125. Stavropoulos C., Spyropoulou M., Koumantaki Y., Kappou I., Kaklamanis P.V., Linos A. *et al.* HLA-DRB1* genotype and rheumatoid in Greek rheumatoid arthritis patients: Association with disease characteristics, sex, and age at onset. *Br J Rheumatol*, 1997;36:141–2.

126. Hong G.H., Park M.H., Takeuchi F., Oh M.D., Song Y.W., Nabeta H. *et al.* Association of specific amino acid sequence of HLA-DR with rheumatoid arthritis in Koreans and its diagnostic value. *J Rheumatol*, 1996;23:1699–703.

127. MacGregor A., Ollier W., Thomson W., Jawaheer D., Silman A. HLA-DRB1 *0401/0404 genotype and rheumatoid arthritis: Increased association in men, young age at onset, and disease severity. *J Rheumatol*, 1995;22:1032–6.

128. Seglias J., Li E.K., Cohen M.G., Wong R.W.S., Potter P.K., So A.K. Linkage between rheumatoid arthritis susceptibility and the presence of HLA-DR4 and DRB allelic third hypervariable region sequences in Southern Chinese persons. *Arthritis Rheum*, 1992;35:163–7.

129. Koh W., Chan S., Lin Y., Boey M. Association of HLA-DRB1 *0405 with extraarticular manifestations and erosions in Singaporean Chinese with rheumatoid arthritis. *J. Rheumatol*, 1997;24:629–32.

130. Yelamos J., García-Lozano J.R., Moreno I., Aguilera I., Gonzales M.F., García A. *et al.* Association of HLA-DR4-Dw15 (DRB1*0405) and DR10 with rheumatoid arthritis in Spanish population. *Arthritis Rheum*, 1993;36:811–4.

131. McDonagh J.E., Dunn A., Ollier W.E., Walker D.J. Compound heterozygosity for the shared epitope and the risk and severity of rheumatoid arthritis in extended pedigrees. *Br J Rheumatol*, 1997;36:322–7.

132. Willkens R.F., Nepom G.T., Marks C.R., Nettles J.W., Nepom B.S. Association of HLA-Dw16 with rheumatoid arthritis in Yakima Indians. Further evidence for the 'Shared Epitope' hypothesis. *Arthritis Rheum*, 1991;34:43–7.

133. van der Horst-Bruinsma I.E., de Vries R.R., Hazes J.M., Breedveld F.C., Verduyn W., Schreuder G.M. *et al.* Reevaluating the role of HLA in rheumatoid arthritis: some DRB1 alleles prevent disease onset. *Arthritis Rheum*, 1997;40:S156.

134. Zanelli E., Gonzalez-Gay M.A., David C.S. Could HLA-DRB1 be the protective locus in rheumatoid arthritis? *Immunol Today*, 1995;16:274–8

135. Larsen B.A., Alderdice C.A., Hawkins D., Martin J.R., Mitchell D.M., Sheridan D.P. Protective HLA-DR phenotypes in rheumatoid arthritis. *J Rheumatol*, 1989;16:455–8.

136. Voskuyl A.E., Hazes J.M., Schreuder G.M., Schipper R.F., de Vries R.R., Breedveld F.C. HLA-DRB1, DQA1, and DQB1 genotypes and risk of vasculitis in patients with rheumatoid arthritis. *J Rheumatol*, 1997;24:852–5.

137. Perdriger A., Chales G., Semana G., Guggenbuhl P., Meyer O., Quillivic F. *et al.* Role of HLA-DR-DR and DR-DQ associations in the expression of extraarticular manifestations and rheumatoid factor in rheumatoid arthritis. *J Rheumatol*, 1997;24:1272–6.

138. Moxley G., Meyer J., Han J. Microsatellite haplotypes of tumor necrosis factor (TNFab) show linkage disequilibrium with shared-epitope DRB1 alleles (TNFa2b1-bearing HLA haplotypes may contribute to rheumatoid arthritis risk). *Arthritis Rheum*, 1997;40:S125.

139. Lacaile D., Khani-Hanjani A., Horne C., Hoar D., Beattie C, Rnagno K. *et al.* HLA-DRB1 frequency, TNF gene polymorphism and disease severity in patients with rheumatoid arthritis. *Arthritis Rheum*, 1997;40:S77.

140. Mataran L., Vinasco J., Beraun Y., Nieto A., Fraile A., Pareja E. *et al.* Association of TNF-a polymorphism with outcome of rheumatoid arthritis. *Arthritis Rheum*, 1997;40:S77.

141. Vinasco J., Beraun Y., Nieto A., Fraile A., Mataran L., Pareja E. *et al.* Polymorphism at the TNF loci in rheumatoid arthritis. *Tissue Antig*, 1997;49:74–8.

142. Field M., Gallagher G., Eksdale J., McGarry F., Richards S.D., Munro R. *et al.* Tumor necrosis factor locus polymorphisms in rheumatoid arthritis. *Tissue Antig*, 1997;50:303–7.

143. Gallagher G., Eksdale J., Steven M., Wordsworth P., Field M. No role for the TNF gene cluster in the genetic predisposition to rheumatoid arthritis or systemic lupus erythematosus. *Arthritis Rheum*, 1997;40:S77.

144. Auger I., Roudier J. Influence of the QKRAA/QRRAA/RRRAA motifs of the third hypervariable region of HLA-DRB1 in the development of rheumatoid arthritis. *J Rheumatol*, 1997;41:1131–2.

145. Ford D.K. Understanding rheumatoid arthritis. *J Rheumatol*, 1997;24:1464–6.

146. McKendry R.J.R. Is rheumatoid arthritis caused by an infection? *Lancet*, 1995;345:1319–20.

147. Wilder R.L. Hypothesis for retroviral causation of rheumatoid arthritis. *Curr Opin Rheumatol*, 1994;6:295–9.

148. Cole P., MacMahon B. Attributable risk percent in case-control studies. *Brit J Prev Soc Med*, 1971;25:242–4.

149. Nikkari S., Roivainen A., Hannonen P., Mottonen T., Luukkainen R., Yli-Jama T. *et al.* Presistence of parvovirus B19 in synovial fluid and bone narrow. *Ann Rheum Dis*, 1995;54:597–600.

150. Woolfe A.D., Cohen B.J. Parvovirus B19 and chronic arthritis—causal or casual association? *Ann Rheum Dis*, 1995;54:533–6.

151. Barthold S.W. Globalization of Lyme borreliosis. *Lancet*, 1996;348:1603.

152. Le Guenno B. Haemorrhagic fevers and ecological perturbations. *Arch Virol Suppl*, 1997;13:191–9.

153. Albani S., Keystone E.C., Nelson J.L., Ollier W.E., La Cava A., Montemayor A.C. *et al.* Positive selection in autoimmunity: abnormal immune responses to a bacterial dnaJ antigenic determinant in patients with early rheumatoid arthritis. *Nat Med*, 1995;1:448–52.

154. Baum H., Staines N.A. MHC-derived peptides and the CD4+ T-cell repertoire: implications for autoimmune disease. *Cytokines Cell Mol Ther*, 1997;3:115–25.

155. La Cava A, Nelson J.L., Ollier W.E., MacGregor A, Keystone E.C., Thorne J.C. *et al.* Genetic bias in immune responses to a cassette shared by different microorganisms in patients with rheumatoid arthritis. *J Clin Invest*, 1997;**100**:658–63.

156. Wilder R.L. Adrenal and gonadal steroid hormone deficiency in the pathogenesis of rheumatoid arthritis. *J Rheumatol*, 1996;**44**:1–2.

157. Hench P.S. The ameliorating effect of pregnancy on chronic atrophic (infectious rheumatoid) arthritis, fibrositis and intermittent hydarthrosis. Proc Staff Meeting Mayo Clin, 1988;March16:161–7.

158. Buyon J.P. The effects of pregnancy on autoimmune diseases. *J Leukoc Biol*, 1998;**63**:281–7.

159. Nelson J.L. Ostensen M. Pregnancy and rheumatoid arthritis. *Rheum Dis Clin North Am*, 1997;**23**:195–212.

160. Roberts R.M., Xie S., Nagel R.J., Low B., Green J., Beckers J. F. Glycoproteins of the aspartyl proteinase gene family secreted by the developing placenta. *Adv Exp Med Biol*, 1995;**362**:231–40.

161. Perdriger A., Chales G. Influence on non-HLA factors in rheumatoid arthritis: Role of enzyme abnormalities in joint destruction. *Rev Rhum Engl Ed*, 1997;**64**:523–6.

162. Rademacher T.W,. Williams P., Dwek R.A. Agalactosyl glycoforms of IgG autoantibodies are pathogenic. *Proc Natl Acad Sci*, 1994;**91**:6123–7.

163. Rook G.A., Steele J., Brealey R., Whyte A., Isenberg D., Sumar N. *et al.* Changes in IgG glycoform levels are associated with remission of arthritis during pregnancy. *J Autoimmun*, 1991;**4**:779–94.

164. Cuchacovich M., Gatica H., Grigg D.M., Pizzo S.V., Gonzalez-Gronow M. Potential pathogenicity of deglycosylated IgG cross reactive with streptokinase and fibronectin in the serum of patients with rheumatoid arthritis. *J Rheumatol*, 1996;**23**:44–51.

165. Nelson J.L., Hughes K.A., Smith A.G., Nisperos B.B., Branchaud A.M., Hansen J.A. Maternal-fetal disparity in HLA class II alloantigens and the pregnancy. Induced amelioration of rheumatoid arthritis. *N Engl J Med*, 1993;**329**:466–71.

166. Dugowson C.E., Nelson J.L., Koepsell T.D., Voigt L.F. Is nulliparity a risk factor for rheumatoid arthritis? *Arthritis Rheum* 1991;**34**:S48.

167. Anonymous. Reduction in incidence of rheumatoid arthritis associated with oral contraceptives. Royal College of General Practitioners' Oral Contraception Study. *Lancet*, 1978;**1**:569–71.

168. Spector T.D., Hochberg M.C. The protective effect of the oral contraceptive pill on rheumatoid arthritis: An overview of the analytic epidemiological studies using meta-analysis. *J Clin Epidemiol*, 1990;**43**:1221–30.

169. Bruce I.N., Laskin C.A. Sex hormones in systemic lupus erythematosus: A controversy for modern times. *J Rheumatol*, 1997;**24**:1461–3.

170. Dequeker J., Westhovens R. Low dose corticosteroid associated osteoporosis in rheumatoid arthritis and its prophylaxis and treatment: bones of contention. *J Rheumatol*, 1995;**22**:1013–9.

171. Koepsell T.D., Dugowson C.E., Nelson J.L., Voigt L.F., Daling J.R. Non-contraceptive hormones and the risk of rheumatoid arthritis in menopausal women. *Int J Epidemiol*, 1994;**23**:1248–55.

172. James W.H. Further evidence that low androgen values are a cause of rheumatoid arthritis: the response of rheumatoid arthritis to serious life events. *Ann Rheum Dis*, 1997;**56**:566.

173. Cutolo M., Masi A.T. Do androgens influence the pathophysiology of rheumatoid arthritis? Facts and hypothesis. *J Rheumatol*, 1998;**25**:1041–7.

174. Cutolo M. Do sex hormones modulate the synovial macrophages in rheumatoid arthritis? *Ann Rheum Dis*, 1997;**56**:281–4.

3 | *Infection in the pathogenesis of rheumatoid arthritis*

Gabrielle Kingsley

Historical background

The idea that rheumatoid arthritis (RA) might be caused by infection, and more specifically a focus of infection in a distant part of the body, is far from new. Osler[1], in his classical medical textbook of the 1920s, suggested that RA was secondary to a focus of infection somewhere: 'the possible sources are many but infections of the mouth and throat probably take first place'. Such ideas remained popular up to the Second World War and resulted in patients with arthritis being subjected to total dental clearances, appendectomies, and other surgical interventions in the hope of eradicating the supposed source of infection. The theory that RA was caused by mycobacterial infection underpinned the use of gold, one of the earliest antirheumatic drugs, because it was known to be effective *in vitro* against these organisms[2].

Advances in immunology, and in particular the discovery of rheumatoid factor, led to an emphasis on the autoimmune nature of systemic rheumatic diseases and theories relating pathogenesis to infection fell into disrepute. Over the next four decades, the treatment of RA focused on the use of anti-inflammatory and immunosuppressive agents to inhibit an apparently overactive immune system. Similarly, research into the pathogenesis of the disease targeted abnormalities of the humoral and later the cellular immune system. Recently, these therapeutic and pathogenetic ideas have come together in the use of biologics targeting specific arms of the immune system, such as the cytokine TNFα or the CD4[+] T cell. Though some of these approaches have resulted in clinical improvement, they have not led to a long-term remission or cure. One possible explanation is that the immune abnormalities seen in RA are not the primary cause of disease but secondary to an underlying etiological agent.

Interest in infection as a trigger for these immune aberrations, has been rekindled by the demonstration, both in animal models and human diseases, that a number of microbes, both viruses and bacteria, can induce arthritis. In some cases, this is associated with immune alterations which resemble those seen in RA. The aim of this chapter is to review the evidence that either bacterial or viral infection may play a role in the initiation or perpetuation of RA.

Identifying potential infectious triggers of disease

It may appear a relatively simple task to demonstrate that a disease is due to infection. The classical method has been to use Koch's postulates which require that:

(1) the proposed causative infectious agent can be identified in all cases of the disease in a distribution that corresponds to the relevant pathology;

(2) the agent can be isolated and obtained in pure culture;

(3) experimental subjects inoculated with the proposed agent develop the disease; and

(4) the agent can be found in this experimentally-induced disease.

While this approach might be appropriate for classical acute bacterial and viral diseases, where a clinically characteristic condition develops shortly after exposure and affects the majority of those exposed, it has a number of limitations where chronic diseases are concerned. First, the agent might only be present early in the disease or even before pathology appears. Second, the microbe might only be cultivable with extreme difficulty, if at all *in vitro*. Third, the disease might only develop fully in sub-section of the population, such as those who are genetically predisposed; for example, in reactive arthritis, infection in the majority leads to uncomplicated gastroenteritis or urethritis and only a minority develop joint disease. Fourth, if a tissue has a relatively limited pathological repertoire, an apparently similar disease pattern may be induced by a number of different infectious agents. The relative pathological similarity of many forms of arthritis suggests that this may apply to the joint. Fifth, the latter two of Koch's postulates usually depend on having an appropriate animal model of the disease since the induction of experimental disease is generally considered unethical in humans. However, some researchers have used this approach in volunteers, often themselves, as illustrated by Marshall's attempt to establish a pathogenic role for *Helicobacter pylori* in gastric ulceration[3].

Additional forms of evidence, some not available in Koch's era, may partially help to resolve these problems. Exposure to an infectious agent may be demonstrated indirectly, for example

RA because of the proliferation of the synovium, the upregulation of pro-inflammatory cytokines and T-cell involvement, and has prompted a careful search for retroviruses in human disease.

Evidence of bacterial or viral involvement in the pathogenesis of RA

Although classical epidemiological observations, such as the lack of clustering in time or space, do not support the concept that RA is an infectious illness, they cannot rule out this possibility. As discussed earlier in this chapter, there are many mechanisms by which infection can induce disease. Several of these situations would not be amenable to classical epidemiological analysis, for example because of a long time interval between the initiating infection and the onset of arthritis or because there is a strong genetic element in susceptibility to arthritis. For similar reasons, the lack of a clear clinical association between infection and RA does not provide conclusive evidence against the possibility of an infectious trigger. To examine the possibility that infection is involved in the pathogenesis of RA, therefore, recourse must be made to other forms of analysis. These have included looking for evidence of exposure to infectious agents by serology, of specific immune responses to infectious agents in the synovium, and of persistence of the infectious agent within the joint. Additionally, data from antibiotic and sulfasalazine studies, despite the hazards alluded to above, has sometimes been interpreted as suggesting a role for infection in pathogenesis. This data will be critically examined, initially for bacteria and then for viruses (Table 3.3).

Bacteria as a cause for RA

As noted at the beginning of this chapter, the idea that bacterial infection might trigger RA is very old indeed yet there is, to date, relatively little convincing evidence for this hypothesis. The improvement in RA seen with antimicrobial drugs has often been interpreted as suggesting that the disease is associated with continuing bacterial infection. The early idea that gold was effective in the disease because of its *in vitro* antimycobacterial properties[2] has already been mentioned. The early development of sulfasalazine resulted from a deliberate attempt to combine the antibacterial action of sulfapyridine and the anti-inflammatory effect of salicy-

late; its antiarthritic activity appears to result from sulfapyridine moiety though the exact mechanism remains unknown (reviewed in reference 5). Several antibiotics, including rifampicin, sulfonamides other than sulfapyridine, dapsone, metronidazole, and ciprofloxacin, have been studied in RA but the most extensive analysis has been undertaken with tetracyclines.

Rifampicin was initially reported to have an antiarthritic effect when used systemically in an open study[63] but this was not confirmed in later work[64,65] although intra-articular injections might have some efficacy[66]. Early open or single-blind studies of several non-sulfapyridine sulfonamides gave positive results but later work suggested that improvement was confined to sulfapyridine[67]. Similarly, dapsone showed early promise but later work showed the beneficial effect to be small[68]. Both metronidazole[69] and ciprofloxacin[70] have been shown to be ineffective in RA. Many studies of tetracyclines, most recently minocycline[71,72], have been undertaken over several years. In summary (reviewed in reference 5), these have shown benefit, at least in the short-term, but concurrent research has confirmed the extensive effects these drugs have on the immune system and also on matrix metalloproteinase activity. Antibacterial agents, therefore, do not display a general effect on RA and the two specific agents which are beneficial, sulfasalazine and tetracyclines, both have other potentially relevant modes of action. Although these data cannot be used to support the concept that RA is due to continuing bacterial infection, neither do they rule out a role for microbes as has been shown by the experience of antimicrobial therapy in reactive arthritis[32].

An enduring idea about RA is that there may be some abnormality of the gastrointestinal tract. Support for a role of the gut in the development of inflammatory arthritis is provided by the examples of arthritis related to inflammatory bowel disease, enteric reactive arthritis, and Whipple's disease and by the somewhat confusing data on diet and fasting in RA[73]. Interestingly, in most of these examples, bacteria play a definite (reactive arthritis, Whipple's disease) or presumptive role (alteration of intestinal flora by diet). Differences in intestinal flora between rheumatoid and control subjects have been demonstrated[74] but the significance of these observations remains uncertain[75]. One possible mechanism by which such changes could induce disease is suggested by the identification of bacterial flora-derived antigen in synovial tissue macrophages and dendritic cells where it could presumably induce a synovial T-cell response[76].

Another line of evidence has come from studies examining serological responses to bacteria. *Proteus mirabilis* was first proposed as a cause for RA many years ago[77] and has been extensively studied since. The evidence for its involvement in RA (reviewed in reference 78) can be summarized as follows. There is an increase in anti-*Proteus* antibodies, especially in patients with active disease[79] though the differences are relatively small; these levels fall with improvement of RA induced by dietary treatment[73]. Some studies have found an increased frequency of *Proteus* infections in RA[80,81] but others have not[82]. Finally, sequence similarities identified between *Proteus mirabilis* hemolysin and the RA-associated HLA antigen, HLA-DR4, and between *Proteus* urease and the $\alpha2$ chain of type XI collagen,

Table 3.3 Gathering evidence about the role of microbes in disease pathogenesis

Clinical evidence	Laboratory evidence
Clinically apparent preceding infection	Persistent organism in joint on culture, PCR or within immune complexes
Epidemiological evidence of disease clustering	Specific antimicrobial T-cell or antibody response in the joint
Response to antimicrobial therapy	Serological evidence of recent infection

PCR—polymerase chain reaction.

have been interpreted as suggesting that molecular mimicry between *Proteus* proteins and self-antigens might play a role in RA pathogenesis[83]. Many problems remain with this hypothesis. For instance, the changes in antibody level with disease activity would be unusual if RA represented arthritis due to *Proteus* infection since antibodies to bacteria normally remain elevated for some time after an infection resolves and are persistently elevated in continuing infection. This variation with activity suggests elevated *Proteus* antibody levels are more likely to be induced by some aspect of the immune-inflammatory response in RA. A second set of problems lies with the molecular mimicry explanation for pathogenesis. It has not been shown whether the anti-*Proteus* antibody response in RA actually recognizes either of the mimicking sequences. Conversely, hemolysins from *Serratia, Pseudomonas,* and *Escherichia* also have the HLA-mimicking determinant yet antibodies to these three organisms are not elevated in RA[83,84]. Finally, there is a more basic problem. The similarities identified between self-antigens and proteins are for short linear peptide sequences (the type of epitope recognized by T-cells). However, the abnormal immune response demonstrated is an elevation in antibody titers to *Proteus* (antibodies recognize conformational not linear determinants); T-cell responses have not, so far, been investigated. Convincing evidence for the involvement of *Proteus mirabilis* in RA will require further research at a fundamental level, rather than further repetition, in other patient groups, of the now well-described antibody findings.

Immune responses to other agents have been much less extensively examined in RA. As described above, there is no increase in the antibody response to *Klebsiella, Serratia, Pseudomonas,* and *E. Coli*[77,81,83]. Other workers have shown no increase in antibodies to *Borrelia burgdorferi*, the agent responsible for Lyme disease[85]. The synovial lymphocyte response, as a diagnostic tool for RA, has been championed by Ford[49] despite the known limitations of response to more than one organism, definition of positive responses, and absence of response in the presence of bacteria which have been so clearly demonstrated in reactive arthritis[43,49]. Ford has described small numbers of RA patients who have persistent, synovial T-cell responses to *Chlamydia trachomatis* or to *Salmonella* but, as mentioned in the section on reactive arthritis above, the interpretation of such responses as indicating causation is fraught with problems. They could merely represent the migration of irrelevant, systemically-infecting organism or bystander lymphocytes into an inflamed knee joint.

Perhaps the most exciting, recent approach to the problem has been to use specific or broad-spectrum PCR techniques to identify bacterial DNA within the joint. However, just as with the other techniques examined above, the limitations of such analyses must be borne in mind[47]. The absence of bacteria in the synovium does not rule out a role in pathogenesis since the organism might act only as transient trigger or be present in the lesion only in the earliest stages of disease. Conversely, the presence of bacterial DNA in the joint does not necessarily imply persisting infection with an etiological role. Although less stable than bacterial antigen, which can clearly persist within cells for years, it is possible that DNA could be transported from elsewhere; this is much less likely for the very short-lived messenger RNA species. Even if bacterial DNA does represent living bacteria, caution must be exercised as to what the presence of such bacteria might mean. Microbial DNA, at least from viruses, has been shown to persist in the joint long after resolution of the infection and the same might well be true of intracellular organisms[86]. Irrelevant microbes might also enter the joint as part of a systemic infection, especially in chronic arthritis where the synovium is hypertrophied and vascular. Such bacteria might not be entirely irrelevant since, as discussed briefly below, they might be involved in disease exacerbation and it is clear that bacterial DNA can stimulate immune responses[87]; nonetheless their presence would not imply causation. Once the presence of bacteria is established, further studies will need to be undertaken to try to ascertain whether they have a triggering role in disease and it is here that measurement of the T-cell response and other circumstantial immune response data may, as in reactive arthritis, play a helpful role[47,49]. To fulfill Koch's postulates will be even more difficult, probably involving the use of animal models provided that the organism is not host-specific.

Initial PCR studies in RA employed organism-specific PCRs to look for a variety of agents previously suspected, for various reasons, to be involved in RA. Two groups have failed to find any evidence of *Mycobacterium tuberculosis* DNA in the joint[88,89]. Some groups have been able to find *Mycoplasma* DNA in synovial fluid[90,91] while others, even using ultrasensitive assays, have not[92]. Even those authors who did find the organism found it in only 10–20 per cent of RA patients and, disappointingly, were not able to find any evidence of the bacteriophage MAV1 which is arthritogenic in rodents[93]. A few patients with RA have been reported as having *Chlamydia trachomatis*[94] or *Chlamydia pneumoniae* DNA in their joints[27,95] but these findings are infrequent and cannot represent major causes of RA; more likely they represent intercurrent infections with these common organisms.

An alternative PCR approach, which is capable of detecting both unknown bacteria and those not previously suspected of being associated with RA as well as identifying known candidate bacteria, is the broad-spectrum or pan-bacterial PCR. This technique requires the development of a PCR targeting a highly-conserved bacterial gene which is not found in eukaryotic DNA; the 16S ribosomal RNA gene has been a common choice. These PCRs will amplify almost any bacterial material though it is important to check sensitivity over a wide range of organisms as certain bacteria, especially those which diverge a little from the mainstream, such as mycoplasmas, may not be detected with the appropriate degree of sensitivity[31]. The identity of the bacterial material amplified is then confirmed by sequencing. The earliest attempt at this technique in arthritis failed to amplify any bacterial DNA from 26 RA synovial fluid samples[96] but later studies have been successful in several idiopathic inflammatory arthritides[31,48] including RA[31]. In the study by Wilkinson *et al.* 8/19 RA patients were found to have bacterial DNA in their synovial fluid. A single known pathogenic organism was isolated in two of these patients (in one case *Haemophilus influenzae* and in the other, *Bordetella pertussis*). *Acinetobacter sp.* (a low virulence organism) was found in one other RA patient, *Bacillus* (considered of uncertain pathogenicity since it is a common airborne contaminant) in two, and multiple PCR products (so far not cloned out to separate them) in three. While this work is very preliminary and requires study of a much larger number of patients as well as confirmation by other, it illustrates the enormous potential of this technique.

Overall, there is little direct evidence for any particular bacterial pathogen as a causative agent in RA but further work with the newly-developed pan-bacterial PCR techniques may shed more light on the situation. The role of the intestinal flora also needs further examination.

Viruses as a cause for RA

The idea that RA might be caused by viral infection is supported by the evidence that various viruses can induce arthritis in humans and by the existence of RA-like naturally-occurring and model arthritides in animals. Rubella causes an inflammatory polyarthritis much like early RA[51] but it is self-resolving and non-destructive. Grahame et al.[52] reported a small group of patients with chronic arthritis in whom rubella virus could be persistently isolated from the synovial fluid but these patients did not appear to have classical RA. Ford[49] reported on several patients whose synovial fluid lymphocyte responses were maximal to rubella; one of these patients was shown to lack responses to the neutralizing rubella antigen, E1. Again these subjects did have chronic arthritis but it was not typical RA. Taken together, this data suggests that in patients who fail to respond to the rubella neutralizing antigen, rubella virus may persist in the joint and perhaps induce an immune/inflammatory response but not classical RA.

Parvovirus can cause arthritis, especially in infected adults, but it is usually transient[50]. The work of Saal et al.[97], showing that parvovirus DNA could be detected in 75 per cent of RA synovial membranes but in only 16 per cent of controls, suggested a pathogenetic role for the virus. However this idea was not supported by subsequent work[98] demonstrating parvovirus DNA in 40 per cent of RA and osteoarthritis synovia, and others who found parvoviral DNA only very rarely in RA.[99] The demonstration by Soderlund et al.[86] that parvoviral DNA was present in the joints of patients with traumatic arthritis casts further doubt on the concept that persistent parvoviral DNA has a pathogenetic role in inflammatory arthritis.

The herpes viruses have been suggested as candidates for involvement in RA pathogenesis because of their propensity to persist within lymphocytes for long periods. They can also induce arthralgia, and rarely arthritis, in human though it is not one of their major manifestations. Newkirk et al.[100] demonstrated that Epstein–Barr virus (EBV) and human herpes virus type 6 (HHV-6) were found at increased frequency in salivary cells from RA patients compared to controls but there was no difference in peripheral blood cells between the two groups. This was interpreted as suggesting a local immune abnormality allowing salivary viral persistence rather than an etiopathogenic role for these viruses in RA. Zhang et al.[101] examined synovial fluid from RA and a variety of other rheumatic diseases for the presence of DNA from several herpes viruses including EBV, HSV-1, HSV-2, and HHV-6. Only EBV DNA was detected and

that was equally frequent in both groups, again arguing against a pathogenetic role for any of these herpes viruses in RA. Newkirk et al.[100] also examined RA patients for cytomegalovirus (CMV) DNA but did not find an increase over normal controls nor was the level of anti-CMV antibodies different between the groups. Tamm et al.[102] showed that CMV DNA was equally frequently found in RA synovial fluid and synovial fluid from other rheumatic diseases, again not favoring a causative role for the virus in RA. In contrast, Einsele et al.[103] found that CMV DNA was found in 11/83 RA synovial samples but only 2/64 samples from other rheumatic diseases. However, although this difference is statistically significant, only 13 per cent of the RA samples are positive suggesting CMV can only be relevant, if at all, in a small proportion of RA patients.

Adenoviruses are known to induce arthralgia and even arthritis in a small proportion of affected humans. Against a role for these viruses in RA, a search for adenoviral DNA in the RA synovium was negative[104]. Ford[49], however, found adenoviral DNA in one of five patients in whom he had demonstrated maximal synovial T-cell responses were to that virus. Clearly adenovirus infection is common and the pathogenetic relevance to RA of such a finding must be in doubt. One study has also looked for DNA from papillomaviruses in the RA synovium but failed to find it[105]. Overall, these results do not support the concept that RA is due to triggering infection by one of the viruses known to cause transient arthritis in humans although a role for any or all of them as one of several disease triggers cannot be excluded.

The idea that exogenous retroviruses might be involved in the pathogenesis of RA has engendered considerable research interest[106]. HTLV-1 can induce a chronic destructive arthritis in humans[54] and an RA-like disease in HTLV-1 transgenic mice[56]. The relationship between HIV and arthritis remains uncertain, as discussed above[57]. Another retrovirus, the lentivirus CAEV, is the cause of a naturally-occurring chronic erosive arthritis in sheep and goats[58]. Is there any evidence that RA itself is due to retroviral infection? Attempts to detect HTLV-1, a type C oncornavirus, or HIV in patients with RA, Felty's syndrome, and a number of other rheumatic diseases have proved unsuccessful although some patients showed serological responses to HTLV-1[107-109]. There is one report of an atypical type C-retrovirus-like particle in synovial fluid[110].

Another association of interest is between endogenous retroviruses, which are vertically transmitted through germline DNA, and rheumatic disease (reviewed references 106 and 111). Human endogenous retroviruses constitute 0.1–1.6 per cent of the human genome. While they are usually stable genetic elements, some of their murine counterparts have been shown to induce autoimmunity in mice by transposing and integrating near a gene of interest. Healthy humans express RNA from many endogenous retroviruses so that interpretation of their expression in patients with rheumatic diseases is seriously problematic. In a recent study, Nakagawa et al.[112] found multiple endogenous retroviruses were expressed in all normal and diseased synovia; however, specific transcripts could be differentially expressed in RA.

Infection in the course of RA

Even if infection is not associated with the initiation of RA, it clearly is relevant in the course of the disease. First, infection is much more common in RA patients and is one of the major causes of death[113,114]. Second, and more interestingly, intercurrent infections are often associated with flares of RA as in many chronic immune-mediated diseases.

Discussion of these two observations is largely outside the scope of this chapter which focuses on the etiological role of infection in RA. However, just as infection might initially trigger autoimmunity in RA by breaking self-tolerance via molecular mimicry or bystander activation, it could similarly lead to increase immunopathology during a disease exacerbation. Disease exacerbations are very important in determining the progression of disease since patients with persistently active disease tend to deteriorate more rapidly. In this sense, the disease trigger is only the first part of the story and it is possible that many different infectious agents could, over the years, contribute to the ultimate outcome of RA.

Summary

There is no doubt that both bacteria and viruses can induce arthritis in humans and animal models; some of these diseases bear considerable resemblance to RA. Although there is no convincing direct evidence that RA is due to any particular infectious agent, yet there are tantalizing hints that infection may play a role in triggering or perpetuating the disease. One possibility, which does not lend itself to an easily testable hypothesis, is that a variety of infectious agents may be able to trigger the syndrome we currently term RA. Perhaps the current state of play is best summed up in the words of the Scottish legal verdict 'not proven'. Further fundamental research in this area is eagerly awaited.

References

1. Osler, W. and McCrae, T. (eds). *The principles and practice of medicine*, (9th edn). Appleton and Co, New York.
2. Forestier, J. (1934). Rheumatoid arthritis and its treatment by gold salts. *Lancet*, 1920;ii:646–8.
3. Marshall, B.J., Armstrong, J.A., McGechie, D.B., and Glancy, R.J. Attempt to fulfil Koch's postulates for pyloric campylobacter. *Medical Journal of Australia*, 1985;142:436–9.
4. Relman, D.A., Loutit, J.S., Schmidt, T.M., Falkow, S., and Tompkins, L.S. Identification of uncultured bacillus of Whipple's disease. *New England Journal of Medicine*, 1992;327:292–301.
5. Kloppenburg, M., Dijkmans, B.A.C., and Breedveld, F.C. Antimicrobial therapy for rheumatoid arthritis. *Baillere's Clinical Rheumatology*, 1995;9:759–69.
6. Behar, S.M. and Porcelli, S.A. Mechanisms of autoimmune disease induction: the role of the immune response to microbial pathogens. *Arthritis & Rheumatism*, 1995;38:458–476.
7. Krause, A., Kamradt, T., and Burmester, G.R. Potential infectious agents in the induction of arthritides. *Current Opinion in Rheumatology*, 1996;8:203–9.
8. Hasunuma, T., Kato, T., Kobata, T., and Nishioka, K. Molecular mechanism of immune response, synovial proliferation and apoptosis in rheumatoid arthritis. *Springer Seminars in Immunopathology*, 1998;20:41–52.
9. Sieper, J. and Kingsley, G. Recent advances in the pathogenesis of reactive arthritis. *Immunology Today*, 1996;17:160–3.
10. Benoist, C. and Mathis, D. The pathogen connection. *Nature*, 1998;394:227–8.
11. Zhao, Z-S., Granucci, F., Yek, L., Schaffer, P.A., and Cantor, H. Molecular mimicry by herpes simplex virus-type 1: autoimmune disease after viral infection. *Science*, 1998;279:1344–7.
12. Horwitz, M.S. Bradley, L.M., Harbertson, J., Krahl, T., Lee, J., and Sarvetnick, N. Diabetes induced by Coxsackie virus: initiation by bystander damage and not molecular mimicry. *Nature Medicine*, 1998;4:781–5.
13. Kingsley, G. and Panayi, G. Joint destruction in rheumatoid arthritis: biological bases. *Clinical and Experimental Rheumatology*, 1997;15 (Supplement 17), S3–S14.
14. Verheijden, G.F., Rijnders, A.W., Bos, E., Coenen-de Roo, C.J., van Starveren, C.J., Miltenburg, A.M. Meijerink, J.H. Elewaut, D., de Keyser, F., Veys, E., and Boots, A.M. Human cartilage glycoprotein-39 as a candidate autoantigen in rheumatoid arthritis. *Arthritis & Rheumatism*, 1997;40:1115–25.
15. Keat, A., Thomas, B., Dixey, J., Osborn, M., Sonnex, C., and Taylor-Robinson, D. *Chlamydia trachomatis* trachomatis and reactive arthritis; the missing link. *Lancet*, 1987;i:72–4.
16. Granfors, K., Jalkanen, S., von Essen, R., Lahesmaa-Rantala, R., Isomaki, O., Pekkola-Heino, K., Merilahti-Palo, R., Saario, R., Isomaki, H., and Toivanen, A. Yersinia antigens in synovial fluid-cell from patients with reactive arthritis. *New England Journal of Medicine*, 1989;320:216–21.
17. Granfor, K., Jalkanen, S., Lindberg, A.A., Maki-Ikola, O., von Essen, R., Lahesmaa-Rantala, R., Isomaki, H., Saario, R., Arnold, W.J., and Toivanen, A. Samonella lipopolysaccharide in synovial cells from patients with reactive arthritis. *Lancet*, 1990;335:685–8.
18. Granfors, K., Jalkanen, S., Toivanen, P., Koski., and Lindberg, A.A.Bacteral lipopolysaccharide in synovial fluid cells in Shigella triggered reactive arthritis. *Journal of Rheumatology*, 1992 ;19:500.
19. Gaston, J.S.H., Life, P.F., Granfors, K., Merilahti-Palo, R., Bailey, L., Consalvey, S., Toivanen, A., and Bacon, P.A. Synovial T lymphocyte recognition of organisms that trigger reactive arthritis. *Clinical and Experimental Immunology*, 1989;76:348–53.
20. Sieper, J., Kingsley, G., Palacios-Boix, A., Pitzalis, C., Treharne, J., Hughes, R., Keat, A., and Panayi, G.S. Synovial T lymphocyte specific immune response to *Chlamydia trachomatis* in Reiter's disease. *Arthritis & Rheumatism*, 1991;34:588–98.
21. Ford, D.K. (1991). Lymphocytes from the site of disease in reactive arthritis indicate antigen-specific immunopathology. *Journal of Infectious Diseases*, 164, 1032–3.
22. Campbell, F., Mygind, P., Birkelund, S., Holm, A., Travers, P., Panayi, G.S., and Kingsley, G.H. Sexually-acquired reactive arthritis (SAReA) synovial T cell clones respond to *Chlamydia trachomatis* (Ct) 60kD heat shock protein: identification of CD4+ Tcell epitopes (abstract). *Arthritis & Rheumatism*, 1998;41 (Supplement), S148.
23. Mertz, A., Wu, P., Rudwaleit, M., Braun, J., and Sieper, J.Synovial T cell response to the heat shock protein 60 of *Yersinia enterocolitica* in yersinia arthritis patients: epitope analysis and cytokine secretion profile (abstract). *Arthritis & Rheumatism*, 1998;41 (Supplement), S131.
24. Rudwaleit, M., Mertz, A., Wu, P., Lauster, R., Ugrinovic, S., Schauer-Petrowskaja, C., Distler, A., and Sieper, J. Synovial proliferation to *Yersinia enterocolitica* 19kD differentiates yersinia-triggered reactive arthritis (ReA) from other ReA and oligoarthritides (abstract). *Arthritis & Rheumatism*, 1998;41 (Supplement), S244.
25. Taylor-Robinson, D., Gilroy, C.B., Thomas, B.J., and Keat, A.C. Detection of *Chlamydia trachomatis* DNA in the joints of reactive arthritis patients by polymerase chain reaction. *Lancet*, 1992;340, 81–2.

26. Bas, S., Griffais, R., Kvien, T.K., Glennas, A., Melby, K., and Vischer, T.L. Amplification of plasmid and chromosome Chlamydia DNA in the synovial fluid of patients with reactive arthritis and undifferentiated seronegative arthritis. *Arthritis & Rheumatism*, 1995;**38**:1005–13.

27. Wilkinson, N.Z., Kingsley, G.H., Sieper, J., Braun, J., and Ward, M.E. Lack of correlation between the detection of *Chlamydia trachomatis* DNA in synovial fluid from patients with a range of rheumatic disease and the presence of an antichlamydial immune response. *Arthritis & Rheumatism*, 1998;**41**:845–54.

28. Gerard, H.C., Branigan, P.J., Schumacher, H.R. Jr., and Hudson, A.P. Synovial Chlamydia trachomatis in patients with reactive arthritis/Reiter's syndrome are viable but show aberrant gene expression. *Journal of Rheumatology*, 1998;**25**:734–42.

29. Braun, J., Tuszewski, M., Eggens, U., Mertz, A., Schauer-Petrowskaja, C., Doring E., Laitko, S., Distler, A., Sieper, J., and Ehler, S. Nested polymerase chain reaction strategy simultaneously targeting DNA sequences of multiple bacterial species in inflammatory joint diseases. I. Screening of synovial fluid samples of patients with spondyloarhropathies and other arthritides. *Journal of Rheumatology*, 1997;**24**:1092–100.

30. Pacheco-Tena, C., Alvarado de la Barrera, C., Lopez-Vidal, Y., Vasquez-Mellado, J., Richaud-Patin, Y., Llorente, L., Amieva, R.I., Martinez, A., Ramos, J., Cifuentes, M., and Burgos-Vargas, R. Bacterial DNA in synovial fluid (SF) cells of patients (pts) with juvenile-onset spondyloarthropathies (JO-SpA) (abstract). *Arthritis & Rheumatism*, 1998;**41** (Supplement), S150.

31. Wilkinson, N.Z., Kingsley, G.H., Jones, H.W., Sieper, J., Braun, J., and Ward, M.E. The detection of DNA from a range of bacterial species in the joints of patients with a variety of arthritides using a nested, broad-range PCR. *Rheumatology*. 1999;**38**:260–6

32. Sieper, J. and Braun, J. Treatment of reactive arthritis with antibiotics. *British Journal of Rheumatology*, 1998;**34**:717–720.

33. Propert, A.J., Gill, A.J., and Laird, S.M. A prospective study of Reiter's syndrome. An interim report on the first 82 cases. *British Journal of Venereal Diseases*, 1964;**40**:160–5.

34. Fryden, A., Bengtsson, A., and Foberg, U. Early antibiotic treatment of reactive arthritis associated with enteric infections; clinical and serological study. *British Medical Journal*, 1990;**301**:1299–302.

35. Lauhio, A., Leirisalo-Repo, M., Lahdevirta, J., Saikku, P., and Repo, H. Double-blind placebo-controlled study of three-month treatment with lymecycline in reactive arthritis, with special reference to Chlamydia arthritis. *Arthritis & Rheumatism*, 1991;**34**:6–14.

36. Toivanen, A., Yli Kerttula, T., Luukainen, R., Merilahti-Palo, R., Granfors, K., and Seppala, J. Effect of antimicrobial treatment on chronic reactive arthritis. *Clinical and Experimental Rheumatology*, 1993;**11**:301–7.

37. Sieper, J., Fendler, C., Eggens, U., Laitko, S., Sorenso, H., Keitel, W., Hiepe, and F., Braun, J. Long-term antibiotic treatment in reactive arthritis (REA) and undifferentiated oligoarthritis (UOA): results of a double-blind placebo-controlled randomized study (abstract). *Arthritis & Rheumatism*. 1997;**40** (Supplement), S227.

38. Wollenhaupt, J., Hammer, M., Pott, H.G., and Zeidler, H. A double-blind placebo-controlled comparison of 2 weeks versus 4 months treatment with doxycycline in Chlamydia-induced arthritis (abstract). *Arthritis & Rheumatism*, 1997;**40** (Supplement):S143.

39 Snydman, D.R., Schenkein, D.P., Berardi, V.P., Lastavica, C.C., and Pariser, K.M. *Borrelia Burgdorferii* in joint fluid in chronic Lyme arthritis. *Annals of Internal Medicine*, 1986;**104**:798–800.

40. Nocton, J.J., Dressler, F., Rutledge, B.J., Rys, P.N., Persing, D.H., and Steere, A.C. Detection of *Borrelia burgdorferii* DNA by polymerase chain reaction in synovial fluid from patients with Lyme arthritis. *New England Journal of Medicine*, 1994;**330**:229–34.

41. Sigal, L.H., Steere, A.C., Freeman, D.H., and Dwyer, J.M. Proliferative response of mononuclear cells in Lyme disease; reactivity to *Borrelia Burgdorferii* is greater in joint fluid than in blood. *Arthritis & Rheumatism*, 1986;**29**:761–9.

42. Kalish, R. (1993). Lyme disease. *Rheumatic Disease Clinics of North America*, **19**, 399–426.

43. Burmester, G.R., Daser, A., Kamradt, T., Krause, A., Mitchison, N.A., Sieper, J., and Wolf, N. Immunology of reactive arthritides. *Annual Reviews of Immunology*, 1995;**13**:229–50.

44. Gross, D.M., Forsthuber, T., Tary-Lehmann, M., Etling, C., Kouichi, I., Nagy, Z.A., Field, J.A., Steere, A.C., and Huber, B.T. Identification of LFA-1 as a candidate autoantigen in treatment-resistant Lyme arthritis. *Science*, 1998;**281**:703–6.

45. Muller, B., Gimsa, U., Mitchison, N.A., Radbruch, A., Sieper, J., Yin, Z. Modulating the Th1/Th2 balance in inflammatory arthritis. *Springer Seminars in Immunopathology*. 1998;**20**:181–96.

46. Yin, Z., Braun, J., Neure, L., Wu, P., Liu, L., Eggens, U., and Sieper J. Crucial role of interleukin-10/interleukin-12 balance in the regulation of the type 2 T helper cytokine response in reactive arthritis. *Arthritis Rheumatism*, 1997;**40**:1788–97.

47. Kingsley, G. Microbial DNA in the synovium—a role in etiology or a mere bystander? *Lancet*, 1997;**349**:1038–9.

48. Wilbrink, B., van der Heijden, I.M., Schouls, L.M., van Embden, J.D.A., Hazes, J.M.W., Breedveld, F.C., and Tak, P.P. Detection of bacterial DNA in joint samples from patients with undifferentiated arthritis and reactive arthritis, using polymerase chain reaction with universal 16S ribosomal RNA primers. *Arthritis & Rheumatism*, 1998;**41**:535–43.

49. Ford, D.K. Understanding rheumatoid arthritis. *Journal of Rheumatology*, 1997;**24**:1464–5.

50. Naides, S.J.Viral arthritis. In *Rheumatology* (eds Klippel, J.H. and Dieppe, P.A.) (2nd edn), 1998;6.6.1–8. Mosby, London

51. Mitchell, L.A., Tingle, A.J., Shukin, R., Sangeorzan, J.A., McCune, J., and Braun, D.K. Chronic rubella vaccine-associated arthropathy. *Archives of Internal Medicine*, 1993;**153**:2268–74.

52. Grahame, R., Armstrong, R., Simmons, N., Wilton, J.M.A., Dyson, M., Laurent, R., Millis, R., and Mims, C.A Chronic arthritis associated with the presence of intrasynovial rubella virus. *Annals of the Rheumatic Diseases*, 1983;**42**:2–13.

53. Naides, S.J., Scharosch, L.L., Foto, F., and Howard, E.J. Rheumatologic manifestations of human parvovirus B19 infection in adults. Initial two year clinical experience. *Arthritis & Rheumatism*, 1990;**33**:1297–1309.

54. Guerin, B., Arfi, S., Numeric, P., Jean Baptiste, G., Le Parc, J.M., Smadja, D., and Grollier Bois, L. Polyarthritis in HTLV-1 infected patients: a review of 17 cases. *Revue du Rhumatisme (English Edition)*, 1995;**62**:21–8.

55. Nishioka, K., Nakajima, T., Hasunuma, T., and Sato, K. Rheumatic manifestations of human leukaemia virus infection. *Rheumatic Disease Clinics of North America*, 1993;**19**:489–503.

56. Iwakura, Y., Tosu, M., Yoshida, E., Takiguchi, M., Sato, K., Kitajima, I., Nishioka, K., Yamamoto, K., Takeda, T., Hatanaka, M., *et al.* Induction of inflammatory arthropathy resembling rheumatoid arthritis in mice transgenic for HTLV-1. *Science*, 1991;**253**:026–8.

57. Calabrese, L.H. Rheumatic aspects of human immunodeficiency virus infection and other immunodeficient states. In *Rheumatology* (eds Klippel, J.H. and Dieppe, P.A.). Mosby, London (2nd edn), 1998;6.7.1–12.

58. Haase, A.T. Pathogenesis of lentivirus infections. *Nature*, 1986;**322**:130–136. Mosby, London

59. Wilkerson, M.J., Davis, W.C., and Cheevers, W.P. Peripheral blood and synovial fluid mononuclear cell phenotypes in lentivirus-induced arthritis. *Journal of Rheumatology*, 1995;**22**:8–15. Mosby, London

60. Lechner, F., Vogt, H.R., Seow, H.F., Bertoni, G., Cheevers, W.P., von Bodungen, U., Zurbriggen, A., and Peterhans E. Expression of cytokine mRNA in lentivirus-induced arthritis. *American Journal of Pathology*, 1997;**151**:1053–65. Mosby, London

61. Perry, L.L.,Wilkerson, M.J., Hullinger, G.A., and Cheevers, W.P. Depressed CD4+ T lymphocyte proliferative response and enhanced antibody response to viral antigen in chronic lentivirus-induced arthritis. *Journal of Infectious Diseases,* 1995;**171**:328–34.

62. Davies, J.M., Robinson, W.F., Carnegie, P.R., Davies, J.M., Robinson, W.F., and Carnegie, P.R. Antibody reactivity to the transmembrane protein of the caprine arthritis encephalitis virus correlates with severity of arthritis: no evidence for the involvement of epitope mimicry. *Veterinary Immunology Immunopathology* 1997;**60**:131–47.

63. McConkey, B. and Situnayake, R.D. Effects of rifampicin with and without isoniazid in rheumatoid arthritis. *Journal of Rheumatology,* 1988;**15**:46–50.

64. Gabriel, S.E., Conn, D.L., and Luthra, H. Rifampin therapy in rheumatoid arthritis. *Journal of Rheumatology,* **17**, 163–6.

65. Cox, N.L., Prowse, M.V., Maddison, M.C. and Maddison, P.J. Treatment of early rheumatoid arthritis with rifampicin. *Annals of the Rheumatic Diseases,* 1992;**51**:32–4.

66. Lindblad, S., Hedfors, E., and Malmborg, A.S. Rifamycin SV in local treatment of synovitis. Arthroscopic and pharmacologic evaluation. *Journal of Rheumatology,* 1985;**12**:900–3.

67. Astbury, C., Hill, J., and Bird, H.A. Co-trimoxazole in rheumatoid arthritis: a comparison with sulfapyridine. *Annals of the Rheumatic Diseases,* 1988;**47**:323–7.

68. Swinson, D.R., Zlosnick, J., and Jackson, L. Double-blind trial of dapsone against placebo in the treatment of rheumatoid arthritis. *Annals of the Rheumatic Diseases,* 1981;**40**:235–9.

69. Marshall, D.A.S., Hunter, J.A., and Capell, H.A. Double-blind, placebo-controlled study of metronidazole as a disease-modifying agent in the treatment of rheumatoid arthritis. *Annals of the Rheumatic Diseases,* 1992;**51**:758–60.

70. Mortiboy, D. and Palmer, R.G. Ciprofloxacin and rheumatoid arthritis. Lack of effect. *British Journal of Rheumatology,* 1989;**28**:272.

71. Kloppenburg. M., Breedveld, F.C., Terwiel, J., Mallee, C., and Djikmans, B.A.C. Minocycline in rheumatoid arthritis. A 48-week double-blind placebo-controlled trial. *Arthritis & Rheumatism,* 1994;**37**:629–36.

72. Tilley, B.C., Alarcon, G.S., Heyse, S.P., Trentham, D.E., Neuner, R., Kaplan, D.A., Clegg, D.O., Leisen, J.C., Buckley, L., Cooper, S.M., *et al.* Minocycline in rheumatoid arthritis. A 48-week, double-blind, placebo-controlled trial. MIRA Trial Group. *Annals of Internal Medicine,* 1995;**122**:81–9.

73. Kjeldsen-Kragh, J., Rashid, T., Dybwad, A., Sioud, M., Haugen, M., Forre, O., and Ebringer, A. Decrease in anti-Proteus mirabilis but not anti-Escherichia coli antibody levels in rheumatoid arthritis patients treated with fasting and a one year vegetarian diet. *Annals of the Rheumatic Diseases,* 1995;**54**:221–4.

74. Eerola, E., Mottonen, T., Hannonen, P., Luukkainen, R., Kantola, I., Vuori, K., Tuominen, J., and Toivanen, P. Intestinal flora in early rheumatoid arthritis. *British Journal of Rheumatology,* 1994;**33**:1030–4.

75. Hazenberg, M.P. Intestinal flora bacteria and arthritis: why the joint? *Scandinavian Journal of Rheumatology,* 1995;**101** (**Supplement**), 207–11.

76. Melief, M.J., Hoijer, M.A., Van Paassen, H.C., and Hazenberg, M.P. Presence of bacterial flora-derived antigen in synovial tissue macrophages and dendritic cells. *British Journal of Rheumatology,* 1995;**34**:1112–6.

77. Ebringer, A., Ptaszynska, T., Corbett, M., Wilson, C., Macafee, Y., Avakian, H., Baron, P., and James, D.C. Antibodies to proteus in rheumatoid arthritis. *Lancet,* 1985;**2**:305–7.

78. Gaston, H. Proteus—is it a likely etiological factor in chronic polyarthritis? *Annals of the Rheumatic Diseases,* 1995;**54**:157–8.

79. Deighton, C.M., Gray, J., Bint, A.J., and Walker, D.J. Anti-Proteus antibodies in rheumatoid arthritis same-sexed sibships. *British Journal of Rheumatology,* 1992;**31**:241–5.

80. Wilson C., Corbet M., and Ebringer A. Increased isolation of Proteus mirabilis species from rheumatoid arthritis patients compared with osteoarthritis patients and healthy controls (abstract). *British Journal of Rheumatology,* 1990;**29** (**supplement 2**), 99.

81. Wilson, C., Thakore, A., Isenberg, D., and Ebringer, A. Correlation between anti-Proteus antibodies and isolation rates of P. mirabilis in rheumatoid arthritis. *Rheumatology International,* 1997;**16**:187–9.

82. McDonagh, J., Gray, J., Sykes, H., Walker, D.J., Bint, A.J., and Deighton, C.M. Anti-proteus antibodies and proteus organisms in rheumatoid arthritis: a clinical study. *British Journal of Rheumatology,* 1994;**33**:32–5.

83. Wilson, C., Ebringer, A., Ahmadi, K., Wrigglesworth, J., Tiwana, H., Fielder, M., Binder, A., Ettelaie, C., Cunningham, P., Joannou, C. *et al.* Shared amino acid sequences between major histocompatibility complex class II glycoproteins, type XI collagen and Proteus mirabilis in rheumatoid arthritis. *Annals of the Rheumatic Diseases,* 1995;**54**:216–20.

84. Tiwana, H. Wilson, C., Cunningham, P., Binder, A., and Ebringer, A. Antibodies to four gram-negative bacteria in rheumatoid arthritis which share sequences with the rheumatoid arthritis susceptibility motif. *British Journal of Rheumatology,* 1996;**35**:592–4.

85. Chary-Valckenaere, I., Guillemin, F., Pourel, J., Schiele, F., Heller, R., and Jaulhac, B. Seroreactivity to *Borrelia burgdorgeri* antigens in early rheumatoid arthritis: a case control study. *British Journal of Rheumatology,* 1997;**36**:945–9.

86. Soderlund, M., von Essen, R., Haapasaari, J., Kiistala, U., Kiviluoto, O., and Hedman, K. Persistence of parvovirus B19 DNA in synovial membranes of young patients with and without chronic arthropathy. *Lancer,* 1997;**349**, 1063–5.

87. Klinman, D.M., Yi, A–K., Beaucage, S.L., Conover, J., and Krieg, A.M. CpG motifs in bacterial DNA rapidly induce lymphocytes to secrete interleukin-6, interleukin-12 and interferon-γ. *Proceedings of the National Academy of Sciences* (USA), 1996;**93**:2879–83.

88. Jalal, H., Millar, M., Linton, C., and Dieppe, P. Absence of *mycobacterium tuberculosis* DNA in synovial fluid from patients with rheumatoid arthritis. *Annals of Rheumatic Disease,* 1994;**53**:695–8.

89. Pras, E., Schumacher, H.R., Kastner, D.L., and Wilder, R.L. Lack of evidence of mycobacteria in synovial tissue from patients with rheumatoid arthritis. *Arthritis & Rheumatism,* 1996;**39**:2080–1.

90. Schaeverbeke, T., Gilroy, C.B., Bebear, C., Dehais, J., and Taylor-Robinson, D.Mycoplasma fermentans, but not M penetrans, detected by PCR assays in synovium from patients with rheumatoid arthritis and other rheumatic disorders. *Journal of Clinical Pathology,* 1996 ;**49**:824–8.

91. Schaeverbeke, T., Renaudin, H., Clerc, M., Lequen, L., Vernhes, J.P., De Barbeyrac, B., Bannwarth, B., Bebear, C., and Dehais, J. Systematic detection of mycoplasmas by culture and polymerase chain reaction (PCR) procedures in 209 synovial fluid samples. *British Journal of Rheumatology,* 1997;**36**:310–4.

92. Hoffman, R.W., O'Sullivan, F.X., Schafermeyer, K.R., Moore, T.L., Roussell, D., Watson-McKown, R., Kim, MF., and Wise, K.S. Mycoplasma infection and rheumatoid arthritis: analysis of their relationship using immunoblotting and an ultrasensitive polymerase chain reaction detection method. *Arthritis & Rheumatism,* 1997;**40**:1219–28.

93. Schaeverbeke, T., Clerc, M., Lequen, L., Charron, A., Bebear, C., de Barbeyrac, B., Bannwarth, B., Dehais, J., and Bebear, C. Genotypic characterization of seven strains of Mycoplasma fermentans isolated from synovial fluids of patients with arthritis. *Journal of Clinical Microbiology,* 1998;**36**:1226–31.

94. Bulbul, R., Davis, J., Yarboro, C., Gourley, M., Klippel, J, Arayssi. T., Branigan, P., Hudson, A., Rothfuss, S., and Schumacher, H.R. Treatment responses in chlamydia trachomatis-associated arthritis; an observational study (abstract). *Arthritis & Rheumatism,* 1996;**39** (**Supplement**), S184.

95. Saaibi. D.L., Arayssi. T., Gowin, K.M., Branigan, P.J., Gerard, H.C., Hudson, A.P., Klippel, J.H., and Schumacher, H.R. Clinical spectrum of arthritis associated with chlamydia pneumoniae in synovium, (abstract). *Arthritis & Rheumatism*, 1996;**39 (Supplement)**, S183.

96. Gray, J., Marsh, P.J., and Walker, D.J., A search for bacterial DNA in RA synovial fluid using the polymer chain reaction. *British Journal of Rheumatology*, 1994;**33**:997–8.

97. Saal, J.G., Steidle, M., Einsele, H., Muller, C.A., Frits, P., and Zacher, J. Persistence of B19 parvovirus in synovial membrances of patients with rheumatoid arthritis. *Rheumatology International*, 1992;**12**:147–51.

98. Kerr, J.R., Cartron, J.P, Curran, M.D, Moore, J.E., Elliott, J.R., and Mollan, R.A. A study of the role of parvovirus B19 in rheumatoid arthritis. *British Journal of Rheumatology*, 1995;**34**:809–13.

99. Nikkari, S., Roivainen, A., Hannonen, P., Mottonen, T., Luukkainen, R., Yli-Jama, T., and Toivanen P. (1995). Persistence of parvovirus B19 in synovial fluid and bone marrow. *Annals of the Rheumatic Diseases*, **54**, 597–600.

100. Newkirk, M.M., Watanabe Duffy, K.N., Leclerc, J., Lambert, N., and Shiroky, J.B. Detection of cytomegalovirus, Epstein-Barr virus and herpes virus-6 in patients with rheumatoid arthritis with or without Sjogren's syndrome. *British Journal of Rheumatology*, 1994;**33**:317–22.

101. Zhang, L., Nikkari, S., Skurnik, M., Ziegler, T., Luukkainen, R., Mottonen, T., and Toivanen P. Detection of herpesviruses by polymerase chain reacion in lymphocytes from patients with rheumatoid arthritis. *Arthritis & Rheumatism*, 1993;**36**:1080–6.

102. Tamm, A., Ziegler, T., Lautenschlager, I., Nikkari, S., Mottonen, T., Luukkainen, R., Skurnim, M., and Toivanen, P. Detection of cytomegalovirus DNA in cells from synovial fluid and peripheral blood of patients with early rheumatoid arthritis. *Journal of Rheumatology*,1993; **20**:1489–93.

103. Einsele, H., Steidle, M., Muller, C.A., Frots, P., Zacer, J., Schmidt. H., and Saal, J.G. Demonstration of cytomegalovirus (CMV) DNA and anti-CMV response in the synovial membrane and serum of patients with rheumatoid arthritis. *Journal of Rheumatology*, 1992;**19**:677–81.

104. Nikkari, S., Luukkainen, R., Nikkari, L., Skurnik, M., and Toivanen, P. No evidence of adenoviral hexon regions in rheumatoid synovial cells and tissue. *Journal of Rheumatology*, 1994;**21**:2179–83.

105. Berthelot, J.M., Besse, B., Bilaudel, S., Delecrin, J., Letenneur, J., Youinou, P., Maugars, Y., Prost A. Search of papillomavirus genome in synovial membranes and rheumatoid nodules. *Revuede Rhumatisme (Edition Francaise)*, 1994;**61**:491–6.

106. Nelson, P.N. Retroviruses in rheumatic diseases. *Annals of the Rheumatic Diseases*, 1995;**54**:441–2.

107. Bailer, R.T., Lazo, A., Harisdangkul, V., Ehrlich, G.D., Gray, L.S., and Whisler, R.L., Blakeslee, J.R. Lack of evidence for human T cell lymphotrophic virus type I or II infection in patients with systemic lupus erythematosus or rheumatoid arthritis. *Journal of Rheumatology*, 1994;**21**:2217–24.

108. Nelson, P.N., Lever, A.M., Bruckner, F.E., Isenberg, D.A., Kessaris, N., and Hay, F.C. Polymerase chain reaction fails to incriminate exogenous retroviruses HTLV-I and HIV-1 in rheumatological diseases although a minority of sera cross react with retroviral antigens. *Annals of the Rheumatic Diseases*, 1994;**53**:749–54.

109. Nelson, P.N., Bowman, S.J., Hay, F.C., Lanchbury, J.S., Panayi, G.S., and Lever, A.M. Absence of exogenous retroviruses in Felty's syndrome. *British Journal of Rheumatology*, 1995;**34**:185–7.

110. Stransky, G., Vernon, J., Aicher, W.K., Moreland, L.W., Gay, R.E., and Gay, S. Virus-like particles in synovial fluids from patients with rheumatoid arthritis. *British Journal of Rheumatology*, 1993;**32**:1044–8.

111. Kalden, J.R. and Gay, S. Retroviruses and autoimmune rheumatic diseases. *Clinical and Experimental Immunology*, 1994;**98**:1–5.

112. Nakagawa, K., Brusic, V., McColl, and G., Harrison, L.C. Direct evidence for the expression of multiple endogenous retroviruses in the synovial compartment in rheumatoid arthritis. *Arthritis & Rheumatism*, 1997;**40**:627–38.

113. Hernandez-Cruz, B., Cardiel, M.H., Villa, A.R., and Alcocer-Varela, J. Development, recurrence and severity of infections in Mexican patients with rheumatoid arthritis. A nested case-control study. *Journal of Rheumatology*, 1998;**25**:1900–7.

114. Symmons, D.P.M. Mortality in rheumatoid arthritis. *British Journal of Rheumatology*, 1988;**27 (Supplement 1)**, 44–54.

4 | *Experimental models for rheumatoid arthritis*

Rikard Holmdahl

Introduction

To understand the complexity of the pathogenesis of RA, animal models are a necessity. Obviously a disease identical to RA cannot develop in any experimental animal since they are different species with different genetics and live in a different environment, compared with humans.

The advantages of using animal models are mainly:

1. The animals can be genetically controlled. Laboratory mouse and rat strains have been inbred which dramatically facilitate genetic studies.

2. Their environment can be better controlled

3. Manipulative experiments can be performed. The genome of inbred strains can be changed by mutations, insertions, and deletions. The environment can also be changed in a controlled way; they can be immunized or infected which may lead to arthritis.

To be able to evaluate and select proper animal models for RA it is of value to be able to reproduce some of the basic features of RA.

Such hallmarks of RA are:

- *Tissue-specificity*: RA is characterized by a tissue-specific, inflammatory attack affecting diarthrodial joints. Although systemic manifestations can be prominent, the predominant inflammatory attack is directed towards peripheral joints.
- *Chronicity*: the disease is chronic and occurs in tissues in which no causative infectious pathogens have been demonstrated. Acute joint inflammation has common manifestations in both physiological responses to infections and connected with other inflammatory disorders, but in RA chronicity is an essential characteristic. The disease course may proceed with identifiable relapses, but there is usually steady progression of joint destruction
- *Class II MHC association*: the genetic influence is significant but not prominent and the genetic control defined so far points towards an important role of class II genes in the major histocompatibility complex. In particular, certain structures near the peptide-binding pocket of HLA-DR4 molecules are highly associated with RA.

Taken together, these findings suggest that immune-mediated inflammation directed to peripheral joints plays a role in the disease process. The closest explanation for such a response is the occurrence of an infectious agent persisting in the joint. However, so far it has not been possible to identify such an agent as an explanation for RA. Alternatively, the immune reaction could be directed to the joint structure, that is cartilage-specific proteins. Another explanation could relate to a defect in a gene related to peripheral joints, for example leading to cartilage fragility or a gene affecting immune recognition. However, such a genetic defect has not been found. Thus, the cause and driving forces are polygenic and multifactorial, and understanding the disease will require a detailed basic analysis of disease mechanisms.

Animal models are excellent tools for such an analysis. With animals, controlled experiments can be performed in which one can control environmental and genetic factors. Recent advances in animal models mimicking different aspects of human diseases, as well as the improvement in genetic techniques, has dramatically increased their usefulness. Here, an overview of the large number of different animal models for arthritis will be provided. This will include not only models that most closely mimic RA, but also models similar to arthritides such as Reiter's disease, ankylosing spondylitis, Lyme disease, and septic arthritis (summarized in Table 4.1).

Arthritis caused by live infectious agents

Several infectious agents may invade and persist in joints, thereby causing arthritis. As with most persistent infectious agents, a balance between the parasite and the host is usually achieved. Thus, inflammatory consequences might not only be caused directly by the parasite but also by an aberrant inflammatory response of the host. When live organisms are present in the target tissue, chronic autoimmunity could be maintained by different mechanisms such as superantigens directly activating T cells, a cross-reactive immune response, or the presence of adjuvant material enhancing autoantigen presentation. Several such arthritogenic agents have been described in experimental animals and some of these mimic a corresponding infectious disease in humans.

joint manifestations do not occur, showing the importance of an as yet undefined infectious agent[17]. A similar phenomenon occurs in B27 transgenic mice[18], in which arthritis occurs only in conventional animal facilities. Inoculation of LEW but not DA rats with *Yersinia* induces an arthritis that persists in the peripheral joints[19]. A contributing factor could be the collagen adhesion protein YadA expressed on arthritogenic *Yersinia* strains[20,21]. These models are more reminiscent of Reiter's disease and ankylosing spondylitis rather than RA and offer excellent possibilities for elucidating the mechanisms of these diseases. However, the link between B27 expression and arthritis induction by bacteria remains unclear.

Arthritis caused by fragments derived from infectious agents persisting in joints

Postinfectious arthritis may develop after bacterial infections. The occurrence of this arthritis seems to be related to the spreading of the bacterial cell wall fragments to the reticuloendothelial system, that is they are ingested by macrophages throughout the body. Bacterial cell wall fragments are difficult to degrade and may cause prolonged activation of macrophages and arthritis.

Mycobacterium cell wall-induced arthritis

The first animal model for RA to be described was the so-called adjuvant arthritis induced in rats after injection of mycobacteria cell walls suspended in mineral oil, that is complete Freund's adjuvant (CFA)[22]. Surprisingly, so far only rats (and not mice or primates) have been shown to develop arthritis after mycobacteria challenge[23], although it has been reported that joint-related granuloma formation has occurred in humans treated with BCG[24]. CFA is a potent adjuvant that stimulates both cellular and humoral immunity. Subcutaneous injection of CFA in rates leads to granulomatous inflammation in many organs, including the spleen, liver, bone marrow, skin, and eyes, and causes profound inflammation in peripheral joints[22].

The adjuvant-induced disease is severe but self-limited and the rat recovers within a few months (Fig. 4.1). It was earlier suggested that the mycobacteria cell wall was disseminated throughout the body and engulfed by tissue macrophages that had difficulty degrading the bacterial cell wall structures and were therefore transformed into an activated state. In this process, T cells are essential since the disease can be abrogated by the elimination of T cells[25,26]. The specificity of such T cells has, however, not been reproducibly demonstrated, although some studies have suggested cross reactive bacterial structures and cartilage components[27,28]. While a role for heat shock proteins in the induction of the disease has not been confirmed, they clearly play an important regulatory role for the development of arthritis[29]. In the search for the minimal arthritogenic epitope in mycobacterium, it was observed that one of the essen-

tial structural elements of the mycobacterium peptidoglycan, muramyl dipeptide, could induce arthritis[30]. Interestingly, T cells do not recognize this structure but it has potent adjuvant capacity indicating that it stimulates antigen presenting cells or innate immune recognition. Whatever the causes of the inflammatory disease triggered by mycobacterium in oil is, it will not explain why joints are specifically inflamed, such as in RA, since the mycobacteria-induced disease is systemic.

Streptococcal cell wall-induced arthritis

Postinfectious arthritis has been observed to occur following streptococcal infection in humans. Similarly, a rapidly developing form of arthritis occurs after injection of streptococcal cell wall fragments in rats[31] and mice[32] but not in primates[23]. Severe systemic polyarthritis develops in many rat strains after systemic inoculation of streptococcal fragments. Peptidoglycans from the cell wall rapidly disseminate throughout the rat, including the joints[33]. These structures are difficult to degrade and as a consequence synovial macrophages are persistently activated. T cells are necessary for the initiation and perpetuation of the chronic arthritis[34] but their precise role is still unclear. However, mechanisms other than peptidoglycan-mediated activation of macrophages are likely to participate since the injection of only peptidoglycan induces a milder and less chronic disease. There are also a number of streptococcal proteins that clearly skew the immune response and may be of additional importance.

Other adjuvant-induced models of arthritis

The induction of arthritis in rats is not only dependent on the mycobacteria cell walls but also the oil into which the mycobacteria fragments are suspended. Interestingly, some oils support the induction of arthritis whereas others do not[35]. Many years later it was noted that the oils supporting the induction of arthritis were in fact arthritogenic themselves depending on the rat strain used[36,37]. It was also found that adjuvant compounds, such as avridine and pristane, which bear no relation to bacteria cell walls, were highly effective in inducing arthritis in rats[37,38]. As these adjuvant compounds, in most cases, produce inflammation confined to the joints, they potentially offer better experimental models for RA than the earlier, commonly used 'adjuvant arthritis' or mycobacterium in oil-induced arthritis models.

Mineral oil-, pristane-, and avridine-induced arthritis in rats

Mineral oil-induced arthritis (OIA)[36], avridine-induced arthritis (AvIA)[37], and pristane-induced arthritis (PIA) in the rat[38] share many common features and differ mainly in the severity and chronicity of the disease. They are induced with adjuvant compounds lacking immunogenic capacity, that is, no specific immune responses are elicited towards them after injection. Instead they are rapidly and widely spread throughout the body after a single subcutaneous injection and penetrate through cell membranes into cells. After a delay of at least one or two weeks, arthritis suddenly ensues (Fig. 4.2). The arthritis appears in the peripheral joints, with a distribution similar to RA, and is mainly symmetrical. Occasionally other joints are involved, but systemic manifestations in other tissues have so far not been reported.

In certain rat strains, especially in the AvIA and PIA models, acute arthritis develops along a chronic relapsing disease course. Surprisingly, no immune response to cartilage proteins has been observed although rheumatoid factors are present in serum. A role for cartilage proteins in regulating disease activity is possible as the disease can be prevented and even therapeutically ameliorated by nasal vaccination with various cartilage proteins[39]. Another way to both prevent and therapeutically decrease disease severity in the established phase is by blocking $\alpha\beta$T cells[38,40]. Together with the observation that the chronic disease course in associated with the MHC region[38,40], this could implicate the activation of T cells recognizing cartilage proteins. However, such T cells have not been observed and T-cell transfer of the disease has so far failed to identify antigen-specific T cells[41,42].

The inducing agents are all small molecular structures unable to bind to class II MHC molecules or recognized by T cells. A role for environmental infectious agents is not likely since no difference in disease susceptibility could be seen in germ-free rats, although only conventional rats respond to heat shock proteins[43]. There is no evidence for recognition by lymphocyte receptors or receptors involved in the innate immune system. Surprisingly, some of the arthritogenic adjuvants are in fact components already present in the body before injection. For example, pristane is a component of chlorophyll and is normally ingested by all mammals including laboratory rats. Pristane is taken up through the intestine and spread throughout the body. However, they all share the capacity to penetrate into cells where they could change membrane fluidity and modulate transcriptional regulation[44,45]. The injection route and doses are critical, that is, it is, most likely to be of importance which cell is first activated and to what extent.

The arthritis is genetically controlled, not only by the major histocompatibility complex but also by genes outside the MHC. In fact, recently published studies indicate the location of major regions controlling different phases of the disease such as arthritis onset, clinical severity, joint erosion, and chronicity[46,47]. A challenge for the future will be to determine the genes controlling the transformation of an acute arthritis into a chronic disease, which occurs 3–4 weeks after disease onset.

Pristane-induced arthritis in mice

Surprisingly, adjuvant arthritis is not easily inducible in species other than rats. Of the above mentioned adjuvants, only pristane-induced arthritis (PIA) has been described in the mouse[48,49]. The induction of PIA in mouse requires repeated intraperitoneal injections of pristane that triggers an inflammatory disease with a late and insidious onset. The disease is clearly different from PIA in the rat; the same inducing protocol does not induce disease in the other species and the disease course and characteristics are different. In the mouse, a role for an induced recognition of heat shock proteins has been observed although such experiments have not been performed using germ-free animals[50,51].

However, there are also similarities, such as to the chronicity of arthritis, the T-cell dependency, and perhaps the MHC association[49]. The difference between rats and mice is surprising but may be related to the specific effects of pristane in the mouse, with its capacity to induce tumours after intraperitoneal injections[52].

Cartilage protein-induced arthritis

Collagen-induced arthritis (CIA) was first demonstrated in 1977 in the rat[53] and was later reported using other species such as mouse[54] and primates[55]. Immunization with the major collagen restricted to cartilage, type II collagen (CII), leads to an autoimmune response and, as a consequence, sudden onset of severe arthritis. Although it is necessary to emulsify the CII in adjuvant, such as mineral oil in the rat and complete Freund's adjuvant in the mouse, the disease can be distinguished from the various forms of adjuvant arthritis.

Arthritis is caused by a specific immune attack on cartilage in peripheral joints. Not surprisingly, several other cartilage proteins, such as aggrecan[56], CXI[57], gp39[58], and COMP[59] have subsequently been shown to be arthritogenic in different animal strains. These various models have different characteristics and genetics but the CIA induced with CII is still the most commonly used model and is a prototype of cartilage protein-induced disease.

Collagen II-induced arthritis

The CIA model is perhaps the most commonly used model for rheumatoid arthritis today. However, the model varies considerably depending on the experimental animal species and on whether the type II collagen (CII) used is of self or non-self origin.

In both rats and mice immunized with heterologous CII, a severe, erosive polyarthritis suddenly develops 2–3 weeks after immunization (Fig. 4.3). The inflammation usually subsides within 3–4 weeks although in certain strains a few animals may develop a chronic relapsing disease. The disease is critically dependent on both a strong T- and B-cell response to CII and a significant part of the inflammatory attack on the joints is most likely to be mediated by pathogenic antibodies[60,61]. These CII-specific antibodies bind to cartilage surface, fix complement, attract neutrophilic granulocytes, and activate macrophages. The disease induced with homologous CII in both rats and mice is not as easily inducible but once started is as severe; however, it tends to be more chronic than the disease induced with heterologous CII[62, 63]. The pathogenic events in the chronic disease phase are largely unknown but are most likely to be dependent on both autoreactive B- and T-cell activity. Nevertheless, the CIA model is the most extensively investigated model for RA and has

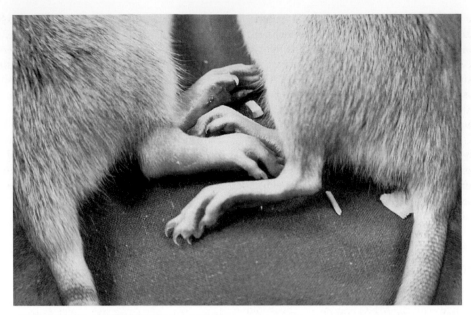

Fig. 4.2 The left paw is from a DA rat injected with 150 μl mineral oil in the back of the skin. The arthritis is severe but non-erosive and acute, and does not become chronic. See also Plate 2.

given valuable insights into the genetic control of arthritics and of autoimmune interactions with cartilage. It has also proven useful for the development of new therapeutic approaches and for drug screening.

Genetic control of CIA; the role of the major histocompatibility complex

Early observations using the CIA model in both mice and rats induced with heterologous CII indicated a role for the major histocompatibility complex region[64,65]. It was later found that the MHC association of CIA induced with homologous CII was even more limited to certain haplotypes. Immunization of rats with homologous (rat) CII leading to arthritis development is associated with class II MHC genes, with the a haplotype as the most permissible, u, f and l intermediate, and n resistant[63]. In the mouse, CIA induced with both heterologous and homologous CII is most strongly associated with H-2q and H-2r haplotypes although most other haplotypes, such as b, s, d, and p, are not totally resistant to disease induced with heterologous CII[54,64,66]. Of interest is that it has been possible to map further the MHC association of CIA to the genes coding for the MHC class II A molecule[67] (Table 4.2). Moreover, the immunodominant peptide derived from the CII molecule bound to the arthritis-associated q variant of the A (A^q) molecule has been found to be located between positions 256 and 270 of CII[68,69]. This is a glycopeptide with an oligosaccharide pointing towards the T-cell receptor and is recognized by many of CII-reactive T cells[70]. Interestingly, the peptide binding pocket of the A^q molecule is very similar to that of the DR4 (DRB1*0401/DRA) and DR1 molecules that are associated with RA[71]. Furthermore, mice transgenically expressing DR4 or DR1 are susceptible to CIA and respond to a peptide from the same CII region[72,73] (Table 4.2). This

Table 4.2 MHC class II molecules associated with CIA in the mouse

MHC class II	CII peptide	MHC binding	T-cell activation	CIA	Reference
A_q	259–270	++	++	+	67
A_p	259–270	+	+	−	67
DR4*0401	260–270	++	++	+	73
DR1*0101	260–270	++	++	+	72
DQ6	?	?	?	−	121
DQ8	?	?	++	+	122

finding provides a model for studies of RA displaying some critical structural similarities to the human disease.

Autoimmune recognition of cartilage

It is important to emphasize that the identified structural interaction between MHC class II+peptide complexes and T cells does not give us the answer to the pathogenesis of CIA (or RA), but rather a better tool for further analysis. An important question is how the immune system in fact interacts with the peripheral joints, that is how autoreactive T and B cells are normally tolerized and what happens in the pathologic situation after their activation by CII immunization. Most of the T cells reactive with the CII256-270 peptide do not cross-react with the corresponding peptide from mouse CII. The difference between the heterologous and the homologous peptide is position 266, in which the rat has a glutamic acid (E) and the mouse an aspartic acid (D). The importance of this minor difference was demonstrated in transgenic mice expressing CII mutated to express a glutamic acid at this position. When mutated CII was expressed in cartilage the T-cell response to CII was partially but not completely tolerized. The mice were susceptible to arthritis but the incidence was lower—similar to what is seen in mice immunized with homologous CII. This finding shows that a normal interaction between cartilage and T cells leads to tolerance manifested by an impaired capacity to give rise to a recall proliferative response to CII. However, the tolerance is not complete since the T cells can still produce effector cytokines such as γ interferon and give help to B cells. Partially tolerized T cells may, under extreme circumstances (such as CII immunization), mediate arthritis. In contrast, B cells reactive with CII are not tolerized and as soon as the T cells are activated, even in a partially tolerized state, they help B cells to produce autoreactive, and most probably pathogenic, antibodies. It is possible that a similar situation may exist in humans, which could explain the difficulties in isolating CII reactive T cells compared with the relative ease in which CII reactive B cells can be detected in the joints.

Development of new therapeutic approaches using the CIA model

The reproducibility and basic characterization of the CIA model has laid ground for its usefulness in the development of new therapies.

Mucosal vaccination

CIA was the first autoimmune disease to be ameliorated by oral vaccination[74]. High doses of CII given orally to rats before immunization with CII suppressed the development of CIA. It was later found that treatment through the nasal route required somewhat lower doses to be effective[75]. It has also been found that the immunodominant CII peptide itself is a nasal tolerogen for CIA[75,76]. However, so far only preventive and no therapeutic effects have been achieved in the CIA model, although recent experiments using the PIA model in the rat show that nasal vaccination could be therapeutic[39]. A disturbing finding is that reverse effects have been observed with higher doses of CII; the nasal or oral treatment may enhance or induce arthritis development[77,39]. Nevertheless, the initial results from the animal models encouraged initiation of several human trials of oral treatment with peptide antigens like CII.

T-cell modulation

It was earlier found that *in vivo* treatment with antibodies reactive with CD4+ T cells or the T-cell receptor prevented development of heterologous CIA in the mouse but had no therapeu-

tic effects[78,79]. In homologous CIA in DA rats, treatment with antibodies to the T-cell receptor was also effective after disease onset[80]. The most pronounced effects were observed if the antibodies modulated T-cell function, either through the CD4 receptor or the T-cell receptor, rather than depleting the T cells[80,81]

Inflammatory cytokines

IL-1 and TNF-α are among the most important cytokine mediators of joint inflammation. Blocking these cytokines results in pronounced therapeutic effects in the CIA model[82–84], showing that these cytokines represent key regulatory sites in the inflammatory attack on the joints.

Angiogenesis inhibition

The development of synovial inflammation in both RA and CIA is associated with pronounced angiogenesis with growth of high endothelial venules. Not surprisingly, inhibitors of angiogenesis have profound effects on CIA[85] and also represent an interesting therapeutic possibility in RA.

Deviation of the autoimmune response towards a Th2 type

Circumstantial evidence suggests that the pathogenic inflammation is dependent on Th1 cells rather than Th2. Accordingly, Th2 cytokines such as IL-4 and IL-10[86–88] and blockage of Th1 cytokines such as IL-12 and interferon γ[89] may have ameliorative effects on the disease.

Induction of arthritis with other cartilage and joint related proteins

Type XI collagen-induced arthritis

The type XI collagen (CXI) is structurally similar to CII and is, to a large extent, colocalized. In contrast to CII, it is a heterotrimer with three different α-chains where one is shared with CII (the α3 chain). Heterologous CXI has been reported to induce arthritis in rat strains[57,90]. The disease is similar to CII-induced arthritis but appears later and with a milder disease course. Surprisingly, the arthritogenic immune recognition primarily involves the α1 or α2 chains, and not the CII homologous α3 chain, showing that the disease is not the same as type II collagen-induced arthritis.

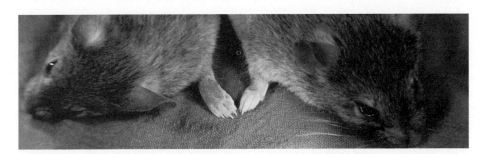

Fig. 4.3 Collagen-induced arthritis in mice expressing an A^q transgene compared with littermate controls. See also Plate 1.

COMP-induced arthritis

Another cartilage-specific protein is cartilage oligomeric matrix protein (COMP). Homologous COMP induces arthritis in rats. In comparison with CIA, it has a more self-limited disease course, is less erosive, and is under different genetic control[59]. The most susceptible MHC haplotype for homologous COMP-induced arthritis is the RT1[u] whereas the RT1[a] is more strongly associated with homologous CIA.

Proteoglycan (aggrecan)-induced arthritis

Other major components of joint cartilage are proteoglycans, of which the largest is aggrecan. Repeated immunization of Balb/c mice with fetal human aggrecan induces chronic arthritis[56]. Both B and T cells are involved in the pathogenesis. Autoreactive T cells have been isolated and respond to the G1-domain of aggrecan in which neo epitopes are created[91]. A pathogenic role for T cells was highlighted by the demonstration that a cloned T-cell hybridoma, specific for aggrecan, induced arthritis after transfer into Balb/c mice[92].

gp39-induced arthritis in mice

A protein produced by stressed synoviocytes and chondrocytes and normally expressed by hepatocytes, named gp39[93], has recently been shown to induce mild arthritis in Balb/c mice[58]. Only Balb/c mice are susceptible to arthritis with gp39 indicating that pristane-induced arthritis, aggrecan-induced arthritis, and gp39-induced arthritis might share some common genetics that differ from CIA.

C1q-induced arthritis in rats

An interesting observation was recently made using the initiator molecule of the classical complement cascade, C1q. C1q binds to the Fc-regions of immunoglobulin when they are aggregated on cell surfaces or on immune complexes and is clearly a critical event in the development of CIA. Part of the C1q molecule consists of collagen structures and antibodies reactive with CII sometimes cross-react with C1q[94]. The structure of C1q is changed upon binding and oxidation, and it was recently demonstrated that oxidized C1q induces severe arthritis in rats[95]. If the C1q molecule can present arthritogenic epitopes at the site of inflammation, this could be one of the mechanisms for the prolongation of chronic arthritis.

Antigen-induced arthritis

Antigen-induced arthritis is a classical model of RA that is induced by immunizing animals with a foreign antigen, usually bovine serum albumin, and subsequently injecting the same antigen into a joint. As a result, a pronounced T cell-dependent immune complex-mediated arthritis develops that is severe but self-limited. The advantage of this model is that a defined part of the pathogenesis leading to arthritis is addressed.

Spontaneous disease in genetically defective animals

Some of the classical inbred mouse strains can spontaneously develop arthritis[96–98]. In some strains, such as DBA/1, the grouping of males induces inter-male aggressiveness and such stress seems to be associated with arthritis development[97]. This stress-induced arthritis is not likely to be immune-mediated and is perhaps not an optimal model for RA, but the findings are important to take into consideration when performing animal experiments.

There are, however, a number of genetically-defective mouse and rat strains that spontaneously develop arthritis. One such strain is the MRL/lpr mouse, which develops arthritis as part of a severe lupus-like disease promoted, in part, by a mutation in the Fas gene (giving the lpr defect)[99]. Spontaneous arthritis has also been observed in a number of different transgenic mouse strains. One such example is a mouse in which TNFα is over-expressed leading to inflammation in tissues with elevated TNFα[100]. Another is a T-cell receptor transgene expressed in the NOD mouse in which the TCR recognizes a self-peptide derived from the ubiquitous enzyme glucose-6-phosphate isomerase bound to the H-2g7 class II molecule. This autoreactivity leads to severe immune complex arthritis[101]. The inflammatory attack is restricted to the joints in which arthritis develops at an early age and with high penetrance. Immune complexes are also found in viscera and the disease is dependent on B cell activity. Another transgenic model in which spontaneous arthritis has been observed is mice and rats transgenic for the envelope protein of human T cell leukemia virus 1[102,103]. In this case, there is not only joint inflammation but also widespread inflammatory infiltrates in skin, salivary glands, and blood vessels. In these transgenic models, the spontaneous penetrance of disease is high and therefore is reminiscent of monogenic and highly penetrant diseases in humans such as the APECED syndrome[104].

These models are most likely to represent various aspects of the processes leading to arthritis, which will be determined by the transgene or defective gene. They are useful and efficient to work with and will give answers to specific questions but are not likely to be optimal models for RA, which is not a spontaneous disease with high penetrance and is not believed to be dependent on a dominant genetic defect.

Using animal models

Understanding the pathogenesis of arthritis

The most important use of animal models is to extend our knowledge of the key elements of the cause and the perpetuation of arthritis. Questions that need to be addressed include:

1. How does the immune system interact with cartilage in the physiological state?

2. Why is a normal inflammatory response transformed into a chronic relapsing disease?

3. Which effector arms causing the erosive inflammation of a joint are most important?

4. How can various environmental agents, including pathogens, cause and modulate arthritis?

These are basic questions and are relevant to ask in any model regardless of whether it resembles a particular human disease. It is important to accept that the solutions to these basic questions can be sought only when addressed in the context of the particular species or model; a comparison to humans in pathogenic details will not always be productive. Recent advances in genetic methodology have highlighted the usefulness of animal models. Today it is possible to add, delete, and specifically mutate genes, thereby analyzing their role in the pathogenesis of arthritis. However, these studies address the gene in a specific mouse strain that might differ considerably from other strains in an environment that may also differ. Thus, although these techniques dramatically increase our knowledge it is also important to evaluate the results in the context of a different strain or a specific model. The development of techniques to find genes associated with disease is another breakthrough for studies on arthritis. This will enable us to investigate the genetic context of a mouse that allows the transformation of a physiological response to a pathological one, resulting in chronic erosion of the joints. The identification of such genes and the elucidation of their role and interactions will be an important step towards understanding the basic mechanisms leading to arthritis. It will be possible to compare and transform the results between the human disease and the animal model, thus facilitating the process of developing better diagnostics and therapy for RA.

Developing new therapeutic strategies

The basis for the development of new therapeutic strategies is clearly the result of basic research in various areas investigating biological pathways. Knowledge gained can be applied in the different animal models for RA. Clinical experiences are of particular importance for prioritizing different projects in terms of what will be clinically useful for diagnosis, prevention, and therapy. The application of new therapeutic possibilities in the animal models also increases our basic knowledge of them that will further help to improve our knowledge about mechanisms as discussed above.

To test new drugs and therapies it will be necessary to select from the different models available. Obviously there is no optimal model for RA and there will never be one. The models described, however, are useful since they represent different aspects of RA pathogenesis. Thus, depending on the questions to be asked or symptoms to be treated, different models may be used. Recapitulating the three hallmarks for RA discussed above—tissue specificity, chronicity, and MHC association—reasonable criteria should be that the animal models should display these hallmarks. A common mistake is to use only acute models and to use only disease prevention as a read out. More relevant for RA would be to use chronic models and to determine therapeutic effects. Another common mistake is the experimental

Table 4.3 Some environmental effects on mouse CIA

Environmental effect	Effect on arthritis	Reference
Inter-male stress	+	97
Pregnancy	−	114
Postpartum	+	107
Estrogen	−	115
Darkness	+	108

+ = increased arthritis, − = decreased arthritis.

Table 4.4 Some environmental effects on rat arthritis

Environmental effect	Effect on arthritis	Reference
Noise stress	++	116
Predator stress	−	117
Estrogen	−	118
Testosterone	−	118
Infections	−/+	43, 119, 120

+ = increased arthritis, − = decreased arthritis.

design. Arthritis models (as humans) are very sensitive to environmental factors (see Tables 4.3 and 4.4). Of particular importance are stress effects which are easily produced by mixing mice from different litters in the same cage and which will lead to cage-dependent effects[97]. Other important factors are sex hormones[105–107] and probably also neurohormones[108] that play an important role modulating disease activity—seen as effects by estrous cycling, pregnancy, and light effects. Clearly, not only environmental effects need to be controlled but also genetic effects. The control of genetics is usually achieved by testing standardized inbred strains. The problem is that these vary considerably between different colonies, mainly due to genetic contamination. Moreover, with the introduction of transgenic mice the genetic homogeneity is often spurious since these techniques usually involve gene-segregating crosses. In spite of these problems, there is no question that both environment and genetics can be better controlled in experimental animal models than can be achieved in studies directly involving the human population.

Ethical considerations

One important drawback of using experimental models for RA is the use of animals. However, in light of the various human activities that use animals, their application to research seems to be easy to defend. In fact, it would be unethical not to use them since it would prohibit further understanding of human diseases, thereby letting people suffer from something that will be possible to cure or prevent. It should also be emphasized that the recent development of animal models for RA has refined them to be of more specific use, which has decreased animal suffering. For example the most commonly used model for RA used to be mycobacterium-induced adjuvant arthritis, which is a systemic and severe inflammatory disease, whereas the collagen-induced arthritis, which is the most common model used today, is a much more specific disease of the joints.

Conclusions

Experimental animal models are essential tools not only for investigating the basic mechanisms leading to RA but also for the development of new therapies. Many models have been described and each represents different aspects of the disease and it is therefore important to use different models. The models for RA described so far can be divided into three principal groups: (1) adjuvant-induced, (2) cartilage protein-induced, and (3) spontaneous. It has been emphasized that the models used should reflect essential hallmarks of rheumatoid arthritis such as tissue specificity, chronicity, and class II MHC gene association, and they should reflect the fact that RA is a polygenic disease triggered by unknown and multifactorial environmental factors.

References

1. Franz A., Webster A.D., Furr P.M., Taylor-Robinson D. Mycoplasmal arthritis in patients with primary immunoglobulin deficiency: clinical features and outcome in 18 patients. *Br J Rheumatol*, 1997;36:661–668.
2. Cole B.C., Ward J.R., Jones R.S., Cahill J.F. Chronic proliferative arthritis of mice induced by Mycoplasma arthritidis. I. Induction of disease and histopathologic characteristics. *Infect Immun*, 1971;4:344–355.
3. Berglöf A., Sandstedt K., Feinstein R., Bölske G., Smith C.I. B cell-deficient muMT mice as an experimental model for Mycoplasma infections in X-linked agammaglobulinemia. *Eur J Immunol*, 1997;27:2118–21.
4. Cole B.C., Knudtson K.L., Oliphant A., et al. The sequence of the Mycoplasma arthritidis superantigen, MAM: identification of functional domains and comparison with microbial superantigens and plant lectin mitogens. *J Exp Med*, 1996;183:1105–1110.
5. Gross D.M., Forsthuber T., Tary-Lehmann M., et al. Identification of LFA-1 as a candidate autoantigen in treatment-resistant Lyme arthritis. *Science*, 1998;281:703–706.
6. Schaible E.E., Kramer M.D., Wallich R., Tran T., Simon M.M. Experimental Borrelia burgdorferi infection in inbred mouse strains: antibody response and association of H-2 genes with resistance and susceptibility to development of arthritis. *Eur J Immunol*, 1991;21:2397–2405.
7. Yang L., Weis J.H., Eichwald E., Kolbert C.P., Persing D.H., Weis J.J. Heritable susceptibility to severe Borrelia burgdorferi-induced arthritis is dominant and is associated with persistence of large numbers of spirochetes in tissues. *Infect Immun*, 1994;62:492–500.
8. Zhong W., Stehle T., Museteanu C., et al. Therapeutic passive vaccination against chronic Lyme disease in mice. *Proc Natl Acad Sci USA*, 1997;94:12533–12538.
9. Bremell T., Lange S., Yacoub A., Ryden C., Tarkowski A. Experimental *Staphylococcus aureus* arthritis in mice. *Infect Immun*, 1991;59:2615–2623.
10. Bremell T., Lange S., Holmdahl R., Ryden C., Hansson G.K., Tarkowski A. Immunopathological features of rat Staphylococcus aureus arthritis. *Infect Immun*, 1994;62:2334–2344.
11. Patti J.M., Bremell T., Krajewska-Pietrasik D., et al. The Staphylococcus aureus collagen adhesin is a virulence determinant in experimental septic arthritis. *Infect Immun*, 1994;62:152–161.
12. Verdrengh M., Tarkowski A. Role of neutrophils in experimental septicemia and septic arthritis induced by Staphylococcus aureus. *Infect Immun*, 1997;65:2517–2521.
13. Zhao Y.X., Abdelnour A., Holmdahl R., Tarkowski A. Mice with the xid B cell defect are less susceptible to developing Staphylococcus aureus-induced arthritis. *J Immunol*, 1995;155:2067–2076.
14. Abdelnour A., Zhao Y-X., Holmdahl R., Tarkowski A. Major histocompatibility complex class II region confers susceptibility to *Staphylococcus aureus* arthritis. *Scand J Immunol*, 1997;45:301–307.
15. Abdelnour A., Bremell T., Holmdahl R., Tarkowski A. Clonal expansion of T lymphocytes causes arthritis and mortality in mice infected with toxic shock syndrome toxin-1-producing staphylococci. *Eur J Immunol*, 1994;24:1161–1166.
16. Hammer R.E., Maika S.D., Richardson J.A., Tang J.P., Taurog J.D. Spontaneous inflammatory disease in transgenic rats expressing HLA-B27 and human beta2m: An animal model of HLA-B27-associated human disorders. *Cell*, 1990;63:1099–1112.
17. Taurog J.D., Richardson J.A., Croft J.T., et al. The germfree state prevents development of gut and joint inflammatory disease in HLA-B27 transgenic rats. *J Exp Med*, 1994;180:2359–64.
18. Khare S.D., Hansen J., Luthra H.S., David C.S. HLA-B27 heavy chains contribute to spontaneous inflammatory disease in B27/human beta2-microglobulin (beta2m) double transgenic mice with disrupted mouse beta2m. *J Clin Invest*, 1996;98:2746–2755.
19. Hill J.L., Yu D.T. Development of an experimental animal model for reactive arthritis induced by Yersinia enterocolitica infection. *Infect Immun*, 1987;55:721–726.
20. Gripenberg-Lerche C., Skurnik M., Zhang L., Söderström K.O., Toivanen P. Role of YadA in arthritogenicity of Yersinia enterocolitica serotype O:8: experimental studies with rats. *Infect Immun*, 1994;62:5568–5575.
21. Schulze Koops H., Burkhardt H., Heesemann J., von der Mark K., Emmrich F. Characterization of the binding region for the Yersenia enterocolitica adhesin YadA on types I and ii collagen. *Arthritis Rheum*, 1995;38:1283–1289.
22. Pearson C.M., Wood F.D. Studies of polyarthritis and other lesions induced in rats by injection of mycobacterial adjuvant. I. General clinical and pathologic characteristics and some modifying factors. *Arthritis Rheum*, 1959;2:440–459.
23. Bakker N.P.M., Van Erck M.G., Zurcher C., et al. Experimental immune mediated arthritis in rhesus monkeys. A model for human rheumatoid arthritis? *Rheumatol Int*, 1990;10:21–29.
24. Torisu M., Miyahara T., Shinohara N., Ohsato K., Sonozaki H.A new side effect of BCG immunotherapy-BCG-induced arthritis in man. *Cancer Immunol Immunother*, 1978;5:77–83.
25. Pearson C.M., Wood F.D. Passive transfer of adjuvant arthritis by lymph node or spleen cells. *J Exp Med*, 1964;120:547–573.
26. Yoshino S., Schlipkoter E., Kinne R., Hunig T., Emmrich F. Suppression and prevention of adjuvant arthritis in rats by a monoclonal antibody to the alpha/beta T cell receptor. *Eur J Immunol*, 1990;20:2805–2808.
27. Van Eden W., Holoshitz J., Nevo Z., Frenkel A., Klajman A., Cohen I.R. Arthritis induced by a T-lymphocyte clone that responds to Mycobacterium tuberculosis and to cartilage proteogycans. *Proc Natl Acad Sci USA*, 1985;82:5117–5120.
28. Van Eden W., Thole J.E.R., van der Zee R., et al. Cloning of the mycobacterial epitope recognized by T lymphocytes in adjuvant arthritis. *Nature*, 1988;334:171–173.
29. Anderton S.M., van der Zee R., Prakken B., Noordzij A., van Eden W. Activation of T cells recognizing self 60-kD heat shock protein can protect against experimental arthritis. *J Exp Med*, 1995;181:943–952.
30. Kohashi O., Pearson C.M., Watanabe Y., Kotani S. Preparation of arthritogenic hydrosoluble peptidoglycans from both arthritogenic and non-arthritogenic bacterial cell walls. *Infect Immun*, 1977;16:861–866.
31. Cromartie W.J., Craddock J.G., Schwab J.H., Anderle S.K., Yang C.H. Arthritis in rats after systemic injection of streptococcal cells or cell walls. *J Exp Med*, 1977;146:1585–602.
32. Koga T., Kakimoto K., Hirofuji T., et al. Acute joint inflammation in mice after systemic injection of the cell wall, its peptidoglycan,

and chemically defined peptidoglycan subunits from various bacteria. *Infect Immun*, 1985;50:27–34.

33. Dalldorf F.G., Cromartie W.J., Anderle S.K., Clark R.L., Schwab J.H. The relation of experimental arthritis to the distribution of streptococcal cell wall fragments. *Am J Pathol*, 1980;100: 383–402.

34. Yoshino S., Cleland L.G., Mayrhofer G., Brown R.R., Schwab J.H. Prevention of chronic erosive streptococcal cell wall-induced arthritis in rats by treatment with a monoclonal antibody against the T cell antigen receptor alpha beta. *J Immunol*, 1991;146: 4187–4189.

35. Whitehouse M.W., Orr K.J., Beck F.W.J., Pearson C.M. Freund's adjuvants: Relationship to arthritogenicity and adjuvanticity in rats to vehicle composition. *Immunology*, 1974;27:311–330.

36. Holmdahl R., Goldschmidt T.J., Kleinau S., Kvick C., Jonsson R. Arthritis induced in rats with adjuvant oil is a genetically restricted, alpha beta T-cell dependent autoimmune disease. *Immunology*, 1992;76:197–202.

37. Chang Y.H., Pearson C.M., Abe C. Adjuvant polyarthritis. IV. Induction by a synthetic adjuvant: Immunologic, histopathologic, and other studies. *Arthritis Rheum*, 1980;23:62–71.

38. Vingsbo C., Sahlstrand P., Brun J.G., Jonsson R., Saxne T., Holmdahl R. Pristane-induced arthritis in rats: a new model for rheumatoid arthritis with a chronic disease course influenced by both major histocompatibility complex and non-major histocompatibility complex genes. *Am J Pathol*, 1996;149:1675–1683.

39. Lu S., Holmdahl R. Therapeutic nasal vaccination of chronic arthritis in rats. *Clin Immunol Immunopathol*, 1998; in press.

40. Vingsbo C., Jonsson R., Holmdahl R. Avridine-induced arthritis in rats; a T Cell-dependent chronic disease influenced both by MHC genes and by non-MHC genes. *Clin Exp Immunol*, 1995;99:359–363.

41. Taurog J.D., Sandberg G.P., Mahowald M.L. The cellular basis of adjuvant arthritis. II. Characterization of the cells mediating passive transfer. *Cell Immunol*, 1983;80:198–204.

42. Svelander L., Mussener A., Erlandsson-Harris H., Kleinau S. Polyclonal Th1 cells transfer oil-induced arthritis. *Immunology*, 1997;91:260–5.

43. Björk J., Kleinau S., Midtvedt T., Klareskog L., Smedegård G. Role of the bowel flora for development of immunity to hsp 65 and arthritis in three experimental models. *Scand J Immunol*, 1994;40:648–652.

44. Bly J.E., Garrett L.R., Cuchens M.A. Pristane induced changes in rat lymphocyte membrane fluidity. *Cancer Biochem Biophys*, 1990;11:145–54.

45. Lee S.H., Ackland B.C., Jones C.J. The tumor promoter pristane activates transcription by a cAMP dependent mechanism. *Mol Cell Biochem*, 1992;110:75–81.

46. Vingsbo-Lundberg C., Nordquist N., Sundvall M., et al. Genetic analysis of pristane induced arthritis in the rat. *Nat Gen*, 1998;20:401–4.

47. Lorentzen J.C., Glaser A., Jacobsson L., et al. Identification of rat susceptibility loci for adjuvant-oil induced arthritis. *Proc Natl Acad Sci USA*, 1998;95:6383–6387.

48. Hopkins S.J., Freemont A.J., Jayson M.I.V. Pristane-induced arthritis in Balb/c mice. I. Clinical and histological features of the arthropathy. *Int Rheumatol*, 1984;5:21–28.

49. Wooley P.H., Seibold J.R., Whalen J.D., Chapdelaine J.M. Pristane-induced arthritis. The immunologic and genetic features of an experimental murine model of autoimmune disease. *Arthritis Rheum*, 1989;32:1022–1030.

50. Thompson S.J., Francis J.N., Siew L.K., et al. An immunodominant epitope from mycobacterial 65-kDa heat shock protein protects against pristane-induced arthritis. *J Immunol*, 1998;160:4628–34.

51. Thompson S.J., Rook G.A.W., Brealey R.J., Van der Zee R., Elson C.J. Autoimmune reactions to heat shock proteins in pristane-induced arthritis. *Eur J Immunol*, 1990;20:2479–2484.

52. Potter M., Wax J.S. Genetics of susceptibility to pristane-induced plasmacytomas in BALB/cAn: reduced susceptibility in BALB/cJ with a brief description of pristane-induced arthritis. *J Immunol*, 1981;127:1591–1595.

53. Trentham D.E., Townes A.S., Kang A.H. Autoimmunity to type II collagen: an experimental model of arthritis. *J Exp Med*, 1977;146:857–868.

54. Courtenay J.S., Dallman M.J., Dayan A.D., Martin A., Mosedal B. Immunization against heterologous type II collagen induces arthritis in mice. *Nature*, 1980;283:666–667.

55. Yoo T.J., Kim S.Y., Stuart J.M., et al. Induction of arthritis in monkeys by immunization with type II collagen. *J Exp Med*, 1988;168:777–782.

56. Glant T.T., Mikecz K., Arzoumanian A., Poole A.R. Proteoglycan-induced arthritis in Balb/c mice. *Arthritis Rheum*, 1987;30:201–212.

57. Cremer M.A., Ye X.J., Terato K., Owens S.W., Seyer J.M., Kang A.H. Type XI collagen-induced arthritis in the Lewis rat. Characterization of cellular and humoral immune responses to native types XI, V, and II collagen and constituent alpha-chains. *J Immunol*, 1994;153:824–32.

58. Verheijden G.F., Rijnders A.W., Bos E., et al. Human cartilage glycoprotein-39 as a candidate autoantigen in rheumatoid arthritis. *Arthritis Rheum*, 1997;40:1115–1125.

59. Carlsen S., Olsson H., Heinegå D., Holmdahl R. Induction of arthritis with autologous cartilage oligomeric matrix protein. *Clin Exp Immunol*, 1998; in press.

60. Stuart J.M., Cremer M.A., Townes A.S., Kang A.H. Type II collagen induced arthritis in rats. Passive transfer with serum and evidence that IgG anticollagen antibodies can cause arthritis. *J Exp Med*, 1982;155:1–16.

61. Stuart J.M., Dixon F.J. Serum transfer of collagen induced arthritis in mice. *J Exp Med*, 1983;158:378–392.

62. Holmdahl R., Jansson L., Larsson E., Rubin K., Klareskog L. Homologous type II collagen induces chronic and progressive arthritis in mice. *Arthritis Rheum*, 1986;29:106–113.

63. Holmdahl R., Vingsbo C., Hedrich H., et al. Homologous collagen-induced arthritis in rats and mice are associated with structurally different major histocompatibility complex DQ-like molecules. *Eur J Immunol*, 1992;22:419–424.

64. Wooley P.H., Luthra H.S., Stuart J.M., David C.S. Type II collagen induced arthritis in mice. I. Major histocompatibility complex (I-region) linkage and antibody correlates. *J Exp Med*, 1981;154:688–700.

65. Griffiths M. Immunogenetics of collagen-induced arthritis in rats. *Intern Rev Immunol*, 1988;4:1–15.

66. Holmdahl R., Jansson L., Andersson M., Larsson E. Immunogenetics of type II collagen autoimmunity and susceptibility to collagen arthritis. *Immunology*, 1988;65:305–310.

67. Brunsberg U., Gustafsson K., Jansson L., et al. Expression of a transgenic class II Ab gene confers susceptibility to collagen-induced arthritis. *Eur J Immunol*, 1994;24:1698–1702.

68. Michaëlsson E., Andersson M., Engström A., Holmdahl R. Identification of an immunodominant type-II collagen peptide recognized by T cells in H-2q mice: self tolerance at the level of determinant selection. *Eur J Immunol*, 1992;22:1819–25.

69. Brand D.D., Myers L.K., Terato K., et al. Characterization of the T cell determinants in the induction of autoimmune arthritis by bovine alpha 1(II)-CB11 in H-2q mice. *J Immunol*, 1994;152:3088–97.

70. Corthay A., Bäcklund J., Broddefalk J., et al. Epitope glycosylation plays a critical role for T cell recognition of type II collagen in collagen-induced arthritis. *Eur J Immunol*, 1998;28:2580–2590.

71. Fugger L., Rothbard J.B., Sonderstrup-McDevitt G. Specificity of an HLA-DRB1*0401-restricted T cell response to type II collagen. *Eur J Immunol*, 1996;26:928–933.

72. Rosloniec E.F., Brand D.D., Myers L.K., et al. An HLA-DR1 transgene confers susceptibility to collagen-induced arthritis elicited with human type II collagen. *J Exp Med*, 1997;185:1113–1122.

73. Andersson E.C., Hansen B.E., Jacobsen H., *et al*. Definition of MHC and T cell receptor contacts in the HLA-DR4 restricted immunodominant epitope in type II collagen and characterization of collagen-induced arthritis in HLA-DR4 and human CD4 transgenic mice. *Proc Natl Acad Sci USA*, 1998;**95**:7574–7569.

74. Thompson H.S.G., Staines N.A. Gastric administration of type II collagen delays the onset and severity of collagen-induced arthritis in rats. *Clin Exp Immunol*, 1986;**64**:581–586.

75. Staines N.A., Harper N., Ward F.J., Malmström V., Holmdahl R., Bansal S. Mucosal tolerance and suppression of collagen-induced arthritis (CIA) induced by nasal inhalation of synthetic peptide 184-198 of bovine type II collagen (CII) expressing a dominant T cell epitope. *Clin Exp Immunol*, 1996;**103**:368–375.

76. Myers L.K., Seyer J.M., Stuart J.M., Kang A.H. Suppression of murine collagen-induced arthritis by nasal administration of collagen. *Immunology*, 1997;**90**:161–4.

77. Terato K., Ye X.J., Miyahara H., Cremer M.A., Griffiths M.M. Induction by chronic autoimmune arthritis in DBA/1 mice by oral administration of type II collagen and Escherichia coli lipopolysaccharide. *Br J Rheumatol*, 1996;**35**:828–838.

78. Ranges G.E., Sriram S., Cooper S.M. Prevention of type II collagen-induced arthritis by in vivo treatment with anti-L3T4. *J Exp Med*, 1985;**162**:1105–1110.

79. Maeda T., Saikawa I., Hotokebuchi T., *et al*. Exacerbation of established collagen-induced arthritis in mice treated with an anti-T cell receptor antibody. *Arthritis Rheum*, 1994:**37**:406–413.

80. Goldschmidt T.J., Holmdahl R. Anti-T cell receptor antibody treatment of rats with established autologous collagen-induced arthritis. Suppression of arthritis without reduction of anti-type II collagen autoantibody levels. *Eur J Immunol*, 1991;**21**:1327–1330.

81. Mauri C., Chu C.Q., Woodrow D., Mori L., Londei M. Treatment of a newly established transgenic model of chronic arthritis with nondepleting anti-CD4 monoclonal antibody. *J Immunol*, 1997;**159**:5032–5041.

82. Williams R., Feldmann M., Maini R. Anti-tumor necrosis factor ameliorates joint disease in murine collagen-induced arthritis. *Proc Natl Acad Sci USA*, 1992;**89**:9784–9788.

83. Wooley P.H., Whalen J.D., Chapman D.L., *et al*. The effect of an interleukin-1 receptor antagonist protein on type II collagen-induced arthritis in mice. *Arthritis Rheum*, 1993;**36**:1305–1314.

84. van den Berg W.B., Joosten L.A., Helsen M., van de Loo F. Amelioration of established murine collagen-induced arthritis with anti-IL- 1 treatment. *Clin Exp Immunol*, 1994;**95**:237–243.

85. Peacock D., Banquerigo M., Brahn E. Angiogenesis inhibition suppresses collagen arthritis. *J Exp Med*, 1992;**175**:1135–1138.

86. Walmsley M., Katsikis P.D., Abney E., *et al*. Interleukin-10 inhibition of the progression of established collagen-induced arthritis. *Arthritis Rheum*, 1996;**39**:495–503.

87. Persson S., Mikulowska A., Narula S., O'Garra A., Holmdahl R. Interleukin-10 suppresses the development of collagen type II-induced arthritis and ameliorates sustained arthritis in rats. *Scand J Immunol*, 1996;**44**:607–614.

88. Horsfall A.C., Butler D.M., Marinova L., *et al*. Suppression of collagen-induced arthritis by continuous administration of IL-4. *J Immunol*, 1997;**159**:5687–96.

89. Joosten L.A., Lubberts E., Helsen M.M., van den Berg W.B. Dual role of IL-12 in early and late stages of murine collagen type II arthritis. *J Immunol*, 1997;**159**:4094–4102.

90. Morgan K., Evans H.B., Firth S.A., *et al*. $1\alpha,2\alpha,3\alpha$ collagen is arthritogenic. *Ann Rheum Dis*, 1983;**42**:680–683.

91. Zhang Y., Guerassimov A., Leroux J.Y., *et al*. Arthritis induced by proteoglycan aggrecan G1 domain in BALB/c mice. Evidence for T cell involvement and the immunosuppressive influence of keratan sulfate on recognition of T and B cell epitopes. *J Clin Invest*, 1998;**101**:1678–1686.

92. Buzas E.I., Brennan F.R., Mikecz K., *et al*. A proteoglycan (aggrecan)-specific T cell hybridoma induces arthritis in BALB/c mice. *J Immunol*, 1995;**155**:2679–2687.

93. Hakala B.E., White C., Recklies A.D. Human cartilage gp-39, a major secretory product of articular chondrocytes and synovial cells, is a mammalian member of a chitinase protein family. *J Biol Chem*, 1993;**268**:25803–25810.

94. Heinz H.R., Rubin K., Laurell A.B., Loos M. Common epitopes in C1q and collagen type II. *Mol Immunol*, 1989;**26**:163–169.

95. Trinder P.K.E., Maeurer M.J., Stoerkel S.S., Loos M. Altered (oxidized) C1q induces a rheumatoid arthritis- like destructive and chronic inflammation in joint structures in arthritis-susceptible rats. *Clin Immunol Immunopathol*, 1997;**82**:149–156.

96. Bouvet J.P., Couderc J., Bouthillier Y., Franc B., Ducailar A., Mouton D. Spontaneous rheumatoid-like arthritis in a line of mice sensitive to collagen-induced arthritis. *Arthritis Rheum*, 1990;**33**:1716–1722.

97. Holmdahl R., Jansson L., Andersson M., Jonsson R. Genetic, hormonal and behavioral influence on spontaneously developing arthritis in normal mice. *Clin Exp Immunol*, 1992;**88**:467–472.

98. Nakamura K., Kashiwasaki S., Takagishi K., *et al*. Spontaneous degenerative polyarthritis in male New Zealand Black/KN mice. *Arthritis Rheum*, 1991;**34**:171–179.

99. Hang L., Theofilopoulos A.N., Dixon F.J. A spontaneous rheumatoid arthritis-like disease in MRL/l mice. *J Exp Med*, 1982;**155**:1690–1701.

100. Keffer J., Probert L., Cazlaris H., *et al*. Transgenic mice expressing human tumour necrosis factor: a predicitive genetic model of arthritis. *EMBO J*, 1991;**10**:4025–4031.

101. Kouskoff V., Korganow A.S., Duchatelle V., Degott C., Benoist C., Mathis D. Organ-specific disease provoked by systemic autoimmunity. *Cell*, 1996;**87**:811–822.

102. Iwakura Y., Tosu M., Yoshida E., *et al*. Induction of inflammatory arthropathy resembling rheumatoid arthritis in mice transgenic for HTLV-I. *Science*, 1991;**253**:1026–1028.

103. Yamazaki H., Ikeda H., Ishizu A., *et al*. A wide spectrum of collagen vascular and autoimmune diseases in transgenic rats carrying the env-pX gene of human T lymphocyte virus type I. *Int Immunol*, 1997;**9**:339–346.

104. Aaltonen J., Björses P., Perheentupa J., *et al*. An autoimmune disease, APECED, caused by mutations in a novel gene featuring two PHD-type zinc-finger domains. *Nat Genet*, 1997;**17**:399–403.

105. Jansson L., Mattsson A., Mattsson R., Holmdahl R. Estrogen induced suppression of collagen arthritis. V: Physiological level of estrogen in DBA/1 mice is therapeutic on established arthritis, suppresses anti-type II collagen T-cell dependent immunity and stimulates polyclonal B-cell activity. *J Autoimmunity*, 1990;**3**:257–270.

106. Holmdahl R., Jansson L., Andersson M. Female sex hormones suppress development of collagen-induced arthritis in mice. *Arthritis Rheum*, 1986;**29**:1501–1509.

107. Mattsson R., Mattsson A., Holmdahl R., Whyte A., Rook G.A.W. Maintained pregnancy levels of oestrogen afford complete protection from post-partum exacerbation of collagen-induced arthritis. *Clin Exp Immunol*, 1991;**85**:41–47.

108. Mattsson R., Hansson I., Holmdahl R. Pineal gland in autoimmunity: melatonin-dependent exaggeration of collagen-induced arthritis in mice [letter]. *Autoimmunity*, 1994;**17**:83–86.

109. Wilder R.L., Calandra G.B., Garvin A.J., Wright K.D., Hansen C.T. Strain and sex variation in the susceptibility to streptococcal cell wall-induced polyarthritis in the rat. *Arthritis Rheum*, 1982;**25**:1064–1072.

110. Holmdahl R., Kvick C. Vaccination and genetic experiments demonstrate that adjuvant oil induced arthritis and homologous type II collagen induced arthritis in the same rat strain are different diseases. *Clin Exp Immunol*, 1992;**88**:96–100.

111. Remmers E.F., Longman R.E., Du Y., *et al*. A genome scan localizes five non-MHC loci controlling collagen-induced arthritis in rats. *Nat Gen*, 1996;**14**:82–85.

112. Jirholt J., Cook A., Sundvall M., *et al*. Evidence for a susceptibility locus to collagen induced arthritis on mouse chromosome 3: a common susceptibility locus in multiple autoimmune disorders. *Eur J Immunol*, 1998;in press.

113. Butler D.M., Malfait A.M., Mason L.J., *et al.* DBA/1 mice expressing the human TNF-alpha transgene develop a severe, erosive arthritis: characterization of the cytokine cascade and cellular composition. *Biochem J*, 1997;**326**:763–772.

114. Waites G.T., Whyte A. Effect of pregnancy on collagen-induced arthritis in mice. *Clin Exp Immunol*, 1987;**67**:467–476.

115. Holmdahl R., Jansson L., Meyerson B., Kalreskog L. Oestrogen induced suppression of collagen arthritis: I. Long term oestradiol treatment of DBA/1 mice reduces the severity and incidence of arthritis and decrease the anti-type II collagen immune response. *Clin Exp Immunol*, 1987;**70**:372–378.

116. Rogers M.P., Trentham D.E., Dynesius-Trentham R., Daffner K., Reich P. Exacerbation of collagen arthritis by noise stress. *J Rheumatol*, 1983;**10**:651–654.

117. Rogers M.P., Trentham D.E., McCune W.J., *et al.* Effect of psychological stress on the induction of arthritis in rats. *Arthritis Rheum*, 1980;**23**:1337–1341.

118. Holmdahl R. Female preponderance for development of arthritis in rats is influenced by both sex chromosomes and sex steroids. *Scand J Immunol*, 1995;**42**:104–109.

119. Taurog J.D., Leary S.L., Cremer M., Mahowald M.L., Sandberg G.P., Manning P.J. Infection with mycoplasma pulmonis modulates adjuvant- and collagen-induced arthritis in Lewis rats. *Arthritis Rheum*, 1984;**27**:943–946.

120. Kohashi O., Kohashi Y., Takahashi T., Ozawa A., Shigematsu N. Suppressive effect of Escherichia Coli on adjuvant-induced arthritis in germ-free rats. *Arthritis Rheum*, 1986;**29**:547–553.

121. Bradley D.S., Nabozny G.H., Cheng S., *et al.* HLA-DQB1 polymorphism determines incidence, onset, and severity of collagen-induced arthritis in transgenic mice. Implications in human rheumatoid arthritis. *J Clin Invest*, 1997;**100**:2227–34.

122. Nabozny G.H., Baisch J.M., Cheng S., *et al.* HLA-DQ8 transgenic mice are highly susceptible to collagen-induced arthritis: a novel model for human polyarthritis. *J Exp Med*, 1996:**183**:27–37.

Mechanisms of inflammation

5 | *Examination of the synovium and synovial fluid*

Paul-Peter Tak

Introduction

The synovium lines the non-cartilaginous surfaces of the diarthrodial joints and provides nutrients to avascular structures such as cartilage. Synovial tissue (ST) is also found in tendon sheaths and bursae[1,2]. Since rheumatoid arthritis (RA) is an inflammatory disease that primarily involves the synovium examination of ST might provide insight into the pathogenesis of the disease. Thus, descriptive studies of rheumatoid synovium contribute to an understanding of the events that take place *in vivo* and complement experimental animal studies and *in vitro* studies. Recently, there has been an enormous upsurge in investigations of the pathological changes of the rheumatoid synovium because of the availability of new methods to obtain synovial biopsy specimens and because of the development of immunohistological methods, *in situ* hybridization, and the polymerase chain reaction for analysis of the tissue.

Systematic comparison of RA ST with tissue from patients with other forms of arthritis has made it possible to identify specific features of the cell infiltrate in RA. This chapter will describe these pathological changes in early and in chronic RA. The main focus is to define the cell infiltrate *in situ* to provide a morphological background for understanding the role of various cell types in the pathogenesis of RA. Furthermore, the relationship between characteristics of the synovium and disease activity and the diagnostic value of ST analysis will be discussed.

Studies of ST will increasingly be the subject of scientific communication and ST analysis might become a diagnostic tool in clinical practice. Since standardization of the methodology is mandatory, several questions remain to be answered; for instance questions concerning the optimal technique to obtain synovial biopsy specimens, sampling errors, the most efficient and reliable systems to evaluate the sections, and quality control. Therefore, the methods to obtain and to evaluate synovial biopsy specimens will be reviewed briefly.

Synovial fluid (SF) is in direct contact with the synovium and the articular cartilage. Analysis of SF is generally less relevant than ST analysis except, for example, neutrophils and platelets. However, by examination of its characteristics one can learn about the cellular events within the synovium and cartilage. SF analysis may also provide information about the presence of soluble mediators at the site of inflammation. Moreover, SF analysis plays an important role in the diagnostic work-up of patients with arthritis. Hence, this chapter will also deal with some of the features of RA SF, although this will not be the main focus.

Rheumatoid synovial tissue

The synovium consists of the intimal lining layer or synovial lining layer, which comprises normally only one to three cell layers without an underlying basement membrane, and the synovial sublining or subsynovium, which merges with the joint capsule (Fig. 5.1). The intimal lining layer consists mainly of intimal macrophages and fibroblast-like synoviocytes (FLS). The intimal macrophages are often referred to as macrophage-like synoviocytes or type A synoviocytes, while the FLS are also called type B synoviocytes. The synovial sublining is normally relatively acellular, containing scattered blood vessels, fat cells, and fibroblasts. Since the intimal lining layer is discontinuous, SF is in direct contact with cells in both the intimal lining layer and the synovial sublining.

In RA, the synovium is hypertrophic and edematous (Fig. 5.2). Villous projections of ST protrude into the joint cavity, where it overgrows and invades the underlying cartilage and bone. Proliferating ST at the synovium–cartilage junction is often referred to as pannus. Rheumatoid ST is characterized by marked intimal lining hyperplasia and by accumulation of T cells, plasma cells, macrophages, B cells, mast cells, natural killer cells, and dendritic cells in the synovial sublining (Table 5.1)[3–7]. There is large variability in synovial inflammation between

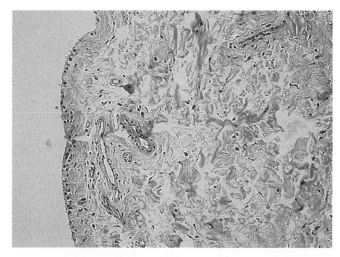

Fig. 5.1 Normal synovial tissue consisting of the intimal lining layer of one to three cell layers and the synovial sublining that contains scattered blood vessels, fat cells, and fibroblasts. See also Plate 3.

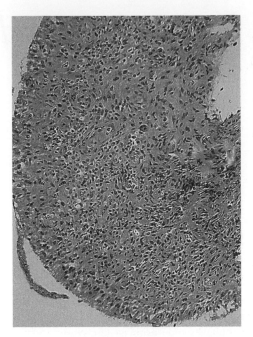

Fig. 5.2 Rheumatoid synovial tissue, showing intimal lining hyperplasia and infiltration of the synovial sublining by mononuclear cells. See also Plate 4.

Table 5.1 The cell infiltrate in rheumatoid synovial tissue

Intimal lining layer
Intimal macrophages
Fibroblast-like synoviocytes

Synovial sublining
Macrophages
T cells
Plasma cells
B cells
Interdigitating dendritic cells
Follicular dendritic cells
Natural killer cells
Mast cells
Neutrophils

individuals, joints, and even within joints[4]. At the pannus--cartilage junction, so-called pannocytes have been identified, which exhibit phenotypic and functional features of both FLS and chondrocytes[8,9]. These cells have distinctive rhomboid morphology and very strong expression of vascular cell adhesion molecule-1 (VCAM-1). It is unclear whether pannocytes represent a separate lineage of cells. In addition, cells with features of osteoclasts have recently been identified at the synovium--cartilage junction[10]. These cells are probably derived from the monocyte/macrophage lineage.

Recruitment of inflammatory cells, local retention, and cell proliferation contribute to the increased cellularity of the rheumatoid synovium. Recent studies suggest that impaired apoptosis, or programmed cell death, could also enhance hyperplasia in rheumatoid ST[11,12]. Very few apoptotic cells are found in the synovium of RA patients[13,14], despite the presence of fragmented DNA in the intimal lining layer[11,13]. Thus, increased cel-

lularity could be the result of immunological factors that enhance the influx of inflammatory cells into the synovium and of non-immunological factors, such as mutations of the p53 suppressor gene[15,16] and deficient Fas ligand expression[17], that could cause reduced apoptosis.

The intimal lining layer

The thickened intimal lining layer in RA consists mainly of intimal macrophages (Fig. 5.3) and FLS (Fig. 5.4). Two-thirds or more of the synoviocytes are macrophages (Fig.5.3). Hyperplasia of the intimal lining layer is often focal. Both intimal macrophages and FLS appear highly activated and secrete a variety of cytokines[18–20] as well as matrix metalloproteinases[21–23] (see Chapters 6 and 9). FLS can also produce other factors such as proteoglycans and arachidonic acid metabolites[24]. Other cells that can occasionally be detected in association with the intimal lining layer include multinucleated giant cells, which form as a consequence of fusion of macrophages[25], and T cells, in case of severe hyperplasia of the intimal lining layer[26].

Fibroblast-like synoviocytes

The FLS are peculiar to the synovium and have secretory features as well as an active Golgi apparatus. They appear to be of mesenchymal origin[27], although the relationship with fibroblasts in the synovial sublining and with other fibroblasts is, at present, unclear. The increased number of FLS in RA synovium is thought to be caused in part by impaired apoptosis[12,14]; the overall frequency of morphologically-defined apoptotic fibroblasts in rheumatoid ST is only about 3 per cent of the synovial sublining fibroblasts and the intimal lining layer FLS show no

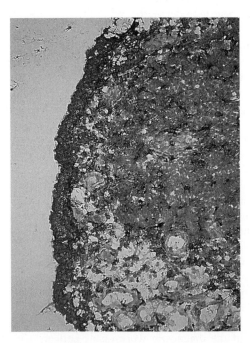

Fig. 5.3 CD68+ macrophages (red-brown) in the intimal lining layer and in the synovial sublining of rheumatoid synovial tissue. See also Plate 5.

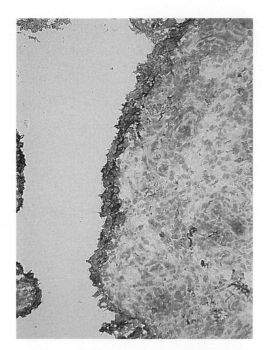

Fig. 5.4 CD55+ fibroblast-like synoviocytes (red-brown) in the intimal lining layer of rheumatoid synovial tissue. See also Plate 6.

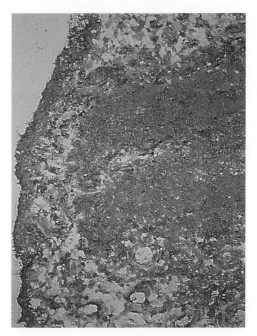

Fig. 5.5 Rheumatoid synovial tissue stained with a monoclonal antibody directed against CD97. Note prominent staining (red-brown) on intimal macrophages and on leukocytes in the synovial sublining. See also Plate 7.

signs of apoptosis[14]. *In situ* proliferation also contributes to some extent, although rates of cell division within the intimal lining layer are low[28,29]. Furthermore, it is conceivable that mesenchymal cells migrate from the synovial sublining into the intimal lining layer, where they could differentiate into FLS. They can be distinguished from other fibroblasts by the marked expression of CD55 or complement decay accelerating factor (DAF) (Fig. 5.4)[30–32] and VCAM-1[33–35]. CD55 is a regulatory protein of the complement cascade that protects cells from complement-mediated damage by inhibiting C3 convertases[36]. Of interest, CD55 can also act as a cellular ligand for the sevenspan-transmembrane molecule 7-TM CD97[37], which is expressed by nearly all intimal macrophages (Fig. 5.5)[32]. The microarchitecture of the intimal lining layer suggests that intimal macrophages and FLS may specifically interact via the CD97/CD55, the VCAM-1/$\alpha 4 \beta 1$ integrin, and the intercellular adhesion molecule (ICAM)-1/leukocyte function antigen (LFA)-1 ligand pairs[32,35,38]. Others molecules, such as CD40 and $\beta 1$ integrins can also be detected on FLS, but at lower levels. In addition, FLS exhibit increased activity of the enzyme uridine diphosphoglucose dehydrogenase (UDPGD)[38,39], which converts UDP-glucose into UDP-glucuronate. This is one of the substrates for hyaluron polymer synthesis. FLS exhibit relatively low human leukocyte antigen (HLA) class II expression compared with macrophages[40,41].

Intimal macrophages

Macrophages are present in the intimal lining layer, particularly in the more superficial parts of the synovial lining layer[42], and in the synovial sublining (Fig. 5.3). The intimal macrophages have phagocytic capacity and endocytic vacuoles. The increased number of intimal macrophages in RA is mainly the result of

recruitment of bone marrow-derived mononuclear phagocytes. The circulating monocytes are thought to pass through endothelial cells and enter the synovial sublining[43]. Relatively little is known about the factors that influence the subsequent migration into the intimal lining layer. The macrophages can be identified immunohistochemically on the basis of their strong expression of CD68, a marker probably associated with lysosomes, and the high activity of non-specific esterase[42]. FLS can also express CD68, but at lower levels. Of interest, intimal macrophages exhibit stronger expression of FcγRIIIa, non-specific esterase and CD97, and lower expression of CD14, than macrophages in the synovial sublining, illustrating the highly activated phenotype of the intimal macrophages in rheumatoid ST[37,42,43]. Although monocytes could be activated prior to entry into the joint[44], these data suggest that further activation of macrophages also takes place within the synovium. In addition to the markers mentioned above, synovial macrophages exhibit strong expression of HLA class II molecules, ICAM-1, and CD11b.

The synovial sublining

Edema, blood vessel proliferation, and increased cellularity of the second layer of the synovium, the synovial sublining, lead to a marked increase in ST volume in RA. The predominant cell types are T cells, plasma cells, and macrophages. Lymphocyte aggregates (Table 5.2) are observed in 50–60 per cent of RA patients and can be surrounded by coronas of plasma cells[4]. In addition, the areas between the lymphocyte aggregates, often referred to as the diffuse leukocyte infiltrate, are infiltrated mainly by macrophages and lymphocytes[4]. In some patients,

Table 5.2 Lymphocyte aggregates in rheumatoid synovial tissue

T cells (mainly CD4+CD45RO+CD27+)
Interdigitating dendritic cells and macrophages
B cells
Follicular dendritic cells

areas with granulomatous necrobiosis are apparent[45]. These areas are characterized by regions with fibrinoid necrosis lined by a collar of epithelioid histiocytes and granulation tissue. Moreover, fibrin deposition and fibrosis can be observed.

Sublining macrophages

The sublining contains large numbers of cells capable of antigen presentation, such as macrophages, interdigitating dendritic cells, and other cells that express HLA class II molecules[46–48]. However, it is as yet a matter of debate which cells serve as primary antigen-presenting cells in the synovium. The macrophages, which are derived from circulating monocytes and can be identified on the basis of their strong expression of CD68, often constitute the majority of the inflammatory cells in rheumatoid ST[4]. Macrophage infiltration occurs preferentially in areas adjacent to the articular cartilage[49]. Of interest, most cells in areas where synovial cells display tumor-like morphology are macrophages[50]. They have an activated phenotype and secrete a variety of cytokines and other proinflammatory mediators[4,51–55]. The preferential accumulation of macrophages at the pannus–cartilage junction is probably related to the expression of a range of adhesion molecules by macrophages[56–58] and to the effects of selective chemotactic factors[52,59,60].

Interdigitating dendritic cells

Interdigitating dendritic cells (IDC) are potent antigen-presenting cells. The advent of relatively specific markers, such as RFD1, in combination with markers to exclude macrophages, made it possible to detect substantial numbers of IDCs in rheumatoid ST. They are located in proximity to CD4+ T cells in the perivascular lymphocyte aggregates and near the intimal lining layer[46,61–63]. Cytokines, including granulocyte macrophage colony stimulating factor (GM-CSF) and tumor necrosis factor (TNF-α), play an important role in the differentiation of precursor cells from the myeloid lineage into the mature activate IDCs that are observed in the rheumatoid synovium[64,65]. In addition to HLA class II molecules, the costimulatory molecule CD86 (B7-2), which has an important role in antigen presentation, is also expressed on these cells[66–68]. Thus, the morphological data suggest that IDCs can undergo full functional differentiation in the cytokine milieu of the rheumatoid synovium, where they might present antigen to CD4+ T cells, especially in the perivascular lymphocyte aggregates. Whether this involves mainly endogenous autoantigens[69–70] or exogenous agents such as bacteria[71] and viruses[72], remains to be elucidated.

Follicular dendritic cells

Follicular dendritic cells (FDC) play an important role in the accumulation of B cells by stimulatory effects on migration and

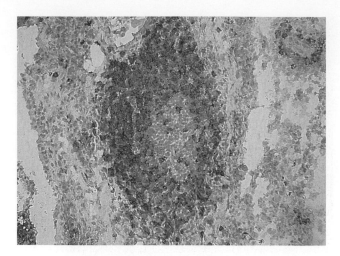

Fig. 5.6 CD22+ B cells (red-brown) in a lymphocyte aggregate in rheumatoid synovial tissue. See also Plate 8.

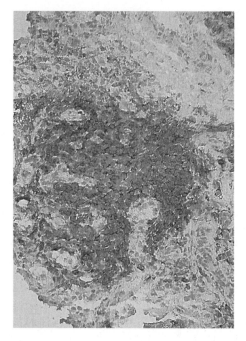

Fig. 5.7 CD4+ T cells (red-brown) in a lymphocyte aggregate in rheumatoid synovial tissue. See also Plate 9.

proliferation[73] and by inhibition of apoptosis[74]. Moreover, they are thought to play a crucial role in isotype switching and final differentiation of B cells towards plasma cells or memory B cells[75,76]. The FDCs may be derived from fibroblastic reticulum cells rather than from bone marrow-derived cells[73]. Of interest, FDCs are observed in the synovium in proximity to proliferating B cells in lymphocyte aggregates and close to B cells near the intimal lining layer[63–75]. When the perivascular lymphocyte aggregates are large, substantial numbers of B cells (Fig. 5.6) can be found in close association with CD4+ cells (Fig. 5.7) and FDCs[3,4]. These areas may be surrounded by large fields of plasma cells (Fig. 5.8). These aggregates of mainly CD4+ T cells and B cells resemble germinal centers, although they are mor-

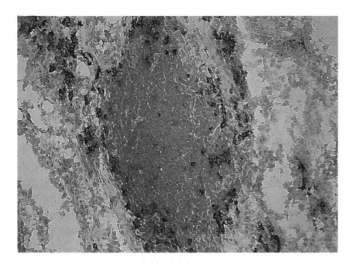

Fig. 5.8 CD38⁺ plasma cells (red-brown) surrounding a lymphocyte aggregate in rheumatoid synovial tissue. See also Plate 10.

phologically not identical to germinal centers in lymphatic organs[63,77]. The microenvironment suggests a close functional relationship between FDCs and B cells in RA synovium, allowing activation and maturation of the humoral immune response.

T cells

Large numbers of T cells are present in rheumatoid synovium (Fig. 5.9). Compared with peripheral blood, the overall CD4/CD8 ratio in ST is increased[61], but this ratio differs depending on the area within the synovium[78]. There are two basic patterns of T cell infiltration. First, perivascular lymphocyte aggregates can be found, as discussed above. These aggregates consist predominantly of CD4⁺ cells in association with B cells, few CD8⁺ cells, and dendritic cells[61,62]. The endothelial cells of the postcapillary venules adjacent to the aggregates tend to be tall and may resemble high endothelial venules[79]. The second pattern of T cell infiltration is the diffuse infiltrate of T

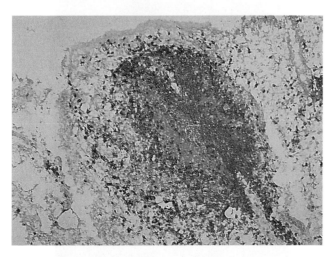

Fig. 5.9 CD3⁺ T cells (red-brown) in a perivascular lymphocyte aggregate and in the diffuse leukocyte infiltrate in rheumatoid synovial tissue. See also Plate 11.

cells scattered throughout the ST; in particular CD8⁺ T cells have this diffuse distribution at the periphery of the lymphocyte aggregates. Based on the overall paucity of CD8⁺ cells compared to CD4⁺ cells, the resultant lack of suppressor activity could contribute to increased stimulation of B cell and immunoglobulin synthesis in the synovium.

CD4⁺ T cells can be divided into two largely reciprocal subsets: CD45RA⁺–CD45RO⁻ naive cells and CD45RA–CD45RO⁺ memory cells[80]. Synovial T cells are primarily of the CD4⁺ CD45RO⁺ subset[81], which suggests previous antigen exposure. These cells exhibit greater migratory capacity than CD45RO- T cells, resulting in accumulation at the site of inflammation[82]. The preferential recruitment of memory cells may largely explain the presence of the multitude of T cells in the synovium, where only minimal proliferating T cells are found[47,83]. The CD45RO⁺ cells in rheumatoid synovial tissue consist mainly of the CD45RO⁺ CD45RB^dim subset, which is more differentiated than the CD45RO⁺ CD45RB^bright early memory cells[84]. These mature memory cells have enhanced capacity to provide B cell help.

The CD4⁺ CD45RO⁺ memory cells can also be divided on the basis of the surface expression of a recently-defined activation and differentiation antigen termed CD27, a member of the TNF-receptor superfamily[85]. Differentiation of CD4⁺ T cells is reflected in the change from the CD45RO-CD27⁺ phenotype' via CD45RO⁺ CD27⁺' to the CD45RO⁺ CD27⁻ phenotype. The interaction between CD27 and its ligand, CD70, plays a role in T cell proliferation[86] and in providing B cell help[87–90]. Interestingly, the large majority of the CD4⁺ T cells in the lymphocyte aggregates, where the T cells can be found in close association with B cells and FDCs, are CD27⁺ memory cells[88]. This supports the view that these regions play an important in the activation and maturation of antibody-producing cells. In line with this notion, there is a positive correlation between the levels of soluble CD27 in SF (produced by CD27⁺ cells) and the levels of rheumatoid factors in serum and SF of RA patients[88]. In the diffuse leukocyte infiltrate[88] and in the SF[88,91'] there is a relative increase in the percentage of terminally differentiated CD27⁻ memory T cells.

A subset of the CD4⁺ T cells in ST displays phenotypic evidence of prior activation, as indicated by the decreased density of CD3 and CD4 and the increased expression of activation antigens such as HLA class II antigens, very late activation antigen-1 (VLA-1), CD69, and CD27[88,92,93]. However, many of the T cells are small and few of them express activation molecules such as transferrin and the interleukin (IL)-2 receptor[83,94,95]. Moreover, the percentage of interferon (IFN-γ) producing T cells[83,96] and the detectable levels of T cell receptor-ζ (TCR ζ) protein[97] are significantly lower in RA synovium than in a chronic T cell mediated immunological reaction, such as tonsillitis or tuberculous pleuritis. Thus, the morphological data indicate that T cells in RA synovium are in a peculiar activation state.

B cells and plasma cells

B cells constitute a small proportion of the total amount of lymphocytes in rheumatoid synovium. When the perivascular within the joint, including the cartilage–pannus junction. A recent study compared the measures of inflammation in ST samples selected under direct vision at arthroscopy with those in biopsy specimens obtained blindly from the suprapatellar pouch by needle biopsy at the same time from the same joint[49]. The results show that it is not useful to know the macroscopic appearance of the rheumatoid synovium in order to predict the microscopic features[49,140]. Moreover, most measures of inflammation in needle biopsies are similar to those selected at arthroscopy. However, the intensity of macrophage infiltration may be underestimated in some patients when blind needle biopsies are used.

Microscopic analysis of synovial tissue

There are essentially three methods to quantify the features of synovial inflammation: semiquantitative analysis, quantitative analysis, and computer-assisted analysis[141,142]. Semiquantitative analysis involves assigning one of a limited number of scores, quantitative analysis involves counting of cells, and image analysis uses computerized digital image processing techniques to extract numerical information from visual images.

Because semiquantitative analysis is time-efficient, it offers the opportunity to evaluate sections from many biopsy specimens, which minimizes sampling error, and from many patients. This is an important advantage in light of the variation of synovial inflammation that can be found within the joint[137,140,143] and between individuals within one diagnostic group[4,35]. Reliable results can be obtained by evaluating sections from six different biopsy specimens, which results in a variability of less than 10 per cent[144]. Semiquantitative analysis is a sensitive and reproducible tool to assess differences between patient groups and to evaluate the effects of therapeutic interventions[6,7,35,54,145]. Furthermore, it is possible to detect highly significant correlations between semiquantitative scores for cell infiltration and expression of cytokines on the one hand and scores for local disease activity on the other[4,129].

Quantitative analysis appears to be accurate, but is more laborious and time-consuming than semiquantitative analysis. A recent study suggested that reliable, quantitative microscopic measurement may be obtained from a limited number of microscopic fields, which makes it more practical[146]. However, a complete evaluation of one patient with this limited quantitative analysis takes about four times longer than with semiquantitative methods. A recent, cross-sectional comparison of semiquantitative with quantitative analysis showed a highly significant correlation between the two methods for the evaluation of infiltration by macrophages and T cells[141]. This suggested that both methods can be used for the analysis of the cell infiltrate. In some patients exhibiting a decrease in serum levels of C-reactive protein and global subjective scores, quantitative analysis showed reduced cell numbers, whereas the semiquantitative scores were unchanged[141]. Whether the higher sensitivity to change of the quantitative method is an advantage remains to be determined. To date, there are no examples of studies showing a significant beneficial effect of treatment without a concomitant decrease in semiquantitative scores for synovial inflammation. The fact that even a significant reduction in synovial inflammation is not necessarily associated with clinical improvement[132] cautions against methods that are too sensitive.

Computer-assisted image analysis appears to be more sophisticated than semiquantitative analysis or quantitative analysis, although its marginal value still has to be determined. Until now there are no studies that demonstrate that computer-assisted image analysis produces data in a more objective or efficient way than other methods. However, it is likely that image analysis will be increasingly important with the use of more advanced computer systems. The major advantage is probably the ability to quantify the concentration of the antigen of interest, which may be important, for instance in the evaluation of cytokine expression[142].

Rheumatoid synovial fluid

SF is in direct contact with the synovium and the articular cartilage. The fluid contains a significant amount of extravasated plasma supplemented with high molecular molecules, in particular hyaluronan, which accounts for the viscoelastic features of SF[147]. SF analysis plays an important role in the diagnostic work-up in patients with arthritis, because it is easily accessible for aspiration and may help to differentiate between inflammatory and non-inflammatory arthropathies. Such a distinction is mainly made according to its appearance at the time of aspiration and the cell count. SF analysis is important to exclude infections and crystal-induced arthritis.

Many different cell types, such as neutrophils, plasma cells, lymphocytes, macrophages, fibroblasts, and platelets, are found in rheumatoid SF. In contrast with their paucity in the synovium, neutrophils are the predominant cell type. Neutrophil counts in RA SF are variable, but can exceed 10^5 mm^{-3}. The turnover rate can be more than a billion cells per day[148]. These neutrophils are activated and contain a variety of proteinases and other enzymes, such as collagenase, elastase, gelatinase, and myeloperoxidase. They also release proteins, such as fibronectin, and cytokines, such as IL-1. Thus, neutrophils can be of primary importance in inflammation and destruction of the joint[149]. As noted above, plasma cells in the synovium produce autoantibodies and the immune complexes formed by these antibodies may activate complement. This leads to generation of C5a, which serves as a chemotactic factor for neutrophils. Of interest, articular cartilage of RA patients contains immune complexes[150] that could enhance adherence and invasion by neutrophils. The migration of neutrophils is also influenced by adhesion molecules, chemokines, and cytokines, as discussed elsewhere in this book.

Platelets are also a potent source of a variety of soluble mediators[151]. The mean platelet count in rheumatoid SF is about 15 000 mm^{-3} and may be as high as 65 000 mm^{-3} [152]. During platelet activation vasoactive, chemotactic, and bactericidal substances can be released into the fluid. In addition, cell membrane-derived metabolites from arachidonic acid, platelet activating factor (PAF), and growth factors, such as platelet derived growth factor (PDGF) and transforming growth factor

Table 5.3 Cytokines, soluble cytokine-inducible adhesion molecules, and other soluble activation-related molecules that are elevated in rheumatoid synovial fluid

Cytokines	Surface membrane antigens
IL-1β	IL-2 receptor
TNF-α	CD27
IL-6	CD97
IL-8	CD80
TGF-β	CD14
Adhesion molecules	**Serine proteinases**
ICAM-1	granzyme A
VCAM-1	granzyme B
E-selectin	

(TGF-β), may be derived form platelets[151]. Thus, platelets can be considered as inflammatory cells that are capable of enhancing synovial inflammation.

Many cytokine-inducible adhesion molecules and other activation-related molecules are released from the cell surface and can be measured in soluble form in SF (Table 5.3). RA patients have, for instance, high levels of soluble ICAM-1, VCAM-1, E-selectin[153], CD27[88], IL-2 receptor[154], CD80 (B7–1)[155], granzymes A and B, CD97[32] and CD14[156]. The increased levels of these molecules in SF represent activation of various cell types, such as T cells, macrophages, and cytotoxic cells, in the synovium. In addition, almost every known cytokine has been detected in SF from RA patients[157]. In line with the observations of rheumatoid ST, high levels of cytokines derived for macrophages and FLS, such as IL-1-β, TNF-α, IL-6, IL-8, and TGF-β are present in the fluid. The levels of T-cell-derived cytokines, such as IL-2, IL-4, TNF-β, and IFN-λ are much lower[157].

The levels of molecules involved in the kallikrein–kinin system are also elevated in rheumatoid SF[158]. Activation of this system by, for example coagulation pathways and immune complexes, could cause release of other mediators, such as prostaglandins, histamine, and proinflammatory cytokines. This system is probably involved in the development of pain and swelling of the joints. Finally, joint matrix molecules or fragments of the matrix molecules can be released into the SF[159]. Measurement of these molecular markers may provide insight into the mechanisms underlying the process of destruction of bone and articular cartilage.

References

1. Henderson B., Pettipher E.R. The synovial lining cell: biology and pathobiology. *Semin Arthritis Rheum*, 1985;**15**:1–32.
2. Palmer D.G. The anatomy of the rheumatoid lesion. *Br Med Bull*, 1995;**51**:286–95.
3. Yanni G., Whelan A., Feighery C., Bresnihan B. Analysis of cell populations in rheumatoid arthritis synovial tissues. *Semin Arthritis Rheum*, 1992;**21**:393–9.
4. Tak P.P., Smeets T.J.M., Daha M.R., Kluin P.M., Meijers K.A.E., Brand R., Meinders A.E., Breedveld F.C. Analysis of the synovial cellular infiltrate in early rheumatoid synovial tissue in relation to local disease activity. *Arthritis Rheum*, 1997;**40**:217–25.
5. De Paulis A., Marino I., Ciccarelli A., De Crescenzo G., Concardi M., Verga L., Arbustini E., Marone G. Human synovial mast cells. 1. Ultrastructural in situ and in vitro immunologic characterization. *Arthritis Rheum*, 1996;**39**:1222–33.
6. Tak P.P., Kummer J.A., Hack C.E., Daha M.R., Smeets T.J.M., Erkelens G.W., Meinders A.E., Kluin P.M., Breedveld F.C. Granzyme positive cytotoxic cells are specifically increased in early rheumatoid synovial tissue. *Arthritis Rheum*, 1994;**37**:1735–43.
7. Smeets T.J.M., Dolhain R.J.E.M., Breedveld F.C., Tak P.P. Analysis of the synovial infiltrates and expression of cytokines in synovial tissue from patients with rheumatoid arthritis and from patients with reactive arthritis. *J Pathol*, 1998;**186**:75–81.
8. Zvaifler N.J., Tsai V., Alsalameh S., Vonkempis J., Firestein G.S., Lotz M. Pannocytes: Distinctive cells found in rheumatoid arthritis articular cartilage erosions. *Am J Pathol*, 1997;**150**:1125–38.
9. Xue C., Takahashi M., Hasunuma T., Aono H., Yamamoto K., Yoshino S., Sumida T., Nishioka K. Characterisation of fibroblast-like cells in pannus lesions of patients with rheumatoid arthritis sharing properties of fibroblasts and chondrocytes. *Ann Rheum Dis*, 1997;**56**:262–7.
10. Gravallese E.M., Harada Y., Wang J.T., Gorn A.H., Thornhill T.S., Goldring S.R. Identification of cell types responsible for bone resorption in rheumatoid arthritis and juvenile rheumatoid arthritis. *Am J Pathol*, 1998;**152**:943–51.
11. Firestein G.S., Yeo M., Zvaifler N.J. Apoptosis in rheumatoid arthritis synovium. *J Clin Invest*, 1995;**96**:1631–8.
12. Firestein G.S. Invasive fibroblast-like synoviocytes in rheumatoid arthritis. Passive responders or transformed aggressors? *Arthritis Rheum*, 1996;**39**:1781–90.
13. Nakajima T., Aono H., Hasunuma T., Yamamoto K., Shirai T., Hirohata K., Nishioka K. Apoptosis and functional Fas antigen in rheumatoid arthritis synoviocytes. *Arthritis Rheum*, 1995;**38**:485–91.
14. Matsumoto S., Muller-Ladner U., Gay R.E., Nishioka K., Gay S. Ultrastructural demonstration of apoptosis, Fas and Bcl-2 expression of rheumatoid synovial fibroblasts. *J Rheumatol*, 1996;**23**:1345–52.
15. Firestein G.S., Echeverri F., Yeo M., Zvaifler N.J., Green D.R. Somatic mutations in the p53 tumor suppressor gene in rheumatoid arthritis synovium. *Proc Natl Acad Sci USA*, 1997;**94**:10895–900.
16. Reme T., Travaglio A., Gueydon E., Adla L., Jorgensen C., Sany J. Mutations of the p53 tumour suppressor gene in erosive rheumatoid synovial tissue. *Clin Exp Immunol*, 1998;**111**:353–8.
17. Cantwell M.J., Hua T., Zvaifler N.J., Kipps T.J. Deficient Fas ligand expression by synovial lymphocytes from patients with rheumatoid arthritis. *Arthritis Rheum*, 1997;**40**:1644–52.
18. Koch A.E., Kunkel S.L., Burrows J.C., Evanoff H.L., Haines G.K., Pope R.M., Strieter R.M. Synovial tissue macrophage as a source of the chemotactic cytokine IL-8. *J Immunol*, 1991;**147**:2187–95.
19. Koch A.E., Kunkel S.L., Chensue S.W., Haines G.K., Strieter R.M. Expression of interleukin-1 and interleukin-1 receptor antagonist by human rheumatoid synovial tissue macrophages. *Clin Immunol Immunopathol*, 1992;**65**:23–9.
20. Taketazu F., Kato M., Gobl A., Ichijo H., Tendijke P., Itoh J.P., Kyogoku M., Ronnelid J., Miyazono K., Heldin C.H., *et al.* Enhanced expression of transforming growth factor-beta s and transforming growth factor-beta type II receptor in the synovial tissues of patients with rheumatoid arthritis. *Lab Invest*, 1994;**70**:620–30.
21. Firestein G.S., Paine M.M., Littman B.H. Gene expression (collagenase, tissue inhibitor of metalloproteinases, complement, and HLA-DR) in rheumatoid arthritis and osteoarthritis synovium. Quantitative analysis and effect of intraarticular corticosteroids. *Arthritis Rheum*, 1991;**34**:1094–105.
22. McCachren S.S. Expression of metalloproteinases and metalloproteinase inhibitor in human arthritic synovium. *Arthritis Rheum*, 1991;**34**:1085–93.
23. Gravallese E.M., Darling J.M., Ladd A.L., Katz J.N., Glimcher L.H. In situ hybridization studies of stromelysin and collagenase messenger RNA expression in rheumatoid synovium. *Arthritis Rheum*, 1991;**34**:1076–84.
24. Cisar LA, Schimmel RJ, Mochan E. Interleukin-1 stimulation of arachidonic acid release from human synovial fibroblasts;

cells in synovia from patients with rheumatoid arthritis. *Rheumatol Int*, 1997;**17**:169–74.

101. Melbye O.J., Vartdal F., Pahle J., Mollnes T.E. IgG and IgA subclass distribution of total immunoglobulin and rheumatoid factors in rheumatoid tissue plasma cells. *Scand J Rheumatol*, 1990;**19**:333–40.

102. Otten H.G., Dolhain R.J., de Rooij H.H., Breedveld F.C. Rheumatoid factor production by mononuclear cells derived from different sites of patients with rheumatoid arthritis. *Clin Exp Immunol*, 1993;**94**:236–40.

103. Hakoda M., Ishimoto T., Hayashimoto S., Inoue K., Taniguchi A., Kamatani N., Kashiwazaki S.. Selective infiltration of B cells committed to the production of monoreactive rheumatoid factor in synovial tissue of patients with rheumatoid arthritis. *Clin Immunol Immunopathol*, 1993;**69**:16–22.

104. Williams D.G., Taylor P.C. Clonal analysis of immunoglobulin mRNA in rheumatoid arthritis synovium: characterization of expanded IgG3 populations. *Eur J Immunol*, 1997;**27**:476–85.

105. Clausen B.E., Bridges S.L., Jr., Lavelle J.C., Fowler P.G., Gay S., Koopman W.J., Schroeder H.W., Jr. Clonally-related immunoglobulin VH domains and nonrandom use of DH gene segments in rheumatoid arthritis synovium. *Mol Med*, 1998;**4**:240–57.

106. Reinitz E., Neighbour P.A., Grayzel A.I. Natural killer cell activity of mononuclear cells from rheumatoid patients measured by a conjugate-binding cytotoxicity assay. *Arthritis Rheum*, 1982;**25**:1440–4.

107. Combe B., Pope R., Darnell B., Talal N. Modulation of natural killer cell activity in the rheumatoid joint and peripheral blood. *Scand J Immunol*, 1984;**20**:551–8.

108. Thoen J., Waalen K., Forre O. Natural killer (NK) cells at inflammatory sites of patients with rheumatoid arthritis and IgM rheumatoid factor positive polyarticular juvenile rheumatoid arthritis. *Clin Rheumatol*, 1987;**6**:215–25.

109. Mueller C., Gershenfeld H.K., Lobe C.G., Okada C.Y., Bleackley R.C., Weissman IL. A high proportion of T lymphocytes that infiltrate H-2-incompatible heart allografts in vivo express genes encoding cytotoxic cell-specific serine proteases, but do not express MEL-14-defined lymph node homing receptor. *J Exp Med*, 1988;**167**:1124–36.

110. Hendrich C., Kuipers J.G., Kolanus W., Hammer M., Schmidt R.E. Activation of CD16+ effector cells by rheumatoid factor complex. Role of natural killer cells in rheumatoid arthritis. *Arthritis Rheum*, 1991;**34**:423–31.

111. Goto M., Zvaifler N.J. Characterization of the natural killer-like lymphocytes in rheumatoid synovial fluid. *J Immunol*, 1985;**134**:1483–6.

112. Griffiths G.M., Issaz S. Granzymes A and B are targeted to the lytic granules of lymphocytes by the mannose-6-phosphate receptor. *J Cell Biol*, 1993;**120**:885–96.

113. Liu C.C., Young L.H.Y., Young J.D.E. Mechanisms of disease: Lymphocyte-mediated cytolysis and disease. *N Engl J Med*, 1996;**335**:1651–9.

114. Froelich C.J., Dixit V.M., Yang X.H., Yang X. Lymphocyte granule-mediated apoptosis: matters of viral mimicry and deadly proteases. *Immunol Today*, 1998;**19**:30–6.

115. Muller-Ladner U., Kriegsmann J., Tschopp J., Gay R.E., Gay S. Demonstration of granzyme A and perforin messenger RNA in the synovium of patients with rheumatoid arthritis. *Arthritis Rheum*, 1995;**38**:477–84.

116. Tak P.P., Spaeny-Dekking E.H.A., Kraan M.C., Breedveld F.C., Froelich C.J., Hack C.E. The levels of soluble granzyme A and B are elevated in plasma and synovial fluid of patients with rheumatoid arthritis. *Clin Exp Immunol*, 1999;**116**:366–70.

117. Crisp A.J., Chapman C.M., Kirkham S.E., Schiller A.L., Krane S.M. Articular mastocytosis in rheumatoid arthritis. *Arthritis Rheum*, 1984;**27**:845–51.

118. Gotis-Graham I., McNeil H.P. Mast cell responses in rheumatoid synovium. Association of the MCtc subset with matrix turnover and clinical progression. *Arthritis Rheum*, 1997;**40**:479–89.

119. Bromley M., Woolley D.E. Histopathology of the rheumatoid lesion. Identification of cell types at sites of cartilage erosion. *Arthritis Rheum*, 1984;**27**:857–63.

120. Tetlow L.C., Woolley D.E. Mast cells, cytokines, and metalloproteinases at the rheumatoid lesion: Dual immunolocalisation studies. *Ann Rheum Dis*, 1995;**54**:896–903.

121. Arnason J.A., Malone D.G. Role of mast cells in arthritis. *Chem Immunol*, 1995;**62**:204–38.

122. Qu Z.H., Huang X.N., Ahmadi P., Andresevic J., Planck S.R., Hart C.E., Rosenbaum J.T. Expression of basic fibroblast growth factor in synovial tissue from patients with rheumatoid arthritis and degenerative joint disease. *Lab Invest*, 1995;**73**:339–46.

123. Kiener H.P., Baghestanian M., Dominkus M., Walchshofer S., Ghannadan M., Willheim M., Sillaber C., Graninger W.B., Smolen J.S., Valent P. Expression of the C5a receptor (CD88) on synovial mast cells in patients with rheumatoid arthritis. *Arthritis Rheum*, 1998;**41**:233-45.

124. Youssef P.P., Cormack J., Evill C.A., Peter D.T., Roberts-Thomson P.J., Ahern M.J., Smith M.D. Neutrophil trafficking into inflamed joints in patients with rheumatoid arthritis, and the effects of methylprednisolone. *Arthritis Rheum*, 1996;**39**:216–25.

125. Koch A.E., Kunkel S.L., Shah M.R., Hosaka S., Halloran M.M., Haines G.K., Burdick M.D., Pope R.M., Strieter R.M. Growth-related gene product alpha—A chemotactic cytokine for neutrophils in rheumatoid arthritis. *J Immunol*, 1995;**155**:3660–6.

126. Gao J.X., Issekutz A.C. The beta 1 integrin, very late activation antigen-4 on human neutrophils can contribute to neutrophil migration through connective tissue fibroblast barriers. *Immunology*, 1997;**90**:448–54.

127. Schumacher H.R., Jr., Kitridou R.C. Synovitis of recent onset. A clinicopathologic study during the first month of disease. *Arthritis Rheum*, 1972;**15**:465–85.

128. Konttinen Y.T., Bergroth V., Nordstrom D., Koota K., Skrifvars B., Hagman G., Friman C., Hamalainen M., Slatis P. Cellular immuno-histopathology of acute, subacute, and chronic synovitis in rheumatoid arthritis. *Ann Rheum Dis*, 1985;**44**:549–55.

129. Kraan M.C., Versendaal H., Jonker M., Bresnihan B., Post W., 't Hart B.A., Breedveld F.C., Tak P.P. Asymptomatic synovitis precedes clinically manifest arthritis. *Arthritis Rheum*, 1998;**41**:1481–8.

130. Mulherin D., FitzGerald O., Bresnihan B. Synovial tissue macrophage populations and articular damage in rheumatoid arthritis. *Arthritis Rheum*, 1996;**39**:115–24.

131. Yanni G., Farahat M.N.M.R., Poston R.N., Panayi G.S. Intramuscular gold decreases cytokine expression and macrophage numbers in the rheumatoid synovial membrane. *Ann Rheum Dis*, 1994;**53**:315–22.

132. Tak P.P., Van der Lubbe P.A., Cauli A., Daha M.R., Smeets T.J.M., Kluin P.M., Meinders A.E., Yanni G., Panayi G.S., Breedveld F.C. Reduction of synovial inflammation after anti-CD4 monoclonal antibody treatment in early rheumatoid arthritis. *Arthritis Rheum*, 1995;**38**:1457–65.

133. Tak P.P., Taylor P.C., Breedveld F.C., Smeets T.J.M., Daha M.R., Kluin P.M., Meinders A.E., Maini R.N. Decreases in cellularity and expression of adhesion molecules by anti-tumor necrosis factor alpha treatment in patients with rheumatoid arthritis. *Arthritis Rheum*, 1996;**39**:1077–81.

134. Dolhain R.J.E.M., Tak P.P., Dijkmans B.A.C., De Kuiper P., Breedveld F.C., Miltenburg A.M.M. Methotrexate treatment reduces inflammatory cell numbers, expression of monokines and of adhesion molecules in synovial tissue of patients with rheumatoid arthritis. *Br J Rheumatol*, 1998;**37**:502–8.

135. Kraan M.C., Haringman J.J., Post W., Versendaal J., Breedveld F.C., Tak P.P. Immunohistologic analysis of synovial tissue for differential diagnosis in early arthritis. *Rheumatology (Oxford)* 1999;**38**:1074–80.

136. Tak P.P., Lindblad S., Klareskog L., Breedveld F.C. Synovial biopsies for analysis of the synovial membrane: new perspectives. *Newslett Eur Rheumatol Res*, 1994;**2**:27–9.

137. Lindblad S., Hedfors E. Intraarticular variation in synovitis. Local macroscopic and microscopic signs of inflammatory activity are significantly correlated. *Arthritis Rheum*, 1985;**28**:977–86.

138. Reece R., Emery P. Needle arthroscopy. *Br J Pheumatol*, 1995;34:1102–4.

139. Ike R.W. Diagnostic arthroscopy. *Baillieres Clin Rheumatol*, 1996;10:495–517.

140. Rooney M., Condell D., Daly L., Whelan A., Feighery C., Bresnihan B. Analysis of the histologic variation of synovitis in rheumatoid arthritis. *Arthritis Rheum*, 1988;31:956–63.

141. Youssef P.P., Smeets T.J.M., Bresnihan B., Cunnane G., FitzGerald O., Breedveld F.C., Tak P.P. Microscopic measurement of inflammation in the rheumatoid arthritis synovial membrane: a comparison of semiquantitative and quantitative analysis. *Br J Rheumatol* 1998;37:1003–7.

142. Youssef P.P., Triantafillou S., Parker A., Coleman M., Roberts-Thomson P.J., Ahern M.J., Smith M.D., Robertsthomson P.J. Variability in cytokine and cell adhesion molecule staining in arthroscopic synovial biopsies: quantification using color video image analysis. *J Rheumatol*, 1997;24:2291–8.

143. Hutton C.W., Hinton C., Dieppe P.A. Intra-articular variation of synovial changes in knee arthritis: biopsy study comparing changes in patellofemoral synovium and the medial tibiofemoral synovium. *Br J Rheumatol*, 1987;26:5–8.

144. Dolhain R.J.E.M., Terhaar N.T., Dekuiper R., Nieuwenhuis I.G., Zwinderman A.H., Breedveld F.C., Miltenburg A.M.M. Distribution of T cells and signs of T-cell activation in the rheumatoid joint: Implications for semiquantitative comparative histology. *Br J Rheumatol*, 1998;37:324–30.

145. Tak P.P., Breedveld F.C. Analysis of serial synovial biopsies as a screening method for predicting the effects of therapeutic interventions. *J Clin Rheumatol*, 1997;3:186–7.

146. Bresnihan B., Cunnane G., Youssef P.P., Yanni G., FitzGerald O., Mulherin D. Microscopic measurement of synovial membrane inflammation in rheumatoid arthritis: proposals for the evaluation of tissue samples by quantitative analysis. *Br J Rheumatol*, 1998;37:636–42.

147. Simkin P.A. Synovial perfusion and synovial fluid solutes. *Ann Rheum Dis*, 1995;54:424–8.

148. Hollingsworth J.W., Siegel E.R., Creasey W.A. Granulocyte survival in synovial exudate of patients with rheumatoid arthritis and other inflammatory joint diseases. *Yale J Biol Med*, 1967;39:289–96.

149. Pillinger M.H., Abramson S.B. The neutrophil in rheumatoid arthritis. *Rheum Dis Clin North Am*, 1995;21:691–714.

150. Jasin H.E. Autoantibody specificities of immune complexes sequestered in articular cartilage of patients with rheumatoid arthritis and osteoarthritis. *Arthritis Rheum*, 1985;28:241–8.

151. Endresen G.K., Forre O. Human platelets in synovial fluid. A focus on the effects of growth factors on the inflammatory responses in rheumatoid arthritis. *Clin Exp Rheumatol*, 1992;10:181–7.

152. Farr M., Wainwright A., Salmon M., Hollywell C.A., Bacon P.A. Platelets in the synovial fluid of patients with rheumatoid arthritis. Rheumatol Int, 1984;4:13–7.

153. Haskard D.O. Cell adhesion molecules in rheumatoid arthritis. *Curr Opin Rheumatol*, 1995;7:229–34.

154. Carotti M., Salaffi F., Ferraccioli G.F., Binci M.C., Sartini A., Cervini C. Soluble interleukin-2 receptor in sera and synovial fluids of rheumatoid patients: correlations with disease activity. *Rheumatol Int*, 1994;14:47–52.

155. McHugh R.S., Ratnoff W.D., Gilmartin R., Sell K.W., Selvaraj P. Detection of a soluble form of B7-1 (CD80) in synovial fluid form patients with arthritis using monoclonal antibodies against distinct epitopes of human B7-1. *Clin Immunol Immunopathol*, 1998;87:50–9.

156. Yu S., Nakashima N., Xu B.H., Matsuda T., Izumihara A., Sunahara N., Nakamura T., Tsukano M., Matsuyama T. Pathological significance of elevated soluble CD14 production in rheumatoid arthritis: in the presence of soluble CD14, lipopolysaccharides at low concentrations activate RA synovial fibroblasts. *Rheumatol Int*, 1998;17:237–43.

157. Houssiau F.A. Cytokines in rheumatoid arthritis. *Clin Rheumatol*, 1995;14 (Suppl 2):10–3.

158. Sharma J.N., Buchanan W.W. Pathogenic responses of bradykinin system in chronic inflammatory rheumatoid disease. *Exp Toxicol Pathol*, 1994;46:421–33.

159. Saxne T. Differential release of molecular markers in joint disease. *Acta Orthop Scand Suppl*, 1995;266:80–3.

6 | *The role of macrophages in rheumatoid arthritis*

Raimund W. Kinne, Bruno Stuhlmüller, Ernesta Palombo-Kinne, and Gerd-R. Burmester

Introduction

Activated macrophages are critical in rheumatoid arthritis (RA), due not only to the predominance of macrophage-derived cytokines in the synovial compartments[1], but also because of their localization in strategic sites within the destructive pannus tissue[2,3]. In addition, not only tissue macrophages, but also circulating monocytes and other cells of the myelomonocytic lineage contribute to disease[1,4-6]. More importantly, several conventional or experimental therapeutic trials have documented a clear link between marked clinical response and down-regulation of the mononuclear phagocyte system[5,7,8]. Indeed, the radiological progression of joint damage appears to be proportional to the degree of macrophage infiltration in the synovial tissue[9]. All these observations indicate that, until the etiology of RA is proven and therapy can be specifically shaped on the causing agent/factor, suppressing the activated mononuclear phagocyte system remains the most promising means of reducing inflammation and arresting tissue destruction. Indeed, the rapidly growing knowledge of the specific effects of conventional antirheumatic drugs on macrophages[10] is determining a major re-evaluation of their classification and administration criteria[11,12]. In parallel, considerable research is now aimed at defining soluble or juxtacrine stimuli that favor the amplifying role of macrophages in disease[13,14].

Differentiation of the mononuclear phagocyte system in RA

The myelomonocytic lineage, outlined in Fig. 6.1A, gives rise to several cell types involved in disease, that is monocytes/macrophages, osteoclasts, and dendritic cells, and is characterized by a certain degree of plasticity. Interestingly, several steps along the differentiation pathway are affected by particular pathophysiological stimuli (for example an excess/imbalance of cytokines or growth factors, including some derived from activated macrophages), which result in altered differentiation or maturation (Fig. 6.1B). In RA, some of these alterations with potential pathophysiological implications already have been localized in inflamed joints, peripheral blood, and bone marrow, as described below (Fig. 6.1B; Table 6.1).

Table 6.1 Potential sites of macrophage activation in RA

Joint compartments:	Synovial membrane
	Cartilage–pannus junction
	Subchondral bone
	Synovial fluid
	Vascular endothelium
Extra-articular compartments:	Peripheral blood
	Bone marrow
	Subendothelial macrophages
	Rheumatoid nodules
	Alveolar macrophages

Local terminal differentiation of macrophages in the RA synovial membrane

Under inflammatory conditions, macrophages undergo local differentiation which may become pathogenic if regulatory mechanisms fail. In the RA synovial membrane, a first differentiation step is that from early to mature macrophages[15]. These subsets differentially colonize the synovial sublining and lining layer, respectively, as well as the superficial and deep layers of the lining[9]. The diversity of these areas is documented by expression patterns of activation markers and adhesion molecules[16]. The importance of this 'segregation' is immediately evident when considering that macrophage subtypes may differentially contribute to disease progression[9].

Another relevant differentiation step is that into stimulatory versus inhibitory macrophage subpopulations, which may critically influence the T-cell reactivity in RA[17,18]. In experimental models of arthritis, for example, immunoregulatory macrophages have been clearly identified[19], which greatly affect T-cell responses to arthritogenic proteins[20] and, upon non-selective targeting, influence clinical and histopathological improvement of arthritis[20].

In RA, macrophage subpopulations may well be responsible for separate (patho)physiological functions, including the separate synthesis of proinflammatory or regulatory cytokines[14,21]. Consistently, IL-1 and TNF-α may be produced by macrophage subsets different from those that produce IL-10[22]. In contrast, IL-1 and its receptor antagonist (IL-1Ra) are probably produced by the same synovial macrophages[14]. A subset of synovial macrophages may also exert a predominant role in angiogenesis[23].

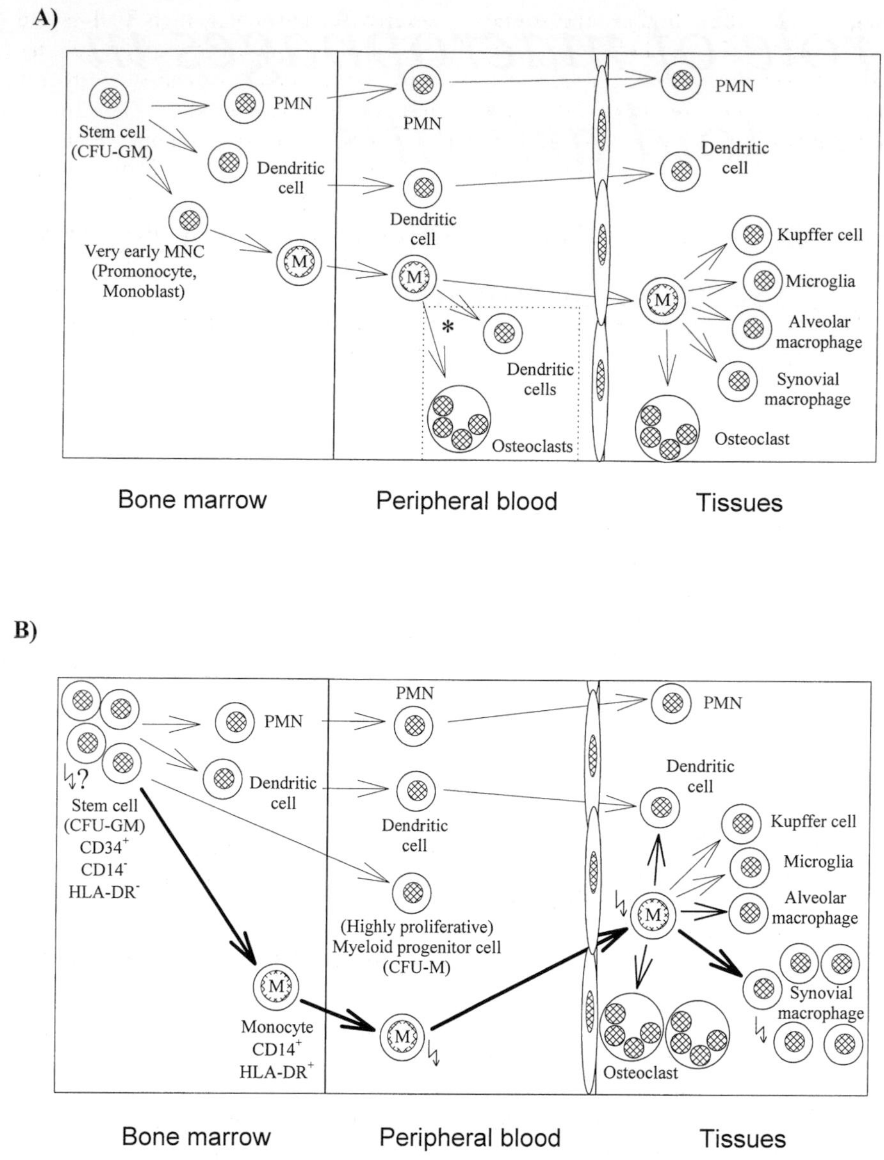

A)

Bone marrow Peripheral blood Tissues

B)

Bone marrow Peripheral blood Tissues

Fig. 6.1 A Differentiation of the mononuclear phagocyte system (MPS). In the human system, monocytes differentiate from a CD34+ stem cell via an intermediate step of monoblasts. Monocytes (**M**) leave the bone marrow and remain in circulation for about 3 days. Upon entering various tissues, they differentiate into various types of resident macrophages, including synovial macrophages. It is believed that these mature cells do not recirculate, surviving for several months in their respective tissues until they senesce and die. Some circulating monocytes retain the potential for differentiating into dendritic cells and osteoclasts 171 (* in the insert). The steady-state myeloid differentiation involves many factors, including GM-CSF, IL-1, IL-6, and TNF-α, which are produced by resident bone marrow macrophages.
B Plasticity of myeloid differentiation and its possible role in RA. The differentiation of the myeloid lineage is characterized by some plasticity[172]. Human bone marrow intermediate cells can differentiate into macrophages or dendritic cells in the presence of c-kit ligand, GM-CSF, and TNF-α. TNF-α, in turn inhibits the differentiation of monocytes into macrophages *in vitro*, and, together with GM-CSF, directs the differentiation of precursor cells into dendritic cells, another important arm of the accessory cell system[173]. Also, IL-11[174], or vitamin D3 and dexamethasone, induce the differentiation of bone marrow cells or mature macrophages into osteoclasts, cells involved in the destruction of subchondral bone in RA[6]. Osteoclasts and dendritic cells can also be derived from circulating monocytes upon stimulation with M-CSF or IL-4 *plus* GM-CSF[171]. This plasticity, and its dependence on growth factors or cytokines that are clearly elevated in peripheral blood[29,35,58,75] and bone marrow of RA patients[63,68,69], may explain some differentiation anomalies in the disease[45–47,65], and also the efficacy of some antirheumatic drugs. Non-specific enhancement of monocyte maturation and tissue egression, in turn, are consistent with the known alterations in inflammation. The differentiation paths potentially relevant to RA are indicated by bold arrows. The jagged arrows represent possible sites of cell activation.

Local terminal differentiation of macrophages in subcutaneous nodules

A particular example of terminal differentiation is that of granulomas present in subcutaneous rheumatoid nodules (and in the synovial membrane of some RA patients)[24,25]. In these lesions, monocytes are actively and continuously recruited, differentiating into epithelioid cells and multinucleated giant cells (the latter fusion products of the former), both of which surround a necrotic center[25]. Functionally, these palisading cells display poorer phagocytosis, but higher lysosomal activity, than 'regular' macrophages[26]. Skin and synovial granulomatous lesions in RA are interesting not only because they may obey common systemic stimuli, but also because they are associated with severe RA[25], thus pointing to a possible link between engagement of extra-articular macrophages and disease severity.

Activation of the mononuclear phagocyte system in RA

Synovial compartments

Synovial membrane

In the normal synovial membrane, macrophages predominate in the lining layer, which usually consists of two to three cell layers. These cells scavenge debris released from articular structures, and eliminate micro-organisms entering the joints via the blood stream or upon traumatic injury. While critically needed for the smooth functioning of the joints, these functions might also create the basis for excessive production of inflammatory mediators and/or entry of micro organisms/antigenic material into the joint structures.

In RA, two primary types of non-lymphoid cells are present in the hyperplastic synovial membrane: Type A cells, lysosome-rich macrophages frequently filled with phagocytosed material and strongly MHC-II+ and CD14+; and type B cells, fibroblast-like cells with a well-developed rough endoplasmic reticulum, negative for the above markers, however able to express MHC-II *in vitro* upon activation with IFN-γ[27–29].

The degree of macrophage infiltration bears direct consequences for the development of RA. Indeed, its intensity correlates not only with the clinical status of the disease[27], including joint pain[30], but also with the radiological progression of permanent joint damage[9]. Also, the degree of macrophage activation in the synovial membrane is correlated with the general inflammatory status of the patients[31].

Rheumatoid macrophages often show a unique distribution. The joint space is lined by a layer of HLA-DR+, CD14+, and CD68+ macrophages[9,27], followed by a layer of fibroblasts that lack these markers. Below the lining layer, macrophages are distributed in different histological areas: they are most numerous adjacent to activated lymphoid cells in diffuse infiltrates, especially near CD8+ T cells[32], suggesting active participation of these macrophages in immune processes.

In chronic inflammatory diseases, the prevalence of certain histological configurations can be associated with different courses of disease. Thus, the tissue microheterogeneity might also represent an important variable in the course of RA, especially in view of the resulting cytokine milieu or cell–cell interactions. While some recent analyses deny that the patterns of cytokine gene expression correlate with the degree of macrophage- or T-cell infiltration[33], other studies suggest that the gene expression of cytokines TNF-α, IL-4, and IL-10 defines certain histological subsets of rheumatoid synovitis and disease

severity. In particular, high TNF-α and IL-1β production may be associated with the rare granulomatous synovitis, which is more frequently associated with subcutaneous rheumatoid nodules[24,34]. Conversely, these cytokines appear modestly elevated in diffuse synovitis, which may be associated with seronegative RA[24]. These features may also explain some variability among studies on the abundance of TNF-α and/or TNF-α receptor expression in the RA synovial membrane[35].

The activated state of synovial monocytes/macrophages in RA and its link to disease has been long recognized[1,2,8,27]. This is documented by the over-expression of at least five classes of products:

(1) Class II MHC molecules[27,28], which may be implicated in the presentation of antigens relevant to disease initiation or severity[36];

(2) cytokines and growth factors mediating or regulating inflammation, i.e. IL-1, IL-6, IL-10, IL-13, TNF-α, and GM-CSF[1,24,27,33];

(3) chemokines and chemoattractants, i.e. IL-8, MIP-1, and MCP-1[23,37,38,39], relevant to cell migration and exudation processes;

(4) metalloproteinases[40,41]; and

(5) neopterin[5,7].

Many of these products show correlations with disease activity or severity, as will be discussed below.

Cartilage–pannus junction (CPJ)

Macrophages close to the articular cartilage are of special interest in RA, since they are in the position to invade cartilage. At the CPJ, macrophages produce significant amounts of the inflammatory cytokines IL-1, TNF-α, and GM-CSF[27]. Together with fibroblasts and endothelial cells, CPJ macrophages are considerable sources of the metalloproteinases, collagenase, stromelysin, gelatinase B, as well as leukocyte elastase[42,43]. Indeed, gelatinase B levels positively correlate with disease progression and severity[44]. However, the potential of macrophages to degrade cartilage matrix components may be modest compared to that of synovial fibroblasts[42,43]. Thus, macrophages might represent the amplifier of the pathogenetic cascade (especially via activation of fibroblasts) rather than the primary effector of tissue destruction.

Subchondral bone

In contrast to the indirect role of macrophages at the CPJ, osteoclasts and macrophages may exert a much more direct role in the destruction of subchondral bone[6]. At this site, mononuclear cells with ultrastructural, intracellular, and surface characteristics of macrophages (cathepsin L- and CD68-positivity) have been described in association with bone degradation areas[45,46]. Also, functionally efficient bone-resorbing osteoclasts can be clearly derived from RA synovial macrophages cocultured with passaged RA synovial fibroblast[47] (Fig. 6.1B). Indeed, studies of experimental arthritis show a significant reduction of subchondral bone loss upon systemic administration of liposomes laden with clodronate, a means that selectively targets activated osteoclasts and macrophages[48].

Synovial fluid

In acute RA, the cellular composition of the synovial fluid is distinct from that of the synovial tissue, that is polymorphonuclear cells (PMN) largely predominate in the synovial fluid, whereas macrophages predominate in the synovial tissue. The mechanisms for this dichotomy are unclear. On the one hand, the synovial fluid contains complement molecules which, through monocyte autocrine or paracrine mechanisms, inhibit monocyte chemotaxis and exudation into the synovial fluid. On the other hand, lining macrophages are the main producers of IL-8 and epithelial neutrophil-activating peptide-78 (ENA-78), which are powerful PMN attractants[23,49,50]. Thus, RA monocytes/macrophages are active participants in the mechanisms that determine the fluid/tissue dichotomy. Combinations of the macrophage-derived molecules IL-15, IL-8, MCP-1, and MIP-1α, also seem to favor the preferential exudation of memory T cells into the synovial fluid[51].

RA synovial fluid, notably, possesses stimulatory activity for monocytes, documented by their increased FcγR I/III and HLA-DR expression following exposure to synovial fluid *in vitro*[29,52]. This process is mediated by a member of the signal transducer and activator of transcription (STAT) family, proceeds in an IFN-γ-independent manner, and may involve GM-CSF or IL-6.

Vascular endothelium

The over-representation of monocytes/macrophages in the RA SM implies the existence of mechanisms that favor the infiltration of these cells, possibly based on the use of select receptor/ligand adhesion molecules[53]. While the extracellular matrix composition in RA does not differ from that of OA, differences in the recruitment of monocytes on the basis of altered expression of integrins/selectin pairs on monocytes and endothelial cells remains an interesting possibility[16]. On the endothelial side, P-selectin (CD62) appears to be a powerful molecule for binding of monocytes to arthritis synovial samples[54], with a moderate contribution of E-selectin. On the side of the RA monocytes, in turn, there is clear up-regulation of the integrins CD11b[55], CD18, and CD62-ligand[55]. Also, while *in vitro* studies point to the general importance of CD11/CD18 or VLA-4 for monocyte migration, RA lining and sublining macrophages preferentially coexpress the α_d/CD18 integrin and its counter-receptor ICAM-3[53], suggesting a monocyte-selective role for this adhesion pair. *In vitro* studies with mature macrophages suggest also that the pattern of integrin expression on monocytes may change depending upon exposure to cytokines, particularly TNF-α[16].

Recent animal studies also indicate a potential role for osteopontin, a bone matrix protein mediating macrophage migration in wound healing, whose over-expression in chemotactically activated macrophages accounts for more than 60 per cent of macrophage migration[56]. In addition to activation of the adhesion machinery, a subpopulation of RA monocytes may adhere to endothelium by virtue of a strong negative charge[55].

Extra-articular compartments

In RA, important pathophysiological alterations of the macrophage lineage can be found not only at the primary site of pathology, but also in circulation and in the bone marrow. Whether a cytokine spill-over from the inflamed synovial membrane influences precursor myeloid cells with residual plasticity (Fig. 6.1B), or whether an inherent change characterizes the 'rheumatoid' myelomonocytic lineage, remains to be clarified. Indeed, other activated cells of the myeloid lineage, that is, dendritic cells and osteoclasts, appear to contribute to disease, suggesting systemic involvement of the whole lineage.

Peripheral blood

The activation of circulating monocytes in RA, is documented by several findings:

(1) spontaneous production of several proinflammatory molecules, i.e. prostanoids and PGE$_2$[4,57], cytokines[5,27,29,58], soluble CD14[7], and neopterin[7], a molecule exclusively produced by human mononuclear phagocytes whose urinary levels correlate with disease activity[59];

(2) increased phagocytic activity;

(3) increased integrin expression and monocyte adhesiveness[54,55]; and

(4) presence of activated suppressor monocytes[17,18].

New aspects of the active participation of blood monocytes in RA are also emerging in the acute phase response (see below) or in the production of matrix-degrading enzymes. The high plasma levels of gelatinase B[44,60], for instance, thought to derive from a spill-over from the inflamed joint[60], may be at least partially due to intrinsic production by RA blood monocytes, which also produce the metalloproteinase-inhibitor TIMP-1[61]. Likewise, the Mn-superoxido-dismutase, a critical enzyme for the control of oxygen radicals, is also actively expressed by these cells[61].

Revealing features are also emerging from differential analysis of gene patterns in RA monocytes, for example in samples collected at the beginning and at the end of therapeutic leukapheresis[27], a procedure that induces clinical remission in some patients with severe RA[27a] and reduces the degree of macrophage activation[5], or from the comparison between RA and Crohn's disease[61]. In addition to the expected cytokine gene activation, RA monocytes display gene activation for the chemokine GRO (or melanoma growth activity factor) and thrombospondin-1. Notably, these molecules are also over-expressed in the RA joints, suggesting that RA monocytes are imprinted with a 'rheumatoid' phenotype before entry in the inflamed tissue. Immigration into the inflamed synovial membrane may thus accentuate, but not initiate, disease-related activation of macrophages.

Novel or functionally undefined genes are also over-expressed in RA monocytes, for example the glycoprotein gp39[62], which is associated with late stages of monocyte differentiation and is also over-expressed in RA tissue macrophages[62]. These findings suggest that the pathogenetic potential of RA blood monocytes, and perhaps that of macrophages altogether, requires exploration.

Bone marrow

Because of the systemic nature of RA and the lack of a clear etiology, research is also directed at evaluating a potential role for extrasynovial compartments (Fig. 6.1B; Table 6.1). In the bone marrow of RA patients with active or severe disease, for example, the generation of CD14[+] myelomonocytic cells and their differentiation into HLA-DR[+] cells is faster than in controls[63]. The number of myeloid precursors is also elevated in the bone marrow adjacent to rheumatoid joints[64] (Fig. 6.1B). While both features are consistent with the inflammatory status of disease, the differentiation of precursor cells *in vitro* becomes insensitive to GM-CSF[63], suggesting intrinsic alterations. A possible bone marrow defect is also suspected to underlie the presence of highly proliferative potential colony forming cells (HPP-CFC) in the peripheral blood of RA patients[65,66], which form large macrophage colonies *in vitro*. Since this alteration is associated with higher incidence of interstitial pulmonary involvement[66], a contributor to poor prognosis in RA, monocyte precursors may play a role in disease severity. Finally, bone marrow stromal cells also over-express BST-1, a pre-B-cell growth factor which is significantly elevated in the sera of patients with severe RA[67] and has growth inhibition effects on monocytes/macrophages.

While it is unclear how all these aspects contribute to RA, a common potential trigger for bone marrow alterations could be the altered monokine (e.g. IL-1, IL-6, TNF-α) or growth factor milieu (e.g. GM-CSF) which builds up not only in circulation[4,29] but also in the bone marrow of RA patients[68,69]. The involvement of the myelopoietic system in RA, indeed, may also partially explain the mode of action of slow-acting antirheumatic drugs, which probably target altered precursors and/or differentiation mechanisms, or that of stem cell transplantation therapy.

Macrophages in the sub-endothelial space and the incidence of cardiovascular diseases in RA

Patients with active disease display not only increased serum levels of lipid peroxidation products[70], but also a form of dyslipoproteinemia which, due to high lipoprotein lipase activity and fast removal of lipids, leads to low plasma levels of cholesterol and triglycerids[71]. The paradoxical coexistence of low risk factors with high mortality for cardiovascular diseases, thus, might be due to a mechanism whereby partially degraded lipoproteins are increasingly cleared by macrophages through scavenger receptors. This excessive removal may lead to formation of foam cells and development of atherosclerotic plaques. The link between disease activity and activation of subendothelial macrophages, in turn, may be the high TNF-α, IL-1, and IL-6 levels in circulation[71].

Synovial–hepatic axis and systemic acute phase response (APR)

The APR in RA is part of a complex local/systemic network between macrophages, fibroblasts, and hepatocytes. The activation of this network contributes to at least three aspects of RA:

(1) the systemic pattern of inflammation;

(2) the severity of joint inflammation[72]; and

(3) the degree of radiological progression of the joint damage[73].

The macrophage-derived IL-1 and TNF-α, and the mostly fibroblast-derived IL-6 are sufficient to stimulate hepatocytes into the production of AP proteins in a hormone-like fashion[74], with IL-6 clearly representing the most important systemic AP mediator[75]. Interestingly, RA monocytes contribute to the acute phase response by producing not only IL-6, but also the AP proteins α_1-antitrypsin and apoferritin[27,61].

The synovial/systemic communication network may also have an efferent arm: the AP protein C-reactive protein (CRP) may directly stimulate macrophages through specific CRP macrophage receptors. Indeed, human macrophages exposed to CRP increase their mRNA expression for IL-1 and TNF-α[76]. Likewise, serum amyloid A can not only induce monocyte recruitment *in vivo*, but also potentiate the collagenase production by synovial fibroblasts. These effects may be the basis for the observed correlation between the APR (i.e. CRP levels) and radiological progression of joint damage[73]. However, CRP can also induce the protective IL-1Ra[76], suggesting a parallel involvement in autocrine regulatory loops.

Cellular and molecular aspects of monocyte/macrophage involvement in RA

In RA, the interplay of monocytes/macrophages with other inflammatory cells and/or their products is multifaceted, heavily depending on the balance of different factors:

(1) the abundance of physiological stimuli acting on mononuclear phagocytes (whether soluble or membrane-bound, stimulatory or suppressive;

(2) the number of different receptors involved in such stimulation; and

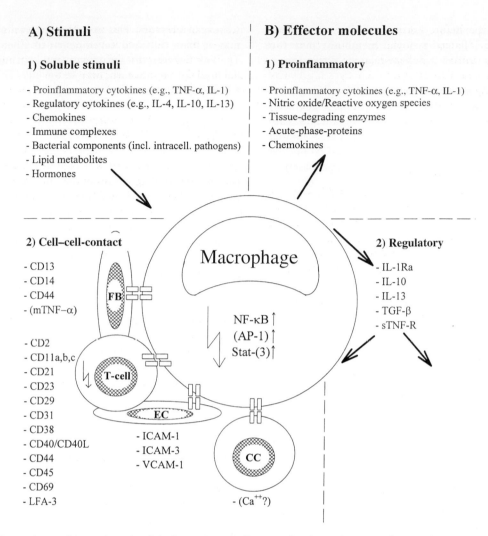

A) Stimuli

1) Soluble stimuli

- Proinflammatory cytokines (e.g., TNF-α, IL-1)
- Regulatory cytokines (e.g., IL-4, IL-10, IL-13)
- Chemokines
- Immune complexes
- Bacterial components (incl. intracell. pathogens)
- Lipid metabolites
- Hormones

2) Cell–cell-contact

- CD13
- CD14
- CD44
- (mTNF-α)

- CD2
- CD11a,b,c
- CD21
- CD23
- CD29
- CD31
- CD38
- CD40/CD40L
- CD44
- CD45
- CD69
- LFA-3

- ICAM-1
- ICAM-3
- VCAM-1

- (Ca^{++}?)

Macrophage

NF-κB ↑
(AP-1) ↑
Stat-(3) ↑

FB
T-cell
EC
CC

B) Effector molecules

1) Proinflammatory

- Proinflammatory cytokines (e.g., TNF-α, IL-1)
- Nitric oxide/Reactive oxygen species
- Tissue-degrading enzymes
- Acute-phase-proteins
- Chemokines

2) Regulatory

- IL-1Ra
- IL-10
- IL-13
- TGF-β
- sTNF-R

Fig. 6.2 Paracrine, juxtacrine, and autocrine stimuli (**column A**) and effector molecules (**column B**) of macrophage activation in RA. Most of the regulatory products of activated macrophages act on macrophages themselves, creating autocrine regulatory loops whose dysregulation possibly promotes disease severity and chronicity. **FB**: fibroblasts; **EC**: endothelial cells; **CC**: chondrocytes. The jagged arrow in the T cell indicates the necessity of preactivating T cells for effective juxtacrine stimulation of macrophages.

(3) the variety of cells infiltrating the inflamed synovial membrane, with their plethora of potential macrophage stimuli.

Likewise, the macrophage response to these stimuli must be considered from the viewpoint that macrophages exert not only proinflammatory functions, but also powerful anti-inflammatory and tissue repair functions. Finally, macrophage stimuli and macrophage responses rely heavily on autocrine regulatory mechanisms, which makes it difficult to differentiate the cause from the effect (Fig. 6.2).

Macrophage functions and their role in RA

The monocyte/macrophage system is an integral part of the natural immunity system, contributing to the first-line response against infectious agents. Also crucial to the body's

homeostasis is the scavenging function of any debris generated by physiological or pathological processes. Recognition and incorporation of the material to be cleared occurs through a number of complex surface and intracellular processes, some of which are described below in view of their pathogenetic relevance in RA.

Clearance of immune complexes

Clearance of immune complexes is triggered by Ig binding to several types of Fc receptors present on the surface of synovial macrophages[77], some of which show affinity for monomeric IgG and others for high-molecular weight immune complexes[78]. While in RA the removal of rheumatoid factor could prevent its pathogenic deposition, the cross-linking of Fc-R is also a powerful macrophage-activation stimulus[79,80]. This may result on the one hand in protective responses (e.g. reduction of T-cell stimulation by inhibiting the CD80/CD86 second signal system), but on the other hand in aggravating responses, such as the production of the proinflammatory cytokines IL-1, IL-6, IL-8, TNF-α, MCP-1 and GM-CSF[78], thereby, tilting the balance towards a predominant proinflammatory and chemotactic milieu.

Immune complexes can also be opsonized by complement factors, thereby binding to macrophage complement receptors (CR1, CR3, and CR4) and inducing release of proinflammatory cytokines, another mechanism whereby the synovial cytokine milieu can be affected.

Phagocytosis of particulate agents

Macrophages ingest particulate matter in two possible ways. In conventional (or *Fc-mediated*) phagocytosis, two cell processes engulf the foreign material and incorporated it by a zipper-like mechanism involving Fc and complement receptors, leading to phagolysosomal formation. The antigens derived from lysosomal degradation are typically processed for class-II-MHC-restricted presentation. In *coiling phagocytosis*, in contrast, only one process sticks out of the cell and wraps the foreign material. In this case, the ingested material is disintegrated in a lysosome-independent fashion, leading to class-I-MHC-restricted antigen presentation[82]. Given the strict correspondence between class-I MHC system and CD8+ T-cells versus class-II MHC system and CD4+ T cells[36], and owing to the influence that this correspondence exerts on the cytokine milieu at the antigen presentation site[36], macrophages may strongly affect the development of arthritis. Interestingly, both conventional and coiling and mechanisms are used in the phagocytosis of *Borrelia burgdorferi*, the causative agent of Lyme arthritis[83].

Clearance of intracellular pathogens

More generally, in view of the unifying hypothesis that viral/bacterial infections might trigger autoimmune arthritis, macrophages could prove critical in RA[84] since several agents under suspicion are obligate or facultative intracellular pathogens. On the one hand, the prolonged persistence and replication of pathogens in macrophages can directly lead to the development of arthritis. This is the case in human epidemic polyarthritis, caused by the Ross River virus[85], or in caprine-arthritis encephalitis, caused by a lentivirus that highly replicates in synovial tissue and does not elicit an antibody response. In the latter case, notably, viral replication within macrophages correlates with the severity of tissue pathology[86]. On the other hand, the host immune reaction against viral proteins present in macrophages may suffice to cause or sustain arthritis. This is the case in arthritis of the HIV-1-associated diffuse infiltrative syndrome, which, as in all other organ manifestations in this disease, is due to virus tropism for macrophages. Another example is the chronic arthritis associated with lymphotropic virus-1 (HTLV-1), which also harbors in macrophage-like synovial cells[87]. In general, the pathogen/host interaction critically influences the local pattern of cytokine synthesis, including:

(1) TNF-α and IFN-γ, which are essential for the differentiation of macrophages capable of destroying ingested bacteria; or

(2) IL-12, which is differentially elicited by different bacterial components.

Because of the differentiation effects towards Th1-like or Th2-like response, the direction of the macrophage response following bacterial or viral infection may become decisive for the potential development of autoimmunity[88].

Indeed, a recent study of multicase RA families suggested a link between RA and bacterial activation of macrophages, through the over-expression of the natural resistance-associated macrophage protein (NRAMP1) gene. This gene, located on chromosome 2q35 and critical for the handling of intracellular pathogens, appears to be linked to RA susceptibility[89]. This genetic link does not exclude, but rather is compatible with the known genetic association between HLA-DR genes and RA. In fact, while non-MHC genes may determine susceptibility to disease *per se*, class-II-MHC genes may determine disease severity, through modulation of epitope-specific responses of CD4+ T cells[36].

In spite of considerable research aimed at finding microorganism(s) responsible for the etiopathogenesis of RA, the list of which includes at least *Mycobacterium tuberculosis*[90], intestinal bacteria[91], and several viruses (for instance parvovirus B19[92]), or novel retroviruses[93], and in spite of the pathogenic influence of Mycobacteria in experimental models of arthritis[36], there is as yet no conclusive evidence on this subject. The analysis of early-diagnosed RA, before the infectious agent becomes serodetectable, might be required for this purpose.

Antigen processing/presentation

Macrophages as antigen-processing and presenting cells (APC) may be engaged in the very central aspects of autoimmunity. Since thymic class II MHC+ APC contribute to T-cell education for self- and non-self recognition[36], macrophages can already influence the physiological repertoire of tolerance to self constituents. Also, during the process of antigen recognition, macrophages can exert important cognate functions (signal 2), without which formation of the trimolecular complex MHC/antigenic epitope/T-cell receptor (signal 1) does not proceed to effector responses, but rather to tolerance[36]. Indeed, mononuclear phagocytic cells are at least capable of presenting antigen in the synovial membrane. Besides class II MHC molecules[32], the second signal molecules CD40, CD54, CD80, CD86, and ICAM-3 are all expressed on synovial macrophage-like cells adjacent to T cells[94,95]. Also, murine macrophages transfected with human class II MHC molecules linked to RA susceptibility (i.e., HLA-DR4) successfully present antigen, stimulating DR4-restricted T-cell clones[96].

In spite of the experimental evidence, the mechanisms of antigen presentation in the RA synovial membrane remain a matter of speculation. The lack of unequivocal oligoclonal T-cell expansion[36], as well as the failure to detect any candidate antigens, has questioned the significance of local antigen presentation. Also, while macrophages are the elective APC of arthritogenic epitopes in murine collagen-induced arthritis[97], in human RA it is unclear which APC is most relevant for the processing of putative antigen(s), since synovial fibroblasts and chondrocytes also become capable of antigen presentation *in vitro*[27,36]. Furthermore, well differentiated dendritic cells expressing second signal molecules are also enriched in the rheumatoid synovial tissue, clustered with activated T cells[95,98].

In principle, potential antigens may be incorporated at sites distant from the synovial membrane, for example by circulating monocytes or by dendritic cells. In this fashion, antigen could be imported to the synovial tissue via homing to the joints. Alternatively, activated monocytes located distant from the primary site of pathology may release mediators that cause synovial inflammation. Indeed, it is unclear which factors prime monocytes to locate in specific organs. Two mechanisms appear possible: monocytes may receive a 'stamp' in the bone marrow directing them to their designated sites; or monocytes may recognize their target by selective binding of their leukointegrins to paired selectins in the respective tissues[16].

Wound healing

Some of the features displayed by macrophages in chronic RA are very similar to those observed in wound repair models[99]. Sustained monocyte recruitment at the wound injury site is mediated through secretion of the monocyte chemoattractant MIP-1α[99]. Newly immigrated macrophages phagocytose matrix debris, including collagen fragments—a process that stimulates endogenous production of IL-1, TNF-α, and several growth factors. These induce fibroblasts (or macrophages themselves) to produce collagenase, stromelysin, and elastase, necessary for postinjury tissue remodeling and resolution of the fibrin clot. In parallel, macrophages also produce TIMP, providing a self-containing control mechanism against excessive tissue destruction, as well as TGF-β and growth factors, which activate endothelial cells and fibroblasts for tissue reconstruction. Granulation tissue, a loose connective tissue with a dense capillary network, is then formed and gradually replaced by healing fibrous tissue. The above features, similar to those observed in the RA synovial membrane, suggest that sustained macrophage and fibroblast activation may be partially driven by the necessity for repairing damaged synovial or cartilage tissue, as in RA. At the same time, the repair stimuli may be opposed by persistent inflammatory stimuli.

Chemotaxis and angiogenesis

Several studies have documented the existence of a positive feedback between macrophage-derived cytokines (for example TNF-α and IL-1) and several chemotactic factors for monocytes, for example IL-8 and monocyte chemoattractant protein 1 (MCP-1), which are produced by synovial macrophages in an autocrine fashion (Fig. 6.2)[38]. The highest levels of secreted IL-8 are observed in patients with seropositive RA, indicating a correlation with a particularly vigorous macrophage activation[37]. Significantly, IL-8 derived from synovial macrophages is a powerful promoter of angiogenesis, thus providing a link between macrophage activation and the often impressive neovascularization of the RA synovial membrane[100]. In addition, angiogenesis in the synovial membrane is promoted by soluble forms of adhesion molecules, such as VCAM-1 and ELAM-1[101], both of which are present on cells in the synovial lining of RA patients[102]. Since adhesion molecules such as VCAM-1 are upregulated by macrophage-derived cytokines, or by cocultivation of synovial fibroblasts and macrophages *in vitro*, it seems likely that macrophages play a pivotal role in inducing angiogenesis in the rheumatoid synovium.

Lipid metabolism

Lipid metabolism in macrophages involves multiple receptors and complex biochemical pathways which lead to the synthesis of prostaglandins (PG) and leukotrienes. While the proinflammatory activity of these molecules in RA is long defined, renewed attention has recently arisen from the discovery of nuclear receptor family transcription factors, the peroxisome proliferator-activated receptors-α and -γ (PPAR-α and -γ)[103,104], that bind endogenous PG and leukotriene metabolites. Upon activation, macrophages up-regulate these receptors; however, *in vitro* exposure to self-produced PGD$_2$ metabolites down-regulates several parameters of macrophage activation, including the production of TNF-α, IL-1β, and IL-6, as well as that of inducible nitric oxide synthase (iNOS) and gelatinase B. This provides an autocrine mechanism with negative feed-back, whereby activated cells control for their own degree of activation. Ligand binding to PPAR receptors also down-regulates the expression of the scavenger receptor A, which is responsible for the uptake of oxdized low-density lipoprotein, the process involved in altered lipid metabolism and cardiovascular alterations in RA (see above). Since some non-steroidal anti-inflammatory drugs (NSAIDs) act as PPAR-γ receptor agonists, the development of more specific, highly potent NSAID derivatives might also be promising for the pharmacological modulation of macrophage activation.

A link between lipid metabolism, macrophage function, and inflammation in RA may be represented by the effects of polyunsaturated fatty acids in the diet. Indeed, linoleic acid-rich n-6 polyunsaturated fatty acids (corn oil) enhance the production of IL-1, whereas oleic-rich n-3- or n-9 polyunsaturated fatty acids (fish or olive oil) down-modulate IL-1. These effects may underlie the observation that fish-based diets are associated with clinical improvement of human and experimental arthritis[105].

Stimuli of monocyte/macrophage activation in RA

Cell–cell interaction

Research in recent years has documented that a significant part of macrophage effector responses occurs in the absence of soluble stimuli, through cell contact-dependent signaling[13] (Fig. 6.2). In RA, the physical interaction of macrophages with neighboring cells of the inflamed synovial membrane has quickly become an active area of research[106,107] aimed at clarifying the signals underlying cell interaction, at dissecting the outcome of simplified interactions, and also at establishing the hierarchy of interactions relevant to arthritis. Several cell interaction models have been devised for this purpose[108,109].

T cell–macrophage interaction

All known macrophage functions, that is accessory, inflammatory, effector, and inhibitory, can be stimulated by paraformaldehyde-fixed, preactivated T cells or by plasma membranes of activated T cells[13]. As T-cell preactivation is an absolute requirement, surface molecules induced by the activation of T cells are assumed to mediate their stimulatory action on macrophages[13]. Cell–cell contact between fixed T cells and monocytes, for example, or the mere interaction of T-cell membrane fragments and monocytes, activates synovial macrophages to produce metalloproteinases[107]; this process involves the CD69 molecule, expressed on recently activated T cells. Contact between anti-CD3 preactivated T cells and monocytes is a potent stimulus for IL-1α and IL-1β mRNA production[110]. In addition, T cells prestimulated in an antigen-mimicking fashion stimulate TNF-α and IL-10 production once in contact with monocytes; interestingly, T-cell-bound membrane-TNF-α appears to play an important role in this process. Conversely, fixed T cells stimulated in an antigen-independent fashion (i.e. with IL-15, IL-2, or a combination of IL-6 and TNF-α), induce monocyte production of TNF-α but not IL-10[111].

Based on these findings, one hypothesis suggests that the early phase of RA could represent an antigen-specific T-cell–macrophage interaction. Conversely, an antigen-independent interaction may become more prominent in chronic phases of RA, dominated by an exuberant cytokine milieu. This model would also explain the paucity of IL-10 in the RA synovial membrane (see below), as well as the relative inefficacy of antigen- or T-cell-receptor-directed therapies in chronic RA.

Fibroblast–macrophage interaction

Because macrophages and fibroblasts are the most active cells in the RA synovium, their interaction is particularly interesting in view of the resulting effector responses and their relevance to cartilage destruction. Indeed, *in vitro* model systems show significant cartilage degradation by cocultures of mouse fibroblasts and macrophages, which markedly exceeds the degradation observed with each culture alone[106]. Also, the mere contact of these two cell types elicits the production of IL-6, GM-CSF, and IL-8, but not that of IL-1, IL-10, and TNF-α[108]. Cytokine output can be enhanced or down-modulated not only by addition of proinflammatory or regulatory cytokines (e.g. IL-4, IL-10, IL-13, or IL-1Ra), but also by neutralization of the LPS/LAM receptor CD14[108] (see below). More recently, purified synovial fibroblasts cocultured with myelomonocytic cell lines have been shown to induce cartilage degradation *in vitro*. The mechanism of this response, however, seems to be paracrine- and not cell-contact-mediated, since cartilage degradation is most effectively blocked by a mixture of anti-IL-1 and anti-TNF-α mAbs[112].

Soluble stimuli

Proinflammatory cytokines

While in infectious diseases the main macrophage activator is IFN-γ, in RA this cytokine is conspicuously scarce[1], as is IL-2[1]. In view of the antigen-driven T-cell hypothesis of RA, therefore, other T-cell products with powerful macrophage-activating effects (for example GM-CSF, IL-15 or IL-17[113–115]) are likely to operate in the synovial membrane.

Interleukin 15 IL-15, an IL-2-like cytokine with chemoattractant properties for memory T cells[116], might play a leading role in the interaction between T cells and macrophages. IL-15 is highly expressed in the RA synovial fluid, produced by lining layer cells, including macrophages[116] (see below). Notably, IL-15-stimulated peripheral blood or synovial T cells induce macrophages to produce IL-1β, TNF-α, IL-8, and MCP-1[111,114,117] but not IL-10[111]. This stimulation proceeds via obligatory cell–cell contact. The IL-15 produced by macrophages, in turn, may (re)stimulate T cells, creating a self-perpetuating proinflammatory cycle[117].

Interleukin 17 The newly described T-cell cytokine IL-17 appears to possess powerful stimulating properties on macrophages, documented by the increased production of IL-1 and TNF-α (apparently NF-κB-mediated), as well as of IL-10 and IL-1Ra[115]. The induction of TNF-α production can be completely reversed by addition of IL-10.

Bacterial components

The ability of bacterial factors (toxins or superantigens) to initiate proinflammatory responses characterized by secretion of macrophage-derived cytokines is under intense scrutiny, in view of the possible micro-organism etiology of RA. The prototype of these factors is lipopolysaccharide (LPS), which binds to macrophages through the CD14 receptor and which, *in vitro*, stimulates these cells to produce IL-1β, TNF-α, and MIP-1α. Staphylococcal enterotoxin B (SEB), also a potent macrophage-activating factor *in vitro* and *in vivo*, enhances arthritis features in MRL-*lpr/lpr* mice. Anti-TNF-α therapy, in this case, reverses both the severe wasting effects of SEB and the incidence of arthritis, indicating that TNF-α is central in this system[118].

Lipoarabinomannan (LAM), a mycobacterial lipoglycan with biological activities ranging from attenuating host immune responses to mediating the entry of mycobacteria into macrophages[119], interacts with macrophages in two ways. On the one hand it binds to macrophages via LPS receptors, inducing CD14-mediated monocyte chemotaxis. On the other hand it can bind via mannose receptors, inducing selective IL-12 production and subsequent differentiation of T cells towards a Th1-like phenotype. Furthermore, LAM stimulates macrophages (but not T cells) to produce TNF-α, GM-CSF, IL-1, IL-6, IL-8, and IL-10[119].

Hormones

The common observations that: (1) RA is more frequent in women in reproductive age than in men of corresponding age; (2) clinical fluctuations occur during the menstrual cycle; and (3) disease improves during pregnancy, point to a pathophysiological basis in the expression of sex hormone receptors on RA synovial macrophages[120]. Indeed, physiological concentrations of androgens inhibit, and estrogens stimulate the production of the proinflammatory cytokine IL-1 by RA macrophages. Conversely, higher concentrations of estrogens inhibit IL-1 production, perhaps mimicking the clinical improvement during pregnancy[120].

Regulation of monocyte/macrophage activation in RA

Regulatory cytokines

Interleukin 4

The prototypic anti-inflammatory cytokines. IL-4, is also believed to play a protective role in arthritis, although its virtual absence from synovial samples points rather to the lack of protective mechanisms than to the presence of active regulation[121]. Produced by Th2-like cells, this cytokine down-modulates monocyte/macrophage cytotoxicity and cytokine production, including TNF-α and TNF-α receptors[122], as well as IL-15-induced chemokine production[114]. Notably, IL-4 decreases IL-1β production while increasing the IL-1Ra production, thus offering a 'co-ordinated' anti-inflammatory approach[123]. IL-4 also decreases the mRNA production of COX-2 and cytosolic phospholipase A2, thereby reducing the levels of PGE$_2$[124]. In RA, IL-4 decreases the monokine production in *ex vivo* synovial specimens[121], or the TNF-α receptor expression by synovial fluid macrophages[122]. Importantly, IL-4 reduces bone resorption[121] as well as synovial proliferation *in vitro*. Consistent with all these macrophage regulatory effects, experimental therapy with IL-4 suppresses streptococcal cell wall-induced arthritis, a strongly macrophage-dependent model[123].

Interleukin 10

IL-10 is a clear example of a macrophage-derived cytokine affecting macrophage functions in an autocrine fashion (Fig. 6.2). IL-10 reduces HLA-DR expression and antigen presentation in monocytes and inhibits the production of proinflammatory cytokines, including TNF-α, by synovial fluid macrophages. Accordingly, IL-10 has a suppressive effects in experimental arthritis, based also on chemokine down-regulation[125]. Exposure of RA synovial mononuclear cells to IL-10 induces a major decrease of TNF-α, IL-1, and GM-CSF, as well as of HLA-DR molecules and Fc-γ receptors.

In spite of IL-10 elevation in serum and synovial compartments of RA patients, some studies suggest a relative deficiency of IL-10[126]. This deficiency, combined with that of IL-4, may therefore tilt the cytokine balance to a proinflammatory predominance. Because of the autocrine regulatory effects of IL-10, this imbalance may thus further enhance the 'rheumatoid' macrophage imprint.

Interleukin 13

Similar to IL-4 and IL-10, IL-13 exerts suppressive effects in experimental arthritis[127], probably through a selective effect on monocytes/macrophages, since B and T cells do not carry IL-13 receptors. In RA, IL-13 can be produced by synovial fluid mononuclear cells, which, exposed to exogenous IL-13, diminish in turn their production of IL-1 and TNF-α. IL-13, therefore, may also be part of macrophage autocrine circuits (Fig. 6.2). Much the same can be said for IL-1Ra, as described below.

Monocyte/macrophage effector molecules in RA

Proinflammatory cytokines

Tumor necrosis factor-α

TNF-α is a pleiotropic cytokine which increases the expression of cytokines, adhesion molecules, PGE$_2$, collagenase, and collagen by synovial cells. In RA, TNF-α is mostly produced by macrophages[1] and is believed to be a critical cytokine in the inflammatory cascade. The importance of TNF-α is documented by several *in vivo* observations:

(1) lymph node TNF-α production precedes clinical synovitis in experimental arthritides[128,128a];

(2) neutralization of TNF-α suppresses collagen-induced arthritis;

(3) combinations of IL-1 and TNF-α are potent inducers of synovitis[129]; and

(4) transgenic, deregulated expression of TNF-α alone can cause the development of chronic arthritis, however disease can be completely reversed by anti-IL-1-receptor treatment[130].

In RA, TNF-α^+ macrophages are found not only in the synovial membrane, but also at the cartilage–pannus junction. Also, the TNF-α levels in the synovial fluid correlate with the number of lining macrophages and with the degree of radiologically assessed bone erosion[131]. While an average of 5 per cent of synovial cells express TNF-α mRNA *in situ*[1], the degree of TNF-α expression in the synovial tissue seems to depend upon the prevailing histological configuration[24] (see above).

While soluble TNF-α can act at a distance from its release site, membrane-bound TNF-α seems involved in locally restricted, cell-contact-mediated processes, and appears the prime stimulator of the p75 receptor[132]. Interestingly, the transgenic expression of this form alone is sufficient to induce chronic arthritis[133], likewise, a mutant membrane-TNF-α, which utilizes both p55 and p75 receptors, can also cause arthritis[134]. Conversely, the soluble form of TNF-α, which primarily stimulates the p55 receptor, seems to mediate more transient effects[132]. Consistent with the activating role of TNF-α in leukocyte extravasation[135], anti-TNF-α treatment reduces endothelial E-selectin and VCAM-1 in synovial samples, as well as the levels of E-selectin, ICAM-1, IL-8, and VEGF in circulation[130]. this down-modulation may lead to deactivation of the vascular endothelium and suppression of angiogenesis, as substantiated by animal studies[136].

TNF-α receptors

TNF-receptors are highly expressed in synovial tissue and fluid of RA patients[35,135], especially in more severe disease[135]. There are 2 known TNF-receptors, the p55 (TNF-R1; high-affinity receptor) and the p75 (TNF-R2; low affinity receptor). The resulting stable or transient character of the ligand/receptor complex, respectively, mediates different cellular responses to soluble and trans-membrane-TNF-α. TNF-receptors can also be shed, binding to soluble TNF-α and hence acting as natural inhibitors in disease[138].

Interleukin-1

In addition to its proinflammatory properties, IL-1 induces proteoglycan degradation and inhibition of proteoglycan synthesis in cartilage[139]. At the same time, IL-1 induces the production of the metalloproteinases stromelysin and collagenase[14], and enhances bone resorption[140]. In RA, IL-1 mRNA is found predominantly in CD14+ macrophages[1,141], and IL-1 levels in the synovial fluid significantly correlate with the joint inflammatory activity[14]. Significantly, the balance between IL-1 and its physiological inhibitor IL-1Ra is shifted in favor of IL-1[21], indicating a dysregulation in the cytokine network which may be crucial in promoting chronicity.

Anti-inflammatory/regulatory cytokines

Macrophages also generate anti-inflammatory cytokines (Fig. 6.2), most notably IL-Ra and IL-10 (the latter described above), both cytokines utilizing autocrine regulatory loops for the control of macrophage function (Fig. 6.2).

Interleukin-1 receptor antagonist

Differentiated macrophages constitutively express IL-1Ra, which binds to IL-1 receptors without evoking physiological responses[14]. This protein is up-regulated by proinflammatory cytokines, including IL-1 itself or GM-CSF, and induces strong anti-inflammatory effects[14]. By means of this feedback mechanism, macrophages can contribute to the termination of inflammatory reactions. The critical relevance of IL-1 in chronic RA[14], as well as the imbalance between IL-1 and IL-1Ra[21], constitute the rationale for therapy with IL-1Ra[142].

Cytokines with a dual role in arthritis

Interleukin-6

In RA, IL-6 is the most strikingly elevated cytokine, especially in the synovial fluid during acute disease[143]. The acute rise is consistent with its role in acute phase responses (see above). IL-6 levels in the synovial fluid correlate with the degree of radiological joint damage, and IL-6 and soluble IL-6 receptors promote the generation of osteoclasts[144]. While IL-6 is mostly produced by synovial fibroblasts and only partially by macrophages[1], two findings suggest that the striking IL-6 rise is a prominent outcome of macrophage activation:

(1) the co-localization of IL-6-expressing fibroblasts with CD14+ macrophages in the RA synovial tissue; and

(2) the *in vitro* and coculture studies showing that IL-1 stimulates IL-6 production.

In experimental arthritis, IL-6 is clearly necessary for disease development[145]. During the course of arthritis, however, this cytokine may exert a dual role, protecting cartilage in acute disease but promoting excessive bone formation in chronic disease[146]. A dual role for IL-6 is conceivable also in human RA, since:

(1) unexpected elevations of IL-6 have been observed in patients undergoing clinical improvement; and

(2) IL-6 elevations coincide not only with acute arthritis but also with histological signs of chronic synovitis.

Transforming growth factor-β

In RA, different TGF-β molecules and TGF-β receptors are expressed by lining and sublining macrophages[147], as well as at the cartilage–pannus junction[148] and in the synovial fluid. TGF-β is a main regulator of connective tissue remodeling, controlling both matrix production and degradation. In experimental animals, TGF-β can induce synovial inflammation but it can also suppress acute and chronic arthritis. In the latter case, TGF-β can act as a regulatory molecule, especially by contrasting some IL-1 effects, that is, lymphocyte proliferation, metalloproteinase production, and phagocytosis of collagen. On the other hand, synovial fluid TGF-β induces the expression of Fc-γRIII macrophage receptor, whose stimulation induces release of tissue-damaging reactive oxygen species[149]. Likewise, TGF-β is a potent chemotactic factor for leukocytes, promoting monocyte adhesion and possibly resulting in excessive inflammatory infiltration in chronic disease[150]. Another deleterious effect can be that of enhancing the proliferation of synovial fibroblasts, which may limit the therapeutic potential of TGF-β.

The inhibiting effects on metalloproteinases are also controversial. While the inhibition of gelatinase B and collagenase suggest a protective role of TGF-β in tissue destruction[151], the increase of collagenase 3 production by chondrocytes may aggravate cartilage damage[152]. Indeed, the TGF-β regulation of MMP and TIMP may depend on different tissue domains (superficial versus deep cartilage layers) and may also vary for intra- or extracellular digestion of collagen (although in all cases in clear antagonism to IL-1)[152]. Metalloproteinases themselves can also affect TGF-β, by regulating the shedding of latent TGF-β attached to decorin[153] and thereby creating a loop that may enhance disease.

Nitric oxide (NO) and reactive oxygen species (ROS)

In RA, variable numbers of synovial lining macrophages express inducible nitric oxide synthase (iNOS), representing a source of NO[154]. Synovial cells exposed to NO increase their TNF-α production[154], possibly adding to the mechanisms that promote synovitis. NO may also be relevant to arthritis for its effects on bone remodeling[155]. However, it is becoming increasingly clear that NO can also exert protective effects in experimental autoimmunity[156], limiting perhaps the antiarthritic impact of selective antagonists for human iNOS.

RA macrophages also produce ROS[157], which are involved in distal inflammatory processes. Their enhanced mitochondrial production in RA blood monocytes correlates indeed with plasma levels of TNF-α, confirming the stimulatory effect of this cytokine on ROS production[157].

Studies of experimental models of arthritis

Experimental arthritides with histological similarities to human RA confirm the role(s) of macrophages and/or their products in synovitis[27], including:

(1) macrophage infiltration and activation patterns;

(2) migration mechanisms of bone marrow-derived monocytes;

(3) maturation into effector and immunoregulatory subpopulations;

(4) activation of circulating monocytes and extra-articular macrophages;

(5) leading role of TNF-α;

(6) sensitivity to cytokine-based therapy, including gene therapy approaches; and

(7) sensitivity to reduction of monocyte recruitment or depletion of activated macrophages/osteoclasts.

In addition to the TNF-α transgenic models of arthritis (see above), two recent transgenic manipulations are worth mentioning. The first is a back-cross of TNF-α transgenic mice with arthritis-susceptible DBA/1 mice, which resulted in arthritis with enhanced production of TNF-α, IL-1, and IL-6 in the synovial membrane, but with remarkable paucity of macrophage and lymphocyte infiltration[158]. The second is the back-cross of a T-cell receptor (TCR) transgene with the non-obese diabetes (NOD) strain[159], which results in arthritis achieved through chance TCR allorecognition of a NOD-derived class II MHC molecule. This model is remarkable, first, in demonstrating how erosive arthritis can result from a general breakdown of tolerance rather than from autoimmunity to a joint-specific antigen. Also, at odd with the above TNF-α/DBA/1 model, this model is characterized by predominant macrophage infiltration and, notably, by other striking similarities to human RA—Synovitis of the distal joints, lymphocyte clustering close to macrophage infiltrates, and predominant PMN exudation in the synovial fluid. Also, IL-6 is produced at very high levels and TNF-α at high levels, whereas IFN-γ, IL-2, and IL-4 are barely detectable. The comparative study of these two models may thus possibly shed light on the general mechanisms of macrophage involvement in arthritis.

Treatment of human RA with conventional anti-macrophage approaches

The definition of the role of macrophage-derived cytokines in the perpetuation of RA[27], of the pathophysiological and therapeutic dichotomy between inflammation and cartilage destruction, and of the crucial significance of activated macrophages in the synovial membrane in relationship to permanent joint damage[9], has prompted a radical re-evaluation of the concepts underlying the current regimens of anti-inflammatory and disease-modifying treatments. While the cytokine and adhesion molecule studies have generated seminal studies on the effects of IL-1Ra, anti-TNF-α, and anti-ICAM-1 in RA patients (Fig. 6.3), research concerning currently used agents with antimacrophage actions is now aimed at potentiating such effects.

Disease-modifying antirheumatic therapy

Empirically introduced disease-modifying antirheumatic drugs (DMARDs) possess a broad array of antimacrophage effects[10].

Gold compounds

Administration of gold compounds to RA patients results in gold accumulation in the lysosomes of synovial macrophages, especially in lysosome-rich sublining macrophages[160]. In monocytes, gold compounds inhibit Fc and C3 receptor expression, oxygen radical generation, and IL-1 production[27]. Through their effects on macrophages as accessory cells, gold compounds also inhibit T-cell proliferation in response to antigen or mitogen[27]. Gold compounds inhibit the production of IL-1, IL-8, and MCP-1[161] and decrease monocyte chemotaxis *in vitro*[27]. In the synovial lining, this is paralleled by a significant decrease in macrophage numbers and IL-1, IL-6, and TNF-α production[8,10]. *In vitro*, gold salts inhibit angiogenic properties of macrophages, probably through their thiol moiety[162], which colocalizes in macrophage lysosomes together with gold[160]. In experimental arthritis, gold salts seem much more effective as long-term disease-modifying-drugs than anti-inflammatory agents, also hardly reducing the incidence of synovitis. Thus, their antirheumatic effects are compatible with the multiple influence on arthritis-perpetuating features of monocytes/macrophages.

Methotrexate (MTX)

One of the most effective DMARDs, MTX, also impairs chemotaxis of blood monocytes[27] and monokine production[163], while increasing the production of cytokine inhibitors, including soluble TNF-receptor p75[163]. Because MTX shifts the IL-1/IL-1Ra balance in favor of IL-1Ra, this drug may pharmacologically correct the imbalance between these two mediators[163,164]. A change in the monokine balance, including TNF-α, may indirectly cause the significant, selective decrease of collagenase production in the synovial tissue following MTX treatment[164].

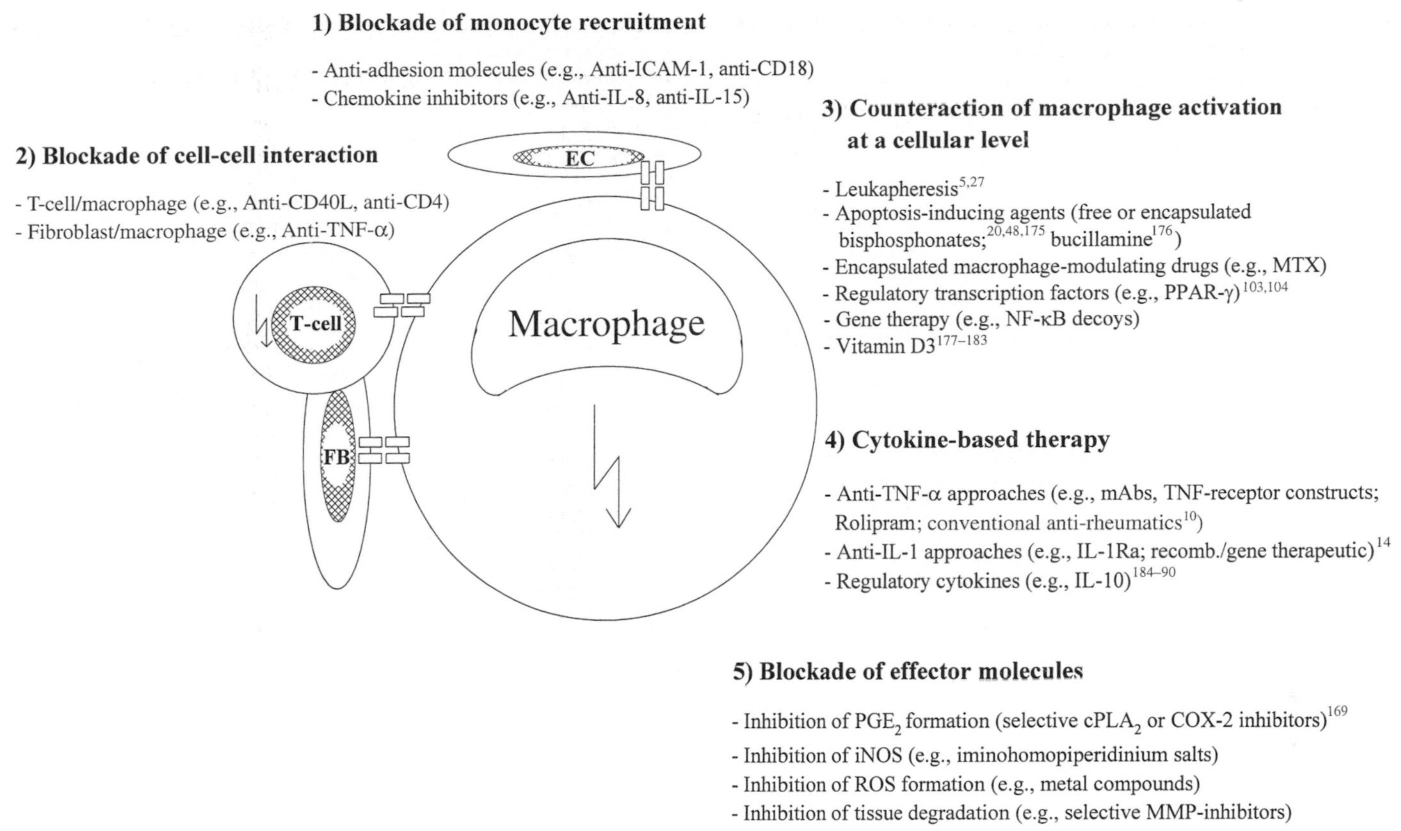

1) Blockade of monocyte recruitment

- Anti-adhesion molecules (e.g., Anti-ICAM-1, anti-CD18)
- Chemokine inhibitors (e.g., Anti-IL-8, anti-IL-15)

2) Blockade of cell-cell interaction

- T-cell/macrophage (e.g., Anti-CD40L, anti-CD4)
- Fibroblast/macrophage (e.g., Anti-TNF-α)

3) Counteraction of macrophage activation at a cellular level

- Leukapheresis[5,27]
- Apoptosis-inducing agents (free or encapsulated bisphosphonates;[20,48,175] bucillamine[176])
- Encapsulated macrophage-modulating drugs (e.g., MTX)
- Regulatory transcription factors (e.g., PPAR-γ)[103,104]
- Gene therapy (e.g., NF-κB decoys)
- Vitamin D3[177–183]

4) Cytokine-based therapy

- Anti-TNF-α approaches (e.g., mAbs, TNF-receptor constructs; Rolipram; conventional anti-rheumatics[10])
- Anti-IL-1 approaches (e.g., IL-1Ra; recomb./gene therapeutic)[14]
- Regulatory cytokines (e.g., IL-10)[184–90]

5) Blockade of effector molecules

- Inhibition of PGE_2 formation (selective $cPLA_2$ or COX-2 inhibitors)[169]
- Inhibition of iNOS (e.g., iminohomopiperidinium salts)
- Inhibition of ROS formation (e.g., metal compounds)
- Inhibition of tissue degradation (e.g., selective MMP-inhibitors)

Fig. 6.3 Modulation of monocyte/macrophage functions in RA. FB: Fibroblasts; EC: endothelial cells.

Antimalarials

Endowed with significant antirheumatic effects in early RA, but apparently less effective than gold, antimalarials are attractive because of their limited toxicity. Their tropism for lysosomes[165] is probably the cause for their slow accumulation in macrophages, in which they inhibit the release of arachidonate and the production of PGE2 via phospholipase A_2 inhibition[166]. At high concentrations, antimalarials also inhibit the production of IL-1 and TNF-α in LPS-stimulated macrophages[167].

Corticosteroids

At pharmacological doses, corticosteroids exert potent anti-inflammatory effects in RA, which can be at least partially explained by transcriptional down-regulation of the inflammatory cytokines IL-1 and IL-6, or, as recently reported, transcriptional and post-transcriptional TNF-α down-regulation in monocytes[168]. Corticosteroids may also potentially affect the balance of membrane-bound and soluble TNF-α, which exert different functions[132]. Interestingly, *in vitro* studies suggest that addition of low doses of IL-4 and IL-10 decreases the dose of corticosteroids necessary to down-modulate TNF-α, possibly via a co-ordinated attack on activated macrophages. If applicable in RA, such optimization may reduce the degree of corticosteroid side-effects. Another interesting corticosteroid effect is the decreased production of IL-8 and MCP-1[38,161], which, once opti-

mally exploited, may limit the self-perpetuating ingress of these cells in the inflamed joint.

Non-steroidal anti-inflammatory drugs (NSAIDs)

Aspirin, the most classic anti-inflammatory drug, reduces the production of PGE_2 through acetylation of the isoforms 1 and 2 of the cyclooxygenase (COX). While its use has been limited by the gastric side-effects (mostly COX-1-dependent), a new wave of interest may arise from the discovery that some aspirin derivatives potently and selectively inactivate the inducible COX-2 isoform, both in isolated macrophages and in an *in vivo* model of local inflammation[169]. In RA, the potential of COX-2 selective drugs is particularly interesting, since COX-2-dependent mechanisms selectively induce the production of IL-6. Aspirin may also affect macrophages by decreasing the TNF-α production via NF-κB mechanisms[170].

Conclusions

The variety and extent of macrophage-derived cytokines in RA and their reverberating effects (including those directed to other cells of the myeloid lineage), indicate that macrophages are local and systemic amplifiers of disease severity and perpetuation. The main *local* mechanisms include:

(1) self-perpetuating, chemokine-mediated recruitment of inflammatory cells;

(2) cytokine-mediated activation of newly immigrated inflammatory cells;

(3) cell-contact-mediated activation of neighboring inflammatory cells;

(4) cytokine- and cell-contact-mediated secretion of matrix degrading enzymes;

(5) activation of mature dendritic cells, *plus* cytokine-mediated differentiation of B cells, T cells, macrophages, fibroblasts, and chondrocytes into antigen-presenting cells, with possible effects on spreading of autoimmunity to cryptic epitopes;

(6) neovascularization, with potentiation of cellular and exudatory mechanisms;

(7) differentiation of macrophages into osteoclasts involved in subchondral bone damage.

At a *systemic* level, amplification of disease can proceed at least through the following mechanisms:

(1) acute phase response network;

(2) systemic production of TNF-α;

(3) bone marrow differentiation anomalies; and

(4) chronic activation of circulating monocytes.

Although uncovering the etiology of disease remains the ultimate means to silence the whole pathogenetic process, the efforts currently being made in understanding how activated macrophages influence disease are generating new concepts of how conventional treatments can be optimized to target macrophages selecctively, and of how new agents can be devised on the basis of specific features of macrophage activation in RA. This approach has at least two advantages:

(1) striking the very cell population that mediates/amplifies most of the irreversible cartilage destruction; and

(2) minimizing adverse effects on other cells that may have no (or marginal) effects on joint damage.

Reducing the numbers of activated macrophages by means of selective apoptosis-inducing agents, inhibiting activation signals and/or their specific macrophage receptors, or selectively counteracting the macrophage products that act as disease amplifiers (Fig. 6.3), are but a few possibilities.

References

1. Firestein G.S., Alvaro-Gracia J.M., Maki R., Alvaro-Garcia J.M. Quantitative analysis of cytokine gene expression in rheumatoid arthritis. *J Immunol*, 1990;**144**:3347–3353.

2. Palmer D.G. The anatomy of the rheumatoid lesion. *Br Med Bull* 1995;**51**:286–295.

3. Youssef P.P., Kraan M., Breedveld F., Bresnihan B., Cassidy N., Cunnane G., *et al.* Quantitative microscopic analysis of inflammation in rheumatoid arthritis synovial membrane samples selected at arthroscopy compared with samples obtained blindly by needle biopsy. *Arthritis Rheum*, 1998;**41**:663–669.

4. Seitz M., Hunstein W. Enhanced prostanoid release from monocytes of patients with rheumatoid arthritis and active systemic lupus erythematosus. *Ann Rheum Dis*, 1985;**44**:438–445.

5. Hahn G., Stuhlmuller B., Hain N., Kalden J.R., Pfizenmaier K., Burmester G.R. Modulation of monocyte activation in patients with rheumatoid arthritis by leukapheresis therapy. *J Clin Invest*, 1993;**91**:862–870.

6. Gravallese E.M., Harada Y., Wang J.T., Gorn A.H. Thornhill T.S., Goldring S.R. Identification of cell types responsible for bone resorption in rheumatoid arthritis and juvenile rheumatoid arthritis. *Am J Pathol* 1998;**152**:943–951.

7. Horneff G., Sack U., Kalden J.R., Emmrich F., Burmester G.R. Reduction of monocyte-macrophage activation markers upon anti-CD4 treatment. Decreased levels of IL-1, IL-6, neopterin and soluble CD14 in patients with rheumatoid arthritis. *Clin Exp Immunol*, 1993;**91**:207–213.

8. Yanni G., Nabil M., Farahat M.R., Poston R.N., Panayi G.S. Intramuscular gold decreases cytokine expression and macrophage numbers in the rheumatoid synovial membrane. *Ann Rheum Dis*, 1994;**53**:315–322.

9. Mulherin D., Fitzgerald O., Bresnihan B. Synovial tissue macrophage populations and articular damage in rheumatoid arthritis. *Arthritis Rheum*, 1996;**39**:115–124.

10. Bondeson J. The mechanisms of action of disease-modifying antirheumatic drugs: a review with emphasis on macrophage signal transduction and the induction of proinflammatory cytokines. *Gen Pharmacol*, 1997;**29**:127–150.

11. Salmon S.E., Dalton W.S. Relevance of multidrug resistance to rheumatoid arthritis: development of a new therapeutic hypothesis. *J Rheumatol Suppl*, 1996;**44**:97–101.

12. Buttgereit F., Wehling M., Burmester G.R. A new hypothesis of modular glucocorticoid actions: steroid treatment of rheumatic diseases revisited. *Arthritis Rheum*, 1998;**41**:761–767.

13. Stout R.D., Suttles J. T cell signaling of macrophage function in inflammatory disease. *Front Biosci*, 1997;**2**:d197–206.

14. Arend W.P., Malyak M., Guthridge C.J., Gabay C. Interleukin-1 receptor antagonist: role in biology. *Annu Rev Immunol*, 1998;**16**:27–55.

15. Hogg N., Palmer D.G., Revell P.A. Mononuclear phagocytes of normal and rheumatoid synovial membrane identified by monoclonal antibodies. *Immunology*, 1985;**56**:673–681.

16. Pirila L., Heino J. Altered integrin expression in rheumatoid synovial lining type B cells: *in vitro* cytokine regulation of alpha 1 beta 1, alpha 6 beta 1, and alpha v beta 5 integrins. *J Rheumatol*, 1996;**23**:1691–1698.

17. Zembala M., Lemmel E.M. Inhibitory factor(s) of lymphoproliferation produced by synovial fluid mononuclear cells from rheumatoid arthritis patients: the role of monocytes in suppression. *J Immunol*, 1980;**125**:1087–1092.

18. Okawa-Takatsuji M., Aotsuka S., Uwatoko S., Yokohari R., Inagaki K. Monocyte-mediated suppression of rheumatoid factor production in normal subjects. *Clin Immunol Immunopathol*, 1988;**46**:195–204.

19. van den Berg T.KD.I., van D.I., de Lavalette C.R., Dopp E.A., Smit L.D., van der Meide P.H., *et al.* Regulation of sialoadhesin expression on rat macrophages. Induction by glucocorticoids and enhancement by IFN-beta, IFN-gamma, IL-4, and lipopolysaccharide. *J Immunol*, 1996;**157**:3130–3138.

20. Kinne R.W., Schmidt-Weber C.B., Hoppe R., Buchner E., Palombo-Kinne E., Nürnberg E., *et al.* Long-term amelioration of rat adjuvant arthritis following systemic elimination of macrophages by clodronate-containing liposomes. *Arthritis Rheum*, 1995;**38**:1777–1790.

21. Firestein G.S., Boyle D.L., Yu C., Paine M.M., Whisenand T.D., Zvaifler N.J., *et al.* Synovial interleukin-1 receptor antagonist and interleukin-1 balance in rheumatoid arthritis. *Arthritis Rheum,* 1994;37:644–652.

22. van den Berg W.B., van Lent P.L. The role of macrophages in chronic arthritis. *Immunobiology,* 1996;195:614–623.

23. Koch A.E. Review: angiogenesis: implications for rheumatoid arthritis. *Arthritis Rheum,* 1998;41:951-962.

24. Klimiuk P.A., Goronzy J.J., Bjor N.J., Beckenbaugh R.D., Weyand C.M. Tissue cytokine patterns distinguish variants of rheumatoid synovitis. *Am J Pathol,* 1997;151:1311–1319.

25. Palmer D.G., Hogg N., Highton J., Hessian P.A., Denholm I. Macrophage migration and maturation within rheumatoid nodules. *Arthritis Rheum,* 1987;30:728–736.

26. Duke O.L., Hobbs S., Panayi G.S., Poulter L.W., Rasker J.J., Janossy G. A combined immunohistological and histochemical analysis of lymphocyte and macrophage subpopulations in the rheumatoid nodule. *Clin Exp Immunol,* 1984;56:239–246.

27. Burmester G.R., Stuhlmuller B., Keyszer G., Kinne R.W. Mononuclear phagocytes and rheumatoid synovitis. Mastermind or workhorse in arthritis? *Arthritis Rheum,* 1997;40:5–18.

27a. Stuhlmöller, B., Ungethüm, U., Scholze., Martinez L., Backhaus M., Kraetsch H.-G., Kinne R.W., Burmester G.R. Identification of known and novel genes in activated monocytes from patients with rheumatoid arthritis. *Arthritis Rheum* (Press).

28. Burmester G.R., Jahn B., Rohwer P., Zacher J., Winchester R.J., Kalden J.R. Differential expression of la antigens by rheumatoid synovial lining cells. *J Clin Invest,* 1987;80:595–604.

29. Firestein G.S., Zvaifler N.J. Peripheral blood and synovial fluid monocyte activation in inflammatory arthritis. II. Low levels of synovial fluid and synovial tissue interferon suggest that gamma-interferon is not the primary macrophage activating factor. *Arthritis Rheum,* 1987;30:864–871.

30. Tak P.P., Smeets T.J., Daha M.R., Kluin P.M., Meijers K.A., Brand R., *et al.* Analysis of the synovial cell infiltrate in early rheumatoid synovial tissue in relation to local disease activity. *Arthritis Rheum,* 1997;40:217–225.

31. Sack U., Stiehl P., Geiler G. Distribution of macrophages in rheumatoid synovial membrane and its association with basic activity. *Rheumatol Int,* 1994;13:181–186.

32. Iguchi T., Kurosaka M., Ziff M. Electron microscopic study of HLA-DR and monocyte/marcophage staining cells in the rheumatoid synovial membrane. *Arthritis Rheum,* 1986;29:600–613.

33. Wagner S., Fritz P., Einsele H., Sell S., Saal J.G. Evaluation of synovial cytokine patterns in rheumatoid arthritis and osteoarthritis by quantitative reverse transcription polymerase chain reaction. *Rheumatol Int,* 1997; 16:191–196.

34. Kahle P., Saal J.G., Schaudt K., Zacher J., Fritz P., Pawelec G. Determination of cytokines in synovial fluids: correlation with diagnosis and histomorphological characteristics of synovial tissue. *Ann Rheum Dis,* 1992;51:731–734.

34a. Feldmann M., Brennan F.M., Maini R.N. Role of cytokines in rheumatoid arthritis. *Annu Rev Immunol,* 1996;14:397–440.

35. Alsalameh S., Winter K., Al-Ward R., Wendler J., Kalden J.R., Kinne R.W. Distribution of TNF-α, TNF-R55, and TNF-R75 in the rheumatoid synovial membrane: TNF-receptors are localised preferentially in the lining layer; TNF-α is distributed mainly in the vicinity of TNF-receptors in the deeper layers. *Scand J Immunol,* 1999;49:278–85.

36. Kinne R.W., Palombo-Kinne E., Emmrich F. T-cells in the pathogenesis of rheumatoid arthritis: Villains or accomplices? *Biochim Biophy Acta,* 1997;1360:109–141.

37. Seitz M., Dewald B., Gerber N., Baggiolini M. Enhanced production of neutrophil-activating peptide-1/interleukin-8 in rheumatoid arthritis. *J Clin Invest,* 1991;87:463–469.

38. Loetscher P., Dewald B., Baggiolini M., Seitz M. Monocyte chemoattractant protein 1 and interleukin 8 production by rheumatoid synoviocytes. Effects of anti-rheumatic drugs. *Cytokine,* 1994;6:162–170.

39. Koch A.E., Kunkel S.L., Harlow L.A., Mazarakis D.D., Haines G.K., Burdick M.D., *et al.* Macrophage inflammatory protein-1 alpha. A novel chemotactic cytokine for macrophages in rheumatoid arthritis. *J Clin Invest,* 1994;93:921–928.

40. Firestein G.S., Paine M.M., Littman B.H. Gene expression (collagenase, tissue inhibitor of metalloproteinases, complement, and HLA-DR) in rheumatoid arthritis and osteoarthritis synovium. Quantitative analysis and effect of intraarticular corticosteroids. *Arthritis Rheum,* 1991;34:1094–1105.

41. Gravallese E.M., Darling J.M., Ladd A.L., Katz J.N., Glimcher L.H. *In situ* hybridization studies of stromelysin and collagenase messenger RNA expression in rheumatoid synovium. *Arthritis Rheum,* 1991;34:1076–1084.

42. Tetlow L.C., Lees M., Woolley D.E. Comparative studies of collagenase and stromelysin-1 expression by rheumatoid synoviocytes *in vitro.* *Virchows Arch,* 1995;425:569–576.

43. Tetlow L.C., Lees M., Ogata Y., Nagase H., Woolley D.E. Differential expression of gelatinase B (MMP-9) and stromelysin-1 (MMP-3) by rheumatoid synovial cells *in vitro* and *in vivo.* *Rheumatol Int,* 1993;13:53–59.

44. Ahrens D., Koch A.E., Pope R.M., Stein-Picarella M., Niedbala M.J. Expression of matrix metalloproteinase 9 (96-kd gelatinase B) in human rheumatoid arthritis. *Arthritis Rheum,* 1996;39:1576–1587.

45. Fujikawa Y., Shingu M., Torisu T., Itonaga I., Masumi S. Bone resorption by tartrate-resistant acid phosphatase-positive multinuclear cells isolated from rheumatoid synovium. *Br J Rheumatol,* 1996;35:213–217.

46. Iwata Y., Mort J.S., Tateishi H., Lee E.R. Macrophage cathepsin L., a factor in the erosion of subchondral bone in rheumatoid arthritis. *Arthritis Rheum,* 1997;40:499–509.

47. Takayanagi H., Oda H., Yamamoto S., Kawaguchi H., Tanaka S., Nishikawa T., *et al.* A new mechanism of bone destruction in rheumatoid arthritis: synovial fibroblasts induce osteoclastogenesis. *Biochem Biophys Res Commun,* 1997;240:279–286.

48. Oelzner P., Brauer R., Henzgen S., Thoss K., Wünsche B., Hersmann G., *et al.* Periarticular bone alterations in chronic antigen-induced arthritis: Free and liposome-encapsulated clodronate prevent loss of bone mass in the secondary spongiosa. *Clin Immunol Immunopathol,* 1999;90:79–88.

49. Koch A.E., Kunkel S.L., Harlow L.A., Mazarakis D.D., Haines G.K., Burdick M.D., *et al.* Epithelial neutrophil activating peptide-78: a novel chemotactic cytokine for neutrophils in arthritis. *J Clin Invest* 1994;94:1012–1018.

50. Walz A., Schmutz P., Mueller C., Schnyder-Candrian S. Regulation and function of the CXC chemokine ENA-78 in monocytes and its role in disease. *J Leukoc Biol,* 1997;62:604–11.

51. al-Mughales J., Blyth T.H., Hunter J.A., Wilkinson P.C. The chemoattractant activity of rheumatoid synovial fluid for human lymphocytes is due to multiple cytokines. *Clin Exp Immunol,* 1996;106:230–236.

52. Sengupta T.K., Chen A., Zhong Z., Darnell J.E.J., Ivashkiv L.B. Activation of monocyte effector genes and STAT family transcription factors by inflammatory synovial fluid is independent of interferon gamma. *J Exp Med,* 1995;181:1015–1025.

53. El-Gabalawy H., Canvin J., Ma G.M., Van der Vieren M., Hoffman P., Gallatin M., *et al.* Synovial distribution of alpha d/CD18, a novel leukointegrin. Comparison with other integrins and their ligands. *Arthritis Rheum,* 1996;39:1913–1921.

54. Grober J.S., Bowen B.L., Ebling H., Athey B., Thompson C.B., Fox D.A., *et al.* Monocyte-endothelial adhesion in chronic rheumatoid arthritis. *In situ* detection of selectin and integrin-dependent interactions. *J Clin Invest,* 1993;91:2609–2619.

55. Mazure G., Fernandes T., McCarthy D.A., Macey M., Perry J.D., Taub N.A., *et al.* Blood monocytes in rheumatoid arthritis are highly adherent to cultured endothelium. *Int Arch Allergy Immunol,* 1995;108:211–223.

56. Giachelli C.M., Lombardi D., Johnson R.J., Murry C.E., Almeida M. Evidence for a role of osteopontin in macrophage infiltration in response to pathological stimuli *in vivo.* *Am J Pathol,* 1998;152:353–358.

57. Bomalaski J.S., Clark M.A., Zurier R.B. Enhanced phospholipase activity in peripheral blood monocytes from patients with rheumatoid arthritis. *Arthritis Rheum*, 1986;29:312–318.

58. Schulze-Koops H., Davis L.S., Kavanaugh A.F., Lipsky P.E. Elevated cytokine messenger RNA levels in the peripheral blood of patients with rheumatoid arthritis suggest different degrees of myeloid cell activation. *Arthritis Rheum*, 1997;40:639–647.

59. Reibnegger G., Egg D., Fuchs D., Gunther R., Hausen A., Werner E.R., *et al.* Urinary neopterin reflects clinical activity in patients with rheumatoid arthritis. *Arthritis Rheum*, 1986;29:1063–1070.

60. Gruber B.L., Sorbi D., French D.L., Marchese M.J., Nuovo G.J., Kew R.R., *et al.* Markedly elevated serum MMP-9 (gelatinase B) levels in rheumatoid arthritis: a potentially useful laboratory marker. *Clin Immunol Immunopathol*, 1996;78:161–171.

61. Heller R.A., Schena M., Chai A., Shalon D., Bedilion T., Gilmore J., *et al.* Discovery and analysis of inflammatory disease-related genes using cDNA microarrays. *Proc Natl Acad Sci USA*, 1997;94:2150–2155.

62. Kirkpatrick R.B., Emery J.G., Connor J.R., Dodds R., Lysko P.G., Rosenberg M. Induction and expression of human cartilage glycoprotein 39 in rheumatoid inflammatory and peripheral blood monocyte-derived macrophages. *Exp Cell Res*, 1997;237:46–54.

63. Hirohata S., Yanagida T., Itoh K., Nakamura H., Yoshino S., Tomita T., *et al.* Accelerated generation of CD14+ monocyte-lineage cells from the bone marrow of rheumatoid arthritis patients. *Arthritis Rheum*, 1996;39:836–843.

64. Kotake S., Higaki M., Sato K., Himeno S., Morita H., Kim K.J., *et al.* Detection of myeloid precursors (granulocyte/macrophage colony forming units) in the bone marrow adjacent to rheumatoid arthritis joints. *J Rheumatol*, 1992;19:1511–1516.

65. Santiago-Schwarz F., Sullivan C., Rappa D., Carsons S.E. Distinct alterations in lineage committed progenitor cells exist in the peripheral blood of patients with rheumatoid arthritis and primary Sjogren's syndrome. *J Rheumatol*, 1996;23:439–46.

66. Horie S., Nakada K., Masuyama J., Yoshio T., Minota S., Wakabayashi Y., *et al.* Detection of large macrophage colony forming cells in the peripheral blood of patients with rheumatoid arthritis. *J Rheumatol*, 1997;24:1517–1521.

67. Lee B.O., Ishihara K., Denno K., Kobune Y., Itoh M., Muraoka O., *et al.* Elevated levels of the soluble form of bone marrow stromal cell antigen 1 in the sera of patients with severe rheumatoid arthritis. *Arthritis Rheum*, 1996;39:629–637.

68. Tanabe M., Ochi T., Tomita T., Suzuki R., Sakata T., Shimaoka Y., *et al.* Remarkable elevation of interleukin 6 and interleukin 8 levels in the bone marrow serum of patients with rheumatoid arthritis. *J Rheumatol*, 1994;21:830–835.

69. Jongen-Lavrencic M., Peeters H.R., Wognum A., Vreugdenhil G., Breedveld F.C., Swaak A.J. Elevated levels of inflammatory cytokines in bone marrow of patients with rheumatoid arthritis and anemia of chronic disease. *J Rheumatol*, 1997;24:1504–1509.

70. Winyard P.G., Tatzber F., Esterbauer H., Kus M.L., Blake D.R., Morris C.J. Presence of foam cells containing oxidised low density lipoprotein in the synovial membrane from patients with rheumatoid arthritis. *Ann Rheum Dis*, 1993;52:677–680.

71. Wallberg-Jonsson S., Dahlen G., Johnson O., Olivecrona G., Rantapaa-Dahlqvist S. Lipoprotein lipase in relation to inflammatory activity in rheumatoid arthritis. *J Intern Med*, 1996;240:373–380.

72. Mallya R.K., de Beer F.C., Berry H., Hamilton E.D., Mace B.E., Pepys M.B. Correlation of clinical parameters of disease activity in rheumatoid arthritis with serum concentration of C-reactive protein and erythrocyte sedimentation rate. *J Rheumatol*, 1982;9:224–228.

73. Larsen A. The relation of radiographic changes to serum acute-phase proteins and rheumatoid factor in 200 patients with rheumatoid arthritis. *Scand J Rheumatol*, 1988;17:123–129.

74. McNiff P.A., Stewart C., Sullivan J., Showell H.J., Gabel C.A. Synovial fluid from rheumatoid arthritis patients contains sufficient levels of IL-1 beta and IL-6 to promote production of serum amyloid A by Hep3B cells. *Cytokine*, 1995;7:209–219.

75. Okamoto H., Yamamura M., Morita Y., Harada S., Makino H., Ota Z. The synovial expression and serum levels of interleukin-6, interleukin-11, leukemia inhibitory factor, and oncostatin M in rheumatoid arthritis. *Arthritis Rheum*, 1997;40:1096–1105.

76. Tilg H., Vannier E., Vachino G., Dinarello C.A., Mier J.W. Antiinflammatory properties of hepatic acute phase proteins: preferential induction of interleukin 1 (IL-1) receptor antagonist over IL-1 beta synthesis by human peripheral blood mononuclear cells. *J Exp Med*, 1993;178:1629–1636.

77. Broker B.M., Edwards J.C., Fanger M.W., Lydyard P.M. The prevalence and distribution of macrophages bearing Fc gamma R I, Fc gamma R II, and Fc gamma R III in synovium. *Scand J Rheumatol*, 1990;19:123–135.

78. Jarvis J.N., Wang W., Moore H.T., Zhao L., Xu C. *in vitro* induction of proinflammatory cytokine secretion by juvenile rheumatoid arthritis synovial fluid immune complexes. *Arthritis Rheum*, 1997;40:2039–2046.

79. Burmester G.R., Beck P., Eife R., Peter H.H., Kalden J.R. Induction of a lymphotoxin-like mediator in peripheral blood and synovial fluid lymphocytes by incubation with synovial fluid from patients with rheumatoid arthritis. *Rheumatol Int*, 1981;1:139–143.

80. MacKinnon S.K., Starkebaum G. Monocyte Fc receptor function in rheumatoid arthritis. Enhanced cell-binding of IgG induced by rheumatoid factors. *Arthritis Rheum*, 1987;30:498–506.

81. Edwards J.C., Blades S., Cambridge G. Restricted expression of Fc gamma RIII (CD16) in synovium and dermis: implications for tissue targeting in rheumatoid arthritis (RA). *Clin Exp Immunol*, 1997;108:401–406.

82. Rittig M.G., Haupl T., Burmester G.R. Coiling phagocytosis: a way for MHC class I presentation of bacterial antigens? *Int Arch Allergy Immunol*, 1994;103:4–10.

83. Rittig M.G., Haupl T., Krause A., Kressel M., Groscurth P., Burmester G.R. Borrelia burgdorferi-induced ultrastructural alterations in human phagocytes: a clue to pathogenicity? *J Pathol*, 1994;173:269–282.

84. Rook G., McCulloch J. HLA-DR4, mycobacteria, heat-shock proteins, and rheumatoid arthritis. *Arthritis Rheum*, 1992;35:1409–1412.

85. Linn M.L., Aaskov J.G., Suhrbier A. Antibody-dependent enhancement and persistence in macrophages of an arbovirus associated with arthritis. *J Gen Virol*, 1996;77:407–411.

86. Wilkerson M.J., Davis W.C., Baszler T.V., Cheevers W.P. Immunopathology of chronic lentivirus-induced arthritis. *Am J Pathol*, 1995;146:1433–1443.

87. Hasunuma T., Nakajima T., Aono H., Sato K., Matsubara T., Yamamoto K., *et al.* Establishment and characterization of synovial cell clones with integrated human T-cell leukemia virus type-I. *Clin Immunol Immunopathol*, 1994;72:90–97.

88. Finkelman F.D. Relationships among antigen presentation, cytokines, immune deviation, and autoimmune disease. *J Exp Med*, 1995;182:279–282.

89. Shaw M.A., Clayton D., Atkinson S.E., Williams H., Miller N., Sibthorpe D., *et al.* Linkage of rheumatoid arthritis to the candidate gene NRAMP1 on 2q35. *J Med Genet*, 1996;33:672–677.

90. Pras E., Schumacher H.R.J., Kastner D.L., Wilder R.L. Lack of evidence of mycobacteria in synovial tissue from patients with rheumatoid arthritis. *Arthritis Rheum*, 1996;39:2080–2081.

91. Eerola E., Mottonen T., Hannonen P., Luukkainen R., Kantola I., Vuori K., *et al.* Intestinal flora in early rheumatoid arthritis. *Br J Rheumatol*, 1994;33:1030–1038.

92. Takahashi Y., Murai C., Shibata S., Munakata Y., Ishii T., Ishii K., *et al.* Human parvovirus B19 as a causative agent for rheumatoid arthritis. *Proc Natl Acad Sci USA*. 1998;95:8227–8232.

93. Griffiths D.J., Venables P.J., Weiss R.A., Boyd M.T. A novel exogenous retrovirus sequence identified in humans. *J Virol*, 1997;71:2866–2872.

94. Ranheim E.A., Kipps T.J. Elevated expression of CD80 (B7/BB1) and other accessory molecules on synovial fluid mononuclear cell subsets in rheumatoid arthritis. *Arthritis Rheum*, 1994;37:1637–1646.

95. Liu M.F., Kohsaka H., Sakurai H., Azuma M., Okumura K., Saito I., *et al.* The presence of costimulatory molecules CD86 and CD28 in rheumatoid arthritis synovium. *Arthritis Rheum*, 1996;**39**:110–114.

96. Daubenberger C., Lang B., Nickel B., Willcox N., Melchers I. Antigen processing and presentation by a mouse macrophage-like cell line expressing human HLA class II molecules. *Int Immunol*, 1996;**8**:307–315.

97. Michaelsson E., Holmdahl M., Engstrom A., Burkhardt H., Scheynius A., Holmdahl R. Macrophages, but not dendritic cells, present collagen to T cells. *Eur J Immunol*, 1995;**25**:2234–2241.

98. Thomas R., Quinn C. Functional differentiation of dendritic cells in rheumatoid arthritis: role of CD86 in the synovium. *J Immunol*, 1996;**156**:3074–3086.

99. DiPietro L.A., Burdick M., Low Q.E., Kunkel S.L., Strieter R.M. MIP-1 alpha as a critical macrophage chemoattractant in murine wound repair. *J Clin Invest*, 1998;**101**:1693–1698.

100. Koch A.E., Polverini P.J., Kunkel S.L., Harlow L.A., DiPietro L.A., Elner V.M., *et al.* Interleukin-8 as a macrophage-derived mediator of angiogenesis. *Science*, 1992;**258**:1798–1801.

101. Koch A.E., Halloran M.M., Haskell C.J., Shah M.R., Polverini P.J. Angiogenesis mediated by soluble forms of E-selectin and vascular cell adhesion molecule-1. *Nature*, 1995;**376**:517–519.

102. Kriegsmann J., Keyszer G.M., Geiler T., Lagoo A.S., Lagoo-Deenadayalan S., Gay R.E., *et al.* Expression of E-selectin messenger RNA and protein in rheumatoid arthritis. *Arthritis Rheum*, 1995;**38**:750–754.

103. Jiang C., Ting A.T., Seed B. PPAR-gamma agonists inhibit production of monocyte inflammatory cytokines. *Nature*, 1998;**391**:82–86.

104. Ricote M., Li A.C., Willson T.M., Kelly C.J., Glass C.K. The peroxisome proliferator-activated receptor-gamma is a negative regulator of macrophage activation. *Nature*, 1998;**391**:79–82.

105. Leslie C.A., Gonnerman W.A., Ullman M.D., Hayes K.C., Franzblau C., Cathcart E.S. Dietary fish oil modulates macrophage fatty acids and decreases arthritis susceptibility in mice. *J Exp Med*, 1985;**162**:1336–1349.

106. Janusz M.J., Hare M. Cartilage degradation by cocultures of transformed macrophage and fibroblast cell lines. A model of metalloproteinase-mediated connective tissue degradation. *J Immunol*, 1993;**150**:1922-1931.

107. Lacraz S., Isler P., Vey E., Welgus H.G., Dayer J.M. Direct contact between T lymphocytes and monocytes is a major pathway for induction of metalloproteinase expression. *J Biol Chem*, 1994;**269**:22027–22033.

108. Chomarat P., Rissoan M.C., Pin J.J., Bancherau J., Miossec P. Contribution of IL-1, CD14, and CD13 in the increased IL-6 production induced by *in vitro* monocyte-synoviocyte interactions. *J Immunol*, 1995;**155**:3645–3652.

109. Schultz O., Keyszer G., Zacher J., Sittinger M., Burmester G.R. Development of *in vitro* model systems for destructive joint diseases: novel strategies inflammatory pannus. *Arthritis Rheum*, 1997;**40**:1420–1428.

110. Landis R.C., Friedman M.L., Fisher R.I., Ellis T.M. Induction of human monocyte IL-1 mRNA and secretion during anti-CD3 mitogenesis requires two distinct T cell-derived signals. *J Immunol*, 1991;**146**:128–135.

111. Sebbag M., Parry S.L., Brennan F.M., Feldmann M. Cytokine stimulation of T lymphocytes regulates their capacity to induce monocyte production of tumor necrosis factor-alpha, but not interleukin-10: possible relevance to pathophysiology of rheumatoid arthritis. *Eur J Immunol*, 1997;**27**:624–632.

112. Khalkhali-Ellis Z., Seftor E.A., Nieva D.R., Seftor R.E., Samaha H.A., Bultman L., *et al.* Induction of invasive and degradative phenotype in normal synovial fibroblasts exposed to synovial fluid from patients with juvenile rheumatoid arthritis: role of mononuclear cell population. *J Rheumatol*, 1997;**24**:2451–2460.

113. Alvaro-Gracia J.M., Zvaifler N.J., Brown C.B., Kaushansky K., Firestein G.S. Cytokines in chronic inflammatory arthritis. VI. Analysis of the synovial cells involved in granulocyte-macrophage colony-stimulating factor production and gene expression in rheumatoid arthritis and its regulation by IL-1 and tumor necrosis factor-alpha. *J Immunol*, 1991;**146**:3365–3371.

114. Badolato R., Ponzi A.N., Millesimo M., Notarangelo L.D., Musso T. Interleukin-15 (IL-15) induces IL-8 and monocyte chemotactic protein 1 production in human monocytes. *Blood*, 1997;**90**:2804–2809.

115. Jovanovic D.V., DiBattista J.A., Martel-Pelletier J., Jolicoeur F.C., He Y., Zhang M., *et al.* IL-17 stimulates the production and expression of proinflammatory cytokines, IL-1 beta and TNF-alpha, by human macrophages. *J Immunol*, 1998;**160**:3513–3521.

116. McInnes I.B., Al-Mughales J., Field M., Leung B.P., Huang F.P., Dixon R., *et al.* The role of interleukin-15 in T-cell migration and activation in rheumatoid arthritis. *Nat Med*, 1996;**2**:175–182.

117. McInnes I.B., Leung B.P., Sturrock R.D., Field M., Liew F.Y. Interleukin-15 mediates T cell-dependent regulation of tumor necrosis factor-alpha production in rheumatoid arthritis. *Nat Med*, 1997;**3**:189–195.

118. Edwards C.K., Zhou T., Zhang J., Baker T.J., De M., Long R.E., *et al.* Inhibition of superantigen-induced proinflammatory cytokine production and inflammatory arthritis in MRL-lpr/lpr mice by a transcriptional inhibitor of TNF-alpha. *J Immunol*, 1996;**157**:1758–1772.

119. Chatterjee D., Khoo K.H. Mycobacterial lipoarabinomannan: an extraordinary lipoheteroglycan with profound physiological effects. *Glycobiology*, 1998;**8**:113–120.

120. Cutolo M. Do sex hormones modulate the synovial macrophages in rheumatoid arthritis? *Ann Rheum Dis*, 1997;**56**:281–284.

121. Miossec P., Naviliat M., Dupuy DA., Sany J., Banchereau J. Low levels of interleukin-4 and high levels of transforming growth factor beta in rheumatoid synovitis. *Arthritis Rheum*, 1990;**33**:1180–1187.

122. Hart P.H., Hunt E.K., Bonder C.S., Watson C.J., Finlay-Jones J.J. Regulation of surface and soluble TNF receptor expression on human monocytes and synovial fluid macrophages by IL-4 and IL-10. *J Immunol*, 1996;**157**:3672–3680.

123. Allen J.B., Wong H.L., Costa G.L., Bienkowski M.J., Wahl S.M. Suppression of monocyte function and differential regulation of IL-1 and IL-1Ra by IL-4 contribute to resolution of experimental arthritis. *J Immunol*, 1993;**151**:4344–4351.

124. Kuroda A., Sugiyama E., Taki H., Mino T., Kobayashi M. Interleukin-4 inhibits the gene expression and biosynthesis of cytosolic phospholipase A2 in lipopolysaccharide stimulated U937 macrophage cell line and freshly prepared adherent rheumatoid synovial cells. *Biochem Biophys Res Commun*, 1997;**230**:40–43.

125. Kasama T., Strieter R.M., Lukacs N.W., Lincoln P.M., Burdick M.D., Kunkel S.L. Interleukin-10 expression and chemokine regulation during the evolution of murine type II collagen-induced arthritis. *J Clin Invest*, 1995;**95**:2868–2876.

126. Katsikis P.D., Chu C.Q., Brennan F.M., Maini R.N., Feldmann M. Immunoregulatory role of interleukin 10 in rheumatoid arthritis. *J Exp Med*, 1994;**179**:1517–1527.

127. Bessis N., Boissier M.C., Ferrara P., Blankenstein T., Fradelizi D., Fournier C. Attenuation of collagen-induced arthritis in mice by treatment with vector cells engineered to secrete interleukin-13. *Eur J Immunol*, 1996;**26**:2399–2403.

128. Mussener A., Klareskog L., Lorentzen J.C., Kleinau S. TNF-alpha dominates cytokine mRNA expression in lymphoid tissues of rats developing collagen- and oil-induced arthritis. *Scand J Immunol*, 1995;**42**:128–134.

128a. Schmidt-Weber C.B., Pohlers D., Siegling A., Schädlich H., Buchner E., Volk H.-D., Palombo-Kinne E., Emmrich F., Kinne R.W. Cytokine gene activation in synovial membrane regional lymph nodes, and spleen during the course of rat adjuvant arthritis. *Cell Immunol*. 19999;**195**:53–65.

129. Henderson B., Pettipher E.R. Arthritogenic actions of recombinant IL-1 and tumour necrosis factor alpha in the rabbit: evidence for synergistic interactions between cytokines *in vivo*. *Clin Exp Immunol*, 1989;**75**:306–310.

130. Probert L., Plows D., Kontogeorgos G., Kollias G. The type I interleukin-1 receptor acts in series with tumor necrosis factor

(TNF) to induce arthritis in TNF-transgenic mice. *Eur J Immunol*, 1995;**25**:1794–1797.

131. Neidel J., Schulze M., Lindschau J. Association between degree of bone-erosion and synovial fluid-levels of tumor necrosis factor alpha in the knee-joints of patients with rheumatoid arthritis. *Inflamm Res*, 1995;**44**:217–221.

132. Grell M., Douni E., Wajant H., Lohden M., Clauss M., Maxeiner B., *et al*. The transmembrane form of tumor necrosis factor is the prime activating ligand of the 80 kDa tumor necrosis factor receptor. *Cell*, 1995;**83**:793–802.

133. Georgopoulos S., Plows D., Kollios G., Transmembrane TNF is sufficient to induce localized tissue toxicity and chronic inflammatory arthritis in transgenic mice. *J Inflamm*, 1996;**46**:86–97.

134. Alexopoulou L., Pasparakis M., Kollias G. A murine transmembrane tumor necrosis factor (TNF) transgene induces arthritis by cooperative p55/p75 TNF receptor signaling. *Eur J Immunol*, 1997;**27**:2588–2592.

135. Mackay F., Loetscher H., Stueber D., Gehr G., Lesslauer W. Tumor necrosis factor alpha (TNF-alpha)-induced cell adhesion to human endothelial cells is under dominant control of one TNF receptor type, TNF-R55. *J.Exp.Med.* 1993;**177**:1277–1286.

137 Roux-Lombard P., Punzi L., Hasler F., Bas S., Todesco S., Gallati H., *et al*. Soluble tumor necrosis factor receptors in human inflammatory synovial fluids. *Arthritis Rheum*, 1993;**36**:485–489.

138. Su X., Zhou T., Yang P., Edwards C.K., Mountz J.D. Reduction of arthritis and pneumonitis in motheaten mice by soluble tumor necrosis factor receptor. *Arthritis Rheum*, 1998;**41**:139–149.

138. Paleolog E. Target effector role of vascular endothelium in the inflammatory response: insights form the clinical trial of anti-TNF alpha antibody in rheumatoid arthritis. *Mol Pathol*, 1997;**50**:225–233.

139. von den Hoff H., de Koning M., van Kampen J., van der Korst J. Interleukin-1 reversibly inhibits the synthesis of biglycan and decorin in intact articular cartilage in culture. *J Rheumatol*, 1995;**22**:1520–1526.

140. Assuma R., Oates T., Cochran D., Amar S., Graves D.T. IL-1 and TNF antagonists inhibit the inflammatory response and bone loss in experimental periodonitis. *J Immunol*, 1998;**160**:504–409.

141. Wood N.C., Dickens E., Symons J.A., Duff G.W. *In situ* hybridization of interleukin-1 in CD14-positive cells in rheumatoid arthritis. *Clin Immunol Immunopathol*, 1992;**62**:295–300.

142. Campion G.V., Lebsack M.E., Lookabaugh J., Gordon G., Catalano M. Dose-range and dose-frequency study of recombinant human interleukin-1 receptor antagonist in patients with rheumatoid arthritis. The IL-1Ra Arthritis Study Group. *Arthritis Rheum*, 1996;**39**:1092–1101.

143. Houssiau F.A., Devogelaer J.P., Van Damme J., de Deuxchaisnes C.N., Van Snick J. Interleukin-6 in synovial fluid and serum of patients with rheumatoid arthritis and other inflammatory arthritides. *Arthritis Rheum*, 1988;**31**:784–788.

144. Kotake S., Sato K., Kim K.J., Takahashi N., Udagawa N., Nakamura I., *et al*. Interleukin-6 and soluble interleukin-6 receptors in the synovial fluids from rheumatoid arthritis patients are responsible for osteoclast-like cell formation. *J Bone Miner Res*, 1996;**11**:88–95.

145. Alonzi T., Fattori E., Lazzaro D., Costa P., Probert L., Kollias G., *et al*. Interleukin 6 is required for the development of collagen-induced arthritis. *J Exp Med*, 1998;**187**:461–468.

146. Van De Loo F.A., Kuiper S., van Enckevort F.H., Arntz O.J., van den Berg W.B. Interleukin-6 reduces cartilage destruction during experimental arthritis. A study in interleukin-6-deficient mice. *Am J Pathol*, 1997;**151**:177–191.

147. Szekanecz Z., Haines G.K., Harlow L.A., Shah M.R., Fong T.W., Fu R., *et al*. Increased synovial expression of transforming growth factor (TGF)-beta receptor endoglin and TGF-beta 1 in rheumatoid arthritis: possible interactions in the pathogenesis of the disease. *Clin Immunol Immunopathol*, 1995;**76**:187–194.

148. Chu C.Q., Field M., Abney E., Zheng R.Q., Allard S., Feldmann M., *et al*. Transforming growth factor-beta 1 in rheumatoid synovial membrane and cartilage/pannus junction. *Clin Exp Immunol*, 1991;**86**:380–386.

149. Wahl S.M., Allen J.B., Welch G.R., Wong H.L. Transforming growth factor-beta in synovial fluids modulates Fc gamma RIII (CD16) expression on mononuclear phagocytes. *J Immunol*, 1992;**148**:485–490.

150. Wahl S.M., Allen J.B., Weeks B.S., Wong H.L., Klotman P.E. Transforming growth factor beta enhances integrin expression and type IV collagenase secretion in human monocytes. *Proc Natl Acad Sci USA*, 1993;**90**:4577–4581.

151. Suto T.S., Fine L.G., Shimizu F., Kitamura M. *in vivo* transfer of engineered macrophages into the glomerulus: endogenous TGF-beta-mediated dense against macrophage-induced glomerular cell activation. *J Immunol*, 1997;**159**:2476–2483.

152. Moldovan F., Pelletier J.P., Hambor J., Cloutier J.M., Martel-Pelletier J. Collagenase-3 (matrix metalloprotease 13) is preferentially localized in the deep layer of human arthritic cartilage *in situ*: in vitro mimicking effect by transforming growth factor beta. *Arthritis Rheum*, 1997;**40**:1653–1661.

153. Imai K., Hiramatsu A., Fukushima D., Pierschbacher M.D., Okada Y. Degradation of decorin by matrix metalloproteinases: indetification of the cleavage sites, kinetic analyses and transforming growth factor-beta-1 release. *Biochem J*, 1997;**322**:809–814.

154. McInnes I.B., Leung B.P., Field M., Wei X.Q., Huang F.P., Sturrock R.D., *et al*. Production of nitric oxide in the synovial membrane of rheumatoid and osteoarthritis patients. *J Exp Med*, 1996;**184**:1519–1524.

155. Chae H.J., Park R.K., Chung H.T., Kang J.S., Kim M.S., Choi D.Y., *et al*. Nitric oxide is a regulator of bone remodelling. *J Pharm Pharmacol*, 1997;**49**:897–902.

156. Bogdan C. The multiplex function of nitric oxide in (auto)immunity. *J Exp Med*, 1998;**187**:1361–1365.

157. Miesel R., Murphy M.P., Kroger H. Enhanced mitochondrial radical production in patients which rheumatoid arthritis correlates with elevated levels of tumor necrosis factor alpha in plasma. *Free Radic Res*, 1996;**25**:161–169.

158. Butler D.M., Malfait A.M., Mason L.J., Warden P.J., Kollias G., Maini R.N., *et al*. DBA/1 mice expressing the human TNF-alpha transgene develop a severe, erosive arthritis: characterization of the cytokine cascade and cellular composition. *J Immunol*, 1997;**159**:2867–2876.

159. Kouskoff V., Korganow A.S., Duchatelle V., Degott C., Benoist C., Mathis D. Organ-specific disease provoked by systemic autoimmunity. *Cell*, 1996;**87**:811–822.

160. Nakamura H., Igarashi M. Localization of gold in synovial membrane of rheumatoid arthritis treated with sodium aurothiomalate. Studies by electron microscope and electron probe x-ray microanalysis. *Ann Rheum Dis*, 1977;**36**:209–215.

161. Seitz M., Loetscher P., Dewald B., Towbin H., Baggiolini M. *in vitro* modulation of cytokine, cytokine inhibitor, and prostaglandin E release from blood mononuclear cells and synovial fibroblasts by antirheumatic drugs. *J Rheumatol*, 1997;**24**:1471–1476.

162. Koch A.E., Burrows J.C., Polverini P.J., Cho M., Leibovich S.J. Thiol-containing compounds inhibit the production of monocyte/macrophage-derived angiogenic activity. *Agents Actions*, 1991;**34**:350–357.

163. Seitz M., Loetscher P., Dewald B., Towbin H., Rordorf C., Gallati H., *et al*. Methotrexate action in rheumatoid arthritis: stimulation of cytokine inhibitor and inhibition of chemokine production by peripheral blood mononuclear cells. *Br J Bheumatol*, 1995;**34**:602–609.

164. Firestein G.S., Paine M.M., Boyle D.L. Mechanisms of methotrexate action in rheumatoid arthritis. Selective decrease in synovial collagenase gene expression. *Arthritis Rheum*, 1994;**37**:193–200.

165. MacIntyre A.C., Cutler D.J. Role of lysosomes in hepatic accumulation of chloroquine. *J Pharm Sci*, 1988;**77**:196–199.

166. Angel J., Colard O., Chevy F., Fournier C. Interleukin-1-mediated phospholipid breakdown and arachidonic acid release in human synovial cells. *Arthritis Rheum*, 1993;**36**:158–167.

167. Jeong J.Y., Jue D.M. Chloroquine inhibits processing of tumor necrosis factor in lipopolysaccharide-stimulated RAW 264.7 macrophages. *J Immunol*, 1997;**158**:4901–4907.

168. Amano Y., Lee S.W., Allison A.C. Inhibition by glucocorticoids of the formation of interleukin-1 alpha, interleukin-1 beta, and interleukin-6: mediation by decreased mRNA stability. *Mol Pharmacol*, 1993:**43**:176–182.

169. Kalgutkar A.S., Crews B.C., Rowlinson S.W., Garner C., Seibert K., Marnett L.J. Aspirin-like molecules that covalently inactivate cyclooxygenase-21211. *Science*, 1998;**280**:1268–1270.

170. Shackelford R.E., Alford P.B., Xue Y., Thai S.F., Adams D.O., Pizzo S. Aspirin inhibits tumor necrosis factor alpha gene expression in murine tissue macrophage. *Mol Pharmacol*, 1997;**52**:421–429.

171. Akagawa K.S., Takasuka N., Nozaki Y., Komuro I., Azuma M., Ueda M., *et al.* Generation of CD1⁺Rel8⁺: dendritic cells and tartrate-resistant acid phosphatase-positive osteoclast-like multinucleated giant cells from human nonocytes. *Blood*, 1996;**88**:4029–4039.

172. Inaba K., Inaba M., Deguchi M., Hagi K., Yasumizu R., Ikehara S., *et al.* Granulocytes, macrophages, and dendritic cells arise form a common major histocompatibility complex class II-negative progenitor in mouse bone marrow. *Proc Natl Acad Sci USA*, 1993;**90**:3038–3042.

173. Sallusto F., Lanzavecchia A. Efficient presentation of soluble antigen by cultured human dendritic cells is maintained by granulocyte/macrophage colony-stimulating factor plus interleukin 4 and downregulated by tumor necrosis factor alpha. *J Exp Med*, 1994; **179**:1109–1118.

174. Girasole G., Passeri G., Jilka R.L., Manolagas S.C. Interleukin-11: a new cytokine critical for osteoclast development. *J Clin Invest*, 1994;**93**:1516–1524.

175. Schmidt-Weber C.B., Rittig M., Buchner E., Hauser I., Schmidt I., Palombo-Kinne E., *et al.* Apoptotic cell death in activated monocytes following incorporation of clodronate-liposomes. *J Leukoc Biol*, 1996;**60**:230–244.

176. Sawada T., Hashimoto S., Furukawa H., Tohma S., Inoue T., Ito K. Generation of reactive oxygen species is required for bucillamine, a novel anti-rheumatic drug, to induce apoptosis in concert with copper. *Immunopharmacology*, 1997;**35**:195–202.

177. Mawer E.B., Hayes M.E., Still P.E., Davies M., Lumb G.A., Palit J., *et al.* Evidence for nonrenal synthesis of 1,25-dihydroxyvitamin D in patients with inflammatory arthritis. *J Bone Miner Res*, 1991;**6**:733–739.

178. Yuan J.Y., Freemont A.J., Mawer E.B., Hayes M.E. Regulation of 1 alpha, 25-dihydroxyvitamin D3 synthesis in macrophages from arthritic joints by phorbol ester, dibutyryl-cAMP and calcium ionophore (A23187). *FEBS Lett*, 1992;**311**:71–74.

179. Oelzner P., Muller A., Deschner F., Huller M., Abendroth K., Hein G., *et al.* Relationship between disease activity and serum levels of vitamin D metabolites and PTH in rheumatoid arthritis. *Calcif Tissue Int*, 1998;**62**:193–198.

180. DeLuca H.F., Zierold C. Mechanisms and functions of vitamin D. *Nutr Rev* 1998;**56**:S4–10.

181. Cantorna M.T., Hayes C.E., DeLuca H.F. 1,25-Dihydroxycholecalciferol inhibits the progression of arthritis in murine models of human arthritis. *J Nutr* 1998;**128**:68–72.

182. Cantorna M.T., Woodward W.D., Hayes C.E., DeLuca H.F. 1,25-dihydroxyvitamin D3 is a positive regulator for the two anti-encephalitogenic cytokines TGF-beta 1 and IL-4. *J Immunol*, 1998;**160**:5314–5319.

183. Ito S., Nozawa S., Ishikawa H., Tohyama C., Nakazono K., Murasawa A., *et al.* Renal stones in patients with rheumatoid arthritis. *J Rheumatol*, 1997;**24**:2123–2128.

184. Geoethe R., Loc P.V. The far upstream chicken lysozyme enhancer at −6.1 kilobase, by interacting with NF-M, mediates lipopolysaccharide-induced expression of the chicken lysozyme gene in chicken myelomonocytic cells. *J Biol Chem*, 1994;**269**:31302–31309.

185. Foxwell B., Browne K., Bondeson J., Clarke C., de Martin R., Brennan F., *et al.* Efficient adenoviral infection with IkappaB alpha reveals that macrophage tumor necrosis factor alpha production in rheumatoid arthritis is NF-kappaB dependent. *Proc Natl Acad Sci USA*, 1998;**95**:8211–8215.

186. Handel M.L., McMorrow L.B., Gravallese E.M. Nuclear factor-kappa B in rheumatoid synovium. Localization of p50 and p65. *Arthritis Rheum*, 1995;**38**:1762–1770.

187. Donnelly R.P., Crofford L.J., Freeman S.L., Buras J., Remmers E., Wilder R.L., *et al.* Tissue-specific regulation of IL-6 production by IL-4. Differential effects of IL-4 on nuclear factor-kappa B activity in monocytes and fibroblasts. *J Immunol*, 1993;**151**:5603–5612.

188. Chomarat P., Banchereau J., Miossec P. Differential effects of interleukins 10 and 4 on the production of interleukin-6 by blood and synovium monocytes in rheumatoid arthritis. *Arthritis Rheum*, 1995;**38**:1046–1054.

189. Wang P., Wu P., Siegel M.I., Egan R.W., Billah M.M. Interleukin (IL)-10 inhibits nuclear factor kappa B (NF kappa B) activation in human monocytes. IL-10 and IL-4 suppress cytokine synthesis by different mechanisms. *J Biol Chem*, 1995;**270**:9558–9563.

190. Bogdan C., Paik J., Vodovotz Y., Nathan C. Contrasting mechanisms for suppression of macrophage cytokine release by transforming growth factor-beta and interleukin-10. *J Biol Chem*, 1992;**267**:23301–23308.

7 | *The role of T lymphocytes in rheumatoid arthritis*

David A. Fox

Introduction

The concept that T cells might be important to the pathogenesis of RA is relatively recent. It was little more than 20 years ago that initial evidence was provided that the preponderance of lymphocytes in synovial tissue were in fact T cells, and not antibody producing cells. A detailed understanding of T-cell biology began to take shape in the 1980s, in large part due to the development of monoclonal antibodies against a variety of lymphocyte surface structures. In parallel with these advances in basic immunology, the hypothesis for a central role of T lymphocytes in a variety of immune-mediated diseases, such as rheumatoid arthritis, begin to take shape[1]. Data from animal models and from genetic studies were also important factors in the development of a 'T cell hypothesis' for the pathogenesis of RA.

It was not long, however, before elements of this T-cell hypothesis came under skeptical scrutiny, and at the present time a central role for T cells in RA seems less well accepted than it was 10 years ago.

This chapter will begin with a review of some basic rules that help define our current understanding of T-cell development and T-cell function. Evidence both for and against the central role of T cells in RA will be presented. Specific aspects of immune mechanisms that are related to the function of T cells in RA will be emphasized, including the role of MHC determinants, evidence for T-cell oligoclonality in RA, the nature of antigen driven T-cell responses in RA, activation pathways for T lymphocytes relevant to joint inflammation, aspects of cytokine biology that control T-cell behaviour in RA, and cell–cell interactions involving T lymphocytes in the joint.

In considering the role of T lymphocytes in RA, it is appropriate to bear in mind that definitions of autoimmunity and autoimmune disease are in flux, and that there is no universally agreed, comprehensive model of autoimmunity. Whether or not one regards rheumatoid arthritis as an 'autoimmune disease', with a potential key role for T cells, depends in part on one's definition of autoimmunity. If such a definition requires that a disease be driven by defined lymphocyte responses to a specific autoantigen, the notion that RA is an autoimmune disease remains an unproven hypothesis. If a less narrow definition, such as dysfunction of immune responses resulting in organ-specific tissue damage were acceptable, one might be able to designate RA as an autoimmune disease.

Overview of T-cell biology

T-cell development, activation, and function have become some of the most intensively studied processes in mammalian biology, and space permits only a brief summary of a few key points.

- T lymphocyte development occurs primarily in the thymus, following migration of precursor cells to that organ from the bone marrow. Thymic development is accompanied by (in part mediated through) the sequential appearance and disappearance of critical functional cell membrane glycoproteins, that define stages of thymic selection.
- The T-cell receptor (TCR) for antigen is expressed during this developmental process in the thymus, in association with a glycoprotein complex termed CD3.
- Most mature lymphocytes (more than 95 per cent of circulating T cells) express the $\alpha\beta$ TCR, while the remainder express the $\gamma\delta$ TCR.
- The α and γ genes are composed of V, J, and C segments while the β and δ chains are composed of V, D, J, and C segments.
- TCR diversity is achieved by several mechanisms which include: combinatorial rearrangement of germ line gene segments, addition and deletion of nucleotides at junctions of these segments, and variable pairing of α and β chains.
- Most T cells express only one TCR but rare T cells with two distinct TCRs can be found.
- The majority of T cells that develop in the thymus are subject to negative selection and do not form part of the mature T cell repertoire (this is likely to be very important in limiting autoreactivity of the immune system).
- Positive and negative selection both occur in the thymus and are regulated by antigen presenting MHC molecules expressed in that organ, and by the affinity and abundance of antigens presented to developing T cells by those MHC molecules.
- Unlike B lymphocytes, T lymphocytes do not recognize free antigen, but instead respond to antigenic material displayed by specialized antigen presenting cells.
- Most T cells recognize processed antigens presented in the peptide binding cleft of MHC molecules; in general CD4+ T cells recognize antigen on class II MHC due to coreceptor function of CD4 for class II molecules, and CD8+ T cells

recognize antigen on class I MHC due to CD8 coreceptor function for class I molecules.

- Some T cells recognize non-peptide antigens, including lipid and carbohydrate containing molecules, which are presented by non-MHC structures such as CD1.

- Superantigens are larger than conventional peptide antigens and do not require the same degree of antigen processing. Superantigens are also presented to the TCR by MHC structures, but through binding sites distinct from the peptide-binding MHC cleft.

- Activation of T cells requires one or more costimulatory signals in addition to ligation of the TCR; CD28 is the best studied example of a molecule that can deliver such a second signal, but a variety of cell surface glycoproteins may be able to serve a similar function, including cytokine receptors and receptors that recognize cell membrane determinants on antigen presenting cells.

- T-cell activation is accompanied by a complex and rapid sequence of signal transduction events, which leads to changes in gene expression and ultimately proliferation and effector function; a key series of steps involve expression of interleukin 2 (IL-2), the high affinity IL-2 receptor, and delivery of a mitogenic signal by IL-2 binding to the IL-2 receptor.

- T lymphocyte trafficking to and from specialized lymphoid organs and inflamed tissues is a regulated process, depending in part on expression of specific adhesion receptors on the T-cell surface.

- T cells carry out effector functions through a variety of mechanisms including direct interactions with other cells, (such as lysis of virally infected target cells by cytotoxic T lymphocytes), as well as by secretion of a range of cytokines that regulate the function of other components of the immune response.

- Profiles of cytokine secretion and surface receptor expression have been useful in defining functional subsets of T lymphocytes; Th cells have a functional program that includes production of γ-interferon while TH$_2$ cells produce IL4 and other cytokines.

T-cell hypothesis for RA

The foundation for the view that T cells are central to the pathogenesis of RA was first laid in the 1970s, when it was demonstrated that the majority of lymphocytes in the synovial compartment formed rosettes with sheep erythrocytes, at that time the best method for identifying lymphocytes as T cells[2,3]. In the early 1980s the hypothesis of RA as a T-cell driven disease was formally articulated[1]. Several impressive lines of evidence support this view of RA (Table 7.1). Use of monoclonal antibodies that identify T lymphocyte-specific lineage differentiation markers has confirmed that the great majority of lymphocytes in RA synovial tissue and synovial fluid are T cells[4–7]. Far smaller numbers of B lymphocytes, plasma cells, and natural killer cells are present. The preponderance of T cells is not unique to RA, but instead is also typical for synovial lesions in other forms of

Table 7.1   Evidence for a central role for T cells in RA

Large numbers of T cells and antigen-presenting cells are present in synovial tissue and fluid.

Synovial T cells express activation and memory markers.

T-cell subsets, and possibly clonal T-cell populations, accumulate in RA joints in a non-random manner.

RA is associated with specific MHC class II alleles (DR and/or DQ).

T cells and specific clonal T-cell populations are central to the induction and regulation of several animal models of RA.

T cell-directed therapeutic interventions may be effective in RA, and are clearly effective in animal models.

T-cell cytokines, such as γ-IFN and IL-17, that are present in RA joints, can mediate biological effects highly relevant to the pathogenesis of joint inflammation and damage.

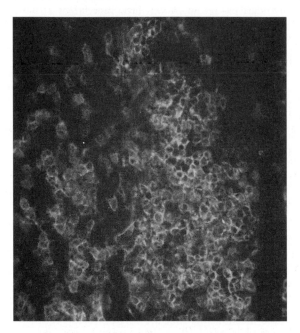

Fig. 7.1   Immunoflourescent micrograph of a frozen section of RA synovial tissue showing a perivascular cluster of T lymphocytes (green fluorescence). The section has been stained with antibody to the CD3 complex, which is associated with the T-cell antigen receptor. (Reprinted with permission from Ref. 7). See also Plate 15.

inflammatory arthritis. T cells in synovial tissue form clusters around vascular structures and are most densely distributed in these regions (Fig. 7.1)[7]. However, T cells are also scattered widely throughout the entire RA synovium, ranging from the sublining layers to the deeper, less cellular regions of RA pannus. Typically, the majority of cells are CD4$^+$, but the number of CD8$^+$ cells is more nearly equal to the number of CD4$^+$ cells than is the case in RA peripheral blood[7,8]. Synovial tissue also contains large numbers of antigen-presenting cells (Fig. 7.2). Furthermore, synovial T cells are distinct in many respects from peripheral blood T cells. Most synovial tissue and synovial fluid T cells bear the CD45 isoforms associated with T-cell memory, such as CD45RO, rather than those associated with the 'naïve' T cell subset[9–11]. Moreover, a large proportion of synovial T

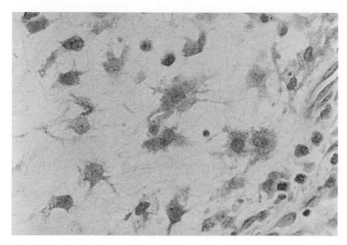

Fig. 7.2 High-power view of a section of fixed, parrafin-embedded synovial tissue, showing T lymphocytes (smaller, rounded cells), in proximity to and interacting with various antigen-presenting cells, including dendritic cells, macrophages, and fibroblasts. (Reprinted with permission from Laboratory Investigation, vol 73, p334, 1995). See also Plate 16.

cells, especially CD8[+] lymphocytes, express class II MHC antigens on the cell surface[4,5], which are only expressed on T cells as a consequence of prior activation. Comparable expression of class II MHC on T cells is only rarely found in RA peripheral blood. Relatively few synovial T cells (generally no more than a few per cent) express high affinity IL-2 receptors on their surface[7], indicating that a relatively small subset of synovial T cells has recently been activated. Paradoxically, many synovial T cells express CD69, also a marker of recent cell activation. Various explanations for this incomplete activation phenotype of synovial T cells have been proposed, but full clarification of this issue is not yet available.

Most T cells express the $\alpha\beta$ TCR but a minor subset expresses the $\gamma\delta$ TCR. The repertoire of antigens recognized, the mechanisms of antigen presentation, some aspects of receptor stimulation, and intracellular signaling all have unique properties in $\gamma\delta$ T cells[12-15]. Some studies have suggested that this subset is expanded in RA synovial fluid and synovial tissue[16-18]. In RA, the role of $\gamma\delta$ T cells, which can be either pathogenic or regulatory in animal models of inflammatory arthritis[19,20], is not yet clear.

One of the most powerful bodies of evidence for the central role of T cells in RA draws from the extensive investigation of animal models of RA. In many of these models, T-cell responses are central to the initiation and maintenance of disease (see Chapter 4). Particularly impressive are studies from the adjuvant arthritis model, in which T-cell clones of appropriate specificity can transfer disease to naïve recipients[21]. Moreover, attenuated, arthritogenic T-cell clones can be used as vaccines that protect naïve animals. Although the data are quite convincing concerning specific animal models, a major limitation is that no animal model appears to be a perfect replica of human RA. Nonetheless, these models point out the great potential of T cells to initiate immune-mediated mechanisms that lead to joint destruction.

Effects of various therapeutic agents on RA and on animal models also attest to the role of T cells in RA. One example is cyclosporin, which blocks T-cell activation by inhibiting transcription of the IL-2 gene through mechanisms that affect activation of essential transcription factors[22]. Other disease modifying antirheumatic drugs also have been postulated to have direct or indirect effects on T-cell activation. In the case of antimalarials and gold salts this may be at the level of antigen-presenting cells. Azathioprine clearly depletes lymphocytes and affects lymphocyte function (reviewed in ref. 23). Methotrexate has a variety of anti-inflammatory effects, and it is not yet clear that the lymphocyte is the major target for this drug. Therefore, although a variety of the conventional pharmaceutical agents used to treat RA can be shown to affect T-cell function, it is not proven that successful treatment of RA requires interference with the action of T lymphocytes.

Challenges to the T-cell hypothesis for RA (Table 7.2)

By the mid 1980s, following the elucidation of the structure of the T-cell antigen receptor, it seemed that a full understanding of the pathogenesis of RA might be close at hand. The underline premises were:

1. RA is an autoimmune disease.

2. Autoimmunity arises from a breakdown in normal self/nonself discrimination by the immune system.

3. It would therefore (it was hoped) be possible to identify specific T-cell clones targeted to self antigen that would be principal pathogenic effectors of autoimmunity.

Such concepts derived largely from elegant studies of autoimmune models in inbred rodent strains, in which specific organ-

Table 7.2 Evidence against a central role for T cells in RA

RA has not been proven to be an autoimmune disease.

T-cell responses to specific antigens have not been shown to trigger or perpetuate RA.

Demonstration of oligoclonal T cells in RA synovial tissue and fluid has been difficult, and different oligoclonal populations appear in different patients.

T cell-derived cytokines are less abundant in the joint than are cytokines produced by other cell types, especially when compared to other chronic T cell-mediated diseases.

Erosion of cartilage and bone does not always correlate with inflammation, and may become independent of regulation by T cells.

Depletion of T cells by monoclonal antibodies may not be therapeutic in RA.

Association of RA with the HLA-DR 'shared epitope' is not consistently strong in all ethnic or racial groups.

targeted lesions could be induced by autoantigen or by foreign antigen that cross-reacted with autoantigen, in the setting of a defined, homogeneous genetic background.

Unfortunately, none of these three premises has proven to be correct in understanding human autoimmune disease. The difficulties in defining specific pathogenic, or even oligoclonally-expanded, populations of lymphocytes in RA are discussed later in this chapter. The ongoing changes in our understanding of autoimmunity have been alluded to earlier. Furthermore as noted above, it cannot be considered formally proven that RA is indeed an autoimmune disease. With all three premises in doubt, it still would be possible to support a central role for T cells in RA by successful specific targeting of T cells using therapy such as anti-T cell monoclonal antibodies. Earlier, experimental approaches such as lymphocyte depletion by thoracic duct drainage[23] or total lymphoid radiation[25,26] had supported the concept that RA was a lymphocyte dependent, and probably T lymphocyte dependent, disease. On this basis and in light of very favorable effects of anti-T cell monoclonal antibodies in various animal models, numerous studies using cell-depleting monoclonal antibodies specific for T lymphocyte surface markers were conducted in RA patients from the late 1980s through the mid 1990s. In general, the results of such studies have been disappointing[27]. Findings that emerge from this body of work that would challenge the T-cell hypothesis of RA include:

1. The extent of T-cell depletion in peripheral blood by anti-T cell monoclonal antibodies does not differ between 'responders' and non-responders to such treatment[28].

2. In general, controlled studies have not shown consistent benefit of anti-T cell antibody treatment of RA[27].

3. Prolonged T cell lymphopenia does not always lead to remission of RA. In addition, despite prior concepts that RA and HIV infection were absolutely incompatible, sporadic reports of co-existence of AIDS and RA have appeared.

A further challenge to the role of T cells in RA arose from analysis of the cytokine profile within the joint. In general, monocyte-derived cytokines, such as tumor necrosis factor (TNF)-α and interleukin 1 (IL-1), are very abundant and have readily discernible inflammatory and tissue destructive properties[29]. In contrast, T-cell cytokines are either absent or present in low levels compared with other lesions that contain T cells, like tuberculous pleuritis or chronic tonsilitis[30]. Interferon γ can generally be demonstrated in the joint, but at very low levels, while IL-2 is inconsistently detected and IL-4 is generally absent. On the other hand IL-10, which tends to suppress Th1, responses, is abundant[31]. These findings, and others, have led to the hypothesis that RA is largely mediated by activated macrophages and synovial fibroblasts, with a restricted role for T lymphocytes at specific points in the evolution of the disease[32]. In contrast to disappointing findings with anti-T cell antibodies, experimental treatment with cytokine blockade, notably neutralization of TNF-α, has been clearly successful in patients with established disease[33]. Although T cells can also make this cytokine, the primary source in RA synovium is the macrophage. The role of membrane bound T-cells cytokines such as TNF-α has been more difficult to assess, although low mRNA levels suggest a minor contribution.

The following sections will explore specific mechanisms of T cell participation in the pathogenesis of RA in order to evaluate further the evidence for and against a central role for T cells in this disease.

Immune mechanisms and the role of T cells in RA

MHC predisposition – what does this tell us about the etiology and pathogenesis of RA?

The MHC locus contains genes that encode the antigen-presenting molecules for most T-cell responses. Also clustered in the same region are other genes relevant to immune and inflammatory responses, such as the genes for TNF and some complement components. RA, at least in Caucasian patients with seropositive disease, is associated with HLA-DR4 and related DR alleles, that contain a five amino acid sequence from residues 70–74 of the DR β chain termed the 'shared epitope'[34]. This sequence, consisting of amino acids QKRAA or QRRAA, is associated with both susceptibility to RA and severity of RA[35-38]. Since the molecules that contain the 'shared epitope' present peptide antigens to CD4$^+$ T cells, it seems straight forward to conclude that the shared epitope is associated with RA because it presents an arthritogenic peptide to specific clones of T cells. However, the situation is likely to be considerably more complicated. There is evidence that other genes in the class II locus, such as HLA-DQ[39,40] and perhaps HLA-DM, also play a role in RA susceptibility. Even in Caucasian patients with seropositive disease, a small subset do not have MHC alleles that contain the shared epitope. Thus far, attempts to isolate unique arthritogenic peptides from RA-associated MHC alleles have not yielded conclusive insights. On the one hand, it has been found that there are distinctions between the peptides that can be externally inserted into molecules bearing the shared epitope compared with other DR molecules, and such distinctions include some peptides derived from potential autoantigens such as type II collagen and heat shock proteins[41,42]. However, most peptides presented by MHC antigens are loaded on these molecules intracellularly, not inserted externally from the extracellular milieu. Analyses of intracellularly-loaded peptides eluted from HLA molecules have not shown unique peptides that are selectively displayed by those MHC structures that bear the shared epitope. However, peptides that are displayed only by non-shared epitope DR molecules have been identified[43].

Some data also suggests that the presence of two copies of the shared epitope confers greater risk of disease and augmented disease severity compared with one copy[35-38]. It would be expected that presentation of an arthritogenic antigen should be a dominant rather than an codominant characteristic. Taken together, these lines of evidence raise the possibility that the shared epitope could augment risk for RA by failing to present

Table 7.3 Possible mechanisms for the association of RA with class II MHC polymorphisms

Presentation of arthritogenic antigens CD4[+] T cells by RA-associated class II MHC alleles

Linkage to other genes in or near the class II MHC locus

Altered T-cell selection in thymic development, leading to expanded populations of potentially arthritogenic T cells

Cross-reactivity between foreign antigen and MHC peptide sequences, particularly the 'shared epitope'

Differences in surface expression and intracellular trafficking of specific MHC alleles

Aberrant signaling through MHC alleles

'Holes' in the T-cell repertoire that lead to inability to respond to an antigen that would protect against the development of RA:

- absence of a particular set of T-cell receptors due to negative
- selection
- absence of MHC molecules capable of presenting a critical antigen
- to a particular set of T-cell receptors

an antigen that the immune system must recognize in order to prevent RA, perhaps by clearing a microbial pathogen. In such a model, non-RA-associated DRB1 alleles would be protective, while arthritogenic antigens might be presented by non-DR MHC molecules such as DQ, DP, or class I MHC[44]. This possible model has interesting parallels in a transgenic rodent system in which mice that expresses HLA-DQ8 are susceptible to collagen induced arthritis, while some alleles of the polymorphic H-2E locus (homologous to HLA-DR) suppress disease[39,40].

Presentation of an arthritogenic antigen or failure to present a protective antigen are only two of the possible explanations for MHC association with rheumatoid arthritis. These and other possible mechanisms are listed in Table 7.3. MHC can shape the T-cell repertoire, not only in presentation of antigen within the mature immune system, but importantly during thymic development, during which negative and positive selection are controlled by MHC molecules. Examination of the TCR repertoire expressed by naïve CD4[+] peripheral blood T cells (presumably representing cells positively selected in the thymus) suggests that the shared epitope molds the expressed TCR repertoire[45]. In addition, shared epitope-positive RA patients differ from normal individuals. It is difficult to prove conclusively that these findings directly represent intrathymic events, and the unique features of the RA T-cell repertoire observed in these studies have not yet been linked to responses to specific arthritogenic antigens.

Other explanations center on interesting sequence homology between the QKRAA sequence and microbial antigens, including bacterial heat shock proteins. Synovial fluid T cells from patients with early RA can recognize peptides containing QKRAA[46]. It has been suggested that positive selection of T cells reactive with the shared epitope might occur during thymic development, yielding lymphocytes that could create an arthritogenic response later, after an appropriate microbial challenge. Yet another possible mechanism relates to a recent observation that the shared epitope may alter intracellular trafficking of class II molecules, with potential consequences for the loading or presenta-tion of particular antigens or for the extent of surface expression of the MHC molecules[47]. Overall therefore, no firm conclusion about the mechanism for a link between predisposing MHC alleles and the etiology or pathogenesis of RA has yet emerged, but several unique and fascinating possibilities deserve further exploration.

RA T lymphocytes—heterogeneous or clonal?

Over the past decade, analysis of the expressed T-cell receptor repertoire in RA has attracted enormous attention and effort[48-64] (reviewed in ref. 64). Much of this work has been motivated by the hypothesis that it may be possible to identify expanded clones of antigen-specific T cells that are of central importance in the pathogenesis of RA. Initial techniques used to study TCR rearrangements in populations of synovial and peripheral T cells, such as Southern blot analysis, were relatively insensitive. However, more recent approaches have involved precise methods to amplify, measure, clone, and sequence T cell receptor gene segments, using quantitative polymerase chain reaction techniques, gel electrophoresis of PCR products, and direct sequencing of TCR gene segments. In patients with RA, there are many problems inherent in attempts to analyze the TCR repertoire. Control subjects should ideally be of similar age, gender, and MHC background. It seems possible that changes in the TCR populations found in blood or joints could either be a part of the cause of RA or be a consequence of inflammation, so that study of patients with early disease might be important. However, identifying such patients and obtaining synovial specimens is often difficult. Additional issues arise in comparison between peripheral blood and synovial tissue or fluid, since the subsets present in the lesional samples are distinct from those in peripheral blood, particularly the expanded proportion with memory markers. Additionally, the effects of medications used in the treatment of RA may be important in altering the pool of lymphocytes available for study.

Nevertheless, more than 50 studies of the expressed T-cell repertoire in RA have been published[48-64]. Most of these examine the $\alpha\beta$ TCR, particularly Vβ gene segment usage, while fewer studies examine $\gamma\delta$ chain usage. Table 7.4 illustrates the results of some of the larger studies of the Vβ repertoire in RA (selected and adapted form more than 50 studies described in ref. 64).

The results of these studies may be summarized as follows:

(1) Selective expansion of use of specific TCR V region genes has been frequently observed in the synovial compartment. This is often termed 'skewing' or 'bias' in TCR repertoire expression.
(2) The specific V genes over-expressed differ among different studies.
(3) There is no evidence yet that TCR expression is distinctive in early versus late RA.
(4) There is no evidence yet for functionally significant TCR expression that is unique to RA, compared with other forms of arthritis.

6. Hemler, M.E., Glass, D., Coblyn, J.S., and Jacobson, J.G., Very late activation antigens on rheumatoid synovial fluid T lymphocytes. Association with stages of T cell activation. *J Clin Invest*, 1986;78:696–702.

7. Fox, D.A., Millard, J.A., Kan, L., Zeldes, W.S., Davis, W., Higgs, J., Emmrich, F., and Kinne, R.W., Activation pathways of synovial T lymphocytes. Expression and function of the UM4D4/CDw60 antigen. *J Clin Invest*, 1990;86:1124–36.

8. Veys, E.M., Hermanns, P., Verbruggen, G., Schindler, J., and Goldstein, G., Evaluation of T cell subsets with monoclonal antibodies in synovial fluid in rheumatoid arthritis. *J Rheumatol*, 1982;9:821–6.

9. Emery, P., Gentry, K.C., Mackay, I.R., Muirden, K.D., and Rowley, M., Deficiency of the suppressor inducer subset of T lymphocytes in rheumatoid arthritis. *Arthritis Rheum* 1987;30:849–54.

10. Morimoto, C., Romain, P.L., Fox, D.A., Anderson, P., DiMaggio, M., Levine, H., and Schlossman, S.F., Abnormalities in CD4+ T lymphocyte subsets in inflammatory rheumatic diseases. *Am J Med*, 1988;84:817–25.

11. Kohem, C.L., Wisbey, H., Tortorella, C., Lipsky, P.E., and Oppenheimer-Marks N., Enrichment of differentiated CD45RB dim, CD27-memory T cells in the peripheral blood, synovial fluid, and synovial tissue of patients with rheumatoid arthritis. *Arthritis Rheum*, 1996;39:844–54.

12. Holoshitz, J., Vila, L.M., Keroack, B.J., McKinley, D.R., and Bayne, N.K., Dual antigenic recognition by cloned γδ T cells. *J Clin Invest*, 1992;89:308–14.

13. Tanaka, Y., Mariata C.T., Tanaka, Y., Nieves, E., Brenner, M.B., and Bloom, B.R., Natural and synthetic non-peptide antigens recognized by human gamma delta T cells. *Nature*.

14. Haftel, H.M., Chung, Y., Hinderer, R., Hanash, S., and Holoshitz, J., Induction of the autoantigen proliferating cell nuclear antigen in T lymphocytes by a mycobacterial antigen. *J Clin Invest*, 1994;94:1365–72.

15. Vila, L.M., H.H., Park, H.S., Lin, M.S., Romzek, N.C., Hanash, S.M., and Holoshitz, J., Expansion of mycobacteria-reactive gamma delta T cells by a subset of memory helper T cells. *Infect Immun*, 1995;63:1211–7.

16. Lunardi, C., Marguerie, C., Walport, M.J., and So, A.K., T γδ cells and their subsets in blood and synovial fluid from patients with rheumatoid arthritis. *Br J Rheumatol*, 1992;31:527–30.

17. Bucht, A., Soderstrom, K., Hultman, T., Uhlen, M., Nilsson, E., Kiessling, R., and Gronberg, A., T cell receptor diversity and activation markers in the Vδ1 subset of rheumatoid synovial fluid and peripheral blood T lymphocytes. *Eur J Immunol* 1992;22:567.

18. Meliconi, R., Uguccioni, M., D'Errico, A., Cassisa, A., Frizziero, L., and Facchini, A., T-cell receptor γδ positive lymphocytes in synovial membrane. *Br J Rheumatol*, 1992;31:59–61.

19. Peterman, G.M., Spencer, C., Sperling, A.I., and Bluestone, J.A., Role of γδ T cells in murine collagen-induced arthritis. *J Immunol*, 1993;151:6546–58.

20. Pelegri, C., Kuhnlein, P., Buchner, E., Schmidt, C.B., Franch, A., Castell, M., Hunig, T., Emmrich, F., and Kinne, R.W., Depletion of γδ T cells does not prevent or ameliorate, but rather aggravates, rat adjuvant arthritis. *Arthritis Rheum*, 1996;39:204–15.

21. Cohen, I.R., Holoshitz, J., van Eden, W., and Frenkel, A., T lymphocyte clones illuminate pathogenesis and affect therapy of experimental arthritis. *Arthritis Rheum*, 1985;28:841–15.

22. Schreiber, S.L., and Crabtree, G.R., The mechanisms of action of cyclosporin A and FK506. *Immunol Today* 1992;13:136–42.

23. Fox, D.A., and McCune, W.J., Immunologic and clinical effects of cytotoxic drugs used in the treatment of rheumatoid arthritis and systemic lupus erythematosus. *Concepts in Immunopathology*, 1989;7:20–78.

24. Ueo, T., Tanaka, S., Tominaga, Y., Ogawa, H., and Sakurami, T., The effect of thoracic duct drainage on lymphocyte dynamics and clinical symptoms in patients with rheumatoid arthritis. *Arthritis Rheum*, 1979;22:1405–12.

25. Kotzin, B.L., Strober, S., Engleman, E.G., Calin, A., Hoppe, R.T., Kansas, G.S., Terrell, C.P., and Kaplan, H.S., Treatment of intractable rheumatoid arthritis with total lymphoid irradiation. *N Eng J Med*, 1981;305:969–76.

26. Trentham, D.E., Belli, J.A., Anderson, R.J., Buckley, J.A., Goetzl, E.J., David, J.R., and Austen, K.F., Clinical and immunologic effects of fractionated total lymphoid irradiation in refractory rheumatoid arthritis. *N Engl J Med*, 1981;305:976–82.

27. Fox, D.A., Biological therapies: A novel approach to the treatment of autoimmune disease. *Am J Med*, 1995;99:82–8.

28. Moreland, L.W., Bucy, R.P., Tilden, A., Pratt, P.W., LoBuglio, A.F., Khazaeli, M., Everson, M.P., Daddona, P., Ghrayeb, J., Kilgarriff, C., *et al.*, Use of a chimeric monoclonal anti-CD4 antibody in patients with refractory rheumatoid arthritis. *Arthritis Rheum*, 1993;36:307–18.

29. Feldmann, M., Brennan, F.M., and Maini, R.N., Role of cytokines in rheumatoid arthritis. *Ann Rev Immunol* 1996;14:397–44.

30. Firestein, G.S., and Zvaifler, N.J., How important are T cells in chronic rheumatoid synovitis?. *Arthritis Rheum*, 1990; 33:768–73.

31. Katsikis, P., Chu, C.Q., Brennan, F.M., Maini, R.N., and Feldmann, M., Immunoregulatory role of interleukin 10 in rheumatoid arthritis. *J Exp Med*, 1994;179:1517–27.

32. Nguyen, K.H.Y., and Firestein, G.S., T cells as secondary players in rheumatoid arthritis. In: *T Cells in Arthritis* (Miossec, P., van den Berg, W.B., Firestein, G.S. eds), p. 1–18. Birkhauser, Basel. (1998).

33. Elliott, M.J., Feldmann, M., Kalden, J.R., Antoni, C., Smolen, J.S., Leeb, B., Breedveld, F.C., Macfarlane, J.D., Biji, H., and Woody, J.N., Randomized double blind comparison of a chimaeric monoclonal antibody to tumor necrosis factor alpha (cA2) versus placebo in rheumatoid arthritis. *Lancet*, 1994;344:1105–10.

34. Gregersen, P.K., Silver, J., and Winchester, R.J., The shared epitope hypothesis: an approach to understanding the molecular genetics of susceptibility to rheumatoid arthritis. *Arthritis Rheum*, 1987;30:1205–13.

35. Weyand, C.M., Xie, C., and Goronzy, J.J., Homozygosity for the HLA-DRB1 allele selects for extra-articular manifestations in rheumatoid arthritis. *J Clin Invest*, 1992;89:2033–9.

36. Weyand, C.M., Hicok, C., Conn, D., and Goronzy, J.J., The influence of HLA-DRB1 genes on disease severity in rheumatoid arthritis. *Ann Intern Med*, 1992;117:801–6.

37. Evans, T.I., Han, J., Singh, R., and Moxley, G., The genotypic distribution of shared-epitope DRB1 alleles suggests a recessive mode of inheritance of the rheumatoid arthritis disease-susceptibility gene. *Arthritis Rheum*, 1995;38:1754–61.

38. Moreno, I., Valenzuela, A., Garcia, A., Yelamos, J., Sanchez, B., and Hernanz, W., Association of the shared epitope with radiological severity of rheumatoid arthritis. *J Rheumatol*, 1996;23:6–9.

39. Zanelli, E., Gonzalez-Gay, M.A., and David, C., Could HLA-DRB1 be the protective locus in rheumatoid arthritis? *Immunol Today*, 1995;16:274–8.

40. Nabozny, G.H., Baisch, J.M., Cheng, S., Cosgrove, D., Griffiths, M.M., Luthra, H.S., David, C.S., HLA-DQ8 transgenic mice are highly susceptible to collagen-induced arthritis: A novel model for human polyarthritis. *J Exp Med*, 1996;183:27–37.

41. Woulfe, S.L., Bono, C.P., Zacheis, M.L., Kirschmann, D.A., Baudino, T.A., Swearingen, C., Karr, R.W., and Schwartz, B.D., Negatively charged residues interacting with the p4 pocket confer binding specificity to DRB1 *0401. *Arthritis Rheum*, 1995;38:1744–53.

42. Hammer, J., Gallazzi, F., Bono, E., Karr, R.W., Guenot, J., Valsasnini, P., Nagy, Z.A., and Sinigaglia, F., Peptide binding specificity of HLA-DR4 molecules: correlation with rheumatoid arthritis association. *J Exp Med*, 1995;181:1847–55.

43. Kirschmann, D.A., Duffin, K.L., Smith, C.E., Welply, J.K., Howard, S.C., Schwartz, B.D., and Woulfe, S.L., Naturally processed peptides from rheumatoid arthritis associated and non-associated HLA-DR alleles. *J Immunol*, 1995; 155:5655–62.

44. Fox, D.A. Rheumatoid arthritis—heresies and speculations. *Perspectives in Biology and Medicine*, 1997;40:479–91.

45. Walser-Kuntz, D.R., Weyand, C.M., Weaver, A.J., O'Fallon, W.M., and Goronzy, J.J., Mechanisms underlying the formation of the T cell receptor repertoire in rheumatoid arthritis. *Immunity*, 1995;2:597–605.

46. Albani, S., Keystone, E.C., Nelson, J.L., Ollier, W.E.R., La Cava, A., Montemayor, A.C., Weber, D.A., Montecucco, C., Martini, A., and Carson, D.A., Positive selection in autoimmunity: Abnormal immune responses to a bacterial dnaJ antigenic determinant in patients with early rheumatoid arthritis. *Nat Med*, 1995;1:448–52.

47. Auger, I., Escola, J.M., Gorvel, J.P., and Roudier, J., HLA-DR4 and HLA-DR10 motifs that carry susceptibility to rheumatoid arthritis bind 70-kD heat shock proteins. *Nature Med*, 1996;2:306–10.

48. Brennan, F.M., Allard, S., Londei, M., Savill, C., Boylston, A., Carrel, S., Maini, R.N., and Feldmann, M., Heterogeneity of T cell receptor idiotypes in rheumatoid arthritis. *Clin Exp Immunol*, 1988;73:417–23.

49. Gudmundsson, S., Ronnelid, J., Karlsson-Parra, A., Lysholm, J., Gudbjornsson, B., Widenfalk, B., Janson, C.H., and Klareskog, L., T-cell receptor V-gene usage in synovial fluid and synovial tissue from RA patients. *Scand J Immunol*, 1992;36:681–8.

50. Williams, W.V., Fang, Q., Demarco, D., VonFeldt, J., Zurier, R.B., and Weiner, D.B., Restricted heterogeneity of T cell receptor transcripts in rheumatoid synovium. *J Clin Invest*, 1992;90:326–33.

51. Jenkins, R.N., Nikaein, A., Zimmermann, A., Meek, K., and Lipsky, P.E., T cell receptor Vβ gene bias in rheumatoid arthritis. *J Clin Invest*, 1993;92:2688–701.

52. Struyk, L., Kurnick, J.T., Hawes, G.E., van Laar, J.M., Schipper, R., Oksenberg, J.R., Steinman, L., de Vries, R.R., Breedveld, F.C., and van den Elsen, P., T-cell receptor Vβ gene usage in synovial fluid lymphocytes of patients with chronic arthritis. *Hum Immunol*, 1993;37:237–51.

53. Zagon, G., Tumang, J.R., Li, Y., Friedman, S.M., and Crow, M.K., Increased frequency of Vβ 17-positive T cells in patients with rheumatoid arthritis. *Arthritis Rheum*, 1994;37:1431–40.

54. Alam, A., Lule, J., Coppin, H., Lambert, N., Mazieres, B., De Preval, C., and Cantagrel, A., T-cell receptor variable region of the β-chain gene use in peripheral blood and multiple synovial membranes during rheumatoid arthritis. *Human Immunol*, 1995;42:331–9.

55. Fitzgerald, J.E., Ricalton, N.S., Meyer, A.C., West, S.G., Kaplan, H., Behrendt, C., and Kotzin, B.L., Analysis of clonal CD8+ T cell expansions in normal individuals and patients with rheumatoid arthritis. *J Immunol*, 1995;154:3538–47.

56. Huchenq, A., Champagne, E., Sevin, J., Riond, J., Tkaczuck, J., Mazieres, B., Cambon-Thomsen, A., and Cantagrel, A., Abnormal T cell receptor Vβ gene expression in the peripheral blood and synovial fluid of rheumatoid arthritis patients. *Clin Exp Rheumatol*, 1995;13:29–36.

57. Melchers, I., Peter, H.H., and Eibel, H., The T and B cell repertoire of patients with rheumatoid arthritis. *Scand J Rheumatol Suppl*, 1995;101:153–62.

58. Jenkins, R.N., and McGinnis, D.E., T-cell receptor Vβ gene utilization in rheumatoid arthritis. *Ann N Y Acad Sci*, 1995;756:159–72.

59. Hingorani, R., Monteiro, J., Pergolizzi, R., Furie, R., Chartash, E., and Gregersen, P.K., CDR3 length restriction of T-cell receptor β chains in CD8+ T-cells of rheumatoid arthritis patients. *Ann N Y Acad Sci*, 1995;756:179–82.

60. Alam, A., Lule, J., Lambert, N., Coppin, H., Mazieres, B., De Preval, C., and Cantagrel, A., Use of T-cell receptor V genes in synovial membrane in rheumatoid arthritis. *Ann N Y Acad Sci*, 1995;756:199–200.

61. Gonzalez-Quintial, R., Baccala, R., Pope, R.M., and Theofilopoulos, A.N., Identification of clonally expanded T cells in rheumatoid arthritis using a sequence enrichment nuclease assay. *J Clin Invest*, 1996;97:1335–43.

62. Hingorani, R., Monteiro, J., Furie, R., Chartash, E., Navarrete, C., Pergolizzi, R., and Gregersen, P.K., Oligoclonality of Vβ3 TCR chains in the CD8+ T cell population of rheumatoid arthritis patients. *J Immunol*, 1996;156:852–8.

63. Rittner, H.L., Zettl, A., Jendro, M.C., Bartz-Bazzanella, P., Goronzy, J., and Weyand, C., Multiple mechanisms support oligoclonal T cell expansion in rheumatoid synovitis. *Mol Med*, 1997;3:452–65.

64. Fox, D.A., and Singer, N., T cell receptor rearrangements in arthritis. In: *T Cells in Arthritis* (Miossec, P., van den Berg, W.B., and Firestein, G.S. eds), p. 19–53. Birkhauser, Basel. (1998).

65. Bonneville, M., Scotet, E., Peyrat, M.A., Lim, A., David-Ameline, J., and Houssaint, E., T cell reactivity to Epstein-Barr virus in rheumatoid arthritis. In: *T Cells in Arthritis* (Miossec, P., van den Berg, W.B., and Firestein, G.S. eds), p. 149–167. Birkhauser, Basel. (1998).

66. Rosloniec, E.F., Brand, D.D., Myers, L.K., Whittington, K.B., Gumanovskaya, M., Zaller, D.M., Woods, A., Altmann, D.M., Stuart, J.M., and Kang, A.H., An HLA-DR1 transgene confers susceptibility to collagen-induced arthritis elicited with human type II collagen. *J Exp Med*, 1997;185:1113–22.

67. Cuesta, I.A., Sud, S., Song, Z., Affholter, J.A., Karvonen, R.L., Fernandez-Madrid, F., and Wooley, P.H., T cell receptor (Vβ) bias in the response of rheumatoid arthritis synovial fluid T cells to connective tissue antigens. *Scand J Rheumatol*, 1997;26:166–73.

68. Snowden, N., Reynolds, I., Morgan, K., and Holt, L., T cell responses to human type II collagen in patients with rheumatoid arthritis and healthy controls. *Arthritis Rheum*, 1997;40:1210–10.

69. Londei, M., Savill, C.M., Verhoef, A., Brennan, F., Leech, Z.A., Duance, V., Maini, R.N., and Feldmann, M., Persistence of collagen type II-specific T-cell clones in the synovial membrane of a patient with rheumatoid arthritis. *Proc Natl Acad Sci USA*, 1989;86:36–40.

70. Verheijden, G.F.M., Rijinders, A.W.M., Bos, E., Coenen-de Roo, C.J., van Staveren, C.J.J., Miltenburg, A.M.M., Meijerink, J.H., Elewaut, D., de Keyser, F., Veys, E. *et al.*, Human cartilage glycoprotein-39 as a candidate autoantigen in rheumatoid arthritis. *Arthritis Rheum*, 1997;40:1115–25.

71. Cannons, J.L., Karsh, J., Birnboim, H.C., and Goldstein, R., HRPT-Mutant T cells in the peripheral synovial tissue of patients with rheumatoid arthritis. *Arthritis Rheum*, 1998;41:1772–82.

72. Firestein, G.S., Yeo, M., and Zvaifler, N.J., Apoptosis in rheumatoid arthritis synovium. *J Clin Invest*, 1995;96:1631–8.

73. Liu, M., Kohsaka, H., Sakurai, H., Azuma, M., Okumura, K., Saito, I., and Miyasaka, N., The presence of costimulatory molecules CD86 and CD28 in rheumatoid arthritis synovium. *Arthritis Rheum*, 1996;39:110–4.

74. Sfikakis, P.P., Zografou, A., Viglis, V., Iniotaki-Theodoraki, A., Piskontaki, I., Tsokos, G.C., Sfikakis, P., and Choremi-Papadopoulou, H., CD28 expression on T cell subsets *in vivo* and CD28-mediated T cell response in vitro in patients with rheumatoid arthritis. *Arthritis Rheum*, 1995;38:649–511.

75. Schmidt, D., Goronzy, J., and Weyand, C.M., CD4+ CD7⁻ CD28⁻ T cells are expanded in rheumatoid arthritis and are characterized by autoreactivity. *J Clin Invest*, 1996;97:2027–37.

76. Bott, C.M., Doshi, J.B., Morimoto, C., Romain, P.L., and Fox, D.A., Functional effects of a novel anti-CD6 monoclonal antibody and definition of four epitopes of the CD6 glycoprotein. *Int Immunol*, 1993;5:783–92.

77. Singer, N.G., Richardson, B.C., Powers, D., Hooper, F., Lialios, F., Sanders, J., Bott, C.M., and Fox, D.A., Role of the CD6 glycoprotein in antigen-specific and autoreactive responses of cloned human T lymphocytes. *J Immunol*, 1995;88:537–43.

78. Bowen, M.A., Patel, D.D., Li, X., Modrell, B., Malacko, A.R., Wang, W.C., Marquardt, H., Neubauer, M., Pesando, J.M., Francke, U., *et al.*, Cloning, mapping, and characterization of activated leukocyte-cell adhesion molecule [ALCAM], a CD6 ligand. *J Exp Med*, 1995;181:2213–20.

79. Higgs, J.B., Zeldes, W., Kozarsky, K., Schteingart, M., Kan, L., Bohlke, P., Krieger, K., Davis, W., and Fox, D.A., A novel pathway of human T lymphocyte activation. Identification by a monoclonal antibody generated against a rheumatoid synovial T cell line. *J Immunol*, 1988;140:3758–65.

80. Wagner, U.G., Kurtin, P.J., Wahner, A., Brackertz, M., Berry, D.J., Goronzy, J.J., and Weyand, C.M., The role of CD8+ CD40L+ T

rich in histamine and react with basic dyes while eosinophil granules contain cationic granule proteins with high affinity for eosin and other acid stains. Neutrophils, the predominant granulocyte in blood and synovial fluid, are important sources of inflammatory mediators. As they participate in inflammatory reactions, they respond to microbial products as well as to mediators of both the innate and acquired immune systems[53]. These mediators include myeloid and lymphoid-derived cytokines, lipid-based mediators, immunoglobulin aggregates, and complement split-products (especially C3 and C5 derived products).

Degranulation

The neutrophil has four distinct intracellular granular organelles,—the primary (azurophilic), secondary (specific), tertiary (gelatinase) granules, and the secretory vesicle[54-56]. The primary granules appear first during neutrophil maturation and comprise approximately one-third of the granule content in mature neutrophils. Primary granules contain hydrolases, proteases, peroxidases, and a diverse group of cationic antimicrobial proteins. In addition to secretion of contents through exocytosis, these granules fuse with the intracellular phagolysosomal vacuole formed during phagocytosis and facilitate the killing and degradation of internalised micro-organisms. Myeloperoxidase, a major constituent of primary granules and the enzyme responsible for the characteristic yellow-green color of pus, is critical for the conversion of hydrogen peroxide to microbiocidal hypochlorous acid. Primary granules also include elastase, cathepsins D and G, and proteinase 3, each of which has been implicated in inflammatory tissue damage: elastase can cleave collagen cross-linkages, proteoglycans, and the elastin components of vessels and supporting tissues; cathepsin G is a broad spectrum protease that activates latent collagenase; and proteinase 3 is a potent serine protease.

Secondary granules appear later in neutrophil maturation at the metamyelocyte stage and contain leukocyte-specific proteins, lactoferrin, and vitamin B_{12}-binding protein. These granules are more easily mobilized for exocytosis than primary granules and their contents have an important role in regulating the inflammatory response[54-56]. In this regard, specific granules contain numerous cell-surface-associated proteins including the $\beta 2$ integrin CD11b/CD18, which is also a receptor of the C3 split product iC3b, and receptors for laminin, vitronectin, thrombospondin, tumor necrosis factor, and formyl peptides. An important component of the NADPH oxidase complex, cytochrome b558, is also contained within specific granule membranes. Specific granules also contain procollagenase, heparanase, plasminogen activator, and the chitinase YKL-40 (HC gp-39) that is also expressed in articular cartilage[41,42]. Procollagenase, when activated by oxidants or cathepsins, can degrade type I and type II collagen and, to a lesser degree, type III collagen[11,57]. Collagen breakdown products have chemotactic activity towards neutrophils, monocytes, and fibroblasts[11].

At times, constituents of granules may be the target of an acquired immune response[38-40,58]. The occurrence of antineutrophil cytoplasmic antibodies (ANCA) with specificity for granule proteins provides an additional novel mechanism for neutrophil activation[59,60]. In patients with RA, the most common ANCA target is the secondary (specific) granule component lactoferrin. Given the recent insight that the HC gp-39 (YKL-40) chitinase is also expressed in neutrophil secondary granules and in human cartilage[41,42], acquired immune responses to this protein may result in a specific anticartilage reaction leading to cartilage destruction as well as an antineutrophil reaction promoting neutrophil activation[59,60].

Some constituents are found in several different types of granules. For example CD11b/CD18 is found in secondary granules, tertiary granules, and secretory vesicles. Nonetheless, differential regulation of the granule organelles in the degranulation response is an important determinant of the neutrophil response at sites of inflammation. This regulation is determined by the nature and intensity of the activation signal and can be modified by counterbalancing receptor-specific negative signals[61]. Variations in the intensity of both the activating and de-activating signals may reflect genetic polymorphisms in membrane-associated receptors[50,51].

The oxidative burst

The neutrophil respiratory burst is characterized by increased consumption of oxygen and the generation of multiple proinflammatory and cytotoxic products (reviewed in ref. 62,63). Activated through cell surface receptors for Fc region of immunoglobulin, complement activation (C5a, C1q), lipid mediators (PAF, LTB_4), or bacterial products (LPS, fMLP), the respiratory burst starts with the assembly of the NADPH oxidase complex. This complex is composed of the membrane-associated cytochrome b558 which contains an α-chain (gp91^{phox}) and a β-chain (p22^{phox}). This flavin (FAD)-binding complex also binds NADPH and contains two heme groups. Upon proper activation, three cytosolic proteins (p67^{phox}, p47^{phox}, and p21^{rac}) associate with flavocytochrome b558 to form the complete oxidase. Once assembled, NADPH is the electron donor for the oxidase that converts O_2 to superoxide (O_2^-) with the generation of $NADP + H^+$. Superoxide can be transported across membranes via anion channels, and while it probably does not have direct toxic effects, it is a precursor or substrate for formation of other toxic products including singlet oxygen, hydroxyl radical, OH$^\bullet$, and hydrogen peroxide and peroxynitrite[16]. Hydrogen peroxide can also be produced directly from divalent oxygen through the action of glucose oxidase or from dismutation of superoxide generated by xanthine oxidase. In a reaction catalysed by myeloperoxidase, hydrogen peroxide may be used as a substrate for the generation of hypochlorous acid (HOCl), a regulator of protease activity. The most toxic of all of these compounds may be the hydroxyl radical, a powerful one-electron oxidant capable of reacting with a wide range of compounds to form new radicals that can then oxidize other substrates.

Soluble mediators of inflammation

Lipid-derived inflammatory mediators produced by neutrophils include eicosanoids and leukotrienes (reviewed in ref. 64). Activation of neutrophils by cell surface receptors can induce phospholipase activity. Phospholipase A_2 releases arachidonic acid from the sn-2 position of membrane phospholipids which then can be metabolized by the cyclo-oxygenase and lipoxygenase pathways. Prostaglandins and thromboxanes (particularly PGE_2 and PGI_2), products of the cyclo-oxygenases, enhance vascular permeability, can potentiate the effects of agents such as histamine and bradykinin, and enhance pain perception. In some models, however, PGE_2 can have an anti-inflammatory effect, probably through increased cAMP production. Metabolism of arachidonic acid by the lipoxygenase pathway can lead to the production of mono-, di-, and trihydroxyeicosatetraenoic acids (HETEs), precursors of leukotrienes. These lipid-derived mediators can also have potent proinflammatory effects. 5,12-HETE is proinflammatory through its leukocyte chemoattractant activity, and LTB4, in addition to being chemoattractant, stimulates cell adhesion, superoxide anion generation, and degranulation. Generation of these lipid mediators, by both the cyclo-oxygenase and lipoxygenase pathways, are important mechanisms for perpetuation of the chronic inflammatory reaction typically observed in the affected joints of patients with RA. Recently, expression of the inducible form of cyclo-oxygenase 2, COX-2, was described in stimulated neutrophils suggesting that neutrophils may also actively influence the eicosanoid composition of the acute inflammatory milieu[65,66].

While the release of degradative enzymes and the generation of reactive oxygen intermediates by neutrophils is widely appreciated, the role of neutrophils in modulating the inflammatory reaction through production of cytokines is less clear. Careful analysis of the biosynthetic capacity of neutrophils has shown that these cells can activate transcription in response to stimulation and can thus play an important role in shaping the inflammatory response through the synthesis and secretion of cytokines[34–36] (reviewed in ref. 67). Of the cytokines typically found in rheumatoid synovial fluid, IL-1β, IL-6, IL-8, TNF-α, TGF-β, and IL-1ra can all be released by neutrophils. The ability of neutrophils to be transcriptionally active should not come as a great surprise given the ample evidence of receptor-mediated activation of intracellular signaling cascades known to lead to the activation of transcription factors in other cell types. For example both the ras pathway and the MAP kinase pathways are active in neutrophils[11,68] and probably play a key regulatory role in the ability of neutrophils to modulate inflammation through the secretion of cytokines.

Neutrophil surface receptors

Neutrophils respond to inflammatory mediators through cell surface receptors, and there has been a tremendous increase in our knowledge of the mechanisms by which these receptors regulate neutrophil function. For instance the complexity in the signaling cascades initiated by neutrophil surface receptors extends beyond G-protein-mediated signals to networks of phosphorylation/dephosphorylation reactions and formation of lipid-based signaling intermediates. Furthermore, there is increased recognition of the role of antigen non-specific pattern recognition systems in regulating inflammatory reactions[2–6].

The range of stimuli that a neutrophil encounters includes chemotactic factors and chemokines, adhesion receptors/counter-receptors, immunoglobulin and complement breakdown products in the context of immune complexes, cytokines and lymphokines, lipid-based mediators such as prostaglandins and leukotrienes, and reactive oxygen/nitrogen based compounds. While a detailed consideration of all of the receptors for these agonists and the mechanisms by which they activate neutrophils is well beyond the scope of this chapter, there are a number of general principles and new avenues of research.

Chemokine receptors

The ability of neutrophils to migrate to sites of inflammation is regulated by a variety of chemotactic factors that include bacterially-derived peptides such as fMLP, complement fragments (especially C5a), and chemokines. These agonists can also initiate degranulation and the oxidative burst. Neutrophils express three chemokine receptors, CXCR1, CXCR2, and CXCR4, which bind to CXC chemokines such as IL-8, melanoma growth stimulatory activity (GROα/β/γ), neutrophil activating peptide 2 (NAP-2), epithelial activating peptide 78 (ENA78), granulocyte chemotactic protein 2 (GCP-2), and stromal-derived factor (SDF-1)[69,70]. Intense investigation of chemokines and chemokine receptors has identified structural polymorphisms both in chemokines and their receptors[71–73]. The 32 bp deletion in CCR5, which has an allele frequency approaching 0.10, blocks the uptake of HIV, and is associated with delay in HIV disease progression, provides a compelling example of an association between a polymorphism and clinical phenotype[72,73]. Such findings open up the possibility that polymorphisms in the chemokine receptor family or in chemokines themselves may also play a role in chronic inflammatory diseases such as RA. Indeed, preliminary data suggest that homozygosity of the CCR5$^-$ allele might protect against RA.[73a] Insight into mechanisms of functional blockade of receptor binding or inhibition of receptor function may also be fruitful areas of future investigation.

Perhaps not surprisingly given the common functional responses elicited by chemotactic agents, the receptors for each of these factors share many common structural and functional features[11,69,70,74,75]. All members of the superfamily of seven-transmembrane-domain family of receptors signal through heterotrimeric GTP-binding proteins. Typically, upon ligand binding, a *Bordetella pertussis*-toxin-sensitive G-protein, usually of the Gα_{i2} type, initiates a signaling cascade leading to activation of a phosphatidyl-inositol-specific phospholipase C, small GTPases, Src-family protein tyrosine kinases, and phosphatidyli-nositol-3-OH (PI-3) kinases. Phospholipase C activation leads to the production of IP$_3$ which releases intracellular Ca^{2+}, leading to a transient rise in cytosolic Ca^{2+} concentration and diacylglycerol which activates protein kinase C. The rise in cytosolic Ca^{2+} is required for granule release and superoxide production but is probably not required for cytoskeletal reorganization. PI-3 kinases can be activated by the β/γ subunit of G proteins, small GTPases or Src-family tyrosine kinases. The small GTPases are particularly important in the formation of the oxidase complex and for regulation of cytoskeletal rearrangements involving adhesion and chemotaxis. They can also activate phospholipase D. If specificity can be achieved, therapeutic targeting of neutrophil chemotaxis and activation by IL-8, C5a or other chemoattractants represents an attractive goal in RA.

Adhesion receptors

After initial neutrophil interaction with chemotactic agonists, adhesion receptors play an important role in altering neutrophil activation. The process of neutrophil margination in the vessel, adherence to endothelial cells, and transmigration are all active processes that are mediated by specific adhesion receptor interactions[76]. Initial interactions between neutrophils and activated endothelial cells involve binding of L-selectin on the neutrophil with its receptor on endothelial cells. This interaction promotes rolling of neutrophils along the endothelial cells leading to firm adhesion mediated by the β_2 integrin CD11b/CD18 binding to ICAM-1 on the endothelial cell. The initial L-selectin-mediated binding may also upregulate CD11b/CD18 expression on neutrophils[77]. Engagement and cross-linking of CD11b by its counter-receptor can activate neutrophils at the same time that it leads to an enhanced rate of apoptosis through CD11b-mediated oxidant production[78,79]. This may be a mechanism by which the neutrophil can limit their own proinflammatory potential and suggests that interruption of the carefully orchestrated interplay of adhesion molecules may have some unanticipated results. For example murine models of arthritis in P-selectin knock-out mice may have a more severe, rather than less severe, phenotype (D. Bullard, personal communication).

Receptors for immunoglobulins

Another class of receptors that are potent activators of neutrophils are the receptors for the Fc region immunoglobulin.

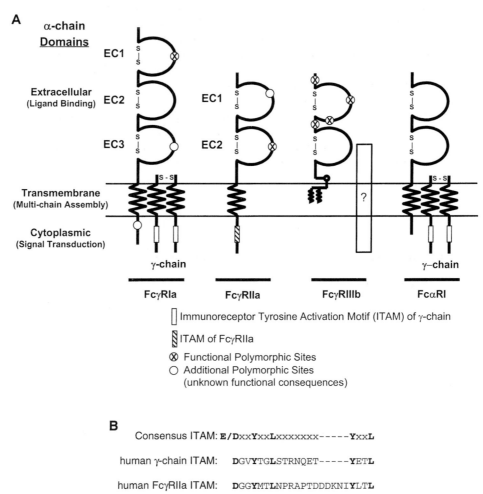

Fig. 8.1 Immunoglobulin receptors expressed on human neutrophils. A. Human neutrophils constitutively express two receptors for IgG (FcγRIIa and FcγRIIIb) and a receptor for IgA FcαRI. Upon stimulations with IFNγ or IL-10, neutrophils can also express the FcγRIa IgG receptor. These homologous receptors share certain structural and functional domains and motifs. In the extracellular ligand binding domains, all of these receptors have two or three immunoglobulin-like domains. In the cytoplasmic domain (except FcγRIIIb), an ITAM is necessary for receptor-induced cell activation. The Fcγ receptors are most homologous and form a group of gene families on the q arm of chromosome 1. FcαRI is also homologous to the Fcγ receptors but more distantly related than the Fcγ receptors are to each other. The gene for FcαRI has been mapped to the q arm of chromosome 19 and it probably diverged from a common ancestor gene early in the evolution of immunoglobulin receptors. B. The ITAM expressed in the cytoplasmic domains of γ-chain and FcγRIIa are similar but distinct. The primary sequence differences in these ITAMs can lead to distinct activation phenotypes.

Most important for RA are the receptors for the Fc region of IgG (FcγR) and for the Fc region of IgA (FcαR) (reviewed in ref. 49–51,80). Neutrophils constitutively express two distinct FcγR, FcγRIIa (CD32) and FcγRIIIb (CD16), and a receptor of IgA (FcαRI) (Fig. 8.1). Activation of neutrophils can lead to the appearance of another IgG receptor (FcγRIa) and upregulation of FcαRI. Engagement of Fc receptors, upon cross-linking by immune complexes, by ANCA or by surface absorbed Ig, results in activation of neutrophils, triggering the respiratory burst, degranulation, and phagocytosis (or frustrated phagocytosis on surfaces) (Fig. 8.2). While the mechanisms by which each of these receptors signal are distinct, there are a number of common themes[81]. These receptors do not use G protein signaling pathways, but they do engage tyrosine kinase-dependent signaling pathways, first involving a Src-family kinase (such as fgr) and then activation of the p72 syk kinase and PI-3 kinase. Unlike FcγRIIIb, neutrophil FcγRIa and FcγRIIa receptors use an immunoreceptor tyrosine activation motif (ITAM) that is required for the initial activation steps. FcγRIIIb is an extremely interesting receptor due to its linkage to the outer leaflet of the membrane through a glycosyl-phosphatidyl inositol (GPI) linkage and its lack of any transmembrane or cytoplasmic domains. This receptor is clearly an active participant in neutrophil activation[82,83] and current models of signaling by GPI-anchored proteins involve the partitioning of these receptors to distinct lipid domains in the membrane that are enriched for other lipid-associated Src-kinases on the inner leaflet of the membrane[84,85].

Both constitutive neutrophil Fcγ receptors are polymorphic, and the FcγRIIa-H131/R131 and FcγRIIIb-NA1/NA2 polymorphisms open the possibility of functionally different IgG-induced responses between individuals[49–51]. In fact, the polymorphisms of these receptors have been correlated with risk to certain bacterial infections (reviewed in ref. 86). Precedent for the importance of FcγR allelic polymorphisms in human autoimmune disease has been established by association of alleles of FcγRIIa and FcγRIIIa with SLE[51,86–89]. While corresponding association studies have not yet been reported in patients with RA, the allelic distribution in patients with RA may alter the magnitude or vigor of IgG-induced neutrophil activity in patients with disease.

The H131/R131 polymorphism of FcγRIIa, the result of a single nucleotide change in the second extracellular immunoglobulin-like domain changing histidine to arginine at amino acid 131, alters the binding of IgG2 (reviewed in ref. 50,51). The H131 allele is the only FcγR that binds IgG2 and is associated with an increased risk of heparin induced thrombocytopenia in patients with autoimmune antiphospholipid syndrome. Conversely, the R131 allele, which binds IgG2 poorly, has been associated with certain bacterial infections and with SLE in some ethnic groups. Another polymorphic site is found at residue 27 in the first extracellular Ig-like domain and predicts a glutamine to tryptophan change but there is no known functional significance associated with this polymorphism. A rare substitution in codon 127, changing a glutamine to lysine, restores moderate IgG2 binding in the context of the low-binding R131 allele. The H131 allele may have increased affinity for IgG3.

The two commonly recognized allelic forms of FcγRIIIb, NA1 and NA2, were originally defined serologically. More recently,

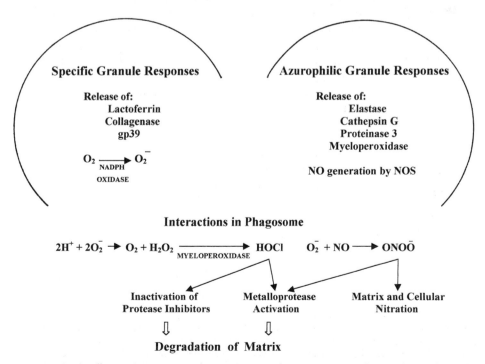

Fig. 8.2 Neutrophil responses to tissue-adherent immune complexes. Ligation of Fc receptors results in release of specific and azurophilic granule proteinases into phagolysosomes in concert with activation of oxidant-generating enzymes. Oxidative modification of enzymes and regulatory proteins by phagosome reaction products promotes the enzymatic degradation of adjacent tissue matrix. Oxidants derived from superoxide and nitric oxide may furthermore modify cellular functions or engender somatic mutations.

sequencing of the genes encoding the alleles has revealed five polymorphic residues. Systematic analysis of FcγRIIIb sequence from donors of the two allotypes indicates that there are two predominant genotypes that differ from each other by four amino acids in the first extracellular Ig-like domain. Combinatorial grouping of these sites to yield a larger number of alleles does not occur. The NA1 and NA2 alleles have different quantitative levels of function despite comparable binding of IgG-opsonized erythrocytes (reviewed in ref. 50,51). Donors homozygous for the NA1 allele demonstrate a larger FcγR-mediated phagocytic response owing, at least in part, to quantitative differences in the ability of this allele to elicit a larger oxidative burst and/or degranulation response. Although the molecular basis for the higher level of function of the NA1 allele has not been determined, the NA1 and NA2 alleles have different numbers of glycosylation sites and are differentially glycosylated *in vivo*. These post-translational modifications may mediate interactions between FcγRIIIb and the β2 integrin, CD11b/CD18, in the neutrophil membrane[90] and as a result alter net receptor function. The NA1/NA2 alleles appear to have clinical significance[86]. Donors homozygous for the NA1 allele are more resistant to certain bacterial infections. In addition, donors homozygous for NA2 may be more likely to have severe infection especially in the context of the low IgG2-binding R131-allele of FcγRIIa. Theoretically, these polymorphisms may govern the intensity of the neutrophil contribution to disease in patients with RA.

Complement receptors

In addition to a seven-transmembrane-domain receptor for C5a, neutrophils express two distinct receptors for opsonic fragments of complement. Complement receptor type 1 (CR1, CD35) has highest affinity for C3b but can also bind iC3b while CR3 (CD11b/CD18) binds iC3b[91,92]. CR1 is a member of the regulator of complement activation (RCA) family. Members of this family share a common extracellular structural domain, the short consensus motif (SCR). Multiple SCRs are grouped into larger repeating structures called long homologous repeats (LHR). In contrast to CR1, CR3 is a β2 integrin composed of two structurally distinct chains, $α_M$ and β2. In addition to binding iC3b, CD11b/CD18 (CR3) also binds to ICAM-1, fibrinogen, β-glucan, and possibly LPS. Functionally, CR3 is important in the transendothelial migration of neutrophils and monocytes[76]. There is also increasing evidence that CR3 is associated in the membrane with many other cell surface receptors such as CD14 (receptor for LPS), CD87 (the uPA receptor) and Fcγ receptors (both FcγRIIa and FcγRIIIb)[90]. These associations may alter the biology of these receptors.

It has long been appreciated that complement opsonization of immune complexes results in more effective stimulation of neutrophils, suggesting that complement receptors and Fc receptors interact in some way[93]. The ability of CR3 to synergize with FcγR in stimulation of phagocytosis and the respiratory burst has now been directly documented[82,83] and, as mentioned above, some studies have suggested physical association in the membrane between FcγR and CR3[90]. While association may

occur between these receptor systems, distinct signaling pathways are activated[94]. Synergism might result by convergence of these pathways on common signaling intermediates. More importantly, these results demonstrate the complexity of neutrophil biology and show that analysis of single receptors systems might not reflect the full functional capacity of the cell.

More intriguing is the recent observation that engagement of CR1 selectively down modulates IgG-induced release of azurophilic granules[47]. Treatment of cells with the protein kinase C activator PMA leads to threonine and/or serine phosphorylation of CR1[95], but the mechanism(s) by which CR1 specifically alters the azurophilic degranulation response is not well characterized. The absence of tyrosine residues in the cytoplasmic domain of CR1 suggests, at least, that tyrosine phosphorylation pathways are not important. However, the ability of CR1 to attenuate IgG-induced primary granule release indicates that the interaction between complement opsonization and Fc receptors is more complex than synergism for activation.

Cytokine receptors

Activation of neutrophils can lead to the synthesis and/or secretion of cytokines, and, given the expression of receptors for multiple cytokines by the neutrophil, both autocrine and paracrine regulation of responses are possible[67]. Of particular importance in the pathogenesis of RA, neutrophils have receptors for cytokines such as IL-8 (discussed above), IL-1 (reviewed in ref. 96), and TNF-α (see below).

TNF-α has attracted particular attention given the clinical efficacy of anti-TNF therapy in RA[97]. TNF-α can prime neutrophils, facilitate neutrophil adhesion through $β_2$ integrins, induce neutrophil secretion of both IL-1β and TNF, and stimulate oxidase activity[12,98-99]. The two structurally distinct high affinity receptors for TNF-α (p55 and p75) on neutrophils may mediate different functional responses[100]. The p55 TNFRI is able to induce all of the known responses, and mAb inhibition studies indicate a role for the p75 TNFRII in the induction of the oxidative burst. TNFRII may be required for a full neutrophil response to TNF-α perhaps through co-operative binding of TNF-α by the two receptors. This observation suggests a model in which the p75 receptor is the initial TNF-α capture receptor that facilitates presentation of the cytokine to TNFRI, especially at low concentrations of TNF-α. Nonetheless, the ability of TNF-α to induce oxidase activity and cytokine secretion and to prime neutrophils for enhanced responses to other stimuli (such as chemotactic factors and IgG[101,102]) underscores the complexity of neutrophils responses in the inflammatory milieu and demonstrates the inter-relationship between the many receptor systems that are likely to be important for neutrophil in inflammatory diseases.

Rheumatoid synovial fluid can also contain GM-CSF which can prime neutrophils and retard apoptosis[103]. In fact, most agents that can prime neutrophils also retard the induction of apoptosis resulting in more sustained functional responses[104]. This delay in cell death could be an important mechanism by which chronic inflammatory reactions are perpetuated. Certainly, prolonged neutrophil survival could lead to more sustained release of IL-8, IL-1β, and TNF-α, thereby facilitating cellular transmigration and infiltration.

Receptors for lipopolysaccharide

One of the most potent neutrophil activators is lipopolysaccharide (LPS). While this bacterial product may not be of primary importance in the pathogenesis of RA, the study of the mechanisms by which LPS activates neutrophils is nonetheless instructive. Indeed, recent studies on the mechanisms of LPS stimulation of leukocytes has led to the recognition of the importance of an entirely new receptor system, the Toll-like receptors[8-10].

LPS is a potent stimulus that can elicit cytokine secretion, adhesion, degranulation, and an oxidative burst[7,105,106]. Paradoxically, we know little about the LPS recognition system(s) at the membrane that are necessary for these varied and robust responses[7]. The ability of LPS to activate neutrophils at low concentrations of $\leq$ 1ng ml^{-1} is dependent on the GPI-anchored protein CD14 on the surface of the cells. However, LPS binds most effectively to CD14 after first binding to a serum lipopolysaccharide binding protein (LBP) and/or soluble CD14. Until very recent studies of the mammalian homologues of the *Drosophila* Toll receptor protein, the mechanism of CD14 activation of the intracellular signaling events has remained unclear. Toll is directly involved in host defense in *Drosophila*, and cross-linking the mammalian Toll-like receptor can induce cell activation leading to production of proinflammatory cytokines[9,107]. There are now five known human homologues of the Toll protein, and the link between LPS binding and the Toll-like receptors has now been established[8-10]. The resultant activation is further enhanced by the addition of CD14, and while expression of Toll-like receptors in human neutrophils has not yet been examined, it is likely that the same or a similar pathway will be important. The role of the Toll-like family of receptors in chronic inflammatory diseases such as RA is now an open question and a clear reminder that much remains to be learned.

Neutrophils in rheumatoid arthritis

Neutrophils in rheumatoid synovial fluid

Neutrophils that have emigrated into rheumatoid joints retain the ability to engage immune complexes and respond to inflammatory cytokines. The constitutively expressed Fc receptors, FcγRIIa and FcγRIIIb, show some variability in expression levels, reflecting activation and shedding of FcγRIIIb[108-110], and FcγRIa is upregulated on synovial fluid neutrophils[108,108a]. In response to ligation of Fc receptors, synovial-fluid-derived neutrophils produce superoxide derived oxidants and release both specific and azurophilic granule enzymes. These cells also retain the capacity for liberation of lipid mediators such as LTB$_4$[111,112], but the extent to which IL-1, IL-8, and other inflammatory cytokines are synthesized and secreted by rheumatoid synovial fluid neutrophils has not been established[113,114].

Alteration and degradation of articular cartilage

The consequences of neutrophil activation within the joint depend upon the activating ligand(s), cytokine milieu, site of activation, and genetic factors governing the neutrophil response. In response to fluid phase ligands, release of azurophilic granule constituents including elastase, cathepsin G, and myeloperoxidase may be limited[115]. Furthermore, the abundance of proteinase inhibitors present in normal as well as inflamed synovial fluids probably inactivate proteinases released by fluid phase neutrophils. However, immunoglobulins of the IgG and IgA classes on and within the surface layers of articular cartilage[31,116] can engage neutrophil Fc receptors and result in neutrophil activation with alteration of subjacent articular cartilage[30,117].

Surface-adherent immunoglobulins are potent stimuli for the release of both specific and azurophilic granule proteinases and for the generation of oxidants such as HOCl which can activate procollagenase[115,118]. IgG and IgA-triggered production of superoxide and release of specific granule-derived metalloporteinases (including collagenase) into phagolysosomes accompanied by myeloperoxidase derived from azurophilic granules favors the generation of HOCl and activation of latent metalloproteinases[119,120]. Other azurophilic-granule-derived enzymes, including cathepsin G and possibly nitric oxide synthase, are also capable of enhancing the activity of latent metalloproteinases[121-123]. Furthermore, by inactivating tissue or synovial fluid proteinase inhibitors, HOCl generated within the phagolysosome promotes the activity of neutrophil serine proteases such as cathepsin G and elastase[124]. In a variety of *in vitro* models, neutrophil engagement of immunoglobulins adherent to matrix proteins results in degradation of adjacent matrix, even within the milieu of proteinase inhibitors or synovial fluid[125,126]. This model has been extended to explants of human articular cartilage pretreated with immunoglobulins derived from RA synovial fluid, whereby degradation of collagens and proteoglycans in the explant occurs during incubation with neutrophils in synovial fluids[127].

Histological studies of rheumatoid joints and studies with cartilage explants provide compelling evidence that neutrophils engage and are capable of altering the articular surface. Cartilage-adherent neutrophils have been observed at the cartilage–pannus interface, and neutrophils have been shown to adhere to rheumatoid cartilage explants[30,128,129]. Immunohistochemical studies, enzymatic assays, and assays for enzyme-inhibitor complexes identifying the presence of neutrophil granule constituents, including elastase in the superficial layers of rheumatoid cartilage and at sites of erosion by synovial pannus, all provide 'footprint' evidence of neutrophil activation on the articular surface of rheumatoid joints in vivo[117,130].

Footholds: the evolution of the synovial pannus

Degradation of the superficial layers of articular cartilage by elastase and collagenase promotes binding of immunoglobulins to articular cartilage, including the specific binding of autoantibodies to type II collagen[131]. The binding of such autoantibodies may reflect the unmasking of 'hidden' collagen epitopes, and the alteration of articular surfaces by neutrophils may be a critical early step in the pathogenesis of RA. Through reactions catalyzed by myeloperoxidase, neutrophil-derived oxidants promote covalent cross-linking of cartilage-associated immunoglobulins, rendering them relatively insoluble to extraction[132,133]. Superoxide radicals may interact with nitric oxide generated by neutrophils or adjacent chondrocytes to generate species that oxidize and cross-link immune complexes on articular surfaces[134]. Although not yet formally proven, oxidative modification and nitration of articular structures may result in the generation of immunogenic neoepitopes, resulting in antigen-driven production of autoantibodies. Indeed, the presence of antibodies to modified lipoproteins has established the precedent for production of antibodies to oxidized proteins[135,136]. Such oxidative modification of immune complexes and articular structures may lead to self-perpetuating immune responses and inflammation within the joint.

Degradation of the articular surface by neutrophils also promotes the attachment of rheumatoid synovial fibroblasts to cartilage *in vitro*[137] Both neutrophil serine protease and metalloproteinase-mediated alterations in cartilage facilitate fibroblast attachment[131,137] which suggests that alteration of the articular surface and enhancement of synoviocyte attachment to cartilage might be a critical event in the evolution of erosive anthropathy[138].

Oxidants and synovial cell and synovial fluid biology

Neutrophil activation within inflamed joints may also impact upon the properties of synovial fluid. Oxidants such as HOCl are capable of degrading proteoglycans and hyaluronate via oxidation of N-acetyl groups on chondroitin sulfate, hyaluronic acid and N-acetylglucosamine[139,140]. Since high molecular weight polymers of hyaluronic acid have been shown to attenuate neutrophil phagocytic responses and inhibit release of proteoglycan from cartilage explants, depolymerization and breakdown of hyaluronate mediated by neutrophil-derived oxidants may further promote the degradation of articular cartilage[141,142]. Depolymerization of hyaluronate polymers within synovial fluid may also result in heightened nociceptive processes within rheumatoid joints. Indirect evidence for increased joint pain in RA as a result of the loss of hyaluronate polymerization is provided by at least one pilot study in which sequential injection of high molecular hyaluronate (normally used for management of knee osteoarthritis) into rheumatoid knees resulted in pain relief[143].

Although the impact of neutrophil activation directly on synovial tissues has received less attention, oxidants and the release of granule constituents can create a potent, toxic microenvironment. Somatic mutations in the p53 tumor suppressor gene have recently been described in the synovial lining cells of the rheumatoid pannus[44] and mutations of this and other genes regulating cell growth and adhesion may account for the invasive/proliferative phenotype of rheumatoid pannus.

Although the mechanism(s) whereby such mutations occur have not been elucidated, products of nitration reactions have demonstrated mutagenic capacity[144], and we have found abundant evidence of nitration reactions within rheumatoid synovium (W. Chatham, unpublished observations). In addition to generating chlorinated oxidants such as HOCl, myeloperoxidase released from neutrophil granules can promote nitration reactions capable of altering cellular function[16,134]. It is certainly conceivable that neutrophils activated within or adjacent to the synovium may promote mutagenic events in the synovium by:

(1) producing superoxide which than reacts with NO (generated by the neutrophils or adjacent monocyte/macrophages and chondrocytes) to form reactive $ONOO^-$ species;

(2) generating HOCl which can react with $ONOO^-$ to form mutagenic nitrosyl chloride species; and

(3) releasing myeloperoxidase which catalyzes nitration events.

The interplay between neutrophils, their reaction products and synovial biology should provide a fertile area of investigation for elucidating mechanisms of disease in RA.

References

1. Steinman, L. Escape from 'horror autotoxicus': pathogenesis and treatment of autoimmune disease. *Cell,* 1995;**80**:7–10.
2. Medzhitov, R., Janeway, C.A. Jr. Innate immunity: the virtues of a nonclonal system of recognition. *Cell,* 1997;**91**:295–298.
3. Fearon, D.T., Locksley, R.M. The instructive role of innate immunity in the acquired immune response. *Science,* 1996;**272**:50–54.
4. Fearon, D.T. Seeking wisdom in innate immunity. *Nature,* 1997;**388**:323–324.
5. Medzhitov, R., Janeway, C.A., Jr. Innate immunity: impact of the adaptive immune response. *Current Opinion Immunol,* 1997;**9**:4–9.
6. Matzinger, P. Tolerance, danger, and the extended family. *Annu Rev Immunol,* 1994;**12**:991–1045.
7. Ulevitch, R.J., Tobias, P.S. Receptor-dependent mechanisms of cell stimulation by bacterial endotoxin. *Annu Rev Immunol,* 1995;**13**:437–457.
8. Kirschning, C.J., Wesche, H., Ayres, T.M., Rothe, M. Human Toll-like receptor 2 confers responsiveness to bacterial lipopolysaccharide. *J Exp Med,* 1998;**188**:2091–2097.
9. Yang, R.B., Mark, M.R., Gray, A., Huang A., Xie, M.H., Zhang, M., Goddard, A., Wood, W.I., Gurney, A.L., Godowski, P.J. Toll-like receptor-2 mediates lipopolysaccharide-induced cellular signaling. *Nature,* 1998;**17**:284–288.
10. Poltorak, A., He, X., Smirnova, I., Liu, M.Y., van Huffel, C., Du, X., Birdwell, D., Alejos, E., Silva, M., Galanos, C., Freudenberg, M., Ricciardi-Castagnoli, P., Layton, B., Beutler, B. Defective LPS signaling in C3H/HeJ and C57L/10ScCr mice: Mutations in Tlr4 gene. *Science,* 1998;**282**:2085–2088.
11. Pillinger, M.H., Abramson, S.B. The neutrophil in rheumatoid arthritis. *Rheum Dis Clin North Am,* 1995;**21**:691–714.
12. Edwards, S.W., Hallett, M.B. Seeing the wood for the trees: the forgotten role of neutrophils in rheumatoid arthritis. *Immunol Today,* 1997;**18**:320–324.
13. Ogilvie, A.C., Hack, C.E., Wagstaff, J., van Mierlo, G.J., Erenberg, A.J., Thomsen, L.L., Hoekman, K., Rankin, E.M. IL-1 beta does not cause neutrophil degranulation but does lead to IL-6, IL-8 and nitrite/nitrate release when used in patients with cancer. *J Immunol,* 1996;**156**:389–394.

14. Evans, T.J., Buttery, L.D., Carpenter, A., Springhall, D.R., Polak, J.M., Cohen, J. Cytokine-treated human neutrophils contain inducible nitric oxide synthase that produces nitration of ingested bacteria. *Proc Natl Acad Sci USA*, 1996;93:9553–9558.

15. Domigan, N.M., Charlton, T.S., Duncan, M.W., Winterbourn, C.C., Kettle, A.J. Chlorination of tyrosyl residues in peptides by myeloperoxidase and human neutrophils. *J Biol Chem*, 1995;270:16542–16548.

16. Eiserich, J.P., Hristova, M., Cross, C.E., Jones, A.D., Freeman, B.A., Halliwell, B., van der Vliet, A. Formation of nitric oxide-derived inflammatory oxidants by myeloperoxidase in neutrophils. *Nature*, 1998;391:393–397.

17. Sampson, J.B., Ye, Y., Rosen, H., Beckman, J.S. Myeloperoxidase and horseradish peroxidase catalyze tyrosine nitration in proteins from nitrite and hydrogen peroxide. *Arch Biochem Biophys*, 1998;356:207–213.

18. Gagnon, C., Leblond, F.A., Filep, J.G. Peroxynitrite production by human neutrophils, monocytes and lymphocytes challenged with lipopolysaccharide. *FEBS Letters*, 1998;431:107–110.

19. Farrell, A.J., Blake D.R., Palmer, R.M.J., Moncada, S. Increased concentrations of nitrite in synovial fluid and serum samples suggest increased nitric oxide synthesis in rheumatic diseases. *Ann Rheum Diseases*, 1992;51:1219–1222.

20. Kaur, H., Halliwell, B. Evidence for nitric oxide-mediated oxidative damage in chronic inflammation. Nitrotyrosine in serum and synovial fluid from rheumatoid patients. *FEBS Lett*, 1994;350:9–12.

21. Stichtenoth, D.O., Fauler, J., Zeidler, H., Frolich, J.C. Urinary nitrate excretion is increased in patients with rheumatoid arthritis by prednisolone. *Ann Rheum Dis*, 1995;54:820–824.

22. Grabowski, P.S., England, A.J., Dykhuizen, R., Copland, M., Benjamin, N., Reid, D.M., Ralston, S.H. Elevated nitric oxide production in rheumatoid arthritis. Detection using the fasting urinary nitrate: creatinine ratio. *Arthritis Rheum*, 1996;39:643–647.

23. Wigand, R., Meyer, J., Busse, R. Hecker, M. Increased serum NG-hydroxy-L-arginine in patients with rheumatoid arthritis and systemic lupus erythematosus as an index of an increased nitric oxide synthase activity. *Ann Rheum Dis*, 1997;56:330–332.

24. Hilliquin, P., Borderie, D., Hervann, A., Menkes, C.J., Ekindjian, O.G. Nitric oxide as S-nitrosoproteins in rheumatoid arthritis. *Arthritis Rheum*, 1997;40:1512–1517.

25. Okamoto, T., Akaike, T., Nagano, T., Miyajima, S., Suga, M., Ando, M., Ichimori, K., Maeda, H. Activation of human neutrophil procollagenase by nitrogen dioxide and peroxynitrite: a novel mechanism for procollagenase activation involving nitric oxide. *Arch Biochem Biophys*, 1997;342:261–274.

26. Menninger, H., Putzier, R., Mohr, W., Wessinghage, D., Tillmann, K. Granulocyte elastase at the site of cartilage erosion by rheumatoid synovial tissue. *Z Rheumatol*, 1980;39:145–146.

27. Mohr, W., Westerhellweg, H., Wessinghage, D. Polymorphonuclear granulocytes in rheumatic tissue destruction. III. An electron microscopic study of PMNs at the pannus cartilage junction in rheumatoid arthritis. *Ann Rheum Dis*, 1981;40:396–399.

28. Mohr, W. Cartilage destruction via the synovial fluid in rheumatoid arthritis. *J Rheumatol*, 1995;22:1436–1438.

29. Ugai, K., Ziff, M., Jasin, H.E. Interaction of polymorphonuclear leukocytes with immune complexes trapped in joint collagenous tissues. *Arthritis Rheum*, 1979;22:353–364.

30. Ugai, K., Ishikawa, H., Hirohata, K., Shirane, H. Interaction of polymorphonuclear leukocytes with immune complexes trapped in rheumatoid articular cartilage. *Arthritis Rheum*, 1983;26:1434–1441.

31. Jasin, H.E. Autoantibody specificities of immune complexes sequestered in articular cartilage of patients with rheumatoid arthritis and osteoarthritis. *Arthritis Rheum*, 1985;28:241–248.

32. Staite, N.D., Messner, R.P., Zoschke, D.C. Inhibition of human T lymphocyte E rosette formation by neutrophils and hydrogen peroxide. Differential sensitivity between helper and suppressor T lymphocytes. *J Immunol*, 1987;139: 2424–2430.

33. Hirohata, S., Yanagida, T., Yoshino, Y., Miyashita, H. Polymorphonuclear neutrophils enhance suppressive activities of anti-CD3 induced CD4+ suppressor T cells. *Cellular Immunol*, 1995;160:270–277.

34. Romani, L., Bistoni, F., Puccetti, P. Initiation of T-helper cell immunity to Candida albicans by IL-12H: the role of neutrophils. *Chemical Immunol*, 1997;68:110–135.

35. Romani, L., Mencacci, A., Cenci, E., Del Sero, G., Bistoni, F., Puccetti, P. An immunoregulatory role for neutrophils in CD4+ T helper subset selection in mice with candidiasis. *J Immunol*, 1997;158:2356–2362.

36. Romani, L., Mencacci, A., Cenci, E., Spaccapelo, R., Del Sero, G., Nicoletti, I., Trinchieri, G., Bistoni, F., Puccetti, P. Neutrophil production of IL-12 and IL-10 in candidiasis and efficacy of IL-12 therapy in neutropenic mice. *J Immunol*, 1997;158: 5349–5356.

37. Mencacci, A., Del Sero, G., Cenci, d'Ostiani, C.F., Bacci, A., Montagnoli, C., Kopf, M., Romani, L. Endogenous interleukin 4 is required for development of protective CD4+ T helper type 1 cell responses to Candida albicans. *J Exp Med*, 1998;187:307–317.

38. Bosch, X., Llena, J., Collado, A., Font, J., Mirapeix, E., Ingelmo, M., Munoz-Gomez, J., Urbano-Marquez, A. Occurrence of anti-neutrophil cytoplasmic and antineutrophil (peri)nuclear antibodies in rheumatoid arthritis. *J Rheumatol*, 1995;22:2038–2045.

39. Braun, M.G., Csernok, E., Schmitt, W.H., Gross, W.L. Incidence, target antigens, and clinical implications of antineutrophil cytoplasmic antibodies in rheumatoid arthritis. *J Rheumtol*, 1996;23:826–830.

40. Rother, E., Schocbat, T., Peter, H.H. Antineutrophil cytoplasmic antibodies (ANCA) in rheumatoid arthritis: a prospective study. *Rheumatol Int*, 1996;15:231–217.

41. Volck, B., Price, P.A., Johansen, J.S., Sorensen, O., Benfield, T.L., Nielsen, H.J., Calafat, J., Borregaard, N. YKL-40, a mammalian member of the chitinase family, is a matrix protein of specific granules in human neutrophils. *Proc Assoc Am Physicians*, 1998;110:351–360.

42. Baeten, D, DeKeyser, F., Elewaut, D., Rijnders, A.M.W., Verheijden, G.F., Miltenburg, A.M.W., Steenbakkers, P., Verbruggen, G., Boots, A.M.H., Veys, E.M. HC gp-39 expression is synovial lining is correlated with joint destruction in RA. *Arthritis Rheum*, 1998;41:S365.

43. Nakamura, N., Nakamura, K., Yodoi, J. Redox regulation of cellular activation. *Ann Rev Immunol*, 1997;15:351–369.

44. Firestein, G.S., Echeverri, F., Yeo, M., Zvaifler, N.J., Green, D.R. Somatic mutations in the p53 tumor suppressor gene in rheumatoid arthritis synovium. *Proc Natl Acad Sci USA*, 1997;94:10895–10900.

45. Bharadwaj D., Stein M.P., Volzer M., Mold C., Du Clos T.W. The major receptor for C-reactive protein on leukocytes is Fcg Receptor II. *J Exp Med*, 1999;190:85–590.

46. Marnell, L.L., Mold, C., Volzer, M.A., Burlingame, R.W., Du Clos, T.W. C-reactive protein binds to Fc gamma RI in transfected COS cells. *J Immunol*, 1995;155:2185–2193.

47. Sambandam, T., Chatham, W.W. Ligation of CR1 attenuates Fc receptor-mediated myeloperoxidase release and HOCl production by neutrophils. *J Leukocyte Biology*, 1998;63:477–485.

48. Chatham, W.W., Blackburn, W.D. Jr. Fixation of C3 to IgG attenuates neutrophil HOCl generation and collagenase activation. *J Immunol*, 1993;151:949–958.

49. Edberg, J.C., Salmon, J.E., Kimberly, R.P. Functional capacity of Fc gamma receptor III (CD16) on human neutrophils. *Immunologic Research*, 1992;11:239–251.

50. Kimberly, R.P., Salmon, J.E., Edberg, J.C. Receptors for immunoglobulin G. Molecular diversity and implications for disease. *Arthritis Rheum*, 1995;38:306–314.

51. Gibson, A.W., Wu, J. Edberg, J.C., R.P. Kimberly. 1999. Diversity in Fc receptors. In: Tsokos, G., Kammer, G. (eds). *Lupus: cellular and molecular pathogenesis*. Humana Press, p. 557–573.

52. Henson, P.M., Henson, J.E., Fittschen, C., Bratton, D.L., Riches, D.W.H. 1992. Degranulation and secretion ny phagocytic cells. In:

Gallin JI, Goldstein IM, Synderman R (eds). *Inflammation: basic principles and clinical correlates* NY, NY, Raven, p. 511–539.

53. Abramson, J.S., Wheeler, J.G. 1993. *The neutrophil.* IRL Press at Oxford Univ. Press, Oxford.

54. Borregarrd, N., Cowland, J.B. Granules of human neutrophilic polymorphonuclear leukocytes. *Blood,* 1997;**89**:3503–3521.

55. Gullsberg, U., Andersson, E., Garwicz, D., Lindmark, A., Olsson, I. Biosynthesis, processing and sorting of neutrophil proteins: Insights into neutrophil granule development. *Eur J Haemat,* 1997;**58**:137–153.

56. Khanna-Gupta, A., Zibello, T., Berliner, N. Coordinate regulation of neutrophil secondary granule protein expression. *Curr Topics Micro Immunol,* 1996;**211**:165–171.

57. Muller-Ladner, U., Gay, R.E., Gay, S. Molecular biology of cartilage and bone destruction. Current Opin Rheum, 1998;**10**:212–219.

58. Csernok, E., Trabandt, A., Gross, W.L. Immunogenetic aspects of ANCA-associated vasculitides. *Exp Clin Immunogenetics,* 1997;**14**:177–182.

59. Kocher, M., Edberg, J.C., Fleit, H.B., Kimberly, R.P. Antineutrophil cytoplasmic antibodies preferentially engage FcγRIIIb on human neutrophils. *J Immunol,* 1998 ;**161**:6909–6914.

60. Edberg, J.C., Wainstein, E., Wu, J., Csernok, E., Sneller, M.C., Hoffman, G.S., Keystone, E.C., Gross, W.L., Kimberly, R.P. Analysis of FcγRII gene polymorphisms in Wegener's granulomatosis. *Exp Clin Immunogenetics,* 1997;**14**:183–195.

61. Scharenberg, A.M., Kinet, J.P. The emerging field of inhibitory signaling: SHP or SHIP? *Cell,* 1996;**87**:961–964.

62. Hampton, M.B., Kettle, A.J., Winterbourn, C.C. Inside the neutrophil phagosome: Oxidants, myeloperoxidase, and bacterial killing. *Blood,* 1998;**92**:3007–3017.

63. Klebanoff, S.J. 1992. Oxygen metabolites from phagocytes. In: Gallin, J.I., Golstein, I.M., Snyderman, R. (eds). *Inflammation: basic principles and clinical correlates.* NY, NY, Raven, p. 541–588.

64. Davies, P., MacIntyre, D.E. 1992. Prostaglandins and inflammation. In Gallin, J.I., Goldstein, I.M., Snyderman, R. (eds). *Inflammation: basic principles and clinical correlates.* NY, NY, Raven, p.123–138.

65. Maloney, C.G., Kutchera, W.A., Albertine, K.H., McIntyre, T.M., Prescott, S.M., Zimmerman, G.A. Inflammatory agonists induce cyclooxygenase type 2 expression in human neutrophils. *J Immunol,* 1998;**160**:1402–1410.

66. Poiliot, M., Gilbert, C., Borgeat, P., Poubelle, P.E., Bourgoin, S., Creminon, C., Maclouf, J., McColl, S.R., Naccache, P.H. Expression and activation of prostaglandin endoperoxide synthase-2 in agonist-activated human neutrophils. *FASEB J,* 1998;**612**:1109–1123.

67. Cassatella, M.A. 1996. *Cytokines produced by polymorphonuclear neutrophils: molecular and biological aspects.* Chapman and Hall, NY.

68. Nick, J.A., Avdi, N.J., Gerwins, P., Johnson, G.L., Worthen, G.S. Activation of a p38 mitogen-activated protein kinase in human neutrophils by lipopolysaccharide. *J Immunol,* 1996;**156**:4867–4875.

69. Baggiolini, M. Chemokines and leukocyte traffic. *Nature,* 1998;**392**:565–568.

70. Baggiolini, M., Dewald, B., Moser, B. Human chemokines: An update. *Ann Rev Immunol,* 1997;**15**:675–705.

71. Lee, B., Doranz, B.J., Rana, S., Yi, Y., Mellado, M., Frade, J.M., Martinez, A.C., O'Brien, S.J., Dean, M., Collman, R.G., Doms, R.W. Influence of the CCR2-V64I polymorphism on human immunodeficiency virus type 1 coreceptor activity and on chemokine receptor function of CCR2b, CCR3, CCR5, and CXCR4. *J Virol,* 1998;**72**:7450–7458.

72. Mummidi, S., Ahuja, S.S., Gonzalez, E., Anderson, S.A., Santiago, E.N., Stephan, K.T., Craig, F.E., O'Connell, P., Tryon, V., Clark, R.A., Dolan, M.J., Ahuja, S.,K. Genealogy of the CCR5 locus and chemokine system gene variants associated with altered rates of HIV-1 disease progression. *Nature Med,* 1998;**4**:786–793.

73. Winkler, C., Modi, W., Smith, M.W., Nelson, G.W., Wu, X., Carrington, M., Dean, M., Honjo, T., Tashiro, K., Yabe, D., Buchbinder, S., Vittinghoff, E., Goedert, J.J., O'Brien, T.R., Jacobson, L.P., Detels, R., Donfield, S., Willoughby, A., Gomperts, E., Vlahov, D., Phair, J., O'Brien, S.J. Genetic restriction of AIDS pathgenesis by an SDF-1 chemokine gene variant. ALIVE Study, Hemophilia Growth and Development Study (HGDS), Multicenter AIDS Cohort Study (MACS), Multicenter Hemophilia Cohort Study (MHCS), San Francisco City Cohort (SFCC). *Science,* 1998;**279**:389–393.

73a. Gomez-Reino J.J., Pablos J.L., Carreira P.E., Santiago B., Serrano L., Vicario J.L., Balsa A., Figueroa M., de Juan M.D. Association of rheumatoid arthritis with a functional chemokine receptor, CCR5. Arthritis Rheum 1999;**42**:989–92.

74. Philips, M.R., Pillinger, M.H., Staud, R., Volker, C., Rosenfeld, M.G., Weissmann, G., Stock, J.B. Carboxyl methylation of Ras-related proteins during signal transduction in neutrophils. *Science,* 1993;**259**:977–80.

75. Bokoch, G.M. Chemoattractant signaling and leukocyte activation. *Blood,* 1995;**86**:1649–1660.

76. Springer, T.A. Traffic signals for lymphocyte recirculation and leukocyte emigration: The multistep paradigm. *Cell,* 1994;**76**:301–314.

77. Gopalan, P.K., Smith, C.W., Lu, H., Berg, E.L., McIntire, L.V., Simon, S.I. Neutrophil CD18-dependent arrest on intracellular adhesion molecule 1 (ICAM-1) in shear flow can be activated through L-selectin. *J Immunol,* 1997;**158**:367–375.

78. Schnitzler, N., Haase, G., Podbielski, A., Lutticken, R., Schweizer, K.G. A co-stimulatory signal through ICAM-β2 integrin-binding potentiates neutrophil phagocytosis. *Nature Med,* 1999;**5**:231–235.

79. Coxon, A., Rieu, P., Barkalow, F.J., Askari, S., Sharpe, A.H., von Andrian, U.H., Arnaout, M.A., Mayadas, T.N. A novel role for the β2 integrin CD11b/CD18 in neutrophil apoptosis: a homeostatic mechanism in inflammation. *Immunity,* 1996;**5**:653–666.

80. Hulett, M.D., Hogarth, P.M. Molecular basis of Fc receptor function. *Adv Immunol,* 1994;**57**:1–127.

81. Daeron, M. Fc receptor biology. *Ann Rev Immunol,* 1997;**15**:203–234.

82. Edberg, J.C., Kimberly, R.P. Modulation of Fcγ and complement receptor function by the glycosyl-phosphatidylinositol-anchored form of FcγRIII. *J Immunol,* 1994;**152**:5826–5835.

83. Zhou, M.J., Brown, E.J. CR3 (Mac-1, αMβ2, CD11b/CD18) and FcγRIII cooperate in generation of a neutrophil respiratory burst: Requirement for FcγRIII and tyrosine phosphorylation. *J Cell Biol,* 1994;**125**:1407–1416.

84. Green, J.M., Schreiber, A.D., Brown, E.J. Role for a glycan phosphoinositol anchor in Fcγ receptor synergy. *J Cell Biol,* 1997;**139**:1209–1218.

85. Brown, D.A., London, E. Functions of lipid rafts in biological membranes. *Ann Rev Cell Dev Biol,* 1998;**14**:111–136.

86. van der Pol, W., van de Winkel, J.G. IgG receptor polymorphisms: risk factors for disease. *Immunogenetics,* 1998;**48**:222–232.

87. Duits, A.J., Bootsma, R.H., Derksen, R.H.W., Spronk, P.E., Kater, L., Kallenberg, C.G.M., Capel, P.J.A., Westerdaal, G.T., Spierenburg, F.H., Gmelig-Meyling, F.H., van de Winkel, J.G.J. Skewed distribution of IgG Fc receptor IIa (CD32) polymorphisms is associated with renal disease in systemic lupus erythematosus patients. *Arthritis Rheum,* 1995;**39**:1832–1836.

88. Salmon, J.E., Millard, S., Schachter, L.A., Arnett, F.C., Ginzler, E.M., Gourley, M.F., Ramsey-Goldman, R., Peterson, M.G., Kimberly, R.P. FcγRIIA alleles are heritable risk factors for lupus nephritis in African Americans. *J Clin Invest,* 1996;**97**:1348–1354.

89. Wu, J., Edberg, J.C., Redecha, P.B., Bansal, V., Guyre, P.M., Coleman, K., Salmon, J.E., Kimberly, R.P. A novel polymorphism of FcγRIIIa (CD16) alters receptor function and predisposes to autoimmune disease. *J Clin Invest* 1997;**100**:1059–1070.

90. Petty, H.R., Todd, R.F. Receptor–receptor interactions of complement receptor type 3 in neutrophil membranes. *J Leuk Biol*, 1993;**54**:492–494.

91. Ahearn, J.M., Fearon, D.T. Structure and function of complement receptors CR1 (CD35) and CD2 (CD21). *Adv Immunol*, 1989;**46**:183–219.

92. Ross, G.D., Vetvicka, V. CR3 (CD11b, CD18): a phagocyte and NK cell membrane receptor with multiple ligand specificities and functions. *Clin Exp Immunol*, 1993;**92**:181–184.

93. Miller, G.W., Nussenzweig, V. Complement as a regulator of interactions between immune complexes and cell membranes. *J Immunol*, 1974;**113**:464–469.

94. Edberg, J.C., Moon, J.M., Chang, D.J., Kimberly, R.P. Differential regulation of human neutrophil FcγRIIa (CD32) and FcγRIIIb (CD16)-induced Ca^{2+} transients. *J Biol Chem*, 1998;**273**:8071–8079.

95. Changelian, P.S., Fearon, D.T. Tissue-specific phosphorylation of complement receptors CR1 and CR2. *J Exp Med*, 1986;**163**: 101–115.

96. Dinarello, C.A. Interleukin-1, interleukin-1 receptors and interleukin-1 receptor antagonist. *Internatl Rev Immunol*, 1998;**16**:457–499.

97. Moreland, L.W. Soluble tumor necrosis factor receptor (p75) fusion protein (ENBREL) as a therapy of rheumatoid arthritis. *Rheum Dis Clinics N Am*, 1998;**24**:579–591.

98. Naismith, J.H., Sprang, S.R. Modularity in the TNF-receptor family. *Trends Biochem Sci*, 1998;**23**:74–79.

99. Darnay, B.G., Aggarwal, B.B. Early events in TNF signaling: a story of associations and dissociations. *J Leuk Biol*,1997; **61**:559–566.

100. Peschon, J.J., Torrance, D.S., Stocking, K.L., Glaccum, M.B., Otten, C., Willis, C.R., Charrier, K., Morrissey, P.J., Ware, C.B., Mohler, K.M. TNF receptor-deficient mice reveal divergent roles for p55 and p75 in several models of inflammation. *J Immunol*, 1998;**160**:943–952.

101. Simms, H.H., Gaither, T.A., Fries L.F., Frank M.M. Monokines released during short-term Fc gamma receptor phagocytosis up-regulate polymorphonuclear leukocytes and monocyte-phagocytic function. *J Immunol*, 1991 ;**147**:265–272.

102. Gresham, H.D., Zheleznyak A., Mormol J.S., Brown E.J. Studies on the molecular mechanisms of human neutrophil Fc receptor–mediated phagocytosis. Evidence that a distinct pathway for activation of the respiratory burst results in reactive oxygen metabolite-dependent amplification of ingestion. *J Biol Chem*, 1990;**265**:7819–7826.

103. Wei, S., Liu, J.H., Epling-Burnette, P.K., Gamero, A.M., Ussery, D., Pearson, E.W., Elkabani, M.E., Diaz, J.I., Djeu, J.Y. Critical role of Lyn kinase in inhibition of neutrophil apoptosis by granulocyte-macrophage colony–stimulating factor. *J Immunol*, 1996 **157**:5155–5162.

104. Homburg, C.H., Roos, D. Apoptosis of neutrophils. *Curr Opin Hematol*, 1996;**3**:94–99.

105. Haslett, C., Savill, J.S., Meagher, L. The neutrophil. *Curr Opin Immunol*, 1989;**2**:10–18.

106. Smedly, L.A., Tonnesen, M.G., Sandhaus, R.A., Haslett, C., Guthrie, L.A., Johnston, R.B., Henson, P.M., Worthen, G.S. Neutrophil–mediated injury to endothelial cells. Enhancement by endotoxin and essential role of neutrophil elastase. *J Clin Invest*, 1986;**77**:1233–1243.

107. Medzhiton, R., Preston-Hurlbut, P., Janeway, C.A. A human homologue of the Drosophila Toll protein signals activation of adaptive immunity. *Nature*, 1991;**388**:394–397.

108a. Quayle, J.A., Watson, F., Bucknall, R.C., Edwards, S.W. Neutrophils from the synovial fluid of patients with rheumatoid arthritis express the high affinity immunoglobulin G receptor, FcγRI (CD64): role of immune complexes and cytokines in induction of receptor expression. *Immunol*, 1997;**91**: 266–273.

108. Felzmann, T., Gadd, S., Majdic, O., *et al.* Analysis of function-associated receptor molecules on peripheral blood and synovial fluid granulocytes from patients with rheumatoid and reactive arthritis. *J Clin Immunol*, 1988;**11**:205–212.

109. Watson, F., Robinson, J.J., Phelan, M., *et al.* Receptor expression in synovial fluid neutrophils from patients with rheumatoid arthritis. *Ann Rheum Dis*, 1993;**52**:354–359.

110. Goulding, N.J., Guyre, P.M. Impairment of neutrophil Fcγ receptor mediated transmembrane signaling in active rheumatoid arthritis. *Ann Rheum Dis*, 1992;**51**:594–559.

111. Jobin, D. Kreis, C., Gauthier, J., *et al.* Differential synthesis of 5-lipoxygenase in peripheral blood and synovial fluid neutrophiols in rheumatoid arthritis. *J Immunol*, 1991;**146**:2701–2707.

112. Poubelle, P.E., Bourgoin, S., McColl, S.R., *et al.* Altered formation of leukotriene B$_4$ in vitro by synovial fluid neutrophils in rheumatoid arthritis. *J Rheum*, 1989;**16**:280.

113. Lord, P.C.W., Wilmoth, L.M.G., Mizel, S.B., *et al.* Expression of interleukin-1α and β genes by human blood polymorphonuclear leukocytes. *J Clin Invest*, 1991;**87**:1312–1321.

114. Marucha, P.T., Zeff, R.A., Kreutzer, D.L. Cytokine regulation of IL-1β gene expression in the human polymorphonuclear leukocyte. *J Immunol*, 1990;**145**:2932–2937.

115. Chatham, W.W., Turkiewicz, A., Blackburn, W.D., Jr. Determinants of neutrophil HOCl generation: ligand-dependent responses and the role of surface adhesion. *J Leuk Biol*, 1994;**56**:654–660.

116. Veto, A.A., Mannik, M., Zatavain-Rios, E., Wener, M.H. Immune deposits in articular cartilage of patients with rheumatoid arthritis have a granular not seen in osteoarthritis. *Rheumatol Int*, 1990;**10**:13.

117. Velvart, M., Fehr, K. Degradation in vivo of articular cartilgate in rheumatoid arthritis and juvenile chronic arthritis by cathepsin G and elastase from polymorphonuclear leukocytes. *Rheumatol Int*, 1987;**7**:195–202.

118. Henson, P.M. The immunologic release of constituents from neutrophil leukocytes—I. The role antibody and complement on nonphagocytosable surfaces or phagocytosable particles. *J Immunol*, 1971;**107**:1535.

119. Weiss, S.J., Peppin, G. Ortiz, X. Ragsdale, C. Oxidative autoactivation of latent collagenase by human neutrophils. *Science* 1985;**227**:747.

120. Chatham, W.W., Heck, L.W., Blackburn, W.D. Jr. Ligand-dependent release of active neutrophil collagenase. *Arthritis Rheum*, 1990;**33**:328.

121. Capodici, C., Mathukumaran, G., Amorosu, M., Berg, R.A. Activation of neutrophil collagenase by cathepsin G. *Inflammation*, 1989;**13**:245–258.

122. Chatham, W.W., Blackburn, W.D. Jr., Heck, L.W. Addictive enhancement of neutrophil collagenase by HOCl and cathepsin G. *Biochem Biophys Res Commun*, 1992;**184**:560–567.

123. Chatham, W.W., Sampson, J., Beck, J., Blackburn, W.D. Jr. Activation of neutrophil collagenase by peroxynitrite—evidence for nitric oxide production during neutrophil activation with surface bound IgG. *Arthritis Rheum*, 1996;**39**:S37.

124. Ossanua, P.J., Test, S.T., Mathesen, N.R., Regiani, S., Weiss, S.J. Oxidative regulation of neutrophil elastase-alpha-1-proteinase inhibitor interactions. *J Clin Invest*, 1986;**77**:1939.

125. Weiss, S.J., Regiani, S. Neutrophils degrade subendothelial matrices in the presence of alpha-1 protease inhibitor. *J Clin Invest*, 1984;**73**:1297–1303.

126. Chatham, W.W., Heck, L.W., Blackburn, W.D. Jr. Lysis of fibrillar collagen by neutrophils in synovial fluid—a role for surface bound immunoglobulins. *Arthritis Rheum*, 1990;**33**:1333–1339.

127. Chatham, W.W., Swaim, R.S., Frohsin, H., Jr., Heck, L.W., Miller, E.J., Blackburn, W.D., Jr. Degradation of human articular cartilage by neutrophils is synovial fluid. *Arthritis Rheum*, 1993;**36**:51–58.

128. Mohr, W., Menninger, H. Polymorphonuclear granulocytes at the pannus–cartilage junction in rheumatoid arthritis. *Arthritis Rheum*, 1980;**33**:228–234.

129. Bromley, M., Woolley, D.E. Histopathology of the rheumatoid lesion: Identification of cell types at sites of cartilage erosion. *Arthritis Rheum*, 1984;**27**:857–863.

130. Momohara, S. Kashiwazaki, S., Inoue, K., Saito, S., Nakagawa, T. Elastase from polymorphonuclear leukocytes in articular cartilage

and synovial fluids of patients with rheumatoid arthritis. *Clin Rheumatol*, 1997;**16**:133–140.

131. Jasin, H.E., Taurog, J.D. Mechanisms of disruption of the articular cartilage surface in inflammation: neutrophil elastase increases the availability of collagen type II epitopes for binding with antibody on the surface of articular cartilage. *J Clin Invest*, 1991;**87**:1531–1536.

132. Jasin, H.E. Oxidative cross-linking of immune complexes by human polymorphonuclear leukocytes. *J Clin Invest*, 1988;**81**:6.

133. Jasin, H.E. Oxidative modification of inflammatory syniovial fluid immunoglobulin G. *Inflammation*, 1993;**17**:167.

134. Uesugi, M., Hayashi, T., Jasin, H.E. Covalent cross-linking of immune complexes by oxygen radicals and nitrite. *J Immunol*, 1998;**161**:1422–1427.

135. Bui, M.N., Sack, M.N., Moutsatsos, G. *et al*. Autoantibody titers to oxidized low-density lipoprotein in patients with coronary atherosclerosis. *Am Heart J*, 1996;**131**:663–667.

136. Horkko, S., Miller, E., Dudl, E. *et al*. Antiphospholipid antibodies are directed against epitopes of oxidized phospholipids. Recognition of cardiolipin by monoclonal antibodies to epitopes of oxidized low density proteins. *J Clin Invest*, 1996; **98**:815–825.

137. McCurdy, L., Chatham, W.W., Blackburn, W.D., Jr. Rheumatoid synovial fibroblast adhesion to human articular cartilage—enhancement by neutrophil proteases. *Arthritis Rheum*, 1995;**38**:1694–1699.

138. Harris, E.D., Jr. Rheumatoid Arthritis—pathophysiology and implications for therapy. *N Eng J Med*, 1989;**322**:1277–1289.

139. Greenwarld, R.A., Moi, W.W. Effect of oxygen-derived free radicals on hyaluronic acid. *Arthritis Rheum*, 1980;**23**:455–463.

140. Schiller, J., Arnhold, J., Sonntag, K., Arnold K. NMR studies on human, pathologically change synovbial fluids: role of hypochlorous acid. *Magn Reson Med*, 1996;**35**:848–853.

141. Shimazu, A., Jikko, A., Iwamoto, M., *et al*. Effects of hyaluronic acid on the release of proteoglycan from the cell matrix in rabbit chondrocyte cultures in the presence and absence of cytokines. *Arthritis Rheum*, 1993;**36**:247–253.

142. Tamoto, K., Tada, M., Shimada, S. *et al*. Effects of high molecular weight hyaluronates on the functions of guinea pig polymorphonuclear leukocytes. *Semin Arthritis Rheum*, 1993;**22** (suppl):4–8.

143. Goto, M., Hosako, Y., Katayama, M., Yamada, T. Biochemical analysis of rheumatoid synovial fluid after serial intra-articular injection of high molecular weight sodium hyaluronate. *Int J Clin Pharmacol Res*, 1993;**13**:161–166.

144. Nguyen, T., Brunson, D., Crespi, C.L., Penman, B.W., Wishnok, J.S., Tannenbaum, S.R. DNA damage and mutation in human cells exposed to nitric oxide in vitro. *Proc Natl Acad Sci USA*, 1992;**89**:3030–3034.

9 | *The role of fibroblast-like synoviocytes in rheumatoid arthritis*

Pércio S. Gulko, Tetsunori Seki, and Robert Winchester

Introduction

The joint is a functionally unique structure primarily formed from mesenchymal cells. Its distinctive cavity is mainly lined by specialized cells belonging to the fibroblast lineage that are designated as **fibroblast-like intimal synoviocytes**. Through their unique and increasingly defined pattern of gene expression, the fibroblast-like intimal synoviocytes appear to be differentiated to perform a series of functions critical to the biological function of the normal joint. The characteristics of fibroblast-like intimal synoviocytes and their pattern of gene expression suggest that this cell type might be closer to a mesenchymal stem cell than to a normal fibroblast. This phenotype also appears to confer the potential for a special role in fostering the development and synovial localization of the immune response underlying rheumatoid arthritis, and to participate in joint destruction.

In addition to the fibroblast-like intimal synoviocytes[1,2] that account for approximately two-thirds of the lining cells in an uninflamed joint, the intima contains a second intercalated cell type determined by their morphology, phenotype, and function to be derived from the CD14[+] branch of the monocyte lineage[3]. This latter cell is designated the **macrophage-like intimal synoviocyte**. These two types of lining cells were originally named 'type B' and 'type A' respectively according to their appearance in electron microscopy[4], but referring to them by their lineage derivation is more descriptive. The macrophage-like intimal synoviocyte, with its equally specialized phenotype that distinguishes it from the typical monocyte, exhibits some features found in certain types of dendritic cells.

The monocyte progenitors of the macrophage-like intimal synoviocyte enter the intima after leaving blood vessels and differentiate into their mature form in response to guidance clues and interactions apparently provided by the fibroblast-like intimal synoviocytes. The molecules that are responsible for this critical phase of joint histogenesis are beginning to be identified. The function, and especially the interactions of these two cell types, is of special importance in understanding both the biology of the normal joint in the inflammation of rheumatoid arthritis. The macrophage-like lineage cells are covered in detail in Chapter 6.

Beneath the intimal lining layer composed of these two cell types lies a thin zone of vascular connective tissue, the **subin-**

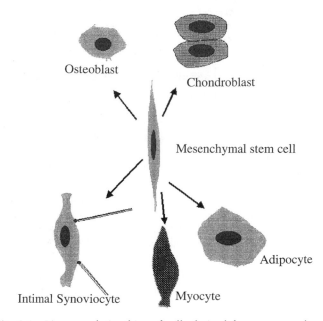

Fig. 9.1 Lineage relationships of cells derived from a mesenchymal stem cell. This cell also gives rise to fibroblasts, including those in the subintima. See also Plate 18.

tima, that may also contain variable numbers of adipocytes. In contrast to the fibroblast-like intimal synoviocyte, the subintimal synoviocytes appear to be more typical connective tissue fibroblasts. The inter-relationships of the various members of the mesenchymal cell lineage is depicted in Figure 9.1.

The goal of this chapter is to summarize interpretively some insights into the biology of the intimal and subintimal synoviocyte regarding their role in the afferent and effector pathways of the pathogenesis of rheumatoid arthritis, and the potential that alleles of genes selectively expressed in these cells have to influence susceptibility to this disease. These insights primarily came from the efforts to identify the genes responsible for the distinctive phenotype exhibited by fibroblast-like synoviocytes obtained in rheumatoid arthritis and certain other synovitides in culture and *in situ*. Certain mechanisms involved in synovial fibroblast gene regulation will also be discussed. Since the majority of the newly-identified genes, including those constitutively expressed at high levels in cultured synoviocytes, appeared very likely to be performing physiological functions, our view of the events in the normal and diseased synovium have been influenced by this perspective. The result is an emphasis on attempting to incorporate the pattern of expression of these genes into schemes that reflect on the normal biology of the joint. For a more detailed and comprehensive treatment, the reader is referred to several comprehensive reviews of the synoviocyte and synovitis[5–7]. Accompanying chapters in this book will also expand some of the related topics mentioned briefly herein.

Synovial fibroblast function and behavior in arthritis

Synovial fibroblast function in the joint and role in joint histogenesis

Because the function of the joint is to permit weight-bearing motion on avascular cartilage, the lining cells appear to be specialized for performing a series of physiological roles aimed at maintaining the integrity of the joint. These functions (Table 9.1) include responsibility for maintaining cartilage viability and function, removal of cartilage debris resulting from impact and weight bearing stresses, and co-ordinating the immunological surveillance of this relatively large fluid space. Interestingly, in the instance of the fibroblast-like intimal synoviocyte, these functions require a degree of spatial polarization and organization unusual for a fibroblast and more commonly encountered in an epithelium. One face of the synoviocyte interacts with extracellular matrix fibers and the lining cells, while the other face interacts with the hyaluronate-rich synovial fluid (Figure 9.2). The intimal lining, however, has none of the structural features of an epithelium such as a basement membrane or tight junctions.

The functions of fibroblast-like intimal synoviocytes, and their presence in early stages of the development of the joint suggest

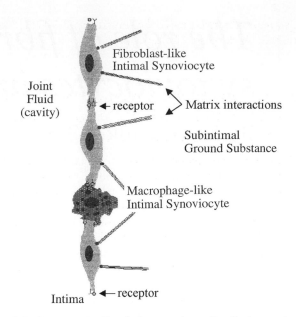

Fig. 9.2 Receptor-mediated homotypic cell–cell interaction of fibroblast-like intimal synoviocytes with each other and their heterotypic interaction with macrophage-like intimal synoviocytes. The polarized state of the intimal cells is indicated by their interaction of one surface, on the right, with the subintimal connective tissue matrix and on the left with the hyaluronate-rich synovial fluid. See also Plate 19.

that these fibroblast-like intimal synoviocytes are responsible for attracting circulating monocyte lineage cells to become resident phagocytic cells in the intima. It is likely that the specific accumulation of monocyte lineage cells in the joint reflects the need for specialized innate immune surveillance and debris removal in this vulnerable mesenchymal cavity. Furthermore, interactions between the monocyte and synoviocyte are responsible for patterning the histogenesis of the normal joint[2]. Similarly, it is possible that the fibroblast-like intimal synoviocyte provides an enhanced recruitment of T and B cells into the joint cavity to

---

Table 9.1　Partial list of fibroblast-like intimal synoviocyte functions

---

Surface specialization for:
a) synovial fluid interface
b) extra-cellular matrix interface with subintima
c) receptors for
　　1. homotypic (fibroblast–fibroblast)
　　2. heterotypic (fibroblast–monocyte/macrophage)
Synthesis of components of the synovial fluid and factors for cartilage nutrition and function

Histogenic functions
guidances clues to monocyte entrance

Immune surveillance

Matrix remodeling
a) metalloproteinases and other proteinases
b) synthesis of matrix components

---

perform more effectively parallel cognitive immune surveillance functions in this large extracellular space.

Genes essential to physiological synoviocyte function form the basis of the role of the synoviocyte in disease

Based on the identification of certain genes expressed in fibroblast-like intimal synoviocytes, the argument will be advanced in this chapter that the basis for the role of the fibroblast-like intimal synoviocytes in inflammation is a direct consequence of their physiological role. This is especially evident in the function of genes potentially involved in patterning the histogenesis of the normal joint and the functional adaptations required of fibroblast lineage cells to maintain joint integrity.

An exaggeration of this patterning process, perhaps in part attributed to genetic polymorphisms, is involved in the entrance of large numbers of monocytes, macrophages, and lymphocytes into the milieu of the rheumatoid arthritis joint, accounting in part for the feedback loops between these cells evident in chronic arthritis. Indeed this potentially proinflammatory surveillance may suffice to attract autoimmune responses into the joint without the requirement of postulating a drive by a joint-specific autoantigen[8]. We similarly envisage that the gene programs that are involved in the extensive structural and matrix modifications invoked during embryogenesis of the joint are also involved in the development of some of the seemingly aberrant destructive events involving the synoviocytes in rheumatoid arthritis apparently under the paracrine drive of the immune response underlying rheumatoid arthritis.

Lineage disposition, and cell–cell interactions of fibroblast-like intimal synoviocytes

The fibroblast-like intimal synoviocytes appears to be as distinct from a fibroblast as are the other members of this lineage, such as osteocytes and chondrocytes that originate from the same mesenchymal progenitor, as illustrated in Figure 9.1. One feature of this differentiation discussed above is that fibroblast-like intimal synoviocytes exhibit a polarization unusual for a typical connective tissue fibroblast, as illustrated in Figure 9.2. It is likely that the various surfaces of the intimal synoviocyte are specialized to perform these disparate functions, although this point has not been the subject of much attention. However, it is probable that the receptors for interaction with collagen and other elements of the subintimal ground are disposed only on the abluminal surface of the cell, and that the lateral margins of the intimal synoviocyte exhibit a density of receptors for cell–cell contact not found on the luminal or abluminal surfaces.

Another lineage feature is that there are two types of cell–cell interactions exhibited by the fibroblast-like intimal synoviocyte. One is the homotypic cell–cell interaction of fibroblast-like intimal synoviocytes with each other and the second is the heterotypic interaction of the fibroblast-like intimal synoviocytes with macrophage-like intimal synoviocytes. In electron microscopic studies, tight junctions or desmosomes, characteristic of epithelial cells, are not seen suggesting that homotypic and heterotypic cellular interactions during the continued histogenesis of the synovial lining are perhaps entirely receptor-mediated. Evidence for the presence of various receptor–counter receptor interactions that could mediate these interactions will be reviewed below. Additionally, matrix components such as collagen VI have been implicated in maintaining cells attached to each other and to the matrix[9]. The expression of these receptors and/or their ligands in the cell are also likely to be polarized.

A third feature is that the fibroblast-like intimal synoviocytes appear responsible for the localization and guidance clues that result in the entrance and differentiation of monocytes in the intima. The property of forming a cell–cell relationship with monocytes is another feature that distinguishes the synoviocyte from typical fibroblasts in this lineage. Candidate molecules that could mediate these functions will be discussed. The fibroblast-like intimal synovial lining cell exhibits a phenotype that suggests it also provides receptors for the engagement of counter receptors on the entering monocytoid cells, and that receptor engagement involved in this interaction results in both monocyte adherence and their subsequent differentiation into macrophage-like macrophage-like intimal synovial lining cells. In view of the terminal differentiation state of macrophages, there is probably continual repopulation of the intima by newly entering monocyte lineage cells from the blood.

This patterning, histogenesis, and organization of the intimal membrane in joint organogenesis is of particular interest. In fact, it is possible that some of the mechanisms involved in joint development might also be involved in tissue injury during inflammation. During fetal development, cavitation occurs within the primitive skeleton along planes destined to become the articular surfaces of synovial joints. Evidence suggesting that joint cavitation is dependent on the behavior of fibroblastic cells and/or adjacent chondrocytes, rather than macrophages, has been presented in a histochemical study of human fetal limbs[2]. Macrophages are found in the site of the future joint prior to cavitation in the periphery of joint interzones but not at the presumptive joint line in the central interzone, suggesting that macrophages are not actively involved in the process of cavity formation[2].

Uridine diphosphoglucose dehydrogenase (UDPGD) activity was increased in a narrow band of cells at the presumptive joint line prior to cavitation. Since UDPGD activity is involved in hyaluronan synthesis, Edwards has proposed that joint cavitation is facilitated by a rise in local hyaluronan concentration in an area of tissue where cohesion is dependent on the interaction between cellular CD44 and extracellular hyaluronan. It is possible that an early role of macrophages in the histogenesis of the joint is removal of cells that may undergo apoptosis in the formation of the joint cavity, and dysfunction in apoptosis could contribute to synovial hyperplasia, as discussed below.

At a more fundamental level, the genes involved in the regulation of these and earlier events in joint formation are beginning to be delineated. The mouse brachypodism locus encodes a bone morphogenetic protein called growth/differentiation factor 5. Transcripts of this gene are expressed in a pattern of transverse stripes within many skeletal precursors in the developing limb, corresponding to the sites where joints will later form between skeletal elements. Null mutations in this gene disrupt the formation of many synovial joints in the limb, leading to complete or partial fusions between particular skeletal elements, and changes in the patterns of repeating structures in the digits, wrists, and ankles[10]. Particular bone morphogenetic protein family members may also play an essential role in the segmentation process that cleaves skeletal precursors into separate elements. This process helps determine the number of elements in repeating series in both limbs and sternum, and is required for normal generation of the functional articulations between many adjacent structures in the vertebrate skeleton. Whether these genes play a role in predisposition to synovitis has not been explored.

Potential role for genes expressed in fibroblast-like intimal synoviocytes as candidates of the genetic susceptibility to rheumatoid arthritis

In terms of the relationship between disease pathogenesis and genetic susceptibility, several of the genes differentially expressed in fibroblast-like synoviocytes from rheumatoid arthritis as compared to osteoarthritis map to non-MHC chromosomal regions where both susceptibility loci for rheumatoid arthritis and experimental arthritis in rodents are located. This point will be discussed below in greater detail. This makes these genes candidate susceptibility genes whose expression may be regulated differently in alternate gene forms. It is a distinct possibility that normal down-regulatory pathways that operate to protect the joint from going into a state of persistent inflammatory and local immune response are deficient in patients with rheumatoid arthritis. The normal functions of the fibroblast-like intimal synoviocytes, and how these physiological functions can favor, initiate, or perpetuate the inflammatory process will also be reviewed, including how possible abnormalities identified in the expression of genes involved in the regulation of transcription, cellular replication, cellular survival, and cytokines and chemokines expression can be implicated in the pathogenesis of rheumatoid arthritis.

Problems in the study of synoviocytes

The two fundamental questions asked of the fibroblast-like intimal synoviocyte are: 1) What genes are expressed that enable it to perform its distinctive functions and how does this pattern of gene expression differ from that of the typical fibroblast and from the subintimal fibroblast-like synoviocyte? 2) How is this pattern of gene expression altered in inflammation and what are

the functional consequence of this change? The answers to these questions are still quite incomplete, in part because it has been relatively difficult to study the properties of the fibroblast-like intimal synoviocytes. This, because of several features of the biology of both the normal and the inflamed joint, including the fact that the single layer of fibroblast-like intimal synoviocytes is not separated from the subintima by a basement membrane (Figure 9.2), making the isolation of fibroblast-like intimal synoviocytes from the normal joint a difficult problem.

Accordingly, because of the uncertainty as to whether a given fibroblast-like cell propagated in tissue culture originated from the intima or subintima, cells cultured from the joint are referred to as **fibroblast-like synoviocytes**. In rheumatoid arthritis and many other chronic arthritides, the synovial intimal membrane becomes highly hyperplastic, forming multiple layers of cells that in short-term cultures exhibit a stellate or dendritic-like phenotype. However, despite the greatly increased number of fibroblast-like intimal synoviocytes, the same anatomical problem persists of the inability to reliably distinguish the origin of a cultured cell from the intima or subintima.

The second major problem is that the inflammatory state has induced additional alterations in phenotype by what is likely to be paracrine mechanism. These cytokines and growth factors may be either directly derived from infiltrating lymphocytes or reflect additional activation pathways involving monocytes and/or fibroblast-like cells. By definition, these paracrine effects are short lived and disappear in culture after several days. It however has been hypothesized, but not established, that a consequence of prolonged exposure to these paracrine effects may persist leaving a 'phenotypic immunological imprinting' that could account for a significant percentage of the phenotypic behavior of these cells in culture[11,12].

Nevertheless, many studies use inflammatory synoviocytes as a starting point, particularly after they have been cultured in an attempt to isolate them from the short-lived macrophage-like cells and allow their phenotype to recover from most, if not all, of the paracrine effects of exposure to the products of an immune response. This chapter will adopt this latter perspective, largely derived from a series of studies on established cultures[8,11,15]. It is a fundamental postulate in the approach of this chapter, though an unproven one, that the findings made on these cultured cells may be directly extrapolated to provide insights into the nature of the intimal synoviocyte.

Distinctive phenotype of cultured synoviocytes from inflammatory synovitis

In freshly enzyme-dissociated preparations of cells obtained from rheumatoid arthritis synovia and those from other inflammatory arthritides, many fibroblast-like lineage cells are found that have a striking stellate or dendritic morphology. HLA-DR expression[15,16] and the morphological phenotype of the fibroblast-like synoviocyte freshly isolated from a rheumatoid synovium has sometimes warranted the term **dendritic cell** although this cell is also referred to as a **stellate cell** (Figure 9.3). The use of the term dendritic brings up the question of whether

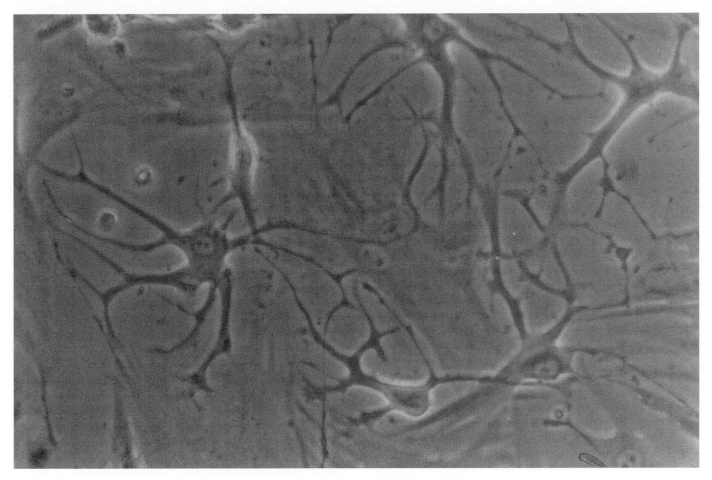

Fig. 9.3 Fibroblast-like intimal synoviocyte exhibiting stellate or 'dendritic' morphology in culture. See also Plate 21.

these cells exhibit a functional relationship to the dendritic cells of the myeloid and lymphoid lineages that are increasingly being recognized as playing a key role in the early events of the immune response. These cells lack the property of enhanced endocytosis or phagocytosis, expression of CD14, Fc receptors, and the leukocyte common antigen, CD45[17], making it very likely that they belong to the fibroblast lineage and are most probably fibroblast-like intimal synoviocytes. When preparations of these cells are placed into culture, the preponderance of these cells lose expression of HLA-DR, but the stellate morphology remains. However, the precise lineage and fate of the cells that express HLA-DR molecules have not been carefully traced, particularly with their relationship to the stellate synoviocytes that characterize rheumatoid arthritis samples and are most likely to be fibroblast-like intimal synoviocytes. Moreover, it is not known whether these cells are efficient antigen-presenting cells. Zvaifler *et al.* have also emphasized the increased percentages of true dendritic cells in the joint[18].

During the first three passages of these cells many of the marked phenotypic alterations such as the expression of MHC class II molecules greatly diminishes, emphasizing the role of paracrine and cell interaction factors in inducing some of the phenotypic alterations found in the freshly isolated synovio-

cytes[17,19]. However, the synoviocytes obtained from synovial tissue of individuals with rheumatoid arthritis[4,20,21] and other disorders with marked degrees of intimal hyperplasia do not revert to an entirely typical fibroblast-like morphology and behavior, maintaining a complex phenotype that includes varying degrees of 'stellate' morphology, enhanced growth, increased glucose consumption, altered adherence behavior, constitutive overproduction of metalloproteinases, and the elaboration of proinflammatory cytokines[14,15,22,23], as well as loss of contact inhibition[20], features suggestive of a mesenchymal stem cell.

The distinctive, but not entirely uniform, phenotype of the remaining cultured rheumatoid synoviocytes is not found in similarly cultured synoviocytes obtained from osteoarthritis synovia that have been shown to lack lining cell hyperplasia and any inflammatory cell infiltration[14,24] (Winchester unpublished observations). We and others have postulated that the distinctive changes in synoviocyte phenotype observed in these cultured cell lines mirror certain similar events occurring in the inflamed synovium itself[11,13,22,23,25].

The pattern of gene expression in these cultured cells has been characterized in a series of studies[8,11,14,26]. Two features of the cells exhibiting the distinctive phenotype were identified: the first is that cells exhibiting this phenotype are not specific for rheumatoid arthritis, as it is also demonstrable in cultures initiated from a number of different entities characterized by chronic inflammation, including psoriatic arthritis and cases of what was termed 'osteoarthritis', but presented considerable degrees of inflammation[13,14]. The second feature is that the pattern of gene expression is similar, but not at all identical among samples from different inflammatory synovia.

Explanations for the distinctive phenotype and function of the long-term cultured synoviocytes

There are four possible explanations for the distinctive phenotype and functions of these long-term cultured cells (Table 9.2). Each of these possibilities has a different implication in terms of whether the genes found to be over-expressed in these cultures are identifiable in the normal synovium.

First, the phenotype could be a consequence of a disease-specific sustained modulation in gene expression in the intimal and subintimal fibroblast lineage cells of the joint that developed as a response to prolonged paracrine signaling through products of a local immune response, as has been postulated in earlier work[11,13,14,27]. This sustained modulation, analogous to a phenotypic imprinting process, would be clearly distinct from the paracrine-mediated activation phenotype in that it does not decay quickly in culture. Rather, the phenotype would be maintained as a sustained pattern of altered gene expression through many months of culture. The implication of this pattern is that neither normal fibroblast-like intimal synoviocytes, nor subintimal synoviocytes, would have increased expression of genes in both of these cell types in rheumatoid arthritis. This is a philosophically appealing notion, but no direct evidence has been advanced to support it.

A second possibility is that the cells are primarily 'transformed' as suggested by Gay and colleagues[28], where there would be a disease specific nature of the distinctive phenotype. This viewpoint considers the disease of rheumatoid arthritis to result from an immune response against the agent responsible for the transformation, or a possible innate abnormal regulation of oncogene expression leading to a hyperproliferating cell. The lack of disease specificity for the phenotype renders this otherwise attractive possibility more remote. The implication of this model is that normal fibroblast-like intimal synoviocytes and subintimal synoviocytes would not express these genes, and that it is likely that the over-expression pattern is specific for rheumatoid arthritis and not other chronic arthritides.

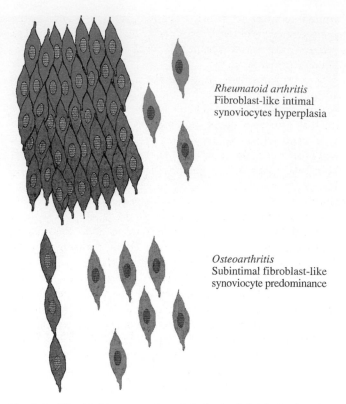

Rheumatoid arthritis
Fibroblast-like intimal synoviocytes hyperplasia

Osteoarthritis
Subintimal fibroblast-like synoviocyte predominance

Fig. 9.4 The third interpretation of the basis of the distinctive phenotype of cultured rheumatoid arthritis synoviocytes. This is the lineage model that bases the distinctive phenotype on the fact that the starting point of the culture differs greatly in the proportion of intimal and subintimal synoviocytes in rheumatoid arthritis and osteoarthritis. This model postulates that the intimal and subintimal synoviocytes have different phenotypes based on their differentiation lineages and that the difference in the phenotype of the cultured cells simply reflects the varying starting proportions of the two cell types. See also Plate 20.

Thirdly, the distinctive phenotype observed in these cultures could be the normal phenotype of the fibroblast-like intimal synoviocyte found in the normal joints of all individuals[8]. The differences in cultural phenotype between inflammatory and non-inflammatory synovitis would simply reflect the increased proportion of fibroblast-like intimal synoviocytes compared to subintimal synoviocytes in the starting culture material obtained from a joint with intimal hyperplasia, as illustrated in Figure 9.4. By parsimony, this more prosaic concept is the simplest of the explanations. The implication here is that normal fibroblast-like intimal synoviocytes, but not subintimal synoviocytes, would express the genes found to be constitutively increased in

Table 9.2 Four possible explanations for the distinct phenotype of rheumatoid arthritis cultured synovial fibroblasts

Disease-specific sustained modulation in gene expression
    Local paracrine regulation
    Phenotypic 'imprinting'
Transformed cells
    Secondary to unidentified viral infection
Normal intimal cell phenotype
    Differences represent different percentages of intimal versus subintimal cells in the synovial tissue
Normal intimal cell phenotype and is dependent on genetic polymorphisms in arthritis susceptibility genes

cultured rheumatoid arthritis synoviocytes. In synovitis, the hyperplasia of fibroblast-like intimal synoviocytes would lead to a relatively increased expression of genes normally characteristic of mesenchymal stem cells.

The fourth possibility is essentially a variation of the third, with the important distinction that while the over-expression phenotype reflects the starting phenotype of the individual's pre-arthritis intimal synoviocytes, this phenotype of genetically determined increased expression is intrinsically abnormal because of the presence in the allele of a regulatory polymorphism that predisposes to immunologically-mediated arthritis. Thus, genes that are over- or under-expressed in the intimal synoviocyte in arthritic disease are candidate genes for genetic polymorphisms defining the susceptibility state. A variation on this last possibility is the situation where the genetic abnormality arises somatically through mutation, rather than through the inheritance of alternate forms of germline genes. This implication of this model is that in the patient, unaffected joints containing normal fibroblast-like intimal synoviocytes would over-express these genes before arthritis developed, but that the over-expression of these genes would be lacking, or reduced, in entirely normal individuals without rheumatoid arthritis. Based on gene identification work presented below, we currently favor the third and fourth of these possibilities as the simplest explanation of the basis of the distinctive phenotype.

Strategy for the identification of genes responsible for the distinctive phenotype and their relationship to intimal and subintimal synoviocytes lineages

To identify the genes responsible for the distinctive phenotype of the cultured synoviocytes obtained from a rheumatoid arthritis patient, a gene discovery approach has been taken that involves identifying genes similarly and differently expressed compared to a line derived from a selected osteoarthritis sample. One recent approach was based on the construction of representational difference libraries[29,30] that had been used to clone the differences between two complex genomes. It involves a cloning procedure with PCR amplification of cDNA to generate simplified representations of the expressed genes followed by a modified subtraction step and subsequent screening to facilitate the gene identification.

A number of genes were identified in cultured synoviocytes obtained from both rheumatoid arthritis and osteoarthritis that were expressed at approximately the same or similar levels in each parent cell line northern or equivalent analyses. In light of the possibilities explaining the basis of the distinctive phenotype, these genes are likely expressed in both fibroblast-like intimal and in subintimal synoviocytes. In contrast, other genes exhibited increased expression by northern analysis in only the rheumatoid arthritis synoviocytes (Figure 9.5). Hence, the genes found constitutively over-expressed in the rheumatoid arthritis synoviocyte culture appear to be expressed at high levels in fibroblast-like intimal synoviocytes and appear to be primary markers of the phenotype of this lineage (Table 9.3).

Considering the pattern of gene expression to reflect cell lineage is the least biologically complex of the possible interpretations. However, whether this interpretation is correct for some or all of the identified genes will be determined by the results of studies designed to characterize their expression on normal and inflamed joint tissue samples, specifically distinguishing intimal from subintimal cells. Immunophenotypic distinction between these two cell lines, or a simple method to differentiate them, remains the subject of ongoing studies.

Gene identification

Genes likely to be expressed constitutively in fibroblast-like intimal synoviocytes

The specialized functions of the fibroblast-like intimal synoviocytes are mediated by either quantitative differences in the expression of genes found on other members of the fibroblast-like lineage, or the qualitative expression of genes unique to the synoviocyte sublineage. The genes identified by the subtraction library method as differentially expressed in rheumatoid arthritis synoviocyte cultures are likely candidates for the fibroblast-like intimal synoviocyte phenotype[8]. These include differentially expressed chemokines such as SDF-1, connective tissue matrix components such as biglycan and lumican, adhesion molecules such as VCAM-1, and other molecules of a less clear function in the synovial tissue such as semaphorin VI, Mac2-binding protein, IGF-BP5, interferon-inducible 56 kD protein, and interferon-induced 71 kD 2'5' oligoadenylate synthetase (Table 9.3). Additionally, two genes that were

RA OA   RA OA   RA OA   RA OA   RA OA   RA OA   RA OA

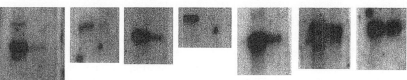

ML2122   ML2115 lumican   IGFBP5 SDF-1α   sem VI   collagenase IV

Fig. 9.5 Northern analysis of lumican, IGFBP5, SDF-1α, semaphorin VI, collagenase type IV, and the two novel transcripts of yet unidentified genes ML2122 and ML2115, indicating that stem cell-like cells in RA have a distinctive pattern of gene expression.

Table 9.3 Genes identified through a subtraction method differentially expressed in RA and OA fibroblast-like synovial cultures and correlation with their possible lineage origin

Genes preferentially expressed in RA synovial cultures: intimal origin	Genes expressed in both RA and OA synovial fibroblast cultures: intimal and subintimal origin
Biglycam	Adrenomodulin
IFN-induced 56 kD	α subunit of GsGTP binding protein
IFN-induced 71 kD 2′5′-oligoadenylate synthetase	α-B-crystallin
IGF-BP5	B94 protein
Lumican	beta subunit of prolyl-4-hydroxylase
Mac2-binding protein	Candidate sulphatase
ML2115	Cathepsin B
ML2122	Collagen alpha 1 type III
SDF-1α	Collagenase IV
Semaphorin VI/E	Complement C1r
VCAM-1	Complement C1s
	Complement factor B
	DNA-binding protein TAXREB10
	Elongation factor 2
	Epithelin
	Extracellular protein (SI-5)
	HLA-E heavy chain
	Interferon-γ IEF SSP 5111
	Manganese superoxide dismutase
	Milk fat globule protein
	Muscle fatty acid binding protein
	NMB protein
	Osteoblast specific factor 2 (OSF-2)

not homologous to any known genes were over-expressed in rheumatoid arthritis synovial fibroblast-like cultures (ML2122 and ML2115).

VCAM-1 had previously been identified as being expressed by normal fibroblast-like intimal synoviocytes[2,6], and this observation supports the interpretation that the remaining genes found by the subtraction method are characteristic of fibroblast-like intimal synoviocytes. In addition, several other genes have been identified as being selectively, or more highly, expressed by fibroblast-like intimal synoviocytes, either from staining patterns in normal or diseased synovial membranes or from cultured cells. These include other chemokines such as IL-8, RANTES, MCP-1[8,32–33], cytokines such as TNF-α, IL-1, IL-6, GM-CSF[14,34,35], IL-11[36,37], metalloproteinases and other proteinases[13,38,39], adhesion molecules such as ICAM-1[40–44], integrins[45] and CD44[43,46,47], and costimulatory molecules such as CD40[48] (Winchester R., unpublished observations) (Table 9.4).

Genes expressed both in fibroblast-like intimal and subintimal synoviocytes

A number of genes were similarly expressed in the rheumatoid arthritis and osteoarthritis synovial fibroblast cultures, and are likely to be genes expressed by both cultured fibroblast-like intimal and subintimal synoviocytes. Among these genes are some involved in cellular and matrix turn-over such as collagenase IV, genes involved in the inflammatory response such as manganese superoxide dismutase, complement factor B, interferon-γ IEF SSP 5111, and HLA-E heavy chain, and other genes with unknown function in the synovium such as NMB protein, α-B crystallin, B94 protein, and muscle fatty-acid-binding

protein. Other genes have been shown to be either similarly expressed in synovial fibroblasts from patients with a variety of diseases or specifically expressed in both the intimal and subintimal layer by *in situ* hybridization or staining with monoclonal antibodies (Tables 9.3 and 9.5).

Role of molecules identified in fibroblast-like intimal synoviocytes in afferent reactions leading to intensification of synovitis

Chemokines, cytokines, and growth factors

Chemokines

The finding that a number of chemokines have been identified as likely to be over-expressed by the fibroblast-like intimal synoviocytes, including IL-8[49], Gro-α[50], MCP-1[31,49], MIP-1α[51], and SDF-1[8] directs attention to the role of these molecules in the normal synovium. Moreover, it is of interest whether they could participate in fostering the localization or intensification of an autoimmune or immune response into the joint.

Expression of chemokines and their receptors has been demonstrated to have a critical role in the regulation of the attachment of leukocytes and endothelial cells, and in their passage into the tissues[52,53]. For instance leukocyte egress from blood vessels occurs in four identifiable stages[54] (Figure 9.6). During most of these stages, chemokine receptor expression in the leukocytes is critical in regulating leukocyte egress.

Table 9.4 Genes differentially expressed in cultured rheumatoid fibroblast-like intimal cells, their chromosomal location, their relationship with susceptibility loci mapped in rheumatoid arthritis and with homologous loci regulating experimental arthritis in rats.

Genes	Human chromosome	RA susceptibility loci[e]	Arthritis loci in rats[a]
Cytokines			
IL-1	2q12		
IL-6	7p14		Cia3, Aia3
IL-11	19q13.3-q13.4		Cia2
IL-15	4q31		
TNF-α	6p21.3-21.1	Cornelis	Cia1, Aia1, Oia1
GM-CSF	5q23.1-23.3		
TGF-β	6p11.1		
Chemokines			
SDF-1	10q11.1		
RANTES	17q11.2-q12		
MCP-1	17q11.2-q12		
MIP-1α	17q11-q21		Cia5, Oia3
IL-8	17q24.2-24.3		Cia5, Oia3
MMP[d], proteases and inhibitors			
MMP-1 (collagenase 1)	11q14.2		Cia2
MMP-2 (gelatinase A)	16q12.1		
MMP-3 (stromelysin 1)	11q14.2		Cia2
MMP-10 (stromelysin 2)	11q14.2		Cia2
MMP-13 (collagenase 3)	11q14.2		Cia2
Cathepsin B	3p21.1		
Cathepsin L	9q21.2		
Cathepsin S	1q21.1		
TIMP-1	Xp11.4-q11.2		
TIMP-2	17q25		
Oncogenes and transcription factors			
Myc	8q24, 12-q24,13		Cia3
Fos	14q22-q23		
Jun	1p31.1-22.3		
NF-κB p50/p65	4q24/11q13		
Matrix compounds			
Biglycam	Xq28	Cornelis	
Lumicam	12q21.3		Cia8[f]
Adhesion Molecules			
VCAM-1	1p13.3-p11		Cia10[c]
CD44	11pter-p13		
Others			
CD40	20q12-q13.2		
HLA-E	6p21.3-p21.1	Cornelis	Cia1, Aia1, Oia1
IGF-bp5	2q33-q34		
Mac-2BP	17q25		
Semaphorin VI/E	7q21		Aia2
IFN-inducible 56kd[b]	10q22.3		
IFN-inducible 71kd 2'5' oligo a.s.[b]	12q21.3-q22		Cia8[f]

a Cia = collagen-induced arthritis; Aia = adjuvant-induced arthritis; Oia = oil-induced arthritis.
b IFN = interferon; oligo a.s. = oligoadenylate synthetase.
c Suggestive of linkage;
d MMP = matrix metalloproteinase, TIMP = tissue inhibitor of metalloproteinase.
e Cornelis = Cornelis *et al.* 1998;
f = Dracheva *et al.*, unpublished observations.

Among chemokines, SDF-1 is one of the most efficacious in T cell and monocyte migration[52]. Both CD4+ and CD8+ cells, as well as CD45RA+ näive and, less effectively, CD45RO+ memory T-lymphocyte subsets in peripheral blood are subject to SDF-1 chemoattractive effects[55]. Similarly, monocyte-lineage dendritic cells acquire CXCR4 upon induction with GM-CSF and IL-4[56]. Additionally, SDF-1 is an important B-cell developmental and maturation factor, as revealed by the observation that mice lacking SDF-1 show defects on B-cell lymphopoiesis and bone marrow myelopoiesis[57].

The SDF-1 receptor, CXCR4, is a seven-transmembrane-spanning, G-protein-coupled receptor and is a coreceptor for T-cell-line tropic human immunodeficiency virus HIV-1. CXCR-4 is constitutively expressed by quiescent, resting endothelial cells.

Table 9.5 Partial list of genes expressed by fibroblast-like synoviocytes[a]

Matrix components	*Co-stimulatory molecules*
Collagen I	CD40
Collagen III	
Collagen IV	*Complement*
Biglycam	Complement C1r
Laminin	Complement C1s
Lumicam	Complement factor B
Perlecam	
Hyaluronan	*HLA genes and activation markers*
Fibronectin	HLA-A, B, C
Proteoglycans	HLA-DR
Glycosaminoglycans	HLA-DQ
	HLA-E heavy chain
Metalloproteinases, other proteinases and inhibitors	Interferon-gamma IEF SSP 5111
MMP-1 (collagenase 1)	IFN-induced 71 kDa 2'5'-oligoadenylate synthetase
MMP-2 (gelatinase A, collagenase 4)	IFN-induced 56 kDa
MMP-3 (stromelysin 1)	
MMP-10 (stromelysin 2)	*Oncogenes and transcription factors*
MMP-13 (collagenase 3)	NF-κB
Cathepsin B	c-Jun
Cathepsin L	c-Fos
TIMP-1	Sis
TIMP-2	c-Myc
	Egr-2
Cell–cell, cell–matrix interactions, receptors	Ras
Mac2-binding protein	
VCAM-1	*Apoptosis regulatory genes*
ICAM-1	p53
ICAM-2	Fas
$\alpha1$–$\alpha6$ integrins	Bcl-2
$\beta1$, $\beta4$ integrins	
PECAM/CD31	*Other inflammation-related genes*
CD44	Manganese superoxide dismutase
IGF-BP5	COX1
Cadherin-11	COX2
Plasminogen receptor	PGE-2
Cytokines and growth factors	*Neurohormones*
IL-1	Substance P
IL-6	Parathyroid hormone
IL-15	
IL-11	*Others with unclear function in the synovium*
TNF-α	Adrenomodulin
GN-CSF	α subunit of GsGTP binding protein
bFGF	α-B-crystalline
TGFb	B94 protein
PDGF	β subunit of prolyl-4-hydroxylase
Semaphorin VI/E	Candidate sulfatase
Oncostatin M	DNA-binding protein TAXREB10
LIF	Elongation factor 2
	Epithelin
Chemokines	Extracellular protein (SI-5)
SDF-1	Milk fat globule protein
MIP-1α	ML2115
MCP-1	ML2122
IL-8	Muscle fatty acid binding protein
RANTES	NMB protein
GRO-α	Osteoblast specific factor 2 (OSF-2)

a The character of this chapter does not permit the coverage of all the genes expressed by synovial fibroblasts. Most of these genes are referenced in the text.

A similar phenotype was identified in both SDF-1 and CXCR4 knock-out mice[57,58]. Cytokine stimulation studies revealed that bFGF upregulates endothelial CXCR4 expression, whereas TNF-α down-regulates it. In addition to the abnormalities seen in the SDF-1 knock-out, mice lacking CXCR4 also have defec-

tive formation of the large vessels supplying the gastrointestinal tract, defective vascular development, and show many proliferating granule cells invading the cerebellar anlage, suggesting the involvement of the SDF-1/CXCR4 system in neuronal cell migration and patterning in the central nervous system.

The chemokine receptors CXCR3 and CCR5, recently described to be preferentially expressed in Th1 T cells[59], are expressed in the majority of the synovium infiltrating T cells in rheumatoid arthritis[60]. In contrast, CXCR4, the SDF-1 receptor, does not appear to be preferentially expressed in Th1 or Th2 cells, but is preferentially expressed on naïve cells. IP-10, one of the chemokine ligands for CXCR3, is produced by synovial fibroblast cultures in response to IL-1 and TNF-α[61]. Mig, another CXCR3 binding chemokine, has not been studied in the rheumatoid synovium. The CCR5 chemokine ligands RANTES[33,62], MIP-1α[51,62], and MIP-1β[62] have been described as over-expressed in the rheumatoid arthritis synovium. Furthermore, antibodies to RANTES ameliorated adjuvant-induced arthritis in rats[63]. The production of chemokines by synovial fibroblasts, the fact that the infiltrating lymphocytes express the corresponding receptors and are likely to be Th1 cells, and the improvement of arthritis in experimental animal models using antichemokine therapy support the concept that chemokines have an important role in the localization of T cells and the inflammatory process to the synovial membrane.

We speculate that the production of SDF-1 by fibroblast-like intimal synoviocytes in the normal joint could act as a guidance cue for the continual entrance into the intimal synovial membrane of monocyte lineage precursors committed to differentiation into phagocytic lining cells or to progress through normal differentiation pathways[8]. Similarly SDF-1 and other chemokines elaborated by the normal synoviocytes may act to enhance the ingress of lymphocytes into the joint tissues to facilitate increasing innate and acquired immune surveillance in the synovial cavity. These same mechanisms may be relevant to the immune response of rheumatoid arthritis in two ways: first, the chemokines may attract an autoimmune response in the synovial intima, although it is not driven by an antigen uniquely expressed there. Second, the chemokines may modify the responsiveness and organization of the ongoing autoimmune response and cells related to it such as dendritic cells. Furthermore, since these genes are constitutively expressed as part of normal physiological properties of the cells, it is likely that regulatory or suppressor mechanisms exist normally to protect the joint from developing a chronic inflammatory process. Abnormalities in these regulatory pathways, especially those that occur through genetic polymorphisms, could have a fundamental role in disease susceptibility.

Cytokines and growth factors

Cytokine networks in rheumatoid arthritis are discussed in detail in Chapter 11. Several groups have demonstrated increased expression of several cytokines including TNF-α, IL-1, IL-6, IL-11, IL-15, GM-CSF, TGF-β, PDGF, and bFGF by fibroblast-like intimal synoviocytes[13,14,35–37,64–69].

Cytokines have key functions in altering the pattern of gene expression and consequently cell function at several levels in the activation of the endothelium, in the regulation of the immune response, including immune deviation between Th1 and Th2, and on cells in the area of an ongoing immune response. Some of these effects are on cell–cell and cell–matrix interactions, while other effects may affect different cell functions. Some of these alterations mediate cartilage damage. The migration of a given inflammatory cell into the synovium is not a random event but one determined by the prior immunological history of the particular cell as well as that of the endothelium. The increased production of certain cytokines such as IL-1 and TNF-α has been shown to activate the endothelium and to initiate over-expression of certain adhesion molecules. This would affect phases 2, 3, and possibly 4 in the diagram of directed cellular egress (Figure 9.6). Accordingly the increased activation status of the endothelium in concert with increased chemokine production could greatly facilitate the localization of inflammatory and autoimmune cells to the synovial membrane, further perpetuating the disease process and tissue injury. A similar failure in the normal suppressor regulatory pathways proposed above could also operate to release an unopposed proinflammatory cytokine production. Some selected examples follow:

IL-1 induces the expression of more IL-1α and IL-1β, in a positive feedback loop[70]. IL-1 also induces transcriptional activation of protein kinase C, and, by a separate pathway, induces the synthesis of PGE$_2$[71]. This latter response is much greater when rheumatoid arthritis fibroblast-like cells are used instead of cells from osteoarthritis synovia and the response is potentiated by PDGF and certain other polypeptide growth factors, suggesting that fibroblast-like intimal synoviocytes are the source of increased amounts of this cytokine[72]. These two pathways initiated by IL-1 also converge to regulate the transcriptional activation of stromelysin. IL-1 induces fibroblast-like synovial cell lines to increase IL-6 gene expression, by an incompletely defined pathway that is suppressed by corticosteroids[68]. Similarly IL-8 is induced by the addition of IL-1 or TNF-α[73], although to much lower levels than those elaborated by synovial

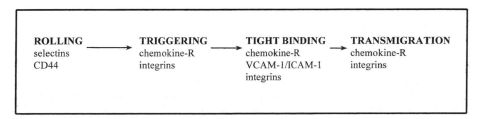

Fig. 9.6 Four stages of leukocyte egress. Cytokines act in the endothelium and chemokines act in the leukocyte to regulate their efflux from blood vessels.

monocyte-like cells from rheumatoid arthritis samples. IL-1 induces the expression of GM-CSF mRNA with a maximum at 4 h[66]. IL-1 also induces the production of fibronectin and types I and III collagen[74].

TNF-α is produced by fibroblast-like intimal and subintimal synoviocytes, and by synovial monocytes/macrophages, and among several functions it is capable of inducing fibroblast-like intimal synoviocytes cellular proliferation, matrix metalloproteinases (MMP)[75], and cathepsin production[76]. As with IL-1, the addition of TNF-α to fibroblast-like cell cultures induces the expression of GM-CSF[66]. A number of studies have documented the importance of TNF-α in the development of arthritis, including a TNF-transgenic mouse that develops chronic arthritis[77], and the significant improvement of disease with agents targeting TNF[78–80].

IL-6, a cytokine with effects on B-cell differentiation, is constitutively expressed in synovial fibroblasts obtained from rheumatoid arthritis patients[14,34]. This cytokine appears critical to the development of a pathway leading to arthritis in mice, as gene-targeted mutation prevents disease[81]. IL-6, particularly in the presence of soluble IL-6 receptor, induces synovial fibroblast proliferation and IL-1 production[82]. However, IL-6 does not appear to induce directly MMP expression[83]; On the contrary, IL-6 can be a potent inducer of TIMP-1[84,85]. IL-6 regulates osteoclast activity and through this mechanism perhaps participates in the bone loss and in the erosive process seen in RA. Other molecules of the IL-6 family, such as oncostatin M, leukemia inhibitory factor (LIF), and IL-11, have been reported by other groups to be differentially expressed in synovial fibroblasts of rheumatoid arthritis compared to osteoarthritis[67,86], again suggesting that they are constitutively produced by fibroblast-like intimal synoviocytes. Oncostatin M, but not IL-6 or LIF, increased MMP-1[87], particularly in the presence of IL-1[88]. In addition, oncostatin M[88] and LIF, like IL-6, are able to induce TIMP-1 expression in synovial fibroblasts[85]. Interestingly, both IL-6R and LIFR map in the human genome to a region syntenic to an interval where a non-MHC arthritis severity regulatory locus has been mapped in collagen-induced arthritis, suggesting that these genes are candidate susceptibility/severity genes[89].

IL-15 is another cytokine produced by synovial fibroblasts (I. McInnes, personal communication) capable of activating T cells in the absence of IL-2, as well as inducing TNF-α production[90]. Furthermore, it is a potent chemotactic factor for leukocytes to migrate into the synovial membrane[69,90]. GM-CSF, a growth factor produced by fibroblast-like intimal synoviocytes, is important for the maturation and homing of macrophages and dendritic cells, and it is produced by normal and rheumatoid arthritis fibroblast-like intimal synoviocytes[13,91]. A recent study of collagen-induced arthritis in GM-CSF knock-out mice described significant resistance to disease, despite evidence for T and B cell-mediated autoimmune reponses[92]. This suggests that GM-CSF, like SDF-1 and other cytokines and chemokines produced by fibroblast-like intimal synoviocyte, may not necessarily be directly involved in the genesis of the autoimmune response, but instead, operate to localize this systemic autoimmune response to the joint.

TGF-β is widely distributed in the rheumatoid synovium, predominantly located in the lining cell layer and in the perivascular lymphoid aggregates. Both fibroblast-like and macrophage-like lineage cells expressed this growth and immunoregulatory factor[93]. If TGF-β is synthesized in an attempt to down-regulate the inflammatory and destructive processes, it apparently does not fully succeed in this task.

The over-expression of the semaphorin VI human homologue of mouse semaphorin E by synovial fibroblasts[8,94] is intriguing because the semphorins are a family of transmembrane signaling and secreted guidance glycoprotein molecules that are implicated in directing axonal extension and operate broadly in neuronal patterning[95]. However, in view of the relatively small number of axons in the synovium, it seems unlikely that the physiological role of the semaphorin VI molecule is to signal through an axonal receptor. Indeed its expression has been observed in a wide variety of tissues such as the heart, skeletal muscle, colon, small intestine, ovary, testis, and prostate. This suggests strongly that the semaphorins may have a function other than in guidance of axon, and preliminary evidence suggests that semaphorin VI plays some role in chemataxis of monocytes and their differentiation. Its function on fibroblast-like cells is to be determined. It is noteworthy that neuropilin, a receptor for semaphorin, is expressed on vascular endothelial cells. Neuropilin expression is upregulated by TNF-α and implicated in angiogenesis as a coreceptor of VEGF. Previously, other molecules initially identified in the central nervous system were found in the synovium and described as having proinflammatory properties, such as substance P, CRH, and others[96]. Therefore, it seems reasonable to speculate that in addition to chemotaxis, semaphorin VI may have a direct role in the local inflammatory process. Semaphorin may, however, play other roles as its identity as a multidrug resistance element and loss in certain tumors suggests[97,98].

Cell–cell interaction receptors potentially involved in macrophage-like–fibroblast-like and fibroblast-like–fibroblast-like synoviocyte interactions

Several molecules expressed by fibroblast-like intimal synoviocytes appear to be candidates for mediating cell–cell interactions involved in the histogenesis of the normal synovium. These include macrophage-like–fibroblast-like and fibroblast-like–fibroblast-like synoviocyte interactions. Some of these genes have a well-defined role in cell–cell interaction, while others have the potential to act as cell interaction receptor–ligand systems, but also have other actions.

Among the well-recognized adhesion molecules and receptors are differentially expressed in the rheumatoid fibroblast-like intimal synoviocytes are VCAM-1, a 110 kD a member of the immunoglobulin gene superfamily, and Mac-2 binding protein (Mac-2BP), also termed '90k tumor associated protein'. Both VCAM-1 and Mac-2BP exhibit properties that suggest they could mediate heterotypic and homotypic binding of macrophage-lineage intimal synoviocytes to fibroblast-like intimal synoviocytes. VCAM-1 has been previously described as markedly increased on rheumatoid arthritis synoviocytes[6,25] and it binds circulating monocytes and lymphocytes expressing the $\alpha4\beta1$ (VLA-4) integrin.

Mac-2BP, a heavily N-glycosylated secreted protein which binds stoichiometrically to the macrophage-associated lectin Mac-2 (galectin-3)[99,100], has been shown to increase in the serum of cancer and HIV-positive patients, suggesting that it participates in some aspects of immune reaction. Mac-2BP also binds to the monocyte CD14 structure in the presence of LPS and LPS-binding protein[101]. Binding of Mac-2BP to these receptors initiates monocyte lineage cells to secrete IL-1[102].

Similarly, these molecules could attract and facilitate interaction with, and activation of, monocytes. For example, Mac-2BP that induces homotypic monocyte aggregation and activation[100] could be a factor present in supernatants from cultured rheumatoid arthritis synoviocytes that induces blood monocytes to form giant cells[103]. Thus, along with the variety of genes that mediate the well-recognized effector functions of matrix remodeling and tissue destruction[74], the genes expressed by the mesenchymal cells of the joint may affect antigen non-specific immune localization or amplification mechanisms that could play a role in the puzzling phenomenon of why localized joint inflammation develops in many disparate diseases in the setting of immune responses that apparently have little to do with the joint.

Cadherin-11 was recently reported to be expressed in rheumatoid arthritis synovial fibroblasts[104]. Cadherin may participate in the mediation of homophilic adhesion between synoviocytes. All of the cell–cell interactions have the important potential of reverse signaling which could influence synovial proliferation and pannus invasion into cartilage or could engage in a heterophilic interaction that anchors lymphocytes within the synovial membrane.

Molecules involved in cell–matrix interaction of fibroblast-like intimal synoviocytes

In view of the unusual situation of the intimal synoviocyte, delimiting a fluid environment from a typical connective tissue matrix, the typical fibroblast–matrix interactions with collagen and other fixed fibrillar structures occur in a polarized manner on one side of the cell, and are likely to necessitate a polarized localization of the gene products. Although the precise polarization of gene products has not been studied, several matrix component genes exhibited a pattern of expression suggesting that they are constitutively produced by fibroblast-like intimal synoviocytes. Lumican was identified as likely to be constitutively expressed by fibroblast-like intimal synoviocytes.[8]. Lumican's role in the synovium is not understood. However, its role in corneal transparency[105], and in inhibition of macrophage adhesion to intact corneal keratan proteoglycans are of interest. Keratan sulfate chains modulate the biological activity of this molecule. After the removal of the keratan sulfate chains, macrophages rapidly attach to the lumican core protein[106]. Although the state of the keratan sulfate chains in the synovial lumican molecule is unknown, this observation suggests some species of lumican could also act to localize macrophages to sites in the synovium.

Biglycan, another gene likely to be constitutively expressed by fibroblast-like intimal synoviocytes, is a dermatan sulfate-proteoglycan. It is both induced by TGF-β and binds TGF-β[107] suggesting that biglycan may down-regulate TGF-β activity by sequestering this growth factor in the extracellular matrix. IL-6 stimulates the expression of biglycan, while TNF-α depresses its expression[108].

Hyaluronan is an abundant constituent of the extracellular matrix and is especially increased in the synovial fluid. Both high and low (fragments) molecular weight forms bind to CD44. Recent studies have demonstrated that in alveolar macrophages lower molecular weight hyaluronan fragments induce the production of chemokines such as IL-8 and MIP-1α through its receptor CD44, while the high molecular weight form inhibits chemokine production[109]. CD44 is predominantly expressed by intimal, as opposed to subintimal, fibroblast-like synoviocytes[46,47]. Although this pathway has not been extensively studied in fibroblast-like intimal synoviocytes, one could envision similar effects in the synovium. It is also conceivable that a similar concept may apply to other matrix components. For instance, if infact and large matrix components predominate in the synovium, representing absence of injury, a chemokine/cytokine inhibitory signal would predominate. On the other hand, when traumatic or inflammatory injury occur, signaling through hyaluronan fragments-CD44, and maybe through biglycan, lumican, or other component fragments and other receptors, would activate a proinflammatory response to remove cellular debris, or fight an infection.

IGFBP5 (insulin-like growth factor binding protein-5) appears to be very strongly expressed by fibroblast-like intimal synoviocytes[8]. It is an important regulator of fibroblast growth that increases IGF-1 binding to the fibroblast membrane by attaching to the extracellular matrix proteins, types III and IV collagen, laminin, and fibronectin[110]. IGFBP5 may have an anti-inflammatory role that opposes the effect exhibited by IL-1 and TNF-α of stimulating proteoglycan degradation and decreasing proteoglycan synthesis[111]. The observation that IGFBP5 is further induced by exposure of cells to prostaglandin E2[112] is of interest with respect to the pattern of morphological changes and gene activation observed in synoviocyte cultures after the addition of this agent[74].

Of interest, a novel gene in the sulfatase family, not previously identified in any libraries, primarily prepared from non-synovial sources, was identified in both fibroblast-like intimal synoviocytes and sub intimal synoviocytes[8]. This gene has a high degree of homology with a chondroitin sulfatase found in *C. elegans* and could have an interesting role in synovial matrix biology. Other proteoglycans and glycosaminoglycans are produced by the synovial fibroblast, and the reader is referred to comprehensive book chapters or review articles[5].

Activation-related genes

The level of tyrosine phosphorylation is elevated in rheumatoid arthritis synovia compared to that found in osteoarthritis synovia, suggesting that these cells are experiencing a high degree of activation of diverse signaling pathways. These pathways are analogous to that induced by *src. c-fos* expression is elevated[113] and so are several other activation-related genes (see Table 9.5). Two recently-described genes that are differentially expressed in rheumatoid arthritis synovial fibroblast cultured cells are interferon-induced and markers of cellular activation. One is the 71 kD 2'–5' oligoadenylate synthase, a subunit of one of several interferon-induced enzymes that, when activated by double-stranded RNA, converts ATP into 2'–5' linked oligomers of adenosine[114]. The second is the interferon-inducible 56 kD protein, which has unknown function, but in common with 2'–5' oligoadenylate synthetase is strongly induced by interferons[115].

The expression of these two genes directs attention to the presence of activation-like features in the phenotype of the rheumatoid arthritis synoviocytes. Whether the expression of these genes is found in quiescent, normal fibroblast-like intimal synoviocytes, whether they reflect a type of 'memory' of being harvested from a site of immune inflammation, or whether this is a lineage-specific response of fibroblast-like intimal synoviocytes to *in vitro* culture conditions remains to be studied. We favor the last possibility as the most likely explanation, reflecting a higher degree of responsiveness in these cells to environmental effects that could parallel their response of hyperplasia in joint injury and inflammation. Although some genes related to cell activation continue to be expressed in cultured synoviocytes, others such as HLA-DR appear to be more dependent on the synovial tissue proinflammatory environment, and become greatly reduced after two to three passages[116].

Matrix-modifying enzymes: metalloproteinases, proteases, and their inhibitors

There are many differences in the levels of mRNA for a variety of genes between whole synovial tissues obtained from rheumatoid arthritis and osteoarthritis patients. In previous studies, a dot blot assay using a labeled cDNA probe based on total tissue mRNA enabled parallel quantitation of the amount of message from multiple MMP and other Zn-independent protease genes. mRNA levels for stromelysin, collagenase, and cathespin D along with TIMP-1 are elevated in the representative rheumatoid arthritis sample[13,14]. Normally, these enzymes can attack all of the elements of connective issue, participating in histogenesis, physiological remodeling, or pathological destruction[117]. All are synthesized as proenzymes that are activated by proteolytic cleavage. They are of particular interest to the mechanism of synovitis because firstly they are induced from very low basal levels by a variety of cytokines and growth factors but are also constitutively expressed by a variety of transformed cells. The mesenchymal cell variety of collagenase has been strongly implicated in synovitis by the finding that its mRNA is expressed at high levels in the synovial lining[118]. The identification of abundant collagenase at the protein level in the vicinity of erosions but not in equivalent abundance in other regions of the synovium suggests that it may play a special role at these sites[119]. As with other metalloproteinases, especially stromelysin, collagenases are a major product of fibroblast-like intimal synoviocytes[120]. The primary action of stromelysin is to cleave proteoglycan core and link proteins, fibronectin, elastin, and

procollagens I, II and III, thereby remodeling of most of the matrix components other than collagen. Stromelysin also participates in collagenase activation[121]. Stromelysin mRNA is strongly expressed in rheumatoid arthritis fibroblast-like intimal synoviocytes cells[118]. Although the gene is primarily expressed in the intimal lining, immunohistochemical staining reveals that stromelysin protein is present in fibroblasts and endothelial cells[71], as well as in monocyte lineage lining cells using *in situ* probing[39]. Using *in situ* hybridization, collagenase mRNA was colocalized with that for stromelysin suggesting that the production of these two metalloproteinases is co-ordinated[39,118].

The cysteine proteinase cathepsin L, which is one of the major Ras-induced proteins in Ras-transformed cells, is also identifiable in half of rheumatoid synovia, being localized to the fibroblast-like intimal cells[28]. In contrast, cathepsin B was identified in both fibroblast-like intimal synoviocytes and subintimal synoviocytes[8].

The activated metalloproteinases bind stoichiometrically to α_2-macroglobulin in the plasma, but their major regulation after activation is through the two tissue inhibitors of metalloproteinases, TIMP-1 and TIMP-2[122,123]. These are two homologous molecules that are secreted in a highly regulated manner by cells elaborating metalloproteinases. The TIMPs also stoichiometrically bind to the metalloproteinases[122]. The expression TIMP was found in the same regions where stromelysin and collagen are expressed, but was greater in the osteoarthritis synovial tissue compared to rheumatoid synovial tissue[39,124]. It appears that the ratio of synthesis of TIMP to specific metalloproteinase is a critical index of the potential of a tissue to mediate matrix remodeling. In cultured synoviocytes from osteoarthritis patients, there is a much higher average ratio of TIMP to stromelysin than is found in rheumatoid arthritis[125]. This suggests that fibroblast-like intimal synoviocytes are likely to be characterized by a higher ratio of MMP to TIMP than subintimal synoviocytes.

Operation of genes in the normal synovium to attract an immune response into the joint

Taken together, the phenotype of the fibroblast-like intimal synoviocyte contains an intriguing array of gene products. Some of these are shared with subintimal synoviocytes, while others are differentially or selectively expressed in the intimal synoviocyte. Many of these gene products have the potential to be involved in normal joint histogenesis and organizing immune surveillance of the joint cavity. However, the other face of this pattern of gene expression is that these same molecules could foster localization of an ongoing immune response to the joint. Some of these gene products could deviate the immune response as well as intensify it. Macrophage-like intimal synoviocytes could serve as antigen-presenting cells with functions that might verge on those provided by dendritic cells. Moreover, this combination of cell types could provide the milieu appropriate for a form of secondary lymphoid aggregation outside the regulatory structure of the normal lymphoid organ. Thus, taken together, the phenotype of the lining cells could act powerfully in the afferent limb of disease development by converting an autoimmune response into an autoimmune disease.

Interestingly, the chemokine receptors expressed by T cells infiltrating the rheumatoid synovium have been described as markers for Th1 cells and naïve T cells as well as certain dendritic cell subsets. It is conceivable that in the normal synovium similar T cells and dendritic cells would be trafficking through the joint as a part of normal immunosurveillance and remain because the lining cell environment is favorable for continued stimulation of the clone.

Additionally some of the genes required for germinal center formation, such as VCAM-1, an important ligand for B cells, are expressed by synovial fibroblasts and may have a role in the formation of germinal centers in the inflammatory synovium. Based on these data it appears that normal fibroblast-like intimal synoviocytes can support the development of germinal centers, B cell migration, and affinity maturation. For example, an additional action of SDF-1 at higher concentrations could be the facilitation of earlier stages of peripheral B-cell development in the synovial milieu that are relevant to the presence and maturation of abundant B-cells in the rheumatoid synovium and to their production of rheumatoid factors[126]. Furthermore, several additional molecules produced by the synoviocyte can interact to facilitate other aspects of B-cell development. IL-6, a cytokine with effects on B-cell differentiation, is constitutively increased in synoviocytes obtained from rheumatoid arthritis patients[14] and its synthesis by monocytes is induced by Mac-2BP, as described above. Interleukin 7-dependent proliferation of pre-B cells is also enhanced upon exposure to biglycan[127].

Hyperlasia and tissue injury mediated by fibroblast-like intimal synoviocytes

Hyperplasia

In addition to the likely role of the fibroblast-like intimal synoviocyte in facilitating the afferent limb of the development of the autoimmune response underlying synovitis, the intima also plays a major part in the loss of function and joint destruction that characterize fully developed rheumatoid arthritis. A feature of the rheumatoid synovium is the marked hyperplasia of the lining layer and the apparent invasion and destruction of cartilage and other joint structures by the mesenchymally-derived fibroblasts and the bone marrow derived monocyte-like lineage cells. The cell biology is covered in Chapters 12 and 14. The changes in the lining during hyperplasia include a massive increase in the number of fibroblast-like intimal synoviocytes and altered cell–cell relationship with the monocyte-like lineage synoviocytes. In fact, in a parallel to synovial hyperplasia there is also loss of contact inhibition of rheumatoid arthritis cultured synovial fibroblasts with disorganized accumulation of cells[4,20,24]. This could be a reflection of the normal biology of the fibroblast-like intimal synoviocyte revealed by its response to culture conditions.

In rheumatoid arthritis, it is unknown whether initiation of the autoimmune response and its localization to the joint occurs in the setting of entirely normal intima, or whether minor degrees of non-specific hyperplasia could play a role in localizing an immune response into the joint through the repertoire of immunologically relevant molecules expressed by these cells. Hyperplasia could be initiated by a non-specific, minor traumatic event or even driven by a local immune response to a common pathogen, and the constitutive production of such chemokines might provide a non-antigen-specific mechanism for localizing pathogenic immune responses to the joint. In other words, the production of such chemoattractant molecules would be part of the normal function of the fibroblast-like intimal synoviocytes and would have increased transcription when either activated or subjected to an inflammatory 'imprinting', or when the number of cells increase. The unusual behavior of fibroblast-like intimal synoviocytes in culture may reflect this response.

Hyperplasia appears to be an intrinsic response of intimal synoviocytes to injury and healing. Apparently, in responses to the events initiated within the T-cell compartment of the joint tissues, the synovial membrane undergoes this striking change in its form and in its pattern of gene expression. It is transformed from a nutritive tissue into one that is the central agent of joint destruction, most notably focused on causing injury to the cartilage through expression of enhanced levels of degradative enzymes and through secretion of cytokines that can act to alter the pattern of gene expression in the chondrocyte. This alteration in the synovium involves a massive influx of monocyte-lineage cells and extensive neovascularization as well as marked hyperplasia of the intimal synoviocytes, likely mediated, in part, by genes described above. Three sets of biological events are evident:

(1) the intrinsic biology of the fibroblast-like intimal synoviocyte, where increased cell number simply is reflected as increased local concentration of mediators and cell surface molecules;

(2) the pathways of mutual interaction of fibroblast-like and macrophage-like intimal synoviocytes;

(3) paracrine influences of the products of the immune response on the intimal synoviocytes.

It is possible that the loss of normal cell matrix signals due to hyperplasia and its replacement by more extensive cell–cell receptor interactions result in reverse signaling that leads to a perpetuation of the hyperplasia.

However, the question remains as to why is that this physiological process performed by the synovial fibroblasts gets out of control leading to massive cell proliferation and invasion of cartilage? Although a definitive response for this question is not at hand, it has been recently considered that these cells not only are activated and have increased proliferation rate, but also that their cellular turnover through apoptosis is decreased, further contributing to the cellular accumulation and hyperlasia seen in rheumatoid arthritis fibroblast-like intimal synoviocytes. This could well be a feature of cells of the synoviocyte lineage. Several genes over-expressed in these cells and involved in the increased cytokine expression, as well as in the regulation of cell proliferation and/or survival in the rheumatoid synovium, provide clues to the regulation of hyperplasia. Among these genes, recent studies suggest that NF-κB has a key role in the regulation of synovial fibroblast apoptosis and gene expression (discussed below). NF-κB is highly expressed in the rheumatoid synovium and synovial fibroblasts[128], and its inhibition has been demonstrated to render these cells more susceptible to both TNF-α and Fas-L mediated apoptosis[129]. Furthermore, its inhibition greatly decreases IL-1, IL-6, TNF-α and VCAM-1 expression in both streptococcal cell wall- and pristane-induced arthritis in rats, thus not only regulating local and systemic mediators of joint injury, but also decreasing the expression of critical molecules involved in homing of lymphocytes to the joint[129].

Proliferation and increased oncogene expression

Whether these events found in hyperplastic synoviocytes in rheumatoid arthritis are specific, unique changes that lead to the joint destruction in this disease, or whether they are simply a reflection of the intrinsic hyper-responsiveness of these cells to signaling circuits remains to be established. Fibroblast-like intimal synoviocytes from rheumatoid arthritis and other inflammatory arthropathies survive and continue to proliferate after several passages in culture. These cells have increased expression of oncogenes and proteins involved in cell cycle regulation, mitosis, and production of growth factor and cytokines. It is our perspective that this is a reflection of the intrinsic property of the fibroblast-like intimal synoviocytes. Increased expression of some of these molecules, including a number of oncogenes, mediate cell proliferation and hyperplasia. Both autocrine and paracrine factors are involved in the regulation of these genes (reviewed in ref. 130). Among the genes over-expressed in rheumatoid arthritis synovium and cultured synovial fibroblasts is *egr-1*[131,132] which regulates the transcription of *ras* and *sis* and is down-regulated by p53. *c-fos* and *c-jun* regulate the transcription of IL-1, IL-6, TNF, and MMPs, and both oncogenes have their expression increased in rheumatoid arthritis fibroblast-like synoviocytes[113,131,133]. In fact, inhibition of *c-fos* reduced synovial fibroblast proliferation in culture[134], and ameliorated collagen-induced arthritis in mice[135]. *C-myc*[13,28], like *ras*[28], is sometimes highly expressed in fibroblast-like intimal synoviocytes. *Ras* is involved in the regulation of cathepsin L expression, a protease involved in cartilage degradation[28]. Additionally, *H-ras* point mutations of as yet unknown significance have been recently described in rheumatoid arthritis and osteoarthritis synovium[136]. Other oncogenes and proteins involved in cellular proliferation have been identified in rheumatoid arthritis synovial fibroblasts including PCNA, NOR[137], and *c-sis*/PGDF[138]. The question remains as to whether the primary defect is an abnormal proliferation that must occur through the well-known pathways involving oncogenes, or alternatively, if the fundamental defect in rheumatoid arthritis is altered oncogene expression with increased proliferation being a consequence.

The expression of oncogenes and their down-stream regulatory functions in cellular replication and production of proteolytic enzymes such as MMP, cathepsin, and others is a critical in the cartilage and bone damage caused by the infiltrating fibroblast-like intimal synoviocytes, and is discussed in more details in a separate chapter. Additionally, these genes interact with several genes and gene products regulating apoptosis, however, little of those interactions have been studied in the rheumatoid arthritis synovium.

Abnormalities in synovial apoptosis

Chapter 12 discusses synovial apoptosis in greater depth. This section will concentrate on the synovial fibroblast as it pertains to hyperplasia. It has been suspected that not only the fibroblast-like intimal synoviocytes proliferation is increased, but also its longevity is increased, possibly due to defects in the regulation of apoptosis. Independent groups described abnormalities in apoptosis of rheumatoid arthritis fibroblast-like intimal synoviocytes, with increased number of apoptotic figures along the lining layer[139,140]. Although increased numbers of apoptotic figures are seen in the fibroblast-like intimal synoviocytes, it is probably still an insufficient rate proportional to the high rate of proliferation of those cells. The imbalance between proliferation and cell death would lead to an increased accumulation of these cells[139,140]. Increased Fas expression was identified in the rheumatoid fibroblast-like intimal synoviocytes[139–141]. Not only Fas was expressed, but also apoptosis could be induced with anti-Fas antibodies, demonstrating that the Fas-mediated apoptosis pathway was preserved in these cells[139,140]. Subsequently, animal studies demonstrated that anti-Fas antibodies significantly ameliorate arthritis in mice[142,143] raising the possibility of using proapoptotic strategies to eliminate the proliferating fibroblast-like intimal synoviocytes. However, despite the apparent integrity of the Fas-mediated pathway in rheumatoid fibroblast-like intimal synoviocytes, it was recently demonstrated that several proinflammatory molecules abundant in the rheumatoid synovium, such as IL-1, IL-6, IL-8, TNFα,[144] and TGFβ[145], are capable of down-regulating Fas expression, thereby potentially preventing Fas-mediated apoptosis *in vivo*, and contributing to increased accumulation of the proliferating cells.

Other genes involved in cellular proliferation and apoptosis have also been studied. Among those, p53 expression was increased in rheumatoid arthritis fibroblast-like intimal synoviocytes as determined by immunohistochemistry in synovial tissue and in cultured cells[146]. Firestein *et al.* hypothesized that the increase p53 expression could be secondary to inflammation and increased numbers of somatic mutations in the synovial tissue caused by local injury, for example due to oxygen radicals, and possibly even mutations on p53 leading to an inefficient induction of apoptosis. These investigators identified somatic mutations on the *p53* gene in the majority of rheumatoid arthritis patients' synovial fibroblasts[147]. The same group subsequently demonstrated that inhibiting p53 function in rheumatoid arthritis and normal fibroblast-like synoviocytes could change cellular survival, susceptibility to apoptosis, and cartilage invasiveness[148]. Although at least 5 per cent of the total p53 cDNA pool appears to contain mutations, it is not clear how many cells contain those mutations and whether a mutation rate of 1 to 100 synovial fibroblasts would still be biologically relevant. Despite the presence of p53 mutations, cancer does not develop in the rheumatoid arthritis synovium, perhaps due to the absence of other mutated genes required for cancer development, or maybe due to some unknown synovial protective factor[147]. Semaphorin may also play a role in view of its identity as a multidrug resistance element and possible role in tumorgenesis[97,98].

An alternative mechanism of regulation of apoptosis is through TNF-mediated pathways. TNF-α is abundant in the joint, and activation of its receptors leads to increase levels of NF-κB, a transcription factor that is involved in the regulation of cellular proliferation which has an antiapoptotic effect[149]. NF-κB is highly expressed in rheumatoid arthritis fibroblast-like intimal synoviocytes and inhibition of its activity with N-acetyl-L-cysteine dramatically reduced the rate of cellular proliferation *in vitro*[128]. Recently, Makarov *et al.* studying streptococcal cell wall and pristane-induced arthritis in rats demonstrated that NF-κB is expressed early during the development of arthritis, and that the inhibition of NF-κB rendered synovial fibroblasts susceptible to TNF and Fas-mediated apoptosis[129]. Interestingly some of the drugs used to treat RA, such as gold salts and glucocorticoids, have also been demonstrated to interfere with NF-κB activity[150-152], although it is not known how much of the effects of these drugs is due to an action on fibroblast-like intimal synoviocytes.

Conflicting findings have been described regarding the expression of the antiapoptosis gene Bcl-2 in rheumatoid arthritis synovial fibroblasts[140,153,154]. However, its expression appears to be upregulated by the same proinflammatory molecules present in the rheumatoid synovium that down-regulate Fas expression, thereby favoring antiapoptosis, prosurvival stimuli[144].

Strategies aimed at modifying the rheumatoid fibroblast-like intimal synoviocytes cell turn-over, either by increasing fibroblast-like intimal synoviocytes or decreasing the cellular proliferation rate may prove helpful in managing RA, and the identification of such genes, and the better understanding of their function should lead to the development of new therapeutic agents.

Cartilage Injury

The ultimate clinically relevant consequences of joint inflammation in rheumatoid arthritis are the pain, tenderness, and loss of function of synovitis and the destruction of cartilage mediated by the synovial events. Cartilage injury is likely to proceed by two distinct mechanisms. An indirect one in which cytokines released by the synovial lining cells and infiltrating mononuclear cells activate chondrocytes to a pattern of gene expression that results in remodeling and degradation of the cartilage matrix. For example, IL-1 stimulates chondrocytes to release degradative enzymes[155,156]. A direct mechanism in which metalloproteinases and other enzymes released by the fibroblast-like intimal synoviocytes, and perhaps the infiltrating monocytes, directly act to digest the matrix[157,158]. The junction between the hyperplastic synovium and the cartilage appears to be the principal site of interaction between these former biologi-

cal allies and members of the same lineage. Assessment of the rate and character of cartilage injury has been determined by measuring the fine structure of the products of proteoglycan fragmentation. The glysosaminoglycan-rich region of the core protein predominates during the early phase of cartilage injury before there is significant damage evident on conventional radiographs[159]. Later, when frank radiographic changes are evident, the joint fluid contains an abundance of hyaluronan-binding domains and lesser amounts of the glycosaminoglycan-rich region of the core protein. The fact that the disruption of the stromelysin-1 (MMP-3) gene did not protect mice from developing cartilage destruction in CIA suggests that redundant or compensatory functions exist among MMPs or between MMPs and other genes[160].

Recent studies have demonstrated that some types of cartilage injury occur without the presence of T cells, likely reflecting the constitutive release of cytokines, such as IL-1, described above. In experimental models where rheumatoid synovial fibroblasts were implanted together with cartilage in SCID mice, cartilage erosions occurred despite the absence of T cells[161,162], suggesting that fibroblast-like intimal synoviocytes have the intrinsic potential to mediate this matrix remodeling. Additionally, H2-*c-fos* transgenic mice develop chronic arthritis, and the synovial proliferation and joint erosion occur in the absence of infiltrating lymphocytes in the synovium[163]. Scott *et al.*[164] also demonstrated that the cartilage degradation depended on a critical fibroblast-like intimal synoviocyte–macrophage interaction which was IL-1, IL-6, TNF-α, and CD44 dependent.

Different susceptibility genes regulating various stages of disease development

It is very likely that the development of rheumatoid arthritis proceeds through a variety of stages from susceptibility, through the development of autoreactive T-cell clones, to overt disease as shown in Fig. 9.7. In particular, macrophages and fibroblast-like intimal synoviocytes may have a more important role in localizing the autoimmune process to joints and in its perpetuation, as discussed earlier.

Genes regulating cellular functions at each one of these stages of disease development could be candidate susceptibility/severity genes and potential targets for therapy. One approach for additional gene discovery efforts could be the use of subtraction libraries[8,12,13], or the use of hybridization membranes, SAGE[165], or cDNA/EST hybridization microarrays[166], to study fibroblast-like intimal synoviocyte gene expression in very early RA. In a similar fashion, gene expression on patterns in macrophages or T cells derived from the synovium of patients with normal tissue, osteoarthritis, or established RA could be studied. This approach would shed additional light on the contribution of different genes products at each stage of disease. A similar strategy could be used to determine which genes' down or up regulation are critical for clinical improvement and response to drug therapy. It was first postulated by Dayer *et al.*[167] that the lymphocytic response initi-

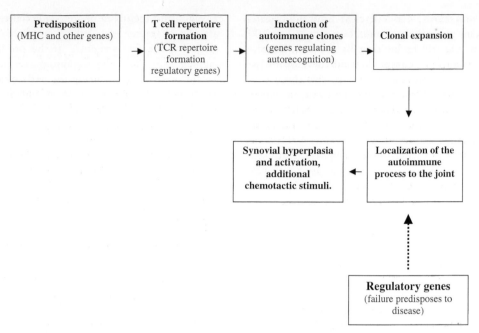

Fig. 9.7 Proposed stages in the development of rheumatoid arthritis.

ates the cascade of immune interactions and cytokine production by acting directly on the target fibroblast cells and indirectly on them by activating monocyte lineage cells to release additional cytokines. Thus, T cells may be more involved in the early stages of disease, while in chronic stages the inflammatory drive would be more macrophage and fibroblast-like intimal synoviocytes-dependent.[35,168].

Genomic dissection of the fibroblast-like intimal synoviocyte phenotype

Because of the possibility that some of the genes that are the topic of this chapter may differentially regulate cellular functions at each stage of disease development, they are assuming increasing importance as non-MHC genes involved in the definition of susceptibility. This is especially so in the context of the paradigm underlying this chapter that distinguishes between an autoimmune response and the localization of the response to the joint that results in disease. Linkage studies have been done in both rheumatoid arthritis and in experimental models of arthritis in rodents to identify novel non-MHC genes. This type of analysis tries to identify the cosegregation between phenotype and genotype without prior knowledge of the trait causing/regulating genes. Linkage analysis is a powerful tool to identify new genes and new pathways involved in the regulation of a particular phenotype. Several susceptibility loci have been identified both in rodents and humans. It is not known which genes account for those susceptibility loci, however, several of them map to genomic regions containing some of the genes discussed in this chapter (Table 9.4). Therefore, some of these genes are candidate susceptibility genes. In fact, some may be involved in the regulation of disease severity as well[89,169–171] (Dracheva *et al.*

unpublished observations). How much of this differential gene expression is regulated at the germ line genetic level versus determination at the somatic level is unknown.

Among these candidate genes, one of the genes differentially expressed (biglycan) is located in genomic intervals where a rheumatoid arthritis susceptibility locus has been mapped[172] (Table 9.4). Four other differentially expressed genes (semaphorin, VCAM-1, lumican, interferon-induced 71kD 2'5' oligoadenylate synthetase) map to human chromosomal intervals syntenic with rat regions where loci regulating experimental animal erosive arthritis have been mapped[89,170–172] (Dracheva *et al.* unpublished observations).

For linkage analysis it is critical to have a well-defined phenotype to be mapped. Rheumatoid arthritis is a heterogenous disease with manifestations that may vary from one patient to the other, creating potentially confusing factors. Different clinical and laboratory manifestations may be regulated by different genes. One approach that may facilitate the genetic dissection of rheumatoid arthritis is to study subphenotypes of the disease, such as whether allelic genes are responsible for particular elements in the distinctive fibroblast-like intimal synoviocytes phenotype. For example a certain gene may be more important to the capacity of a fibroblast-like intimal synoviocytes to degrade cartilage than it is to the complete phenotype that is RA. By subphenotyping disease we may obtain more 'clean' phenotypes and increase the likelihood of identifying linkage.

Conclusion

This chapter makes the hypothesis that the synovial fibroblast, particularly the intimal cells, have a central role in localizing the autoimmune response in rheumatoid arthritis to the joint, and further, that this role in the afferent arm of the development of autoimmune disease may be in part an extension of the normal function of these cells seen during development, embryogenesis, and in normal synovial physiology. It was also proposed that part of the differential gene expression seen in cultured rheumatoid arthritis synovial fibroblast is lineage-dependent and related to the initial proportion of intimal to subintimal cells in the biopsy or surgical specimens, with the differential expression representing increased number, or hyperplasia, of intimal cells. Thus, much of the distinctive phenotype of cultured rheumatoid arthritis synoviocytes could be a combination of the intrinsic pattern of gene expression in this stem-cell-like sublineage and its pattern of response to culture *in vitro*. The synovial intimal fibroblast expresses certain genes also seen in mesenchymal progenitor cells, suggesting that this cell might respresent a form of less-differentiated fibroblast[173].

The synovial fibroblast gene products operate in an autocrine and paracrine pattern futher favoring the programmed constitutive functions of this intriguing cell. However, it is possible that among what we are considering as lineage differences there may be critical allelic differences governing gene expression that confer enhanced susceptibility for the development of rheumatoid arthritis. This possibility needs to be tested. Abnormalities in the expression of genes involved in the regulation of cell proliferation, such as oncogenes, transcription factors critical for cytokine production and regulation of apoptosis, as well as other apoptosis regulatory genes, cytokines, and chemokines could be a factor fostering either the afferent function of fibroblast-like intimal synoviocytes or their efferent effector function. Part of these abnomalities may relate to somatic mutations in the synovium, and part of this effect may be under germ line genetic regulation. It was proposed that some of the genes regulating the fibroblast-like intimal synoviocyte, in the presence of other genes required in the earlier stages in the development of autoimmunity, would culminate in disease. In fact, several of the genes differentially expressed in rheumatoid arthritis as compared to osteoarthritis fibroblast-like synoviocytes in culture are located in chromosomal regions previously described to contain arthritis susceptibility and severity regulatory genes.

The combined study of gene expression, perhaps by cDNA microarray technologies, and function in synovial fibroblasts and linkage analysis may facilitate the gene discovery efforts in rheumatoid arthritis by creating simplified phenotypes, and the identification of these regulatory genes is likely to provide new targets for therapy as well as increasing our understanding of the pathogenesis of arthritis.

References

1. Dayer J.M., *et al.* Production of collagenase and prostaglandins by isolated adherent rheumatoid synovial cells. *Proc Natl Acad Sci USA*, 1976;**73**:945–9.
2. Edwards J.C., *et al.* The formation of human synovial joint cavities: a possible role for hyaluronan and CD44 in altered interzone cohesion. J *Anat*, 1994;**185**:355–67.
3. Burmester G.R., *et al.* The tissue architecture of synovial membranes in inflammatory and non-inflammatory joint diseases. I. The localization of the major synovial cell populations as detected by monoclonal reagents directed towards la and monocyte-macrophage antigens. *Rheumatol Int*, 1983;**3**:173–81.
4. Hammerman D., Stephens M., Barland P. Comparative histology and metabolism of synovial tissue in normal arthritic joints. In:

Inflammation and Disease of Connective Tissue. L.C. Mills and J.H. Moyer, Editors. 1961, W.B. Saunders: Philadelphia. p. 158–68.
5. Fox R.I., Kang H., Structure and function of synoviocytes. In: *Arthritis and Allied Conditions*, D.J. McCarthy and W.J. Koopman, Editors. 1993, Lea & Febiger: Malvern. p. 263–78.
6. Edwards J.C., The nature and origins of synovium: experimental approaches to the study of synoviocyte differentiation. J *Anat*, 1994;**184**:493–501.
7. Cush J.J., Lipsky P.E., Cellular basis for rheumatoid inflammation. *Clin Orthop*, 1991;9–22.
8. Seki T., *et al.* Use of differential subtraction method to identify genes that characterize the phenotype of cultured rheumatoid arthritis synoviocytes. *Arthritis Rheum*, 1998;**41**:1356–64.
9. Okada Y., *et al.* Localization of type VI collagen in the lining cell layer of normal and rheumatoid synovium. *Lab Invest*, 1990;**63**:647–56.
10. Storm E.E., Kingsley D.M., Joint patterning defects caused by single and double mutations in members of the bone morphogenetic protein (BMP) family. *Development*, 1996;**122**:3969–79.
11. Ritchlin C.T., Winchester R.J., Potential mechanisms for coordinate gene activation in the rheumatoid synoviocyte: implications and hypotheses. *Springer Semin Immunopathol*, 1989;**11**:219–34.
12. Winchester R., Su F., Ritchlin C., Alteration of synoviocytes by inflammation—the source of a persistent non-immunologic drive in synovitis: analysis of levels of mRNA expression by a simple multi-gene assay. *Clin Exp. Rheumatol*, 1993;**11**(Suppl 8):S87–90.
13. Ritchlin C., *et al.* Sustained and distinctive patterns of gene activation in synovial fibroblasts and whole synovial tissue obtained from inflammatory synovitis. *Scand J Immunol*, 1994;**40**:292–8.
14. Bucala R., *et al.* Constitutive production of inflammatory and mitogenic cytokines by rheumatoid synovial fibroblasts. J *Exp Med*, 1991;**173**:569–74.
15. Winchester R.J., Burmester G.R., Demonstration of la antigens on certain dendritic cells and on a novel elongate cell found in human synovial tissue. *Scand J Immunol*. 1981;**14**:439–44.
16. Klareskog L., *et al.* Immune functions of human synovial cells. Phenotypic and T cell regulatory properties of macrophage-like cells that express HLA-DR. *Arthritis Rheum*, 1982;**25**:488-501.
17. Burmester G.R., *et al.* Identification of three major synovial lining cell populations by monoclonal antibodies directed to la antigens and antigens associated with monocytes/macrophages and fibroblasts. *Scand J Immunol*, 1983;**17**:69–82.
18. Zvaifler N.J., *et al.* Identification of immunostimulatory dendritic cells in the synovial effusions of patients with rheumatoid arthritis. J *Clin Invest*, 1985;**76**:789–800.
19. Burmester G.R., *et al.* Ia+ T cells in synovial fluid and tissues of patients with rheumatoid arthritis. *Arthritis Rheum*, 1981;**24**:1370–6.
20. Smith C.A., Properties of synovial cells in culture. J *Exp Med*, 1971;**134**:306S.
21. Castor C.W., Connective tissue activation. II. Abnormalities of cultured rheumatoid synovial cells. *Arthritis Rheum*, 1971;**14**:55–66.
22. Werb Z., *et al.* Endogenous activiation of latent collagenase by rheumatoid synovial cells. Evidence for a role of plasminogen activator. *N Engl J Med*, 1977;**296**:1017–23.
23. Castor C.W., *et al.* Connective tissue activation. XI. Stimulation of glycosaminoglycan and DNA formation by a platelet factor. *Arthritis Rheum*, 1977;**20**:859–68.
24. Imamura F., *et al.* Monoclonal expansion of synoviocytes in rheumatoid arthritis. *Arthritis Rheum*, 1998;**41**:1979–86.
25. Kriegsmann J., *et al.* Expression of vascular cell adhesion molecule-1 mRNA and protein in rheumatoid synovium demonstrated by in situ hybridization and immunohistochemistry. *Lab Invest*, 1995;**72**:209–14.
26. Ritchlin C., Haas-Smith S., Collagenase and stromelysin expression in rheumatoid synovium and cartilage: comment on the article by Wolfe *et al. Arthritis Rheum*, 1994;**37**:1831–3.

27. Winchester R., Rheumatoid Arthritis, In: *Sampter's Immunological Diseases*, M.M. Frank and K.F. Austen, Editors. 1995, Little, Brown and Company: Boston. p. 699–757.

28. Trabandt A., *et al.* Expression of the collagenolytic and Ras-induced cysteine proteinase cathepsin L and proliferation-associated oncogenes in synovial cells of MRL/I mice and patients with rheumatoid arthritis. *Matrix*, 1990;10:349–61.

29. Hubank M., Schatz D.G., Identifying differences in mRNA expression by representational difference analysis of cDNA. *Nucleic Acids Res*, 1994;22:5640–8.

30. Lisitsyn N., Wigler M., Cloning the differences between two complex genomes. *Science*, 1993;259:946–51.

31. Hachicha M., *et al.* Production of monocyte chemotactic protein-1 in human type B synoviocytes. Synergistic effect of tumour necrosis factor alpha and interferon-gamma. *Arthritis Rheum*, 1993;36:26–34.

32. Villiger P.M., Terkeltaub R., Lotz M., Production of monocyte chemoattractant protein-1 by inflamed synovial tissue and culture synoviocytes. *J Immunol*, 1992;149:722–7.

33. Rathanaswami P., *et al.* Expression of the cytokine RANTES in human rheumatoid synovial fibroblasts. Differential regulation of RANTES and interleukin-8 genes by inflammatory cytokines. *J Biol Chem*, 1993;268:5834–9.

34. Guerne P.A., *et al.* Synovium as a source of interleukin 6 in vitro. Contribution to local and systemic manifestations of arthritis. *J Clin Invest*, 1989;83:585–92.

35. Firestein G.S., *et al.* Quantitative analysis of cytokine gene expression in rheumatoid arthritis. *J Immunol*, 1990;144: 3347–53.

36. Hermann J.A., *et al.* Important imunoregulatory role of interleukin-11 in the inflammatory process in rheumatoid arthritis. *Arthritis Rheum*, 1998;41:1388–97.

37. Mino T., *et al.* Interleukin-1alpha and tumor necrosis factor alpha synergistically stimulate prostaglandin E2-dependent production of interleukin-11 in rheumatoid synovial fibroblasts. *Arthritis Rheum*, 1998;41:2004–13.

38. Firestein G.S., Paine M.M., Stromelysin and tissue inhibitor of metalloproteinases gene expression in rheumatoid arthritis synovium. *Am J Pathol*, 1992;140:1309–14.

39. McCachren S.S., Expression of metalloproteinases and metaloproteinase inhibitor in human arthritic synovium. *Arthritis Rheum*, 1991;34:1085–93.

40. Wicks I.P., *et al.* The effect of cytokines on the expression of MHC antigens and ICAM-1 by normal and transformed synoviocytes. *Autoimmunity*, 1992;12:13–9.

41. Bombara M.P., *et al.* Cell contact between T cells and synovial fibroblasts causes induction of adhesion molecules and cytokines. *J Leuk Biol*, 1993;54:399–406.

42. Chin J.E., *et al.* Role of cytokines in inflammatory synovitis. The coordinate regulation of intercellular adhesion molecule 1 and HLA class I and class II antigens in rheumatoid synovial fibroblasts. *Arthritis Rheum*, 33:1776–86.

43. Demaziere A., Athanasou N.A., Adhesion receptors of intimal and subintimal cells of the normal synovial membrane. *J Pathol*, 1992;168:209–15.

44. Lindsley H.B., *et al.* Regulation of the expression of adhesion molecules by human synoviocytes. *Semin Arthritis Rheum*, 1992;21:330–4.

45. Rinaldi N., *et al.* Increased expression of integrins on fibroblast-like synoviocytes from rheumatoid arthritis in vitro correlates with enhanced binding to extracellular matrix proteins. *Ann Rheum Dis*, 1997;56:45–51.

46. Croft D.R., *et al.* Complex CD44 splicing combinations in synovial fibroblasts from arthritic joints. *Eur J Immunol*, 1997;27:1680–4.

47. Henderson K.J., Edward J.C., Worrall J.G., Expression of CD44 in normal and rheumatoid synovium and cultured synovial fibroblasts. *Ann Rheum Dis*, 1994;53:729–34.

48. Yellin M.J., *et al.* Ligation of CD40 on fibroblasts induces CD54 (ICAM-1) and CD106 (VCAM-1) up-regulation and IL-6 production and proliferation. *J Leukoc Biol*, 1995;58:209–16.

49. Seitz M., *et al.* Production of interleukin-1 receptor antagonist, inflammatory chemotactic proteins, and prostaglandin E by rheumatoid and osteoarthritic synoviocytes–regulation by IFN-gamma and IL-4. *J Immunol*, 1994;154:2060–5.

50. Hogan M., *et al.* Differential expression of the small inducible cytokines GRO alpha and GRO beta by synovial fibroblasts in chronic arthritis: possible role in growth regulation. *Cytokine*, 1994;6:61–9.

51. Koch A.E., *et al.* Macrophage inflammatory protein-1 beta: a C-C chemokine in osteoarthritis. *Clin Immunol Immunopathol*, 1995;77:307–14.

52. Campbell J.J. *et al.* Chemokines and the arrest of lymphocytes rolling under flow conditions. *Science*, 1998;279:381–4.

53. Moser B., *et al.* Lymphocyte responses to chemokines. *Int Rev Immunol*, 1998;16:323–44.

54. Dunon D., L. Piali, Imhof B.A., To stick or not to stick: the new leukocyte homing paradigm. *Curr Opin Biol*, 1996;8:741–723.

55. Kim C.H., *et al.* CK beta-11/macrophage inflammatory protein-3 beta/EBI1-ligand chemokine is an efficacious chemoattractant for T and B cells. *J Immunol*, 1998;160:2418–24.

56. Delgado E., *et al.* Mature dendritic cells respond to SDF-1, but not to several beta-chemokines. *Immunobiology*, 1998;198:490–500.

57. Nagasawa T., *et al.* Defects of B-cell lymphopoiesis and bone-marrow myelopoiesis in mice lacking the CXC chemokine PBSF/SDF-1. *Nature*, 1996;382:635–8.

58. Zou Y.R., *et al.* Function of the chemokine receptor CXCR4 in haematopoiesis and in cerebellar development. *Nature*, 1998;393: 595–9.

59. Bonecchi R., *et al.* Differential expression of chemokine receptors and chemotactic responsiveness of type 1 T helper cells (Th1s) and Th2s. *J Exp Med*, 1998;187:129–34.

60. Qin S., *et al.* The chemokine receptors CXCR3 and CCR5 mark subsets of T cells associated with certain inflammatory reactions. *J Clin Invest*, 1998;101:746–54.

61. Bedard P.A., Golds E.E., Cytokine-induced expression of mRNAs for chemotactic factors in human synovial cells and fibroblasts. *J Cell Physiol*, 1993;154:433–41.

62. Hosaka S., *et al.* Expression of the chemokine superfamily in rheumatoid arthritis. *Clin Exp Immunol*, 1994;97:451–7.

63. Barnes D.A., *et al.* Polyclonal antibody directed against human RANTES ameliorates disease in the Lewis rat adjuvant-induced arthritis model. *J Clin Invest*, 1998;101:2910–9.

64. Brennan F.M., *et al.* Cytokine production in culture by cells isolated from the synovial membrane. *J Autoimmun*, 1989;2(Suppl):177–86.

65. Buchan G., *et al.* Interleukin-1 and tumour necrosis factor mRNA expression in rheumatoid arthritis: prolonged production of IL-1 alpha. *Clin Exp Immunol*, 1988;73:449–55.

66. Alvaro-Gracia J.M., *et al.* Cytokines in chronic inflammatory arthritis. VI. Analysis of the synovial cells involved in granulocyte-macrophage colony-stimulating factor production and gene expression in rheumatoid arthritis and its regulation by IL-1 and tumor necrosis factor-alpha. *J Immunol*, 1991;146: 3365–71.

67. Okamoto H., *et al.* The synovial expression and serum levels of interleukin-6, interleukin-11, leukemia inhibitory factor, and oncostatin M in rheumatoid arthritis. *Arthritis Rheum*, 1997;40:1096–105.

68. Tan P.L., *et al.* Expression of the interleukin 6 gene in rheumatoid synovial fibroblasts. *J Rheumatol*, 1990;17:1608–12.

69. Mclnnes I.B., *et al.* The role of interleukin-15 in T-cell migration and activation in rheumatoid arthritis. *Nat Med*, 1996;2:175–82.

70. Temime N., *et al.* Autocrine stimulation of interleukin 1 in human adherent synovial lining cells: down regulation by interferon gamma. *Hum Immunol*, 1991;31:261–70.

71. Case J.P. *et al.* IL-1 regulation of transin/stromelysin transcription in rheumatoid synovial fibroblasts appears to involve two antagonistic transduction pathways, an inhibitory, prostaglandin-dependent pathway mediated by cAMP, and a stimulatory, protein kinase C-dependant pathway. *J Immunol*, 1990;145:3755–61.

72. Goddard D.H., Grossman S.L., Moore M.E. Autocrine regulation of rheumatoid arthritis synovial cell growth in vitro. *Cytokine*, 1990;2:149–55.

73. Koch A.E., *et al.* Synovial tissue macrophage as a source of the chemotactic cytokine IL-8. *J Immunol*, 1991;147:2187–95.

74. Krane S.M., *et al.* Mononuclear cell-conditioned medium containing mononuclear cell factor (MCR), homologous with interleukin 1, stimulates collagen and fibronectin synthesis by adherent rheumatoid synovial cells: effects of prostaglandin E2 and indomethacin. *Coll Relat Res*, 19855:99–117.

75. Alvaro-Gracia J.M., Zvaifler N.J., Firestein G.S., Cytokines in chronic inflammatory arthritis. V. Mutual antagonism between interferon-gamma and tumor necrosis factor-alpha on HLA-DR expression, proliferation, collagenase production, and granulocyte macrophage colony-stimulating factor production by rheumatoid arthritis synoviocytes, *J Clin Invest*, 1990;86: 1790–8.

76. Lemaire R., *et al.* Selective induction of the secretion of cathepsins B and L by cytokines in synovial fibroblast-like cells. *Br J Rheumatol*, 1997;36:735–43.

77. Keffer J. *et al.* Transgenic mice expressing human tumour necrosis factor: a predictive genetic model of arthritis. *Embo J*, 1991;10:4025–31.

78. Moreland L.W., *et al.* Treatment of rheumatoid arthritis with a recombinant human tumor necrosis factor receptor (p75)-Fc fusion protein. *N Engl J Med*, 1997;337:141–7.

79. Mori L., *et al.* Attenuation of collagen-induced arthritis in 55-kDa TNF receptor type 1 (TNFR1)-IgG1-treated and TNFR1-deficient mice. *J Immunol*, 1996;157:3178–82.

80. Elliot M.J., *et al.* Randomised double-blind comparison of chimeric monoclonal antibody to tumour necrosis factor alpha (cA2) versus placebo in rheumatoid arthritis. *Lancet*, 1994;344:1105–10.

81. Alonzi T., *et al.* Interleukin 6 is required for the development of collagen-induced arthritis. *J Exp Med*, 1998;187:461–8.

82. Mihara M., *et al.* Interleukin-6 (IL-6) induces the proliferation of synovial fibroblastic cells in the presence of soluble IL-6 receptor. *Br J Rheumatol*, 1995;34:321–5.

83. Ito A., *et al.* Effects of interleukin-6 on the metabolism of connective tissue components in rheumatoid synovial fibroblasts. *Arthritis Rheum*, 1992;35:1197–201.

84. Lotz M., Guerne P.A., Interleukin-6 induces the synthesis of tissue inhibitor of mealloproteinases-1/erythroid potentiating activity (TIMP-1/EPA). *J Biol Chem*, 1991;266:2017–20.

85. Richards C.D., *et al.* Selective regulation of metalloproteinase inhibitor (TIMP-1) by oncostatin M in fibroblasts in culture. *J Immunol*, 1993;150:5596–603.

86. Lotz M., Moats T., Villiger P.M., Leukemia inhibitory factor is expressed in cartilage and synovium and can contribute to the pathogenesis of arthritis, *J Clin Invest*, 1992;90:888–96.

87. Langdon C., *et al.* Oncostatin M stimulates monocyte chemoattractant protein-1-and interleukin-1-induced matrix metalloproteinase-1 production by human synovial fibroblasts in vitro. *Arthritis Rheum*, 1997;40:2139–46.

88. Cawston T.E., *et al.* The role of oncostatin M in animal and human connective tissue collagen turnover and its localization within the rheumatoid joint. *Arthritis Rheum*, 1998;41: 1760–71.

89. Gulko P., *et al.* Identification of a new non-MHC genetic locus on chromosome 2 controlling disease severity in collagen-induced arthritis in rats. *Arthritis Rheum*, 1998;41:2122–31.

90. McInnes I.B., *et al.* Interleukin-15 mediates T cell-dependent regulation of tumor necrosis factor-alpha production in rheumatoid arthritis. *Nat Med*, 1997;3:189–95.

91. Hamilton J.A., *et al.* Cytokine regulation of colony-stimulating factor (CSF) production in cultured human synovial fibroblasts. II. Similarities and differences in the control of interleukin-1 induction of granulocyte-macrophage CSF and granulocyte-CSF production. *Blood*, 1992;79:1413–9.

92. Campbell I.K., *et al.* Protection from collagen-induced arthritis in granulocyte-macrophage colony-stimulating factor-deficient mice. *J Immunol*, 1998;161:3639–44.

93. Chu C.Q., *et al.* Transforming growth factor-beta 1 in rheumatoid synovial membrane and cartilage/pannus junction. *Clin Exp Immunol*, 1991;86:380–6.

94. Mangasser-Stephan K., *et al.* Identification of human semaphorin E gene expression in rheumatoid synovial cells by mRNA differential display. *Biochem Biophys Res Commun*, 1997;234:153–6.

95. Luo Y., *et al.* A family of molecules related to collapsing in the embryonic chick nervous system. *Neuron*, 1995;14:1131–40.

96. Kidd B.L., *et al.* A neurogenic mechanism for symmetrical arthritis [see comments]. *Lancet*, 1989;2:1128–30.

97. Sekido Y., *et al.* Human semaphorins A(V) and IV reside in the 3p21.3 small cell lung cancer deletion region and demonstrate distinct expression patterns. *Proc Natl Acad Sci USA*, 1996;93:4120–5.

98. Yamada T. *et al.* Identification of semaphorin E as a non-MDR drug resistance gene of human cancers. *Proc Natl Acad Sci USA*, 1997;94:14713–8.

99. Koths K., *et al.* Cloning and characterization of a human Mac-2-binding protein, a new member of the superfamily defined by the macrophage scavenger receptor cysteine-rich domain. *J Biol Chem*, 1993;268:14245–9.

100. Inohara H., *et al.* Interactions between galectin-3 and Mac-2-binding protein mediate cell-cell adhesion. *Cancer Res*, 1996;56:4530–4.

101. Yu B., Wright S.D., LPS-dependent interaction of Mac-2-binding protein with immobilized CD14. *J Inflamm*, 1995;45:115–25.

102. Jeng K.C., Frigeri L.G., Liu F.T., An endogenous lectin, galectin-3 (epsilon BP/Mac-2), potentiates IL-1 production by human monocytes. *Immunol Lett*, 1994;42:113–6.

103. Merrill J., *et al.* Synovial fibroblast supernatants induce monocytes to form giant cells via CD18 integrins, *Arthritis Rheum*, 1992;35:S97.

104. Valencia X., *et al.* Identification of cadherin-11 in type B synoviocytes derived from rheumatoid arthritis patients. *Arthritis Rheum*, 1998;41(suppl):S190.

105. Rada J.A., Cornuet P.K., Hassell J.R., Regulation of corneal collagen fibrillogenesis in vitro by corneal proteoglycan (lumican and decorin) core proteins. *Exp Eye Res*, 1993;56: 635–48.

106. Funderburgh J.L., *et al.* Macrophage receptors for lumican. A corneal keratan sulfate proteoglycan. *Invest Ophthalmol Vis Sci*, 1997;38:1159–67.

107. Hildebrand A., *et al.* Interaction of the small interstitial proteoglycans biglycan, decorin and fibromodulin with transforming growth factor beta. *Biochem J*, 1994;302:527–34.

108. Ungefroren H.,. Krull N.B, Transcriptional regulation of the human biglycan gene. *J Biol Chem*, 1996;271:15787–95.

109. McKee C.M., *et al.* Hyaluronan (HA) fragments induce chemokine gene expression in alveolar macrophages. The role of HA size and CD44. *J Clin Invest*, 1996;98:2403–13.

110. Jones J.I., *et al.* Extracellular matrix contains insulin-like growth factor binding protien-5: potentiation of the effects of IGF-1. *J Cell Biol*, 1993;121:679–87.

111. Tyler J.A., Insulin-like growth factor 1 can decrease degradation and promote synthesis of proteoglycan in cartilage exposed to cytokines. *Biochem J*, 1989;260:543–8.

112. Pash J.M., Canalis E., Transcriptional regulation of insulin-like growth factor-binding protein-5 by prostaglandin E2 in osteoblast cells. *Endocrinology*, 1996;137:2375–82.

113. Remmers E.F., Sano H., Wilder R.L., Platelet-derived growth factors and heparin-binding (fibroblast) growth factors in the synovial tissue pathology of rheumatoid arthritis. *Semin Arthritis Rheum*, 1991;21:191–9.

114. Marie I., Hovanessian A.G., The 69-kDa 2-5A synthetase is composed of two homologous and adjacent functional domains. *J Biol Chem*, 1992;267:9933–9.

115. Wathelet M., *et al.* Molecular cloning, full length sequence and preliminary characterization of a 56-kDa protein induced by human interferons. *Eur J Biochem*, 1986;155:11–7.

116. Burmester G.R., *et al.* Differential expression of Ia antigens by rheumatoid synovial lining cells. *J Clin Invest*, 1987;**80**:595–604.

117. Edwards J.C., *et al.* Matrix metalloproteinases in the formation of human synovial joint cavities. *J Anat*, 1996;**188**:355–60.

118. Gravallese E.M., *et al.* In situ hybridization studies of stromelysin and collagenase messenger RNA expression in rheumatoid synovium. *Arthritis Rheum*, 1991;**34**:1076–84.

119. Woolley D.E., Crossley M.J., Evanson J.M., Collagenase at sites of cartilage erosion in the rheumatoid joint. *Arthritis Rheum*, 1977;**20**:1231–9.

120. Goldberg G.I., *et al.* Human fibroblast collagenase. Complete primary structure and homology to an oncogene transformation-induced rat protein. *J Biol Chem*, 1986;**261**:6600–5.

121. Suzuki K., *et al.* Mechanisims of activation of tissue procollagenase by matrix metalloproteinase 3 (stromelysin). *Biochemistry*, 1990;**29**:10261–70.

122. Cawston T.E., *et al.* The interaction of purified rabbit bone collagenase with purified rabbit bone metalloproteinase inhibitor. *Bioch J*, 1983;**211**:313–18.

123. Stetler Stevenson, W.G., *et al.* Tissue inhibitor of metalloproteinases-2 (TIMP-2) mRNA expression in tumor cell lines and human tumor tissues. *J Biol Chem*, 1990;**265**:13933–8.

124. Okada Y., *et al.* Matrix metalloproteinase 2 from human rheumatoid synovial fibroblasts. Purification and activation of the precursor and enzymic properties. *Eur J Biochem*, 1990;**194**:721–30.

125. Ritchlin C., *et al.* Patterns of gene activation in synovial fibroblasts and whole synovial tissue obtained from patients with inflammatory and non-inflammatory synovitis. *Clinical Research*, 1991;**39**:341.

126. Mellors R.C. *et al.* Rheumatoid factor and the pathogenesis of rheumatoid arthritis. *J Ex Med*, 1961;**113**:475.

127. Oritani K., Kincade P.W., Identification of stromal cell products that interact with pre-B cells. *J Cell Biol*, 1996;**134**:771–82.

128. Fujisawa K., *et al.* Activation of transcription factor NF-kappa B in human synovial cells in response to tumor necrosis factor alpha. *Arthritis Rheum*, 1996;**39**:197–203.

129. Miagkov A.V. *et al.* NF-kappa B activation provides the potential link between inflammation and hyperplasia in the arthritic joint. *Proc Natl Acad Sci USA*, 1998;**95**:13859–64.

130. Muller-Ladner U., *et al.* Oncogenes in rheumatoid arthritis. *Rheum Dis Clin North Am*, 1995;**21**:675–90.

131. Trabandt A., *et al.* Spontaneous expression of immediately-early response genes c-fos and egr-1 in collagenase-producing rheumatoid synovial fibroblasts. *Rheumatol Int*, 1992;**12**:53–9.

132. Aicher W.K., *et al.* Overexpression of zinc-finger transcription factor Z-225/Egr-1 in synoviocytes from rheumatoid arthritis patients. *J Immunol*, 1994;**152**:5940–8.

133. Dooley S., *et al.* Constitutive expression of c-fos and c-jun, overexpression of ets-2, and reduced expression of metastasis suppressor gene nm23-H1 in rheumatoid arthritis. *Ann Rheum Dis*, 1996;**55**:298–304.

134. Morita Y., *et al.* Antisense oligonucleotides targeting c-fos mRNA inhibit rheumatoid synovial fibroblast proliferation. *Ann Rheum Dis*, 1998;**57**:122–4.

135. Shiozawa S., *et al.* Studies on the contribution of c-fos/AP-1 to arthritic joint destruction. *J Clin Invest*, 1997;**99**:1210–6.

136. Roivainen A., *et al.* H-ras oncogene point mutations in arthritic synovium. *Arthritis Rheum*, 1997;**40**:1636–43.

137. Qu Z., *et al.* Local proliferation of fibroblast-like synoviocytes contributes to synovial hyperplasia. Results of proliferating cell nuclear antigen/cyclin, c-myc, and nucleolar organizer region staining. *Arthritis Rheum*, 1994;**37**:212–20.

138. Remmers E.F., *et al.* Production of platelet derived growth factor B chain (PDGF-B/c-sis) mRNA and immunoreactive PDGF B-like polypeptide by rheumatoid synovium: coexpression with heparin binding acidic fibroblast growth factor-1. *J Rheumatol*, 1991;**18**:7–13.

139. Nakajima T., *et al.* Apoptosis and functional Fas antigen in rheumatoid arthritis synoviocytes. *Arthritis Rheum*, 1995;**38**:485–91.

140. Firestein G.S., Yeo M., Zvaifler, N.J. Apoptosis in rheumatoid arthrits synovium. *J Clin Invest*, 1995;**96**:1631–8.

141. Hashimoto H., *et al.* Soluble Fas ligand in the joints of patients with rheumatoid arthritis and osteoarthritis. *Arthritis Rheum*, 1998;**41**:657–62.

142. Fujisawa K., *et al.* Therapeutic effect of the anti-Fas antibody on arthritis in HTLV-1 tax transgenic mice. *J Clin Invest*, 1996;**98**:271–8.

143. Zhang H., *et al.* Amelioration of collagen-induced arthritis by CD95 (Apo-1/Fas)-ligand gene transfer. *J Clin Invest*, 1997;**100**:1951–7.

144. Wakisaka S., *et al.* Modulation by proinflammatory cytokines of Fas/Fas ligand-mediated apoptotic cell death of synovial cells in patients with rheumatoid arthritis (RA). *Clin Exp Immunol*, 1998;**114**:119–28.

145. Kawakami A., *et al.* Inhibition of Fas antigen-mediated apoptosis of rheumatoid synovial cells in vitro by transforming growth factor beta 1. *Arthritis Rheum*, 1996;**39**:1267–76.

146. Firestein G.S., *et al.* Apoptosis in rheumatoid arthritis: p53 overexpression in rheumatoid arthritis synovium. *Am J Pathol*, 1996;**149**:2143–51.

147. Firestein G.S., *et al.* Somatic mutations in the p53 tumor suppressor gene in rheumatoid arthritis synovium. *Proc Natl Acad Sci U S A*, 1997;**94**:10895-900.

148. Aupperle K.R., *et al.* Regulation of synoviocyte proliferation, apoptosis, and invasion by the p53 tumor suppressor gene. *Am J Pathol*, 1998;**152**:1091–8.

149. Van Antwerp D.J., *et al.* Suppression of TNF-alpha-induced apoptosis by NF-kappaB. *Science*, 1996;**274**:787–9.

150. Scheinman R.I., *et al.* Role of transcriptional activation of I kappa B alpha in mediation of immunosuppression by glucocorticoids. *Science*, 1995;**270**:283–6.

151. Auphan N., *et al.* Immunosupression by glucocorticoids: inhibition of NF-kappa B activity through induction of I kappa B synthesis. *Science*, 1995;**270**:286–90.

152. Yang J.P., *et al.* Inhibition of the DNA-binding activity of NF-kappa B by gold compounds in vitro. *FEBS Lett*, 1995;**361**:89–96.

153. Isomaki P., *et al.* Expression of bcl-2 in rheumatoid arthritis. *Br J Rheumatol*, 1996;**35**:611–9.

154. Matsumoto S., *et al.* Ultrastructural demonstration of apoptosis, Fas and Bcl-2 expression of rheumatoid synovial fibroblasts. *J Rheumatol*, 1996;**23**:1345–52.

155. Dingle J.T., Heberden oration 1978. Recent studies on the control of joint damage: the contribution of the Strangeways Research Laboratory. *Ann Rheum Dis*, 1979;**38**:201–14.

156. Steinberg J., *et al.* A tissue-culture model of cartilage breakdown in rheumatoid arthritis. Quantitative aspects of proteoglycan release. *Biochem J*, 1979;**180**:403–12.

157. Harris E.D., DiBona Jr., D.R., Krane S.M., A mechanism for cartilage destruction in rheumatoid arthritis. *Trans Assoc Am Physicians*, 1970;**83**:267.

158. Kingsley-Mills W.M., Pathology of the knee joint in rheumatoid arthritis. *J Bone Joint Surg*, 1970;**52**:746.

159. Saxne T., Heinegard D., Synovial fluid analysis of two groups of proteoglycan epitopes distinguishes early and late cartilage lesions. *Arthritis Rheum*, 1992;**35**:385–90.

160. Mudgett J.S., *et al.* Susceptibility of stromelysin 1-deficient mice to collagen-induced arthritis and cartilage destruction *Arthritis Rheum*, 1998;**41**:110–21.

161. Muller-Ladner U., *et al.* Synovial fibroblasts of patients with rheumatoid arthritis attach to and invade normal human cartilage when engrafted into SCID mice. *Am J Pathol*, 1996;**149**:1607–15.

162. Geiler T., *et al.* A new model for rheumatoid arthritis generated by engraftment of rheumatoid synovial tissue and normal human cartilage into SCID mice. *Arthritis Rheum*, 1994;**37**:1664–71.

163. Shiozawa S., *et al.* Destructive arthritis without lymphocyte infiltration in H2-c-fos transgenic mice. *J Immunol*, 1992;**148**:3100–4.

164. Scott B.B., *et al*. Rheumatoid arthritis synovial fibroblast and U937 macrophage/monocyte cell line interaction in cartilage degradation. *Arthritis Rheum*, 1997;40:490–8.

165. Velculescu V.E., *et al*. Serial analysis of gene expression. *Science*, 1995;270:484–7.

166. Heller R.A., *et al*. Discovery and analysis of inflammatory disease-related genes using cDNA microarrays. *Proc Natl Acad Sci U S A*, 1997;94:2150–5.

167. Dayer J.M., *et al*. Participation of monocyte-macrophages and lymphocytes in the production of a factor that stimulates collagenase and postaglandin release by rheumatoid synovial cells. *J Clin Invest*, 1979;64:1386–92.

168. Koch A.E., Polverini P.J., Leibovich S.J.. Stimulation of neovascularization by human rheumatoid synovial tissue macrophages. *Artritis Rheum*, 1986;29:471–9.

169. Lorentzen J.C., *et al*. Identification of rat susceptibility loci for adjuvant-oil-induced arthritis. *Proc Natl Acad Sci USA*, 1998;95:6383–7.

170. Kawahito Y., *et al*. Localization of quantitative trait loci regulating adjuvant induced arthritis in rats: evidence for genetic factors common to multiple autoimmune diseases. *J Immunol*, 1998;161:4411–9.

171. Remmers E.F., *et al*. A genome scan localizes five non-MHC loci controlling collagen-induced arthritis in rats. *Nat Genet*, 1996;14:82–5.

172. Cornelis F., *et al*. New susceptibility locus for rheumatoid arthritis suggested by a genome-wide linkage study. *Proc Natl Acad Sci USA*, 1998;95:10746–50.

173. Zuaifler N.J., *et al*. Mesenchymal stem cells, stromal derived factor-1 and rheumatoid arthritis. *Arthritis Rheum*, 1999; 62(Supple):S250.

10 | *Adhesion, migration, and cell trafficking*

Costantino Pitzalis

Introduction

Adhesion mechanisms play a major role in the generation of the synovitis typical of many chronic arthropathies, including rheumatoid arthritis (RA)[1]. RA synovitis is characterized by new blood vessel formation, hyperplasia of the lining layer, and an inflammatory constituted mainly by mononuclear cell (MNC) consisting of strongly HLA-DR positive antigen presenting cells (APC) in close contact with T lymphocytes, the majority of which express the helper/memory phenotype (CD4+CD45R0+)[2–5]. The inflammatory infiltrate is generated by a series of events that include the recruitment of immune/inflammatory cells from the blood stream into the tissues, their activation to effector cells, and their local retention through interactions with extracellular matrix components (ECM) and resident cells. Adhesion mechanisms are involved in all these phases: first, they mediate the interaction of leukocytes with vascular endothelial cells (EC) during the process of extravasation from the circulation; second, they aid cell contact and deliver costimulatory signals during antigen (Ag) presentation and cell activation; and, third, they allow leukocyte adhesion to extracellular matrix components for local retention[1,6]. Several excellent articles have been published in the field of adhesion and migration[7–11]. This chapter, therefore, will only briefly review the general mechanisms and concentrate on the 'specific' mechanisms involved in the regulation of leukocyte traffic to the joint.

Molecular and signaling events regulating 'general' leukocyte migration

To extravasate from the circulation into the tissues, leukocytes must first recognize and adhere to the vascular endothelium. The first problem that they face to achieve this is how to overcome the shear forces associated with blood flow. In addition, once they have adhered to the endothelium, leukocytes still must penetrate the vessel wall before they can transmigrate into the tissues. Understanding of these processes has grown considerably in the last few years mainly because of studies performed under conditions of flow *in vitro* and *in vivo*[12–15]. These studies illustrated that, in postcapillary venules, some of the flowing leukocytes briefly contact the vascular endothelial cells (EC), slow down, and start rolling along the vessel wall. Some of these cells then disengage and resume physiological flow, while others come to a complete halt. This is followed by a shape change, acquisition of a spread morphology, and, within a few minutes, active migration between EC (diapedesis)[7,10,16]. The molecular processes underlying these observations have been schematically divided into four sequentially co-ordinated phases mediated by a series of cell adhesion molecules (CAM) acting in combination—'multistep model'[7,16]. In the first step (primary adhesion) leukocytes are tethered to the vascular endothelium by means of selectin molecules that bind to their oligosaccharide ligands (Table 10.1)[12,17–19]. This interaction is activation independent

Table 10.1 Selectins and their receptor/ligand molecules in leukocyte–endothelial interactions

Endothelial distribution	Endothelial receptor/ligand	Leukocyte receptor/ligand	Leukocyte distribution
HEV, activated endothelium	GlyCAM-1 CD34	L-selectin/CD62L	Lymphocyte subset Monocyte Neutrophil Eosinophil
Endothelial Weibel–Palate granules Platelet α granule	P-selectin/CD62P	PSGL-1 Sialyl Lewis[x/a]	Neutrophil Monocyte Lymphocyte subset NK
Activated endothelium	E-selectin CD62E	Sialyl Lewis [x/a]	Neutrophil Monocyte, Eosinophil Basophil Lymphocyte subset NK

and, although not very strong, is sufficient to facilitate multiple transient contacts that provide the basis for the phenomenon of rolling. This allows leukocytes to sample the local microenvironment for the potential presence of inflammatory mediators which, if present, will trigger the subsequent steps. If not, the transient nature of selectin binding permits leukocytes to detach and carry on with the flow.

The arrest of leukocytes onto the endothelial surface (secondary adhesion) is mediated by leukocyte integrins, particularly β1 (VLA-4) and β2 (LFA-1 and MAC-1) and their respective endothelial ligands, VCAM-1, ICAM-1, and ICAM-2, that belong to the immunoglobulin super-family (Table 10.2)[20–23]. However, in order to prevent random adhesion in the circulation, integrins are normally expressed in a low-avidity, nonfunctional state requiring an activation step to increase their binding capacity. Therefore, a second triggering/activation step necessarily precedes firm adhesion. Several factors have been described as having triggering/activating properties, including bacterial wall components and complement products. The most important molecules, however, appear to be a family of chemoattractant cytokines (chemokines, CK) of which more than 40 members have been described (Table 10.3)[24,25]. CK mediate their effects by binding specific receptors (CK-R) characterized by a seven-trans-membrane domain structure that signals through heterotrimeric GTP-binding proteins[26–28]. Engagement of CK-R results in activation of phospholipases with downstream formation of inositol triphosphate and intracellular Ca^{2+} mobilization, and of small GTP binding proteins such as the Ras, Rac, and Rho families[29,30].

The third step is mediated by the formation of strong bonds between activated integrins and their endothelial counter-receptors, enabling leukocytes to stop and begin the process of transendothelial migration. The fourth and final step (diapedesis) involves the passage of leukocytes between EC and through the basal membrane. Cell locomotion starts with a directional protrusion of the leading edge, presumably via actin polymerization, to form a lamellipodium, attachment to the substratum, and subsequent forward retraction of the rear of the cell. Although understanding of this process is limited, activated integrins probably play an important role as they appear to connect the external substratum with the cytoskeleton[7,22]. This view is supported by the fact that the integrin cytoplasmic domain, at least *in vitro*, associates with structural proteins present in focal adhesions such as talin and α-actinin[31,32].

Table 10.2   Integrins and their receptor/ligand molecules in leukocyte–endothelial interactions

Subunit	Alternative name	Distribution	Ligand
β_2 *integrins*			
αMβ2	LFA-1, CD11a, CD18	B and T lymphocytes, monocyte, neutrophil	ICAM-1, ICAM-2, ICAM-3
αLβ2	Mac-1, CR3, CD11b/CD18	Monocyte, neutrophil, NK cell	ICAM-1, iC3b, fibrinogen factor X
αXβ2	p150, 95, CD11c/CD18	Monocyte, neutrophil, NK cell	iC3b, fibrinogen
α4 *integrins*			
α4β1	VLA-4, CD49d/CD29	B and T lymphocytes, monoyte, neural crest-derived cells, fibroblast, muscle	VCAM-1, fibronectin
α4β7	LPAM-1, CD49d	B and T lymphocytes subpopulation	MAdCAM-1, VCAM-1 fibronectin

Table 10.3   Chemokines (CK) and chemokine-receptors (CK-R)

Inflammatory CK	Cognate inflammatory CK-R	Constitutive CK	Cognate constitutive CK-R
MIP-1 α	CCR1, CCR5	MDC, TARC	CCR4
MIP-1 β	CCR5	ELC, SLC	CCR7
RANTES	CCR1, CCR3, CCR5	SDF-1α, -1β	CXCR4
MCP-1	CCR2	BCA-1	CXCR5
MCP-2, -3	CCR1, CCR2, CCR3		
MCP-4	CCR2, CCR3		
Eotaxin, Eotaxin-2	CCR3		
LARC	CCR6		
IL-8, GCP-2	CXCR1, CXCR2		
GRO, ENA78, NAP-2	CXCR2		
IP-10, Mig, I-TAC	CXCR3		

Abbreviations: BCA-1, B-cell attracting chemokine 1; DC, dendritic cell; ELC, EBI1 ligand chemokine; DNA78, epithelial-cell-derived neutrophil attractant 78; GCP-2, granulocyte chemotactic protein 2; GRO, growth-related oncogene; IL-8, interleukin 8; IP-10, interferon-inducible protein 10; I-TAC, interferon-inducible T cell alpha chemoattractant; LARC, liver and activation-regulated chemokine; MCP-1, monocyte chemotactic protein 1; MDC, macrophage-derived chemokine; Mig, monokine induced by interferon λ MIP-1α, macrophage inflammation protein 1α; NAP-2, neutrophil-activating peptide 2; SDF-1α, stromal-cell-derived factor 1α SLC, secondary lymphoid tissue chemokine; TARC, thymus and activation-regulated chemokine; Th1, T helper 1 cell.

Furthermore, the integrin receptor complex serves not only as a structural link, but also as a signaling unit since, in addition to the above structural proteins, regulatory proteins such as focal adhesion kinase (FAK), phospholipase Cγ (PLCγ), and phosphoinositide (PI) 3-kinase are also associated with integrins during cell movement[21,33,34].

Although the multistep model of migration remains largely correct, recent studies have highlighted some variations that refine the concepts. For instance it is now clear that the various steps are not rigidly mediated by different adhesion proteins, and the same molecule can be involved in more than one step of the adhesion cascade. Similarly, some adhesion receptors can be equally involved in general as well as organ-specific migration (see below). For instance, $\alpha4$ integrins can regulate both secondary and primary adhesion as indicated by the fact that $\alpha4\beta1$ and $\alpha4\beta7$ integrins can mediate both firm adhesion and tethering/rolling, under conditions of flow, to purified VCAM-1 and MAdCAM1[35,36]. L-selectin, on the other hand, is involved in primary adhesion as well as in näive lymphocyte homing to peripheral lymph nodes (PLN). Likewise, CK are essential molecules both for general migration and specific homing (see below).

In summary, the extravasation process of leukocytes into tissues is a complex phenomenon regulated by multiple adhesion and signaling interactions. These general mechanisms, which apply particularly during acute inflammation (especially to neutrophils) allow the mobilization and concentration of large numbers of inflammatory cells into those tissues affected by various insults. In addition, specific mechanisms must exist to explain the diversity of leukocyte populations found in various tissues in response to different conditions. These latter mechanisms operate particularly in chronic inflammation where there is a preferential recirculation of specific lymphocyte subsets that return to the tissue in which they were originally activated.

Molecular and signaling events regulating 'specific' leukocyte migration

Specific mechanisms regulate the migration of distinct leukocyte populations to permit diversity and specialization in response to different immune/inflammatory conditions such as the stage and type of inflammation and the state of cellular activation/differentiation. In allergic reactions, for example, the prevalent cells that localize in the inflamed tissue are eosinophils, basophils, and Th2 lymphocytes[37,38]. In delayed-type hypersensitivity (DTH) reactions, on the other hand, Th1 lymphocytes predominate[37,38]. The importance of the state of cellular activation/differentiation is illustrated by the dramatic change in the migratory characteristics of lymphocytes following the näive to effector cell transition. Näive/resting (CD45RA+) lymphocytes recirculate mainly through secondary lymphoid organs (peripheral lymph nodes (PLN), Peyer's patches (PP), tonsils, and spleen) in search of various Ag drained from different tissues and displayed by APC in these specialized microenvironments.

Once näive cells differentiate into memory/activated (CD45RO+) lymphocytes, they primarily recirculate to peripheral inflamed tissues where they exert effector functions, although they still maintain the capacity to access lymphoid organs[39]. In addition, further diversity appears to exist between these two major lymphocyte subsets as indicated by the preferential localization of some näive cells to PLN and others to PP[40]. Different subsets of memory/effectors cells have been proposed to preferentially migrate to various inflamed tissues such the skin, the gut, and the joint[39,41]. In addition, Th1 lymphocytes are primarily involved in DTH type responses, while Th2 cells accumulate in allergic reactions[37,38]. The mechanisms involved in controlling this delicate and sophisticated diversity, by the same nature, are complex and not completely understood. However, it is likely that selective leukocyte migration can be regulated by at least three levels working in combination and partially overlapping. The first level relates to the specific interaction of lymphocyte-associated adhesion molecules, called 'homing receptors', with their microvascular endothelial (MVE) tissue-specific counter-receptors, called 'addressins'. The second level, intimately connected to the first, is represented by the selective interaction of CK with their corresponding CK-receptor (CK-R) expressed preferentially by different lymphocyte populations. The third level of regulation takes place in the tissues where it is decided which cells are locally retained and to which specific area immune cells preferentially localize, that is 'microenvironmental homing'.

Selective lymphocyte–MVE adhesive interactions

The engagement of leukocyte receptors with their cognate endothelial ligand represents an essential step for leukocyte extravasation. Although, it has become clear that the molecular control of lymphocyte homing is considerably more complex than implied by the original simple key-and-lock-type model (single homing receptor/addressin pair, single tissue specificity)[42], there is little doubt of the critical importance of specific adhesive interactions in determining preferential tissue localization. Well characterized examples of this are represented by the interaction of L-selectin with GlyCAM molecules[43], which facilitates the migration of näive cells to PLN, and by $\alpha4\beta7$ with MadCAM1[44], which mediates lymphocyte migration to the gut and gut-associated lymphoid tissue (GALT). The crucial functional importance of L-selectin and $\alpha4\beta7$ in mediating specific lymphocyte homing has been confirmed recently by specific gene deletion experiments in mice. As expected, L-selectin knock-out mice have a severe reduction of the size of PLNs[45] while $\beta7$ deficient animals show underdeveloped GALT[46]. Lymphocytes derived from these animals display a decreased capacity to bind to PNL and mucosal HEV respectively. Moreover, in humans, a particular type of non-Hodgkin's lymphoma characterized by multifocal infiltration of the intestinal tract (malignant lymphomatous polyposis) expresses $\alpha4\beta7$, unlike the nodal variety[47]. This suggests that homing receptors are involved not only in normal lymphocyte recirculation but also in determining the pattern of dissemination of malignant cells.

Further support for this hypothesis comes from the fact that, in cutaneous T-cell lymphoma, most lymphocytes infiltrating the skin express the cutaneous lymphocyte Ag (CLA)[48]. CLA is a cell-surface glycosylated protein that contains a CD15 (Lewis[x]) carbohydrate backbone and binds strongly to E-selectin[49]. This has led to the proposal that CLA and E-selectin are the homing receptor/addressin pair specific for the skin[48,50,51]. However, since E-selectin is expressed by many inflamed tissues, including the synovium where CLA[+] cells are virtually absent[52], it is clear that the expression of this moleculae is not sufficient to allow CLA[+] cell extravasation to tissues other than the skin. Nevertheless, since E-selectin is expressed with such high density by dermal MVE, it has been suggested that quantitative as well as the qualitative differences may be important in determining preferential binding and extravasation[8].

Diversity and specificity can be also achieved by post-translational modifications of CAM. For example it has been recently demonstrated that CLA is an inducible glycosylation variant of P-selectin glycoprotein ligand 1 (PSGL-1), a known surface glycoprotein that is expressed constitutively by all peripheral blood T cells[53]. CLA-negative cells bind P- but not E-selectin. In addition, although both Th1 and Th2 lymphocytes express PSGL-1, Th1 but not Th2 lymphocytes express a type of PSGL-1 that binds to P- and E-selectin and allows this subset to migrate to sites of DTH reactions[54,55]. The PSGL-1 form found on Th2 cells does not bind to P- and E-selectin and it is tempting to speculate that it would interact with an as yet unknown ligand preferentially expressed by MVE of tissues involved in allergic reactions.

Finally, it would appear that adhesion receptors contribute to the selective migration of lymphocyte subsets not only by providing adhesive interactions but also by delivering activation signals. For instance, GlyCAM-1 mediates the migration of naïve lymphocytes to PLN, not only because of its preferential expression on PLN-HEV and its interaction with L-selectin, but also because of its capacity to activate specifically CD45RA lymphocytes[56]. The functional integration between adhesion and signaling events will be explored in more detail below.

Preferential migration in response to chemokine signals

Leukocyte migration can be controlled at a second level through activation signals delivered by CK. These are small polypeptides weight molecules (68 to 120 amino acids in size) that share structural similarities, including four conserved cysteine residues which form disulfide bonds in the tertiary structure of the proteins[24,25]. The majority can be incorporated into two large subfamilies: CXC (where X is any amino acid) and CC chemokines, according to whether an intervening residue spaces the first two cysteines in the motif or they remain adjacent. A protein with two instead of four conserved cysteines, lymphotactin[57], and fractalkine, a CK-like molecule characterized by an interposition of three amino acids between the first two cysteines (CX3C)[58], have also been described. CK can be immobilized in a solid phase on the endothelial surface via electrostatic interac-

tions with negatively charged proteoglycans and CD44 molecules or, as in the case of fractalkine, directly via a mucine-like stalk[58–60]. This hypothesis provides a valid model of how, *in vivo*, a high concentration of chemotactic factors is maintained at the luminal surface of blood vessels adjacent to areas of inflammation, preventing them from being washed away by the blood flow. CK are thought to mediate their effects via interactions with seven-membrane-spanning-domain receptors (CK-R), which form a distinct group of structurally related proteins within the superfamily of receptors that signal through heterotrimeric GTP-binding proteins[26–28]. CK-R also have two conserved cysteines (one in the amino-terminal domain and the other in the third extracellular loop) that are assumed to form a disulfide bond critical for the conformation of the ligand-binding pocket. Engagement of CK-R, as discussed above, results in the triggering of various intracellular signaling pathways and leads to surface integrin activation[30].

In addition to the essential role in integrin activation and, therefore, in general migration, CK also play a major role in the regulation of selective leukocyte migration. Although there is a considerable overlap in the capacity of different CK to bind the same CK-R, their 'combinatorial' use and the ability to modulate the expression of different CK and CK-R in response to diverse conditions provides the CK system with the necessary flexibility to determine precisely the migratory pattern of various types of leukocytes. It has been recognized recently that CK can be broadly divided into two categories: inflammatory and constitutive (see Table 10.3). The former category is produced largely in inflamed tissues in response to inflammatory cytokines, the latter is produced physiologically and serves the function of regulating constitutive leukocyte traffic. Likewise, CK-R expression can be distinguished in a similar fashion. Constitutive CK-R are expressed mainly by naïve lymphocytes while inducible CK-R are acquired following activation and differentiation. For example, naïve lymphocytes constitutively express CXCR4, the receptor for stromal cell-derived factor 1 (SDF-1)[61,62] and CCR7 (previously known as EBI1), the receptor for EBI1 ligand chemokine (ELC)[63], as well as an unidentified receptor responsible for the action of dendritic cell chemokine 1 (DC-K1)[64,65]. These CK produced in lymphoid tissues induce rapid arrest of lymphocytes on purified ICAM-1 under condition of flow[66].

Therefore, it highly probable that the interaction of CK with CK-R is instrumental in facilitating the preferential migration of naïve lymphocytes to lymphoid organs where they are exposed to cognate antigens. Mature, antigen-experienced memory cells acquire a new array of cell surface molecule, including adhesion molecules and CK-R. Among these, memory cells display CCR5 and CCR2 which makes them responsive to CK produced in large amounts in inflamed tissues, such as RANTES, monocyte chemoattractant protein 1 (MCP-1), MCP-2 and MCP-3[67]. In addition, in experimental conditions *in vitro* the activation process itself can induce a switch in CK-R expression. For example CXCR3 is preferentially expressed by IL-2 activated T lymphocytes but not resting cells[68]. In turn, expression of CXCR3 is associated with a selective response to interferon γ (IFN-γ) induced CK, such as IFN-γ induced protein 10 (IP-10), monokine induced by IFN-γ (Mig), and IFN-γ inducible T cell alpha chemoattractant (I-TAC)[67,69]. Of course, IFN-γ is one of the major cytokines produced during Th1 type reactions, and CK might also direct the migration of various lymphocyte subsets according to the pattern of immune response. Indeed, CXCR3 is expressed at much higher levels on Th1 than on Th2 cells[69,70]. Accordingly, Th1 cells respond to ten-fold lower concentrations of IP-10 compared with Th2 cells. Two studies have reported that Th1 cells are also characterized by the expression of CCR5[71,72]. However, it has also been reported that CCR5, although expressed by Th1 but not Th2 clones, is equally present in 'recently activated' T cells, independent of their functional polarization[73]. In contrast, Th2 cells preferentially express CCR4[71,73], the receptor for TARC (thymus and activation-regulated chemokine)[74] and CCR3, a receptor for eotaxin, eotaxin 2, RANTES, MCP-2, MCP-3, and MCP-4, originally described on eosinophils and basophils[75,76]. All these cell types are recruited concomitantly to sites of allergic reactions and it is remarkable that the pathophysiologically-relevant leukocytes share the same CK-R and respond to the same CK. In summary, there is an impressive body of evidence to indicate that the CK/CK-R system functionally integrates adhesion mechanisms in directing the selective traffic of different leukocyte subpopulations in response to the different pathophysiological situations.

Preferential localization in diverse areas within tissues

The third level of leukocyte homing regualtion takes place in the extravascular compartment after they have been recruited into the tissues. Here they follow different fates; while neutrophils are terminal cells and die, mononuclear cells may return to the circulation via the lymphatics or may be retained within the tissue where they tend to segregate into specialized microenvironments. The best example of 'microenvironmental homing' is represented by the specific localization of DC, B, and T cells in particular areas of lymphoid tissue. The molecular mechanisms controlling cell locomotion, direction, and retention within tissues are also complex and not completely known. However, there is growing evidence to indicate that chemo- and hapotactic signals are involved. These lead to cell adhesion/de-adhesion to, and migration through extracellular matrix (ECM) constituents such as collagen, proteoglycans, laminin, and fibronectin. In chemotaxis, cells migrate in the direction of the highest concentration of a chemoattractant (typically a soluble molecule). In hapoptaxis, cells move toward the region of highest adhesiveness (increased expression of adhesion ligands).

The recent description that leukocytes can respond sequentially to CK in a multistep navigation mode puts these molecules and their receptors once again at the center of operations[77]. Leukocytes migrate across the endothelium using one receptor/agonist pair, through the interstitium using another pair, and to the target microenvironment using yet another pair. Only cells displaying all three receptors can successfully home to the target region. The same receptors and agonists, displayed in a different pattern and/or in combination with other receptors would provide the necessary diversity and versatility to direct various specific homing pathways. Furthermore, the capacity to down-modulate a receptor in the presence of high concentrations of its agonist (homologous desensitization) and up-regulate a different receptor for another agonist allows cells to change direction and to move in and out of a certain compartment. This is not only important for cell orientation and motility but is instrumental for an efficient immune response. For example immature DC, as well as their immediate monocyte precursors, express various receptors for inflammatory CK, such as CCR1, 2,5, and 6[78-80]. This facilities their migration to inflamed tissues. Once recruited to these sites, DC capture Ag and undergo maturation under the influence of proinflammatory cytokines and bacterial and viral products[81]. The high local concentration of inflammatory CK induces a down-modulation of their cognate CK-R, through a process of homologous desensitization or receptor sequestration, allowing DC to migrate away from this site. This, combined with the maturation process that induces the up-regulation of CK-R for constitutive CK such as CCR4, CCR7, and CXCR4, facilitates the migration of DC into the local lymphatics. CCR7 appears to be important in this process as its cognate ligand, secondary lymphoid tissue chemokine (SLC), is produced by lymphatic endothelial cells[82]. For the lymphatics, DC drain to the regional lymph nodes where their final positioning, within T cell areas, might depend on another CCR7 ligand, ELC, produced by resident mature DC[67].

The regulatory role of CK in controlling näive lymphocyte migration to lymphoid organs has already been described above. Here suffice to say that, once they enter lymph nodes via high endothelial venules (HEV)[83,84], näive cells go easily through the paracortical areas, which are devoid of extracellular matrix[85], where they meet DC. This process is facilitated by CK produced by DC themselves, such as ELC and DC-CK1[64,67]. Similar considerations apply to B cells as suggested by observations in mice lacking BLR-1, a putative CK-R highly expressed by B lymphocytes. Disruption of the BLR-1 gene leads to loss of inguinal lymph nodes and defective formation of primary follicles and germinal centers in the spleen and PP. BLR-1-deficient B cells enter the T-cell areas but fail to migrate into the B-cell areas[86]. The ligand for BLR-1 (now called CXCR5) is a novel CXC chemokine, B-cell attracting chemokine-1 (BCA-1)[86] and its mouse homologue, B lymphocyte chemoattractant (BLC)[87] which is produced in the germinal centers and is selective for B cells. In summary, similar to the events that control cell extravasation from the blood into the tissues, the preferential localization in specific areas within the tissues is regulated by overlapping and combinatorially determined adhesion and activation signals.

Molecular and signaling events regulating leukocyte migration to the joint

Although the idea that specific pathways regulate the recirculation of synovial lymphocytes has been recognized for a number of years, direct proof of the existence of specific receptors or signaling molecules unique to the joint is still lacking. However, there is considerable indirect information to support this concept. Jalkanen and colleagues were among the first to provide indirect evidence for a synovial-specific lymphocyte–endothelial recognition system[88]. Using a lymphocyte *in vitro* binding assay to frozen sections, they demonstrated a differential ability of various lymphoblastoid lines to bind to PLN but not to synovial MVE. Moreover, using the same assay, they estimated that some (although not all) T-cell lines derived from PLN, gut, and synovium preferentially adhere to homotypic tissue sections[89]. Of note, the greatest level of cross-adhesion found in this study was between gut and synovium-derived cells. This, together with the recent report that 62 per cent of synovial lymphocytes express the $\alpha4\beta7$ homing receptor[90] also expressed by gut but not skin lymphocytes[91], revived the hypothesis of a preferential trafficking between the gut and the joint due to the usage of a common pathway of migration. This is thought to be important in the pathogenesis of some inflammatory arthropathies, such as in patients with gastrointestinal infections and inflammatory bowel disease. However, as the ligand for $\alpha4\beta7$, MAdCAM-1, is not expressed by synovial MVE, mucosal lymphocytes could be either binding to another as yet unknown receptor, or interacting through the $\alpha4$ chain with FN peptides (e.g., CS1) detected on the luminal surface of synovial MVE[92]. In addition, small intestinal lymphocytes have been shown to bind strongly to vascular adhesion protein-1 (VAP-1) a novel molecule expressed, among other tissues, by inflamed synovial MVE[93,94].

Further indirect evidence for the existence of migration pathways specific for the joint comes from studies in psoriatic arthritis (PSA)[52]. T cells infiltrating the skin express the cutaneous lymphocyte antigen (CLA) while those found in the joint from the same patients do not. This suggests that lymphocyte localization to two different inflamed tissues within the same individual is not a process simply driven by inflammation, but specific mechanisms allow for the preferential localization of different lymphocytes subsets in the two compartments. Furthermore, using a model of cell migration into epidermal blisters raised over DTH reactions, the skin localization of CLA+ lymphocytes related to active increased migration of such T cells rather than to the local acquisition of the CLA molecule[52]. However, as mentioned above, identification of synovial-specific homing receptors and addressin ligands remains unresolved.

The search for the specific addressers has been hampered by the difficult culturing tissue-specific MVE endothelium *in vitro*. It is know that culture *in vitro* of EC isolated from various tissues leads to dedifferentiation with changes in their original characteristics such as, loss of tight junctions in brain MVE[95]. The recent development of a tissue transplantation model in which human synovium is grafted into severe combined immunodeficient (SCID) mice might facilitate progress in this area. In this model, specific tissue 'factors' and microenvironmental structures, which are thought to be necessary to maintain tissue-specific MVE, are preserved. This is important as synovial MVE, *in vivo*, shows very different characteristic from *in vitro* cultured EC. For instance, in the RA synovium, some of the blood vessels show an HEV-like morphology[96–98]. Interestingly, such specialized vasculature is formed in areas where lymphocytes are organized in aggregates, while in areas where the lymphocyte infiltrate is diffuse the vascular endothelium remains flat[98,99]. This suggests that HEV-like vessels are important in supporting lymphocyte extravasation into the RA synovium, although it is possible that, because of the low flow velocity in this inflamed edematous tissue, migration may also take place in postcapillary venules lined with flat EC. Reciprocally, lymphocyte traffic also appears to be important for the maintenance of the HEV morphology since in lymph nodes HEV convert from a high to a flat endothelia following ligation of the afferent lymphatics[100].

Turning to consideration of the second level of regulation of lymphocyte homing, recently, there has been a great deal of interest in CK production and CK-R expression in the synovium. Large amounts of inflammatory CK are produced by both mononuclear cells[101,102] and synoviocytes[102–104]. In addition, at least part of the synovial fluid chemotactic activity is related to CK[102]. These studies, therefore, suggested that CK might be important in the attraction of specific lymphocyte subsets to joints. Further support for this idea has been provided by the recent report that the majority of synovial T cells express CCR5 and CXCR3 but not CCR3, pointing to specific selective recruitment of memory Th1 but not Th2 lymphocytes[72]. As mentioned before, the CK/CK-R system functionally integrates with adhesion mechanism and the MVE. The importance of the MVE in lymphocyte recruitment to the joint is illustrated by another interesting study that demonstrated the presence of MIP-1α and MIP-1β in RA vessels *in vivo*[105]. In the same study, purified synovial MVE expressed high levels of heparan sulfate proteoglycan which was capable of immobilizing MIP-1α and MIP-1β onto the endothelial surface and increasing T cell-EC binding through GTP-mediated signaling[105]. The functional integration between the CK adhesion molecules and MVE is further illustrated by the notion that EC themselves can produce CK which, in an autocrine fashion, can induce endothelial CAM expression[25,106]. This would place the MVE of various organs in a central position to control entry of specific cells to a given tissue.

Finally, considering the third level of regulation, that is 'microenvironmental homing' RA mononuclear cells can be found either in a diffuse distribution, scattered throughout the synovium, or in large focal aggregates to constitute follicle-like structures similar to those found in lymphoid organs. This long described organization can now be interpreted in the light of current knowledge. Several of the molecules already discussed, such as CK, are likely to be instrumental in providing spatial orientation signals (see above). In addition, cytokines also seem to play a role. For instance, the formation of focal lymphoid aggregates in inflamed tissues appears to be influenced by the local production of TNFα as suggested by the fact that TNFα deficient animals lack proper germinal centers[107]. Transgenic animals over-expressing the human *TNF-*α gene have increased formation of focal lymphoid aggregates and develop a chronic arthritis very similar to RA[108]. On the other hand, the cellular interactions with the ECM and other constituents of the connective tissue must play a major part in the retention of different cell types within the synovium. It is well recognized that, although the synovial fluid is loaded with neutrophils, this cell type is virtually absent in the synovial membrane. This is due to the lack of specific adhesion receptors on neutrophils for important ECM components such as collagen and fibronectin (FN). In contrast mononuclear cells express high levels of these receptors which belong largely to the $\beta1$ integrin subfamily of VLA molecules. Each VLA integrin mediates adhesion to at least one of the three major ECM glycoproteins. In addition, each ligand is recognized by multiple VLA integrins. Lymphocytes adhere to FN mainly via VLA-4 and VLA-5 integrin receptors, which recognize two different binding sites of the FN molecule. VLA-4 binds to the third connecting segment (IIICS) region[109,110], while VLA-5 recognizes the key short peptide sequence, RGDS, within the central cell binding domain[111,112]. The collagen receptors have been identified as VLA-1, VLA-2, and VLA-3. Interestingly VLA-1 and VLA-2 are not present on resting T cells, but are expressed after long term activation *in vitro* and in approximately 60 per cent of RA synovial T cells. The VLA-6 integrin, which was first identified as a laminin receptor on platelets, has recently also been shown to be the laminin receptor on lymphocytes. Therefore, the ECM provides the supporting physical environment in which lymphocytes can come into close contact with other cells such as APC for the initiation of the immune response. Furthermore, ECM proteins have multiple adhesive domains that facilitate a multiplicity of interactions between cells and ECM and provide costimulatory signals for the amplification of the immune/ inflammatory cascade[113-115].

In conclusion, although no specific synovial receptors have been identified yet, it highly likely that selective pathways regulate the localization of a subpopulation of joint-homing immune cells. These would involve a series of integrated adhesion and signaling events acting in combination and including multiple adhesion molecule–ligand and CK/CK-R pairs[7,8,67,116,117]. The identification of joint specific mechanisms may have important therapeutic implications as this would allow the joint to be targeted without the serious risks associated with generalized adhesion blockade[118].

References

1. Pitzalis, C. Role of adhesion mechanisms in the pathogenesis of chronic synovitis. (The Michael Mason Prize Essay 1996). *Br J Rheumatol*, 1996;**35**:1198–215.
2. Koch, A.E. Angiogenesis: implications for rheumatoid arthritis. *Arthritis Rheum*, 1998;**41**:951–62.
3. Firestein, G.S. Invasive fibroblast-like synoviocytes in rheumatoid arthritis. Passive responders or transformed aggressors? [Review] [85 refs]. *Arthrtis Rheum*, 1996;**39**:1781–90.
4. Pitzalis, C., G. Kingsley, J.S. Lanchbury, J. Murphy, and G.S. Panayi. Expression of HLA-DR, DQ and DP antigens and interleukin-2 receptor on synovial fluid T lymphocyte subsets in rheumatoid arthritis: evidence for 'frustrated' activation, *J Rheumatol*, 1987;**14**:662–6.
5. Pitzalis, C., G. Kingsley, J. Murphy, and G. Panayi. Abnormal distribution of the helper-inducer and suppressor-T-lymphocyte subsets in the rheumatoid joint. *Clin Immunol and Immunopath*, 1987;**45**:252–8.
6. Pitzalis, C. Adhesion and migration of inflammatory cells. *Clin Exp Rheumatol* 1993;**11** (Suppl 8):71–6.
7. Springer, T.A. Traffic signals for lymphocyte recirculation and leukocyte emigration: the multistep paradigm.. *Cell*, 1994;**76**:301–7.
8. Butcher, E.C. and L.J. Picker. Lymphocyte homing and homeostasis. *Science*, 1996;**272**:60–6.
9. Haskard, D.O. Cell adhesion molecules in rheumatoid arthritis. *Current Opinion Rheumatol*, 1995;**7**:229–34.
10. Adams, D.H. and S. Shaw. Leukocyte-endothelial interactions and regulation of leukocyte migration. *Lancet*, 1994;**343**:831–6.
11. Salmi, M. and S. Jalkanen. How do lymphocytes know where to go: current concepts and enigmas of lymphocyte homing. *Advan Immunol*, 1997;**64**:139–218.
12. Lawrence, M.B. and T.A. Springer. Leukocytes roll on a selectin at physiologic flow rates: distinction from and prerequisite for adhesion through integrins. *Cell*, 1991;**65**:859–73.
13. von Andrian, U.H., J.D. Chambers, L.M. McEvoy, R.F. Bargatze, K.E. Arfors, and E.C. Butcher. Two-step model of leukocyte-endothelial cell interaction in inflammation: distinct roles for LECAM-1 and the leukocyte beta 2 integrins in vivo. *Proc Nat Acad Sci USA*, 1991;**88**:7538–42.
14. Ley, K. and P. Gaehtgens. Endothelial, not hemodynamic, differences are responsible for preferential leukocyte rolling in rat mesenteric venules. *Circulation Research*, 1991;**69**:1034–5.
15. Ley, K., P. Gaehtgens, C. Fennie, M.S. Singer, L.A. Lasky, and S.D. Rosen. Lectin-like cell adhesion molecule 1 mediates leukocyte rolling in mesentric venules in vivo. *Blood*, 1991;**77**:2553.
16. Butcher, E.C. Leukocyte-endothelial cell recognition: three (or more) steps to specificity and diversity. *Cell*, 1991;**67**:1033.
17. Springer, T.A. and L.A. Lasky. Sticky sugars for selectins. *Nature*, 1991;**349**:196–7.
18. Lasky, L.A.Selectin-carbohydrate interactions and the initiation of the inflammatory response. *Ann Rev Bioch*, 1995;**64**:113–39.
19. Bevilacqua, M.P. and R.M. Nelson. Selectins. *J Clin Invest*, 1993;**91**:379–87.
20. Springer, T.A. Adhesion receptors of the immune system. *Nature*, 1990;**346**:425.
21. Kornberg, L., H.S. Earp, J.T. Parsons, M. Schaller, and R.L. Juliano. Cell adhesion or integrin clustering increases phosphorylation of a focal adhesion-associated tyrosine kinase. *J Biol Chem*, 1992;**267**:23439–42.
22. Hogg, N. and R.C. Landis. Adhesion molecules in cell interactions. [Review]. *Current Opinion Immunol*, 1993;**5**:383–90.
23. Hogg, N., J. Harvey, C. Cabanas, and R.C. Landis. Control of leukocyte integrin activation. *Am Rev Respir Dis*, 1993;**148**:S55–9.
24. Schall, T.J. and K.B. Bacon. Chemokines, leukocyte trafficking, and inflammation. *Current Opinion Immunol* 1994;**6**:865.
25. Baggiolini, M., B. Dewald, and B. Moser. Human chemokines: an update. *Ann Rev Immunol*, 1997;**15**:675–05.
26. Kelvin, D.J., D.F. Michiel, J.A. Johnston, A.R. Lloyd, H. Sprenger, J.J. Oppenheim, and J.M. Wang. Chemokines and serpentines: the molecular biology of chemokine receptors. *J Leukocyte Biol*, 1993;**54**:604–12.
27. Neote, K., D. DiGregorio, J.Y. Mak, R. Horuk, and T.J. Schall. Molecular cloning, functional expression, and signaling characteristics of a C-C chemokine receptor. *Cell*, 1993;**72**:415–25.
28. Premack, B.A. and T.J. Schall. Chemokine receptors: gateways to inflammation and infection. *Nature Med*, 1996;**2**:1174–8.
29. Bargatze, R.F. and E.C. Butcher. Rapid G protein-regulated activation event involved in lymphocyte binding to high endothelial venules. *J Exp Med*, 1993;**178**:367–72.
30. Laudanna, C., J.J. Campbell, and E.C. Butcher. Role of Rho in chemoattractant-activated leukocyte adhesion through integrins. *Science*, 1996271:981–3.
31. Pavalko, F.M., C.A. Otey, K.O. Simon, and K. Burridge. Alpha-actinin: a direct link between actin and integrins. *Bioch Soc Trans*, 1991;**19**:1065–9.

32. Otey, C.A., F.M. Pavalko, and K. Burridge. An interaction between alpha-actinin and the beta 1 integrin subunit in vitro. *J Cell Biol*, 1990;**111**:721–9.

33. Parsons, J.T., M.D. Schaller, J. Hildebrand, T.H. Leu, A. Richardson, and C. Otey. Focal adhesion kinase: structure and signaling. *J Cell Sci* 1994;**18** (suppl.):109–13.

34. Clark, E.A. and J.S. Brugge, Integrins and signal transduction pathways: the road taken. *Science*, 1995;**268**:233–9.

35. Alon, R., P.D. Kassner, M.W. Carr, E.B. Finger, M.E. Hemler, and T.A. Springer. The integrin VLA-4 supports tethering and rolling in flow on VCAM-1. *J Cell Biol*, 1995;**128**:1243–53.

36. Berlin, C., R.F. Bargatze, J.J. Campbell, U.H. von Andrian, M.C. Szabo, S.R. Hasslen., R.D. Nelson, E. L. Berg, S.L. Erlandsen, and E.C. Butcher. Alpha 4 integrins mediate lymphocyte attachment and rolling under physiologic flow. *Cell*, 1995;**80**:413–22.

37. Romagnani, S. Human Th1 and Th2 subsets: 'eppur si muove':. *Eur Cytokine Network*, 1994;**5**:7–12.

38. Romagnani, S. The Th1/Th2 paradigm. *Immunol Today*, 1997;**18**:263–6.

39. Mackay, C.R. Homing of naive, memory and effector lymphocytes. *Current Opinion Immunol*, 1993;**5**:423–7.

40. Abitorabi, M.A., C.R. Mackay, E.H. Jerome, O. Osorio, E.C. Butcher, and D.J. Erle. Differential expression of homing molecules on recirculating lymphocytes from sheep gut, peripheral, and lung lymph. *J Immunol*, 1996;**156**:3111–7.

41. Mackay, C.R., W.L. Marston, L. Dudler, O. Spertini, T.F. Tedder, and W.R. Hein. Tissue-specific migration pathways by phenotypically distinct subpopulations of memory T cells. *Eur J Immunol*, 1992;**22**:887–95.

42. Picker, L.J. Control of lymphocyte homing. *Current Opinion Immunol*, 1994;**6**:394–106.

43. Michie, S.A., P.R. Streeter, P.A. Bolt, E.C. Butcher, and L.J. Picker. The human peripheral lymph node vascular addressin. An inducible endothelial antigen involved in lymphocyte homing. *Am J Pathol*, 1993;**143**:1688–98.

44. Berlin, C., E.L. Berg, M.J. Briskin, D.P. Andrew, P.J. Kilshaw, B. Holzmann, A. Hamann, and E.C. Butcher. Alpha 4 beta 7 integrin mediates lymphocyte binding to the mucosal vascular addressin MAdCAM-1. *Cell*, 1993;**74**:185–95.

45. Arbones, M.L., D.C. Ord, K. Ley, H. Ratech, C. Maynard-Curry, G. Otten, D.J. Capon, and T.F. Tedder. Lymphocyte homing and leukocyte rolling and migration are impaired in L-selectin-deficient mice. *Immunity*, 1994;**1**:247–60.

46. Wagner, N., J. Lohler, E.J. Kunkel, K. Ley, E. Leung, G. Krissansen, K. Rajewsky, and W. Muller. Critical role for beta 7 integrins in formation of the gut-associated lymphoid tissue. *Nature*, 1996;**382**:366–70.

47. Pals, S.T., P. Drillenburg, B. Dragosics, A.I. Lazarovits, and T. Radaszkiewicz. Expression of the mucosal homing receptor alpha 4 beta 7 in malignant lymphomatous polyposis of the intestine. *Gastroenterology*, 1994;**107**:1519–23.

48. Picker, L.J., S.A. Michie, L.S. Rott, and E.C. Butcher. A unique phenotype of skin-associated lymphocytes in humans. Preferential expression of the HECA-452 epitope by benign and malignant T cells at cutaneous sites. *Am J Pathol*, 1990;**136**:1053–68.

49. Koszik, F., D. Strunk, I. Simonitsch, L.J. Picker, G. Stingl, and E. Payer. Expression of monoclonal antibody HECA-452-defined E-selectin ligands on Langerhans cells in normal and diseased skin. *J Invest Dermatol*, 1994;**102**:773–80.

50. Berg, E.L., T. Yoshino, L.S. Rott, M.K. Robinson, R.A. Warnock, T.K. Kishimoto, and E.C. Butcher. The cutaneous lymphocyte antigen is a skin lymphocyte homing receptor for the vascular lectin endothelial cell-leukocyte adhesion molecule 1. *J. Exp Med*, 1991;**174**:1461–6.

51. Picker, L.J. Mechanisms of lymphocyte homing. *Current Opinion Immunol*, 1992;**4**:277–86.

52. Pitzalis, C., A. Cauli, N. Pipitone, C. Smith, J. Barker, A. Marchesoni, G. Yanni, and G. Panayi. Cutaneous lymphocyte antigen-positive T lymphocytes preferentially migrate to the skin but not to the joint in psoriatic arthritis. *Arthritis Rheum*, 1996;**39**:137–45.

53. Fuhlbrigge, R.C., J.D. Kieffer, D. Armerding, and T.S. Kupper. Cutaneous lymphocyte antigen is a specialized form of PSGL-1 expressed on skin-homing T cells. *Nature*, 1997;**389**:978–81.

54. Borges, E., W. Tietz, M. Steegmaier, T. Moll, R. Hallmann, A. Hamann, and D. Vestweber. P-selectin glycoprotein ligand-1 (PSGL-1) on T helper 1 but not on T helper 2 cells binds to P-selectin and supports migration into inflamed skin. *J Exp Med*, 1997;**185**:573–8.

55. Austrup, F., D. Vestweber, E. Borges, M. Lohning, R. Brauer, U. Herz, R. Hallmann, A. Scheffold, A. Radbruch, and A. Hamann. P- and E-selectin mediate recruitment of T-helper-1 but not T-helper-2 cells into inflammed tissues. *Nature*, 1997;**385**:81–3.

56. Hwang, S.T., M.S. Singer, P.A. Giblin, T.A. Yednock, K.B. Bacon, S.I. Simon, and S.D. Rosen. GlyCAM-1, a physiologic ligand for L-selectin, activates beta 2 integrins on naive peripheral lymphocytes. *J Exp Med*, 1996;**184**:1343–8.

57. Kennedy, J., G.S. Kelner, S. Kleyensteuber, T.J. Schall, M.C. Weiss, H. Yssel, P.V. Schneider, B.G. Cocks, K.B. Bacon, and A. Zlotnik. Molecular cloning and functional characterization of human lymphotactin. *J Immunol*, 1995;**155**:203–9.

58. Bazan, J.F., K.B. Bacon, G. Hardiman, W. Wang, K. Soo, D. Rossi, D.R. Greaves, A. Zlotnik, and T.J. Schall. A new class of membrane-bound chemokine with a CX3C motif. *Nature*, 1997;**385**:640–4.

59. Tanaka, Y., D.H. Adams, and S. Shaw. Proteoglycans on endothelial cells present adhesion-inducing cytokines to leukocytes. *Immunol Today*, 1993;**14**:111–5.

60. Tanaka, Y., D.H. Adams, S. Hubscher, H. Hirano, U. Siebenlist, and S. Shaw. T-cell adhesion induced by proteoglycan-immobilized cytokine MIP-1 beta. *Nature* 1993;**361**:79–5.

61. Oberlin, E., A. Amara, F. Bachelerie, C. Bessia, J.L. Virelizier, F. Arenzana-Seisdedos, O. Schwartz, J.M. Heard, I. Clark-Lewis, D.F. Legler, M. Loetscher, M. Baggiolini, and B. Moser. The CXC chemokine SDF-1 is the ligand for LESTR/fusin and prevents infection by T-cell-line-adapted HIV-1. *Nature* 1996;**382**:833–5.

62. Bleul, C.C., R.C. Fuhlbrigge, J.M. Casasnovas, A. Aiuti, and T.A. Springer. A highly efficacious lymphocyte chemoattractant, stromal cell-derived factor 1 (SDF-1). *J Exp Med*, 1996;**184**:1101–9.

63. Yoshida, R., T. Imai, K. Hieshima, J. Kusuda, M. Baba, M. Kitaura, M. Nishimura, M. Kakizaki, H. Nomiyama, and O. Yoshie. Molecular cloning of a novel human CC chemokine EBI1-ligand chemokine that is a specific functional ligand for EBI1, CCR7, *J Biol Chem*, 1997;**272**:13803–9.

64. Adema, G.J., F. Hartgers, R. Verstraten, E. de Vries G. Marland, S. Menon, J. Foster, Y. Xu, P. Nooyen, T. McClanahan, K.B. Bacon, and C.G. Figdor, and CG. A dendritic-cell-derived C-C chemokine that preferentially attracts naive T cells. *Nature*, 1997;**387**:713–7.

65. Hieshima, K., T. Imai, M. Baba, K. Shoudai, K. Ishizuka, T. Nakagawa, J. Tsuruta, M. Takeya, Y. Sakaki, K. Takatsuki, R. Miura, G. Opdenakker, J. Van Damme, O. Yoshie, and H. Nomiyama. A novel human CC chemokine PARC that is most homologous to macrophage-inflammatory protein-1 alpha/LD78 alpha and chemotactic for T lymphocytes, but not for monocytes. *J Immunol*, 1997;**159**:1140–9.

66. Campbell, J.J., J. Hedrick, A. Zlotnick, M.A. Siani, D.A. Thompson, and E.C. Butcher. Chemokines and the arrest of lymphocytes rolling under flow conditions. *Science*, 1998;**279**: 381–4.

67. Sallusto, F., A. Lanzavecchia, and C.R. Mackay. Chemokines and chemokine receptors in T-cell priming and Th1/Th2-mediated responses. *Immunol Today*, 1998;**19**:568–74.

68. Loetscher, M., B. Gerber, P. Loetscher, S.A. Jones, L. Piali, I. Clark-Lewis, M. Baggiolini, and B. Moser. Chemokine receptor specific for IP10 and mig: structure, function, and expression in activated T-lymphocytes. *J Exp Med*, 1996;**184**:963–9.

69. Farber, J.M. Mig and IP-10: CXC chemokines that target lymphocytes. *J Leukocyte Biol*, 1997;**61**:246–57.

70. Cole, K.E., C.A. Strick, T.J. Paradis, K.T. Ogborne, M. Loetscher, R.P. Gladue, W. Lin, J.G. Boyd, B. Moser, D.E. Wood, B.G. Sahagan, and K. Neote. Interferon-inducible T cell alpha chemoattractant (I-TAC): a novel non-ELR CXC chemokine with potent activity on activated T cells through selective high affinity binding to CXCR3. *J Exp Med*, 1998;**187**:2009–21.

71. Bonecchi, R., G. Bianchi, P.P. Bordignon, D. D'Ambrosio, R. Lang, A. Borsatti, S. Sozzani, P. Allavena, P.A. Gray, A. Mantovani, and F. Sinigaglia. Differential expression of chemokine receptors and chemotactic responsiveness of type 1 T helper cells (Th1s) and Th2s. *J Exp Med*, 1998;**187**:129–34.

72. Loetscher, P., M. Uguccioni, L. Bordoli, M. Baggiolini, B. Moser, C. Chizzolini, and J.M. Dayer. CCR5 is characteristic of Th1 lymphocytes [letter]. *Nature*, 1998;**391**:344–5.

73. Sallusto, F., D. Lenig, C.R. Mackay, and A. Lanzavecchia. Flexible programs of chemokine receptor expression on human polarized T helper 1 and 2 lymphocytes. *J Exp Med*, 1998;**187**:875–83.

74. Imai, T., M. Baba, M. Nishimura, M. Kakizaki, S. Takagi, and O. Yoshie. The T cell-directed CC chemokine TARC is a highly specific biological ligand for CC chemokine receptor 4. *J Biol Chem*, 1997;**272**:15036–42.

75. Ponath, P.D., S. Qin, T.W. Post, J. Wang, L. Wu, N.P. Gerard, W. Newman, C. Gerard, and C.R. Mackay. Molecular cloning and characterization of a human eotaxin receptor expressed selectively on eosinophils. *J Exp Med*, 1996;**183**: 2437–48.

76. Uguccioni, M., C.R. Mackay, B. Oshensberger, P. Loetscher, S. Rhis, G.J. LaRosa, P. Rao, P.D. Ponath, M. Baggiolini, and C.A. Dahinden. High expression of the chemokine receptor CCR3 in human blood basophils. Role in activation by eotaxin, MCP-4, and other chemokines. *J Clin Invest*, 1997;**100**:1137–43.

77. Foxman, E.F., J.J. Campbell, and E.C. Butcher. Multistep navigation and the combinatorial control of leukocyte chemotaxis. *J Cell Biol*, 1997;**139**:1349–60.

78. Sozzani, S., F. Sallusto, W. Luini, D. Zhou, L. Piemonti, P. Allavena, J. Van Damme, S. Valitutti, A. Lanzavecchia, and A. Mantovani. Migration of dendritic cells in response to formyl peptides, C5a, and a distinct set of chemokines. *J Immunol*, 1995;**155**:3292–5.

79. Delgado, E., V. Finkel, M. Baggiolini, C.R. Mackay, R.M. Steinmann, and A. Granelli-Piperno. Mature dendritic cells respond to SDF-1, but not to several beta-chemokines. *Immunobiol*, 1998;**198**:490–500.

80. Sallusto, F., P. Schaerli, P. Loetscher, C. Schaniel, D. Lenig, C.R. Mackay, S. Qin, and A. Lanzavecchia. Rapid and coordinated switch in chemokine receptor expression during dendritic cell maturation. *Eur J Immunol*, 1998;**28**:2760–9.

81. Cella, M., F. Sallusto, and A. Lanzavecchia. Origin, maturation and antigen presenting function of dendritic cells. *Current Opinion Immunol*, 1997;**9**:10–6.

82. Gunn, M.D., K. Tangemann, C. Tam, J.G. Cyster, S.D. Rosen, and L.T. Williams. A chemokine expressed in lymphoid high endothelial venules promotes the adhesion and chemotaxis of naive T lymphocytes. *Proc Nat Acad Sci USA*, 1998;**95**:258–63.

83. Marchesi, V.T. and J.L. Gowans. The migration of lymphocytes through the endothelium of venules in lymph nodes. *Proc R Soc Lond Biol Sci*, 1964;**159**:283.

84. Anderson, A.O. and N.D. Anderson. Lymphocyte emigration from high endothelial venules in rat lymph nodes. *Immunology*, 1976;**31**:731–48.

85. Gretz, J.E., A.O. Anderson, and S. Shaw. Cords, channels, corridors and conduits: critical architectural elements facilitating cell interactions in the lymph node cortex. *Immunology Rev*, 1997;**156**:11.

86. Legler, D.F., M. Loetscher, R.S. Roos, I. Clark-Lewis, M. Baggiolini, and B. Moser. B cell-attracting chemokine 1, a human CXC chemokine expressed in lymphoid tissues, selectively attracts B lymphocytes via BLR1/CXCR5. *J Exp Med*, 1998;**187**:655–60.

87. Forster, R., A.E. Mattis, E. Kremmer, E. Wolf, G. Brem, and M. Lipp. A putative chemokine receptor, BLR1, directs B cell migration to defined lymphoid organs and specific anatomic compartments of the spleen. *Cell*, 1996;**87**:1037–47.

88. Jalkanen, S., A.C. Steere, R.I. Fox, and E.C. Butcher. A distinct endothelial cell recognition system that controls lymphocyte traffic into inflamed synovium. *Science*, 1986;**233**:556–8.

89. Salmi, M., K. Granfors, M. Leirisalo-Repo, M. Hamalainen, R. MacDermott, T. Havia, and S. Jalkanen. Selective endothelial binding of interleukin-2-dependent human T-cell lines derived from different tissues. *Proc Nat Acad Sci USA*, 1992;**89**:11436–40.

90. Lazarovits, A.I. and J. Karsh. Differential expression in rheumatoid synovium and synovial fluid of alpha 4 beta 7 integrin. A novel receptor for fibronectin and vascular cell adhesion molecule-1. *J Immunol*, 1993;**151**:6482–9.

91. Picker, L.J., R.J. Martin, A. Trumble, L.S. Newman, P.A. Collins, P.R. Bergstresser, and D.Y. Leung. Differential expression of lymphocyte homing receptors by human memory/effector T cells in pulmonary versus cutaneous immune effector sites. *Eur J Immunol*, 1994;**24**:1269–77.

92. Elices, M.J., V. Tsai, D. Strahl, A.S. Goel, V. Tollefson, T. Arrhenius, F.C. Gaeta, J.D. Fikes, and G.S. Firestein. Expression and functional significance of alternatively spliced CS1 fibronectin in rheumatoid arthritis micorvasculature. *J Clin Invest*, 1994;**93**:405–16.

93. Salmi, M., P. Rajala, and S. Jalkanen. Homing of mucosal leukocytes to joints. Distinct endothelial ligands in synovium mediate leukocyte-subtype specific adhesion. *J Clin Invest*, 1997;**99**:2165–72.

94. Jalkanen, S. and M. Salmi. 1993. Vascular adhesion protein-1 (VAP-1)—a new adhesion molecule recruiting lymphocytes to sites of inflammation. *Research Immunol*, **144**:746–9.

95. Girard, J. and T.A. Springer. High endothelial venules (HEVs): specialized endothelium for lymphocyte migration. *Immunol Today*, 1995;**16**:449–57.

96. Freemonth, A.J., C.J. Jones, M. Bromley, and P. Andrews. Changes in vascular endothelium related to lymphocyte collections in diseased synovia. *Arthritis Rheum*, 1983;**26**:1427–33.

97. Freemont, A.J. Functional and biosynthetic changes in endothelial cells of vessels in chronically inflamed tissues: evidence for endothelial control of lymphocyte entry into diseased tissues. *J Pathol*, 1988;**155**:225–30.

98. Yanni, G., A. Whelan, C. Feighery, O. Fitzgerald, and B. Bresnihan. Morphometric analysis of synovial membrane blood vessels in rheumatoid arthritis: associations with the immunohistologic features, synovial fluid cytokine levels and the clinical course. *J Rheum*, 1993;**20**:634–8.

99. van Dinther-Janssen, A.C., S.T. Pals, R. Scheper, F. Breedveld, and C.J. Meijer. Dendritic cells and high endothelial venules in the rheumatoid synovial membrane. *J. Rheum*, 1990;**17**:11–7.

100. Mebius, R.E., P.R. Streeter, J. Breve, A.M. Duijvestijn, and G. Kraal. The influence of afferent lymphatic vessel interruption on vascular addressin expression. *J Cell Biol*, 1991;**115**:85–95.

101. Robinson, E., E.C. Keystone, T.J. Schall, N. Gillett, and E.N. Fish. Chemokine expression in rheumatoid arthritis (RA): evidence of RANTES and macrophage inflammatory protein (MIP)-1 beta production by synovial T cells. *Clin Exp Immunol*, 1995;**101**:398–407.

102. Koch, A.E., S.L. Kunkel, L.A. Harlow, D.D. Mazarakis, G.K. Haines, M.D. Burdick, R.M. Pope, and R.M. Strieter. Macrophage inflammatory protein-1 alpha. A novel chemotactic cytokine for macrophage in rheumatoid arthritis. *J Clin Invest*, 1994;**93**:921–8.

103. Rathanaswami, P., M. Hachicha, M. Sadick, T.J. Schall, and S.R. McColl. Expression of the cytokine RANTES in human rheumatoid synovial fibroblasts. Differential regulation of RANTES and interleukin-8 genes by inflammatory cytokines. *J Biol Chem*, 1993;**268**:5834–9.

104. Hachicha, M., P. Rathanaswami, T.J. Schall, and S.R. McColl. Production of monocyte chemotactic protein-1 in human type B

synoviocytes. Synergistic effect of tumor necrosis factor alpha and interferon-gamma. *Arthrtis Rheum*, 1993;**36**:26–34.

105. Tanaka, Y., K. Fujii, S. Hubscher, M. Aso, A. Takazawa, K. Saito, T. Ota and S. Eto. Heparan sulfate proteoglycan on endothelium efficiently induces integrin-mediated T cell adhesion by immobilizing chemokines in patients with rheumatoid synovitis. *Arthrtis Rheum*, 1998;**41**:1365–77.

106. Goebeler, M., T. Yoshimura, A. Toksoy, U. Ritter, E.B. Brocker, and R. Gillitzer. The chemokine repertoire of human dermal microvascular endothelial cells and its regulation by inflammatory cytokines. *J Invest Dermatol*, 1997;**108**:445–51.

107. Pasparakis, M., L. Alexopoulou, V. Episkopou, and G. Kollias. Immune and inflammatory responses in TNF alpha-deficient mice: a critical requirement for TNF alpha in the formation of primary B cell follicles, follicular dendritic cell networks and germinal centers, and in the maturation of the humoral immune response. *J Exp Med*, 1996;**184**:1397–11.

108. Keffer, J., L. Probert, H. Cazlaris, S. Goergopoulos, E. Kaslaris, D. Kioussis, and G. Koolias. Transgenic mice expressing human tumour necrosis factor: a predictive genetic model of arthritis. *EMBO J*, 1991;**10**:4025–31.

109. Mould, A.P., L.A. Wheldon, A. Komoriya, E.A. Wayner, K.M. Yamada, and M.J. Humphries. Affinity chromatographic isolation of the melanoma adhesion receptor for the IIICS region of fibronectin and its identification as the integrin alpha 4 beta 1. *J Biol Chem*, 1990;**265**:4020–4.

110. Wayner, E.A., A. Garcia-Pardo, M.J. Humphries, J.A. McDonald, and W.G. Carter. Identification and characterization of the T lymphocyte adhesion receptor for an alternative cell attachment domain (CS-1) in plasma fibronectin. *J Cell Biol*, 1989;**109**:1321–30.

111. Ruoslahti, E. and M.D. Pierschbacher. New perspectives in cell adhesion: RGD and integrins. *Science*, 1987;**238**:491–7.

112. Pierschbacher, M.D., E.G. Hayman, and E. Ruoslahti. The cell attachment determinant in fibronectin. *J Cellular Biochem*, 1985;**28**:115–26.

113. Matsuyama, T., A. Yamada, J. Kay, K.M. Yamada, S.K. Akiyama, and S.F. Schlossman. Activation of CD4 cells by fibronectin and anti-CD3 antibody. A synergistic effect mediated by the VLA-5 fibronectin receptor complex. *J Exp Med*, 1989;**170**:1133–48.

114. Shimizu, Y., G.A. van Seventer, K.J. Horgan, and S. Shaw. Costimulation of proliferative responses of resting CD4+ T cells by the interaction of VLA-4 and VLA-5 with fibronectin or VLA-6 with laminin. *J Immunol*, 1990;**145**:59–67.

115. Yamada, A., T. Nikaido, Y. Nojima, S.F. Schlossman, and C. Morimoto. Activation of human CD4 T lymphocytes. Interaction of fibronectin with VLA-5 receptor on CD4 cells induces the AP-1 transcription factor. *J Immunol*, 1991;**146**:53–6.

116. Schall, T.J. and K.B. Bacon. Chemokines, leukocyte trafficking, and inflammation. *Current Opinion Immunol*, 1994;**6**:865–73.

117. Baggiolini, M. Chemokines and leukocyte traffic. *Nature*, 1998;**392**:565–8.

118. Pitzalis, C., G.H. Kingsley, and G.S. Panayi, Adhesion molecules in rheumatoid arthritis: role in the pathogenesis and prospects for therapy. *Ann Rheum Dis*, 1994;**53**:287–8.

11 | *Cytokine networks*

William P. Arend and Cem Gabay

Concept of cytokine networks

Introduction

Cytokines are important mediators of inflammation and tissue destruction in rheumatoid arthritis (reviewed in Refs 1–10). These small molecules of cell–cell communication include interferons, interleukins, growth factors, colony-stimulating factors, chemotactic factors, and others. Cytokines seldom function alone but comprise a network of synergistic, complementary, antagonist, and inhibitory factors where the net biological response in a particular tissue depends upon the balance between the multiple factors present. These molecules may act on the same cell that produced them (autocrine effect) and adjacent cells in a tissue or organ (paracrine effect), or, less commonly, travel through the circulation to other organs (endocrine effect). In recent studies, some cytokines have been noted to remain in the synthesizing cell and influence function without ever being released, exhibiting so-called intracrine effects.

Cytokines are synthesized by a variety of cells in response to multiple stimuli, are usually secreted, and bind to specific receptors on target cells. Stimulatory cytokines, or agonists, then activate specific intracellular signal transduction pathways leading to gene transcription and production of new proteins. Inhibitory cytokine may compete with an agonist for receptor binding or may function by inducing antagonistic intracellular responses. A greater understanding of the presence and role of cytokines in rheumatoid synovitis has led to the development of new therapeutic approaches to this disease.

This chapter will first summarize the classification of cytokines, induction of cytokine production, and general mechanisms of cytokine effects. Subsequent sections will discuss the role and function of specific cytokine at different stages of rheumatoid arthritis including in the initiation phase, in the establishment of chronic synovitis, and in the systemic manifestations of this disease. Lastly will be summarized the self-regulatory nature of the cytokine network, and new therapeutic agents for rheumatoid arthritis that interfere with cytokine production or effects.

Classification of cytokines and receptors

No classification scheme for cytokines is completely adequate as the primary function of a particular factor in rheumatoid synovitis may differ considerably from its originally-described biological activity. One possible classification scheme would be to group cytokines by their interaction with a common receptor or

Table 11.1 Functional classification of cytokines

Family	Members
Hematopoietic	SCF, IL-3, TPO, EPO, GM-CSF, G-CSF, M-CSF
Growth and differentiation	PDGF, EGF, FGF, IGF, TGF-β, VEGF
Immunoregulatory	TGF-β, IFN-γ, IL-2, 4, 5, 7, 9–16, and 18
Proinflammatory	IL-1α and β, TNF-α, LT, IL-6, LIF, IL-17
Anti-inflammatory	IL-1Ra, IL-4, IL-10, IL-13
Chemotactic	IL-8, MIP-1α, MIP-1β, MCP-1, RANTES

Adapted from Refs 6–9.
Abbreviations: EGF, epidermal growth factor; EPO, erythropoietin; FGF, fibroblast growth factor; G-CSF, granulocyte colony stimulating factor; GM-CSF, granulocyte–macrophage colony stimulating factor; IFN, interferon; IGF, insulin-like growth factor; IL, interleukin; IL-1Ra, interleukin-1 receptor antagonist; LIF, leukemia inhibitory factor; LT, lymphotoxin; MCP, monocyte chemoattractant protein; M-CSF, macrophage colony stimulating factor; MIP, macrophage inflammatory protein; PDGF, platelet-derived growth factor; RANTES, regulated upon activation T cell expressed and secreted; SCF, stem cell factor; TGF transforming growth factor; TNF, tumor necrosis factor; TPO, thrombopoietin; VEGF, vascular endothelial growth factor.

family of receptors. However, to understand better the involvement of cytokines in the pathophysiology of rheumatoid arthritis, a more logical approach is to group cytokines around their main function in this disease process. In Table 11.1, cytokines are categorized as hematopoietic, growth and differentiation, immunoregulatory, proinflammatory, anti-inflammatory, and chemotactic factors. To complicate matters, a particular cytokine may exhibit functions under more than one of these categories, as detailed below.

Cytokine receptors can be grouped by structural similarities, with a further division by the use of identical molecules of signal transduction (Table 11.2). The IL-1 receptor family members share an immunoglobulin domain-like structure and the TNF receptor family is characterized by the presence of cysteine-rich regions that are repeated in the extracellular domains. Some common signal transduction molecules include the IL-2Rγ chain, which is used by the receptors for interleukins 2, 4, 7, and 15, the gp130 molecule which is utilized by the receptors for IL-6 and related molecules (IL-11, oncostatin M, ciliary neurotrophic factor, and leukemia inhibitory factor), and the GM-CSFβ chain used by GM-CSF, IL-3, and IL-5[7]. The relative degree of activity of a particular cytokine may be influenced by which target cells express its receptor and by the level of receptor expression. Up-regulation or down-regulation of

Table 11.2 Cytokine receptor families

Family	Members	Features
Interleukin-1	IL-1RI and II	Ig-like domains
Tumor necrosis factor domains	TNFRI and II, and many others	Cysteine-rich
Interferon	IFN-α, β and γRs, IL-10R	Clustered 4 cysteines
Hematopoietin	IL-2R, IL-3R, IL-4R, IL-5R, IL-6R, IL-7R, IL-9R, IL-13R, IL-15R, G-CSFR, GM-CSFR, EPOR, TPOR	W–S–X–W–S motif in C-terminus
Chemokine	IL-8RA and B, MCPR, MIPR	7-transmembrane-spanning regions
Tyrosine kinase	EGFR, PDGFR, FGFR, M-CSFR, SCFR	Tyrosine kinase

Adapted from Ref. 7.

receptor expression may occur in response to other cytokines or to molecules released during inflammatory reactions.

Induction of cytokine production

Cytokine production can be induced by soluble factors or by direct cell–cell contact. Specific receptor binding by the soluble factor, or by membrane-bound cytokines and other molecules on inducing cells, leads to activation of signal transduction pathways in target cells. The major biological effect is stimulation of transcription, although regulation of cytokine production also can occur at other levels. The stimuli for cytokine production include other cytokines themselves, complement split products, bacterial products such as lipopolysaccharides, viral proteins, immune complexes or adherent IgG, fragments of connective tissue proteins, insolubilized crystals, and acute phase proteins[7,8]. Many of these mechanisms may be operative in the rheumatoid synovium, as inducers of particular cytokines *in vivo* may be multiple and may vary with different stages of the disease process.

Many cytokines are found at high levels in rheumatoid synovial fluids, such as TNF-α, GM-CSF, IL-6, IL-10, IL-15 and IL-1Ra. However, the synovial tissue may be a more important source of cytokines involved in pathophysiological processes. The cytokines that have been identified at the mRNA or protein level in rheumatoid synovial tissue are summarized in Table 11.3. The primary cells producing cytokines in the rheumatoid pannus are macrophages and fibroblasts, with smaller numbers of T cells possibly secreting immunoregulatory cytokines. The relative role of T cells and their products in the rheumatoid disease process is discussed in the other chapters in this text. However, the numbers of T cells present in the rheumatoid synovium may vary between patients and throughout the disease. Small numbers of T cells, with their secreted cytokines, may exert potent stimulatory or regulatory influences on immunological and inflammatory events.

Table 11.3 Cytokine expression in rheumatoid synovial tissues

Cytokine	mRNA	Protein	Cells
IL-1α and β	Yes	Yes	monocytes and fibroblasts
IL-1Ra	Yes	Yes	monocytes and fibroblasts
TNF-α	Yes	Yes	monocytes and fibroblasts
IL-6	Yes	Yes	monocytes and fibroblasts
IL-8	Yes	Yes	monocytes and fibroblasts
IL-10	Yes	Yes	monocytes and T cells
IL-12	Yes	Yes	monocytes and dendritic cells
IL-15	Yes	Yes	monocytes and fibroblasts
GM-CSF	Yes	Yes	monocytes and fibroblasts
PDGF	Yes	Yes	monocytes
FGF	Yes	Yes	monocytes and fibroblasts
VEGF	Yes	Yes	monocytes
TGF-β	Yes	Yes	monocytes and fibroblasts
LIF	Yes	Yes	monocytes and fibroblasts
MCP-1	Yes	Yes	monocytes and fibroblasts
MIP-1α	Yes	Yes	monocytes and fibroblasts
RANTES	Yes	Yes	fibroblasts
(IL-2, IL-4, IL-13 and IFN-γ)	Yes	+/−	T cells

Adapted from Refs 5 and 6.

General mechanisms of cytokine effects

After cytokine binding to specific cell membrane receptors, a series of signal transduction pathways are stimulated. These pathways consist of cascades of kinases with resultant activation and nuclear localization of specific transcription factors. The transcription factor families that have been identified as being activated in the rheumatoid synovium include AP-1 (c-*fos* and c-*jun*), NF-κB (p50 and p65), and STAT (signal transducer and activator of transcription). The p50 and p65 subunits of the NF-κB family have been identified in macrophages in both the lining and sublining regions of the rheumatoid synovium, as well as in endothelial cells[11,12]. The NF-κB family of transcription factors appears to be important in the induction of transcription of the genes for the proinflammatory cytokines TNF-α, IL-1, IL-6, and IL-8.

High DNA binding activity of AP-1 was found in the rheumatoid synovium in both synovial fibroblasts and macrophages, correlating with disease activity[13]. The mRNAs for the proto-oncogenes c-*fos* and c-*jun* also were localized to the synovial fibroblasts and correlated with the degree of AP-1 activation[13]. Collagenase production in rheumatoid synovitis may be due, in large part, to proteins of the AP-1 family, and the AP-1 pathway appears to be selectively activated during Fas-mediated apoptosis of rheumatoid synoviocytes[14]. Inhibition of the c-*fos*/AP-1 pathways through the administration of specific oligonucleotides led to a reduction in joint destruction in mice with collagen-induced arthritis[15]. Similar results have also been observed with inhibition of the NF-κB pathway in animal models of inflammatory arthritis, suggesting a possible novel approach to the treatment of human diseases.

A recent advance in the understanding of the cellular response to cytokines has been the identification and characterization of the Jak-STAT signal transduction pathway[5,16]. An early signaling event in response to many cytokines is activation of the receptor-associated protein tyrosine kinases of the Janus kinase (Jak) family. This leads to activation of STAT proteins, latent cytoplasmic transcription factors, which are then translocated to the nucleus with up-regulation of the transcription of specific genes. STAT3 is constitutively produced by freshly-isolate rheumatoid synovial fluid cells and these synovial fluids induced STAT3 expression in resting peripheral blood cells while inhibiting expression of STAT1[17]. This observation may suggest inhibition of Th1 cells with decreased IFNγ production. However, it remains unclear whether an imbalance in the Jak/STAT pathway truly exists in rheumatoid arthritis and whether intervention in this pathway will be a feasible therapeutic approach.

Initiation of rheumatoid synovitis

Early events

Concepts about the mechanisms initiating rheumatoid synovitis have evolved over the past 20 years. The theory prevalent in the 1970s, that immune complexes were responsible for initiating the steps leading to inflammation and tissue destruction, was supported by early observations on the presence of these materials in rheumatoid synovial fluids and tissues[18]. The identification and initial characterization of T cells in the rheumatoid synovium in the 1980s, coupled with the description of the HLA-DR4 association with the disease, led to the concept that T cells were responsible for the initiation of rheumatoid synovitis. The 'shared epitope hypothesis' implied that antigen-specific responses of CD4+ T cells were involved in initiation of the disease process[19]. These stimulated T cells would then activate macrophages and other cells through both direct contact and the release of cytokines, leading to enzyme production and tissue destruction. However, extensive efforts over the past 10 years have failed to identify a common rheumatological antigen or to find evidence for a restricted clonal response on the part of rheumatoid synovial T cells[20].

The T-cell theory of the pathogenesis of RA has recently been modified to suggest that non-antigen-specific mechanisms may initiate a rather indolent disease process[21]. Antigen-specific T-cell responses may then be responsible for leading to an aggressive stage of perpetuation with intense inflammation, rapid tissue destruction, and extra-articular manifestations. This hypothesis states that early and episodic release of TNF-α and GM-CSF from macrophages and synovial fibroblasts may be induced by a variety of non-antigen-specific processes, such as minor trauma, infections, allergic reactions, vaccinations, or local immune complex deposition[21,22]. These cytokines then differentiate resident dendritic cells into potent antigen-presenting cells, which may selectively present self-antigens for induction of specific T-cell responses. The presence of the shared epitope on HLA-DR4 molecules may decrease the threshold for transformation of a mild reactive synovitis into a rapidly-destructive synovial reaction by enhancing the presentation of self-antigens by the dendritic cells.

The purported key role of dendritic cells in the initiation of rheumatoid synovitis, and the presumed importance of TNF-α and GM-CSF in this process, are supported by indirect evidence. Rheumatoid synovial fluids and tissue are enriched in differentiated dendritic cells that abundantly express HLA-DR and DQ molecules[23,24]. Furthermore, dendritic cells stimulated with these cytokines upregulate expression of the B7 family of costimulatory molecules (CD80/CD86), leading to enhanced antigen presentation. CD86 expression was observed on both macrophages and dendritic cells in the rheumatoid synovium, with the latter cells present in both a perivascular distribution and within T-cell clusters[25]. Autocrine or paracrine production of GM-CSF by dendritic cells in the rheumatoid synovium may contribute to the enhanced expression of CD86. Whether these potent antigen-presenting cells are truly involved in the initiation of rheumatoid synovitis, and the nature of the self-antigens involved in the early presentation to T cells, remain to be established. However, these questions are difficult to address as the disease-initiating mechanisms may evolve before RA is clinically apparent.

A possible primary role for TNF-α and GM-CSF in RA was suggested by early studies on rheumatoid synovial fluids and cultured synovial tissue cells. The high levels of IL-1 produced by synovial cell cultures were inhibited by antibodies to TNF-α, suggesting that TNF-α may be a major inducer of IL-1 in these cells[26]. GM-CSF production by cultured rheumatoid synovial tissue cells also was inhibited by antibodies to TNF-α[27]. High levels of TNF-α (summarized in refs 1 and 2) and of GM-CSF[28–31] were present in rheumatoid synovial fluids and tissues. IL-1 and TNF-α both induced GM-CSF production in rheumatoid synovial fibroblasts and macrophages[31]. Lastly, mice transgenic for human TNF-α expression in macrophages spontaneously developed a chronic inflammatory polyarthritis[32]. However, a neutralizing antibody to the murine IL-1R type I completely prevented the development of arthritis in the TNF-α transgenic mice, suggesting that the pathogenic effects of TNF-α were mediated through the induction of IL-1[33]. These and other observations on the presence and role of IL-1 and TNF-α in RA[1,2] have led to the development and clinical evaluation of therapeutic approaches designed to prevent the production or effects of these cytokines, as discussed below.

Role of adhesion molecules and chemokines in induction of acute inflammation

Rheumatoid synovitis may be initiated by multiple antigen-specific or non-specific mechanisms, probably operating during an early, preclinical stage of the disease. However, the earliest clinical manifestations of joint swelling, erythema, and pain are due to common inflammatory mechanisms largely driven by cytokines released from synovial macrophages and fibroblasts. Up-regulation of adhesion molecule expression on endothelial cells in the postcapillary venules, and on leukocytes with recruitment and migration of these cells into the synovium, are the most important events in this stage of acute inflammation in the joint.

The three major categories of adhesion molecules are the selectins, present primarily on leukocytes and endothelial cells, the integrins, found on a variety of blood and tissue cells, and the Ig superfamily, identified on circulating white blood cells, fibroblasts, endothelial, and epithelial cells[36]. IL-1 and TNF-α are the major cytokines responsible for induction of expression of these adhesion molecules on endothelial cells, macrophages, dendritic cells, synovial fibroblasts, lymphocytes, and neutrophils, although IL-8 and GM-CSF also play important roles. The multiple roles for adhesion molecules in the pathophysiology of RA include:

(1) attachment of inflammatory cells in the postcapillary venule to endothelial cells;

(2) migration of these cells across the endothelium into the synovium;

(3) perivascular interactions between the inflammatory and immune cells;

(4) retention of cells in the synovium;

(5) enhancement of antigen presentation;

(6) facilitation of angiogenesis; and

(7) shedding of soluble adhesion molecules into the synovial fluid or serum[36].

Table 11.4 Chemokines found in the synovial fluids of patients with rheumatoid arthritis

Chemokine	Type	Responsive inflammatory cells	Reference
IL-8	CXC	neutrophils, T cells	41–43
ENA-78	CXC	neutrophils	44
GRO-α	CXC	neutrophils	45
MCAF (MCP)	CC	monocytes, T cells	46–49
MIP-1α	CC	neutrophils, monocytes, T cells	50
RANTES	CC	monocytes, T cells	51

Adapted from Ref. 38.
Abbreviations: ENA, epithelial neutrophil-activating peptide; GRO, growth-related gene product; MCAF, monocyte-chemotactic and -activating factor; MCP, monocyte chemoattractant protein; RANTES, regulated upon activation T cell expressed and secreted.

Recognition of the importance of adhesion molecules in rheumatoid synovitis has led to experimental therapeutic approaches designed to block their expression.

Chemokines are chemotactic 8–10 kD proteins that share between 20 and 70 per cent homology[37–40]. Over 40 chemokines have been identified and have been classified into at least four families. The α and β families contain four cysteines and include most of the common chemokines. The α or CXC chemokines possess one amino acid between the first two cysteine residues, whereas the first two cysteine residues are adjacent in the β or CC chemokines[40]. The CXC family can be divided into two subgroups: those factors containing the sequence glutamic acid–leucine–arginine near the N terminus include IL-8 and other factors chemotactic for neutrophils, whereas CXC chemokines without this sequence act on lymphocytes. The CC chemokines also can be divided into two subgroups but all of these factors act to attract monocytes, eosinophils, basophils, and lymphocytes, although with varying selectivity. Chemokines induce cell migration and activation by binding to a complex family of specific G-protein-coupled receptors on target cell[39,40]. Specific chemokine receptors may be responsible for attracting subsets of lymphocytes into the rheumatoid joint.

The chemokines found in the synovial fluids of patients with RA are summarized in Table 11.4[38]. These factors function to induce the infiltration of monocytes, neutrophils, and T-cells into the synovial fluid and tissue, and also are capable of activating these cells to release various secretory products. Chemokines found in the rheumatoid joint are synthesized by both macrophages and synovial fibroblasts. Although these factors are primarily proinflammatory, some chemokines may selectively attract T-cell subsets into the joint, possibly contributing to the initiation or maintenance of a local immune response. IL-8 is perhaps the major chemokine in rheumatoid arthritis and intervention with its production or effects is a potential therapeutic approach to RA and other acute inflammatory diseases[52].

Establishment of chronic synovitis

Cytokine patterns in rheumatoid synovitis

Numerous studies over the past 10 years have characterized the cytokines found in rheumatoid synovial fluids, or produced by peripheral blood mononuclear cells, in an effort to understand better the role of different cytokines in the pathophysiology of joint inflammation and destruction. However, of greater importance is the pattern of cytokines produced by synovial tissue cells since the damage to cartilage, bone, and periarticular structures is mediated primarily by cells in the proliferative synovium and adjacent cartilage. Early studies failed to identify the mRNA for either IL-2 or IL-3 in the rheumatoid synovium, although M-CSF mRNA was abundantly present[53]. A comprehensive survey for the presence of mRNAs for various cytokines in rheumatoid synovium was then carried out using *in situ* hybridization[54]. The most prominent cytokine mRNAs found were the macrophage and fibroblast products IL-6, IL-1β, TNF-α, GM-CSF, and TGF-β, whereas IFN-γ was only weakly present. These observations led to the hypothesis that T cells were less important to chronic rheumatoid synovitis[55], although this interpretation remains controversial[56].

Newer studies using highly sensitive techniques have examined the cytokine profile in relationship to the duration of the synovitis and the type of histological changes present in the rheumatoid synovium. IL-2 and IFN-γ mRNA were detected in many rheumatoid synovia using the polymerase chain reaction (PCR) method, suggesting that this was primarily a Th1 disease[57]. However, the levels of Th1 cytokines in the rheumatoid joint are far lower than in other chronic Th1 diseases, such as tonsilitisor tuberculous pleuritis. A more detailed analysis using quantitative nested PCR examined synovial specimens from patients with early synovitis (<12 months in duration) and found abundant mRNA for IL-10, IL-15, IL-1β, TNF-α and IFN-γ[58]. Lesser amounts of mRNA for IL-6 and IL-12 were present with absent mRNA for IL-4 and IL-13. These results indicated that macrophage-derived and some Th1 cytokine mRNAs predominated in early rheumatoid synovitis, with decreased levels present in the tissue of patients treated with prednisone or disease-modifying drugs. Other studies suggested that Th1 cytokine production predominated in the peripheral blood and synovial fluid cells of patients with recent-onset synovitis whereas a Th2 pattern was present in those with chronic arthritis[59].

Examination of the synovial biopsies from 21 patients with active RA led to a classification into three distinct histological subsets[60]. Synovial specimens exhibiting diffuse lymphoid infiltrates without further microarrangement demonstrated low level transcription of IFN-γ, IL-4, IL-1β and TNF-α, as determined by semiquantitative PCR. In contrast, synovia exhibiting lymphoid follicles with germinal center formation demonstrated IFN-γ and IL-10 mRNA, but not IL-4. lastly, granulomatous synovitis, the least common pattern, was characterized by high transcription of IFN-γ, IL-4, IL-1β, and TNF-α, clearly different from the other histological patterns. Diffuse synovitis was present primarily in-patients with mild seronegative RA, whereas granulomatous synovitis was observed in rheumatoid factor-positive patients with nodules. Thus, diffuse synovitis in this study corresponded with a pattern of Th0 cytokines, follicular synovitis with a Th1 pattern, and granulomatous synovitis with a mixed Th1/Th2 pattern[60].

These observations, which still require confirmation, emphasize a probable heterogeneity in the pathophysiological mechanisms of rheumatoid synovitis, making the general paradigm of

a Th1 predominance being harmful and Th2 helpful poorly applicable. The recognition of different subsets of RA patients, either by clinical criteria or the pattern of synovial histopathology, indicates that the therapeutic effects of cytokines or their inhibitors may vary depending on the stage of disease, and the localization and timing of their administration[61]. Recognizing this heterogeneity, the following sections will summarize the effects of cytokines on different cells and pathological events in chronic rheumatoid synovitis.

Immune cell differentiation

The synovium of patients with RA is populated with CD4+ T cells that express surface characteristics of mature memory cells (CD45RO+). Most synovial T cells carry the α/β receptor complex but some are γ/δ positive. Numerous cytokines potentially influence and modulate the activity of rheumatoid synovial T cells. The major T-cell-activating cytokine IL-2 was present in only a few rheumatoid synovial fluids. High levels of soluble IL-2R were detected in both the serum and synovial fluids of patients with RA, probably secondary to release by T cell[62]. However, soluble IL-2R binds to IL-2 with low affinity and probably does not inhibit IL-2 function *in vivo*. The relative absence of IFN-γ and IL-2 in the rheumatoid synovium make it unlikely that these cytokines are responsible for the influx of circulating T cells.

The recent description and characterization of IL-15 indicate that this cytokine may play a pivotal role in inflammatory events in the rheumatoid synovium (Fig. 11.1)[63]. IL-15 is produced by

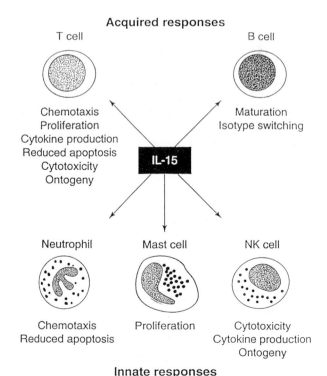

Fig. 11.1 Biological effects of IL-15 with potential relevance to rheumatoid arthritis synovitis. Abbreviation: NK, natural killer. Reproduced with permission from ref. 63.

both macrophages and fibroblasts in the lining layer of the rheumatoid synovium, and in lesser amount by T cells and dendritic cells, and is found in modest concentrations in the synovial fluid[64]. IL-15 exhibits many functional similarities to IL-2, and binds to a receptor that possesses a unique α chain but utilizes the β and γ chains of the IL-2R to transduce signals in target cells. IL-15 was chemotactic for CD45RO+ T cells, and activated these cells in the rheumatoid synovium[64]. Furthermore, IL-15 directly stimulated TNF-α production in synovial T cells, and indirectly led to enhanced TNF-α production by macrophages through direct contact of these cells with IL-15-stimulated T cells[65]. The early activation molecule CD69, as well as the adhesion molecules LFA-1 and ICAM-1, were all involved in the interactions between T cells and macrophages. IL-2 had no effect in this system. IL-15 also functioned as an autocrine regulator of macrophage proinflammatory cytokine production, with enhanced secretion of IL-1, TNF-α, and IL-6 observed at very low concentrations of IL-15[66]. Furthermore, IL-15 was produced by endothelial cells and enhanced the migration of T cells across endothelial cells by activating the binding capacity of LFA-1 and inducing the expression of CD69[67].

It is hypothesized that IL-15 may preferentially activate T cells that have recently encountered exogenous antigens *in vivo*, or that exhibit a suboptimal response to autologous MHC class II molecules[68]. In individuals with susceptible HLA types who develop transient joint inflammation in response to non-specific stimuli, IL-15 may promote the adhesion and activation of memory T cells and macrophages within the synovium. Thus, IL-15 may be important in the transformation of a mild reactive synovitis into an aggressive autoimmune reaction. The mechanisms that stimulate IL-15 production in the rheumatoid synovium are unclear, but mRNA levels for this molecule exceed production of the protein. In fact, IL-15 production is regulated primarily post-transcriptionally at the levels of translation and intracellular protein trafficking[69]. Administration of a soluble IL-15 receptor α chain prevented the development of collagen-induced arthritis in mice, suggesting that IL-15 antagonists may be of value in treating patients with RA[70].

Other T-cell cytokines may play roles in the rheumatoid synovium. The suppressed production of IL-2 and IFN-γ by synovial T cells may be secondary to the abundant presence of IL-10 in the rheumatoid synovial fluid and tissue. In addition, this cytokine exhibits anti-inflammatory effects on synovial macrophages, illustrating the self-regulatory nature of the cytokine network in this disease. Lastly, IL-12 is produced by macrophages and dendritic cells, and promotes a Th1 phenotype by enhancing IFN-γ production by CD4+ T cells and NK cells. However, IL-12 exhibited a dual role in collagen-induced arthritis in mice, stimulating early arthritis expression while suppressing the chronic phase of the disease[71]. Thus, as summarized above, numerous cytokines of T cell origin or acting on T cells are present in the rheumatoid synovium with a resultant heterogenous pattern of effects depending on many factors, including the stage of the disease.

The specific antigens that activate T cells in the rheumatoid synovium, presented in the context of class II MHC, remain unknown but may vary in type and relative importance with the stage of the disease process. In the initiation phase of synovitis, ubiquitous viral and bacterial products, or even the HLA-DR4 shared epitope itself, may be responsible. However, in chronic rheumatoid synovitis T cells may be stimulated by altered self components such as proteoglycan and collagen fragments. Thus, once the disease becomes clinically active, the inducing agents may no longer be present and the T cells are driven by products of tissue destruction. The relative role of T cells versus autonomous macrophage and fibroblast function in the perpetuation of chronic rheumatoid synovitis is discussed briefly below, as well as in other chapters in this text.

Inflammatory cell maturation

Inflammatory cells that are involved in pathophysiological events in rheumatoid synovitis include polymorphonuclear leukocytes (neutrophils), monocytes, and macrophages. Neutrophils predominate in the synovial fluids of patients with chronic RA, and are found in the synovial tissue primarily when necrosis or secondary infection is present. Neutrophils can respond to stimulation by GM-CSF or TNF-α with secretion of small amounts of the proinflammatory cytokines IL-1β, TNF-α, IL-8, and GM-CSF, and of the anti-inflammatory cytokine IL-1Ra. However, the large numbers of neutrophils that may be found in rheumatoid synovial fluids make these cells a potentially important source of IL-8 and IL-1Ra[72].

Monocytes and macrophages in the rheumatoid synovium are derived from bone marrow precursors with a constant renewal through the peripheral blood. These cells do not recirculate but are differentiated and activated in the synovium to assume new phenotypic characteristics. For example, under the influence of GM-CSF, TNF-α, IFN-γ, and IL-4, precursor myeloid cells and monocytes differentiate into potent antigen-presenting dendritic cells[73]. Dendritic cells not only activate lymphocytes, but these cells may also contribute to control of immune responses through tolerizing T cells to self-antigens[74]. The role and function of macrophages in the rheumatoid synovium have been recently reviewed[75]. These cells may play diverse roles in all stages of rheumatoid synovitis from initiation through chronic inflammation and tissue destruction. One of the prime functions of macrophages is phagocytosis and these cells may be important sources of bacterial and viral peptides in the non-specific process of initiation of synovitis discussed above. Macrophages are influenced by the cytokine environment in the rheumatoid synovium in multiple ways.

TGF-β is chemotactic for monocytes and may contribute to the influx of these cells into the inflamed synovium. This cytokine also stimulates macrophage production of IL-1Ra in an autocrine and paracrine fashion through the synthesis and release of IL-1β[76,77]. Monocyte differentiation is enhanced by GM-CSF, leading to increased HLA-DR expression, whereas macrophage activation occurs secondary to IFN-γ. However, given the paucity of IFN-γ in the rheumatoid synovium, it is likely that these cells are activated, at least in part, by direct contact with lymphocytes[78]. In fact, direct contact with Th1 cells preferentially induced IL-β production in human monocytes whereas Th2 cells primarily stimulated IL-1Ra synthesis[79]. The cytokines IL-4, IL-10, and IL-13 all display anti-inflammatory effects through inhibition of IL-1 and TNF-α production in macrophages and enhancement of IL-1Ra.

IL-17 is a recently-characterized Th1 cytokine that may play an important proinflammatory role in the rheumatoid synovium. IL-17 was produced by activated memory CD4+ T cells and induced the production of IL-6, IL-8, and G-CSF by endothelial cells and fibroblasts[80]. Furthermore, IL-1 and IL-17 together exhibited a synergistic effect on IL-6 and LIF production by rheumatoid synovial fibroblasts[81]. The Th2 cytokines IL-4 and IL-13 modestly enhanced the stimulatory effects of IL-1 and IL-17 on synoviocyte production of IL-6, but inhibited that of LIF. Furthermore, IL-17 stimulated the production of IL-1β and TNF-α, as well as that of IL-6, IL-10, IL-12, and IL-1Ra, by human macrophages[82]. Both IL-4 and IL-10 inhibited the IL-17 induction of IL-1β and TNF-α production by these cells. Biologically-active IL-17 was produced by cultured rheumatoid cells[81]. These results establish an important link, through IL-17, between CD4+ T cells in the synovium and induction of production of proinflammatory cytokines by both synovial fibroblasts and macrophages.

One of the major roles of macrophages in the pathophysiology of rheumatoid synovitis is as a source of the proinflammatory cytokines IL-1 and TNF-α[1,2]. Production of these cytokines may be induced in macrophages by multiple agents including direct contact with lymphocytes, lymphocyte products such as IL-17, by IL-1 and TNF-α themselves, immune complexes, bacterial and viral products, and by products of damaged cartilage such as collagen fragments. IL-1 and TNF-α are thought to be key molecules in the mechanisms of tissue destruction through the induction of neutral metalloproteinase synthesis and secretion by transformed fibroblasts in the synovium and chondrocytes in the adjacent articular cartilage. Macrophages at the pannus–cartilage interface are also an important source of these tissue-damaging enzymes[75]. In addition, synovial macrophages are the major source of PDGF and FGF, which have stimulatory effects on fibroblasts, and of GM-CSF and chemokines. Many of the current disease-modifying drugs may be effective in RA in large part because of their inhibitory effects on macrophage function[75].

Fibroblast proliferation and activation

Fibroblast-like synoviocytes play important roles at multiple levels in the pathophysiology of rheumatoid synovitis[83]. The cytokine networks in this inflamed tissue greatly influence the phenotype and functions of these cells. Both IL-1 and TNF-α induce adhesion molecule expression on synovial fibroblasts, enhancing the migration of inflammatory cells from the circulation into the joint. Under the local influence of FGF, PDGF, and other cytokines, synovial fibroblasts develop characteristics of transformed cells, such as adherence-independent growth, expression of oncogenes, and loss of contact inhibition. Furthermore, these cells are the major source in the synovium of IL-6 and angiogenic factors such as FGF, PDGF and VEGF, as well as of IL-8 and GM-CSF which may further activate macrophages. Thus, fibroblasts in the rheumatoid synovium exhibit autocrine and paracrine stimulatory interactions with nearby fibroblasts, as well as with macrophages (Fig. 11.2). These cellular interactions are mediated through cytokines and may lead to autonomous perpetuation of inflammation and tissue destruction.

A distinctive and unusual cell found at the pannus–cartilage junction in the rheumatoid synovitis has been termed 'pannocyte'[84,85]. These cells exhibit characteristics of both fibroblasts and chondrocytes. Cytokine effects on pannocytes include PDGF- and TGF-β-induced proliferation and decreased growth in response to IL-1, characteristics resembling chondrocytes. However, like fibroblasts the pannocytes demonstrated constitutive production of large amounts of collagenase, increased after stimulation with IL-1 and TNF-α[85]. Their rapid growth and prolonged life span *in vivo* suggest that pannocytes may represent a mesenchymal cell in an earlier stage of differentiation.

Regulation of angiogenesis

The growth of new blood vessels is involved in the development of the rheumatoid pannus, and enhanced endothelial cell function is present in this tissue[86,87]. The importance of angiogenesis in inflammatory arthritis was emphasized by prevention of collagen-induced arthritis in mice, or suppression of the ongoing disease, by treatment with a selective angiogenesis inhibitor[88]. Both proan-

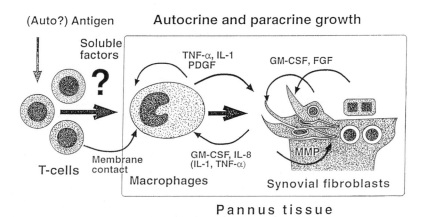

Fig. 11.2   Autocrine and paracrine mechanisms in synovial macrophage activation. Abbreviation: MMP, matrix metalloproteinase. Reproduced with permission from Ref. 75.

giogenic factors and inhibitors, or angiostatic factors, have been found in the rheumatoid synovium with the net effect on capillary growth representing a balance between the two.

Growth factors important in promoting angiogenesis include VEGF, FGF, EGF, IGF-I, AND TGF-β[86]. VEGF is a potent angiogenic factor that possesses structural homology to PDGF and is produced by a variety of cells in sites of neovascularization[89]. High levels of VEGF are present in rheumatoid synovial fluids, with this protein produced primarily by macrophages in the inflamed synovial tissue[90,91]. Both IL-1 and TNF-α stimulated VEGF production by cultured rheumatoid synovial cells[92]. The microvascular endothelial cells of synovial blood vessels strongly expressed the mRNA for VEGF receptors[90]. The mechanism whereby VEGF and other growth factors promote angiogenesis is through stimulation of expression of members of the integrin family of adhesion molecules[87]. Treatment of rheumatoid arthritis patients with monoclonal antibodies to TNF-α, particularly in combination with methotrexate, decreased the elevated serum levels of VEGF[92].

Many other cytokines are also involved in angiogenesis, either as stimulatory agents or as inhibitors. Cytokines that promote angiogenesis include TNF-α, IL-8, and other chemokines. While TNF-α may primarily promote endothelial cell differentiation, rather than proliferation, IL-8 stimulates angiogenesis through attracting macrophages into the synovial tissue and enhancing endothelial cell chemotaxis and proliferation.

In contrast, IFN-γ inhibits angiogenesis both through direct effects on endothelial cells and through inducing production of the angiostatic chemokines interferon-inducible protein 10 (IP-10) and monokine induced by IFN-γ (MIG)[87]. IFN-γ-inducing factors such as IL-12, and theoretically IL-18, may inhibit angiogenesis through upregulating IFN-γ production. IL-18 is a potent IFN-γ inducing factor that is produced by macrophages and other cells as a propeptide, utilizing the IL-1β-converting enzyme (ICE) to generate the active mature protein. In addition to sharing with IL-12 the property of induction of IFN-γ production, IL-18 may exhibit proinflammatory consequences through stimulating TNF-α production in CD4+ T cells and NK cells, with subsequent enhanced production of IL-1β and IL-8 from monocytes[93]. Recently, macrophage-derived IL-18 was demonstrated in RA synovium and synovial fluid. Inhibition of IL-18 by monoclonal antibody ameliorates murine collagen-induced arthritis[93a]. Thus, the cytokine network may contribute either to angiogenesis or angiostasis, depending on the balance of factors locally present in the rheumatoid synovium.

Summary of mechanisms of tissue destruction

Numerous proinflammatory cytokines are involved in the pathogenesis of rheumatoid arthritis. The complexity of some of these cytokine effects on T cells, antigen-presenting cells, macrophages, endothelial cells, fibroblasts, and chondrocytes is summarized in Fig. 11.3. These mediators of cell–cell communication may play

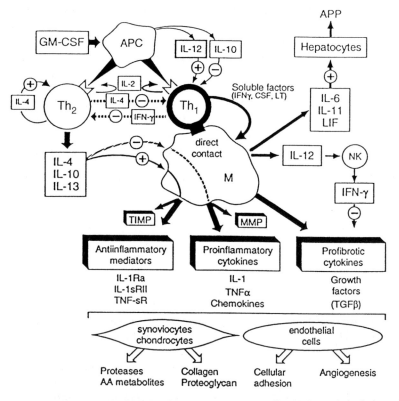

Fig. 11.3 Cells and mediators in chronic inflammation: the role of antigen-presenting cells (APCs) and the balance between lymphocytes (Th1 and Th2) resulting in different cytokine profiles. Activation of monocytes (M) by direct contact or by soluble products leads to the production of matrix metalloproteinases (MMP), tissue inhibitor of MMP (TIMP), and other mediators or cytokines by M. These cytokines then act on synoviocytes, chondrocytes, endothelial cells, natural killer cells (NK), lymphocytes, and hepatocytes, the latter producing acute-phase proteins (APP). Abbreviations: AA, arachadonic acid; LT, lymphotoxin. Reproduced with permission from Ref. 8.

key roles in the initiation of reactive synovitis, in the transformation of this self-limited response into an aggressive and tissue-destructive process, and in the perpetuation of chronic synovitis. In these three stages of the disease process, the same or different cytokines may play changing and complementary roles. However, the cytokine network is self-regulating and, as detailed below, other cytokines, antibodies to cytokines, and soluble cytokine receptors may all act to limit the potentially injurious effects of the proinflammatory members of the cytokine family.

Systemic effects and regulation of cytokine networks

Induction of the acute phase response

The acute phase response is defined as the changes in plasma concentration of many proteins, reflecting alterations in rate of synthesis by hepatocytes, and other biochemical and nutritional changes which accompany inflammation[94,95]. These changes represent adaptations by the organism in an effort to maintain essential functions and survive in the face of overwhelming infection and acute or chronic inflammation. Cytokines are key mediators in both stimulation of production of the acute phase proteins and in the systemic manifestations of the acute phase response, the major cytokines being IL-6, IL-1 and TNF-α (Fig. 11.4)

The plasma proteins whose concentrations increase during the acute phase response include complement factors, proteins of the coagulation and fibrinolytic system, antiproteases, transport proteins, participants in the inflammatory response, and miscellaneous proteins (Table 11.5). The most clinically useful is C-

Table 11.5   Human acute phase proteins

Proteins whose plasma concentrations increase:

Complement system: C3, C4, C9, factor B, C1-inhibitor, C4b-binding protein, mannose-binding lectin

Coagulation and fibrinolytic system: fibrinogen, plasminogen, tissue plasminogen activator, urokinase, protein S, vitronectin, plasminogen activator inhibitor-1

Antiproteases: α-1 protease inhibitor, 1-antichymotrypsin, pancreatic secretory trypsin inhibitor, inter-α-inhibitors

Transport proteins: ceruloplasmin, haptoglobin, hemopexin

Participants in inflammatory responses: secreted phospholipase A2, lipopolysaccharide-binding protein, IL-1 receptor antagonist, granulocyte colony-stimulating factor

Others: C-reactive protein (CRP), serum amyloid A (SAA), α1-acid glycoprotein, fibronectin, ferritin, angiotensinogen

Proteins whose plasma concentrations decrease:
albumin, transferrin, transthyretin, α-2 HS glycoprotein, α-fetoprotein, thyroxine-binding globulin, insulin-like growth factor-1, factor XII

Reproduced from Ref. 95 with permission.

reactive protein, whose levels in plasma are generally the most sensitive indicator of inflammation. The plasma levels of other proteins decrease during the acute phase response (Table 11.5). IL-6 is the most important cytokine in influencing production of the acute phase proteins in the liver; IL-6 is the major inducer of CRP and SAA production by hepatocytes, whereas IL-6 inhibits synthesis of albumin. Depending on the nature of the inflammatory condition, cytokines may exhibit a cascade of effects where TNF-α may induce IL-1 production, which in turn stimulates IL-6 production in a variety of cells.

In addition, combinations of cytokines exhibit varying patterns of stimulation of production of acute phase proteins by hepatoma cell lines, although effects on hepatocytes *in vivo* may not be the same. Either IL-1 or TNF-α may enhance IL-6 induction of CRP and SAA production in these model systems, whereas TNFα or TGF-β may inhibit the stimulatory effects of IL-6 on fibrinogen production by the same cells[96]. The combination of IL-1β and IL-6 was more potent than either cytokine alone in stimulation of IL-1Ra production by HepG2 or cultured human hepatocytes[97]. Furthermore, both IL-4 and IL-13 amplified the stimulatory effect of IL-1β on production of IL-1Ra by these cells, whereas these cytokines exhibited no effects alone or in combination with IL-6[98]. In contrast, IL-4 inhibited the induction of other acute phase proteins by cultured primary human hepatocytes[99]. Thus, depending upon other cytokines present, the effects of IL-6 on stimulation of acute phase protein production may either be enhanced or decreased.

Whether the net effects of IL-6 in rheumatoid synovitis are proinflammatory or anti-inflammatory remains controversial. IL-6 levels are increased in the serum and synovial fluid of patients with rheumatoid arthritis. Rheumatoid synovial fibroblasts constitutively produced large amounts of IL-6 *in vitro*, although synovial macrophages were also capable of producing

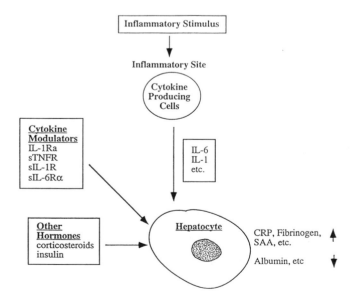

Fig. 11.4   The acute phase response is regulated both directly and indirectly by a complex network of intercellular signaling molecules involving cytokines, cytokine modulators, and other hormones. Inflammation-associated cytokines, produced by cells at the inflammatory site and probably distant cells as well, induce changes in production of acute-phase proteins by hepatocytes. Reproduced with permission from Ref.[94].

this cytokine[100]. Coculture of blood monocytes on rheumatoid synovial fibroblasts led to enhanced production of IL-6, GM-CSF, LIF, and IL-8 by the synoviocytes[101]. Synoviocyte production of IL-6 in this coculture system was inhibited by IL-1Ra, indicating the stimulatory role of endogenous IL-1, and it was also inhibited by IL-4, IL-10, and IL-13. The monocyte appeared to be more important as an inducer of synoviocyte production of cytokines in this model, rather than as a direct source of IL-6 itself. Synoviocyte production of IL-6 was further increased by the addition of IFN-γ, IL-1β, TNF-α, or GM-CSF, thought to be secondary to the ability of these cytokines to increase the expression of adhesion molecules on both cells to enhance their interaction[101].

A proinflammatory role for IL-6 is suggested by its ability to activate endothelial cells to produce chemokines and express adhesion molecules, induce synovial fibroblast proliferation, and stimulate osteoclast formation and activation. Furthermore, complete protection from collagen-induced arthritis, with an absence of inflammatory cell infiltrates in the joints, was observed in mice lacking the IL-6 gene[102]. However, IL-6 stimulates antibody production by B cells[7] and the IL-6 knockout mice in this study demonstrated reduced levels of anticollagen antibodies. Thus, IL-6 in collagen-induced arthritis may be more important in enhancing production of autoantibodies than in acting as a local inflammatory mediator. This possibility is further substantiated by an absence of an effect on arthritis in TNF-α-transgenic mice by ablating IL-6 production[102]. However, in rheumatoid arthritis IL-6 may be responsible for some systemic manifestations such as fever, fatigue, and anorexia, as well as of osteopenia[103].

The anti-inflammatory potential of IL-6 is suggested by the results of many studies (reviewed in Ref. 104. The *in vivo* administration of IL-6 to humans led to enhanced circulating levels of IL-1Ra and soluble TNF receptors, but not of IL-1β or TNF-α. These and other IL-6-induced acute phase proteins have many anti-inflammatory effects. Neutralizing monoclonal antibodies to IL-6 did not reduce the proteoglycan degradation seen in antigen-induced arthritis or zymosan-induced arthritis in mice[105]. Furthermore, proteoglycan depletion was higher in IL-6-deficient mice during zymosan-induced arthritis than in wild-type controls[106]. This observation indicated that IL-6 may be protective for cartilage damage in this model, possibly through inducing the production of cytokine inhibitors and of tissue inhibitors of metalloproteinases. In addition, studies of animal models of endotoxic lung injury indicated that IL-6 played a crucial anti-inflammatory role in both local and systemic acute inflammatory responses by controlling the level of proinflammatory cytokines[107]. Thus, although IL-6 may be involved in some chronic pathophysiological processes, such as the induction of loss of calcium from bone, this cytokine appears to exhibit more protective than injurious effects in animal models of arthritis.

IL-11, a member of the IL-6 family of cytokines, is an important mediator of periarticular osteopenia but also exhibits anti-inflammatory properties. The IL-11 receptor possesses a unique α chain, and, like other members of the IL-6 family, uses the common gp130 molecule to induce intracellular responses[108,109]. IL-11 mRNA and proteins were expressed by human articular chondrocytes and synoviocytes, and were induced in these cells by TGF-β and IL-1β[108]. Endogenous IL-11 produced by rheumatoid synovial cells inhibited TNF-α production, particularly in combination with IL-10[109]. Furthermore, IL-11 directly inhibited spontaneous metalloproteinase production by these cultured cell while upregulating tissue inhibitor of metalloproteinase[109]. Lastly, IL-11 treatment of murine collagen-induced arthritis led to reduced joint inflammation and destruction[110].

Although fever, fatigue, and muscle wasting represent some of the symptomatic effects of cytokines during acute and chronic inflammation, other systemic consequences of the acute phase response may be beneficial to the host[98,99]. CRP may play a role in the clearance of infectious agents, enhancement of phagocytosis, and prevention of neutrophil adherence to endothelial cells. CRP also inhibits the generation of superoxide anions by neutrophils and, along with other acute phase proteins, stimulates the production of IL-1Ra by monocytes. The proteinase inhibitors produced as part of the acute phase response may block the effects of some enzymes released by phagocytic cells. Lastly, the systemic manifestations of acute inflammation may reflect physiological adaptations that enhance the immune response and provide for maintenance of core organ functions, such as the central nervous system. However, failure or overwhelming of these adaptations may lead to physiological collapse, as occurs in severe endotoxemia with septic shock.

Anti-inflammatory effects of cytokines

The major cytokines that exhibit anti-inflammatory effects include IL-4, IL-10, IL-13, TGF-β, and IL-1Ra. In addition to their effects on T cells, IL-4, IL-10, and IL-13 all act on monocytes and macrophages to inhibit production of IL-1 and TNF-α, while enhancing production of the natural antiinflammatory cytokine IL-1Ra. These three cytokines also display additional anti-inflammatory effects. The protective properties of IL-4 include inhibition of bone resorption[111], inhibition of growth factor-induced proliferation of rheumatoid synoviocytes[112], suppression of macrophage production of metalloproteinases[113], suppression of IL-1-induced production of metalloproteinases and PGE$_2$ in human synovial fibroblasts[114], and a decrease in mononuclear cell recruitment to the rheumatoid synovium[115]. In fact, continuous infusion of IL-4 led to a delay in the onset of collagen-induced arthritis in mice and to a suppression of joint damage[116]. A most striking finding in the IL-4-treated mice was a 1000-fold decrease in the production of TNF-α by synovial cells. However, IL-4 and IL-13 appear not to be produced in detectable levels by rheumatoid synovial tissue or fluid cells and probably do not function as natural anti-inflammatory proteins in the joint in this disease.

IL-10 exhibits a similar spectrum of anti-inflammatory properties as IL-4 and IL-13 *in vitro*, but, unlike these cytokines, IL-10 is produced in the rheumatoid synovium and may suppress local inflammation. IL-10 was produced in the joints of mice with collagen-induced arthritis and neutralization of endogenous IL-10 by prophylactic treatment with anti-IL-10 antibodies led to an earlier onset of arthritis with increased severity[117]. Furthermore, IL-10 administration after disease onset in murine collagen-induced arthritis inhibited inflammation and cartilage destruction[118]. The prophylactic administration of viral IL-10 using adenoviral-mediated gene transfer inhibited the onset of collagen-induced arthritis in mice and decreased T cell proliferation *in vitro* induced by collagen type II[119,120]. Although pretreatment with viral IL-10 decreased the severity of joint destruction, treatment of established disease was ineffective.

IL-10 levels are elevated in the serum and synovial fluid of patients with rheumatoid arthritis[121]. In addition, both the mRNA and protein for IL-10 were detected in rheumatoid synovial tissue with production by macrophages and T cells[122]. Furthermore, the IL-10 was functionally important as neutralization of endogenously-produced IL-10 in cultured rheumatoid synovial cells led to three-fold increases in the levels of TNF-α and IL-1β. Normal humans injected with IL-10 exhibited no adverse symptoms and inhibition of LPS-stimulated production of TNF-α and IL-1β by whole blood cells was observed[123]. A four-week phase I trial of IL-10 in patients with rheumatoid arthritis revealed elevations in circulating levels of soluble TNF receptors and IL-1Ra, with some possible early clinical efficacy[124]. An additional clinical trial of IL-10 in rheumatoid arthritis patients is in progress.

TGF-β exhibited either proinflammatory or anti-inflammatory properties in animal models of arthritis, depending on the particular model studied, the route of delivery, and the state of differentiation of the responding cells[125]. Injection of TGF-β into joints of experimental animals generally induced acute and chronic inflammation while systemic delivery was usually anti-inflammatory. TGF-β exhibited a variety of suppressive effects on cell function in vitro, including inhibition of CD4+ T cell proliferation and a reduction in MHC class II expression. This cytokine was present in large amounts in the synovial fluid and tissue of patients with this disease, possibly accounting for the suppressed T cell function present in rheumatoid synovial T cells[126]. Mice rendered deficient in TGF-β production developed wasting and a mixed inflammatory cell infiltration into multiple organs with subsequent tissue necrosis[127]. Furthermore, these mice possessed hyperproliferative lymphocytes and spontaneous production of antibodies to nuclear antigens[128]. The autoimmunity in TGF-β-deficient mice appeared to be dependent upon the excessive expression of MHC class II molecules on CD4+ T cells[129].

Lastly, rats with streptococcal cell wall-induced arthritis who received gene therapy with plasmid DNA for TGF-β by direct injection into muscles exhibited a marked suppression of joint inflammation and destruction[130]. Thus, the major effects of endogenous TGF-β in patients with rheumatoid arthritis may be to suppress fibroblast proliferation and production of tissue-damaging neutral metalloproteinases while enhancing production of the inhibitors of these enzymes[131].

IL-1Ra in the rheumatoid synovium

IL-1Ra is a structural derivative of IL-1 that binds to IL-1 receptors with equal affinity as the agonists IL-1α and IL-1β, but fails to activate target cells[132-134]. The administration of IL-1Ra, either by injection of recombinant protein or by delivery through gene therapy, inhibits the development and severity of arthritis in multiple experimental animal models (reviewed in Refs 133 and 134). Constitutive intra-articular expression of IL-1 following gene transfer to the rabbit synovium led to all of the histopathological changes of the human disease rheumatoid arthritis[135]. Furthermore, some evidence indicated that treatments to block TNF-α in collagen-induced arthritis in mice were primarily anti-inflammatory whereas blocking IL-1 was more inhibitory towards destruction of cartilage and bone[136]. Endogenous IL-1Ra was shown to be an important natural anti-inflammatory protein as neutralizing antibodies to IL-1Ra led to an exacerbation of LPS-induced arthritis in rabbits[137]. Lastly, collagen-induced arthritis was more severe in IL-1Ra knockout mice and was suppressed by the over-expression of IL-1Ra in transgenic mice[138].

IL-1Ra was present in the synovial fluids of patients with rheumatoid arthritis in high levels[139], and the mRNA was abundantly expressed by macrophages and fibroblasts in the synovial lining, particularly at the pannus–cartilage junction[140-142]. However, *in vitro* culture of rheumatoid synovial cells indicated that the amount of IL-1Ra produced was probably not sufficient to inhibit the inflammatory effects of the locally-produced IL-1[143]. The imbalance between IL-1 and IL-1Ra production by rheumatoid synovial cells could be improved in favor of IL-1Ra by culturing with IL-4, and less so with IL-10[144]. The importance of endogenous production of IL-1Ra in patients with inflammatory arthritis was suggested by finding a high ratio of IL-1Ra to IL-1 in the knee synovial fluids of patients with Lyme arthritis who exhibited rapid spontaneous improvements, while the opposite ratio was present in the fluids of patients with more protracted courses[145]. The daily subcutaneous injection of recombinant IL-1Ra in a phase I clinical trial in patients with rheumatoid arthritis was more effective than weekly administration[146]. Patients treated in this manner for 6 months demonstrated a moderate clinical improvement in joint inflammation with radiological evidence of a slowing in progression of joint destruction and a decrease in the rate of development of new bone lesions[147].

Antibodies to cytokines

High affinity antibodies to native IL-1α, IL-6, IL-10, IFN-α, IFN-β, and GM-CSF are present in the sera of normal individuals, possibly developing secondary to a loss T cell tolerance to self[148]. The antibodies against IL-1α, IL-6, IFN-α, and GM-CSF neutralized receptor binding of the respective cytokine *in vitro*. However, the physiological relevance of these naturally-occurring antibodies to cytokines remains unknown. High avidity neutralizing antibodies to IFN-α, IL-1α, IL-6, and GM-CSF were found in pharmaceutical preparations of intravenous gamma globulin (IVIG), with antibody titers present *in vivo* after administration to patients[149,150]. The clinical responses to IVIG may be secondary to these anticytokine antibodies, as well as to antibodies to HLA class I molecules[151] or to anti-idiotypic antibodies also present in these preparations.

Autoantibodies to some cytokines have been described in the sera of patients with rheumatoid arthritis: IL-1α (36 per cent of

49. Harigai, M., Hara, M., Yoshimura, T., Leonard, E.J., Inoue, K., and Kashiwazaki, S. Monocyte chemoattractant protein-1 (MCP-1) in inflammatory joint diseases and its involvement in the cytokine network of rheumatoid synovium. *Clinical Immunology and Immunopathology*, 1993;**69**,83–91.

50. Koch, A.E., Kunkel, S.L., Harlow, L.A., Mazarakis, D.D., Haines, G.K., Burdick, M.D., *et al.* Macrophage inflammatory protein-1α. A novel chemotactic cytokine for macrophages in rheumatoid arthritis. *Journal of Clinical Investigation*, 1994;**93**,921–928.

51. Rathanaswami, P., Hachicha, M., Sadick, M., Schall, T.J., and McColl, S.R. Expression of the cytokine RANTES in human rheumatoid synovial fibroblasts. *Journal of Bioligical Chemistry*, 1993;**268**,5834–5839.

52. Harada, A., Mukaida, N., and Matsushima, K. Interleukin 8 as a novel target for intervention in acute inflammatory diseases. *Molecular Medicine Today*, 1996;**2**:482–489.

53. Firestein, G.S., Xu, W.D., Townsend, K., Broide, D., Alvaro-Gracia, J., Glasebrook, A., *et al.* Cytokines in chronic inflammatory arthritis. I. Failure to detect T cell lymphokines (interleukin 2 and interleukin 3) and presence of macrophage colony-stimulating factor (CSF-1) and a novel mast cell growth factor in rheumatoid synovitis. *Journal of Experimental Medicine*, 1998;**168**,1573–1586.

54. Firestein, G.S., Alvaro-Gracia, J.M., and Maki, R. Quantitative analysis of cytokine gene expression in rheumatoid arthritis. *Journal of Immunology*, 1990;**144**,3347–3353.

55. Firestein, G.S., and Zvaifler, N.J. How important are T cells in chronic rheumatoid synovitis? *Arthritis & Rheumatism*, 1990;**33**,768–773.

56. Panayi, G.S., Lanchbury, J.S., and Kingsley, G.H. The importance of the T cell in initiating and maintaining the chronic synovitis of rheumatoid arthritis. *Arthritis & Rheumatism*, 1992;**35**,729–735.

57. Simon, A.K., Seipelt, E., and Sieper, J. Divergent T-cell cytokine patterns in inflammatory arthritis. *Proceedings of the National Academy of Sciences USA*, 1994;**91**,8562–8566.

58. Kotake, S., Schumacher Jr., H.R., Yarboro, C.H., Arayssi, T.K., Pando, J.A., Kanik, K.S., *et al.* In vivo gene expression of type 1 and type 2 cytokines in synovial tissues from patients in early stages of rheumatoid, reactive, and undifferentiated arthritis. *Proceedings of the Association of American Physicians*, 1997;**109**,286–302.

59. Kanik, K.S., Hagiwara, E., Yarboro, C.H., Schumacher, H.R., Wilder R.L., and Klinman, D.M. Distinct patterns of cytokine secretion characterize new onset synovitis versus chronic rheumatoid arthritis. *Journal of Rheumatology*, 1998;**25**,16–22.

60. Klimiuk, P.A., Goronzy, J.J., Bjornsson, J., Beckenbaugh, R.D., and Weyand, C.M. Tissue cytokine patterns distinguish variants of rheumatoid synovitis. *American Journal of Pathology*, 1997;**151**,1311–1319.

61. Kamradt, T., and Burmester, G.-R. Cytokines and arthritis: is the Th1/Th2 paradigm useful for understanding pathogenesis? *Journal of Rheumatology*, 1998;**25**,6–8.

62. Symons, J.A., Wood, N.C., di Giovine, F.S., and Duff, G.W. Soluble IL-2 receptor in rheumatoid arthritis. Correlation with disease activity, IL-1 and IL-2 inhibition. *Journal of Immunology*, 1988;**141**,2612–2618.

63. McInnes, I.B., and Liew, F.Y. Interleukin 15: a proinflammatory role in rheumatoid arthritis synovitis. *Immunology Today*, 1998;**19**,75–79.

64. McInnes, I.B., Al-Mughales, J., Field, M., Leung, B.P., Huang F.-P., Dixon, R., *et al.* The role of interleukin-15 in T-cell migration and activation in rheumatoid arthritis. *Nature Medicine*, 1996;**2**,175–182.

65. McInnes, I.B., Leung, B.P., Sturrock, R.D., Field, M., and Liew, F.J. Interleukin-15 mediates T cell-dependent regulation of tumor necrosis factor-α production in rheumatoid arthritis. *Nature Medicine*, 1997;**3**,189–195.

66. Alleva, D.G., Kaser, S.B., Monroy, M.A., Fenton, M.J., and Beller, D.I. IL-15 functions as a potent autocrine regulator of macrophage proinflammatory cytokine production. Evidence for dif-

ferential receptor subunit utilization associated with stimulation or inhibition. *Journal of Immunology*, 1997;**159**,2941–2951.

67. Oppenheimer-Marks, N., Brezinsxhek, R.I., Mohamadzadeh, M., and Lipsky, P.E. Interleukin 15 is produced by endothelial cells and increases the transendothelial migration of T cells in vitro and in the SCID mouse–human rheumatoid arthritis model in vivo. *Journal of Clinical Investigation*, 1998;**101**,1261–1272.

68. Carson, D.A. Unconventional T-cell activation by IL-15 in rheumatoid arthritis. *Nature Medicine*, 1997;**3**,148–149.

69. Bamford, R.N., DeFilippis, A.P., Azimi, N., Kurys, G., and Waldmann, T.A. The 5' untranslated region, signal peptide, and the coding sequence of the carboxyl terminus of IL-15 participate in its multifaceted translational control. *Journal of Immunology*, 1998;**160**,4418–4426.

70. Ruchatz, H., Leung, B.P., Wei, X.-Q., McInnes, I.B., and Liew, F.Y. Soluble IL-15 receptor α-chain administration prevents murine collagen-induced arthritis: a role for IL-15 in development of antigen-induced immunopathology. *Journal of Immunology*, 1998;**160**,5654–5660.

71. Joosten, L.A.B., Lubberts, E., Helsen, M.M.A., and van den Berg, W.B. Dual role of IL-12 in early and late stages of murine collagen type II arthritis. *Journal of Immunology*, 1997;**159**,4094–4102.

72. Beaulieu, A.D., and McColl, S. R. Differential expression of two major cytokines produced by neutrophils, interleukin-8 and the interleukin-1 receptor antagonist, in neutrophils isolated from the synovial fluid and peripheral blood of patients with rheumatoid arthritis. *Arthritis & Rheumatism*, 1994;**37**,855–859.

73. Palucka, K.A., Taquet, N., Sanchez-Chapuis, F., and Gluckman, J.C. Dendritic cells as the terminal stage of monocyte differentiation. *Journal of Immunology*, 1998;**160**,4587–4595.

74. Banchereau, J., and Steinmann, R.M. Dendritic cells and the control of immunity. *Nature*, 1998;**392**,245–252.

75. Burmester, G.-R., Stuhlmuller, B., Keyszer, G., and Kinne, R.W. Mononuclear phagocytes and rheumatoid synovitis. Mastermind or workhouse in arthritis. *Arthritis & Rheumatism*, 1997;**40**,5–18.

76. Turner, M., Chantry, D., Katsikis, P., Berger, A., Brennan, F.M., and Feldmann, M. Induction of the interleukin 1 receptor antagonist protein by transforming growth factor-β. *European Journal of Immunology*, 1991;**21**,1635–1639.

77. Wahl, S.M., Costa, G.L., Corcoran M., Wahl, L.M., and Berger, A.E. Transforming growth factor-β mediates IL-1 dependent induction of IL-1 receptor antagonist. *Journal of Immunology*, 1993;**150**,3553–3560.

78. Lacraz, S., Isler, P., Vey, E., Welgus, H.G., and Dayer, J.-M. Direct contact between T lymphocytes and monocytes is a major pathway for induction of metalloproteinase expression. *Journal of Biological Chemistry*, 1994;**269**,22027–22033.

79. Chizzolini, C., Chicheportiche, R., Burger, D., and Dayer, J.-M. Human Th1 cells preferentially induce interleukin (IL)-1β while Th2 cells induce IL-1 receptor antagonist production upon cell/cell contact with monocytes. *European Journal Immunology*, 1997;**27**,171–177.

80. Fossiez, F., Djossou, O., Chomarat, P., Flores-Romo, L., Ait-Yahai, S., Maat, C., *et al.* T cell interleukin-17 induces stromal cells to produce proinflammatory and hematopoietic cytokines. *Journal of Experimental Medicine*, 1996;**183**,2593–2603.

81. Chabaud, M., Fossiez F., Taupin, J.-L., and Miossec, P. Enhancing effect of IL-17 on IL-1 induced IL-6 and leukemia inhibitory factor production by rheumatoid arthritis synoviocytes and its regulation by Th2 cytokines. *Journal of Immunology*, 1998;**161**,409–414.

82. Jovanovic, D.V., Di Battista, J.A., Martel-Pelletier, J., Jolicoeur, F.C., He, Y., Zhang, M., *et al.* IL-17 stimulates the production and expression of proinflammatory cytokines, IL-1β and TNF-α, by human macrophages. *Journal of Immunology*, 1998;**160**,3513–3521.

83. Firestein, G.S. Invasive fibroblast-like synoviocytes in rheumatoid arthritis. Passive responders or transformed aggressors? *Arthritis & Rheumatism*, 1996;**39**,1781–1790.

84. Zvaifler, N.J., and Firestein, G.S. Pannus and pannocytes. Alternative models of joint destruction in rheumatoid arthritis. *Arthritis & Rheumatism*, 1994;37,783–789.

85. Zvaifler, N.J., Tsai, V., Alsalameh, S., von Kempis, J., Firestein, G.S., and Lotz, M. Pannocytes: distinctive cells found in rheumatoid arthritis articular cartilage erosions. *American Journal of Pathology*, 1997;150,1125–1138.

86. Szekanecz, Z., Szegedi, G., and Koch, A.E. Angiogenesis in rheumatoid arthritis: pathogenic and clinical significance. *Journal of Investigative Medicine*, 1998;46,27–41.

87. Koch, A.E. Angiogenesis. Implications for rheumatoid arthritis. *Arthritis & Rheumatism*, 1998;41,951–962.

88. Peacock, D.J., Banquerigo, M.L., and Brahn, E. Angiogenesis inhibition suppresses collagen arthritis. *Journal of Experimental Medicine*, 1992;175,1135–1138.

89. Thomas, K.A. Vascular endothelial growth factor, a potent and selective angiogenic agent. *Journal of Biological Chemistry*, 1996;271,603–606.

90. Fava, R.A., Olsen, N.J., Spencer-Green, G., Yeo, K.-T., Yeo, T.-K., Berse, B., *et al.* Vascular permeability factor/endothelial growth factor (VPF/VEGF): accumulation and expression in human synovial fluids and rheumatoid synovial tissue. *Journal of Experimental Medicine*, 1994;180,341–346.

91. Koch, A.E., Harlow, L.A., Haines, G.K., Amento, E.P., Unemori, E.N., Wong, W.L., *et al.* Vascular endothelial growth factor. A cytokine modulating endothelial function in rheumatoid arthritis. *Journal of Immunology*, 1994;152,4149–4156.

92. Paleolog, E.M., Young S., Stark, A.C., McCloskey, R.V., Feldmann, M., and Maini, R.N. Modulation of angiogenic vascular endothelial growth factor by tumor necrosis factor α and interleukin-1 in rheumatoid arthritis. *Arthritis & Rheumatism*, 1998;41,1258–1265.

93. Puren, A.J., Fantuzzi, G., Gu, Y., Su, M.S.-S., and Dinarello, C.A. Interleukin 18 (IFNγ-inducing factor) induces IL-8 and IL-1β via TNFα production from non-CD14+ human blood mononuclear cells. *Journal of Clinical Investigation*, 1998;101,711–721.

93a. Gracia J.A., Forsey R.J., Chan W.L., Gilmour A., Leung B.P., Greer M.R., Kennedy K., Carter R., Wei X.Q., Xu D., Field M., Foulis A., Liew F.Y., McInnes I.B. A proinflammatory role for IL-18 in rheumatoid arthritis. J. Clin Invest 1999;104:1393–401.

94. Gabay, C., and Kushner, I. (1999) Acute phase proteins. In *Encyclopedia of Life Sciences*. Nature Publishing Group. London.

95. Gabay, C., and Kushner, I. (1998). Acute phase proteins and other systemic responses to inflammation. *New England Journal of Medicine*, 1999;340,448–54.

96. Mackiewicz, A., Speroff, T., Ganapathi, M.K., and Kushner, I. Effects of cytokine combinations on acute phase protein production in two human heptoma cell lines. *Journal of Immunology*, 1991;146,3032–3037.

97. Gabay, C., Smith, Jr., M.F., Eidlen, D., and Arend, W.P. Interleukin 1 receptor antagonist (IL-1Ra) is an acute phase protein. *Journal of Clinical Investigation*, 1997;99,2930–2940.

98. Gabay, C., Porter, B., Guenette, D., Bilir, B., and Arend, W.P. (1998). IL-4 and IL-13 enhance the effect of IL-1 on production of the IL-1 receptor antagonist by human primary hepatocytes and HepG2 hepatoma cells. *Blood*, 1999;93,1299–1307.

99. Loyer, P., Ilyin, G., and Razzak, Z.A. Interleukin 4 inhibits the production of some acute-phase proteins by human hepatocytes in primary culture. *FEBS Letters*, 1993;336,215–220.

100. Miyazawa, K., Mori, A., Yamamoto, K., and Okudiara, H.Constitutive transcription of the human interleukin-6 gene by rheumatoid synoviocytes. *American Journal of Pathology*, 1998 ;152,793–803.

101. Chomarat, P., Rissoan, M.C., Pin, J., Banchereau, J., and Miossec, P. Contribution of IL-1, CD14, and CD13 in the increased IL-6 production induced by in vitro monocyte–synoviocyte interactions. *Journal of Immunology*, 1995;155,3645–3652.

102. Alonzi, T., Fattori, E., Lazzaro, D., Costa, P., Probert, L., Kollias, G., *et al.* Interleukin 6 is required for the development of collagen-induced arthritis. *Journal of Experimental Medicine*, 1998;187,461–468.

103. Papanicolaou, D.A., Wilder, R.L., Manolagas, S.C., and Chrousos, G.P. The pathophysiologic roles of interleukin-6 in human disease. *Annals of Internal Medicine*, 1998;128,127–137.

104. Tilg, H., Dinarello, C.A., and Mier, J.W. IL-6 and APPs: anti-inflammatory and immunosuppressive mediators. *Immunology Today*, 1997;18,428–432.

105. van de Loo, F.A.J., Joosten, L.A.B., van Len, P.L.E.M., Arntz, O.J., and van den Berg, W.B. Role of interleukin-1, tumor necrosis factor α, and interleukin-6 in cartilage proteoglycan metabolism and destruction. Effect of in situ blocking in murine antigen- and zymosan-induced arthritis. *Arthritis & Rheumatism*, 1995;38,164–172.

106. van de Loo, F.A.J., Kuiper, S., van Enckevort, F.H.J., Arntz, O.J., and van den Berg, W.B. Interleukin-6 reduces cartilage destruction during experimental arthritis. *American Journal of Pathology*, 1997;151,177–191.

107. Xing, Z., Gauldie, J., Cox, G., Baumann, H., Jordana, M., Lei, X.-F., *et al.* IL-6 is an antiinflammatory cytokine required for controlling local or systemic acute inflammatory responses. *Journal of Clinical Investigation*, 1998;101,311–320.

108. Maier, R., Ganu, V., and Lotz, M. Interleukin-11, an inducible cytokin in human articular chondrocytes and synoviocytes, stimulates the production of the tissue inhibitor of metalloproteinases. *Journal of Biological Chemistry*, 1993;268,21527–21532.

109. Hermann, J.A., Hall, M.A., Maini, R.N., Feldmann, M., and Brennan, F.M. Important immunoregulatory role of interleukin-11 in the inflammatory process in rheumatoid arthritis. *Arthritis & Rheumatism*, 1998;41,1388–1397.

110. Walmsley, M., Butler, D.M., Marinova-Mutafchieva, L., and Feldmann, M. (1998) An anti-inflammatory role for interleukin 11 is established collagen-induced arthritis. *Immunology*, 1998; 95:31–7.

111. Miossec, P., Chomarat, P., Dechanet, J., Moreau, J.-F., Roux, J.-P., Delmas, P., *et al.* Interleukin-4 inhibits bone resorption through an effect on osteoclasts and proinflammatory cytokines in an ex vivo model of bone resorption in rheumatoid arthritis. *Arthritis & Rheumatism*, 1994;37,1715–1722.

112. Dechanet, J., Briolay, J., Rissoan, M.-C., Chomarat, P., Galizzi, J.-P., Banchereau, J., *et al.* IL-4 inhibits growth factor-stimulated rheumatoid synoviocyte proliferation by blocking the early phases of the cell cycle. *Journal of Immunology*, 1993;151,4908–4917.

113. Lacraz, S., Nicod, L., Galve-de Rochemonteix, B., Baumberger, C., Dayer, J.-M., and Welgus, H.G. Suppression of metalloproteinase biosynthesis in human alveolar macrophages by interleukin-4. *Journal of Clinical Investigation*, 1992;90,382–388.

114. Borghaei, R.C., Rawlings, Jr., P.L., and Mochan, E. Interleukin-4 suppression of interleukin-1-induced transcription of collagenase (MMP-1) and stromelysin 1 (MMP-3) in human synovial fibroblasts. *Arthritis & Rheumatism*, 1998;41,1398–1406.

115. Jorgensen, C., Apparilly, F., Couret, I., Canovas, F., Jacquet, C., and Sany, J. Interleukin-4 and interleukin-10 are chondroprotective and decrease mononuclear cell recruitment in human rheumatoid synovium in vivo. *Immunology*, 1998;93,518–523.

116. Horsfall, A.C., Butler, D.M., Marinova, L., Warden, P.J., Williams, R.O., Maini, R.N., *et al.* Suppression of collagen-induced arthritis by continuous administration of IL-4. *Journal of Immunology*, 1997;159,5687–5696.

117. Kasama, T., Streiter, R.M., Lukacs, N.W., Lincoln, P.M., Burdick, M.D., and Kunkel, S.L. Interleukin-10 expression and chemokine regulation during evolution of murine type II collagen-induced arthritis. *Journal of Clinical Investigation*, 1995;95,2868–2876.

118. Walmsley, M., Katsikis, P.D., Abney, E., Parry, S., Williams, R.O., Maini, R.N., and Feldmann, M. Interleukin-10 inhibition of the progression of established collagen-induced arthritis. *Arthritis & Rheumatism*, 1996;39,495–503.

119. Apparilly, F., Verwaerde, C., Jacquet, C., Auriault, C., Sany, J., and Jorgensen, C. Adenovirus-mediated transfer of viral IL-10

gene inhibits murine collagen-induced arthritis. *Journal of Immunology*, 1998;**160**,5213–5220.

120. Ma, Y., Thornton, S., Duwel, L.E., Boivin, G.P., Giannini, E.H., Leiden, J.M., et al. Inhibition of collagen-induced arthritis in mice by viral IL-10 gene transfer. *Journal of Immunology*, 1998;**161**,1516–1524.

121. Cush, J.J., Splawski, J.B., Thomas, R., McFarlin, J.E., Schulze-Koops, H., Davis, L.S., et al. Elevated interleukin-10 levels in patients with rheumatoid arthritis. *Arthritis & Rheumatism*, 1995;**38**,96–104.

122. Katsikis, P.D., Chu, C.-Q., Brennan, F.M., Maini, R.N., and Feldmann, M. Immunoregulatory role of interleukin 10 in rheumatoid arthritis. *Journal of Experimental Medicine*, 1994;**179**,1517–1527.

123. Chernoff, A.E., Granowitz, E.V., Shapiro, L., Vannier, E., Lonnemann, G., Angel, J.B., et al. A randomized, controlled trial of IL-10 in humans. Inhibition of inflammatory cytokine production and immune responses. *Journal of Immunology*, 1995;**154**,5492–5499.

124. Keystone, E., Wherry, J., and Grint, P. IL-10 as a therapeutic strategy in the treatment of rheumatoid arthritis. *Rheumatic Disease Clinics of North America*, 1998;**24**,629–639.

125. Letterio, J.J., and Roberts, A.B. TGF-β: a critical modulator of immune cell function. *Clinical Immunology and Immunopathology*, 1997;**84**,244–250.

126. Lotz, M., Kekow, J., and Carson, D.A. Transforming growth factor-β and cellular immune responses in synovial fluids. *Journal of Immunology*, 1990;**144**,4189–4194.

127. Shull, M.M., Ormsby, I., Kier, A.B., Pawlowski, S., Diebold, R.J., Yin, M., et al. Targeted disruption of the mouse transforming growth factor-β1 gene results in multifocal inflammatory disease. *Nature*, 1992;**359**,693–699.

128. Yaswen, L., Kulkarni, A.B., Frederickson, T., Mittleman, B., Schiffman, R., Payne, S., et al. Autoimmune manifestations in the transforming growth factor-β1 knockout mouse. *Blood*, 1996;**87**,1439–1445.

129. Letterio, J.J., Geiser, A.G., Kulkarni, A.B., Dang, H., Kong, L., Nakabayashi, T., et al. Autoimmunity associated with TGF-β1-deficiency in mice is dependent on MHC class II antigen expression. *Journal of Clinical Investigation*, 1996;**98**,2109–2119.

130. Song, X.-Y., Gu, M., Jin, W.-W., Klinman, D.M., and Wahl, S.M. Plasmid DNA encoding transforming growth factor-β1 suppresses chronic disease in a streptococcal cell wall-induced arthritis model. *Journal of Clinical Investigation*, 1998;**101**,2615–2621.

131. Wilder, R.L., Lafyatis, R., Roberts, A.B., Case, J.P., Kumkumian, G.K., Sano, H., et al. Transforming growth factor-β in rheumatoid arthritis. *Annals of the New York Academy of Sciences*, 1990;**593**,197–207.

132. Arend, W.P. Interleukin-1 receptor antagonist. *Advances in Immunology*, 1993;**54**,167–227.

133. Arend, W.P., Malyak, M., Guthridge, C.J., and Gabay, C. Interleukin-1 receptor antagonist: role in biology. *Annual Review of Immunology*, 1998;**16**,27–55.

134. Bresnihan, B., and Cunnane, G. Interleukin-1 receptor antagonist. *Rheumatic Disease Clinics of North America*, 1998;**24**,615–628.

135. Ghivizzani, S.C., Kang, R., Georgescu, H.I., Lechman, E.R., Jaffurs, D., Engle, J.M., et al. Constitutive intra-articular expression of human IL-1β following gene transfer to rabbit synovium produces all major pathologies of human rheumatoid arthritis. *Journal of Immunology*, 1997;**159**,3604–3612.

136. Joosten, L.A.B., Helsen, M.M.A., van de Loo, F.A.J., and van den Berg, W.B. Anticytokine treatment of established type II collagen-induced arthritis in DBA/1 mice. *Arthritis & Rheumatism*, 1996;**39**,797–809.

137. Fukumoto, T., Matsukawa, A., Ohkawara, S., Takagi, K., and Yoshinaga, M. Administration of a neutralizing antibody against rabbit IL-1 receptor antagonist exacerbates lipopolysaccharide-induced arthritis in rabbits. *Inflammation Research*, 1996;**45**,479–485.

138. Ma, S., Thornton, S., Boivin, G.P., Hirsh, D., Hirsch, R., and Hirsch, E. Altered susceptibility to collagen-induced arthritis in transgenic mice with aberrant expression of IL-1 receptor antagonist. *Arthritis & Rheumatism*, 1998;**41**,1798–1805.

139. Malyak, M., Swaney, R.E., and Arend, W.P. Levels of synovial fluid interleukin-1 receptor antagonist in rheumatoid arthritis and other arthropathies. *Arthritis & Rheumatism*, 1993;**36**,781–789.

140. Firestein, G.S., Berger, A.E., Tracey, D.E., Chosay, J.G., Chapman, D.L., Paine, M.M., et al. IL-1 receptor antagonist protein production and gene expression in rheumatoid arthritis and osteoarthritis synovium. *Journal of Immunology*, 1992;**149**,1054–1062.

141. Deleuran, B.W., Chu, C.Q., Field, M., Brennan, F.M., Katsikis, P., Feldmann, M., et al. Localization of interleukin-1α, type I interleukin-1 receptor and interleukin-1 receptor antagonist in the synovial membrane and cartilage/pannus junction in rheumatoid arthritis. *British Journal of Rheumatology*, 31,801–809.

142. Koch, A.E., Kunkel, S.L., Chensue, S.W., Haines, G.K., and Strieter, R.M. Expression of interleukin-1 and interleukin-1 receptor antagonist by human rheumatoid synovial tissue macrophages. *Clinical Immunology and Immunopathology*, 1992;**65**,23–29.

143. Firestein, G.S., Boyle, D.L., Yu, C., Paine, M.M., Whisenand, T.D., Zvaifler, N.J., et al. Synovial interleukin-1 receptor antagonist and interleukin-1 balance in rheumatoid arthritis. *Arthritis & Rheumatism*, 1994;**37**,644–652.

144. Chomarat, P., Vannier, E., Dechanet, J., Rissoan, M.C., Banchereau, J., Dinarello, C.A., et al. Balance of IL-1 receptor antagonist/IL-1β in rheumatoid synovium and its regulation by IL-4 and IL-10. *Journal of Immunology*, 1995;**154**,1432–1439.

145. Miller, L.C., Lynch, E.A., Isa, S., Logan, J.W., Dinarello, D.A., and Steere, A.C. Balance of synovial fluid IL-1β and IL-1 receptor antagonist and recovery from Lyme arthritis. *Lancet*, 1993;**341**,146–148.

146. Campion, G.V., Lebsack, M.E., Lookabaugh, J., Gordon, G., and Catalano, M. Dose-range and dose-frequency study of recombinant human interleukin-1 receptor antagonist in patients with rheumatoid arthritis. *Arthritis & Rheumatism*, 1996;**39**,1092–1101.

147. Bresnihan, B., Alvaro-Gracia, J.M., Cobby, M., Doherty, M., Domljan, Z., Emery, P., et al. Treatment of rheumatoid arthritis with recombinant human interleukin-1 receptor antagonist. *Arthritis & Rheumatism*, 1998;**41**,2196–204.

148. Bendtzen, K., Hansen, M.B., Ross, C., and Svenson, M. High-avidity antibodies to cytokines. *Immunology Today*, 1998;**19**,209–211.

149. Ross, C., Svenson, M., Nielson, H., Lundsgaard, C., Hansen, M.B., and Bendtzen, K. Increased in vivo antibody activity against interferon α, interleukin-1α, and interleukin-6 after high-dose Ig therapy. *Blood*, 1997;**90**,2376–2380.

150. Svenson, M., Hansen, M.B., Ross, C., Diamant, M., Rieneck, K., Nielson, H., et al. Antibody to granulocyte-macrophage colony-stimulating factor is a dominant anti-cytokine in human IgG preparations. *Blood*, 1998;**91**,2054–2061.

151. Kaveri, S., Vassilev, T., Hurez, V., Lengagne, R., Lefranc, C., Cot, S., et al. Antibodies to a conserved region of HLA class I molecules, capable of modulating CD8 T cell-mediated function, are present in pooled normal immunoglobulin for therapeutic use. *Journal of Clinical Investigation*, 1996;**97**,865–869.

152. Suzuki, H., Kamimura, J., Ayabe, T., and Kashiwagi, H. Demonstration of neutralizing antibodies against IL-1α in sera from patients with rheumatoid arthritis. *Journal of Immunology*, 1990;**145**,2140–2146.

153. Hansen, M.B., Andersen, V., Rohde, K., Florescu, A., Ross, C., Svenson, M., et al. Cytokine autoantibodies in rheumatoid arthritis. *Scandinavian Journal of Rheumatology*, 1995;**24**,197–203.

154. Jouvenne, P., Fossiez, F., Banchereau, J., and Miossec, P. High levels of neutralizing autoantibodies against IL-1α are associated

with a better prognosis in chronic polyarthritis: a follow-up study. *Scandinavian Journal of Immunology*, 1997;**46**,413–418.

155. Feldmann, M., Elliott, M.J., Woody, J.N., and Maini, R.N. Anti-tumor necrosis factor-α therapy of rheumatoid arthritis. *Advances in Immunology*, 1997;**64**,283–350.

156. Fernandez-Botran, R., Chilton, P.M., and Ma, Y. Soluble cytokine receptors: their roles in immunoregulation and therapy. *Advances in Immunology*, 1996;**63**,269–336.

157. Klein, B., and Brailly, H. Cytokine-binding proteins: stimulating antagonists. *Immunology Today*, 1995;**16**,216–220.

158. Cope, AP., Aderka, D., Doherty, M., Englemann, H., Gibbons, D., Jones, A.C., *et al*. Increased levels of soluble tumor necrosis factor receptors in the sera and synovial fluid of patients with rheumatic diseases. *Arthritis & Rheumatism*, 1992;**35**,1160–1169.

159. Roux-Lombard, P., Punzi, L., Hasler, F., Bas, S., Todesco, S., Gallati, H., *et al*. Soluble tumor necrosis factor receptors in human inflammatory synovial fluids. *Arthritis & Rheumatism*, 1993;**36**,485–489.

160. Moreland, L.W., Baumgartner, S.W., Schiff, M.H., Tindall, E.A., Fleischmann, R.M., Weaver, A.L., *et al*. Treatment of rheumatoid arthritis with a recombinant human tumor necrosis factor receptor (p75)-Fc fusion protein. *New England Journal of Medicine*, 1997;**337**,141–147.

161. Moreland, L.W. Soluble tumor necrosis factor receptor (p75) fusion protein (Enbrel) as a therapy for rheumatoid arthritis. *Rheumatic Disease Clinics of North America*, 1998;**24**,579–591

162. Colotta, F., Dower, S.K., Sims, J.E., and Mantovani, A. The type II "decoy" receptor: a novel regulatory pathway for interleukin 1. *Immunology Today*, 1994;**15**,562–566.

163. Arend, W.P., Malyak, M., Smith, Jr., M.F., Whisenand, T.D., Slack, J.L., Sims, J.E., *et al*. Binding of IL-1α, IL-1β, and IL-1 receptor antagonist by soluble IL-1 receptors and levels of soluble IL-1 receptors in synovial fluids. *Journal of Immunology* 1996;1994;**153**,4766–4774.

164. Drevlow, B.E., Lovis, R., Haag, M.A., Sinacore, J.M., Jacobs, C., Blosche, C., *et al*. Recombinant human interleukin-1 receptor type I in the treatment of patients with active rheumatoid arthritis. *Arthritis & Rheumatism*, **39**,257–265.

165. De Benedetti, F., Massa, M., Pignatti, P., Albani, S., Novick, D., and Martini, A. Serum soluble interleukin 6 (IL-6) receptor and IL-6/soluble IL-6 receptor complexes in systemic juvenile rheumatoid arthritis. *Journal of Clinical Investigation*, 1994;**93**,2114–2119.

166. Gabay, C., Silacci, P., Genin, B., Mentha, G., Le Coultre, C., and Guerne, P.-A. Soluble interleukin-6 receptor strongly increases the production of acute-phase proteins by hepatoma cells but exerts minimal changes on human primary hepatocytes. *European Journal of Immunology*, 1995;**25**,2378–2383.

167. Ye, J., and Young, H.A. Negative regulation of cytokine gene transcription. *FASEB Journal*, 1997;**11**,825–833.

168. Kishimoto, T., Taga, T., and Akira, S. Cytokine signal transduction. *Cell*, 1994;**76**,253–262.

169. Wallis, W.J., Furst, D.E., Strand, V., and Keystone, E. Biologic agents and immunotherapy in rheumatoid arthritis. *Rheumatic Disease Clinics of North America*, 1998;**24**,537–565.

170. Evans, C.H., Ghivizzanni, S.C., Kang, R., Muzzonigro, T., Wasko, M.C., Herndon, J.H., *et al*. Gene therapy for rheumatic diseases. *Arthritis & Rheumatism*, 1999;**42**,1–16.

12 | Apoptosis in rheumatoid arthritis: cause or consequence

Nathan J. Zvaifler

Apoptosis

Physiological cell death is a process by which single cells can be eliminated in the midst of living tissue. The cell deletion is orchestrated by specific proteins encoded in the host's genome (thus programmed cell death—PCD) and has been called apoptosis (the second 'p' is silent), a Greek word used to describe leaves dropping off trees[1]. PCD and apoptosis are used interchangeably although the former refers to the process, and the latter, apoptosis, the morhological appearance of the cells. Apoptosis occurs throughout the life span of complex organisms and is responsible for tissue modeling in verterbrate development, involution, and atrophy that accompanies withdrawal of hormones and growth factors, normal tissue turnover as exemplified by hematopoietic cells in the bone marrow or autoreactive thymocytes in the thymus gland, and the continual loss of cells in tumors in response to chemotherapy or irradiation[2].

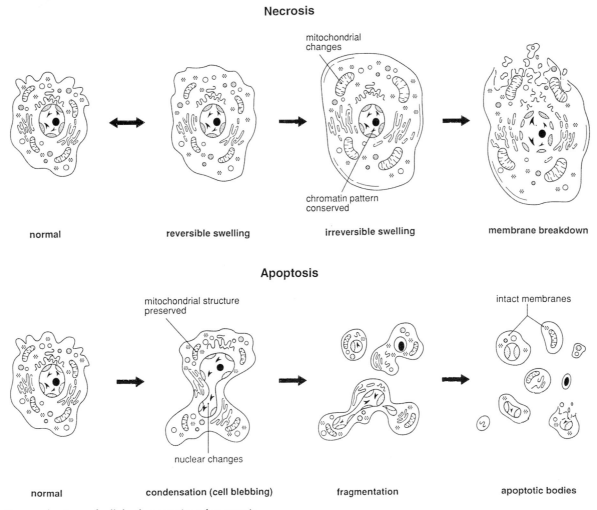

Fig. 12.1 Two mechanisms of cell death: necrosis and apoptosis.

Morphology

The morphological changes that accompany apoptosis are stereotyped and similar in almost all cells from any source. The dying cell separates from its neighbors and membrane structures, such as microvilli and desmosomes, are lost. Affected cells (observed *in vitro*) appear to round up, shrink in size, and the endoplasmic reticulum dilates and forms vesicles that often fuse with the plasma membrane giving rise to an appearance of blebs or bubbling (zeiosis) in electron micrographs. Initially, and in contrast to cells undergoing a pathological cell death (necrosis), cytoplasmic condensation occurs with compaction of organelles and mitochondria that remain near normal in structure[3]. The most impressive change, however, occurs in the nucleus with condensation of the chromatin into dense granular caps and nucleoli splintered into multiple osmophilic particles. Fragmentation of the cell occurs soon thereafter with multiple, small membrane bound segments called apoptotic bodies (Fig. 12.1). This contrasts with the alternative mode of death for nucleated cells, namely necrosis, which occurs through an increased permeability of the cell membrane to fluid, swelling, distortion of cytoplasmic organelles, and eventual cell disrup-

tion (Fig. 12.1). The maintenance of membrane integrity in apoptosis prevents the release of deleterious cytoplasmic elements (lysosomal enzymes and mitochondrial proteins) and the activation of damaging inflammatory responses and scarring[2–4].

In vivo, this sequence is not readily observed because cells undergoing apoptosis generate surface recognition structures that result in their rapid phagocytosis by surrounding cells or macrophages, and digestion within heterophagasomes. This accelerated clearance of apoptotic leukocytes by macrophages may be a physiological process for terminating inflammation (discussed in detail below)[5]. The biochemical counterpart to the morphological changes in the nucleus is the cleavage of chromatin between nucleosomes which reduces the DNA into fragments with multiples of 180 to 200 base pairs[6]. These can be delineated in tissue sections by immunohistochemical techniques that either label the ends of damaged DNA or identify 'nicks' in the DNA, or by extraction and agarose gel electrophoresis with the identification of a ladder-like series of bands of low molecular weight DNA[7]. These approaches allow assessment of *in vivo* PCD at a time prior to the appearance of typical morphological features of apoptosis.

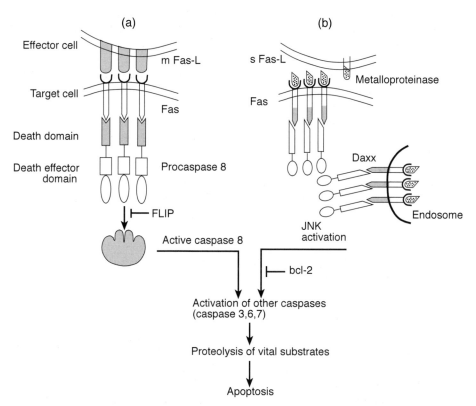

Fig. 12.2 Signaling through membrane-bound Fas ligand (mFas-L). (a) Binding to, and trimerization of Fas receptor gathers FADD/Mort 1 into a death domain. Binding of death effectors lead to caspase 8 transactivation which induces the active caspase 8 tetramer. Subsequent downstream caspases lead to cleavage of vital substrates and apoptosis. Cellular FLIP is an inhibitor of caspase 8 activation.
(b) Signaling through the soluble form of Fas ligand (sFas-L). Cleavage of mFas-L by metalloproteinase forms sFas-L. The sFasL–Fas complex is internalized into endosomes, preventing formation of a death-inducing signaling complex. Instead, jun N-terminal kinase (JNK) is activated through Daxx, leading to activation of other caspases and eventual cleavage of vital substrates and apoptosis (adapted from Strasser, A., and O'Connor, L.O., *Nature Med*, 4:21–22, 1998).

Programmed cell death is often divided into separate phases, beginning with the stimulus-dependent phase, which can be initiated by a variety of events arising from either within the cell (metabolic or cell cycle perturbations, for example toxic oxygen or nitrogen, activation of the p53 tumor suppressor gene, irradiation, cytotoxic drugs, or corticosteroids), or externally by molecules (death receptor ligands) engaging specific cell surface receptors (Fas, TNF, TRAIL, TRAMP)[8,9]. A second common effector phase involves recognition of the stimulus and clustering of membrane proteins into a death effector domain (DED) which converts certain proenzymes (caspases) to their active form. Alternatively, these caspases, which are the orchestrators of apoptotic death, can be actived through mitohondrial events that culminate in the release of cytochrome c. After the death effector machinery is actived, cells enter the third irreversible common degradation phase of cytoskeletal disorganization endonuclease activation, and the lysis of substrated responsible for cellular integrity (Fig. 12.2) Survival proteins provide control of the caspase-drive engine of destruction; the best known are members of the bcl-2 family.

Death factors and surface receptors

Various stimuli can activate apoptosis. An analysis of events that follow the engagement of death factors to their receptors on lymphoid cells provided the orginal insights into the molecular machinery of apoptosis. The best known and characterized are certain members of the tumor necrosis factor (TNF) family; namely Fas ligand (Fas-L) and TNF. Fas-L is synthesized as a 40 kD type II membrane protein (mFas-L), primarily on NK cells and actived lymphocytes[10]. A putative metalloproteinase mediates proteolytic cleavage to generate a smaller (26 kD) soluble form (sFas-L)[11]. Although both can mediate apoptosis, sFas-L is much less potent than mFas-L and may antagonize the action of the protein from which it is cleaved[12]. Soluble Fas-L exists as a trimeric structure; the membrane-bound forms probably have a similar configuration. The receptor for Fas-L, known as Fas (also APO-1 or CD95), is a member of the TNF receptor family and is ubiquitously expressed on most cells. Binding of Fas-L to Fas or cross-linking Fas with agonistic mono-clonal antibodies causes apoptosis in Fas-bearing cells (Fig. 12.2).

When Fas-L engages Fas a trimerization of the receptor is induced resulting in immediate recruitment of several proteins that form a death-inducing signaling complex (DISC) around the cytoplasmic tail (death domain) of the receptor[8]. These proteins bind to each other and the trimerized Fas receptor through a series of head (N terminal) to tail (C terminal) homologous domains. Fas binds to a similar sequence on the C terminus of a protein called FADD (Fas-associated protein with a death domain); FADD contains a distinct N terminal domain (designated the death effector domain) that engages a homologous region in the N terminus of a third protein, FLICE (Fas activated protein like interleukin-1 converting enzyme). The C terminus of FLICE, with structural and functional homology to the caspases, can activate these proteins[13]. Thus, there is a

direct, non-transcriptional coupling between ligand receptors of the TNF receptor family and the activation of caspases. Additional elements modulate this system.

A second approach, genetic analysis of PCD in the tiny round-worm (nematode) *C. elegans*, came to similar conclusions. Almost a dozen genes were found to be directly involved in the cell death pathway and mutations generated abnormalities at different steps in the process. The general significance of this program became evident when homology was identified between two of the genes—ced9 and ced3—with mammalian bcl-2 and ICE (interleukin-1 converting enzyme). ICE is a cysteine protease and it, as well as other homologous mammalian proteins, induces apoptosis when over-expressed in cells and specific inhibitors or knockouts of their genes forestall death. Because they cleave their substrates on the carboxy-terminal side of an aspartic acid residue the group have been called caspases (cysteine-aspases). Caspase-8 (the prototype initiator caspase), when activated, preferentially cleaves the pro-forms of down-stream caspases (executioner caspases) 3, 6, and 7[14]. These, in turn, cause proteolysis of cytoskeletal proteins (actin, fodrin) and critical nuclear constituents (PARP, lamin, DNA-dependent protein kinases, endonucleases, and molecules necessary for membrane integrity—PAK-2, gelsolin) that are responsible for the apoptotic morphological changes in the cell, as well as the characteristic DNA degradation (Fig. 12.2).

Until recently, all Fas-L-induced apoptosis was thought to be similar. However, Tanaka[12] has shown that sFas-L produced by cleavage of mFas-L forms a complex with Fas. The complex, when rapidly internalized into a subcellular compartment, fails to activate the conventional mFas-L-FADD/Mort-1-caspase-8 pathway. Instead, signaling occurs through Daxx-activating jun kinase (JNK) leading to engagement of an unidentified caspase and proteolvis of substrates that induce apoptosis (Fig. 12.3). The potential importance of sFas-L in understanding events in the inflamed RA joint will be discussed below.

PCD can follow by engagement of other members of the receptor family. The best characterized, engagement of the TNF receptor-1, involves either a pathway very similar to Fas (FADD/caspase-8) or the sequential interaction of RIP (receptor interacting protein) with another death-domain-containing protein termed RAIDD (RIP associated Ich-1/CED-3 homologous protein with a death domain) and the recruitment of pro-caspase-2. Subsequent transactivation of other caspase[3,6,7] leads to the final common pathway of cell death[15].

Apoptosis as a cellular response to injury

Programmed cell death is neither limited to lymphoid tissues nor Fas-L and TNF receptors. Apoptosis is a critical component of the response to multiple other causes of cell injury, directed at DNA, cell membranes, or mitochondria. A number of the stimuli to apoptosis involve compromises in the balance between intracellular oxidants and their defense systems. Under aerobic conditions oxygen participating in redox reactions produces a

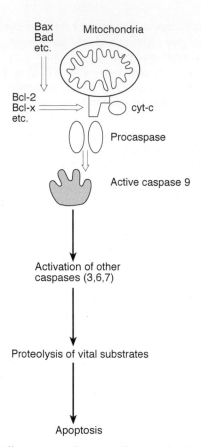

Fig. 12.3 Cell stress pathway with mitochondrial release of cytochrome c (cyt-c). Proapoptotic bcl-2 family members (e.g. bax, bad, etc.) promote and antiapoptotic members (bcl-2, bcl-x, etc.) block cytochrome c release. Procaspases induce active caspase 9 tetramer and subsequent events are similar to the final pathway shown in Fig. 12.2.

variety of very toxic chemicals entities commonly referred to as reactive oxygen intermediate (ROI)[16]. A partial list includes the hydroxyl radical, hydrogen peroxide, nitric oxide, super oxide, and lipid peroxides. The consequences of oxidative stress depend, at least in part, on the severity of the insult; extreme non-physiological concentrations of oxidants cause necrosis, whereas the exposure of cells to low oxygen triggers apoptosis[17]. When the *bcl-2* gene and its product was found to block oxygen-related cell death it was ascribed to its antioxidant and free radical scavenging properties[18]. Later, it was determined to be just one of a number of antiapoptotic proteins[19,20]. Since most, if not all cells, contain caspases, powerful mechanisms must exist to suppress their activation. In the nematode, that suppression is provided by the product of the *ced-9* gene; the homologous molecules in mammals are *bcl-2* and *bcl-x*.

The *bcl-2* gene family is large and includes both death-inducing and death-inhibitory members. Most possess regions of *bcl-2* homology which determine their capacity to interact with each other and unrelated proteins[20]. Many of the proteins encoded by the *bcl-2* gene family are predominately localized in the outer mitochondrial membrane, although *bcl-2* itself is also found in the nuclear membrane and in the endoplasmic reticulum[21,22]. Death antagonists (such as bcl-2, bcl-xL, bcl-w, ncl-1, A1) and agonists (bax, bak, bcl-xs, bad, bid) exist in ratios that

determine how a cell will respond to an apoptotic signal. Competitive dimerization between selective pairs of antagonists and agonists operate as a dynamic equilibrium between homo- and heterodimers and behaves like a death-life rheostat[22].

Among the first manifestations of the apoptotic process, irrespective of either the cell type or the inductive stimulus, is disruption of mitochondrial membrane function specifically through disruption of the mitochondrial trasmembrane potential[23,24]. This results in an opening of mitochondrial permeability transition pores (PT) which are multiprotein complexes formed at the contact sites between the inner and outer membranes of the mithochondria. PT opening causes uncoupling of the respiratory chain, release of matrix Ca^{++}, depletion of reduced glutathione and NAD, and invokes the entire panoply of apoptosis-associated metabolic changes, including caspase activation, redox disequilibria, nuclear DNA fragmentation, and phosphatidylserine exposure on the cell surface[25,26]. Transfection of cells with *bcl-2* or *bcl-x* inhibits the early mitochondrial changes associated with apoptosis[25], but it is not clear whether they directly regulate PT or indirectly influence PT by regulating other mitochondrial functions such as cytochrome-c release. Given the functional importance of bcl-2-related proteins in apoptosis control, they constitute prime targets for therapeutic intervention. On the one hand, cytoprotection can be provided by mimicking bcl-2 effects, while on the other, bcl-2-related proteins can be used to overcome apoptosis resistance, as is the case with cancer chemotherapeutic agents.

DNA injury, p53, and apoptosis

The p53 tumor suppressor gene product is crucial in aspects of DNA damage recognition, DNA repair, cell cycle regulation, and in triggering apoptosis after genotoxic injury. p53 is a DNA-binding phosphoprotein and a transcriptional activator of specific sets of target genes. *In vivo*, p53 is normally rapidly degraded (approximately 20–30 minutes) by ubiquitin-dependent proteolysis. Both post-transcriptional and post-translational mechanisms regulate p53 activity and stability. p53 also negatively regulates its own transcriptional activity through induction of the *mdm-2* oncogene that forms a feedback loop[27-29]. Multiple stimuli can trigger p53, including DNA damage, oncogene activation, the presence or absence of certain cytokines, hypoxia, and heat shock[30]. The apoptosis is both cell type and stimulus specific; for example thymocyte apoptosis triggered by DNA damage is p53 dependent, while dexamethasone triggering is not[31]. Following DNA damage, p53 appears to act at multiple steps, that is sensing DNA damage, binding directly to insertion/deletion mismatches, and DNA strand breaks[32]. Within hours of gamma or UV radiation immunoreactive p53 accumulates within the cell and persists for over 48 hours. *In vitro*, p53 responses can be triggered without changes in protein concentration suggesting that accumulation is not always sufficient or even necessary to initiate downstream events[30]. Once p53 dependent apoptosis is triggered, it does not differ in any way from apoptosis induced by other means and feeds into the caspase effector pathway.

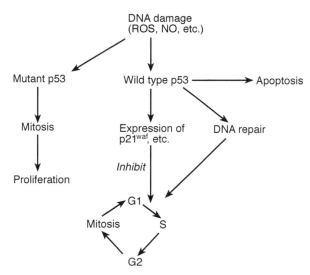

Fig. 12.4 p53 regulates the cell cycle after DNA damage.

Two important inter-related processes are regulated by p53. First, p53 causes cell cycle arrest at the G1/S boundary by inducing expression of a cellular gene (*p21/WAF-1*) that encodes a 21 kD inhibitor of several G1 cycline dependent kinases[33,34]. Second, p53 can induce apoptosis (Fig. 12.4)[27–34]. While the effects of p53 on cell cycle arrest and apoptosis appear to be cyclical functions, it is likely that they both participate in genomic surveillance. Thus, p53 causes the arrest of cycling cells prior to S phase, which allows of repair of damaged DNA prior to DNA replication. In cases where the DNA damage is too severe to be properly repaired, apoptosis ensues[35,36]. Loss or inactivation of p53, as seen in more than half of all tumors, allow malignant cells to replicate their damaged DNA. This fixes errors into the genome and promotes cell survival resulting in the accumulation of genomic alterations with time[37].

At present, it is not clear how p53 induces apoptosis[30]. Of probable relevance, is the finding that p53 is a direct transcriptional activator of the human *bax* gene[38]. Bcl-2 and Bax are homologous proteins with opposing effects on cell life and death. A working model is that intracellular elevations in p53 induced by DNA damaging agents, or other means, lowers the resistance of cells to apoptotic stimuli. Studies with *bcl-2* knockout mice, or by using antibodies to reduce *bcl-2* expression, suggest that lowering the Bax: Bcl-2 ratio may be insufficient by itself to trigger apoptosis, but the cells are relatively more sensitive to induction of cell death by various apoptotic stimuli. Likewise, p53 probably does not induce apoptosis, *per se*, but rather adjusts the relative sensitivity of cells so that apoptosis is triggered more easily.

Rheumatoid arthritis

Inflamed joints demonstrate a complex interaction between multiple types of cells and a variety of soluble factors[39–41]. Moreover, the participants differ in various articular compart-

ments, that is the cells in synovial effusions are predominately polymorphonuclear leukocytes (PMN) and the minority population of lymphocytes have an over-representation of CD8 and NK cells, compared with circulating lymphocytes. In synovial tissues, the PMN leukocytes are sparse, CD4 lymphocytes predominate, B cells and monocyte/macrophages are present, and fibroblastic cells in the synovial lining (FLS = fibroblast-like synoviocytes) are important participants. Apoptosis in each of the players, and in different locations, has been investigated, sometimes with surprisingly disparate findings. Therefore, the results from different kinds of cells will be cataloged before trying to explain their regional differences.

Synovial effusions—Polymorphonuclear (PMN) leukocytes and macrophages

Beginning in the 1960s there was a resurgence of interest in the study of synovial fluid, based on findings compatible with an intra-articular immune complex pathogenesis for RA[41]. Immunoglobulin and rheumatoid factor production was demostrated within the synovium; complexes of IgG, IgM, and complement were present within polymorphonuclear leukocytes in the inflammatory effusion, and hemolytic complement levels in rheumatoid effusions were significantly lower than companion serum samples or when compared to synovial fluid from other

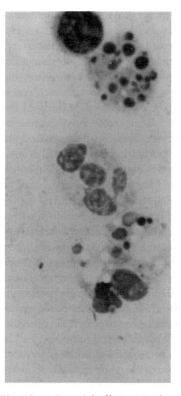 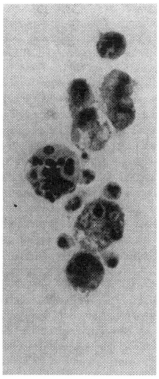

Fig. 12.5 Synovial effusion in rheumatoid arthritis (left) showing an intact leukocyte (center), intact lymphocyte (top), and polymorphonuclear cells undergoing apoptosis (Wright–Gemsa stain, × 1000). Reiters effusion (right) showing a collection of large macrophages with eccentric nuclei and basophilic apoptotic bodies in the cytoplasm. The large size of the macrophages contrasts with the small leukocytes and lymphocytes (Wright-Gemsa stain × 200).

were also detected. In contrast, Fas-L staining was mainly limited to mononuclear cells, primarily of the CD45RO phenotype, suggesting that activated T cells and natural killer cells infiltrating the joint might contribute to apoptosis of FLS through Fas/Fas-L interactions[78]. The predicted outcome of such an interaction should be the elimination of Fas-L-bearing T cells and morphological changes consistent with programmed cell death in the Fas+ synoviocytes. Failure to demonstrate these findings and the overgrowth of the synovial lining suggests that this normal regulatory process is somehow diverted or overcome.

One explanation may lie in the large amounts of TGF-β found in rheumatoid synovial tissue and effusions. *In vitro*, the proliferation of cultured synovial fibroblasts is enhanced by TGF-β in a dose dependent manner, and in addition, TGF-β decrease Fas antigen expression and upregulates Bcl-2 in synoviocytes. Synoviocytes stimulated with TGF-β become markedly resistant to anti-Fas-mediated apoptosis[79].

The role of TNF in synoviocytes apoptosis is controversial. In a few studies, TNF directly induced FLS apoptosis[73], while in most it was only effective in the presence of anti-Fas antibody or protein synthesis inhibitors[77,80,81]. Evidence was reported that TNF sensitizes synoviocytes for Fas-mediated apoptosis through effects on caspase-8 and caspase-3[82]. Similar results were obtained with a specific peptide inhibitor of caspase-3 activation[83]. Furthemore, TGF-β pretreatment of synoviocytes had an opposite effect from TNF in systems that measure activation of caspase-3 and apoptotic cell death.

Ohsima *et al.* confirmed that RA-FLS are susceptible to anti-Fas antibody-mediated apoptotic cell death (ACD), somewhat more than OA-FLS. TNF inhibited ACD of RA synoviocytes treated with Fas antibody in a dose-dependent manner. This effect was neutralized by anti-TNF antibody. Thus, the benefits of anti-TNF treatment of RA could result, in part, from modifying Fas-mediated ACD and reducing synovial hyperplasia[77].

In vitro, some TNF effects are mediated by ceramide, the hydrolytic product of sphingomyelin by sphingomyelinases. Sometimes it promotes cell growth, (e.g. 3T3 fibroblastoid cells), while in others, apoptosis and cell cycle arrest. The addition of C2-ceramide to isolated synovials fibroblasts resulted in sequential changes of cell rounding, nuclear changes, and complete apoptosis in 48 hours. No proliferation was observed. Ceramide had a similar effect on dermal fibroblasts[84].

The death of FLS can be regulated by gene therapy *in vitro*[85] or in animals with experimental arthritis[86,87]. The introduction of large amounts of the gene encoding Fas-L into synovial fibroblasts causes apoptotic death in about 20 per cent of cultured FLS by 20 hours and 80 per cent of the fibroblasts die at 72-96 hours. In murine collagen-induced arthritis, high levels of Fas are expressed on activated lining cells, much as in man, and Fas-L levels in the arthritis joints are extremely low. When a recombinant replication defective adenovirus carrying the Fas-L gene is injected into an inflamed joint, apoptosis is induced in the synovial cells and the collagen induced arthritis is ameliorated[86]. These results imply that modulation of the Fas/Fas-L interaction could be an important therapeutic intervention in RA.

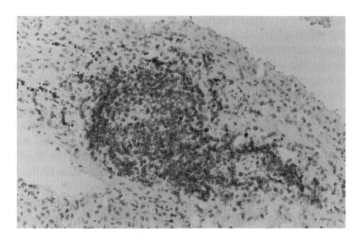

Fig. 12.6 Immunohistology of frozen section of RA synovial tissue stained with antibody to Bcl-2 showing that Bcl-2 is limited mainly to CD45RO lymphocytes in subintimal aggregates (× 200) Ref. 73.

The expression of *bcl-2* in lining cells is sparse when determined with specific antibodies to the protein[73,88]; whereas antisense *bcl-2* riboprobes show strong hybridization[89]. Combined *in situ* hybridization for mRNA and immunohistochemistry determined that synovial lining cells do show abundant *bcl-2* mRNA but there is a corresponding lack of protein expression[90].

Synovial tissue—Lymphoctyes

The very first studies of apoptosis in the RA synovium noted large amounts of Bcl-2 in lymphoid aggregates (Fig. 12.6). Only occasional Bcl-2 staining of cells in other areas, such as the subintimal tissues or lining cells, was found[73]. This original description has been confirmed in a number of subsequent studies[88,90,91]. A double-labeled histomorphological analysis, which distinguishes B and T lymphocytes, revealed that most of the cells in both populations were Bcl-2 protein-positive in the lymphoid aggregates, although in those aggregates that had germinal centers (secondary follicles) the B cells were Bcl-2-negative[91]. Isomaki *et al* made a similar comparison in different lymphocyte subsets in tissues from 13 RA, 7 osteoarthritis, and 12 reactive arthritis patients. Bcl-2-positive lymphocytes were observed in tissue from all the different forms of arthritis, except that in reactive arthritis the positive cells were scattered about the synovium, instead of being situated in aggregates. Interestingly, they also found that in B cell-rich lymphoid follicles the central areas were Bcl-2-negative, whereas the remainder stained positive, a staining pattern similar to that which is seen in normal lymphoid germinal centers[88]. Bcl-2 protein expression by synovial lymphocytes may represent a selection and survival process that could play a role in the persistence of chronic articular inflammation and resistance to therapy. The discordance between the phenotype of RA synovial tissue lymphoctyes (Bcl-2 high) and synovial fluid lymphocytes (Bcl-2 low) means that they are either different cell populations or that different conditions in the two compartments favor the retention and/or downregulation of *bcl-2*. Regardless of the explanation, it is an important reminder that conclusions drawn from analysis of

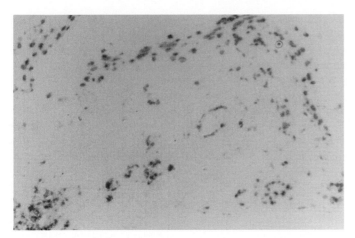

Fig. 12.7 Frozen section of RA synovial tissue showing fragmented DNA (*in situ* end labeling assay) accumulated in the intimal lining and vascular endothelium. The tissue was counter stained only with eosin so that normal nuclei are not visualized, but dark nuclei with fragmented DNA are apparent (×200) Ref. 73.

synovial fluid T cell may not reflect what is going on in the RA synovium. Moreover, the expression of *bcl-2* and the absence of DNA strand breaks in lymphoid aggregates implies that although the T cells appear activated, they may, in fact, have been retained in this location for long periods of time with little turnover or replacement.

Synovial tissue—p53 expression

DNA strand breaks, the hallmark of apoptosis, are common in the lining cells in rheumatoid arthritis and in some samples up to 50 per cent of cells stain positively by *in situ* end labelling (Fig. 12.7). The extent of DNA strand breaks is striking, particularly with the knowledge that only a small number of the lining cells show morphological evidence of complete apoptosis[73]. Because apoptotic cells are cleared very rapidly (usually 1 per cent per hour which extrapolates to 25 per cent of a tissue removed per day) a careful electromicroscopic examination of macrophage-like (type A) synoviocytes was performed, but ingested apoptotic nuclei were not found[74]. An alternative explanation for an inappropriate response to DNA breaks could be an abnormality in the events downstream of DNA damage. An obvious candidate is the p53 tumor suppressor.

Regulatory factors controlling p53 gene expression and/or protein redistribution are not fully understood, but agents that damage DNA (ultraviolet and gamma radiation, hypoxia, oxygen and nitrogen radicals, and oncogene products that control cell proliferation, such as c-myc) all enhance p53 expression[27–29]. The p53 tumor suppressor was named the 'guardian of the genome' because p53 expression increases in response to DNA damage and subsequent cell cycle prolongation permits DNA repair, or if the damage is severe, directs the cell into an apoptotic pathway. Although p53 is a normal constituent of cells, it is rarely detected because of its short half-life (less than 20 minutes). Therefore, in any cross sectional analysis of a tissue, such as the synovium, the protein is rarely demonstrated, unless mutations or other mechanisms of post-translational sta-

bilization prolong its half-life[92,93]. For this reason, the finding of significant quantities of immunoreactive p53 in the rheumatoid synovium was surprising[94,95], although recent data suggest that chronic inflammation can increase p53[96]. The prominent localization to the synovial intimal lining, precisely the region of significant DNA damage, prompted *in vitro* studies of cultured RA synovial fibroblasts. In flow cytometry studies, FLS were shown to express p53 constituitively and western blot analyses for whole synovial tissue and cultured synovial fibroblasts. The RA FLS contain substantially more p53 protein than OA FLS, while dermal fibroblasts show no constitutive p53 expression. Exposure of FLS to reactive oxygen altered intracellular p53 distribution, translocating it from the cytoplasm to the nucleus[94]. Given the abundance of p53 protein in the rheumatoid joint, the modest level of apoptosis in RA is even more surprising. One possible explanation is that p53 persists and is detected because the protein expressed in the joint is abnormal. Similar phenomena are associated with expanded cell populations in tumors, where p53 mutations directly interfere with growth arrest and apoptosis. If this was the case in RA, then p53 mutations could, in combination with other factors, lead to partial transformation of the fibroblast-like synoviocytes (reviewed in Ref. 97).

The synovial fibroblast conundrum

The idea that FLS are 'transformed' in RA is not new[97]. Almost 10 years ago cultured synoviocytes were observed to grow in an anchorage-independent manner and to form foci, reflecting a loss of contact inhibition[98]. Another feature suggesting cell transformation is the expression of immediate early response genes of the jun and fos proto-oncogene families. Cells with a fibroblast morphology expressing high levels of *jun-B* and *c-fos* are found, usually in the synovium within the lining layer. OA and normal joint tissue show similar immunohistological findings, but there are lesser numbers of positive cells and staining is less[97]. Cultured FLS, as well as type B synoviocytes *in situ*, express oncogenes characteristic of cells that have escaped normal growth regulatory mechanisms. One of the most important is *c-myc*, a critical signal that initiates cell proliferation and can independently induce p53 gene expression[99–101].

Transformation of eukaryotic cells refers to their conversion to a state of unrestrained growth in culture. This feature of FLS and the expression of proto-oncogenes does not necessarily imply infection with agents, such as viruses, or mutations in critical genetic material. Rather, there are reports that exposure to pro-inflammatory cytokines can 'imprint' a transformed phenotype on fibroblasts[102,103]. This new phenotype persists through many passages in culture, but the cells are seldom immortalized. Evidence that FLS might be irreversibly altered, long after removal from the articular inflammatory milieu, comes from studies of cell migration and invasion in the absence of exogenous stimulation. When enzymatically-dispersed synovial tissues are injected into the joints of SCID mice[104] or coimplanted with cartilage beneath the renal capsule, there is cartilage invasion which looks like destructive pannus[105]. Since SCID mice lack an immune system and can accept xenografts for long periods of time without introducing their own immune cells, this system allows an analysis of the participation of individual types of cells. Isolated populations of long-term cultured RA FLS cause destruction of cartilage matrix weeks or months later[106]. Synoviocytes from OA patients and normal dermal fibroblasts do not invade the cartilage. Similar results have been observed *in vitro* with articular cartilage explants or artificial matrices[107,108]. For instance long-term cultured RA FLS migrate into such a matrix about four-fold more efficiently than do ligament fibroblasts[107].

The combination of multiple DNA strand breaks, minimal apoptotic morphology in the cells with strand breaks, and over-expression of p53 protein in the same area, led to a hypothesis that alteration in the structure or function of p53 might contribute to the transformed phenotype of RA synoviocytes[109]. By employing a sensitive molecular technique (RNA mismatch detection assay—RMDA) synovial tissues obtained at joint replacement surgery from RA patients with severe and chronic rheumatoid arthritis could be shown to contain mutant p53 transcripts. Similar transcripts were subsequently identified in cultured synoviocytes from rheumatoid joints. Synovium and skin from patients with OA did not have p53 mismatches. The mutations were limited to the joint, because studies of blood samples and skin from the RA patients who provided the joint samples showed no mutant transcripts. When the products of the initial RT-PCR were subcloned and reevaluated by the RMDA technique a variety of mismatch patterns were observed suggesting that more one mutation was present within each RA joint tissue. Because only single clones were studied in the second round, the sensitivity issues due to mixtures of normal and mutant p53 observed in the first round RMDA were not encountered. When the single clones derived in the second round were sequenced, greater than 80 per cent of the mutations identified in both synovium and cultured synoviocytes were G/A and T/C transitions. Such mutations, now reported by others[110], are characteristic of oxidative deamination by NO or oxygen radicals, supporting the proposition that a genotoxic environment in the chronically inflamed RA synovium leads to mutations in the p53 gene[96]. Many of the predicted amino acid substitutions are identical to or in the same location (exons 5–10) as those observed in a variety of tumors[111–113]. Although 40 per cent of the second round mismatches isolated from RA synovium had mutations, this does not mean that a similar frequency of cells in the joints have mutations, because a minority population might produce a disproportionately large fraction of the p53 mRNA.

To test whether specific alterations in the p53 gene (or perhaps other genes that regulate apoptosis or the cell cycle) can contribute to the autonomy of synoviocytes and disease perpetuation, site directed mutagenesis was used to make two transcripts previously identified in RA tissues. Dermal fibroblasts with wild type p53 were transfected with the rheumatoid p53 mutations. They behaved in a dominant negative manner and suppressed endogenous wild type p53. Thus, by analogy, similar mutations could alter the function of synovial cells[114]. This question has also been addressed by transducing cultured RA FLS expressing wild type p53 with a retroviral vector encoding the E6 protein from human papilloma virus (HPV) 18. The E6 protein binds to p53 and inhibits its transcriptional activity and decreases intracellular p53 levels by activating the ubiquitin protease system. Controls included FLS lines transfected with recombinant retrovirus encoding just the neomycin resistance gene and non-treated parental strains. The E6 transfected cells grew faster than the controls, their response to PDGF was significantly greater, and they were less susceptible to dying when exposed to hydrogen peroxide or nitric oxide. E6 FLS invaded more into cartilage extracts than neomycin resistant controls or parental strains[115]. Thus, dysregulation of p53 function in RA synoviocytes could contribute to lining expansion and joint destruction through increased proliferation, invasiveness, and impaired apoptosis.

The p53 mutations in RA synovial fibroblasts are somatic and limited to the joint; therefore, the precipitating factors must also reside in the joint. Repetitive ischemia–reperfusion injury is a characteristic of the inflamed joint[71]. Tissue injury releases iron and copper ions and heme-proteins that are catalytic for free radicals[116]. Electron transport chains are also disrupted in the mitochondria and endoplasmic reticulum leading to leakage of electrons to form superoxide(O_2^-)[116]. Cytokines or bacterial products can substantially increase inducible NO synthase (NOS2) and nitrite levels are elevated in the synovial fluid of RA patients[117,118]. Thus, inflamed joint tissues likely represents a genotoxic environment with resultant DNA damage. One consequence is over-expression of the p53 gene and protein. If the inflammation in RA is severe enough, p53 mutation, and probably mutations in other cell cycle and tumor suppressor genes, will be observed. Such mutations might explain, in part, the high p53 expression, the transformed phenotype of FLS, and inadequate apoptosis in synovial mesenchymal tissues[96]. It remains to be seen whether the clones with p53 mutation and clones that show a transformation phenotype are one and the same and whether a similar paradigm exists in other forms of chronic inflammation.

Synovial fibroblasts are generally considered to be a homogeneous population. Thus their 'transformed' features, namely growth in suspension or in semisolid medium, loss of contact inhibition, invasiveness, and the presence of transcription factors that regulate DNA synthesis, are generally ascribed to all the cells in a culture[94]. However, fibroblasts in general, and FLS in particular, are notoriously difficult to clone, and it is possible that the transformed phenotype might belong to a minority population. For instance, pannus tissue probably contains more than one type of mesenchymal cell. A group of cells that directly erode cartilage can be isolated from RA pannus. They have features of both FLS and chondrocytes and were called pannocytes (PC) because of their location. PC exhibit a distinctive-rhomboid morphology, grow in culture for long periods without becoming senescent, constituitively express large amounts of functional VCAM-1 and are more responsive to factors that favor growth of chondrocytes[119].

Xue identified a similar cell in cultured synoviocytes grown in semisolid agarose medium. By picking those cells that showed loss of contact inhibition a population was isolated that had the morphological appearance of pannocytes and the phenotype of FLS. In addition, they expressed the type II collagen gene and produced proteoglycans, features of chondrocytes. Synovial samples from OA showed no evidence of similar cells[120]. A small percent of the cells growing in soft agar formed clones and proliferated enough to provide DNA for analysis. The DNA of synoviocytes that grew in a monolayer was polyclonal; while the synoviocytes that formed colonies showed a monoclonal expansion. The cells obtained from pannus lesions also produced more TGF-β and PDGF than did synoviocytes from non-pannus areas, perhaps accounting for their growth advantage[121]. Additional support for the idea that FLS are not homogenous comes from the observation that an antibody to bone morphogenetic protein receptors, usually found on primitive mesenchymal cells, stains a small population of large cells in the RA synovial lining and at the carilage pannus junction (Zvaifler, personal observation). In the bone marrow similar cells function as pluripotent mesenchymal stromal cells. Whether marrow stromal cells participate in proliferation of the joint lining and in the destruction of cartilage remains to be shown, but their detection is further evidence that synovial lining cells are not a single population.

References

1. Kerr, J.F., Wyllie, A.H., Currie, A.R. Apoptosis: a basic biological phenomenon with wide-ranging implications in tissue kinetics. *Br J Cancer*, 1972;26:239–257.
2. Wyllie, A.H. Apoptosis: an overview. *Br. Med. Bull*, 1977;53:451–465.
3. Majno, Q., Joris, I. Apoptosis, oncosis and necrosis: An overview of cell death. *Am. J. Pathol*, 1995;146:3–15.
4. Wyllie, A.H. The 1992 Frank Rose Memorial Lecture. *Br J Cancer*, 1993;67:205–208.
5. Haslett, C. Granulocyte apoptosis and inflammatory disease. *Br Med Bull*, 1997;53:669–683.
6. Wyllie, A.H., Morris, R.G., Smith, A.L., Dunlop, D. Chromatin cleavage in apoptosis: association with condensed chromatin morphology and dependence on macromolecular synthesis. *J Pathol*, 1984;142:67–77.
7. McGahon, A.J., Martin, S.J., Bissonnette, R.P. The end of the (cell) line: Methods for the study of apoptosis in vitro. In: Schwartz, L.M., Osborne, B.A., eds., *Methods in Cell Biology, Vol. 46 Cell Death*, New York, Academic Press (1984), p. 153.
8. Vaux, D.L., Strasser, A. The molecular biology of apoptosis. *Proc Natl Acad Sci USA*, 1996;93:2239–2244.
9. Nagata, S. Apoptosis by death factor. *Cell*. 88, 355–365 (1997).
10. Suda, T., Takahashi, T., Golstein, P., Nagata, S. Molecular cloning and expression of the Fas ligand, a novel member of the tumor necrosis factor family. *Cell*, 1993;75:1169–1178.
11. Kayagaki, N., Kawasaki, A., Ebata, T., Ohmoto, H., Ikeda, S., Inoue, S., Yoshino, K., Okumura, K., Yagita, H. Metalloproteinase-mediated release of human Fas ligand. *J Exp Med*, 1995;182:1777–1783.
12. Tanaka, M., Itai, T., Adachi, M., Nagata, S. Downregulation of Fas ligand by shedding. *Nat. Med.*, 1998;4:31–36.
13. Strasser, A, O'Connor, L. Fas ligand—caught between Scylla and Charybdis *Nat. Med*, 1998;4, 21–22.
14. Zou, H., Henzel, W.J., Liu, X., Lutschg, A., Wang, X. Apaf-1, a human protein homologous to C. elegans CED-4, participates in cytochrome c-dependent activation of caspase-3. *Cell*, 1997;90:405-413.
15. Stellar, H. Artifical death switches: Induction of apoptosis by chemically induced caspase multimerization. *Proc. Natl. Acad. Sci. USA*, 1998;95:5421-5422.
16. Halliwell, B., Gutteridge, J.M. *Free Radicals in Biology and Medicine*. Oxford; New York, Clarendon Press; Oxford University Press, (1989).
17. Baggiolini, M., Wymann, M.P. Turning on the respiratory burst. *Trends. Biochem Sci,* 1990;15:69–72.
18. Kane, D.J., Sarafian, T.A., Anton, R., Hahn, H., Gralla, E.B., Valentine, J.S., Ord, T., Bredesen, D.E. Bcl-2 inhibition of neural death: decreased generation of reactive oxygen species. *Science,* 1993;262:1274–1277.
19. Hengarther, M.O., Horvitz, H.R. C. elegans cell survival gene ced-9 encodes a functional homolog of the mammalian proto-oncogene bcl-2. *Cell,* 1994;76:665–676.
20. Kroemer, G. The proto-oncogene Bcl-2 and its role in regulating apoptosis. *Nat. Med,* 1997;3:614–620.
21. Reed, J.C. Bcl-2 and the regulation of programmed cell death. *J Cell Biol,* 1994;124:1–6.
22. Yang, E., Korsmeyer, S.J. Molecular thanatopsis: a discourse on the BCL2 family and cell death. *Blood,* 1996;88,:386–401.
23. Zoratti, M., Szabo, I. The mitochondrial permeability transition. *Biochim Biophys Acta,* 1995;1241:139–176.
24. Kroemer, G., Zamzami, N., Susin, S.A. Mitochondrial control of apoptosis. *Immunol Today,* 1997;18:44–51.
25. Yang, J., Liu, X., Bhalla, K., Kim, C.N., Ibrado, A.M., Cai, J., Peng, T.I., Jones, D.P., Wang, X. Prevention of apoptosis by Bcl-2: release of cytochrome c from mitochondria blocked. *Science,* 1997:275:1129–1132.
26. Kluck, R.M., Bossy-Wetzel, E. Green, D.R., Newmeyer, D.D. The release of cytochrome c from mitochondria: a primary site for Bcl-2 regulation of apoptosis. *Science,* 1997;275:1132–1136.
27. Lane, D.P. Cancer. p53, guardian of the genome. *Nature,* 358:15–16 (1992).
28. Vogelstein, B., Kinzler, K.W. p53 function and dysfunction.*Cell* 1992;70:523–526.
29. Levine, A.J. p53, the cellular gatekeeper for growth and divison. *Cell,* 1997;88:323–331.
30. Sionov, R.V., Haupt, Y. Apoptosis by p53: mechanisms, regulation, and clinical implications. *Springer Semin. Immunopathol,* 1995;195:345–362.
31. Clarke, A.R., Purdie, C.A. Thymocyte apoptosis induced by p53 dependent and independent pathways. *Nature,* 1993;362:849–852.
32. Bates, S., Vousden, K.H. p53 in signaling checkpoint arrest or apoptosis. *Curr. Opin. Genet. Dev.* 6:12–18 (1996).
33. El-Deiry, W.S., Harper, J.W., O'Connor, P.M., Velculescu, V.E., Canman, C.E., Jackman, J., Pietenpol, J.A., Burrell, M., Hill, D.E. WAF1-CIP1 is induced in p53-mediated G-1 arrest and apoptosis. *Cancer Res,* 1994; 54:1169–1174.
34. Gottlieb, T.M., Oren, M. p53 in growth control and neoplasia. *Biochim Biophys Acta* 1287, 77 (1996).
35. Guillouf, C., Grana, X., Selvakumaran, M., De Luca, A., Giordano, A., Hoffman, B., Liebermann, D.A.: Dissection of the genetic programs of p53-mediated G1 growth arrest and apoptosis: blocking p53-induced apoptosis unmasks G1 arrest. *Blood,* 1995;85:2691–2698.
36. Hall, P.A., Meek, D., Lane, D.P. p53-intergrating the complexity [editorial]. *Pathol* 180, 1–5 (1996).
37. Velculescu, V.E., El-Deiry, W.S. Biological and clinical importance of the p53 tumor suppressor gene *Clin Chem* 42, 858–868 (1996).
38. Miyashita, T., Reed, J.C. Tumor suppressor p53 is a direct transcriptional activator of the human bax gene. *Cell,* 1995;80:293–299.
39. Firestein, G.S. Rheumatoid synovitis and pannus. In: Klippel, J.H., Dieppe, P.A., eds., *Rheumatology, Vol 1*, London, Mosby International (1998), p. 1.
40. Harris, E.D., Jr. Rheumatoid arthritis *N Engl J Med,* 1990;322:1277–1289.
41. Zvaifler, N.J. The immunopathology of joint inflammation in rheumatoid arthritis. *Adv. Immunol,* 1973;16:265–336.
42. Malinin, T.I., Pekin, T.J.J., Zvaifler, N.J. Cytology of synovial fluid in rheumatoid arthritis. *Am J Clin Pathol,* 1967;47, 203–208.
43. Pekin, T.J.J., Malinin, T.I., Zvaifler, N.J. Unusual synovial fluid findings in Reiter's syndrome. *Ann Intern Med,* 1967;66: 677–684 .

44. Newman, S.L., Henson, J.E., Henson, P.M. Phagocytosis of senescent neutrophils by human monocyte-dervided macrophages and rabbit inflammatory macrophages. *J Exp Med,* 1982;**156**:430–442.

45. Savill, J.I., Wyllie, A.H., Henson, J.E., Walport, M.J., Henson, P.M., Haslett, C. Macrophage phagocytosis of aging neutrophils in inflammation. Programmed cell death in the neutrophil leads to its recognition by macrophages. *J Clin Invest,* 1989;**83**:865–875 .

46. Jones, S.T., Denton, J., Holt, P.J., Freemont, A.J Possible clearance of effete polymorponuclear leucocytes from synovial fluid by cytophagocytic mononuclear cells: implications for pathogenesis and chronicity in inflammatory arthritis. *Ann Rheum Dis,* 1993;**52**:121–126.

47. Fadok, V.A., Bratton, D.L., Konowal, A, Freed, P.W., Westcott, J.Y., Henson, P.M. Macrophages that have ingested apoptotic cells in vitro inhibit proinflammatory cytokine production through autocrine/paracrine mechanisms involving TGF-beta, PGE2, and PAF. *J Clin Invest,* 1998;**101**:890–898.

48. Voll, R.E., Herrmann, M., Roth, E.A., Stach, C., Kalden, J.R., Girkontaite, I. Immunosuppressive effects of apoptotic cells [letter] . *Nature,* 1997;**390**:350–351.

49. Savill, J. Apoptosis. Phagocytic docking without shocking. *Nature,* 1998;**392**:442–443.

50. Devitt, A., Moffatt, O.D., Raykundalia, C., Capra, J.D., Simmons, D.L., Gregory, C.D. Human CD14 mediates recognition and phagocytosis of apoptotic cells. *Nature,* 1998;**392**:505–509.

51. Mevorach, D., Elkon, K. Complement dependent uptake of apoptotic cells by human macrophages. *Arthritis Rheum.* **41**, S244, (1998)(Abstract).

52. Pekin, T.J.J., Zvaifler, N.J. Hemolytic complement in synovial fluid. *J Clin Invest,* 1964;**43**:1372–1382.

53. Jones, S.T.M., Denton, J. Holt, P.J., Freemont, A.J. Cytophagocytic mononuclear cells in rheumatoid synovial fluid indicate a novel form of reactive arthritis. *Br J Rheumatol* **32**, S-A1-93 (1993) (Abstract).

54. Firestein, G.S., Zvaifler, N.J. Peripheral blood and synovial fluid monocyte activation in inflammatory arthritis. I. A cytofluorographic study of monocyte differentiation antigens and class II antigens and their regulation by gamma-interferon. *Arthritis Rheum,* 1987;**30**:857–863.

55. Salmon, M., Gaston, J.S. The role of T-lymphocytes in rheumatoid arthritis. *Br. Med Bull,* 1995;**51**:332–345.

56. Salmon, M., Pilling, D., Borthwick, N.J., Viner, N., Janossy, G., Bacon, P.A., Akbar, A.N. The progressive differentiation of primed T cells is associated with an increasing susceptibility to apoptosis. *Eur j Immunol,* 1994;**24**:892–899.

57. Fox, D.A. The role of T cells in the immunopathogenesis of rheumatoid arthritis: new perspectives. *Arthritis Rheum,* 1997;**40**:598–609.

58. Struyk, L., Hawes, G.E., Chatila, M.K., Breedveld, F.C., Kurnick, J.T., van den Elsen, P.J. T cell receptors in rheumatoid arthritis. *Arthritis Rheum,*1995; **38**:577–589.

59. Firestein, G.S., Zvaifler, N.J. How important are T cells in chronic rheumatoid synovitis? *Arthritis Rheum,* 1990;**33**:768–773.

60. Cush, J.J., Pietschmann, P., Oppenheimer-Marks, N, Lipsky, P.E. The intrinsic migratory capacity of memory T cells contributes to their accumulation in rheumatoid synovium. *Arthritis Rheum,* 1992;**35**:1434–1444.

61. Salmon, M., Scheel-Toellner, D., Huissoon, A.P., Pilling, D., Shamsadeen, N., Hyde, H., D'Angeac, A.D., Bacon, P.A., Emery, P., Akbar, A.N. Inhibition of T cell apoptosis in the rheumatoid synovium. *J Clin Invest,* 1997;**99**:439–446.

62. Firestein, G.S., Xu, W.D., Townsend, K., Broide, D., Alvaro-Gracia, J., Glasebrook, A., Zvaifler, N.J Cytokineas in chronic inflammatory arthritis. I. Failure to detect T cell lymphokines (interleukin 2 and interleukin 3) and presence of macrophage colony-stimulating factor (CSF-1) and a novel mast cell growth factor in rheumatoid synovitis. *J Exp Med,* 1988;**168**:1573–1586.

63. McInnes, I.B., al-Mughales, J., Field, M., Leung, B.P., Huang, F.P., Dixon, R., Sturrock, R.D., Wilkinson, P.C., Liew, F.Y. The role of interleukin-15 in T-cell migration and activation in rheumatoid arthritis. *Nat. Med,* 1996;**2**:175–182.

64. Boise, L.H., Gonzalez-Garcia, M., Postema, C.E., Ding, L., Lindsten, T., Turka, L.A., Mao, X., Nunez, G., Thompson, C.B. bcl-x, a bcl-2-related gene that functions as a dominant regulator of apoptotic cell death. *Cell,* 1993;**74**:597–608.

65. Cantwell, M.J., Hua. T., Zvaifler, N.J., Kipps, T.J. Deficient Fas ligand expression by synovial lymphocytes from patients with rheumatoid arthritis. *Arthritis Rheum,* 1997;**40**:1644–1652.

66. Suda, T., Hashimoto, H., Tanaka, M., Ochi, T., Nagata, S. Membrane Fas ligand kills human peripheral blood T lymphocytes, and soluble Fas ligand blocks the killing. *J Exp Med,* 1997;**186**:2045–2050.

67. Hashimoto, H., Tanaka, M., Suda, T., Tomita, T., Hayashida, K., Takeuchi, E., Kaneko, M., Takano, H., Nagata, S., Ochi, T. Soluble Fas ligand in the joints of patients with rheumtoid arthritis and osteoarthritis. *Arthritis Rheum,* 1998;**41**:657–662.

68. Nagase, H., Cawston, T.E., De Silva, M., Barrett, A.J. Identification of plasma kallikrein as an activator of latent collagenase in rheumatoid synovial fluid. *Biochim Biophys Acta,* 1982;**702**:133–142.

69. Firestein, G.S., Paine, M.M., Littman, B.H. Gene expression (collagenase, tissue inhibitor of metalloproteinases, complement, and HLA-DR) in rheumatoid arthritis and osteoarthritis synovium. Quantitative analysis and effect of intraarticular corticosteroids. *Arthritis Rheum,* 1991;**34**:1094–1105.

70. Maurice, M.M., Nakamura, H., van der Voort, E.A.M., van Vliet, A.I., Staal, F.J.T., Tak, P.P., Breedveld, F.C., Verweji, C.L. Evidence for the role of an altered redox state in hyporesponsiveness of synovial T cells in RA. *Clin Exp Immunol,* 1997;**158**:1458–1465.

71. Blake, D.R., Merry, P., Unsworth, J., Kidd, B.L., Outhwaite, J.M., Ballard, R., Morris, C.J., Gray, L., Lunec, J. Hypoxic-reperfusion injury in the inflamed human joint. *Lancet,* 1989;**1**:289–293.

72. Mountz, J.D., Wu, J., Cheng, J., Zhou, T. Autoimmune disease. A problem of defective apoptosis. *Arthritis Rheum,* 1994;**37**:1415–1420.

73. Firestein, G.S., Yeo, M., Zvaifler, N.J. Apoptosis in rheumatoid arthritis synovium. *J Clin Invest,* 1995;**96**:1631–1638.

74. Matsumoto, S., Muller-Ladner, U., Gay, R.E., Nishioka, K., Gay, S. Ultrastructural demonstration of apoptosis, Fas and Bcl-2 expression of rheumatoid synovial fibroblasts. *J Rheumatol,* 1996;**23**:1345–1352.

75. Nakajima, T., Aono, H., Hasunuma, T., Yamamoto, K., Shirai, T., Hirohata, K., Nishioka, K. Apoptosis and functional Fas antigen in rheumatoid arthritis synoviocytes. *Arthritis Rheum,* 1995;**38**:485–491.

76. Hasunuma, T., Hoa, T.T., Aono, H., Asahara, H., Yonehara, S., Yamamoto, K., Sumida, T., Gay, S., Nishioka, K. Induction of Fas-dependent apoptosis in synovial infiltrating cells in rheumatoid arthritis. *Int Immunol,* 1996;**8**:1595–1602.

77. Ohshima, S., Saeki, Y., Mima, T. Restoration of Fas mediated apoptosis of rheumatoid synovial cells by a monoclonal anti-tumor necrosis factor antibody (cA2). *Proc Natl. Acad. Sci. U.S.A.* 1999 (In Press).

78. Asahara, H., Hasumuna, T., Kobata, T., Yagita, H., Okumura, K., Inoue, H., Gay, S., Sumida, T., Nishioka, K. Expression of Fas antigen and Fas ligand in the rheumatoid synovial tissue. *Clin Immunol Immunopathol,* 1996;**81**:27–34.

79. Kawakami, A., Eguchi, K., Matsuoka, N., Tsuboi, M., Kawabe Y., Aoyagi, T., Nagataki, S. Inhibition of Fas antigen-mediated apoptosis of rheumatoid synovial cells in vitro by transforming growth factor beta 1. *Arthritis Rheum,* 1996;**39**:1267–1276.

80. Akkoc, N., Geiler, T., State, M., Herrmann, M., Hieronymus, T., Lorenz, H., Kalden, J.R. Fas stimulation induces apoptosis in synovial fibroblasts in the presence of protein synthesis inhibition. *Arthritis Rheum.* **41**, S143 (1998) (abstract).

81. Geiler, T., Akkoc, N., State., M., Herrmann, M., Hieronymus, T., Lorenz, H., Kalden, J.R. TNFα induces apoptosis in synovial fibroblasts. *Arthritis Rheum* **41**, S143 (1998) (abstract).

82. Okamoto, K., Kobayashi, T., Kobata., T., Husunuma, T., Sumida, T., Nishioka, K. FADD/caspase-8/caspase-3/PARP pathway is essential for Fas-mediated apoptosis of rheumatoid synoviocytes. *Arthritis Rheum.* 41, S274 (1998)(abstract).

83. Mizushima, N., Kohsaka, H., Miyasaka., N.: Regulation of synovial cell apoptosis by protesome function. *Arthritis Rheum* 41, S277 (1998) (abstract).

84. Mizushima, N., Kohsaka, H., Miyasaka., N. Ceramide, a mediator of interleukin 1, tumor necrosis factor alpha, as well as Fas receptor signaling, induces apoptosis of rheumatoid arthritis synovial cells. *Ann Rheum Dis*, 1998;7:495–499.

85. Zhang, H., Gao, G., Williams., W.V., Wang, G.F., Wilson, J.M., Schumacher, H.R. Effects of Fas ligand (Fas-L) gene transfer on the apoptosis of synovial fibroblasts from rheumatoid arthritis patients in vitro. *Arthritis Rheum.* 41, S142 (1998)(abstract).

86. Zhang, H., Yang, Y., Horton, J.L., Samoilova, E.B., Judge, T.A., Turka, L.A., Wilson, J.M., Chen, Y. Amelioration of collagen-induced arthritis by CD95 (Apo-1/Fas)-ligand gene transfer. *J Clin Invest*, 1997;100:1951–1957.

87. Kazuyoshi, O., Asahara, H., Kobayashi, T., Matsuno, H., Kobata, T., Hasunuma, T., Sumida, T., Nishioka, K. Induction of apoptosis in the rheumatoid synovium by Fas ligand gene transfer. *Arthritis Rheum.* 41, S274 (1998) (abstract)

88. Isomaki, P., Soderstorm, K.O., Punnonen, J., Roivainen, A., Luukkainen, R., Merilahti-Palo, R., Nikkari, S., Lassila, O., Toivanen, P. Expression of bcl-2 in rheumatoid arthritis. *Br J Rheumatol*, 1996;35:611–619.

89. Liang, H.Y., Jiang, M., Chen, H.M., Wang, Y.C. Overexpression of proto-oncogene bcl-2 in rheumatoid synovium [letter]. *Br J Rheumatol*, 1996;35:803–804

90. Schorpp, C., Gause, A. Overexpressi.on and dysregulation of bcl-2 in lymphocyte subpopulations of synovial membrane (letter). *Br. J Rheumatol*, 1997;6:1335–1336.

91. Zdichavksy, M., Schorpp, C., Nickels, A., Koch, B., Pfreundchuh, M., Gause, A. Analysis of bcl-2+ lymphocyte subpopulations in inflammatory synovial infiltrates by a double-immunostaining technique. *Rheumatol Int*, 1996;16:151–157.

92. Reich, N.C., Oren, M., Levine, A.J. Two distinct mechanisms regulate the levels of a cellular tumor antigen, p53. *Mol Cell Biol*, 1983;3:2143–2150.

93. Finlay, C.A., Hinds, P.W., Tan, T.H., Eliyahu, D., Oren, M., Levine, A.J. Activating mutations for transformation by p53 produce a gene product that forms an hsc70-p53 complex with an altered half-life. *Mol Cell Biol*, 1998;8:531–539.

94. Firestein, G.S., Nguyen, K., Aupperle, K.R., Yeo, M., Boyle, D.L., Zvaifler, N.J. Apoptosis in rheumatoid arthritis: p53 overexpression in rheumatoid arthritis synovium. *Am J Pathol*, 1996;149, 2143–2151.

95. Sugiyama, M., Tsukazaki, T., Yonekura, A., Matsuzaki, S., Yamashita, S., Iwasaki, K. Localisation of apoptosis and expression of apoptosis related proteins in the synovium of patients with rheumatoid arthritis. *Ann Rheum Dis*, 1996;55:442–449.

96. Tak, P.P., Zvaifler, N.J., Green, D.R., Firestein, G.S. Rheumatoid arthritis and p53: How oxidative stress might alter the course of an inflammatory disease. *Immunol Today*, 2000;21:71–82.

97. Firestein, G.S. Invasive fibroblast-like synoviocytes in rheumatoid arthritis. Passive responders or transformed aggressors? *Arthritis Rheum*, 1996;39:1781–1790.

98. Lafyatis, R., Remmers, E.F., Roberts, A.B., Yocum, D.E., Sporn, M.B., Wilder, R.L. Anchorage-independent growth of synoviocytes from arthritis and normal joints. Stimulation by exogenous platelet-derived growth factor and inhibition by transforming growth factor-beta and retinoids. *J Clin Invest*, 1989;83: 1267–1276.

99. Trabandt, A., Gay, R.E., Gay, S. Oncogene activation in rheumatoid synovium. *APMIS*, 1992;100:861–875.

100. Ritchlin, C., Dwyer, E., Bucala, R., Winchester, R. Sustained and distinctive patterns of gene activation in synovial fibroblasts and whole synovial tissue obtained from inflammatory synovitis. *Scand. J Immunol*, 1994;40:292–298.

101. Qu, Z., Garcia, C.H., O'Rourke, L.M., Planck, S.R., Kohli, M., Rosenbaum, J.T. Local profileration of fibroblast-like synoviocytes contributes to synovial hyperplasia. Results of profilerating cell nuclear antigen/cyclin, c-myc, and nucleolar organizer region staining. *Arthritis Rheum*, 1994;37:212–220.

102. Buckingham, R.B., Castor, C.W. Rheumatoid behavior in normal human synovial fibroblasts induced by extracts of Gram-negative bacteria. *J Lab Clin Med*, 1975;85:422–435.

103. Korn, J. Fibroblast prostaglandin E2 synthesis. Persistance of an abnormal phenotype after short term exposure to mononuclear cell products. *J Clin Invest*, 1983;71:1240.

104. Rendt. K.E., Barry, T.S., Jones, D.M., Richter, C.B., McCachren, S.S., Haynes, B.F. Engraftment of human synovium into severe combined immune deficient mice. Migration of human peripheral blood T cells to engrafted human synovium and to mouse lymph nodes. *J Immunol*, 1993;151:7324–7336.

105. Sack. U., Kuhn, H., Ermann, J., Kinne, R.W., Vogt, S., Jungmichel, D., Emmrich, F. Synovial tissue implants from patients with rheumatoid arthritis cause cartilage destruction in knee joints of SCID.bg mice. *J Rheumatol*, 1994;21:10–16.

106. Muller-Ladner, U., Kriegsmann, J., Franklin, B.N., Matsumoto, S., Geiler, T., Gay, R.E., Gay, S. Synovial fibroblasts of patients with rheumatoid arthritis attach to and invade normal human cartilage when engrafted into SCID mice. *Am J Pathol*, 1996;149: 1607–1615.

107. Schultz, O., Keyszer, G., Zacher, J., Sittinger, M., Burmester, G.R. Development of in vitro model systems for destructive joint disease: novel strategies for establishing inflammatory pannus. *Arthritis Rheum*, 1997;40:1420–1428.

108. Frye, C.A., Tuan, R., Yocum, D.E., Hendrix, M.J.C An in vitro model for studying mechanisms underlying cartilage destruction associated with rheumatoid arthritis. *Pathol Oncol Res*, 1996;2: 157–166.

109. Firestein, G.S., Echeverri, F., Yeo, M., Zvaifler, N.J., Green, D.R. Somatic mutations in the p53 tumor suppressor gene in rheumatoid arthritis synovium. *Proc Natl. Acad. Sci. USA* 1997;94, 10895–10900.

110. Reme, T., Travaglio, A., Gueydon, E., Adla, L., Jorgensen, C., Sany, J. Mutations of the p53 tumour suppressor gene in erosive rheumatoid synovial tissue. *Clin Exp ImmunoL*, 1998;111: 353–358.

111. Hollstein, M., Sidrensky, D., Vogelstein, B., Harris, C.C. p53 mutations in human cancers. *Science*, 1998;253:49–53.

112. Wink, D.A., Kasprzak, K.S., Maragos, C.M., Elespuru, R.K., Misra, M., Dunams, T.M., Cebula, T.A., Koch, W.H., Andrews, A.W., Allen, J.S. DNA deaminating ability and genotoxicity of nitric oxide and its progenitors. *Science*, 1991;254:1001–1003.

113. Nguyen, T., Brunson, D., Crespi, C.L., Penman, B.W., Wishnok, J.S., Tannenbaum, S.R. DNA damage and mutation in human cells exposed to nitric oxide in vitro. *Proc Natl. Acad. Sci. USA*, 1992;89:3030–3034.

114. Han, J., Boyle, D.L., Shi, Y., Green, D., Firestein, G.S. Dominant negative p53 mutations in rheumatoid arthritis. *Am J Pathol*. (1999) (In Press).

115. Aupperle, K.R., Boyle, D.L., Hendrix, M., Seftor, E.A., Zvaifler, N.J., Barbosa, M., Firestein, G.S. Regulation of synoviocyte proliferation, apoptosis, and invasion by the p53 tumor suppressor gene. *Am J Pathol*, 1998;152:1091–1098.

116. Halliwell, B. Oxygen radicals, nitric oxide and human inflammatory joint disease. *Ann Rheum Dis*. 54, 505–510 (1995).

117. Sakurai, H., Kohsaka, H., Liu, M.F., Higashiyama, H., Hirata, Y., Kanno, K., Saito, I., Miyasaka, N. Nitric oxide production and inducible nitric oxide synthase expression in inflammatory arthritides. *J Clin Invest*, 1995;96:2357–2363.

118. Farrell, A.J., Blake, D.R., Palmer, R.M., Moncada, S. Increased concentrations of nitrite in synovial fluid and serum samples suggest increased nitric oxide synthesis in rheumatic disease. *Ann Rheum Dis*, 1992;51:1219–1222.

119. Zvaifler, N.J., Tsai, V., Alsalameh, S., von Kempis, J., Firestein, G.S., Lotz, M. Pannocytes: distinctive cells found in rheumatoid

arthritis articular cartilage erosions. *Am J Pathol,* 1997;**150**: 1125–1138.

120. Xue, C., Takahashi, M., Husunuma, T., Aono, H., Yamamoto, K., Yoshino, S., Sumida, T., Nishioka, K. Characterisation of fibroblastlike cells in pannus lesions of patients with rheumatoid

arthritis sharing properties of fibroblasts and chondrocytes. *Ann Rheum Dis,* 1997;**56**:262–267.

121. Imamura, F., Aono, H., Hasunuma, T., Sumida, T., Tateishi, H., Maruo, S., Nishioka, K. Monoclonal expansion of synoviocytes in rheumatoid arthritis. *Arthritis Rheum,* 1998;**41**:1979–1986.

13 | Rheumatoid factor

Diego Kyburz and Dennis A. Carson

Introduction

The term rheumatoid factor (RF) denotes autoantibodies specific for antigenic epitopes on the Fc portion of immunoglobulin G (IgG) antibodies. Generally, rheumatoid factors are associated with rheumatoid arthritis (RA). However, they are not restricted to patients with RA but can also be detected in a variety of other autoimmune and lymphoproliferative disorders and occur in a proportion of normal individuals[1]. Evidence for a physiological function of RF in normal individuals derives from the demonstration that RF specificity can be part of the natural antibody repertoire during early fetal life as well as the fact that RF production is common following immunization.

The rheumatoid factors found in rheumatoid arthritis are, in general, of higher affinity and show specificity for human IgG, whereas the ones associated with other diseases are of lower affinity and polyspecific. Rheumatoid factors are usually of the IgM isotype, however in rheumatoid arthritis IgG, IgA, and IgE RFs can also be detected. Levels of rheumatoid factor may correlate with disease activity and prognosis in rheumatoid arthritis[2].

Antibody structure and Ig genes

Immunoglobulin (Ig) molecules have a tetrameric structure with two identical light and two identical heavy chains. Whereas the light chains are equal for all Ig classes, the heavy chains are different for the five isotypes: IgG, IgA, IgM, IgE, and IgD. IgG, IgD, and IgE are composed of one tetrameric subunit, IgA of two, and IgM of five tetrameric subunits. IgM is therefore decavalent. Each heavy and light chain comprises several structural domains. The domains on the N-terminus of the various chains are called variable since their amino acid sequence varies between antibodies of different specificities. The antigen binding site of an antibody is formed by the combined variable domains of the light and heavy chains. Light chain variable regions exist in two forms, κ and λ, and are generated by recombination between two clusters of gene segments, Vκ or Vλ, and Jκ or Jλ. The heavy chain V regions result from recombination between three gene segment clusters: VH + DH + JH. Each of the clusters contains many different gene segments. By this random recombination process, and the random pairing between kappa or lambda light chain V region genes and heavy chain V region genes, an enormous diversity of the antigen recognition structure is generated. This diversity accounts for the vast range of specificities found in the B-cell repertoire.

Table 13.1 Methods for detection of rheumatoid factor

A IgM RF
1. Agglutination reaction of IgG coated particles
sheep red blood cells (Rose-Waaler test) rabbit IgG coated
latex or bentonite particles human IgG coated
2. Precipitation with soluble aggregated IgG in solution or gel
3. Immunoassays using anti-Ig antibodies
ELISA
RIA
immunofluorescence
4. Immunoabsorption in IgG columns
B IgG RF
1. Analytical ultracentrifugation
2. Same methods as for IgM RF detection after separation from IgM RF by gel filtration, ion exchange chromatography, affinity chromatography, pepsin digestion

Detection methods

The same methods used for measurement of antibodies against exogenous antigens can be applied for the detection of RF (Table 13.1). The first method developed for the detection of IgM RF was the sensitized sheep cell agglutination assay (SSCA), also named Rose–Waaler reaction after its inventors. The assay takes advantage of the fact that the pentameric IgM RFs are efficient agglutinators of antigen-coated particles. The sheep red blood cells used in this assay are coated with subagglutinating quantities of rabbit IgG antibody and are crosslinked in the presence of IgM RF to produce a visible flocculus[3,4]. Although still one of the best methods to detect IgM RF, the SSCA has mostly been replaced by other agglutination tests using latex or bentonite particles passively loaded with aggregated pooled human IgG[5]. The agglutination reactions are semiquantitative tests where the titer of IgM RF in a serum is expressed as the highest dilution yielding a visible agglutination. The development of nephelometry allowed for a more accurate determination of IgM RF titers using agglutination assays[6]. In general, the titers in the SSCA are lower than in the latex fixation because the rabbit IgG used in the SSCA only shares some antigenic determinants with the putative autoantigen human IgG against which RF is directed. Seroepidemiological studies, however, indicated a higher specificity for RA of the SSCA compared to the latex fixation[7,8]. The reason for this might be that rabbit IgG as a cross-reacting antigen binds only to RF of higher affinity and of higher titer and that it does not bear allotypic specificities against which some autoantibodies in normal individuals are directed.

Other techniques capable of detecting RF include immunoassays such as the radioimmunoassay (RIA) and the enzyme linked immunosorbent assay (ELISA)[9]. In both RIA and ELISA, solid phase bound human or rabbit IgG are used which bind to IgM RF in the serum. In the RIA, the bound RF is detected with radiolabelled anti-IgM antibody, and in the ELISA an antibody coupled to an enzyme is used. The immunoassays are much more sensitive than agglutination assays, allowing detection of RF in sera diluted 1000–100 000 fold.

There are several major drawbacks of the common assays for IgM RF. Monomeric, and particularly aggregated IgG, in serum and synovial fluid compete with the IgG detection reagent for binding to RF. Sera can therefore test negative because the binding sites of the RF molecules are saturated with autologous IgG. Such 'hidden' RF can be revealed by separation of the IgM and IgG fractions by gel filtration under dissociating conditions[10]. Similarly the C1q complement component agglutinates IgG-coated particles and should be inactivated prior to the assay[11]. Furthermore, the titers measured depend not only on the concentration of the IgM RF but also on its affinity. Consequently a large number of IgM RF molecules with low affinity or a small number with high affinity may give rise to the same titer in the IgM RF assay.

The detection of IgG RF, which occurs in serum as well as synovial fluids of many patients with severe rheumatoid arthritis[12,13], poses even more difficulties (Table 13.2). Divalent IgG RF is a poor agglutinator compared with the decavalent IgM RF. Also, because of the multivalency, IgM RF has a much higher avidity for aggregated than monomeric IgG, compared with IgG RF. Finally, since the antigenic determinants on the Fc fragment of IgG with which IgG RF react reside in the antibody molecules themselves, the sensitivity of the assay is further decreased by the tendency of IgG RF to self-associate instead of binding aggregated IgG. IgG RF is definitively detected by analytic or preparative ultracentrifugation by their characteristic sedimentation profile as intermediate complexes, which are the actual product of *in vivo* complex formation[14,15]. To determine the IgG RF in routine assays such as ELISA or RIA, IgM RF must be removed or destroyed to avoid false positive results.

This is achieved by gel filtration, ion exchange chromatography, or digestion with the proteolytic enzyme pepsin. The latter destroys the crystallizable Fc portion of IgG, thereby releasing IgG RF from self-associating complexes.

IgA rheumatoid factors can be detected in sera using immuno-electrophoresis, quantitative immunoabsorption, and ELISA and RIA methods by using class-specific anti-immunoglobulin reagents to distinguish them from IgM RF. Because IgA molecules circulate as monomers or dimers they do not bind as efficiently to aggregated IgG as do IgM RF. In rheumatoid arthritis patients and those with sicca syndrome, IgA RF is also found in the saliva[16,17].

It should be noted that IgM RF is the only isotype for which standardized, validated assays exist and for which there is an indication for routine testing. A positive IgM RF is one of several diagnostic criteria for establishing the diagnosis of RA. No indications for a routine testing of IgG RF have been established, although the determination of IgG RF levels can be helpful in monitoring response to therapy in patients with rheumatoid vasculitis or hyperviscosity syndrome[18].

Immunogenetic properties of RF

Antigenic specificities and affinities of RF

Polyclonal IgM RF from rheumatoid arthritis patient sera reacts with diverse antigenic determinants within the CH2 and CH3 domains of the Fc portion of the IgG molecule. Evidence from extensive studies indicates that an isotypic antigen expressed on IgG1, 2, and 4 but not on IgG3, the Ga determinant, represents the main specificity of RF in the serum[19,20]. However, subclass specificities may differ between synovium-derived and serum-derived rheumatoid factors. While serum RF reacts only weakly with IgG3 and most strongly with IgG1, IgG2, and IgG4, synovial antibodies derived from RA patients bind more strongly to IgG3 than to IgG1, IgG2, and IgG4. On the other hand, monospecific RF shows preferential binding to IgG3 and IgG4, whereas polyreactive RF tends to react equally with all subclasses[21]. Comparison of RF specificities by mapping IgG epitopes reveals novel specificities of some RF from RA patients

Table 13.2 Comparison of rheumatoid factors of the IgM and IgG class

Property	IgM RF	IgG RF
Valence for IgG	10	2
Intrinsic affinity for antigen (liters/mole)	1×10^7	$1 \times 10^4 - 5 \times 10^5$
Agglutination of IgG-coated latex particles	strong	weak
Enhanced binding to aggregated IgG	marked	moderate
Usual sedimentation constants in ultracentrifuge	19S–22S	10S–18S
Self-association	no	yes
Binding to IgG after treatment with:		
reducing agents	decreased	unchanged
pepsin	decreased	unchanged or increased

as opposed to healthy immunized donors or individuals with Waldenström's macroglobulinemia[19,22–25]. In one study, clinically severe arthritis was associated with the presence of IgG3-reactive RF[26]. Such antibodies with unique specificities may represent disease-specific autoantibodies in patients with RA.

The affinity of RF for the Fc part of IgG varies between patients with lymphoproliferative diseases and RA patients. In mixed cryoglobulinemia or Waldenström's macroglobulinemia, the monoclonal IgM RF is of low affinity. Dissociation constants (K_d) lie between 10^{-4} and 10^{-5} M[27,28]. In patients with RA, a majority of IgM RF are of higher affinity with (K_d) of 10^{-7} [27,29]. Because of the multivalency of IgM RF, even low affinity RF molecules are able to form stable complexes with IgG antigen if it is in complexed form. In this case, the individual weak bonds of the IgM–IgG aggregate add up to yield a stable complex.

IgG RF, in contrast to all other autoantibodies, has the unique ability to self-associate to form immune complexes even in the absence of exogenous antigen[30,31]. This process depends on the concentration and affinity of the autoantibody and of the ratio of IgG rheumatoid factor to normal IgG. By cross-linking aggregated IgG, IgM RF may additionally enhance the formation of IgG RF complexes.

RF binding is further influenced by the degree of glycosylation. Glycosylation is an important post-translational modification of proteins and has been demonstrated to influence biological properties of proteins such as functional activity, pharmacokinetics, immunogenicity, etc. In normal individuals, the levels of aglycosylated IgG are age-related[32]. A different glycosylation pattern of serum IgG with a shift to the agalactosylated form, where the terminal galactose is not present on the glycosylation site of the CH2 domain, has been described for RA[33]. Agalactosylation early in the disease is associated with a more progressive disease course[34] and may correlate with active disease[35]. In several studies, the absence of galactose on IgG Fc did not influence binding of mono- or polyclonal IgM RF[36–39]. Other studies found increased binding of IgG3 reactive monoclonal and polyclonal RF to agalactosyl IgG3 as opposed to the glycosylated form[23,40]. However, in contrast to the IgG2 and less so the IgG1 and 4 subclasses, there is no difference in glycosylation of the IgG3 subclass between RA patients and normal individuals. Because of preferential binding of RF to agalactosyl IgG3, the resulting immune complexes might be cleared from circulation, thereby accounting for the similar levels of agalacto-IgG3 in normals and RA patients. The influence, if any, of glycosylation on RF binding is not clearly established at the present time and needs further investigation. In this context it is worth mentioning that the X-ray crystallographic analysis of a RF-IgG-Fc complex revealed that the carbohydrate moiety itself does not seem to be involved in the RF recognition of Fc[41].

Idiotypic analysis and immunoglobulin V-region usage

To gain insight into the process of induction and maintenance of RF production, investigators have studied the clonality and mutational patterns of RF V-genes. The aim was to find out whether the genes were in germline configuration, indicating whether the genes were in germline configuration, indicating non-specific polyclonal B cell activation, or whether somatic mutation had occurred, indicating derivation from antigen-selected B cells.

The increased affinity of antibodies to antigen in the course of an immune response is termed affinity maturation. The maturation process consists of mutations of the DNA encoding the antigen binding site of the antibody molecule, resulting in amino acid replacements[42]. Through selection pressure, B cells with high affinity receptors are selected for expansion. The mutations in the V-region genes found in these positively-selected B cells typically show elevated replacement to-silent-ratios [43]. It was possible to determine the influence of somatic mutation on the V gene repertoire of RF by comparing V-region sequences of high affinity RF in RA with low affinity RF derived from patients with lymphoproliferative diseases. Before the development of hybridoma technology, the only RFs that could be studied in humans were the monoclonal IgM RF isolated from patients suffering from the lymphoproliferative disorders Waldenström's macroglobulinemia or mixed cryoglobulinemia. An anti-IgG autoantibody activity of monoclonal IgM is observed in nearly 10 per cent of unrelated patients with Waldenström's macroglobulinemia[44]. Structural studies on these RFs using polyclonal antisera recognizing cross reactive idiotypes (CRI) demonstrated that the variable regions are relatively uniform between unrelated RF autoantibodies[45]. The structural basis of this restricted idiotypic specificity is the preferential usage of certain light chain genes in or near germline configuration. Using murine monoclonal antibodies it was found that high percentages of RFs in paraproteinemias express idiotypes recognized by the monoclonal antibodies 17.109 and 6B6.6, that are markers for the Vκ325 and Vκ328 subgroup genes[28,44,46,47]. These light chains preferentially associate with VH1 and VH4 heavy chains[44,48]. Such natural antibodies display low affinity for human IgG[27,28] and are generally polyspecific, reacting with a wide variety of both self and exogenous antigens[27,28,49,50].

With progress in hybridoma technology in recent years, many monoclonal RFs from RA patient sera or synovial tissues as well as from healthy individuals have been generated. The analysis of V-gene usage of RF in healthy immunized individuals revealed a close resemblance to RF in paraproteinemias with an over-expression of the Vκ3 family and a similar distribution of heavy chain gene segments of the VH1, VH3, and VH4 families[51]. This implies that RF in lymphoproliferative diseases may represent physiological RF having undergone neoplastic transformation[52].

Production of IgM RF in normal individuals can occur following secondary immunization or infection[53,54]. This process requires the presence of immune-complexed antigen and T cells specific for the antigen present in the immune complex[55–57]. Therefore the production of RF in normal individuals is usually transient. Studies of IgM RF-secreting cell lines from patients after secondary immunization demonstrated extensive somatic mutation in the Ig V-region genes. However the affinity of these antibodies was lower than the antibodies found in RA, and had a low replacement-to-silent ratio, suggesting a negative selection of high affinity variants. The lack of evidence of affinity maturation indicated that normal, efficient peripheral mechanisms are able to prevent the expression of higher-affinity, potentially pathological rheumatoid factors[58]. Under conditions of chronic antigenic stimulation monospecific somatically mutated RF could be detected, suggesting that affinity maturation of RF could eventually occur in chronic infections[59].

Although low affinity polyspecific RFs can be derived from rheumatoid arthritis patients, IgM RF with high avidity to human IgG predominates in RA[27,29,60]. The comparison of RF V genes from synovial tissues of RA patients with RF from healthy, immunized individuals or patients with lymphoproliferative diseases revealed a difference in the use of light chain gene segments of the Vκ3 family. Healthy immunized individuals and patients with paraproteinemias express Vκ3 light chains about 90 per cent of the time. However, IgM RF producing lines from RA patients synovial tissue use a wide variety of different VL chain genes, with only a minority expressing Vκ3. In the use of VH gene segments, there is a trend toward VH3 in RF from RA patients synovial tissue[60,61]. Some of the VH and VL gene segments used are also found in low affinity RF but are altered by somatic mutation[62–65]. Analysis of B-cell hybridomas derived from synovial B lymphocyte lines of RA patients revealed predominantly replacement nucleotide changes in RF-producing hybridomas[58,66,67].

In summary, RFs in RA predominantly use VH3 genes and many different VL genes in contrast to the common use of VH1/VH4 and Vκ3 genes in natural antibodies. Overall, the greater diversity in the use of V region genes of monoclonal RF in RA synovial tissue, together with the increased avidity of RF, suggest that RFs in rheumatoid arthritis undergo antigen-induced expansion and affinity maturation (Table 13.3). Further support derives from studies of IgG RF from RA patients, demonstrating an even greater degree of somatic mutation than IgM RF, and indicating a further affinity maturation of the autoantibody response[68,69].

Recently, the crystal structure of a human IgM RF Fab bound to its autoantigen IgG Fc was reported[41]. An important contact residue of the RF was a somatic mutation of germline genes, in the production of pathogenic RF. The X-ray crystallographic analysis further revealed that, unlike other crystal structures of Fab complexes with protein antigens, the RF-Fab complex makes contact with the epitope on the Fc heavy chain on only one side of the potential combining site surface, with a reduced number of contact residues. The remaining accessible combining site could theoretically bind another antigen. This suggests that the RFs might originally have arisen in response to an unknown foreign antigen and that a mutation at the combining site lead to IgG Fc binding.

Isotype switch

Following interaction of B cells with antigen, germline-encoded IgM antibodies are produced. As described above, the immune system adapts to antigenic challenge by affinity maturation, resulting in production of high affinity antibodies. An additional feature of the immune system to increase the efficiency of the humoral immune response is isotype switching. B cells are able to switch from IgM to IgG or IgA isotypes without changing the antibody specificity.

Patients with severe, active RA and extra-articular symptoms characteristically have high levels of IgG RF in the serum[70]. High levels of IgG RF are often associated with circulating immune complexes and complement activation. Large size immune complexes can contribute to the joint inflammation through complement activation. In contrast to RA patients, immunized normal individuals do not produce IgG or IgA RF, indicating that the switch of isotype to IgG and IgA is common in RA but not in normal individuals[68].

Incidence

Although RFs are a characteristic marker for rheumatoid arthritis, these antibodies also occur in a variety of patients with other rheumatic diseases, acute and chronic inflammatory diseases, viral infections, lymphoproliferative diseases, as well as in apparently normal individuals. Table 13.4 lists some of the diseases associated with RF. The exact incidence of RF in a population depends on the titer chosen to separate positive from negative reactors and therefore also varies depending on the assay system. The titer of RF in a population follows a normal distribution but differs among various ethnic groups[7,71]. Mean RF titers of populations tend to increase with age. Studies have shown however, that the prevalence of RF in the general population declines beyond the age of 70 to 80 years[71].

In general, titers of RF in rheumatoid arthritis are higher than in non-rheumatoid conditions. Thus, the specificity of the RF detection assays for RA increases with the RF titer measured. At a serum dilution that excludes 95 per cent of the normal population, 70–80 per cent of RA patients as diagnosed by clinical criteria test positive for RF using the common assay systems. The remaining patients have RF falling in the normal range and are considered seronegative. Some of these may contain hidden IgM RF in their serum, that is IgM RF that is not detected

Table 13.3　Immunogenetic properties of rheumatoid factor in lymphoproliferative disease and rheumatoid arthritis

	Lymphoproliferative diseases	Rheumatoid arthritis
Ig isotypes	IgM	IgM, IgG, IgA
VL-chain gene usage	Vκ3	diverse
VH-chain gene usage	VH1, VH4	VH3
Idiotypes	polyspecific, cross reactive	monospecific
Somatic mutation	limited	extensive
Replacement-silent ratio	low	high
Affinity	low	high
Rheumatoid factor titer	low	high

Table 13.4 Diseases associated with rheumatoid factor

Autoimmune diseases	Rheumatoid arthritis Systemic lupus erythematosus Scleroderma Mixed connective tissue disease Sjögren's syndrome

Infections	Viral: HIV, Hepatitis, Influenza,
	    Mononucleosis after vaccination
	    (may yield falsely elevated titers of
	    antiviral antibodies)
	Parasitic: Trypanosomiasis, Malaria,
	    Schistosomiasis, Filariasis, Kala-azar
	Bacterial: Tuberculosis, Leprosy, Yaws,
	    Syphilis, Brucellosis, Subacute bacterial
	    endocarditis, Salmonellosis

Neoplasms	Tumors after radiation therapy or chemotherapy
Hyperglobulinemias	Hypergammaglobulinemic purpura Cryoglobulinemia Chronic liver disease Sarcoid Chronic pulmonary disease

because of competition for binding by non-specifically aggregated IgG or specific immune complexes[2,11,72]. Some may also have IgG RF in the absence of IgM. Others may convert to seropositive in the course of the disease. Therefore a patient with clinical diagnosis of RA should only be considered seronegative when repetitive testing yields a negative result. A small percentage remains seronegative by the usual criteria. These patients display milder synovitis than the seropositive patients and only rarely develop extra-articular rheumatoid disease[2]. The correlation of disease severity and positivity for RF argues for a role of RF in the pathogenesis of rheumatoid arthritis. The fact that joint disease also develops in the absence of RF, however, indicates that it is not a causative factor for the development of arthritis.

Etiology

RF production in normal individuals can be triggered by various environmental stimuli: for instance the IgG components of antigen–antibody complexes[53,55,73], polyclonal B-cell activation[74,75], and exogenous antigen-bearing cross-reactive determinants to human IgG. RF develops during the course of many acute and chronic inflammatory diseases. Studies in mice revealed that IgM RF is produced regularly in the course of a secondary immune response[76]. Analysis of RF secretion during secondary immune responses in mice demonstrate activation of RF precursor B cells by immune complexes and T cells specific for the carrier protein[55–57]. RF elicited during the secondary immune response is directed against the IgG isotype that is dominant in the antigen–antibody complex. Since RF precursor B cells are able to function as antigen-presenting cells, they can present antigenic peptides derived from antigen–antibody complexes in context of class II MHC and receive help from antigen-

reactive T lymphocytes which, in turn, triggers production of RF. In experimental models, RF is usually only produced as long as there is an appropriate immunological stimulus. For instance, the elimination of bacteria by antibiotics is followed by a decline in RF titer in subacute bacterial endocarditis[54,77].

Polyclonal activators of B lymphocytes can induce RF production. These so called mitogens are able to stimulate lymphocytes to secrete immunoglobulin in the absence of a specific antigen stimulus. A wide variety of substances, including bacterial proteins, lipopolysaccharides, mycoplasma components' and EBV possess the properties of mitogens. Low affinity IgM RF is often produced by normal individuals after mitogenic stimulation by EBV.

Another possible stimulus to induce RF production is represented by cross-reactive epitopes on foreign antigens. Protein A of *Staphylococcus* reacts specifically with human IgG, as well as the streptococcal Fc receptor[78]. Herpes simplex virus and CMV induce Fc receptor expression on infected cells. Some antibodies to these induced Fc receptors may have RF activity[79].

Role of RF in the pathogenesis of autoimmune disease

Physiological role

RF B cells can be involved in a physiological immune response either via cell surface Ig expression or by secreted RF. RF B cells can capture immune complexes and present antigens to T cells[80,81]. Early in a secondary immune response, most antigen probably reaches the draining lymph nodes in immune complexed form due to the small amounts of antigen available. In this situation, IgM-expressing RF B cells might act as antigen-presenting cells (APC) for immune complexed antigen and thereby enhance antigen specific T cell expansion early in a secondary immune response. However, because of the absence of high affinity IgM RF B cells in normal individuals, regulatory elements probably maintain RF at low affinity preventing long-term expression and expansion of higher-affinity RF induced by antigen specific T cells.

IgM RF can usually be detected during acute infections, suggesting they have a physiological function. The ability of IgM RF to cross link low affinity IgG antibodies bound to the surface of micro-organisms could amplify the early response of the humoral immune system by formation of multivalent and multispecific complexes. RFs of the IgM class activate complement efficiently when bound to aggregated IgG[82]. This activation could result in lysis of an invading organism coated with IgG.

The mechanism of RF induction during infections are at present not well understood. Studies analyzing the immune response against immune complexes of viruses and bacteria injected into mice demonstrated that repetitively-arranged epitopes in a paracrystalline structure are able to induce anti-antibodies and, under certain circumstances, also RF[83]. The physiological functions of RF and RF B cells are summarized in Table 13.5.

Table 13.5   Functions of rheumatoid factor and rheumatoid factor B cells

Secreted RF	Immune complex clearance
	Enhancement of opsonization
RF B cells	Accessory cell function
	Processing and presentation of small amounts of antigen, complexed with IgG

Role in rheumatoid arthritis

The hallmark of RA is a chronic inflammatory process in the synovium of affected joints. Eventually, infiltrating macrophages, T and B lymphocytes, form ectopic lymphoid tissue[84]. Plasma cells produce IgG and IgM, including RF[85]. This locally produced RF is presumably of importance in the pathogenesis of RA by virtue of its ability to form immune complexes and bind complement. In fact, compared with the corresponding sera, synovial fluids of RA patients have decreased complement levels[86]. The localized immune complex disease leads to chemotactic recruitment of neutrophils and the release of lysosomal enzymes and inflammatory mediators[87], and may thereby exacerbate joint inflammation and contribute to tissue damage.

How RA is initiated is unknown. T cells might to play a crucial role in the pathogenesis as indicated by the presence of T cell infiltrates in the synovium and by the genetic association with HLA DR1 and DR4 haplotypes[88]. Although T cells in the synovium exhibit an activated phenotype, no specificity for a particular autoantigen has so far been demonstrated. RFs in lymphoproliferative disease, such as chronic lymphocytic leukemia, Waldenström's macroglobulinemia, mixed cryoglobulinemia, and in some cases of Sjögren's syndrome are mono- or oligoclonal nd display cross-reactive idiotypic antigens[89–93]. These properties are not common for an antigen-driven immune response during which the Ig genes should diversify, increasing the affinity of the antibodies with isotype switching, contributing to the heterogeneity of the antibodies. However, such heterogenous RF antibodies are typically found in RA[62]. Sequence analyse indicate that RFs are polyclonal and the corresponding Ig genes contain many somatic mutations[29,47,60–64,68,94,95]. Since these processes are under the control of T cells, the results suggest that RF production in RA is driven by T cells. There is no evidence for the existence of T cells recognizing IgG. However, help by T cells recognizing exogenous antigens contained in the immune complexes may be sufficient to stimulate RF secretion and subsequent affinity maturation of low affinity RFs, which have been demonstrated to present efficiently immune complexed antigen[80,81].

Since high affinity RFs usually do not exist in normal individuals, an efficient peripheral tolerance mechanism must be postulated. In transgenic mouse models, elimination of autoreactive B cells has been shown to involve clonal deletion and functional silencing, termed anergy. Studies with RF transgenic mice have demonstrated that high affinity RFs are centrally deleted in the thymus whereas low affinity RF can escape this process[96]. It has further been demonstrated that high affinity RF-producing cells, upon encountering the autoantigen IgG, undergo cell death in the periphery unless T cell costimulation is provided[97]. Whereas in normal individuals costimulation for RF B cells is lacking, the aforementioned presence of activated T cells, even of different specificity than the RF B cells, might in the inflamed synovium lead to activation of RF B cells and RF production. Because of the abundance and close proximity of the activated T cells with B cells and antigen presenting cells (APC) in the joint, low affinity cell contact via adhesion molecules and short range action of interleukins might be sufficient to provide the necessary costimulation for survival of RF B cells and production and secretion of RF. Such a hypothetical interaction between APC, activated T cells, and RF B cells is depicted in Fig. 13.1. For the

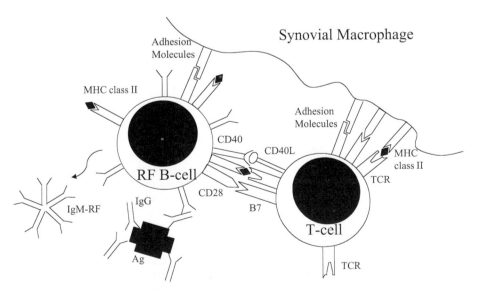

Fig. 13.1   Model for the activation of RF B cells in the rheumatoid synovium. An antigen-specific T helper cell recognizes with its T cell receptor (TCR) the antigen presented in the form of peptides (black diamonds) on MHC class II molecules by a synovial macrophage. Costimulation is provided by CD28-B7 interaction. The RF B cell is activated by the IgG component of an immune complex. The activated T cell provides costimulatory help to the B cell through CD40L-CD40 interaction and interleukins (not shown) and thereby stimulates the production of IgM RF.

sake of simplicity soluble factors are not shown in the figure. It should be noted that the role of antigen in the interaction of T cells and RF B cells is unknown.

Alternative mechanisms explaining the presence of high affinity RF B cells have been proposed. Because of their function as APC, RF B cells may give rise to autoreactive T cells due to presentation of self-components released from damaged joint tissues, such as collagen, proteoglycans, and heat shock proteins. Activated RF B cells in the synovium could thereby promote T-cell-dependent joint inflammation in a vicious circle.

The levels of RF in the serum correlate with a worse prognosis in RA. High titers of RF, particularly IgG RF, are a risk factor for the development of vasculitis[2], whereas IgA RF titers might correlate with bone erosions[98]. Several studies reported an elevation of RF long before clinical onset of disease[99-101], indicating that high affinity RF production is not a secondary phenomenon in RA. On the basis of the current knowledge, however, it is unlikely that high affinity RFs are causally responsible for the joint involvement in RA but rather promote inflammatory processes and thus accelerate tissue destruction.

References

1. Dresner E., Trombly P. The latex-fixation reaction in non-rheumatic diseases. *New Eng J Med*, 1959;261:981–85.
2. Masi A.T., Maldonado-Cocco J.A., Kaplan S.B., Feigenbaum S.L., Chandler R.W. Prospective study of the early course of rheumatoid arthritis in young adults: comparison of patients with and without rheumatoid factor positivity at entry and identification of variables correlating with outcome. *Semin Arthritis Rheum*, 1976;4:299–326.
3. Waaler E. On the occurrence of a factor in human serum activating the specific agglutination of sheep blood corpuscles. *Acta Pathol Microbiol Scand*, 1940;17:172–82.
4. Rose H.M., Ragan C., Pearce E., Lipman M.O. Differential agglutination of normal and sensitized sheep erythrocytes by sera of patients with rheumatoid arthritis. *Proc Soc Exp Biol Med*, 1949;68:1–9.
5. Singer J.M., Plotz C.M. The latex fixation test. I: Application to the serologic diagnosis of rheumatoid arthritis. *Am J Med*, 1956;21:888–94.
6. Jones C.E., Rousseau R.J., Maxwell K.W. Quantitation of rheumatoid factor activity by nephelometry. *Am J Clin Pathol*, 1979;72:432–6.
7. Lawrence J.S. *Rheumatism in populations*. London: William Heinemann, 1977.
8. Bennett P.H., Wood P.H.N. *Population studies of the rheumatic diseases*. Amsterdam: Excerpta Medica, 1968.
9. Gripenberg M., Wafin F., Isomaki H., Linder E. A simple enzyme immunoassay for the demonstration of rheumatoid factor. *J Immunol Methods*, 1979;31:109–18.
10. Allen J.C., Kunkel H.G. Hidden rheumatoid factors with specificity for native γ globulin. *Arthritis Rheum*, 1966;9:758–68.
11. Nykanen M., Palosuo T., Aho K., Sahi T., von Essen R. Improved immunoturbidimetric method for rheumatoid factor testing. *J Clin Pathol*, 1993;46:1065–6.
12. Winchester R.J., Kunkel H.G., Agnello V. Occurrence of γ-globulin complexes in serum and joint fluid of rheumatoid arthritis patients: use of monoclonal rheumatoid factors as reagents for their demonstration. *J Exp Med*, 1971;134 (Suppl):286s.
13. Hannestad K. Presence of aggregated gamma-G-globulin in certain rheumatoid synovial effusions. *Clin Exp Immunol*, 1967;2:511–29.

14. Schrohenloher R.E. Characterization of the γ-globulin complexes present in certain sera having high titers of anti-γ-globulin activity. *J Clin Invest*, 1966;45:501–12.
15. Chodirker W.B.l, Tomasi T.B. Low molecular weight rheumatoid factor. *J Clin Invest*, 1963;42:876–84.
16. Dunne J.V., Carson D., Spiegelberg H.L., Alspaugh M.A., Vaughan J.H. IgA rheumatoid factor in the sera and saliva of patients with rheumatoid arthritis and Sjögren's syndrome. *Ann Rheum Dis*, 1979;38:161–5.
17. Elkon K.B., Delacroix D.L., Gharavi A.E., Vaerman J.P., Hughes G.R. Immunoglobulin A and polymeric IgA rheumatoid factors in systemic sicca syndrome: partial characterization. *J Immunol*, 1982;129:576–81.
18. Scott D.G., Bacon P.A., Allen C., Elson C.J., Wallington T. IgG rheumatoid factor, complement and immune complexes in rheumatoid synovitis and vasculitis: comparative and serial studies during cytotoxic therapy. *Clin Exp Immunol*, 1981;43:54–63.
19. Sasso E.H., Barber C.V., Nardella F.A., Yount W.J., Mannik M. Antigenic specificities of human monoclonal and polyclonal IgM rheumatoid factors. The C gamma 2-C gamma 3 interface region contains the major determinants. *J Immunol*, 1988;140:3098–107.
20. Williams R.C., Jr., Malone CC. Rheumatoid-factor-reactive sites on CH2 established by analysis of overlapping peptide of primary sequence. *Scand J Immunol*, 1994;40:443–56.
21. Robbins D.L., Skilling J., Benisek W.F., Wistar R., Jr. Estimation of the relative avidity of 19S IgM rheumatoid factor secreted by rheumatoid synovial cells for human IgG subclasses. *Arthritis Rheum*, 1986;29:722–9.
22. Bonagura V.R., Artandi S.E., Davidson A., *et al*. Mapping studies reveal unique epitopes on IgG recognized by rheumatoid arthritis-derived monoclonal rheumatoid factors. *J Immunol*, 1993;151:3840–52.
23. Artandi S.E., Canfield S.M., Tao M.H., Calame K.L., Morrison S.L., Bonagura V.R. Molecular analysis of IgM rheumatoid factor binding to chimeric IgG. *J Immunol*, 1991;146:603–10.
24. Artandi S.E., Calame K.L., Morrison S.L., Bonagura V.R. Monoclonal IgM rheumatoid factors bind IgG at a discontinuous epitope comprised of amino acid loops from heavy-chain constant-region domains 2 and 3. *Proc Natl Acad Sci USA*, 1992;89:94–8.
25. Bonagura V.R., Agostino N., Borretzen M., Thompson K.M., Natvig J.B., Morrison S.L. Mapping IgG epitopes bound by rheumatoid factors from immunized controls identifies disease-specific rheumatoid factors produced by patients with rheumatoid arthritis. *J Immunol*, 1998;160:2496–505.
26. Tokano Y., Arai S., Hashimoto H. *et al*. The distinct subgroup of patients with rheumatoid arthritis shown by IgG3-reactive rheumatoid factor. *Autoimmunity*, 1989;5:107–14.
27. Burastero S.E., Casali P., Wilder R.L., Notkins A.L. Monoreactive high affinity and polyreactive low affinity rheumatoid factors are produced by CD5+ B cells from patients with rheumatoid arthritis. *J Exp Med*, 1988;168:1979–92.
28. Chen P.P., Silverman G.J., Liu M.F., Carson D.A. Idiotypic and molecular characterization of human rheumatoid factors. *Chem Immunol*, 1990;48:63–81.
29. Harindranath N., Goldfarb I.S., Ikematsu H. *et al*. Complete sequence of the genes encoding the VH and VL regions of low- and high-affinity monoclonal IgM and IgA1 rheumatoid factors produced by CD5+ B cells from a rheumatoid arthritis patient. *Int Immunol*, 1991;3:865–75.
30. Nardella F.A., Teller D.C., Mannik M. Studies on the antigenic determinants in the self-association of IgG rheumatoid factor. *J Exp Med*, 1981;154:112–25.
31. Pope R.M., Teller D.C., Mannik M. The molecular basis of self-association of antibodies to IgG (rheumatoid factors) in rheumatoid arthritis. *Proc Natl Acad Sci USA*, 1974;71:517–21.
32. Parekh R., Roitt I., Isenberg D., Dwek R., Rademacher T. Age-related galactosylation of the N-linked oligosaccharides of human serum IgG. *J Exp Med*, 1988;167:1731–6.

33. Parekh R.B., Dwek R.A., Sutton B.J., *et al.* Association of rheumatoid arthritis and primary osteoarthritis with changes in the glycosylation pattern of total serum IgG. *Nature*, 1985;**316**:452–7.

34. van Zeben D., Rook G.A., Hazes J.M. *et al.* Early agalactosylation of IgG is associated with a more progressive disease course in patients with rheumatoid arthritis: results of a follow-up study. *Br J Rheumatol*, 1994;**33**:36–43.

35. Parekh R.B., Roitt I.M., Isenberg D.A., Dwek R.A., Ansell B.M., Rademacher T.W. Galactosylation of IgG associated oligosaccharides: reduction in patients with adult and juvenile onset rheumatoid arthritis and relation to disease activity. *Lancet*, 1988;**1**:966–9.

36. Tsuchiya N., Endo T., Matsuta K., *et al.* Effects of galactose depletion from oligosaccharide chains on immunological activities of human IgG. *J Rheumatol*, 1989;**16**: 285–90.

37. Tomana M., Schrohenloher RE, Koopman WJ, Alarcon GS, Paul W.A. Abnormal glycosylation of serum IgG from patients with chronic inflammatory diseases. *Arthritis Rheum*, 1988;**31**:333–8.

38. Newkirk M.M., Lemmo A., Rauch J. Importance of the IgG isotype, not the state of glycosylation, in determining human rheumatoid factor binding. *Arthritis Rheum*, 1990;**33**:800–9.

39. Soltys A.J., Hay F.C., Bond A. *et al.* The binding of synovial tissue-derived human monoclonal immunoglobulin M rheumatoid factor to immunoglobulin G preparations of differing galactose content. *Scand J Immunol*, 1994;**40**:135–43.

40. Bonagura V.R., Artandi S.E., Agostino N., Tao M.H., Morrison S.L. Mapping rheumatoid factor binding sites using genetically engineered, chimeric IgG antibodies. *DNA Cell Biol*, 1992;**11**:245–52.

41. Corper A.L., Sohi M.K., Bonagura V.R. *et al.* Structure of human IgM rheumatoid factor Fab bound to its autoantigen IgG Fc reveals a novel topology of antibody-antigen interaction. *Nat Struct Biol*, 1997;**4**:374–81.

42. Berek C., Ziegner M. The maturation of the immune response. *Immunol Today*, 1993;**14**:400–4.

43. Berek C., Griffiths G.M,. Milstein C. Molecular events during maturation of the immune response to oxazolone. *Nature*, 1985;**316**: 412–8.

44. Crowley J.J., Goldfien R.D., Schrohenloher R.E., *et al.* Incidence of three cross-reactive idiotypes on human rheumatoid factor paraproteins. *J Immunol*, 1988;**140**:3411–8.

45. Kunkel H.G., Agnello V., Joslin F.G., Winchester R.J., Capra J.D. Cross-idiotypic specificity among monoclonal IgM proteins with anti-γ-globulin activity. *J Exp Med*, 1973;**137**:331–42.

46. Chen P.P., Fong S., Goni F., *et al.* Cross-reacting idiotypes on cryoprecipitating rheumatoid factor. *Springer Semin Immunopathol*, 1988;**10**:35–55.

47. Schrohenloher R.E., Accavitti M.A., Bhown A.S., Koopman W.J. Monoclonal antibody 6B6.6 defines a cross-reactive kappa light chain idiotope on human monoclonal and polyclonal rheumatoid factors. *Arthritis Rheum*, 1990;**33**:187–98.

48. Silverman G.J., Schrohenloher R.E., Accavitti M.A., Koopman W.J., Carson D.A. Structural characterization of the second major cross-reactive idiotype group of human rheumatoid factors. Association with the VH4 gene family. *Arthritis Rheum*, 1990;**33**:1347–60.

49. Hardy R.R. Variable gene usage, physiology and development of Ly-1+ (CD5+) B cells. *Curr Opin Immunol*, 1992;**4**:181–5.

50. Nakamura M., Burastero S.E., Notkins A.L., Casal P. Human monoclonal rheumatoid factor-like antibodies from CD5 (Leu-1)+ B cells are polyreactive. *J Immunol*, 1988;**140**:4180–6.

51. Thompson K.M., Borretzen M., Randen I,. Forre O., Natvig J.B. V-gene repertoire and hypermutation of rheumatoid factors produced in rheumatoid synovial inflammation and immunized healthy donors. *Ann N Y Acad Sci*, 1995;**764**:440–9.

52. Mageed R.A., Borretzen M., Moyes S.P., Thompson K.M., Natvig JB. Rheumatoid factor autoantibodies in health and disease. *Ann N Y Acad Sci*, 1997;**815**:296–311.

53. Welch M.J., Fong S., Vaughan J., Carson D. Increased frequency of rheumatoid factor precursor B lymphocytes after immunization of normal adults with tetanus toxoid. *Clin Exp Immunol*, 1983;**51**:299–304.

54. Williams R.C., Kunkel H.G. Rheumatoid factor, complement and conglutinin aberrations in patients with subacute bacterial endocarditis. *J Clin Invest*, 1962;**41**:666.

55. Nemazee D.A., Sato V.L. Induction of rheumatoid antibodies in the mouse. Regulated production of autoantibody in the secondary humoral response. *J Exp Med*, 1983;**158**:529–45.

56. Nemazee D.A. Immune complexes can trigger specific, T cell-dependent, autoanti-IgG antibody production in mice. *J Exp Med*, 1985;**161**:242–56.

57. Coulie P.G., Van Snick J. Rheumatoid factor (RF) production during anamnestic immune responses in the mouse. III. Activation of RF precursor cells is induced by their interaction with immune complexes and carrier-specific helper T cells. *J Exp Med*, 1985; **161**:88–97.

58. Borretzen M., Randen I., Zdarsky E., Forre O., Natvig J.B., Thompson K.M. Control of autoantibody affinity by selection against amino acid replacements in the complementarity-determining regions. *Proc Natl Acad Sci USA*, 1994;**91**:12917–21.

59. Djavad N., Bas S., Shi X., *et al.* Comparison of rheumatoid factors of rheumatoid arthritis patients, of individuals with mycobacterial infections and of normal controls: evidence for maturation in the absence of an autoimmune response. *Eur J Immunol*, 1996;**26**:2480–6.

60. Mantovani L., Wilder R.L., Casali P. Human rheumatoid B-1a (CD5+ B) cells make somatically hypermutated high affinity IgM rheumatoid factors. *J Immunol*, 1993;**151**:473–88.

61. Pascual V, Victor K, Randen I, *et al.* Nucleotide sequence analysis of rheumatoid factors and polyreactive antibodies derived from patients with rheumatoid arthritis reveals diverse use of VH and VL gene segments and extensive variability in CDR-3. *Scand J Immunol*, 1992;**36**:349–62.

62. Youngblood K., Fruchter L., Ding G., Lopez J., Bonagura V., Davidson A. Rheumatoid factors from the peripheral blood of two patients with rheumatoid arthritis are genetically heterogeneous and somatically mutated. *J Clin Invest*, 1994;**93**:852–61.

63. Randen I., Brown D., Thompson K.M., *et al.* Clonally related IgM rheumatoid factors undergo affinity maturation in the rheumatoid synovial tissue. *J Immunol*, 1992;**148**:3296–301.

64. Victor K.D., Randen I., Thompson K., *et al.* Rheumatoid factors isolated from patients with autoimmune disorders are derived from germline genes distinct from those encoding the Wa, Po, and Bla cross-reactive idiotypes. *J Clin Invest*, 1991;**87**:1603–13.

65. Ermel R.W., Kenny T.P., Chen P.P., Robbins D.L. Molecular analysis of rheumatoid factors derived from rheumatoid synovium suggests an antigen-driven response in inflamed joints. *Arthritis Rheum*, 1993;**36**:380–8.

66. Moyes S.P, Brown C.M., Scott B.B., Maini R.N., Mageed R.A. Analysis of V kappa genes in rheumatoid arthritis (RA) synovial B lymphocytes provides evidence for both polyclonal activation and antigen-driven selection. *Clin Exp Immunol*, 1996;**105**: 89–98.

67. Jain R.I., Fais F., Kaplan S., *et al.* IgH and L chain variable region gene sequence analyses of twelve synovial tissue-derived B cell lines producing IgA, IgG, and IgM rheumatoid factors structure/function comparisons of antigenic specificity, V gene sequence, and Ig isotype. *Autoimmunity*, 1995;**22**:229–43.

68. Randen I., Pascual V., Victor K., *et al.* Synovial IgG rheumatoid factors show evidence of an antigen-driven immune response and a shift in the V gene repertoire compared to IgM rheumatoid factors. *Eur J Immunol*, 1993;**23**:1220–5.

69. Deftos M., Olee T., Carson D.A., Chen P.P. Defining the genetic origins of three rheumatoid synovium-derived IgG rheumatoid factors. *J Clin Invest*, 1994;**93**:2545–53.

70. Mageed R.A., Kirwan J.R., Thompson P.W., McCarthy D.A., Holborow E.J. Characterisation of the size and composition of circulating immune complexes in patients with rheumatoid arthritis. *Ann Rheum Dis*, 1991;**51**:231–6.

71. Hooper B., Whittingham S., Mathews J.D., Mackay I.R., Curnow DH. Autoimmunity in a rural community. *Clin Exp Immunol*, 1972;**12**:79–87.

72. Moore T.L., Dorner R.W., Weiss T.D., Baldassare A.R., Zuckner J. Specificity of hidden 19S IgM rheumatoid factor in patients with juvenile rheumatoid arthritis. *Arthritis Rheum*, 1981;**24**:1283–90.

73. Van Snick J., Coulie P. Rheumatoid factors and secondary immune responses in the mouse. I. Frequent occurrence of hybridomas secreting IgM anti-IgG1 autoantibodies after immunization with protein antigens. *Eur J Immunol*, 1983;**13**:890–4.

74. Izui S., Eisenberg R.A., Dixon F.J. IgM rheumatoid factors in mice injected with bacterial lipopolysaccharides. *J Immunol*, 1979;**122**:2096–102.

75. Slaughter L., Carson D.A., Jensen F.C., Holbrook T.L., Vaughan J.H. In vitro effects of Epstein-Barr virus on peripheral blood mononuclear cells from patients with rheumatoid arthritis and normal subjects. *J Exp Med*, 1978;**148**:1429–34.

76. Coulie P., Van Snick J. Rheumatoid factors and secondary immune responses in the mouse. II. Incidence, kinetics and induction mechanisms. *Eur J Immunol*, 1983;**13**:895–9.

77. Carson D.A., Bayer A.S., Eisenberg R.A., Lawrance S., Theofilopoulos A. IgG rheumatoid factor in subacute bacterial endocarditis: relationship to IgM rheumatoid factor and circulating immune complexes. *Clin Exp Immunol*, 1978;**31**:100–3.

78. Nardella FA, Teller DC, Barber CV, Mannik M. IgG rheumatoid factors and staphylococcal protein A bind to a common molecular site on IgG. *J Exp Med*, 1985;**162**:1811–24.

79. Tsuchiya N., Williams R.C., Jr., Hutt-Fletcher L.M. Rheumatoid factors may bear the internal image of the Fc gamma-binding protein of herpes simplex virus type 1. *J Immunol*, 1990;**144**:4742–8.

80. Tighe H., Chen P.P., Tucker R., *et al*. Function of B cells expressing a human immunoglobulin M rheumatoid factor autoantibody in transgenic mice. *J Exp Med*, 1993;**177**:109–18.

81. Roosnek E., Lanzavecchia A. Efficient and selective presentation of antigen-antibody complexes by rheumatoid factor B cells. *J Exp Med*, 1991;**173**:487–9.

82. Sabharwal U.K., Vaughan J.H., Fong S., Bennett P.H., Carson D.A., Curd J.G. Activation of the classical pathway of complement by rheumatoid factors. Assessment by radioimmunoassay for C4. *Arthritis Rheum*, 1982;**25**:161–7.

83. Fehr T., Bachmann M.F., Bucher E., *et al*. Role of repetitive antigen patterns for induction of antibodies against antibodies. *J Exp Med*, 1997;**185**:1785–92.

84. Randen I., Mellbye O.J., Forre O., Natvig J.B. The identification of germinal centres and follicular dendritic cell networks in rheumatoid synovial tissue. *Scand J Immunol*, 1995;**41**:481–6.

85. Munthe E., Natvig J.B. Immunoglobulin classes, subclasses and complexes of IgG rheumatoid factor in rheumatoid plasma cells. *Clin Exp Immunol*, 1972;**12**:55–70.

86. Winchester R.J., Agnello V., Kunkel H.G. Gamma globulin complexes in synovial fluids of patients with rheumatoid arthritis. Partial characterization and relationship to lowered complement levels. *Clin Exp Immunol*, 1970;**6**:689–706.

87. Kitsis E., Weissmann G. The role of the neutrophil in rheumatoid arthritis. *Clin Orthop*, 1991;**265**:63–72.

88. Panayi G.S., Lanchbury JS, Kingsley G.H. The importance of the T cell in initiating and maintaining the chronic synovitis of rheumatoid arthritis. *Arthritis Rheum*, 1992;**35**:729–35.

89. Carson D.A, Chen P.P., Kipps T.J, *et al*. Idiotypic and genetic studies of human rheumatoid factors. *Arthritis Rheum*, 1987;**30**:1321–5.

90. Liu M.F., Robbins D.L., Crowley J.J., *et al*. Characterization of four homologous L chain variable region genes that are related to 6B6.6 idiotype positive human rheumatoid factor L chains. *J Immunol*, 1989;**142**:688-94.

91. Kipps T.J., Tomhave E., Chen P.P., Fox R.I. Molecular characterization of a major autoantibody-associated cross-reactive idiotype in Sjögren's syndrome. *J Immunol*, 1989;**142**:4261–8.

92. Brouet J.C., Clauvel J.P., Danon F., Kleini M., Seligmann M. Biologic and clinical significance of cryoglobulins. A report of 86 cases. *Am J Med*, 1974;**57**:775–88.

93. Fong S., Chen P.P., Gilbertson T.A., Weber J.R., Fox R.I., Carson DA. Expression of three cross-reactive idiotypes on rheumatoid factor autoantibodies from patients with autoimmune diseases and seropositive adults. *J Immunol*, 1986;**137**:122–8.

94. Lee S.K., Bridges S.L., Jr., Koopman W.J., Schroeder H.W., Jr. The immunoglobulin kappa light chain repertoir expressed in the synovium of a patient with rheumatoid arthritis. *Arthritis Rheum*, 1992;**35**:905–13.

95. Soto-Gil R.W., Olee T., Klink B.K., *et al*. A systematic approach to defining the germline gene counterparts of a mutated autoantibody from a patient with rheumatoid arthritis. *Arthritis Rheum*, 1992;**35**:356–63.

96. Wang H., Shlomchik M.J. High affinity rheumatoid factor transgenic B cells are eliminated in normal mice. *J Immunol*, 1997;**159**:1125–34.

97. Tighe H, Warnatz K, Brinson D, *et al*. Peripheral deletion of rheumatoid factor B cells after abortive activation by IgG. *Proc Natl Acad Sci USA*, 1997;**94**:646–51.

98. Arnason J.A., Jonsson T., Brekkan A., Sigurjonsson K., Valdimarsson H. Relation between bone erosions and rheumatoid factor isotopes. *Ann Rheum Dis*, 1987;**46**:380–4.

99. Jonsson T., Thorsteinsson J., Kolbeinsson A., Jonasdottir E., Sigfusson N., Valdimarsson H. Population study of the importance of rheumatoid factor isotypes in adults. *Ann Rheum Dis*, 1992;**51**:863–8.

100. del Puente A., Knowler W.C., Pettitt D.J., Bennett P.H. The incidence of rheumatoid arthritis is predicted by rheumatoid factor titer in a longitudinal population study. *Arthritis Rheum*, 1988;**31**:1239–44.

101. Tuomi T, Palosuo T, Aho K. The distribution of class-specific rheumatoid factors is similar in rheumatoid and pre-illness sera. *Scand J Immunol*, 1986;**24**:751–4.

14 | Mechanisms of joint destruction

Thomas Pap, Renate Gay, and Steffen Gay

Introduction

Rheumatoid arthritis (RA) is a chronic, systematic inflammatory disorder of unknown etiology, that results in the progressive destruction of affected joints. The pathogenesis of RA involves complex changes which include the mutually interacting phenomena of chronic inflammation, altered immune responses, and synovial hyperplasia. The destruction of cartilage and bone represents a unique and prominent feature of this disease, as it clearly distinguishes RA from other arthritides as well as determines its outcome[1]. Intriguingly, recent data provide evidence that the pathological mechanisms of inflammation and articular damage may differ[2], and critical steps that initiate joint destruction occur very early in the course of disease[3].

In the past years, considerable efforts have been expanded to elucidate the molecular and cellular basis of rheumatoid joint destruction as well as to study potential ways of inhibiting this process. Advances in molecular biology, the utilization of novel animal models, and the observation of early disease have provided exciting insights into key mechanisms leading to the destruction of extracellular matrix in RA. It has become clear that these mechanisms are linked to changes occurring predominantly at sites of interaction between rheumatoid synovium and cartilage. Moreover, growing evidence suggests that T-cell-independent mechanisms may play a key role in initiating and perpetuating disease[1,4,5].

Apart from macrophages, considerable interest has focused on fibroblast-like cells within the RA synovial membrane, which substantially differ from normal fibroblasts both in their morphological appearance and in their behavior[6,7]. By investigating the specific properties of these cells it has been understood that **cellular activation** and escape from normal regulation, **attachment** to cartilage and bone, and subsequent **degradation of matrix** components represent critical steps in rheumatoid joint destruction (Fig. 14.1). However, the exact sequence of the cell activation steps as well as the way that the different cell types interact in rheumatoid joint destruction remains to be determined.

In the present chapter we will summarize current concepts in the understanding of rheumatoid joint destruction as well as point to questions still to be answered.

Composition of RA synovium

The observation that the proliferating synovial tissue, often also called the 'pannus', is responsible for joint destruction in RA was recognized over two decades ago[8,9]. However, subsequent research has clearly demonstrated that RA synovium is not a homogenous proliferating mass but rather a highly differentiated tissue with distinct changes in different stages of disease as well as in different areas of the synovial membrane[6,7,10,11].

Thickening of the RA synovium is largely due to hyperplasia in the most superficial layer of cells, which is also called the 'lining layer'. About 25 per cent of lining cells appear to originate from resident synovial cells. These have a fibroblast-like appearance and lack specific surface markers. They have been called fibroblast-like synoviocytes and can be identified by antibodies recognizing prolyl-4-hydroxylase[1,12,13]. By attaching to the cartilage and mediating the progressive destruction of joints, the lining layer plays a central role in the pathogenesis of RA[10].

In the course of RA, deeper areas of the synovial membrane, called the 'sublining', also undergo considerable changes. Highly variable changes in the sublining are characterized by an infiltration with mononuclear cells such as T cells, B cells, and macrophages. Recent data suggest that both accumulation and prolonged survival of T cells within the rheumatoid synovium can be promoted by synovial cells[14,15] and especially fibroblast-derived factors[16,17]. Salmon *et al.* showed that isolated synovial T cells rapidly undergo programmed cell death, whereas coculture with synovial fibroblasts prevented apoptosis[15]. McInnes *et al.* demonstrated that IL-15, which attracts CD4+ T cells and may protect T cells from apoptosis, is also produced by RA synovial lining cells[17]. Even more intriguingly, RA synovial fibroblasts have been identified as the major source for IL-16 within the synovium[16]. In addition to attracting CD4+ cells, IL-16 induces the expression of the IL-2 receptor on resting T cells as well as that of class II MHC molecules. IL-16 also has suppressive properties in so far as it is capable of inducing T-cell anergy[18]. Thus, the properties of IL-15 and -16 may help to explain the paradox between the abundance of T cells in the rheumatoid synovium and the relative lack of T-cell function in the sublining of RA synovial membrane.

Alterations in the architecture of the RA synovium are also accompanied by changes in the vascularization. Increased blood vessel formation appears critical to he hyperplasia of the proliferating synovial membrane[19]. In this context, the high levels of CD146, which is expressed almost exclusively by vascular endothelium and found in the synovial fluid of patients with early RA, indicate increased endothelial activity and angiogenesis[20]. Recent studies have demonstrated that—comparable to malignancies—the formation of new blood vessels results from a complex interaction of synovial cells. Thus, neoangiogenesis is believed to be stimulated mainly by the cells of the activated synovium. For instances, a study showed that soluble forms of both VCAM-1 and E-selectin can induce angiogenesis in RA

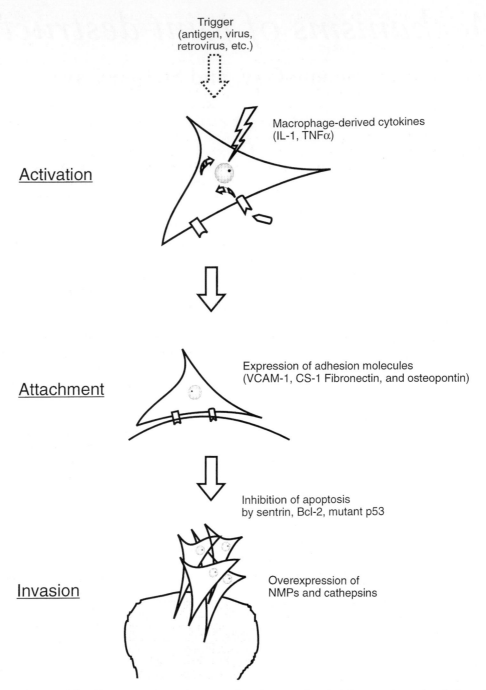

Fig. 14.1 Role of activated synovial fibroblasts in RA. Exogenous or endogenous stimuli, which have not been identified, result in cellular activation and escape from normal regulation of RA synovial fibroblasts. As a consequence, they express a number of adhesion molecules, which mediate the attachment of RA synovium to cartilage and bone. RA synovial fibroblasts produce a broad array of metalloproteinase and cathepsins through which they aggressively invade cartilage and bone. In addition, alterations of apoptotic pathways in RA may lead to an extended life-span of RA synovial fibroblasts which accompanied by a prolonged expression of matrix-degrading enzymes.

synovium[21]. Most interestingly, activated synovial fibroblasts of the lining express significant amounts of VCAM-1[22] which could contribute significantly to blood vessel proliferation in the synovium.

Lessons in joint destruction from animal models

Some important insights into the mechanisms of rheumatoid joint destruction have been obtained from animal models. For instance, MRL-lpr/lpr mice develop RA-like destructive arthritis, and the sequence of events resembles that in human RA.

Histological studies using light and electron microscopy show that initial joint damage in the MRL-lpr/lpr mouse model is mediated by proliferating synovial cells[23,24]. Moreover, cartilage and bone destruction occurs only at sites of synovial attachment. These observations are supported by data from Trabandt *et al.* demonstrating that synovial cells of MRL-lpr/lpr mice constitutively express the collagenase gene[25]. By immunohistochemistry, collagenase was detected *in situ* in proliferating synovial lining cells as well as in chondrocytes of the first stage of pathological changes in the MRL-lpr/lpr mouse arthropathy. Interestingly, collagenase-expressing synovial lining cells from these mice exhibit markedly elevated RNA levels of the *c-fos* proto-oncogene *in vitro*. Inflammatory cells migrate into the synovium and accelerate the process only after cartilage degradation is initiated. Although IL-1 treatment enhances the onset and progression of the spontaneous arthritis in MRL-lpr/lpr mice[26], it is of particular importance that synovial lining cells mediate the initial destructive process in the absence of inflammatory cells, and that autoimmunity to collagen type II occurred as a consequence of cartilage damage rather than preceding it[27].

Injection of various antigens can also lead to the induction of a relapsing, erosive arthritis in rodents. Several models, such as the collagen-induced arthritis (CIA) and the streptococcal-wall antigen-induced arthritis (SCW-A) have been intensively studied as animal models for human RA[28–31]. They have provided us with important insights into molecular mechanisms of joint inflammation and helped elucidate some key aspects of joint destruction. Interestingly, Shiozawa *et al.* could demonstrate that induction of antigen-induced arthritis in *c-fos* transgenic mice leads to a severe destruction characterized by the predominant infiltration of fibroblast-like cells and the absence of lymphocytes[32]. Among the antigen-induced arthritides, the SCW-A model in Lewis rats has been of particular interest, because synovial hyperplasia in this model resembles some important features of human RA. There is a tumor-like proliferation of synovial cells which express high levels of several proto-oncogene products, including *c-fos* and *c-myc*, as well as matrix degrading enzymes such as matrix metalloproteinases MMP-1 and MMP-2[33,34]. In addition, like RA synovial fibroblasts, these cells do not show contact inhibition and can be grown under anchorage-independent conditions[35].

Notably, arthritis in each of these animal models is clearly driven by known antigens. Therefore, it has to be questioned as to what extent their respective pathological processes resemble those of human RA. In addition, most recent studies on the induction of CIA in MMP-3 knock out mice showed that MMP-3 is not required for joint destruction demonstrating the complexity of cartilage and bone degrading enzymes in erosive arthritis[36].

Most recently, the SCID-mouse has been widely used for investigating the molecular and cellular basis of rheumatoid joint destruction. After Mosier *et al.* demonstrated that a functionally intact human immune system can survive in SCID mice recipients[37], the SCID mouse model has been employed to study autoimmune diseases. By implanting rheumatoid synovial tissue under the renal capsule of SCID mice, Adams *et al.*[38] and Rendt *et al.*[39] showed that lymphocyte infiltrates disappear with time, while synoviocytes survive. Moreover, rheumatoid fibroblast-like synoviocytes not only survived in SCID mice but maintained their characteristic biological features. Based on these observation, a novel model for studying molecular mechanisms of rheumatoid joint destruction *in vivo* was developed—the SCID mouse coimplantation model for RA[40]. To imitate the situation in a rheumatoid joint, human RA synovium was coimplanted with normal human cartilage under the renal capsule of SCID mice. Both RA synovial tissue and normal human cartilage could be successfully implanted into SCID mice for more than 300 days, and implanted RA synovium showed the same invasive growth and progressive cartilage destruction as in human RA joints[40]. Intriguingly, the vast majority of synovial cells found at sites of cartilage invasion resembled activated synovial fibroblasts.

To study specifically the molecular properties of these fibroblasts and their contribution to cartilage degradation, normal human cartilage was implanted together with isolated synovial fibroblasts from RA patients to analyze the matrix-degrading properties of these cells in the absence of both lymphocytes and macrophages[41]. Most interestingly, RA synovial fibroblasts maintained their aggressive phenotype, especially at sites of invasion when coimplanted together with normal human cartilage under the renal capsule of SCID mice. In contrast, osteoarthritis (OA) synovial fibroblasts did not exhibit this invasive growth. By using *in situ* hybridization techniques to determine the presence of mRNA for matrix-degrading enzymes, a number of cartilage-degrading proteases could be demonstrated[41]. In contrast, much less or none of these matrix-degrading enzymes could be found, when normal or OA synovial fibroblasts, or dermal fibroblasts were examined in this model. In addition, RA synovial fibroblasts maintained their ability to express VCAM-1[41].

Activated synovial fibroblasts

The hypothesis that activated synovial fibroblasts are critically involved in rheumatoid joint destruction is based on previous observations by Fassbender, which date back to the seventies[6]. By analyzing large numbers of synovial specimens from RA patients he found that invasion of cartilage and subchondral bone by synovial lining cells did not require the presence of inflammatory infiltrates. Moreover, he showed that synovial fibroblasts from RA patients exhibit considerable morphological alterations. They have an abundant cytoplasm, a dense rough endoplasmatic reticulum, and large pale nuclei with several prominent nucleoli[1,6]. Considerable efforts have been undertaken to characterize this 'transformed-appearing' phenotype of synovial fibroblasts. Interest has mainly focused on the characteristics of this phenotype at a cellular and molecular level, and on the mechanisms of activation with respect to their destructive properties.

Up-regulation of proto-oncogenes

Expression of proto-oncogenes and transcription factors in synovial fibroblasts has been described as a major feature indicating the activated nature of these cells[42,43]. The early response gene *egr-1*, coding for a zinc finger protein having DNA binding and transcription regulatory activity, was constitutively over-expressed in RA synovial fibroblasts[44]. Interestingly, egr-1 binding sites were found in promoter regions of several genes, which have been associated with pathogenic mechanisms of RA. Apart from activating other oncogenes, egr-1 has been identified in collagenase-producing rheumatoid synovial fibroblasts[45]. As shown in other studies, oncogenes of the *egr* family are also involved in the activation of the cathepsin L gene[46], a matrix-degrading cysteine proteinase that is up-regulated in RA synovium. These observations are of particular interest as it was shown that joint destruction in RA appears largely mediated by the action of cathepsins and MMPs[45,47,48].

The *c-fos* oncogene which is known to be coexpressed with *egr-1* has also been found to be expressed in RA synovium[45,49,50]. Interestingly, it encodes for a basic leucine zipper transcription factor and is part of the transcriptional activator AP-1(jun/fos). The promoters of several MMP genes, such as *MMP-9*, contain consensus binding sites for the transcription factor AP-1, and the AP-1 site has been shown to be involved in tissue-specific expression of MMPs[51,52]. However, the AP-1 site does not appear to regulate transcription of MMPs alone. Rather, there are essential interactions with other *cis*-acting sequences in the promoters and with certain transcription factors that bind to these sequences[52]. With respect to rheumatoid joint destruction, it is of interest that the proto-oncogene *Fos* has been identified in collagenase-producing rheumatoid synovial fibroblasts[45]. These data suggest *fos*-related proto-oncogenes play an important role in cell activation via AP-1 formation[53].

The oncogenes *ras*, *raf*, *sis*, *myb*, and *myc* have also been detected in RA patients at various levels and are predominantly up-regulated in synovial cells attacking cartilage and bone[43]. Binding sites for the aforementioned early response gene *egr-1* product could be identified in the promoters of the oncogenes *sis* and *ras*. Trabandt *et al.* demonstrated the immunolocalization of Ras and Myc proteins in about 70 per cent of analyzed RA cases. The colocalization of both proteins was restricted to the proliferating synovial lining cells[45]. The cysteine proteinase, cathepsin L, which has been shown to the major Ras-induced protein in *ras*-transformed murine NIH 3T3 cells, was detected in 50 per cent of the RA cases, predominantly in synovial cells[54]. Interestingly, cathepsin L, in these cases, was colocalized with *ras* and *myc*. Most recent data indicate that some of these proto-oncogenes are directly involved in the up-regulation of different MMPs. Gelatinases (MMP-2 and MMP-9) together with MT1-MMP are likely to be regulated by growth factors that mediate their effects through the *ras* proto-oncogene, and c-Ras plays a critical role in the increased expression and proteolytic activation of MMPs in fibroblasts[55,56]. Taken together, these data suggest that pathological expression of proto-oncogenes constitutes an important step leading to the over-expression of matrix-degrading enzymes in RA and consecutive joint destruction.

Alterations in tumor suppressor genes have become of growing interest in explaining some important features of cell activation and survival in RA. Recently, it could be shown that aggressive RA fibroblast-like synoviocyter lack the expression of mRNA for the novel tumor suppressor PTEN, which exhibits tyrosine phosphatase activity as well as extensive homology to the cytoskeletal proteins tensin and auxillin[57]. Firestein, *et al.* have described somatic mutations of the tumor suppressor gene p53 in RA synoviocytes[58]. By producing a non-functional 'cell death suppressor' gene, such mutations could contribute to an extended life span of activated cells aggressively destroying cartilage and bone.

Apoptosis

With respect to synovial cell proliferation, Aicher *et al.* have clearly shown that synovial cells from patients with RA are activated but do not proliferate faster than those from osteoarthritis patients[44]. Using thymidine incorporation, only a small percentage of synovial cells have been found to proliferate[59], and immunohistochemistry for specific proliferation markers such as Ki-67 revealed only a very low number of positive cells[60]. Also, only 1 per cent of fibroblast-like cells expressing proto-oncogenes such as *jun-B* and *c-fos* were concomitantly positive for Ki-67, indicating that the majority of RA synovial fibroblasts do not show accelerated proliferation[61].

In contrast, recent data have provided growing evidence for changes of apoptotic pathways in RA synovium, particularly within the lining layer. When examined by ultrastructural methods, less than 1 per cent of lining cells exhibit morphological features of apoptosis[62,63]. Other studies have reported high expression of antiapoptotic molecules such as Bcl-2 in synovial cells. As mentioned above, somatic mutations of p53 tumor suppressor gene in RA synovial cells may also contribute to reduced apoptosis in these cells[58]. In addition, Franz, *et al.* have demonstrated that the novel antiapoptotic molecule, sentrin, is strongly expressed in RA synovium[64]. Sentrin is found mainly in RA synovial lining cells, whereas normal synovium cells express only very little sentrin mRNA[64,65].

This picture has been confounded by reports on the expression and function of the proapoptotic molecule Fas in synovial lining cells[49,62,66]. To induce apoptosis, specific pathways must be activated, one of which is the ligation of Fas to cell-bound or soluble Fas ligand. However, some recent findings indicate a dual function of the Fas molecule and might shed new light on the role of Fas in the balanced action of pro- and antiapoptotic molecules. Apart from its proapoptotic function, Fas appears to be involved in pathways leading to proliferation[67]. Therefore, intracellular signaling pathways following Fas activation may be modified by additional stimuli that determine whether the affected cell undergoes apoptosis or proliferation. These findings could also explain the fact that cultured synovial fibroblasts are rather resistant to Fas-induced apoptosis, despite the surface expression of Fas molecules[68].

Taken together, these data suggest that apoptosis-suppressing signals outweigh proapoptotic signaling in RA causing a unbalance of pro- and antiapoptotic pathways (Fig. 14.2). This unbalance, subsequently, may lead to an extended life-span of synovial lining cells and result in prolonged expression of matrix-degrading enzymes at sites of joint destruction.

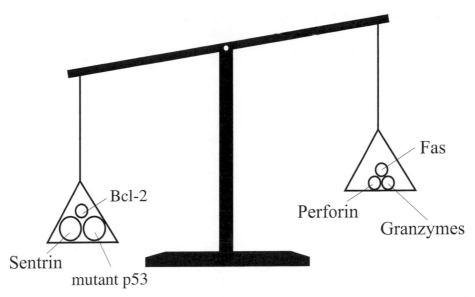

Fig. 14.2 Apoptosis-regulating molecules in RA.

Attachment

Attachment of synovial fibroblasts to the joint cartilage is one of the most prominent features involved in rheumatoid joint destruction. This process appears pivotal for RA as compared with other non-destructive forms of arthritis. Adhesion is mediated by various surface proteins. Three different families have been characterized: selectins, integrins, and the Ig superfamily.

Integrins represent a very complex family of adhesion molecules that contain heterodimers of α and β chains. So far, at least 15 different α and eight different β chains have been described[69]. Integrins have become of general interest for RA not only because of their function as receptor molecules but also because of their interaction with several signaling pathways and cellular proto-oncogenes[70]. Thus, expression of early cell cycle genes such as *c-fos* and *c-myc* is also stimulated by integrin-mediated cell adhesion, and gene expression driven by the *fos* promoter shows strong synergistic activation by integrin-mediated adhesion[71,72]. Recent studies demonstrated that, apart from being displayed on lymphocytes, several β1 integrins such as VLA-3, VLA-4, and VLA-5 are highly expressed on synovial fibroblasts[73,74]. The binding of synovial fibroblasts to extracellular matrix is inhibited, at least in part, by anti-β1 integrin antibodies with the blocking efficacy being significantly higher in RA synovial fibroblasts compared with normal synovial fibroblasts[73]. As a number of integrins function as fibronectin receptors, the fibronectin-rich environment of RA cartilage surface might facilitate the adhesion of RA synovial fibroblasts to the cartilage. In addition to extracellular matrix proteins, the ligands of the integrins may also be cellular surface molecules and some adhesion molecules may bind to more than one ligand. In this respect the recent observations that CS-1, a spliced isoform of fibronectin, is expressed highly in RA synovium[75,76] is of interest. CS-1 appears to be part of a bidirectional adhesion pathway operative in RA as it binds to the integrin VLA-4 (α4β1; CD49d/CD29), which also ligates with vascular cell adhesion molecule 1 (VCAM-1).

VCAM-1 (CD106) is a member of the immunoglobulin gene superfamily and may contain either six or seven immunoglobulin domains of the H type[77]. Several studies have demonstrated increased VCAM-1 expression in RA synovium as compared to normal and OA synovial tissues. While Higashiyama *et al.* suggested macrophage-like cells to be the major source of VCAM-1 in RA synovial tissue[78], most studies revealed high expression of VCAM-1 mainly in synovial fibroblasts but not by macrophage-like cells. Moreover, some recent data suggest that VCAM-1 is particularly up-regulated in the subpopulation of activated lining fibroblasts[22,79,80]. Strong expression of VCAM-1 in the lining layer of RA synovium suggests VCAM-1 is associated with these aggressive cells that are prone to attach, and subsequently invade, articular cartilage[22]. Studies in the SCID mouse coimplantation model revealed sustained-up regulation of VCAM-1 in RA synovial fibroblasts even in the absence of human inflammatory cells for at least 60 days[41]. As mentioned above, VCAM-1 produced by RA activated synovial fibroblasts may not only mediate the attachment to cartilage but may also contribute to T-cell anergy[81] and the induction of angiogenesis[21].

Recently, Petrow *et al.* demonstrated that osteopontin, another extracellular matrix protein that promotes cell attachment, is present in synovial fibroblast-like cells[82]. Most notably in the same study, a stimulatory effect of osteopontin on the secretion of MMP-1 in articular chondrocytes was found. Therefore, osteopontin not only mediates attachment of synovial cells to cartilage but also contributes to perichondrocytic matrix degradation in RA. Moreover, earlier findings demonstrating that osteopontin stimulates B cells to produce immunoglobulins[83] as well as being chemoattractive for macrophages[84] suggest that osteopontin produced by synovial fibroblasts might also play an important role in stimulating B cells to produce rheumatoid factor in the joint and to mediate the influx of macrophages to the synovium in RA.

Taking these data together, the role of adhesion molecules in RA appears not to be restricted to the attachment of synovium to cartilage and bone, but involves the recruitment of inflammatory cells as well as the induction of MMPs.

Cytokine milieu

Although the above mentioned studies indicate clearly that synovial fibroblasts from RA joints maintain their invasive behavior in the absence of human T cells and macrophages, the ability of these cells to stimulate the synovial cells via the production of cytokines must be emphasized[85,86].

Among the cytokines that have been shown to enhance joint destruction in RA, IL-1 and TNF-α are of particular interest. Both cytokines are produced predominantly by macrophage-like synovial lining cells[85,87], and are capable of inducing the variety of other cytokines, chemokines, and prostaglandins. In addition, IL-1 and TNF-α may directly stimulate the production of matrix degrading enzymes such as MMPs[88]. These results indicate that neighboring macrophage-like cells and fibroblast-like cells form a paracrine and autocrine network and that cellular interaction contributes to the perpetuation of chronic synovitis. Data from numerous animal studies, as well as the first promising results from clinical studies using IL-1 and TNF-α inhibitors, highlight the importance of these two cytokines during the course of disease[89-92].

IL-6 is another both fibroblast- and macrophage-derived cytokine that appears to play a role in RA. In IL-6 knock-out mice, the cellular infiltrates within the knee joints were found to be reduced after induction of arthritis by zymosan[93]. However, the loss of cartilage proteoglycan was enhanced, providing further evidence for an uncoupling of inflammatory and destructive pathways[93]. This observation is supported by the finding that IL-6 is also elevated in non-destructive joint diseases.

Matrix degradation

Progressive joint destruction distinguishes RA from other inflammatory joint diseases and is mediated by a concerted action of various proteinases, the most prominent being MMPs[94] and cathepsins[47]. The MMP family consists of at least 20 structurally related members[95]. They are characterized by a zinc cation at the active site and include collagenase (MMP-1), gelatinases (MMP-2 and MMP-9), and stromelysin (MMP-3). Collagenase 3 (MMP-13) is a novel member of the MMP family, that was cloned from mammary carcinoma tissue and, subsequently, from osteoarthritis and rheumatoid synovial tissue[96]. Recently-discovered membrane-type MMPs (MT-MMP) also belong to the MMP family[97]. They are characterized by a transmembrane domain and act on the surface of cells.

MMPs are secreted as inactive proenzymes and are activated proteolyticallly by various enzymes such as trypsin, plasmin, and other proteases. The MMPs differ with respect to their substrate specificities[94]. Whereas MMP-1 degrades collagen types I, II, III, VII, and X only when they are arranged in a triple helical structure, MMP-2 cleaves denatured collagen. MMP-3 is able to activate MMP-1 as well as to degrade proteoglycans. Several reports have implicated MMPs in rheumatoid joint destruction[48,98]. MMP-1 and MMP-3 have been found to be elevated in synovial fluid of patients with RA as compared to OA and are released in large amounts by synovial fibroblast-like cells in culture[48,99]. *In situ* studies revealed strong MMP-1 and MMP-3 expression within rheumatoid synovium, both at the mRNA and protein level[48,100]. Using *in situ* hybridization techniques, other MMPs such as MMP-2 have been localized to the RA synovial membrane. Synovial fibroblast-like cells within the lining layer or at the site of cartilage invasion have been identified as the major source of MMPs. This pattern of distribution is similar to that for proto-oncogenes and is consistent with the notion that proto-oncogenes are involved in the activation of MMP genes[43].

MMP-13 has also been detected at the mRNA[101] and protein level[102] in the rheumatoid synovium, especially in the lining layer. Due to this localization, its substrate specificity for collagen type II, and its relative resistance to known MMP inhibitors, MMP-13 might play an important role in joint destruction. MT-MMPs are also abundantly expressed in cells aggressively destroying cartilage and bone in RA[103]. This is of particular importance because MT1-MMP degrades extracellular matrix components and can activate other disease-relevant MMPs, such as MMP-2 and MMP-13[104,105]. Normally, MMP activity is balanced by the naturally-occurring tissue inhibitors of metalloproteinase (TIMP-1 and TIMP-2). They interact irreversibly with MMPs such as MMP-1 and MMP-3 and are synthesized and secreted by chondrocytes, synovial fibroblasts, and endothelial cells[48,99,106,107]. *In situ* hybridization studies demonstrated striking amounts of TIMP-1 mRNA in the synovial lining of patients with RA[48]. However, the molar ratio of MMPs to TIMP rather than the absolute levels of TIMP are crucial for joint destruction. In RA, the amount of MMPs produced far outweighs than that of the TIMPs, allowing destruction to take place[48].

The expression of MMP genes in RA SFs is regulated by several growth factors and cytokines in a paracrine and autocrine manner. By activating the proto-oncogenes *c-fos* and *c-jun* through receptor-induced intracellular signaling pathways, cytokines are able to influence the level of mRNA for different MMPs. This internal regulation involves several signaling cascades. Thus, *src*-related tyrosine kinases mediate the activation of MMP-1 transcription by IL-1[108], as demonstrated by an inhibition of the increase in MMP-1 mRNA in IL-1-stimulated synovial fibroblasts using herbimycin A, an inhibitor of src-related tyrosine kinases. On the contrary, expression of *v-src* in synovial fibroblasts enhanced both the basal and IL-1-inducible transcription of MMP-1[108].

In cell cultures, IL-1 also had stimulatory effects on the expression of MMP-3[48]. Unstimulated synoviocytes did not express the MMP-3 gene, whereas TIMP was constitutively produced. Addition of IL-1β to cultures significantly induced the expression of MMP-3[48]. As demonstrated in several studies utilizing antigen-induced arthritis in animals, IL-1 not only enhances the production of MMPs but also suppresses the synthesis of proteoglycans (PG)[109]. In some of these studies, anti-IL-1 treatment was able to normalize chondrocyte synthetic function and reduce the activation of MMPs[110]. These data agree with the observations of Müller-Ladner *et al.* showing that over-expression of the IL-1 receptor antagonist (IL-1ra) using retroviral gene transfer significantly reduces perichondrocytic matrix degradation in the SCID mouse model[111]. It has also been suggested that other macrophage-derived proinflammatory cytokines such as TNF-α amplify the destructive processes by stimulating the expression of some MMPs[4,85]. Thus, TNF-α can stimulate the production of MMP-1 in cultured synovial cells[112,113]. However, some recent data indicate a difference in the relative importance of TNF-α and IL-1 with respect to inflammation and joint destruction in animal models of arthritis. While TNF-α appears responsible primarily for the extent of the synovitis, IL-1 seems to have a greater impact on the destruction of cartilage[114]. This hypothesis is supported by data from antigen-induced arthritis and zymosan-induced arthritis in mice, where the suppression of PG synthesis seen by IL-1 was not detected with TNF-α[109]. Related studies using anti-TNF-α treatment in DBA/1 mice with collagen-induced arthritis (CIA) demonstrated efficacy only shortly after onset of the disease, but had little effect on fully established CIA[115]. In contrast, anti-IL-1 α/β treatment ameliorated both early and full-blown CIA. This clear suppression of established arthritis was confirmed by administration of high doses of IL-1Ra[115]. With respect to the up-regulation of MMPs it is of interest that degraded fibronectin also induces MMP-1 and MMP-3 expression in synovial fibroblast-like cells[116,117]. Thus, the synthesis of matrix degrading enzymes in the inflamed joint is not only regulated by proinflammatory cytokines, but also by cleavage products of the destroyed matrix itself.

Cathepsins are the other major group of proteases involved in joint destruction[47]. They are classified by their catalytic mechanism and cleave cartilage types II, IX, and XI as well as proteoglycans[47]. The cysteine proteases cathepsin B and L are up-regulated in RA synovium, especially at sites of cartilage invasion[54,118,119]. In a similar fashion to MMPs, cathepsins are activated by oncogenes. Transfection of fibroblasts with the *ras* proto-oncogene leads to cellular transformation and to the induction of cathepsin L[120]. This is supported by the *in vivo* finding of combined *ras* and cathepsin L expression[25]. Several studies have also shown that proinflammatory cytokines such as IL-1 and TNF-α can stimulate the production of cathepsins B and L by synovial fibroblast-like cells[121,122]. Cathepsin K, a novel cysteinase proteinase, has been suggested to play an important role in osteoclast-mediated bone resorption. Recently, cathepsin K expression by RA synovial fibroblasts and macrophages has been reported, especially at the site of synovial invasion into articular bone, suggesting that it participates in bone destruction in RA[123].

Therapeutic implications

Blocking the action of MMPs and cathepsins is clearly a potential target for the treatment of RA, especially the inhibition of joint destruction. *In vitro* approaches as well as animal models have been used to study the exogenous administration of TIMP and synthetic peptides that inhibit MMPs[124]. Antibiotics such as tetracycline and related compounds, which are inhibitors of MMPs, have been shown to be modestly superior to placebo in controlled trials in RA[124]. In addition, in an animal model, fluoromethylketone-based inhibitors of cathepsins not only inhibited cathepsin L and B activity but also reduced joint destruction[125]. Based on the broad array of different MMPs and cathepsins with different specificities degrading components of extracellular matrix, a combination of inhibitors may be required.

Inhibiting the action of proinflammatory cytokines might also reduce the production of matrix-degrading enzymes[89,111]. Recent studies, surprisingly, suggest that inhibition of single cytokines such as TNF-α might be sufficient to reduce significantly joint destruction in RA. Utilizing the SCID mouse coimplantation model, inhibition of IL-1 by gene transfer with the IL-1Ra reduced the perichondrocytic degradation but had only little effect on the invasiveness of RA synovial fibroblasts into the cartilage[111]. In contrast, transfection of RA synovial fibroblasts with IL-10 resulted in a marked reduction of fibroblast invasion without significant effect on perichondrocytic degradation[126]. Taken together these studies support the development of specific strategies[127], including gene transfer[128], to target the destruction of joints in RA[129].

References

1. Gay S., Gay R.E., Koopman W.J. Molecular and cellular mechanisms of joint destruction in rheumatoid arthritis: two cellular mechanisms explain joint destruction? *Ann Rheum Dis*, 1993;**52** (Suppl 1):S39–47.
2. Mulherin D., Fitzgerald O., Bresnihan B. Clinical improvement and radiological deterioration in rheumatoid arthritis: evidence that the pathogenesis of synovial inflammation and articular erosion may differ. *Br J Rheumatol*, 1996;**35**:1263–1268.
3. Cunnane G., Fitzgerald O., Hummel K.M., Gay R.E., Gay S., Bresnihan B.: Collagenase, cathepsin B and L in the synovial membrane of patients with early inflammatory arthritis. *Br J Rheumatol* 1999;**38**:34–42.
4. Firestein G.S., Wu M., Townsend K., Alvaro-Garcia J., Glasebrook A., Zvaifler N.J.: Cytokines in chronic inflammatory arthritis. I. Failure to detect T cell lymphokines (interleukin 2 and interleukin 3) and presence of macrophage colony-stimulating factor (CSF-1) and a novel mast cell growth factor in rheumatoid synovitis. *J Exp Med*, 1988;**168**:1573–1586.
5. Franz J.K., Pap T., Müller Ladner U., Gay R.E., Burmester G.R., Gay S.: T-cell independent joint destruction in: *T cells in arthritis*. Edited by P Miossec, BW van-den Berg, GS Firestein. Basel, Birkenhäuser, 1998, pp. 55–75.
6. Fassbender H.G.: Histomorphological basis of articular cartilage destruction in rheumatoid arthritis. *Coll Relat Res*, 1983;**3**: 141–155.
7. Firestein G.S.: Invasive fibroblast-like synoviocytes in rheumatoid arthritis. passive responders or transformed aggressors? *Arthritis Rheum*, 1996;**39**:1781–1790.
8. Kobayashi I., Ziff M.: Electron microscopic studies of the cartilage-pannus junction in rheumatoid arthritis. *Arthritis Rheum*, 1975;**18**:475–483.
9. Harris, E.D. Jr., DiBona D.R., Krane S.M.: A mechanism for cartilage destruction in rheumatoid arthritis. *Trans Assoc Am Physicians*. 1970;**83**:267–276.

10. Muller-Ladner U., Gay R.E., Gay S.: Cellular pathways of joint destruction. *Curr Opin Rheumatol.* 9:213–220, 1997.

11. Hamilton J.A.: Hypothesis: in vitro evidence for the invasive and tumor-like properties of the rheumatoid pannus. *J Rheumatol*, 1983;10:845–851.

12. Firestein G.S.: Rheumatoid synovitis and pannus In: *Rheumatology*. Edited by J.H. Klippel, P.A. Dieppe. London, Mosby, 1998;5.13.1.

13. Hoyhtya M., Myllyla R., Piuva J., Kivirikko K.I., Tryggvason K.: Monoclonal antibodies to human prolyl 4-hydroxylase. *Eur J Biochem*, 1984;141:472–482.

14. Shimaoka Y., Attrep J.F., Hirano T., Ishihara K., Suzuki R., Toyosaki T., Ochi T., Lipsky P.E.: Nurse-like cells from bone marrow and synovium of patients with rheumatoid arthritis promote survival and enhance function of human B cells. *J Clin Invest*, 1998;102: 606–618.

15. Salmon M., Scheel Toellner D., Huissoon A.P., Pilling D., Shamsadeen N., Hyde H., D'Angeac A.D., Bacon P.A., Emery P., Akbar A.N.: Inhibition of T cell apoptosis in the rheumatoid synovium. *J Clin Invest*, 1997;99:439–446.

16. Franz J.K., Kolb S., Hummel K.M., Lahrtz F., Neidhart M., Aicher W.K., Pap T., Gay R.E., Fontana A., Gay S.: Interleukin-16 produced by synovial fibroblasts mediates chemoattraction to CD4+ T-cells in rheumatoid arthritis. *Eur J Immunol*, 1998;28:2661–2671.

17. McInnes I.B., al Mughales J., Field M., Leung B.P., Huang F.P., Dixon R., Sturrock R.D., Wilkinson P.C., Liew F.Y.: The role of interleukin-15 in T-cell migration and activation in rheumatoid arthritis. *Nat Med*, 1996;2:175–182.

18. Cruikshank W.W., Lim K., Theodore A.C., Cook J., Fine G., Weller P.F., Center D.M.: IL-16 inhibition of CD3-dependent lymphocyte activation and proliferation. *J Immunol.* 1996;157:5240–5248.

19. Koch A.E.: Angiogenesis: implications for rheumatoid arthritis. *Arthritis Rheum*, 1998;41:951–962.

20. Neidhart M., Wehrli R., Brühlmann P., Michel B.A., Gay R.E., Gay S.: Synovial fluid CD146 (MUC18), a marker for synovial membrane angiogenesis in rheumatoid arthritis. *Arthritis Rheum* 1999;42:622–30.

21. Koch A.E., Halloran M.M., Haskell C.J., Shah M.R., Polverini P.J.: Angiogenesis mediated by soluble forms of E-selectin and vascular cell adhesion molecule-1. *Nature*, 1995;376:517–519.

22. Kriegsmann J., Keyszer G.M., Geiler T., Brauer R., Gay R.E., Gay S.: Expression of vascular cell adhesion molecule-1 mRNA and protein in rheumatoid synovium demonstrated by *in situ* hybridization and immunohistochemistry. *Lab Invest*, 1995;72:209–214.

23. O'Sullivan F.X., Fassbender H.G., Gay S., Koopman W.J.: Etiopathogenesis of the rheumatoid arthritis-like disease in MRL/l mice. I. The histomorphologic basis of joint destruction. *Arthritis Rheum*, 1985;28:529–536.

24. Tanaka A., O'Sullivan F.X., Koopman W.J., Gay S.: Etiopathogenesis of rheumatoid arthritis-like disease in MRL/1 mice: II. Ultrastructural basis of joint destruction. *J Rheumatol*, 1988;15: 10–16.

25. Trabandt A., Gay R.E., Birkedal Hansen H., Gay S.: Expression of collagenase and potential transcriptional factors in the MRL/1 mouse anthropathy. *Semin. Arthritis Rheum*, 1992;21:246–251.

26. Hom J.T., Cole H., Bendele A.M.: Interleukin 1 enhances the development of spontaneous arthritis in MRL/lpr mice. *Clin Immunol Immunopathol*, 1990;55:109–119.

27. Gay S., O'Sullivan F.X., Gay R.E., Koopman W.J.: Humoral sensitivity to native collagen types I-VI in the arthritis of MRL/1 mice. *Clin Immunol Immunopathol*, 1987;45:63–69.

28. Trentham D.E., Townes A.S., Kang A.H.: Autoimmunity to type II collagen an experimental model of arthritis. *J Exp Med*, 1977;146:857–868.

29. Griffiths M.M.: Immunogenetics of collagen-induced arthritis in rats. *Int Rev Immunol*, 19884:1–15.

30. Holmdahl R., Andersson M.E., Goldschmidt T.J., Jansson L., Karlsson M., Malmstrom V., Mo J.: Collagen induced arthritis as an experimental model for rheumatoid arthritis. Immunogenetics, pathogenesis and autoimmunity. *APMIS* 97:575–584.

31. Wilder R.L., Case J.P., Crofford L.J., Kumkumian G.K., Lafyatis R., Remmers E.F., Sano H., Sternberg E.M., Yocum D.E.: Endothelial cells and the pathogenesis of rheumatoid arthritis in humans and streptococcal cell wall arthritis in Lewis rats. *J Cell Biochem*, 1991;45:162–166.

32. Shiozawa S., Tanaka Y., Fujita T., Tokuhisa T.: Destructive arthritis without lymphocyte infiltration in H2-c-fos transgenic mice. *J Immunol.* 148:3100–3104.

33. Case J.P., Sano H., Lafyatis R., Remmers E.F., Kumkumian G.K., Wilder R.L.: Transin/stromelysin expression in the synovium of rats with experimental erosive arthritis. *In situ* localization and kinetics of expression of the transformation-associated metalloproteinase in euthymic and athymic lewis rats. *J Clin Invest*, 1989;84:1731–1740.

34. Yocum D.E., Lafyatis R., Remmers E.F., Schumacher H.R., Wilder R.L.: Hyperplastic synoviocytes from rats with streptococcal cell wall-induced arthritis exhibit a transformed phenotype that is thymic-dependent and retinoid inhibitable. *Am J Pathol*, 1988;132:38–48.

35. Lafyatis R., Remmers E.F., Roberts A.B., Yocum D.E., Sporn M.B., Wilder R.L.: Anchorage-independent growth of synoviocytes from arthritic and normal joints. Stimulation by exogenous plateletderived growth factor and inhibition by transforming growth factor-beta and retinoids. *J Clin Invest*, 1989;83:1267–1276.

36. Mudgett J.S., Hutchinson N.I., Chartrain N.A., Forsyth A.J., McDonnell J., Singer II, Bayne E.K., Flanagan J., Kawka D., Shen C.F., Stevens K., Chen H., Trumbauer M., Visco D.M.: Susceptibility of stromelysin 1-deficient mice to collagen-induced arthritis and cartilage destruction. *Arthritis Rheum*, 1998;41:110–121.

37. Mosier D.E., Gulizia R.J., Baird S.M., Wilson D.B.: Transfer of a functional human immune system to mice with severe combined immunodeficiency. *Nature*, 1988;335:256–259.

38. Adams C.D., Zhou T., Mountz J.D.: Transplantation of human synovium into a SCID mouse as a model for disease activity. *Arthritis Rheum*, 1990;33:S120.

39. Rendt K.E., Barry T.S., Jones D.M., Richter C.B., McCachren S.S., Haynes B.F.: Engraftment of human synovium into severe combined immune deficient mice. Migration of human peripheral blood T cells to engrafted human synovium and to mouse lymph nodes. *J Immunol*, 1993;151:7324–7336.

40. Geiler T., Kriegsmann J., Keyszer G.M., Gay R.E., Gay S.: A new model for rheumatoid arthritis generated by engraftment of rheumatoid synovial tissue and normal human cartilage into SCID mice. *Arthritis Rheum*, 1994;37:1664–1671.

41. Müller-Ladner U., Kriegsmann J., Franklin B.N., Matsumoto S., Geiler T., Gay R.E., Gay S.: Synovial fibroblasts of patients with rheumatoid arthritis attach to and invade normal human cartilage when engrafted into SCID mice. *Am J Pathol*, 1996;149: 1607–1615.

42. Trabandt A., Gay R.E., Gay S.: Oncogene activation in rheumatoid synovium. *APMIS*, 1992;100:861–875.

43. Müller-Ladner U., Kriegsmann J., Gay R.E., Gay S.: Oncogenes in rheumatoid synovium. *Rheum Dis Clin North Am*, 1995;21:675–690.

44. Aicher W.K., Heer A.H., Trabandt A., Bridges S.L., Jr., Schroeder H.W., Jr., Stransk G., Gay R.E., Eibel H., Peter H.H., Siebenlist U., *et al*: Overexpression of zinc-finger transcription factor Z-225/Egr-1 in synoviocytes from rheumatoid arthritis patients. *J Immunol*, 1994;152:5940–5948.

45. Trabandt A., Aicher W.K., Gay R.E., Sukhatme V.P., Fassbender H.G., Gay S.: Spontaneous expression of immediate-early response genes c-fos and egr-1 in collagenase-producing rheumatoid synovial fibroblasts. *Rheumatol Int*, 1992;12:53–59.

46. Ishidoh K., Taniguchi S., Kominami E.: Egr family member proteins are involved in the activation of the cathepsin L gene in v-src-transformed cells. *Biochem Biophys Res Commun*, 1997;238:665–669.

47. Müller-Ladner U., Gay R.E., Gay S.: Cysteine proteinases in arthritis and inflammation. *Perspectives in Drug Discovery and Design* 1996;6:87–98.

48. Firestein G.S., Paine M.M.: Stromelysin and tissue inhibitor of metalloproteinases gene expression in rheumatoid arthritis synovium. *Am J Pathol*, 1992;140:1309–1314.

49. Ashahara H., Hasunuma T., Kobata T., Inoue H., Muller Ladner U., Gay S., Sumida T., Nishioka K.: In situ expression of protooncogenes and Fas/Fas ligand in rheumatoid arthritis synovium. *J Rheumatol*, 1997;24:430–435.

50. Dooley S., Herlitzka I., Hanselmann R., Ermis A., Henn W., Remberger K., Hopf T., Welter C.: Constitutive expression of c-fos and c-jun, overexpression of ets-2, and reduced expression of metastasis suppressor gene nm23- H1 in rheumatoid arthritis. *Ann Rheum Dis*, 1996;55:298–304.

51. Himelstein B.P., Koch C.J.: Studies of type IV collagenase regulation by hypoxia. *Cancer Lett*, 1998.;124:127–133.

52. Benbow U., Brinckerhoff C.E.: The AP-1 site and MMP gene regulation: what is all the fuss about? *Matrix Biol*, 1997;15:519–526.

53. Asahara H., Fujisawa K., Kobata T., Hasunuma T., Maeda T., Asanuma M., Ogawa N., Inoue H., Sumida T., Nishioka K.: Direct evidence of high DNA binding activity of transcription factor AP-1 in rheumatoid arthritis synovium. *Arthritis Rheum*, 1997;40:912–918.

54. Trabandt A., Aicher W.K., Gay R.E., Sukhatme V.P., Nilson H.M., Hamilton R.T., McGhee J.R., Fassbender H.G., Gay S.: Expression of the collagenolytic and Ras-induced cysteine proteinase cathepsin L and proliferation-associated oncogenes in synovial cells of MRL/I mice and patients with rheumatoid arthritis. *Matrix*, 1990;10:349–361.

55. Gum R., Wang H., Lengyel E., Juarez J., Boyd D.: Regulation of 92 kDa type IV collagenase expression by the jun aminoterminal kinase- and the extracellular signal-regulated kinase-dependent signaling cascades. *Oncogene*, 1997;14:1481–1493.

56. Korzus E., Nagase H., Rydell R., Travis J.: The mitogen-activated protein kinase and JAK-STAT signaling pathways are required for an oncostatin M-responsive element-mediated activation of matrix metalloproteinase 1 gene expression. *J Biol Chem*, 1997;272:1188–1196.

57. Pap T., Hummel K.M., Franz J.K., Müller-Ladner U., Gay R.E., Gay S.: Downregulation but no mutation of novel tumor suppressor PTEN in aggressively invading rheumatoid arthritis fibroblasts (RA-SF). *Arthritis Rheum* 1998;41:S239,.

58. Firestein G.S., Echeverri F., Yeo M., Zvaifler N.J., Green D.R.: Somatic mutations in the p53 tumor suppressor gene in rheumatoid arthritis synovium. *Proc Natl Acad Sci U.S.A.* 94:10895–10900, 1997.

59. Nykanen P., Bergroth V., Raunio P., Nordstrom D., Konttinen Y.T.: Phenotypic characterization of 3H-thymidine incorporating cells in rheumatoid arthritis synovial membrane. *Rheumatol Int*, 1986;6:269–271.

60. Petrow P., Theis B. Eckard A., Karbowski A., Eysel P., Salzmann G., Gaumann A., Gay R.E., Gay S., Klein C., Kirkpatrick C., Kriegsmann J.: Determination of proliferating cells at sites of cartilage invasion in patients with rheumatoid arthritis. *Arthritis Rheum*, 1997;40:S251.

61. Kinne R.W., Palombo Kinne E., Emmrich F.: Activation of synovial fibroblasts in rheumatoid arthritis. *Ann Rheum Dis*, 1995;54:501–504.

62. Matsumoto S., Muller Ladner U., Gay R.E., Nishioka K., Gay S.: Multistage apoptosis and Fas antigen expression of synovial fibroblasts derived from patients with rheumatoid arthritis. *J Rheumatol*, 1996;23:1345–1352.

63. Nakajima T., Aono H., Hasunuma T., Yamamoto K., Shirai T., Hirohata K., Nishioka K.: Apoptosis and functional Fas antigen in rheumatoid arthritis synoviocytes. *Arthritis Rheum*, 1995;38:485–491.

64. Franz J.K., Hummel K.M., Aicher W.K., Muller Ladner U., Gay R.E., Gay S.: Sentrin, a novel anti-apoptotic molecule is strongly expressed in synovium of patients with rheumatoid arthritis (RA). *Arthritis Rheum*, 1997;40:S116.

65. Franz J.K., Hummel K.M., Aicher W.K., Pap T., Müller Ladner U., Gay R.E., Gay S.: Invasive synovial fibroblasts express the novel anti-apoptotic molecule sentrin in the SCID mouse model of rheumatoid arthritis. *Arthritis Rheum*, 1998;41:S238.

66. Firestein G.S., Yeo M., Zvaifler N.J.: Apoptosis in rheumatoid arthritis synovium. *J Clin Invest*, 1995;96:1631–1638.

67. Freiberg R.A., Spencer D.M., Choate K.A., Duh H.J., Schreiber S.L., Crabtree G.R., Khavari P.A.: Fas signal transduction triggers either proliferation or apoptosis in human fibroblasts. *J Invest Dermatol*, 1997;108:215–219.

68. Aicher W.K., Peter H.H., Eibel H.: Human synovial fibroblasts are resistant to Fas induced apoptosis. *Arthritis Rheum*, 1996;39:S75.

69. Mojcik C.F., Shevach E.M.: Adhesion molecules: a rheumatologic perspective. *Arthritis Rheum*, 1997;40:991–1004.

70. Schwartz M.A.: Integrins, oncogenes, and anchorage independence. *J Cell Biol*, 1997;139:575–578.

71. Dike L.E., Ingber D.E.: Integrin-dependent induction of early growth response genes in capillary endothelial cells. *J Cell Sci*, 1996.;109:2855–2863

72. Dike L.E., Farmer S.R.: Cell adhesion induces expression of growth-associated genes in suspension-arrested fibroblasts. *Proc Natl Acad Sci USA*, 1998;85:6792–6796.

73. Rinaldi N., Schwarz E.M., Weis D., Leppelmann, J.P., Lukoschek M., Keilholz U., Barth T.F.: Increased expression of integrins on fibroblast-like synoviocytes from rheumatoid arthritis in vitro correlates with enhanced binding to extracellular matrix proteins. *Ann Rheum Dis*, 1997;56:45–51.

74. Ishikawa H., Hirata S., Andoh Y., Kubo H., Nakagawa N., Nishibayashi Y., Mizuno K.: An immunohistochemical and immunoelectron microscopic study of adhesion molecules in synovial pannus formation in rheumatoid arthritis. *Rheumatol Int*, 1996;16:53–60.

75. Muller Ladner U., Elices M.J., Kriegsmann J., Strahl D., Gay R.E., Firestein G.S., Gay S.: Alternatively spliced CS-1 fibronectin isoform and its receptor VLA-4 in rheumatoid synovium demonstrated by in situ hybridization and immunohistochemistry. *J Rheumatol*, 1997;24: 1873–1880.

76. Elices M.J., Tsai V., Strahl D., Goel A., Tollefson V., Arrhenius T., Wayner E., Gaeta F., Fikes J., Firestein G.S.: Expression and functional significance of alternatively spliced csi fibronectin in rheumatoid arthritis microvasculation. *J Clin Invest*, 1994;93:405–416.

77. Osborn L., Hession C., Tizard R., Vassallo C., Luhowskyj S., Chi R.G., Lobb R.: Direct expression cloning of vascular cell adhesion molecule 1, a cytokine-induced endothelial protein that binds to lymphocytes. *Cell*, 1989;59:1203–1211.

78. Higashiyama H., Saito I., Hayashi Y., Miyasaka N.: In situ hybridization study of vascular cell adhesion molecule-1 messenger RNA expression in rheumatoid synovium. *J Autoimmun*, 1995;8:947–957.

79. Morales D.J., Wayner E., Elices M.J., Alvaro G.J., Zvaifler N.J., Firestein G.S.: Alpha 4/beta 1 integrin (VLA-4) ligands in arthritis. Vascular cell adhesion molecule-1 expression in synovium and on fibroblast-like synoviocytes. *J Immunol*, 1992;149:1424–1431.

80. Matsuyama T., Kitani A.: The role of VCAM-1 molecule in the pathogenesis of rheumatoid synovitis. *Hum Cell*, 1996;9:187–192.

81. Kitani A., Nakashima N., Matsuda T., Xu B., Yu S., Nakamura T., Matsuyama T.: T cells bound by vascular cell adhesion molecule-1/CD 106 in synovial fluid in rheumatoid arthritis: inhibitory role of soluble vascular cell adhesion molecule-1 in T cell activation. *J Immunol*, 1996;156:2300–2308.

82. Petrow P., Franz J.K., Muller Ladner U., Hummel K.M., Gay R.E., Prince C.W., Gay S.: Expression of osteopontin mRNA in synovial tissue of patients with rheumatoid arthritis (RA) and osteoarthritis (OA). *Arthritis Rheum*, 1997;39:S36.

83. Lampe M.A., Patarca R., Iregui M.V., Cantor H: Polyclonal B cell activation by Eta-1 cytokine and the development of systemic autoimmune disease. *J Immunol*, 1991;147:2902–2906.

84. Pichler R., Giachelli C.M., Lombardi D., Pippin J., Gordon K., Alpers C.E., Schwartz S.M., Johnson R.J.: Tubulointestinal disease

in glomerulonephritis. Potential role of osteopontin (uropontin). *Am J Pathol*, 1994;**144**:915–926.

85. Burmester G.R., Stuhlmuller B., Keyszer G., Kinne R.W.: Mononuclear phagocytes and rheumatoid synovitis. Mastermind or workhorse in arthritis? *Arthritis Rheum*, 1997;**40**:5–18.

86. Miossec P.: Pro- and antiinflammatory cytokine balance in rheumatoid arthritis. *Clin Exp Rheumatol*, 1995;**13**:S13–16.

87. Wood N.C., Dickens E., Symons J.A., Duff G.W.: In situ hybridization of interleukin-1 in CD14-positive cells in rheumatoid arthritis. *Clin Immunol Immunopathol*, 1992;**62**:295–300.

88. Migita K., Eguchi K., Kawabe Y., Ichinose Y., Tsukada T., Aoyagi T., Nakamura H., Nagataki S.: TNF-alpha-mediated expression of membrane-type matrix metalloproteinase in rheumatoid synovial fibroblasts. *Immunology*, 1996;**89**:553–557.

89. Brennan F.M., Browne K.A., Green P.A., Jaspar J.M., Maini R.N., Fledmann M.: Reduction of serum matrix metalloproteinase 1 and matrix metalloproteinase 3 in rheumatoid arthritis patients following anti-tumour necrosis factor-alpha (cA2) therapy. *Br J Rheumatol*, 1997;**36**:643–650.

90. Maini R.N., Elliott M., Brennan F.M., Williams R.O., Feldmann M.: TNF blockade in rheumatoid arthritis: implications for therapy and pathogenesis. *APMIS*, 1997;**105**:257–263.

91. Evans C.H., Robbins P.D.: The promise of a new clinical trial–intra-articular IL-1 receptor antagonist. *Proc Assoc Am Physicians*, 1996;**108**:1–5.

92. Arend W.P., Dayer J.M.: Inhibition of the production and effects of interleukin-1 and tumor necrosis factor alpha in rheumatoid arthritis. *Arthritis Rheum*, 1995;**38**:151–160.

93. van-de Loo F.A., Kuiper S., van E.F., Arntz O.J., van-den Berg B.W.: Interleukin-6 reduces cartilage destruction during experimental arthritis. A study in interleukin-6-deficient mice. *Am J Pathol*, 1997;**151**:177–191.

94. Krane S.M., Conca W., Stephenson M.L., Amento E.P., Goldring M: Mechanisms of matrix degradation in rheumatoid arthritis. *Am N Y Acad Sci*, 1990;**580**:340–354.

95. Nagase H., Okada Y.: Proteinases and matrix degradation In: *Textbook of Rheumatology*. Edited by W.N. Kelly, E.D. Harris, Jr., S Ruddy, CB Sledge: Saunders, Philadelphia. 1997, p. 323.

96. Mitchell P.G., Magna H.A., Reeves L.M., Lopresti-Morrow L.L., Yocum Sa, Rosner P.J., Geoghegan K.F., Hambor J.E.: Cloning, expression, and type II collagenolytic activity of matrix metalloproteinase-13 from human osteaoarthritic cartilage. *J.Clin.Invest.* 97: 761–768, 1996.

97. d'Ortho M.P., Will H., Atkinson S., Butler G., Messent A., Gavrilovic J., Smith B., Timpl R., Zardi L., Murphy G.: Membrane-type matrix metalloproteinases 1 and 2 exhibit broad-spectrum proteolytic capacities comparable to many matrix metalloproteinases. *Eur J Biochem*, 1997;**250**:751–757.

98. Gravallese E.M., Darling J.M., Ladd A.L., Katz J.N., Glimcher L.: In situ hybridization studies on stromelysin and collagenase mRNA expression in rheumatoid synovium. *Arthritis Rheum*, 1991;**34**:1071–1084.

99. Clark I.M., Powell L.K., Ramsey S., Hazelman B.L., Cawston T.E.: The measurement of collagenase, TIMP and collagenase-TIMP complex in synovial fluids from patients with osteoarthritis and rheumatoid arthritis. *Arthritis Rheum*, 1993;**36**:372–380.

100. Okada Y., Takeuchi N., Tomita K., Nakanishi I., Nagase H.: Immunolocalization of matrix metalloproteinase 3 (stromelysin) in rheumatoid synovioblasts (B cells): correlation with rheumatoid arthritis. *Ann Rheum Dis*, 1989;**48**:645–653.

101. Petrow P., Hummel K.M., Franz J.K., Kriegsmann J., Müller Ladner U., Gay R.E., Gay S.: In-situ detection of MMP-13 mRNA in the synovial membrane and cartilage-pannus junction in rheumatoid arthritis. *Arthritis Rheum*, 1997;**40**:S336.

102. Lindy O., Konttinen Y.T., Sorsa T., Ding Y., Santavirta S., Ceponis A., López-Otín C.: Matrix-metalloproteinase 13 (collagenase 3) in human rheumatoid synovium. *Arthritis Rheum*, 1997;**40**: 1391–1399.

103. Pap T., Kuchen S., Hummel K.M., Franz J.K., Gay R.E., Gay S.: In-situ expression of membrane-type matrix metalloproteinase 1

104. Knauper V., Will H., Lopez O.C., Smith B., Atkinson S.J., Stanton H., Hembry R.M., Murphy G.: Cellular mechanisms for human procollagenase-3 (MMP-13) activation. Evidence that MT1-MMP (MMP-14) and gelatinase a (MMP-2) are able to generate active enzyme. *J Biol Chem*, 1996;**271**:17124–17131.

105. Sato H., Takino T., Okada Y., Cao J., Shinagawa A., Yamamoto E., Seiki M.: A matrix metalloproteinase expressed on the surface of invasive tumour cells. *Nature*, 1994;**370**:61–65.

106. DiBattista J.A., Pelletier J.P., Zafarullah M., Fujimoto N., Obata K., Martel P.J.: Coordinate regulation of matrix metalloproteases and tissue inhibitor of metalloproteinase expression in human synovial fibroblasts. *J Rheumatol*, 1995;**43**(suppl.):123–128.

107. Okada Y., Takeuchi N., Tomita K., Nakanishi I., Nagase H.: Immunolocalization of matrix metalloproteinase 3 (stromelysin) in rheumatoid synovioblasts (B cells): correlation with rheumatoid arthritis. *Ann Rheum Dis*, 1989;**48**:645–653.

108. Vincenti M.P., Coon C.I., White L.A., Barchowsky A., Brinckerhoff CE: src-related tyrosine kinases regulate transcriptional activation of the interstitial collagenase gene, MMP-1, in interleukin-1-stimulated synovial fibroblasts. *Arthritis Rheum*, 1996;**39**:574–582.

109. van-de Loo F.A., Joosten L.A., van Lent P.L., Arntz O.J., van-den Berg B.W.: Role of interleukin 1, tumor necrosis factor alpha, and interleukin-6 in cartilage proteoglycan metabolism and destruction. Effect of in situ blocking in murine antigen- and zymosan-induced arthritis. *Arthritis Rheum*, 1995;**38**:164–172.

110. van-den Berg B.W., Joosten L.A., Helsen M., van-de Loo F.A.: Amelioration of established murine collagen-induced arthritis with anti-IL-1 treatment. *Clin Exp Immunol*, 199495:237–243.

111. Müller-Ladner U., Roberts C.R., Franklin B.N., Gay R.E., Robbins P.D., Evans C.H., Gay S.: Human IL-1Ra gene transfer into human synovial fibroblasts is chondroprotective. *J Immunol*, 1997;**158**: 3492–3498.

112. Dayer J.M., Beutler B., Cerami A.: Cachectin/tumor necrosis factor stimulates collagenase and prostaglandin E2 production by human synovial cells and dermal fibroblasts. *J Exp Med*, 1985;**162**:2163–2168.

113. Brinckerhoff C.E., Auble D.T.: Regulation of collagenase gene expression in synovial fibroblasts. *Ann NY Acad Sci*, 1990.; **580**:355–374

114. Kuiper S, Joosten LA, Bendele AM, Edwards C.K., Arntz O., Helsen M., van de Loo F.A., van-den Berg B.W.: Different roles of TNFα and IL-1 in murine streptococcal wall arthritis. *Cytokine*, 1998;**10**:690–702.

115. Joosten L.A., Helsen M.M., van-de Loo F.A., van-den Berg B.W.: Anticytokine treatment of established type II collagen-induced arthritis in DBA/1 mice. A comparative study using anti-TNF alpha, anti-IL-1 alpha/beta, and IL-1Ra. *Arthritis Rheum*, 1996;**39**:797–809.

116. Werb Z., Tremble P.M., Behrendtsen O., Crowley E., Damsky C.H.: Signal transduction through the fibronectin receptor induces collagenase and stromelysin gene expression. *J Cell Biol*, 1989;**109**: 877–889.

117. Huhtala P., Humphries M.J., McCarthy J.B., Tremble P.M., Werb Z., Damsky C.H.: Cooperative signaling by alpha 5 beta 1 and alpha 4 beta 1 integrins regulates metalloproteinase gene expression in fibroblasts adhering to fibronectin. *J Cell Biol*, 1995;**129**: 867–879.

118. Keyszer G.M., Heer A.H., Kriegsmann J., Geiler T., Trabandt A., Keysser M., Gay R.E.., Gay S: Comparative analysis of cathepsin L, cathepsin D, and collagenase messenger RNA expression in synovial tissues of patients with rheumatoid arthritis and osteoarthritis, by in situ hybridization. *Arthritis Rheum*, 1995;**38**:976–984.

119. Keyszer G., Redlich A., Haupl T., Zacher J., Sparmann M., Engethum U., Gay S., Burmester G.R.: Differential expression of cathepsins B and L compared with matrix metalloproteinases and their respective inhibitors in rheumatoid arthritis and osteoarthritis: a parallel investigation by semiquantitative reverse transcriptase-

polymerase chain reaction and immunohistochemistry. *Arthritis Rheum*, 1998;41:1378–1387.

120. Joseph L., Lapid S., Sukhatme V.: The major ras induced protein in NIH3T3 cells is cathepsin L. *Nucleic Acids Res* 15, 3186, 1987.

121. Lemaire R., Huet G., Zerimech F., Grard G., Fontaine C., Duquesnoy B., Flipo R.M.: Selective induction of the secretion of cathepsins B and L by cytokines in synovial fibroblast-like cells. *Br J Rheumatol*, 1997;36:735–743.

122. Huet G., Flipo R.M., Colin C., Janin A., Hemon B., Collyn dM, Lafyatis R., Duquesnoy B., Degand P.: Stimulation of the secretion of latent cysteine proteinase activity by tumor necrosis factor alpha and interleukin-1. *Arthritis Rheum*, 1993;36:772–780,

123. Hummel K.M., Franz J.K., Petrow P., Muller Ladner U., Aicher W.K., Gay R.E., Brömme D., Gay S.: Cysteine proteinase cathepsin K mRNA is expressed in synovium of patients with rheumatoid arthritis and is detected at sites of synovial bone destruction. *J Rheumatol* 1998;25:1887–94.

124. Moreland L.W., Heck-LWJ, Koopman W.J.: Biologic agents for treating rheumatoid arthritis. Concepts and progress. *Arthritis Rheum*, 1997;40:397–409.

125. Esser R.E., Angelo R.A., Murphey M.D., Watts L.M., Thornburg L.P., Palmer J.T., Talhouk J.W., Smith R.E.: Cysteine proteinase inhibitors decrease articular cartilage and bone destruction in chronic inflammatory arthritis. *Arthritis Rheum*, 1994;37:236–247.

126. Muller Ladner U., Evans C.H., Franklin B.N., Roberts C.R., Gay R.E., Robbins P.D., Gay S.: Gene transfer of cytokine inhibitors into human synovial fibroblasts in the SCID mouse model. *Arthritis Rheum.* (in press): 1998.

127. Hummel K.M., Gay R.E., Gay S.: Novel strategies for the therapy of rheumatoid arthritis. *Br J Rheumatol*, 1997;36:265–267.

128. Jorgensen C., Gay S.: Gene therapy in osteoarticular diseases: where are we? *Immunol Today*, 1998;19:387–91.

129. Firestein G.S.: Novel therapeutic strategies involving animals, arthritis, and apoptosis. *Curr Opin Rheumatol*, 1998;10:236–241.

15 | Pain mechanisms in rheumatoid arthritis

Bruce Kidd, Paul Mapp, and David Blake

Introduction

Pain is the dominant symptom of rheumatoid arthritis. It is a complex phenomenon involving an interaction between physical, psychological, social, and cultural factors. The intensity and character of symptoms arising from inflammatory arthritis vary considerably and are often independent of the underlying disease. In some individuals, pain may occur in the absence of demonstrable pathology whereas in others obviously damaged joints may be relatively symptom-free.

This complexity has been reflected in definitions of pain throughout the ages. Socrates felt that pain and pleasure were closely linked 'passions of the soul', such that the absence of one led inevitably to the other and vice versa[1]. More recent definitions, such as that adopted by the International Association for the Study of Pain, have attempted to encompass the multidimensional character of pain by emphasizing that it is not simply a sensory experience but that it has important emotional and motivational components as well[2].

It is now appreciated that pain depends not only on tissue injury, if any, but also on functional changes within the nervous system. Neural pathways are inherently plastic and may become more (or less) responsive according to different conditions. The extent of this change may well vary between individuals and in some circumstances persist long after the initiating stimulus has resolved.

The first part of this chapter develops a classification of pain based on underlying neurobiological mechanisms. The relevance of these mechanisms to symptoms arising as a consequence of musculoskeletal disease will be explored. Then the process by which sensory nerves not only signal tissue injury but also play an active role in the initiation and maintenance of inflammation are described.

Origins of rheumatic pain

Cutaneous and deep somatic tissues, including joints and muscles, are innervated by primary afferent neurons that synapse with second order neurons in the dorsal horn of the spinal cord[3]. Sensory information is then relayed via spinothalamic and spinoreticular tracts to supraspinal structures including the thalamus and the brainstem (Fig. 15.1). Powerful internal controls are present at all levels, as exemplified by descending

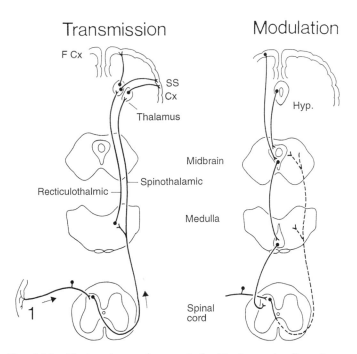

Fig. 15.1 Nociceptive pathways. Left: Noxious stimuli activate primary afferent nociceptors (1) which synapse with second order neurons in the dorsal horn of the spinal cord. Message is then transmitted in the two major ascending pain pathways, the spinothalamic and spinoreticulothalamic, before being relayed in the thalamus to both the fontal (F Cx) and the somatosensory cortex (SS Cx). Right: Inputs from cortex and hypothalamus (hyp) activate cells in the midbrain, which control spinal pain transmission via cells in the medulla. From Fields H.L. *Pain*, (p. 6). McGraw-Hill Book Company, 1987, First Edition.

modulatory systems. Summation and integration of sensory information resulting in pain perception occurs at cortical and subcortical levels. Pain sensation can potentially arise at any point along this pathway, as summarized in Table 15.1.

Tissue injury is a cardinal feature of rheumatoid arthritis and is characterized in other chapters in this book. Although nerve injury at any level may be relatively common in rheumatoid

Table 15.1 Potential causes of rheumatic pain

1. Tissue injury
2. Peripheral nerve injury
3. Spinal injury
4. Altered psychological function

arthritis, it often masked and detection requires a high index of suspicion and help from additional investigations.

Several kinds of peripheral neuropathy may complicate rheumatoid arthritis including polyneuropathy, mononeuropathy (including entrapment neuropathies), and mononeuritis multiplex[4]. The onset is often insidious with pain, paresthesias, or weakness. Carpal tunnel syndrome may be the presenting feature of rheumatoid arthritis, but other neuropathies usually develop in established disease[5]. Entrapment neuropathies are the most frequent and may be multiple. Diagnosis can usually be established using conventional neurophysiological studies, although more sensitive, quantitative sensory testing may be required in early or mild cases.

Although subluxation of the cervical spine is common in rheumatoid arthritis, cervical myelopathy is rare and occurs mostly in those with longstanding disease. Clinical features include progressive neck pain, parethesias or numbness in the limbs or increasing weakness. While plain radiographs, including flexion–extension views, may reveal subluxation, MRI scans generally provide the most useful diagnostic information.

Tissue injury pain

Two principle mechanisms contribute to pain following tissue injury or inflammation: peripheral sensitization and central sensitization. Tissue injury is followed by the release of various mediators from inflammatory cells that serve to sensitize peripheral afferent fibers (i.e. peripheral sensitization). Prolonged activation of peripheral fibers in turn leads to enhanced sensitivity within spinal or central neurons (central sensitization) that modifies pain sensation both at the side of injury and beyond.

Peripheral sensitization

Within deep somatic structures such as the joint, injury or inflammation will inevitably produce sensitization and subsequent activation of articular sensory receptors[3]. It is particularly significant that large numbers of articular nerve fibers are non-responsive under normal conditions and only react following inflammation. Different mediators released either by inflammatory cells or from sympathetic nerve terminals produce varying effects on these receptors. In many, if not all, inflammatory arthropathies the pattern of sensitization and activation in the periphery is likely to be of pivotal importance in determining the character and magnitude of articular symptoms.

Nociceptors

Pain sensations arising from inflamed or damaged joints are mediated in the first instance by primary sensory (afferent) fibers linking peripheral receptors with second order neurons in the spinal cord. Traditionally, these fibers have been regarded as having relatively fixed or static properties and the existance of specialized 'nociceptors' that detect tissue damage or potentially injurious stimuli was first postulated by Sherrington in 1900[6].

It is now reasonably clear that afferent fibers, far from being static as first assumed, are inherently dynamic structures with the ability to vary responses to a broad range of stimuli, including noxious stimuli. There appears to be a critical interaction with the surrounding chemical environment whereby afferent fibers enhance or diminish their capacity to detect and

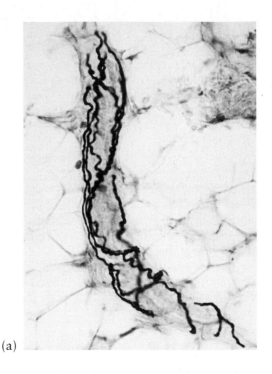

(a)

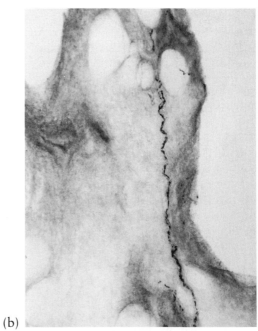

(b)

Fig. 15.2 Unmyelinated nerve fibers within human synovium. (a) CPON-immunoreactive nerve fibers surrounding a blood vessel located deep in normal synovium. (b) CGRP-immunoreactive nerve fiber in the intimal cell layer of the normal synovium. Original material from Paul Mapp.

respond to various stimuli. This is well illustrated in the joint, where inflammatory mediators illicit profound changes in the response properties of afferents to movement and other chemical mediators[3].

Joint innervation

Afferent fibers within peripheral nerves fall within three distinct groups: heavily myelinated $A\beta$ (group II) fibers, thinly myelinated $A\delta$ (group III) fibers and unmyelinated C (group IV) fibers[7]. Synovial joints are innervated with all three groups as well as unmyelinated sympathetic postganglionic fibers[8]. It is notable that the vast majority of articular fibers are unmyelinated comprising sensory C fibers and sympathetic efferent fibers in nearly equal numbers. Only 20 per cent of the fibers in a typical articular nerve are myelinated, mainly comprising $A\delta$ fibers with relatively few of the larger diameter $A\beta$ fibers[9].

The articular capsule of the joint receives an extensive network of nerve fibers with free, complex, or encapsulated nerve endings. A similar innervation has been found in tendons, ligaments, deep fascia, and periosteum. More recent immunohistochemical studies have shown that normal human synovium is also richly supplied with nerves[10,11]. These include fibers containing substance P and calcitonin gene-related peptide (CGRP), which are considered markers of small caliber sensory fibers, as well as nerves containing neuropeptide Y and its C-flanking peptide, found in the majority of sympathetic neurons[11] (Fig. 15.2).

Effects of inflammation

Functional groups of articular afferent fibers can be characterized on the basis of their response to mechanical stimuli[12]. Low-threshold afferents are activated by innocuous stimuli, such as movement within the normal range, which presumably play a role in proprioception. The majority of rapidly conducting $A\beta$ fibers fall into this category. The second group include afferents activated mainly or purely by noxious stimuli such as movement exceeding the normal range. These are $A\delta$ and C fibers and in so far as they respond mainly to potentially damaging events within the joints may be classed as nociceptors. Finally, some fibers do not react to any mechanical stimulus applied to the normal joint whatsoever. These have been termed mechanoinsensitive afferents or silent nociceptors[13].

Several hours after induction of experimental arthritis, the response pattern of articular sensory fibers changes dramatically[14]. The majority become 'sensitized' and show an increased responsiveness to stimuli applied to the joint. Firstly, the highly-threshold sensory fibers become sensitized to movements in the normal range and may have resting activity in the absence of mechanical stimulation. Secondly, a proportion of the initially mechanoinsensitive sensory fibers develop responsiveness to mechanical stimuli. It is relevant that the timecourse of these changes in articular fibers mirrors the development of pain-related behavior in awake animals[3] (Fig. 15.3).

Clinical consequences

In cutaneous tissues, a clear relationship has been demonstrated between pain and peripheral sensitization following a burn[15]. Injury to the skin produces increased pain that correlates strongly with enhanced responses (sensitization) in afferent fibers. It is worth noting that under these circumstances thermal stimuli produce both 'hyperalgesia', defined as an increased response to a

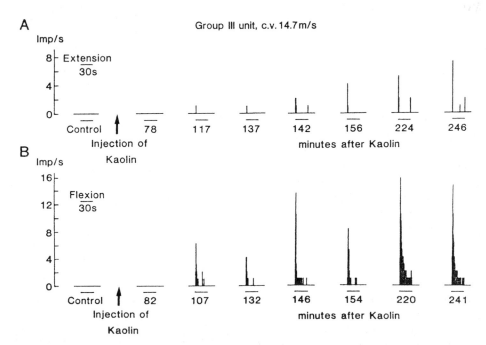

Fig. 15.3 Effects of developing inflammation on high threshold primary afferent fibers in the cat knee. Responses to extension (A) and flexion (B) in the control period and at various times after induction of the arthritis by injection of kaolin (arrows). From Schaible H. and Schmidt R.F. Time course of mechanosensitivity changes in articular afferent s during a developing experimental arthritis. *J Neurophysiol* 1988;60:2180–2195.

stimulus which is normally painful, as well as 'allodynia', defined as pain due to a stimulus that does not normally provoke pain.

Although direct proof in human subjects with inflammatory arthritis is lacking, peripheral sensitization probably underlies use-related or so-called 'incident' pain, experienced only on joint movement and not present at rest. Indirect evidence for the importance of peripheral sensitization in this situation is provided by the relative therapeutic efficacy of peripherally acting non-steroidal anti-inflammatory drugs (NSAIDs). Incident pain arising from peripheral sensitization is often difficult to abolish completely, however, as titration of an adequate dose to provide analgesia during joint movement may result in unacceptable toxicity during pain free periods.

Conversely, it is often wrongly assumed that mechanical hyperalgesia/allodynia originating from deep somatic structures (e.g. joint or muscle tenderness, pain on joint movement) arises exclusively on the basis of peripheral sensitization. Unfortunately, these signs lack specificity and the clinician should be aware that similar findings may well occur in the absence of tissue injury (see below).

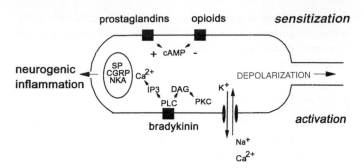

Fig. 15.4 Sensitization and activation of primary afferent C fibers: Prostaglandins (PG) sensitize C fibers probably via a stimulatory G-protein and the cAMP second messenger pathway. Opioids induce formation of inhibitory G-proteins and act to inhibit this pathway. Bradykinin directly activates the C fiber by generation of protein kinase C (PKC) activity and increasing sodium conductance. Heat and mechanical stimuli also increase ion conductance to produce activation although exact mechanisms remain unclear. Release of neuropeptides secondary to changes in intracellular calcium stimulates neurogenic inflammation. From Kidd B.L., Morris V.H. The pathophysiology of joint pain. *Ann Rheum Dis* 1996;55:276–283.

Inflammatory mediators

Many if not all of the chemical mediators found in inflammatory joint fluid have potent and complex effects on afferent fibers with some acting to sensitize their receptors to mechanical and other stimuli while others activate receptors directly. In either case, control of the receptor depends ultimately on the effects of these mediators on membrane ion channels which may be directly coupled to membrane receptors (receptor-gated ion channels) or controlled indirectly through intracellular second messengers[16].

Prostaglandins

Prostanoids, particularly prostaglandin E_2, D_2, and I_2, may activate articular sensory fibers directly, but more usually sensitize fibers to mechanical stimuli and chemicals such as bradykinin[3]. Prostaglandin-induced excitation of sensory membrane receptors leads to a sequence of intracellular events culminating in increased sensitivity, which probably involves a stimulatory G-protein and the cAMP second messenger system[17]. It has long been assumed that the principle site of analgesic activity of non-steroidal anti-inflammatory drugs is in the periphery where they reduce the synthesis of prostaglandins by inhibiting cyclo-oxygenase activity. By reducing prostaglandins it is reasoned that NSAIDs prevent sensitization of articular sensory fibers and thereby inhibit or reduce activation by mechanical and chemical stimuli (Fig. 15.4). While this serves to explain the all-purpose analgesic properties of NSAIDs, other more central analgesic actions for these drugs have been proposed in recent years[18].

Bradykinin

When injected into human skin, bradykinin causes an intense sensation of acute pain. Intra-articular application to the cat knee directly activates a large proportion of group III and IV fibers as well as sensitizing a population of fibers to movement[19].

Although the effects of bradykinin are mediated primarily by bradykinin B2 receptors during acute inflammation, B1 receptors are expressed during chronic disease and may become more important with time[20,21].

Protons

Application of acidic fluid causes pain in experimental situations[22] and protons have been shown to have an excitatory effect on many neurons, which may be of short or relatively prolonged duration[23]. The neuronal activation occurs by the opening of unique ion channels and is distinct from the non-specific effects of protons on membranes observed in many cell types[24]. The overall contribution of protons to pain would be particularly marked within inflamed joints, given the hypoxic environment and extreme acidosis of inflammatory synovial fluid.

Opioids

Opioid receptors have been demonstrated on the terminals of peripheral nerves[25] and local applications of opioid agonists have been shown to reduce hyperalgesia in several experimental and clinical models[26,27] Stein and colleagues have demonstrated that hyperalgesia during adjuvant-induced monarthritis can be reduced in a naloxone-reversible manner following stress-induced release of endogenous opioids. Immunohistochemical studies by the same group have suggested that opioid peptides are produced by many of the cell types commonly found within inflammatory fluids[26].

Central sensitization

Sustained or repetitive activation of peripheral sensory nerves produces substantial changes to the function and activity of central neurogenic pathways, which may, in turn, contribute to symptoms arising from tissue injury. Sensitization of central (spinal) neurons results in exaggerated responses to normal stimuli, expansion of receptive field size, and reduction of the threshold for activation by novel inputs[28].

Referred pain

Local injections of hypertonic saline into interspinous ligaments produces hyperalgesia and referred pain in the abdomen and elsewhere[29]. These effects often occur in areas not sharing the same dermatome and may spread to sites of previous injury or disease[30] Knee pain referred from an osteoarthritic hip is an obvious example. The fact that hyperalgesia and pain spread to areas far removed from the injured region argues strongly against a local process and provides evidence for a central mechanism.

Wind-up and spinal hyperexcitability

The term 'wind-up' was coined to describe changes of activity in dorsal horn neurons whereby sustained or repetitive inputs from C-fibers lead to a progressive increase in the discharge produced by further stimuli[31]. Subsequently, it was shown that acute peripheral injury produced prolonged changes in spinal cord excitability that outlasted the duration of the noxious stimulus[32]. Once wind-up and central hyperexcitability are established, sensory processing within the spinal cord is substantially modified and may produce new sensory modalities such as allodynia, whereby normally innocuous stimuli are perceived as being painful.

Clinical consequences

Dorsal horn neurons receive inputs from various afferent fibers with receptive fields that are not necessarily restricted to one area or even to the same tissue[33]. As an example of this, dorsal horn neurons with receptive fields in the knee also receive inputs from adjacent structures including skin and muscle as well as from remotes sites near the ankle and even the contralateral limb[34]. Under normal circumstances these inputs remain suppressed. However, the development of central hyperexcitibiity allows dorsal horn neurons to respond in an abnormal and exaggerated way[28]. The net effect is that responses to normal stimuli will be increased, the size of the receptive fields will be expanded, and the threshold for activation by novel inputs will be reduced.

Clinically, central sensitization results in enhanced pain perception at the site of injury (primary hyperalgesia) and development of pain and tenderness in normal tissues both adjacent to (secondary hyperalgesia) and removed from (referred pain) the primary site. Furthermore, sensory input from mechanoceptive Aβ fibers may now activate nociceptive pathways, such that innocuous mechanical stimuli such light pressure on the skin produce pains (Aβ fibers allodynia)[35]. Changes within central pathways may be responsible for a history of altered and often bizzare symptoms, while increased numbers of muscle tender points or the presence of trigger points may all indicate the presence of central hyperexcitability.

Spinal neurotransmitters and modulators

Excitatory amino acids

The principal neurotransmitters within the spinal cord are the excitatory amino acids which include glutamine and aspartate. These act via a variety of receptors including the N-methyl-D-aspartate (NMDA) receptor. This receptor belongs to the family of ionotropic glutamate receptors that are coupled to ion channels and are activated by endogenous excitatory amino acids. Their activation evokes long-lasting membrane depolarization and enhanced membrane excitability. Blocking the NMDA receptor blocks the development of wind-up after electrical stimulation[36] and acute inflammation of the knee joint[37]. In keeping with this, Neugebauer and Schaible have shown that sensitization of spinal neurons during acute arthritis is critically dependent on activation of NMDA receptors[38].

Neurokinins

Substance P appears to play an important modulatory role in the spinal dorsal horn. It is released in increased quantities during periods of C-fiber activation[39] and NK-1 receptor anatagonists have proved to be blockers of spinal hyperexcitability evoked by intradermal capsaicin or by acute arthritis in the primate[40]. Consistent with these observations, NK-1 receptor antagonists act as analgesics in animals models of inflammatory pain[41].

Other mediators

A number of endogenous mediators, including prostaglandins, nitric oxide, opioids, and adrenergic agonists have been shown to influence the excitability of spinal neurons. Whereas prostaglandins and nitric oxide appear to facilitate spinal excitibility, alpha$_2$ adrenergic (α2) and μ opioid receptor agonists produce analgesia by presynaptic inhibition of C-fiber neurotransmitter release and post synaptic hyperpolarization of second order neurons[42]. Coadministration of intrathecal morphine and selected α2 agonists or NSAIDs results in substantial analgesic synergy[43] and highlights a role for combination therapy in clinical settings.

Cellular mechanisms

NMDA receptors are activated by glutamate and aspartate which are released in abundance within the spinal cord from both myelinated and unmyelinated primary afferent fibers and also from dorsal horn neurons. NK receptor activation by substance P and neurokinin A receptor enhances the activity of NMDA receptors on both single dorsal horn cells and in isolated spinal cord[44]. The interaction takes place through the activation of protein kinase C which can phosphorylate the NMDA receptor and change its Mg^{2+} binding kinetics. Under normal circumstances, Mg^{2+} binding blocks the NMDA receptor but the alteration of Mg^{2+} binding kinetics allows the release of Mg^{2+} from the receptor and permits glutamate-induced activation and subsequent depolarization of the cell membrane[44].

Nerve injury pain

Dramatic changes to the cell biology of neurons occur when their peripheral axons are severed or damaged. This includes abnormal expression of receptors and transmitters/neuromodulators (primary afferent ectopia), alterations of neural excitability (including central sensitization), and the development of structural changes within the spinal cord (dorsal horn reorganization). These mechanisms will be discussed briefly below.

Primary afferent ectopia

Injury to a peripheral nerve may be followed by alterations in ion channels (most notably sodium channels) leading to abnormal input into the central nervous system from the site of injury and other proximal sites[45]. This ectopic input (ectopia) produces symptoms reflecting those fibers involved (e.g. paresthesias) but may, in the case of abnormal C-fiber input, initiate central sensitization with development of those symptoms and signs discussed previously.

The clinician may obtain a history of nerve injury and, if accessible, the site of injury may be abnormally sensitive to mechanical stimulation (neuroma or Tinel's sign). Nerve conduction studies may demonstrate a major nerve lesion but can miss relatively minor lesions. Quantitive sensory testing may be helpful in these situations[46].

A second consequence of nerve injury is that under some conditions $A\beta$ fiber terminals sprout into lamina II of the dorsal horn making contact with postsynaptic structures that normally receive C-fiber input, leading to the development of tactile (mechanical) allodynia[47]. This has important clinical implications as such structural change may prove refractory to treatment. A further consequence of nerve damage is disinhibition due to down-regulation of inhibitory transmitters/receptors or the loss of interneurons. The development of cold sensitivity may indicate the development of these phenomena.

Norepinephrine sensitivity

Damage to peripheral nerves can also result in the development of adrenosensitivity in injured and adjacent non-injured neurons leading to the development of sympathetically maintained pain. This may be relieved by sympathetic blocks although this is not always the case. The presence of severe, on-going burning pain, touch-evoked pain, and pain evoked by cooling the skin is predictive of a therapeutic response.

The first experimental evidence for interactions between sympathetic and sensory fibers came from observations of neuronal activity in neuromas[48]. In this experimental model, damaged afferent fibers sprout within the neuroma and, unlike undamaged afferent fibers, develop sensitivity to norepinephrine mediated by α-adrenergic receptors[49]. More recent models using subtotal resection or ligature constriction have shown the expression of norepinephrine receptors on the peripheral terminals of those fibers that remain intact[50]. In the context of chronic arthritis, it is relevant that primary sensory fibers activated by prolonged noxious stimulation become sensitized to norepinephrine and sympathetic discharge[51]. The overall conclusion from these and similar studies is that whereas under normal conditions primary sensory nerves do not respond to sympathetic activity, the situation undoubtedly changes following any sort of local injury, including nerve trauma and inflammation. Under these circumstances sensory fibers may be stimulated by ongoing sympathetic activity.

A mechanism-based classification of rheumatic pain

While it is logical to expect that in rheumatoid arthritis inflammatory mediators released from diseased synovium induce peripheral sensitization and hence the development of incident pain, direct proof is lacking. Indirect evidence comes from the response to peripherally-acting NSAIDs and the demonstration that capsaicin-induced axon reflex vasodilatation (reflecting enhanced neurogenic efferent activity—see below) is significantly higher over inflamed wrists, but not control sites, of patients with rheumatoid arthritis when compared with age-matched, normal subjects[52]. Evidence for an important central component is provided by the observation that capsaicin-induced mechanical hyperalgesic responses are higher in rheumatoid patients compared with controls and that the size of the hyperalgesic response (reflecting the degree of central sensitization) correlates with the overall level of pain[53].

Immunohistochemical studies have shown a loss of innervation in inflamed synovium, suggesting the presence of nerve

Table 15.2   Five key neurobiological mechanisms, clinical features and therapy

Site of pathology	Mechanism	Clinical feature	Treatment
Peripheral tissue	Primary afferent sensitization	Heat hyperalgesia	NSAIDs (BK antagonist)
	Central sensitization	$A\beta$ fiber allodynia	Opioids (NMDA, SP antagonist)
Peripheral nerve	Primary afferent ectopia	History, neuroma sign	Nerve block (Na$^+$ channel blockers)
	Adrenergic sensitivity	Vascular instability	SNS blockade

damage[11], while a number of clinical studies suggest an important sympathetic component in some rheumatoid patients[54]. This evidence suggests that at least four different mechanisms may underlie the pain experienced by patients with rheumatoid arthritis: primary afferent sensitization, central sensitization, (possible) primary afferent ectopia, and norepinephrine sensitivity. Recognition of the presence of these mechanisms should allow for a more rational treatment strategies to be developed (Table 15.2). Combination therapy including peripherally and centrally acting analgesics, together with judicious use of sympathetic blocks where appropriate should therefore lead to better symptom control in this disorder. Other clinical syndromes likely lend themselves to a similar analysis.

Neurogenic inflammation

Basic clinical observation indicates that sensory nerves not only signal potential or actual tissue damage but also play an active role in inflammation. Stimulation of unmyelinated sensory fibers produces a local inflammatory response (neurogenic inflammation) characterized in the skin by the familiar wheal and flare reaction[55]. An 'axon reflex' has been proposed whereby activation of sensory fibers following tissue injury results not only in impulse transmission to the central nervous system but also reverse transmission through the extensive network of peripheral nerve fibers known to terminate in close proximity to blood vessels and mast cells.

Neurogenic inflammation is now understood to be mediated through biologically active peptides[56]. These are synthesized within small to medium sized dorsal root ganglion cell bodies and are transported via unmyelinated sensory fibers to peripheral tissues and to synaptic terminals within the superficial laminate (I and II) of the spinal dorsal horn[57]. One of the commonest peptides is substance P, but others, including neurokinin A, calcitonin gene-related peptide (CGRP), vasoactive intestinal polypeptide and somatostatin, have been reported.

A number of clinical studies have provided evidence for altered neurogenic inflammatory responses in musculoskeletal disease. Capsaicin has a selective action on small diameter unmyelinated afferent fibers to produce pain and axon reflex vasodilatation. Although used routinely for a number of years to investigate peripheral sensory function in neuropathic disorders this property has only recently been used to study musculoskeletal disorders. Helme and colleagues have shown that capsaicin-induced skin flares in patients with spinal pain secondary to degenerative disease are significantly smaller than those with pain of non-organic origin[58]. In contrast, a second study by the same group reported increased skin flares in patients with chronic pain syndromes characterized by muscle tender points[59]. A more recent study assessing sensory and autonomic axon reflex responses in rheumatoid arthritis has shown capsaicin-induced axon reflex vasodilatation to be significantly higher over inflamed wrists, but not control sites over the forearms, of patients with rheumatoid arthritis when compared with age-matched, normal subjects[52]. The results suggest selective up-regulation of sensory axon reflex activity in patients with

rheumatoid arthritis but whether this occurs as a result of local mediators or from changes in central control remains unclear.

Neuropeptides

Substance P

This is an 11 amino acid undecapeptide belonging to the tachykinin family of peptides that share a common sequence of six amino acids at the carboxyl terminal[60]. A number of studies have shown increased in mRNA levels of preprotachykinin A, the precursor for substance P, in dorsal root ganglia following induction of arthritis[61,62]. Concomitant with this, substance P levels in the dorsal root ganglia and sciatic nerve have been shown to rise between 40 to 70 per cent following induction of experimental adjuvant-induced arthritis[62,63]. Somewhat paradoxically, levels of substance P in inflamed synovium have been reported to be reduced during the acute stages of short-term inflammation models[63]. This has been taken to reflect rapid degradation of peptides by degradative enzymes known to be present in high concentrations within inflamed tissues. The same explanation may also serve to explain the wide variation in substance P levels reported from synovial fluid removed from arthritic joints[64].

Within the joint, antidromic (reversed) stimulation of unmyelinated articular nerves causes plasma extravasation[65]. This effect appears to be mediated by substance P as it is completely blocked by prior intra-articular administration of a substance P antagonist. Intra-articular injections of substance P produce plasma extravasation[66] (Fig. 15.5) while *in vitro* studies show mast cell degranulation, secretion of PGE_2, and collagenase from synoviocytes and stimulation of IL-1-like activity from macrophages[55]. A role in activation of the immune system has also been suggested. In studies of acute joint inflammation, substance P antagonists significantly inhibit the early articular responses to inflammatory agents such as carrageenan[67].

Calcitonin gene-related peptide

CGRP is a 37-amino acid peptide produced by alternative splicing of the primary transcript of the calcitonin gene. It is particularly abundant in the sensory nervous system, being present in about 50 per cent of primary sensory neurons. It is widely accepted that CGRP, or a closely related peptide, is the major mediator of neurogenic vasodilation in the skin[55]. This effect is mediated by CGRP1 receptors that are coupled to the adenylate cyclase system and arises from a direct action on the vascular smooth muscle, and does not involve nitric oxide or prostaglandins[98]. CGRP may colocalize with substance P in peripheral sensory terminals and simultaneous release produces synergistic interactions (Fig. 15.5).

Growth factors

Nerve growth factor

This is a major regulator of substance P gene expression in adult sensory nerves[69] and may play an important role in the

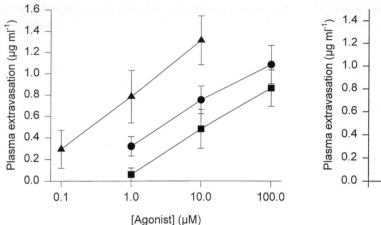
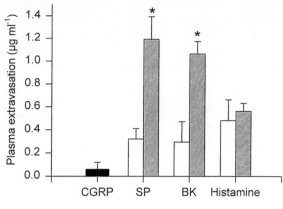

Fig. 15.5   Neuropeptide-induced synovial plasma extravasation. Left: dose response for plasma extravasation into rat knee joints following a 5 min perfusion of bradykinin (triangles), substance P (circles), and histamine (squares). Right: plasma extravasation into rat knee joints following a 5 min perfusion of substance P (SP), bradykinin (BK), and histamine (open columns) and the effects of coperfusion with CGRP (shaded columns). The response to CGRP alone is also illustrated. Values are presented as mean ± standard error. *$p < 0.05$ From Cruwys S.C., Kidd B.L., Mapp P.I., Walsh D.A., Blake D.R. The effects of calcitonin gene-related peptide on formation of intra-articular edema by inflammatory mediators. *Br J Pharmacol* 1992;**107**;116–119.

maintenance of inflammatory pain[70]. Nerve growth factor (NGF) is a member of the neurotrophin family of peptides and is produced by a range of cell types in response to a number of different cytokines including IL-1β and TNF-α[71]. Levels are increased during inflammation[63] and NGF has been identified in synovial fluid of patients with chronic arthritis[72]. In the nervous system, NGF binds to a high affinity trkA receptor where it is internalized and retrogradely transported to the cell body. Systemic administration of anti-NGF neutralizing antibodies in an experimental inflammatory model prevented the up-regulation of neuropeptide, behavioral sensitivity, and development of long-term changes within the spinal cord[71].

Disease outcome

A number of experimental studies have examined the contribution of specific neural components on the expression and outcome of chronic arthritis (Fig. 15.6). In 1983, Colpaert and colleagues reported that capsaicin treatment of adult rats, at doses sufficient to deplete substance P stores, markedly reduced paw swelling and prevented weight loss during adjuvant arthritis[73]. This beneficial effect occurred irrespective of whether capsaicin was given before or after the onset of inflammation. More recent studies have since confirmed and extended these observations by showing that disease outcome as measured by radiographic score was also improved[74,75]. A neurogenic role in the production symmetrical joint disease has been suggested following the observation that inflammation or trauma in one joint can result in a neurogenically-mediated response in the contralateral joint[76,77].

Although neurogenic inflammation has long been thought to be a purely peripheral phenomenon, recent studies suggest that it may be under central control[78,79]. Spinally-administered sensory receptor antagonists significantly reduce joint swelling in kaolin and carrageenan-induced arthritis administered

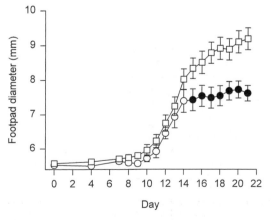
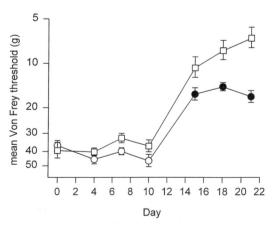

Fig. 15.6   Disease outcome in experimental arthritis. Effect of capsaicin pretreatment on footpad diameter (left) and Von Frey (pain) threshold (right) in adjuvant arthritic rats. Values are expressed as means ± standard error for control (□) and capsaicin pretreated (○) arthritic animals. Statistically significant differences ($p < 0.05$) from the control arthritic group are indicated by the filled circles. From Cruwys S.C., Garrett N.E., and Kidd B.L. Sensory denervation with capsaicin attenuates inflammation and nociception in arthritic rats. *Neurosci Lett* 1995;**193**:205–207.

before[78] or after the onset of disease[80]. A similar effect is shown following dorsal rhizotomy. Of interest, NMDA receptor blockade in the spinal cord also decreases neutrophil migration into peripheral inflamed sites[81]. Therefore, neural loops that regulate chronic pain can directly alter inflammatory responses.

References

1. Rey R. *History of pain*. Editions La Decouverte, Paris 1993.

2. International Association for the Study of Pain Task Force on Taxonomy. IASP Press, Seattle 1994.

3. Schaible H., Grubb B.D. Afferent and spinal mechanisms of joint pain. *Pain*, 1993;**55**:5–54.

4. Bresnihan B. Arthritis and muscle weakness or neuropathy. In: *Rheumatology* (eds J. Klippel, P. Dieppe) Second Edition. Mosby, London. 1998;**4**.1–4.6.

5. Chamberlaine M.A., Corbett M. Carpeal tunnel syndrome in early rheumatoid arthritis. *Ann Rheum Dis*, 1970;**29**:149–52.

6. McMahon S.B., Koltzenburg M. Novel Classes of nociceptors: beyond Sherrington. *TINS*, 1990;**13/6**:199–201.

7. Lynn B. The fibre composition of cutaneous nerves and the classification and response properties of cutaneous afferents, with particular reference to nociception. *Pain Reviews*, 1994;**1**: 172–83.

8. Freeman M.A.R., Wyke B. The innervation of the knee joint. An anatomical and histological study in the cat. *J Anat*, 1967;**101**: 505–32.

9. Heppleman B., Heuss C., Schmidt R.F. Fibre size distribution of myelinated and unmyelinated axons in the medial and posterior articular nerves of the cat's knee joint. *Somatosens Res*, 1988;**5**:267–75.

10. Gronblad M., Konntinen Y.T., Korkala O., Liesi P., Hukkanen M., Polak J. Neuropeptides in the synovium of patients with rheumatoid arthritis and osteoarthritis. *J Rheumatol*, 1988;**15**:1807–10.

11. Mapp P.I., Kidd B.L., Gibson S.J., Terry J.M., Revell P.A., Ibrahim N.B.N, Blake D.R., Polak J.M.I. Substance P-, calcitonin gene-related peptide- and C-flanking peptide of neuropeotide Y-immunoreactive fibres are present in the normal synovium but depleted in patients with rheumatoid arthritis. *Neuroscience*, 1990;**37**:143–53.

12. Schaible H., Schmidt R.F. Responses of fine medial articular nerve afferents to passive movements of knee joint. *J Neurophysiol*, 1983;**49**:1118–26.

13. Schaible H., Schmidt R.F. Time course of mechanosensitivity changes in articular afferents during a developing experimental arthritis. *J Neurophysiol*, 1988;**60**:2180–95.

14. Grigg P., Schaible H., Schmidt R.F. Mechanical sensitivity of group III and IV afferents fromposterior articular nerve in normal and inflamed cat knee. *J Neurophysiol*, 1986;**55**:635–43.

15. Meyer R.A., Cambell J.N. Myelinated nociceptive afferents account for the hyperalgesia that follows a burn to the hand. *Science*, 1981;**72**:305–10.

16. Rang H.P., Bevan S., Dray A. Chemical activation of nociceptive peripheral neurons. *Br Med Bull*, 1991;**47**:534–48.

17. Taiwo Y.O., Bjerknes L., Goetzl E., Levine J.D. Mediation of primary afferent hyperalgesia by the cAMP second messenger system. *Neurosci*, 1989;**32**:577–80.

18. McCormack K. Non-steroidal anti-inflammatory drugs and spinal nociceptive processing. *Pain*, 1994;**59**:9–43.

19. Kanaka R., Schaible H., Schmidt R.F. Activation of the fine articular afferent units by bradykinin. *Brain Res*, 1985;**327**:81–90.

20. Cruwys S.C., Garret N..E., Perkins M.N., Blake D.R., Kidd B.L.. The role of bradykinin B_1 receptors in the maintenance of intra-articular plasma extravasation in chronic antigen-induced arthritis. *Br J Pharmacol*, 1994;**113**:940–4.

21. Dray A., Perkins M. Bradykinin and inflammatory pain. *TINS*, 1993;**13**:99–104.

22. Steen K.H., Reeh P.W., Anton F., Handwerker H.O. Protons selectively induce long lasting excitation and sensitization to mechanical stimulation of nociceptors in rat skin in vitro. *J Neurosci*, 1992;**12**:86–95.

23. Kessler W., Kirchoff C., Reeh P.W., Handwerker H.O. Excitation of cutaneous afferent nerve endings in vitro by a combination of inflammatory mediators and conditioning effect of substance P. *Exp Brain Res*, 1992;**91**:467–76.

24. Bevan S., Geppetti P. Protons: small stimulants of capsaicin-sensitive sensory nerves. *TINS*, 1994;**17**:509–12.

25. Stein C., Hassan A.H.S., Prezewlocki R., Gramsch C., Peter K., Herz. Opioids from immunocytes interact with receptors on sensory nerves to inhibit nociception in inflammation. *Proc Natl Acad Sci* USA, 1990;**87**:5935–9.

26. Stein C. Peripheral mechanisms of opioid analgesia. *Anesth Analg*, 1993;**76**:182–91.

27. Stein C., Comisel K., Haimerl E., Lehrberger K., Yassouridis A., Herz A., Peter K. Analgesic effect of intra-articular morphine after arthroscopic knee surgery. *N Eng J Med*, 1991;**325**:1123–6.

28. Woolf C.J. Generation of acute pain: Central mechanisms. *Br Med Bull*, 1991;**47**:523–33.

29. Lewis T., Kellgren J.H. Observations relating to referred pain, viscero-motor reflexes and other associated phenomena. *Clin Sci*, 1939;**4**:47–71.

30. Coderre T.J., Katz J., Vaccarino A.L., Melzack R. Contribution of central neuroplasticity to pathological pain: review of clinical and experimental evidence. *Pain*, 1993;**52**:259–85.

31. Mendell L.M., Wall P.D. Response of single dorsal cord cells to peripheral cutaneous unmyelinated fibres *Nature*, 1965;**206**:97–9.

32. Woolf C.J. Evidence of a central component of postinjury pain hypersensitivity. *Nature*, 1986;**308**:686–8.

33. Woolf C.J., King A.E. Subthreshold components of the cutaneous mechanoreceptive fields of dorsal horn neurons in the rat lumbar spinal cord. *J Neurophysiol*, 1989;**62**:907–16.

34. Schaible H., Schmidt R.F. Responses of fine medial articular nerve afferents to passive movements of knee joint. *J Neurophysiol*, 1983;**49**:1118–26.

35. Torejork H.E., Lundeberg L., LaMotte R.H. Central changes in processing of mechanoreceptive input in capsaicin-induced secondary hyperalgesia in humans. *J Physiol*, 1992;**448**:765–80.

36. Thompson S.W.N., Gerber G., Sivilotti L.G., Woolf C.J. Long duration ventral root potentials in the neonatal rat spinal cord in vitro; the effects of ionotropic and metabotropic excitatory amino acid receptor antagonists. *Brain Res*, 1992;**595**:87–97.

37. Schaible H.G., Grubb B.D., Neugebauer V., Oppmann M. The effects of NMDA antagonists on neuronal activity in cat spinal cord evoked by acute inflammation in the knee joint *J Neurosci*, 1991;**3**:981–91.

38. Neugebauer V., Lücke T., Schaible H-G. N-methyl-D-aspartate (NMDA) and non-NMDA receptor antagonists block the hyper-excitability of dorsal horn neurons during development of acute arthritis in rat's knee joint. *J Neurophysiol*, 1993;**70**:1365–77.

39. Duggan A.W., Hendry I.A., Morton C.R., Hutchison W.D., Zhao Z.Q. Cutaneous stimuli releasing immunoreactive substance P in the dorsal horn of the cat. *Brain Res*, 1988;**451**:261–73.

40. Dougherty P.M., Palecek J., Paleckova V., Willis W.D. Neurokinin 1 and 2 antagonists attenuate the responses and NK1 antagonists prevent the sensitization of primate spinothalamic tract neurons after intradermal capsaicin. *J Neurophysiol*, 1994;**72**:1464–75.

41. Yamamoto T., Yaksh T.L. Stereospecific effects of a non-peptidic NK1 selective antagonsist, CP-96,345: antionciception in the absence of motor dysfunction. *Life Sci*, 1991;**49**:1955–63.

42. Go V.L., Yaksh T.L. Release of substance P from the cat spinal cord. *J Physiol*, 1987;**391**:141–67.

43. Malmberg A.B., Yaksh T.L. Pharmacology of the spinal action of ketorolac, morphine, ST-91, U50488H, and L-PIA on the formalin test and an isobolographic analysis of the NSAID interaction. *Anesthesiology*, 1993;**79**:270–81.

44. Urban L., Thompson S.W.N., Nagy I., Dray A. Hyperexcitabilty in the spinal dorsal horn: cooperation of neuropeptides and excitatory amino acids. In: Urban L. (ed) *Cellular mechanisms of sensory processing*. Springer, Berlin, 1994;379–99.

45. Devor M. The pathophysiology of damaged peripheral nerves. In: Wall PD, Melzac R (Eds) *Textbook of Pain*, 3rd edn. Churchill Livingstone, Edinburgh: 1994.

46. Bennet G.J. Neuropathic pain. In: Wall PD, Melzac R. (eds) *Textbook of Pain* 3rd edn. Churchill Livingstone, Edinburgh: 1994.

47. Woolf C.J., Shortland P., Coggeshall R.E. Peripheral nerve injury triggers central sprouting of myelinated afferents. *Nature*, 1992;355:75–7.

48. Wall P.D., Gutnick M. Ongoing activity in peripheral nerves: the physiology and pharmacology of impulses originating from a neuroma. *Exp Neurol*, 1974;43:580–93.

49. Devor M. Nerve pathophysiology and mechanisms of pain in causalgia. *J Auton Ner Syst*, 1983;7:371–384.

50. Bennet G.J. The role of the sympathetic nervous system in painful peripheral neuropathy. *Pain*, 1991;45:221–3.

51. Hu S., Zhu J. Sympathetic facilitation of sustained discharges of polymodal nociceptors. *Pain*, 1989;38:85–90.

52. Jolliffee V.A., Anand P., Kidd B.L. Assessment of cutaneous sensory and autonomic axon reflexes in rheumatoid arthritis. *Ann Rheum Dis*, 1995;54:251–5.

53. Morris V.H., Cruwys S.C., Kidd B.L. Characterisation of capsaicin-induced mechanical hyperalgesia as a marker for altered nociceptive processing in patients with rheumatoid arthritis. *Pain*, 1997;71:179–86.

54. Hertford R.A. Extended sympathectomy in the treatment of chronic rheumatoid arthritis. *J Am Geriat Soc*, 1957;5:904–15.

55. Holzer P. Neurogenic vasodilation and plasma leakage in the skin. *Gen Pharmac*, 1998;30:5–11.

56. Holzer P. Local effector functions of capsaicin-sensitive sensory nerve endings: involvement of tachykinins, calcitonin gene-related peptide and other neuropeptides. *Neurosci*, 1988;24:739–68.

57. Foreman J.C. Peptides and neurogenic inflammation. *Br Med Bull*, 1987;43:386–400.

58. LeVasseur S.A., Gibson S.J., Helme R.D. The measurement of capsaisin-sensitive sensory nerve fibre function in elderly patients with pain. *Pain*, 1990;41:19–25.

59. Helme R.D., Littlejohn G.O., Weinstein C. Neurogenic flare responses in chronic rheumatic pain syndromes. *Clin Exp Neurol*, 1987;23:91–4.

60. Pernow B. Substance P. *Pharm Rev*, 1983;35:85–141.

61. Donaldson L.F., Harmar A.J., McQueen D.S., Seckl J.R. Increase expression of preprotachykinin, calcitonin gene-related peptide, but not vasoactive intestinal peptide messenger RNA in dorsal root ganglia during the development of adjuvant monarthritis in the rat. *Mol Brain Res*, 1992;16:143–9.

62. Garrett N.E., Kidd B.L., Cruwys S.C., Tomlinson D.R. Changes in preprotachykinin mRNA expression and substance P levels in dorsal root ganglia of monoarthritic rats: Comparison with changes in synovial substance P levels. *Brain Res*, 1995;675:203–7.

63. Donnerer J., Schuligoi R., Stein C. Increased content and transport of substance P and calcitonin gene-related peptide in sensory nerves innervating inflamed tissue: evidence for a regulatory function of nerve growth factor in vivo. *Neurosci*, 1992;49:693–8.

64. Mapp P.I., Kidd B.L. Substance P in rheumatic disease Sem Arthritis Rheum, 1994;6(S3):3–9.

65. Ferrell W.R., Russell N.J.W. Extravasation in the knee induced by antidromic stimulation of articular C fiber afferents of the anaesthetised cat. *J Physiol (Lond)*, 1986;379:407–16.

66. Cruwys S.C., Kidd B.L., Mapp P.I., Walsh D.A., Blake D.R. The effects of calcitonin gene-related peptide on formation of intra-articular edema by inflammatory mediators. *Br J Pharmacol*, 1992;107:116–19.

67. Lam F.Y., Ferrell. Inhibition of carrageenan induced inflammation in the rat knee joint by substance P antagonist. *Ann Rheum Dis*, 1989;48:928–32.

68. Brain S.D. Sensory neuropeptides in the skin. In: *Neurogenic inflammation* (eds Geppetti P, Holzer P) CRC Press, Boca Raton, FL. 1996;229–44.

69. Lindsay R.M., Harmar A.J. Nerve growth factor regulates expression of neuropeptide genes in adult sensory neurons. *Nature*, 1989;337:362–4.

70. Lewin G.R., Mendell L.M. Nerve growth factor and nociception. *Trends Neurosci*, 1993;16:353–9.

71. Woolf C.J., Safieh-Garabedian B., Ma Q.P., Crilly P., Winters J. Nerve growth factor contributes to the generation of inflammatory sensory hypersensitivity. *Neurosci*, 1994;62:327–31.

72. Aloe L., Turveri M.A., Carcassi U., Levi-Montalcini R. Nerve growth factor in synovial fluid of patients with chronic arthritis. *Arthritis Rheum*, 1992;35:351–5.

73. Colpaert F.C., Donnerer J., Lembeck F. Effects of capsaicin on inflammation and on the substance P content of nervous tissues in rats with adjuvant arthritis. *Life Sci*, 1983;32:1827–34.

74. Levine J.D., Dardick S.J., Roizen M.F., Helms C. Contribution of sensory afferents and sympathetic efferents to joint injury in experimental arthritis. *J Neurosci*, 1986;6:3423–9.

75. Cruwys S.C., Garrett N.E., Kidd B.L. Sensory denervation with capsaicin attenuates inflammation and nociception in arthritic rats. *Neurosci Lett*, 1995;193:205–7.

76. Levine D.J., Dardick S.J., Roizen M.F., Basbaum A.I., Scipio E. Reflex neurogenic inflammation. Contribution of the peripheral nervous system to spatially remote inflammatory responses that follow injury. *J Neurosci*, 1985;5:1380–6.

77. Kidd B.L., Cruwys S.C., Garrett N.E., Mapp P.I., Jolliffe V.A., Blake D.R. Neurogenic influences on contralateral responses during experimental rat monarthritis. *Brain Res*, 1995;688:72–6.

78. Sluka K.A., Westlund K.N. Centrally administered non-NMDA but not NMDA receptor antagonists block peripheral knee joint inflammation. *Pain*, 1993;55:217–25.

79. Sluka K.A., Jordan H.H., Westlund K.N. Reduction in joint swelling and hyperalgesia following post-treatment with a non-NMDA receptor antagonist. *Pain*, 1994;59:95–100.

80. Sluka K.A., Lawand N.B., Westlund K.N. Joint inflammation is reduced by dorsal rhizotomy and not by sympathectomy or spinal cord transection. *Ann Rheum Dis*, 1994;53:309–14.

81. Bong G.W., Rosengren S., Firestein G.S. Spinal cord adenosine receptor stimulation in rats inhibits peripheral neutrophil accumulation: The role of N-methyl-D-aspartate receptors. *J Clin Invest*, 1996;98:2779–85.

SECTION 3 | *Clinical aspects*

16 | Rheumatoid arthritis: clinical picture and its variants

William F. Lems and Ben A.C. Dijkmans

Introduction

Rheumatoid arthritis (RA) is a systemic disease with chronic inflammation of multiple diarthrodial joints as the most prominent feature. The disease is characterized by symmetrical pain and swelling of the joints, which is often accompanied by stiffness and fatigue. The chronic synovitis may lead to joint destruction, deformities, and disabilities. RA has a wide clinical spectrum, which varies from mild joint symptoms to severe inflammation and damage to joints, accompanied by extra-articular symptoms, such as rheumatoid nodules, pericarditis, pulmonary involvement, Felty's syndrome, mononeuritis multiplex, and vasculitis.

Epidemiology

Incidence and prevalence

There is no evidence for the existence of RA in Europe, Asia, or Africa before the 17th century. Findings in skeletal remains in archaic North American Indians suggest that RA originated around 4000 BC in the New World[1]. Based on these findings, the hypothesis was developed that RA originated in the New World and spread to the Old World after Columbus discovered America in 1492[2].

Currently, RA has been identified in all parts of the world, regardless of the ethnic or racial group that has been studied. The prevalence of RA in the community is estimated to be around 1 per cent in the United States[3,4] and in Europe[5], while in Asia and Africa lower prevalence rates are found[2]. In recent, community-based studies from Norway and Italy, prevalence rates of 0.33 and 0.44 per cent were observed[6,7].

The incidence rate of RA varies from 0.89 per cent (Pima Indians) to 0.009 per cent in France[2]. In Pima Indians, the incidence rate decreased from 0.89 per cent in the sixties to 0.39 per cent in the eighties, which supports the idea that incidence and severity are changing in different parts of the world—declining in Europe and the United States and rising in Asia and Africa[2]. Since the decline in incidence of RA parallels the increase in prevalence of atopic disorders, a 'population shift' away from Th1 type immune response and towards a Th2 pattern of response is hypothesized[8]. This hypothesis is supported by a decreased prevalence of hay fever in RA patients and low disease activity in RA patients with hay fever[9].

Hormonal influences

Hormones have an important, though not completely elucidated, influence on RA. Women are affected three times more than men, while the ratio declines to 1 in the elderly. In the majority of women with RA, disease activity is reduced during pregnancy, with rebound of disease activity postpartum[10]. Data on the relationship between the use of oral contraceptives and RA are conflicting[11]: in an European study, the occurrence of RA was decreased in women using oral contraceptives[12], while this could not be confirmed in the United States[13]. Data on the effects of hormonal replacement therapy (HRT) on disease activity of RA in postmenopausal women are also conflicting: positive effects[14] as well as negative effects[15] have been shown. Nevertheless, HRT has a positive effect on bone mass in postmenopausal women with RA[16].

Disease patterns of RA are different in men and women[17]. Erosive disease is more frequent in men than in women and tends to occur earlier. Nodules and rheumatoid lung disease are typical manifestations in men, whereas women more frequently develop sicca syndrome.

Genetics

The genetic component of RA is relatively limited, since the concordance rate, the risk of developing RA in monozygotic twins, is 25 per cent[18]. RA is a genetically complex disease, because of the involvement of multiple predisposing genes and because of variable and incomplete penetrance of these genes[19].

Genetic factors, in particular the HLA-DR genes, do influence the susceptibility and probably also the severity of RA[20]. DR-molecule β chains on antigen-presenting cells present immunogenic proteins to T cells; the shared epitope is located on the DRβ polypeptide. In 80 to 90 per cent of RA patients the shared DRB1 epitope is present. The frequency of the shared epitope in Caucasians is 20 per cent. Since RA will develop in only 1 per cent of the population, the presence of the shared epitope explains only a part of the puzzle. Data on the association between HLA-DR4 and prognosis of RA are not uniform, probably as a result of variation between populations and selection of patients[20]. Although the contribution of the shared epitope to the pathogenesis of RA is limited, the presence of the shared epitope appears to be associated with progressive disease, in some[21,22], but not all[23], populations. Considerable progress has been made in recent years in elucidating the genetic component in RA. However, there is insufficient evidence that genetic information adds substantially to conventional clinical and laboratory parameters in daily practice.

Mortality

RA is not only associated with morbidity, but also with increased mortality[24,25]. In a recent study, the standardized mortality ratio (a comparison with the expected death rate in the general population) for RA patients is 2.7 (95 per cent confidence interval: 2.4–3.1)[26]. Mortality rates are proportionally increased in patients with severe RA[27,28]. The increased mortality is thought to be related to complications of the disease itself, such as vasculitis and cervical myelopathy resulting from C1–C2 subluxation, but also to infectious diseases, cardiovascular diseases, and drug side-effects. The risk of sepsis is increased by the use of immunosuppressive drugs and/or the presence of Felty's syndrome. Increased bleeding tendency and kidney or liver failure may result from the use of non-steroidal anti-inflammatory drugs (NSAIDs) and/or disease modifying antirheumatic drugs (DMARDs).

Clinical picture of RA

History

A careful medical history is essential for the diagnosis RA. Arthritic pain has to be differentiated from non-arthritic pain. In general, non-arthritic pain is absent in the morning and provoked by physical stress; arthritic pain is present throughout the whole day, above all in the morning. The localization and the number of the affected joints contribute to the diagnosis: symmetric polyarthritis with involvement of the small joints of the hands and feet are common presenting symptoms in RA. A history of RA in other members of the family increases the suspicion of RA. Hormonal factors are relevant, for example the risk of RA is increased in a women postpartum.

General manifestations of arthritis

Tenderness and swelling are the key signs of joint inflammation in RA; local heat and limited range of motion are often also present. Redness of joint(s) is hardly seen in RA.

Pain

Pain in the joints is the major symptom. Arthritic pain is caused by elevated intra-articular pressure leading to excessive stresses on the extensively innervated periarticular structures. The correlation between pain and swelling of the joints is limited, which is, at least partly, related to interindividual variation in perception, threshold, and expression of pain. Besides pain on rest, joint tenderness, elicited by direct palpation over the joint, is also an important sign of RA. Testing for joint tenderness is particularly useful for detection of disease activity in wrist, fingers, and toes.

Swelling

Joint swelling may be related to synovial proliferation or increased amount of intra-articular fluid, or both. Effusion may be demonstrated by fluctuation: an increase in fluid tension by pressure in one direction is transmitted equally to other planes. Synovial proliferation may be felt as a doughy texture. Detection of swelling of the shoulders and hips can be difficult, since these joints are not located superficially.

Temperature

Normally, the temperature of a joint is lower than that of surrounding tissue. In arthritic joints, the temperature is equal to or higher than surrounding tissues[29]. Since elevated joint temperature is associated with increased collagen breakdown[29], application of cold ice-packs is, besides other therapeutic interventions, useful in patients with severe arthritis[30].

Stiffness

Morning stiffness lasting more than 1 hour has been included in classification criteria for RA[31]. This symptom is probably related to the accumulation of edema (during sleep) within the synovium and periarticular structures. Since morning stiffness is almost exclusively seen in inflammatory disorders, it is useful as a discriminator from non-inflammatory diseases. Some patients have difficulty in discriminating between pain and stiffness. An important question is to ask the patient for the length of time from waking to maximal improvement[32].

Functio laesa

Limitation of range of joint motion is one of the most important features of RA. In early arthritis, a reversible limitation of the range of motion may be caused through pain or capsular distension from excess synovial fluid or synovial tissue. Proteolytic degradation in chronic arthritis may lead to stretching and weakening of the periarticular ligaments, and to cartilage damage and bone loss[33]. At first presentation, 50 per cent of RA patients show limited mobility of the hand joints. In chronic RA, loss of joint motion is present in 25–35 per cent of the large joints[34].

Muscle strength

In RA patients, loss of muscle strength is very common. In mildly disabled patients, strength of hip and knee muscles is reduced to 50–70 per cent, when compared to age-matched, healthy volunteers[35,36]. In patients with severe RA, the strength of the quadriceps muscles is reduced to 30–45 per cent[37]. Muscle atrophy in patients with RA has usually been attributed to active joint disease, immobilization and antirheumatic drugs. Muscular weakness in RA has an important impact on physical disability[38]. Prevention of muscular wasting by dynamic exercises has not only a positive effect on muscle strength, but also on joint mobility and aerobic capacity, while, in contrast to previous thoughts, dynamic exercises are not associated with a worsening of disease activity[39]. Some DMARDs (d-penicillamine, antimalarials) and corticosteroids have been associated with muscular weakness. Histologically, fiber atrophy of type 2 may be found in patients treated with corticosteroids. In a minority of patients, 'true' polymyositis occurs in the presence of RA[40].

Specific joints

Cervical spine

Cervical involvement in RA patients may lead to serious complications, particularly at the C1–C2 level. Damage of the cervical spine occurs in 30 per cent of RA patients[41,42], predominantly in patients with erosive, deforming RA[42]. Synovitis of the cervical spine may damage periarticular structures leading to instability. Moreover, proliferative synovitis can result in formation of pannus and compression of the spinal cord[43]. Destructive changes are most prominent at the atlantoaxial joint, but may also occur at lower levels of the cervical spine, particularly at C4–C5. The atlantoaxial joint is prone to subluxation in three directions:

1. Anterior subluxation of the atlas, as a result of synovitis induced laxity of the transverse ligament—normally, the space between the odontoid process and the arch of the atlas measures 3 mm or less; in RA patients it may exceed 10 mm. The anterior subluxation is the most common in RA.

2. Posterior subluxation of the atlas is infrequent. It will only occur if the odontoid process has been fractured or destroyed by pannus. Both types of subluxation decrease the anteroposterior width of the cervical canal.

3. Vertical subluxation: destruction of the lateral atlantoaxial joints or of bone around the foramen magnum may cause vertical subluxation.

Patients may present with neck pain on motion, occipital headache, transient episodes of brainstem dysfunction, and cervical myelopathy[44]. Vertebral subluxation may lead to occipital neuralgia and transient episodes of medullary dysfunction: drop attacks, vertigo, nystagmus, and apneas, which can be life-threatening[45]. Pain in occipital neuralgia may be very severe, and may prevent the patient from sleeping. Sensory disturbances, muscle weakness, loss of sphincter control, spontaneous muscle cramps, and Lhermitte's sign, should be regarded as *alarm symptoms* for cervical myelopathy.

The value of physical examination is limited, since the joints of the cervical spine are neither visible nor palpable. In early disease, pain and stiffness throughout the entire arc of motion develops; eventually, generalized loss of motion may occur. A slight rotational tilt of the cervical spine may result from vertical subluxation. Sensory disturbances, absent abdominal reflexes, hyper-reflexia including Babinski's, and muscular weakness of the legs and arms, depending on the level of compression of the myelum, are characteristic of cervical myelopathy.

Unfortunately, the above described symptoms and signs of neurological damage in RA are generally irreversible. Earlier data suggest that, when signs of cervical myelopathy do occur, neurological deterioration progresses rapidly and 50 per cent of the patients die within 1 year, if untreated[46]. It can be difficult to correlate complaints with abnormal structures, since anatomical abnormalities do not necessary lead to symptoms or neurological signs[47]. Neurological abnormalities may be difficult to recognize in RA patients, who also have deformities, muscular atrophy, and peripheral neuropathy. For these reasons, it is difficult to develop a reliable strategy for management of damage to the cervical spine in RA patients. Therefore, these patients should be referred to centers in which a team, consisting of an orthopedic/neurosurgeon, neurologist, and rheumatologist, have a large experience with these patients. In general, RA patients with neck involvement should have careful follow-up, including periodic radiographic and neurological monitoring. In patients with suspected or mild neurological symptoms, radiographs in flexion/extension should only be made if standard radiographs, including an open mouth anteroposterior view, have ruled out a fracture of the odontoid process or large atlantoaxial subluxation[48]. In patients with 'alarm symptoms' and/or neurological signs, MRI is indicated to evaluate the anterior–posterior width of the cervical canal and to look for pannus, both of which may compress the cervical medulla[49].

Cricoarytenoid joints

These small diarthrodial joints rotate with the vocal cords. Pain referred to the ear and fullness aggravated by speaking or swallowing are early symptoms of arthritis. Synovitis of the circoarytenoid joints may lead to hoarseness. Severe inflammation may result in immobilized vocal cords and, when adducted to the midline, to inspiratory stridor, which may require tracheostomy. It is estimated that arthritis of the circoarytenoid joints occurs in 25–50 per cent of RA patients[50,51]. It occurs predominantly in those with long-standing, severe RA. Since hoarseness and stridor occur in a minority of RA patients, cricoarytenoid involvement is asymptomatic in the majority of patients.

Temporomandibular joints

The temporomandibular joints are frequently involved in RA patients. It is estimated that jaw symptoms may occur in 55 per cent of patients at some time during the course of the disease[52]. On radiographs, joint damage is shown in 78 per cent of patients[52]. On physical examination, local tenderness and painful limitation of mouth opening can be observed. In our clinical experience, arthritis of the temporomandibular joint in a patient with polyarthritis, including small joints of hands and feet, is highly suggestive of RA.

Sternoclavicular and manubriosternal joints

These joints, consisting of synovium and a large cartilaginous disc, are often involved in RA[53]. Most patients are asymptomatic, probably because these joints are relatively immobile. In some patients, active synovitis may lead to pain in these joints while lying on their side in bed. In patients with severe pain at the sternoclavicular joint, septic arthritis can be found, particularly in intravenous drug users.

Shoulder

In RA, not only the synovium of the glenohumeral joint may be affected, but also the rotator cuff, the acromioclavicular joint, and several muscles and their tendons around the neck, shoulder, and chest wall. In general, synovitis may lead to decreased joint mobility and weakness and atrophy of muscles. This is easy to observe at the shoulder in RA patients. Weakness of the midthoracic muscles leads to an anterolateral shift of the scapula and decreased stability of the glenohumeral joint. To restore stability, the pectoralis major muscle contracts, resulting in adduction and internal rotation, which limits external rotation.

The function of the rotator cuff is to stabilize the humeral head in the glenoid. Weakening of the cuff, as a result of previous injury and/or aging in combination with the inflammatory process, may result in upward migration of the humeral head, which may eventually lead to complete tears of the tendons of the cuff.

The shoulders are involved in 60–75 per cent of RA patients. On physical examination, abduction and external rotation are limited in patients with synovitis of the shoulder. Although mild glenohumeral swelling is difficult to detect on physical examination, since the shoulder capsule lies beneath the cuff muscles, large shoulder effusions may appear anteriorly below the acromion; these may also occur in patients with chronic bursitis. In patients with acute symptoms, it is generally easy to differentiate between patients with shoulder effusions, in which range of motion is limited, and patients with tendonitis, for whom a painful arc is characteristic. This difference is much more difficult in patients with chronic disease. It is suggested that ultrasound is useful for differentiation between chronic synovitis and bursitis/tendonitis in patients with chronic shoulder complaints. Another advantage of ultrasound is that it may also discriminate between tendonitis and rupture of the cuff, which obviously has an impact on therapeutic intervention[54,55]. Shoulder involvement predominantly occurs in patients with progressive disease. For daily activities, it is often possible to compensate mildly decreased shoulder function in patients with relatively good functional capacity of elbow, wrists, and hands. Radiological damage of the shoulders occurs frequently in RA: erosions have been observed in 69 per cent and superior subluxation in 31 per cent[56].

Elbow

The elbows are frequently involved in RA patients. In patients with persistent synovitis, the interosseous membrane between radius and ulna will be damaged. As a consequence, the head of the radius moves proximal to the capitellum, and may block flexion and extension. While normally a slight hyperextension is possible at the elbows, both active synovitis and degenerative changes may limit extension. Severe RA may have a large impact on elbow function in causing contractures. Since the elbow is located superficially, detection of synovitis is relatively easy by palpation of thickening in the radial–humeral joint. Loss of extension is an early sign. However, it generally does not interfere with daily self-care. Loss of flexion occurs late in the disease, but it may have a severe impact on a patient's self-care activities. The olecranon bursa and proximal extensor surface of the ulna are predilection sites for rheumatoid nodules. Pain and swelling of the olecranon bursa may indicate bursitis as a manifestation of active RA. In the case of a skin break, the physician should be alert to the possibility of a septic bursitis. In patients with large effusions, periarticular cysts may rupture into the forearm. Compression of the ulnar nerve posteromedially to the elbow may result in paresthesias in the fourth and fifth finger.

Wrist and hand

Examination of the wrists and hands is important, since it generally reflects the stage of the disease (early, late, or deforming RA). Synovial proliferation of the wrist may induce the production of degradating enzymes, destroying tendons and ligaments. Weakening of the extensor carpi ulnaris muscle leads to radial deviation of the wrist, and a compensatory ulnar deviation of the fingers. Injury of the distal radioulnar joint with dorsal subluxation of the ulna ('caput ulna syndrome'), may give the impression of pressing a piano key on examination of the ulnar styloid. Further subluxation may induce rupture of the extensor tendons of the fingers, particularly if there is also tenosynovitis. On the volar side, proliferative synovitis may cause carpal tunnel syndrome, an entrapment neuropathy of the median nerve, characterized by decreased sensation on the palmar side of the thumb, index, and long and radial aspect of the ring finger. In RA patients with wrist involvement, the carpal to metacarpal ratio (C:MC ratio) is decreased, as a result of compaction of bone at the radiolunate, lunate–capitate, and capitate–metacarpal joints. The C:MC ratio reflects the progression of RA[57,58].

The two most important deformities at the metacarpophalangeal (MCP) joints are volar subluxation and ulnar deviation[59,60]. Synovitis weakens ligament and tendon insertions around the MCP joint, inducing volar migration of the MCP joint, since the strength of the flexor muscles is greater than that of extensor muscles. Ulnar deviation is also initiated by synovitis of the MCP joints. While the volar plate and collateral ligaments dislocate volar-wards and ulnar-wards, the extensor tendons move ulnar-wards into the cleft between the MCP joints[61]. Thus, a zig-zag deformity results from carpal radial rotation and ulnar drift of the fingers[62].

Synovitis of a proximal interphalangeal (PIP) joint may lead to boutonnière or swan-neck deformity[63]. The boutonnière deformity consists of a flexion and contracture at the PIP joint, combined with hyperextension of the distal interphalangeal (DIP) joint. This deformity is initiated by synovitis of the PIP joint with stretching or rupture of the central extensor tendon. The lateral bands are displaced to the volar side and become flexors of the PIP joint. In the DIP joint, hyperextension will occur, as a result of shortening of the tendons with time. In patients with a swan-neck deformity, there is hyperextension of the PIP joint and flexion of the DIP joint. This deformity occurs when the main extensor forces focus on the base of the proximal phalanx and the lateral bands subluxate to the dorsal side of the terminal phalanx. Although the deformity may be initially reversible, a fixed deformity may develop during the course of the disease. Symmetrical swelling of the MCP joints the PIP joints is characteristic of RA (Figs 16.1 and 16.2). Pain elicited by tangential squeezing of MCP joints is an important diagnostic clue for RA. Although frequently overlooked during physical examination, tenosynovitis in flexion tendon sheats occurs frequently in RA. Initially, crepitus in the hand palm and 'trigger fingers' can be observed during flexion and extension of the fingers. DIP joints are not commonly involved in RA; this is probably related to the fact that these joints have less synovial membrane than other finger joints.

Damage to the thumb may have a severe influence on daily activities. Three types of deformities may affect the thumb: the flail interphalangeal (IP) joint, the boutonnière thumb (S-shaped thumb), and the infrequently occurring duckbill thumb. Synovitis of the IP-joint leads to destruction of the collateral ligaments; pinching pushes the distal phalanx away and the

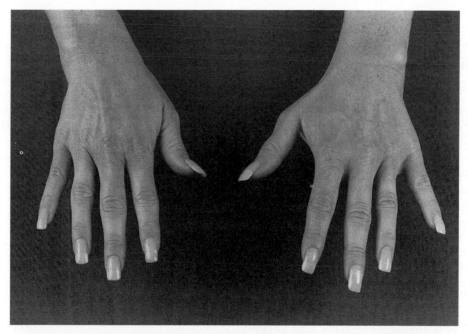

Fig. 16.1 Hands of female patient with early RA: note the discrete swelling of the wrists, MCP joints, and PIP joints.

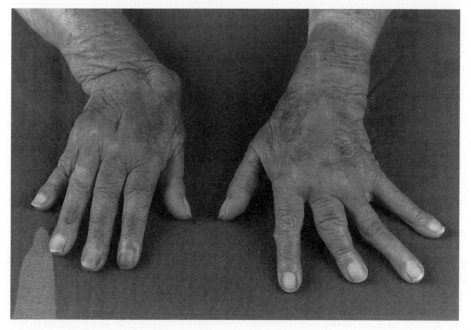

Fig. 16.2 Hands of female patient with deforming RA: ulnar deviation, massive swollen MCP joints, and a boutonnière deformity (digit 3, left hand).

patients needs the proximal phalanx to pinch. The duckbill deformity, hyperextension in MCP joint and flexion in IP joint, parallels the swan-neck deformity of the other fingers; the boutonnière deformity is comparable to that in the other fingers.

It is obvious that arthritis of the wrist and hand has a large influence on daily activities.Radiological damage of the hand and wrists correlates with range of motion, but not with joint tenderness, which suggests that synovitis-induced inflammation and synovitis-induced damage are not the same[64]. Grip is decreased in RA patients, because of:

(1)   active synovitis;

(2)   reflex inhibition of muscular contraction secondary to pain;

(3)   altered joint position sense;

(4)   flexor tenosynovitis;

(5)   muscle weakness;

(6)   edema.

Hip

Hip involvement is often detected late in the disease. This may be related to the paucity of synovial tissue at the hips or to the fact that it is not possible to examine the hips by direct inspection or palpation. Pain in patients with arthritis of the hip is usually felt in the groin but sometimes in the thigh, buttock, or knee. Pain on the lateral aspect of the hips is more often caused by trochanteric bursitis than by synovitis. In patients with coxitis, internal rotation, extension, and abduction are lost earlier than flexion, adduction, and external rotation[65]. In advanced disease, a flexion contracture may be demonstrable, when, during passive flexion of the hip in a supine patient, flexion occurs in the contralateral hip. The initial dysfunction of hip damage is noticed when the patient has some difficulty while putting on shoes. Patients with severe hip involvement have a limp in their walk and have apparent shortening of the leg[66]. Involvement of the large joints, for example the hips is associated with a bad prognosis[67]. On radiographs, loss of joint space is an early sign of hip involvement in RA; collapsed femoral head and/or protrusio acetabuli may occur late in the disease. A collapsed femoral head can be related to prednisone-induced avascular necrosis.

Knee

A moderate to severe synovitis is hard to miss during inspection of the knee joints. Fluctuation confirms the presence of joint effusion. Very small effusions can be detected after stroking the medial or lateral aspect of the knee from above downwards, which elicits some ballooning out of the skin lateral or medial, respectively, to the patella. Since the knee is the largest synovial joint and since it is located superficially, the knee is very suitable for diagnostic procedures such as arthrocentesis and arthroscopy. As in other joints, arthrocentesis is necessary for diagnosing infectious or crystal-induced arthritis. Although some data from the literature suggest that invasive diagnostic

procedures might be useful in differentiating RA from reactive arthritis, it is not common in daily practice. In patients with large knee effusions, the patient tends to assume a more comfortable position with the knee flexed. Eventually, a loss of full knee extension develops, which leads to limitation in walking. Large knee effusions may increase intra-articular pressure and lead to an outpouching of posterior components of the joint space, a Baker's cyst[68]. The intact Baker's cyst may compress superficial venous flow resulting in dilatation of veins and/or leg edema. Rupture of the synovial cyst leads to extravasation of synovial fluid in the calf, which mimics venous thrombosis. If there is doubt, a Baker's cyst can be easily demonstrated by ultrasound[55]. Neuropathy of the posterior tibial nerve with loss of sensation along the plantar aspect of the foot, can be complication of a Baker's cyst[69]. Atrophy of the quadriceps musculature may occur early in the disease, for example after 2 weeks. This atrophy may lead to increased load through the patella to the femoral surface. Severe quadriceps atrophy may increase the risk of falling and of osteoporotic fractures. On radiographs, the thickness of articular cartilage has to be determined with the patient in a standing position. Long-standing RA may lead to laxity of the collateral and cruciate ligaments and to cartilage destruction, which is characterized by joint space narrowing, bony sclerosis, and osteophytes (secondary osteoarthritis).

Ankle, hindfoot, and forefoot

The ankle joint is formed by the distal ends of the tibia and fibula and the proximal aspect of the body of the talus. Its articular capsule is lax on the anterior side but tightly bound laterally. Swelling over the anterior side of the joint is suggestive of synovitis and has to be differentiated from superficial linear swelling of the tendon sheaths. The stability of the ankle decreases if the integrity of ligaments is damaged by the inflammatory process leading to pronation deformities and eversion of the foot. The hindfoot consists of the talus, calcaneus, talonavicular, and calcaneocuboid joint. The talonavicular,joint is most commonly involved in the rheumatoid process; additional subtalar and calcaneocuboid involvement is also observed[70]. Synovitis may lead to pain, stiffness, and peroneus muscle spasm and, eventually, valgus deformity. As valgus deformity increases, progressive flattening of the midfoot may occur. The Achille's tendon is seldom involved in RA. However, this tendon is a predilection site for rheumatoid nodules. The great toe develops medial capsular incompetence that leads to hallux valgus and bunion/callus formation. It may also lead to crossover deformity of the lesser toes. Chronic synovitis of the MTP joints erodes the plantar plate and supportive ligaments that results in downward subluxation of the MTP joints as the metatarsal heads herniate through the plantar plate. This movement will be compensated by flexion of the toes, 'hammer toes'. These joint deformities may result in hypertrophic callus formation under the metatarsal heads and above the PIP joints, and may be complicated by infections, predominantly under the second and third metatarsal head. Although RA is associated with initial foot and ankle involvement in 17 per cent of cases, virtually all patients develop forefoot involvement during the course of the disease[71]. In patients with early RA, radiological damage occurs earlier in the feet than in the hands. Entrapment of the posterior tibial nerve in the tarsal tunnel, posteroinferior to the medial malleolus, may cause burning paresthesias on the sole of the feet.

Course of the disease

Exact data on the frequency of specific joint involvement in RA are lacking since joint involvement is largely dependent on stage of the disease, severity of RA, and treatment. The most commonly involved joints in RA are the wrists and the small joints of the hands and feet. Large joint involvement may occur later in the disease and is associated with moderate to severe disease[67]. The natural course of RA, that is without the use of DMARDs, is not fully known. Between 1930 and 1936, 300 hospitalized RA patients were followed; persisting disease activity was observed in 65 per cent, a disease pattern characterized by remissions and exacerbations in 25 per cent, and remission in the remaining 10 per cent of the patients[2–4]. In controlled studies in RA patients, in which the effect of DMARDs on disease activity was studied, remission was observed in 10 per cent of patients, chronic progressive disease in 40–70 per cent, and a course characterized by remissions and exacerbations in 20–40 per cent[75]. Although these percentages seems to be comparable with data from the thirties, suggesting that effectiveness of antirheumatic treatment has not been increased with the introduction of DMARDs, comparison of the results of these studies is hampered by differences in study design, patient selection, and definition of the course of the disease.

Insidious onset of RA over a period of a few weeks or months occurs in approximately 70 per cent of patients. This gradual onset, in which the disease begins with fatigue and generalized weakness, until the synovitis become apparent, is generally followed by a chronic progressive disease. Abrupt onset of RA may occur in 10–15 per cent of patients. The differential diagnosis in these patients is considerable, since amongst other diagnosis, infections, reactive arthritis, and systemic vasculitis etc., also needs to be considered. In a minority of patients, the onset and course of the disease is 'malignant', which means that the disease cannot be influenced by the use of any antirheumatic drug. In Western countries, the onset of RA is more frequent in winter than in summer. Exacerbations are also more common in winter than in summer[76]. Some data from Finland suggest that a positive rheumatoid factor (RF) test may precede symptoms of RA since the frequency of RF was increased before symptoms of RA began[77]. There is no clear evidence for other precipitating factors, such as physical/emotional trauma and infection, having a causal relationship with RA.

Common extra-articular manifestations

Nodules

Rheumatoid nodules occur in approximately 20 per cent of patients; almost all of these patients are RF positive. Rheumatoid nodules can be considered as a manifestations of

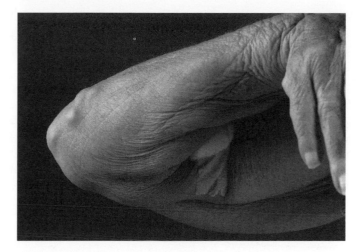

Fig. 16.3 Rheumatoid nodules on the elbow and rupture of extensor tendons at the wrist in a patient with RA.

active disease. Rheumatoid nodules are firm and adherent to the underlying periosteum. They are usually found at the olecranon, finger joints, sacral prominences, and Achille's tendon (Fig. 16.3). Treatment with methotrexate may enlarge these nodules[78].

Heart

At autopsy, pericardial involvement is found in 50 per cent of patients[79]. In ultrasound studies, small pericardial effusions have been found in 20 per cent of patients[80], while actual clinical manifestations of pericarditis are uncommon in RA. Although pericarditis in RA usually follows a benign course, it occasionally progresses to severe constrictive pericarditis, as manifested by pulsus paradoxus, liver enlargement, and ankle edema. Diagnosing coronary insufficiency in RA patients is hampered by their limited exercise tolerance. The risk for coronary insufficiency may be increased in RA patients as a result of prednisone-induced hypercholesterolemia and vasculitis.

Lungs

Pulmonary involvement in RA includes pleural lesions, lung nodules, and interstial lung disease[81,82]. Pleural involvement is the most common manifestation of lung disease in RA: it has been shown in 50 per cent of patients at autopsy. Pulmonary nodules may be found, particularly in RF-positive patients with subcutaneous nodules elsewhere in the body. Pleural involvement and pulmonary nodules are often asymptomatic. Abnormal findings of pulmonary function tests, vital capacity and diffusion capacity, or interstitial infiltrates on radiographs is seen in 32 per cent of patients[83]. Both pack-years of cigarette smoking and disease severity are predictive factors for the development of interstitial lung disease in RA. Severe, clinically manifest pulmonary involvement may occur in RA patients as a result of pleural involvement, pneumoconiosis, fibrosing alveolitis, or methotrexate-induced pneumonitis.

Secundary Sjögren's syndrome

Sicca syndrome is common in patients with RA. It is estimated that it occurs in more than 50 per cent of RF-positive patients. It occurs more often in women than in men[17].

Felty's syndrome

Neutropenia and splenomegaly are characteristic of Felty's syndrome. Usually, these patients are RF positive. Rheumatoid nodules, leg ulcers, hyperpigmentation, serositis, and peripheral neuropathy are frequently found in these patients. Bacterial infections may occur in particular in patients with severe neutropenia.

Vasculitis

The clinical pattern of vasculitis in RA is highly variable[84]. Isolated nail-fold lesions occur in about 5 per cent of patients. They do not alter the prognosis. The clinical pattern of mononeuritis multiplex, polyneuropathy, digital gangrene, severe skin ulcers, purpura, and systemic features (fever in combination with weight loss) strongly suggest systemic vasculitis (Fig. 16.4). The risk of vasculitis is increased in patients of male gender, increased RF titer, joint erosions, rheumatoid nodules, nail-fold lesions, and treatment with corticosteroids[85]. The annual incidence rate for systemic vasculitis is higher in men (15.8/1 000 000) than in women (9.4/1 000 000)[86]. Mortality is increased in patients with RA and systemic vasculitis[87,88].

Osteoporosis

Rheumatologists have become more aware that osteoporosis frequently occurs in RA[89]. It is related to the age of the patient, the use of corticosteroids, and to disease activity[89]. In a longitudinal study of early RA, bone loss in the lumbar spine was greater after 1 year than in healthy controls (–2.4 versus –0.6 per cent), while the decrease in the hips was even more impressive (–4.3 versus –0.4 per cent)[95]. Bone loss in RA patients is related to disease activity and functional capacity[90,91], as shown in

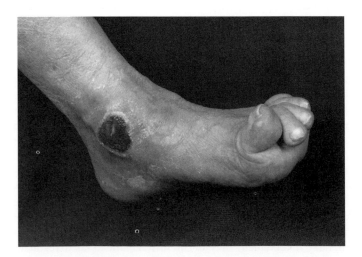

Fig. 16.4 Ulcer on the medial site of the malleolus in a patient with RA and vasculitis. Rheumatoid deformity of the toes.

Table 16.1 Percentage changes in BMD in placebo-arm of a 3-year study with pamidronate versus placebo in patients with RA (Eggelmeijer *et al.* Ref. 91)

	Spine	Femoral neck
ESR ≤ 20 mm/h	+1.4%	–1.4%
ESR > 20 mm/h	0.0%	–6.3%**
HAQ < 1.25	+1.6%	–3.0%
HAQ ≥ 1.25	–2.1%***	–6.6%*

*p<0.05; **p<0.01; ***p<0.005

Table 16.1. Data on fracture incidence in patients with RA are scarce, but it is suggested that the risk of vertebral and peripheral fractures is roughly doubled in RA patients[92,93].

Laboratory values

Inflammation and/or tissue injury may induce elevation of acute phase reactants. In active RA, serum levels of ESR, C-reactive protein (CRP), IL-6, serum amyloid A, transferrin, ferritin, haptoglobin, and platelet count are increased; hemoglobin and serum iron are depressed. Disease activity can be monitored by measurements of ESR or CRP. Both are incorporated in the ACR-core set criteria for improvement of disease activity[94]. A good correlation exists between joint scores, pain and swelling, and the acute phase response[95]. A highly significant correlation was observed between time-integrated, cumulative, values of CRP and radiological progression in patients with early RA during the first 3 years of disease[96].

Anemia is often found in RA patients; it is of great importance to differentiate between iron deficiency anemia (IDA), anemia of chronic diseases (ACD), and a combination of these. In otherwise healthy persons, serum ferritin is useful to detect iron deficiency in patients with anemia. In patients with inflammatory disorders, serum ferritin is increased, acting as an acute phase reactant. The gold standard for differentiation between IDA and ACD is bone marrow examination. In RA patients with anemia, more severe erosive disease occurred[97]. Although thrombocytosis and immobilization are often found in patients with active RA, venous and arterial thromboembolic manifestations do not often occur. It is hypothesized than this is related to the use of NSAIDs.

Recently, new immonoassays for markers of cartilage and bone metabolism have been developed[98]. These markers can be measured in serum or urine. Their release is influenced by the inflammatory process. Serum levels of osteocalcin (bone formation) and urinary levels of pyridinolines (bone resorption) are elevated in patients with active RA indicating high bone turnover[99]. Development of cartilage markers is hampered by the fact that the volume of cartilage in the body is much smaller than that of bone.

Rheumatoid factor

The presence of RF, which is usually positive in less than 5 per cent of healthy controls, is one of the ACR criteria for diagnosis of RA[31]. In a minority of patients, conventional RF tests are negative, 'seronegative RA'. In 50 per cent of these patients, elevated levels of RF could be detected by sensitive methods such as ELISA, but these levels are generally lower than that of patients who are RF positive[100]. RF tests may not only be positive in RA but also in other chronic rheumatic inflammatory diseases, bacterial infections, viral diseases, sarcoidosis, and mixed cryoglobulinemia. The predictive value of a test is related to its pretest probability. The positive predictive value of RF varies from 16 per cent in general practice to 80 per cent at an out-patient rheumatology clinic[101,102]. The negative predictive value of RF in the general population for RA is 89 per cent. This suggests that RF testing is useful for excluding RA in the general population, but that the value of a positive test is limited. Although some data suggest that improvement of disease activity during therapy with NSAIDs[103] or methotrexate[104] is associated with decreases in RF titer, RF testing is not useful for follow-up measurements since measurements of acute phase reactants are cheaper and more widely accessible.

Differential diagnosis of RA and its variants

The 1987 ACR criteria for RA[31] (Table 16.2), are classification criteria. They were developed to identify a homogeneous group of patients that permits comparison of data from different clinical trials. For practical reasons, the classification criteria are often used in daily practice for diagnosing RA.

In a case of polyarthritis, there is a long differential diagnosis to be considered, including spondylarthropathy, polymyalgia rheumatica, crystal-induced synovitis, palindromic rheumatism, RS3PE syndrome, adult-onset Still's disease, systemic lupus erythematosus septic arthritis, reactive arthritis, virus-induced arthritis, hemochromatosis, etc.

RS3PE

This abbreviation stands for Remitting, Seronegative, Symmetrical, Synovitis with Edema. The syndrome is characterized by an abrupt onset of severe swollen dorsum of the hands with edema, synovitis of the wrists, and extensor tenosynovitis. In general, these patients respond very well to NSAIDs. The disease is generally self-limiting after weeks to months[105].

Table 16.2   1987 ACR revised criteria for diagnosis of RA

Synovitis in MCP joints or PIP joints or wrists[a]
Synovitis in ≥ 3 joints areas simultaneously[b]
Symmetric polyarthritis[a]
Morning stiffness > 1 hour[a]
Rheumatoid nodules
Presence of rheumatoid factor
Radiographic changes typical of RA

a Must be present at least 6 weeks.
b The 14 joint areas are: elbows, wrists, MCP joints, PIP joints, knees, ankles, MTP joints.

Polymyalgia rheumatica (PMR)

PMR is characterized by abrupt onset of pain and stiffness in the limb and shoulder girdles in patients over 50 years of age[106]. Fever, weight loss, and malaise may also be present. Discrimination between PMR and RA can be difficult in case of discrete synovitis of the small joints of the hands in combination with malaise and pain in hips and shoulders. It is not unusual for elderly patients to present with signs and symptoms of PMR that gradually develops into classical RA.

Palindromic rheumatism

Palindromic rheumatism is defined as a remitting, recurring, non-destructive, inflammatory arthritis with recurrences over at least 6 months[107]. In palindromic rheumatism the metacarpal, wrist, elbow, shoulder, knee, ankle, and foot may be affected[108]. Generally, each attack involves one joint. The pain in palindromic rheumatism may be severe, as in gout. In about 50 per cent of the patients, the disease will develop into 'classical' RA[108].

Adult-onset still's disease

This disorder is identical to juvenile Still's disease. The disease is characterized by high-spiking fevers and an evanescent rash, which generally occurs in the evening, during episodes of fever. Arthritis, serositis, sore throat, hepatospenomegaly, and lymphadenopathy are also common in this disease. Arthritis is generally localized to the large joints and may be destructive. ANA and RF are present in less than 10 per cent of the patients[109]. Highly elevated levels of ferritin (> 1000 μg 1^{-1}) can be found in these patients[110].

Elderly-onset RA

The average age of onset of RA is around 55 years of age. In elderly-onset RA, defined as RA with onset at age 60 or over, the disease is characterized by RF positivity, more equal gender distribution, an acute onset with high disease activity (often with systemic features), and more radiological and functional deterioration[111,112]. The large joints, in particular the shoulders, are frequently initially involved in these patients. The general prognosis in RF-negative elderly-onset RA is better, resulting from some overlap between RF-negative RA and PMR and RS3PE syndrome, both of which have a more favourable prognosis. The percentage of RA patients who are RF positive is lower in the elderly[113].

Early rheumatoid arthritis

There is little doubt in diagnosing RA in a patient with chronic symmetrical polyarthritis, including wrists and MCP joints, nodules, and erosions and deformities on radiographs. Since development over time is an important diagnostic instrument in RA, diagnosing early RA, for example in the absence of widespread polyarthritis, nodules, and radiological damage, is much more difficult. Early diagnosis of RA is important, since evidence is accumulating that treatment of RA is more effective in the early phase of the disease.

Arguments for treating RA 'aggressively' in early phase of the disease

1. The traditional treatment of RA, the 'pyramid strategy', results in severe deterioration of functional capacity in many patients. In other words, there is no reason to be content with the traditional strategy.

2. Therapy with DMARDs has proven to be superior to NSAIDs in the early phase of RA[114].

3. In an observational study, the use of DMARDs was associated with improved long-term disability, despite a selection bias in which more severely-affected individuals were more frequently prescribed DMARDs[115].

4. Combination therapy, consisting of prednisone, methotrexate, and sulfasalazine, is superior to sulfasalazine alone[116].

5. From observational studies, it appears that a substantial part of erosions occurs in the first 2 years of the disease[117].

ACR criteria

In a group of 135 women with a clinical diagnosis of early RA, 100 fulfilled the 1987 criteria (sensitivity = 73 per cent), while the sensitivity of the 1958 criteria was slightly higher, 86 per cent[118]. Thus, the ACR criteria are not very suitable for diagnosing early RA, probably due to the prerequisite of a minimal 6 weeks symptoms and to the inclusion of criteria such as rheumatoid nodules and radiographic changes that occur particularly in chronic RA.

Since early treatment of RA shows promising results and since reliable criteria for diagnosis and classification of early RA are lacking, new criteria for early RA are needed. In the eighties, it was felt that the 1958 criteria were old-fashioned, because of the long list of exclusion criteria, the need for three invasive tests (synovial fluid aspiration, biopsy of synovium and rheumatoid nodule), and the concepts of possible and probable RA. Since data from synovial biopsies in early RA are promising and since early diagnosis is associated with an increased uncertainty about the diagnosis, it is cannot be excluded that some elements of the 1958 criteria will be useful in criteria for early RA.

Prediction of aggressive disease

Currently, rheumatologists tend to treat RA patients early in the disease with aggressive therapy. However, since aggressive therapy may be accompanied by considerable toxicity, it is only indicated in patients with a bad prognosis. Besides the presence of RF, swelling of two or more large joints and the presence of radiological damage at baseline are associated with an increased risk of radiological damage[119,120]. Although some data suggest that the presence of the shared epitope is associated with a worse prognosis, the value of the presence of the shared epitope varies between different populations[21-23]. Further work is needed to define more accurate and reliable prognostic indicators.

Table 16.3 Criteria for clinical remission in RA (Ref. 122)

5 or 6 of the following requirements must be fulfilled for at least 2 consecutive months

1. duration of morning stiffness not exceeding 15 min
2. no fatigue
3. no joint pain (by history)
4. no joint tenderness or pain on motion
5. no soft tissue swelling in joints or tendon sheaths
6. ESR < 30 mm h^{-1} in women and < 20 min h^{-1} in men

Early Arthritis Clinic

The development of an Early Arthritis Clinic (EAC) is probably useful for early diagnosis and treatment of RA. In a comparison between 241 patients from routine out-patient clinics with 233 patients from EAC duration of symptoms at first visit was much shorter in the EAC patients (31 versus 122 days). Erosions were found on radiographs in 25 per cent of the EAC patients. Both the lag time and the number of patients with erosions are important arguments to justify the start of an EAC as an important instrument for early diagnosis and treatment of RA.

Remission

It is obvious that the percentage of RA patients in remission is strongly related to the definition of remission. Remission suggests total absence of disease activity. Since absence of disease activity hardly occurs, the Pinals criteria are used in most studies (Table 16.3)[122]. It is estimated that during treatment with DMARDs 10 per cent of RA patients are in remission[75]. Theoretically, it may be expected that this percentage will rise with the earlier use of more aggressive antirheumatic drugs. Currently, a well-recognized problem is whether it is useful or not to continue DMARDs in patients in remission. The risk of long-term drug toxicity has to be balanced against the risk of a flare of RA while stopping DMARDs. In a randomized trial, the effect of stopping versus continuing DMARDs was studied[123]. The frequency of flares in 1 year was nearly doubled—22 per cent in those patients on continuous DMARD therapy and 38 per cent of those on placebo.

References

1. Rotschild B.M., Woods R.J., Rotschild C., *et al.* Geographic distribution of RA in ancient North America implications for pathogenesis. *Seminar Arthritis Rheum*, 1992;**22**:181–7.
2. Abdel Nasser A.M., Rasker J.J., Valkenburg H.A. Epidemiological and clinical aspects relating to the variability of RA. *Semin Arthritis Rheum*, 1997;**27**:123–40.
3. Linos A., Worthington J.W., O'Fallon W.M., *et al.* The epidemiology of RA in Rochester, Minnesota: a study of incidence, prevalence, and mortality. *Am J Epidemiol*, 1980;**11**:87–9.
4. Lawrence R.C., Helminck C.G., Arnett F.C., Deyo R.A., Felson D.T., Gianni E.H., *et al.* Estimates of the prevalence of arthritis and selected musculoskeletal disorders in United States. *Arthritis Rheum*, 1998;**41**:778–99.
5. Lawrence J.S. *Rheumatism in populations*, London: Heinemann, 1977.

6. Cimmino M.A., Parisi M., Moggiani G., Mela G.S., Accardo S. Prevalence of RA in Italy: the Chiavari study. *Ann Rheum Dis*, 1998;57:315–18.

7. Kviem T.K., Glennas A., Knudsrod O.G., Smedstad L.M., Mowinckel P., F*yofrre O. The prevalence and severity of RA in Oslo. *Scand J Rheumatol*, 1997;26:412–8.

8. Gaston J.S.H. Will the increasing prevalence of atopy have a favourable impact on RA? *Ann Rheum Dis*, 1998;57:265–67.

9. Verhoef C.M., Roon J.A.G., Vianen M.E., Bruijnzeel-Koomen CAFM, Lafeber F.P.J.G., Bijlsma J.W.J. Mutual antagonism of RA and hay fever; a role for type 1/type 2 T cell balance. *Ann Rheum Dis*, 1998;57:273–80.

10. Nicholas N.S., Panayi G.S. RA and pregnancy. *Clin Exp Rheumatol*, 1988;6:179–82.

11. Vandenbroucke J.P., Hazes J.M.W., Dijkmans B.A.C., Cats A. Oral contraceptives and the risk of RA; the Great Transatlantic Divide? *Br J Rheumatol*, 1989; (suppl 1):1–3.

12. Hazes J.M.W., Dijkmans B.A.C., Vandenbroucke J.P., et al. Reduction of the risk of RA among women with oral contraceptives. *Arthritis Rheum*, 1990;33:173–9.

13. Hernandez-Avila M., Liang M.H., Willet W.C., et al. Exogenous sex hormones and the risk of RA. *Arthritis Rheum*, 1990;33:947–53.

14. Vandenbroucke J.P., Witteman J.C.M., Valkenburg H.A., et al. Noncontraceptive hormones and RA in perimenopausal and postmenopausal women. *JAMA*, 1986;255:1299–1303.

15. Brink H.R. van den, Everdingen A.A. van, Wyk M.J. van, Jacobs J.W.G., Bijlsma J.W.J. Adjuvant oestrogen therapy does not improve disease activity in postmenopausal RA. *Ann Rheum Dis*, 1993;52:862–5.

16. Brink H.R. van den, Lems W.F., Everdingen A.A. van, Bijlsma J.W.J. Adjuvant oestrogen therapy during one year in postmenopausal RA patients increases bone mineral density. *Ann Rheum Dis*, 1993;52:302–5.

17. Weyand C.M., Schmidt D., Wagner U., Goronzy J.J. The influence of sex on the fenotype of RA. *Arthritis Rheum*, 1998;41:817–22.

18. Silman A.J., Mac Gregor A.J., Thomson W., et al. Twin concordace rates for RA: results from a nation wide study. *Br J Rheumatol*, 1993;32: 903–7.

19. Weyand C.M., Gorozny J.J. Pathogenesis of RA. *Med Clin North Am*, 1997;18:785–92.

20. Auger I., Roudier J. HLADR and the development of RA. *Autoimmunity*, 1997;26:123–8.

21. McDonagh J.E., Dunn A., Ollier W.E., Walker D.J. Compound heterozygosity for the shared epitope and the risk and severity of RA. *Br J Rheumatol*, 1997;36:322–7.

22. Wagner U., Kaltenhauser S., Sauer H., Arnold S., Seidel W., Hantzschel H. HLA markers and prediction of clinical course and outcome in RA. *Arthritis Rheum*, 1997;40:341–51.

23. Hameed K., Bowman S., Kondeatis E., Vaughan R., Gibson T. The association of HLADRB genes and the shared epitope with RA in Pakistan. *Br J Rheumatol*, 1997;36:1184–8.

24. Pincus T., Brooks R.H., Callahan L.F. Prediction of long term mortality in-patients with RA according to a simple questionnaire and joint count measures. *Ann Int Med*, 1994;120:26–34.

25. Wolfe F., Mitchell D.M., Sibley J.T., et al. The mortality of RA. *Arthritis Rheum*, 1994;37:481–94.

26. Symmons D.P.M., Jones M.A., Scott D.L., Prior P. Longterm mortality outcome in patients with RA: early presenters continue to do well. *J Rheumatol*, 1998;25:1072–7.

27. Reilly P.A., Cosh J.A., Maddison P.J., Rasker J.J., Silman A.J. Mortality and survival in RA: a 25 year prospective study of 100 patients. *Ann Rheum dis*, 1990;49:363–9.

28. Pincus T., Callahan L.F. Taking mortality in RA seriously. Predictive markers, socioeconomic status and comorbidity. Editorial. *J Rheumatol*, 1984;37:814–20.

29. Oosterveld F.G.J., Rasker J.J. Treating arthritis with locally applied heat or cold. *Sem Arthritis Rheum*, 1994;24:1–10.

30. Oosterveld F.G.J., Rasker J.J., Jacobs J.W.G., Overmars H.J.A. The effect of local heat therapy on the intraarticular and skin surface temperature of the knee. *Arthritis Rheum*, 1992;35:146–51.

31. Arnett F.C., Edworthy S.M., Bloch D.A., et al. The American Rheumatism Association 1987 revised criteria for the classification of RA. *Arthritis Rheum*, 1988;31:315–24.

32. Hazes J.M.W., Hayton R., Burt J. Silman A.J. Consistency of morning stiffness: an analysis of diary data. *Br J Rheumatol*, 1994;33:562–5.

33. Ytterberg S.R., Mahowald M.L., Krug H.E. Exercise for arthritis. *Ballieres Clin Rheum*, 1994;8:161–89.

34. Eberhardt K.B., Fex E. Functional impairment and disability in early RA; development over 5 years. *J Rheumatol*, 1995;22:1037–42.

35. Hakkinen A., Hannonen P., Hakkinen K. Muscle strength in healthy people and in patients suffering from recent-onset inflammatory arthritis. *Br J Rheumatol*, 1995;34:355–60.

36. Ekdahl C., Broman G. Muscle strength, endurance and aerobic capacity in RA: a comparative study with healthy subjects. *Ann Rheum Dis*, 1992;51:35–40.

37. Nordjeso L.O., Nordgren B., Wigren A., Kolstad K. Isometric strength and endurance in patients with severe RA or osteoarthritis in the knee joints. *Scand J Rheumatol*, 1983;12:152–6.

38. Stucki G., Bruhlmann P., Stucki S., Michel B.A. Isometric muscle strength is an indicator of selfreported physical disability in patient with RA. *Br J Rheumatol*, 1998;37:643–8.

39. Ende C.H.M. van den, Hazes J.M.W., le Sessie S., Mulder W.J., Belfor D.G., Breedveld F.C., Dijkmans B.A.C. Comparison of high and low intensity training in well controlled RA. *Ann Rheum Dis*, 1996;55:798–805.

40. Miro O., Pedrol E., Casademont J., Gaccia Carrasco M., Samarti R., Cebrian M., et al. Muscle involvement in RA: clinicopathological study of 21 symptomatic cases. *Sem Arthritis Rheum*, 1996;25:421–8.

41. Kauppi M., Sakaguchi M., Konttinen Y.T., Hamalainen M., Hakala M. Pathogenetic mechanism and prevalence of stable atlantoaxial subluxation in RA. *J Rheumatol*, 1996;23:831–4.

42. Paimela L., Laasonen L., Kankaanpaa E., Leirisalo-Repo M. Progression of cervical spine changes in patients with early RA. *J Rheumatol*, 1997;24:1280–4.

43. Meyers K.A.E., Cats A., Kremer H.P.H., Luijendijk W., Onvlee G.J., Thomeer R.T.W.M. Cervical myelopathy in RA. *Clin Exp Rheumatol*, 1984;2:239–45.

44. Heywood A.W., Learmonth I.D., Thomas M. Cervical spine instability in RA. *J Bone Joint Surg*, 1988;70:702–7.

45. Drossaers Bakker K.W., Spiegel P.I. van, Hamburger H.L., Batchelor D., Bongartz E.B., Soesbergen R.M. van. Sleep apnoe due to rheumatoid cervical myelopathy and/or acquired micrognathia in RA. A life threatening complication. *Br J Rheumatol*, 1988;37:889–94.

46. Agarwal Ak, Peppelman W.C., Kraus D.R., Eisenbeis C.H. The spine in cervical RA. *Br Med J*, 1993;306:79–80.

47. Reijnierse M., Bloem J.L., Dijkmans B.A.C., Kroon H.M., Holscher H.C., Hansen B., Breedveld F.C. The cervical spine in RA: relationship between neurologic signs and morphology of MR imaging and radiographs. *Skeletal Radiology*, 1996;25:113–8.

48. Komusi T., Munro T., Harth M. Radiological review: the cervical spine. *Sem Arthritis Rheum*, 1985;14:187–195.

49. Breedveld F.C., Algra P.R., Vielvoye C.J., Cats A. Magnetic resonance imaging in the evaluation of patients with RA of the cervical spine. *Arthritis Rheum*, 1987;30:624–9.

50. Leicht M.J., Harrington T.M., Davis D.E. Cricoarythenoid arthritis: a cause of laryngeal obstruction. *Ann Emerg Med*, 1987;16:885–8.

51. Lawry G.V., Finerman M.L., Hanafee W.N., Mancuso A.M., Fan P.T., Bluestone R. Laryngeal involvement in RA: a clinical, laryngoscopic and computerized tomographic study. *Arthritis Rheum*, 1984;27:873–82.

52. Ericson S., Lundberg M. Alterations in the temporomandibilar joints at various stages of RA. *Acta Rheumatol Scand*, 1967;12:257–74.

53. Kalliomaki J.L., Viitanen S.M., Virtama P. Radiological findings of sternoclavicular joints in RA. *Acta Rheumatol Scand* **14**:233–40.

54. Olive R.J., Marsh H.E. Ultrasonography of rotator cuff tears. *Clin Orthopedics and Related Research*, 1992;**282**:110–3.

55. Grassi W., Cervini C. Ultrasonography in rheumatology: an evolving technique. *Annals Rheum Dis*, 1998;**57**:268–71.

56. Edeiken J., Hodes P.J. *Roentgen diagnosis of disease of bone* (2nd edn) Baltimore, Willams and Wilkins, 1978: pp. 690–709.

57. Trentham D.E., Masi A.T. Carpo: metacarpal ratio. A new quantitative measure of radiological progression of wrist involvement in RA. *Arthritis Rheum*, 1976;**192**:939.

58. Alarcon G.S., Koopman W.J. The carpometacarpal ration: a useful method for assessing disease progression in RA. *J Rheumatol*, 1985;**12**:846.

59. Eberhardt K., Johnson P.M., Rydgren L. The occurrence and significance of hand deformities in early RA. *Br Rheumatol*, 1991;**30**:211–3.

60. Smith R.J., Kaplan E.B. Rheumatoid deformities at the metacarpophalangeal joints of the fingers. *J Bone Joint Surg*, 1967;**49A**:31–47.

61. Hakstian R.W., Tubiana R. Ulnar deviation of the fingers; the role of joint structure and function. *J Bone Joint Surg*, 1967;**49**:299–316.

62. Read G.O., Solomon L., Biddulph S. Relationship between finger and wrist deformities in RA. *Ann Rheum Dis*, 1983;**42**:619–25.

63. Dreyfus J.N., Schnitzer T.J. Pathogenesis and differential diagnosis of the swanneck deformity. *Sem Arthritis Reheum*, 1983;**13**:200–11.

64. Fuchs H.A., Callahan L.F., Kaye J.J., *et al.*: Radiographic and joint count findings of the hand in RA: related and unrelated findings. *Arthritis Rheum*, 1988;**31**:44–51.

65. Bilka P.J. Physical signs in RA. *Med Clin North Am*, 1968;**52**:493.

66. Buchanan W.W., Kean W.F. Articular and systemic manifestations of RA. In: *Copeman's textbook of rheumatology* (ed Scott J.T.). Churchil Livingstone, Edindurgh, 1986; pp. 653–705.

67. Brennan P., Harrison B., Barret E., *et al.* A simple algoritm to predict the development of radiological erosions in patients with early RA. *Br Med J*, 1996;**313**:471–6.

68. Miller T.T., Staron R.B., Koenigsberg T., Levin T.L., Feldman F. MR Imaging of Baker's cyst: association with internal derangement, effusion, and degenerative arthropathy. *Radiology*, 1996;**201**:247–50.

69. Dash S., Bheemreddy S.R., Tiku N.L. Posterior tibial neuropathy from ruptured Baker's cyst. *Sem Arthritis Rheum*, 1998;**27**:272–6.

70. Selzer S.E., Weismann B.N., Adams D.F. Computed tomography of the hindfoot with RA. *Arthritis Rheum*, 1985;**28**:1234–42.

71. Benson G.M., Johnson E.W. Management of the foot in RA. *Orthop Clin North Am*, 1971;**2**:733–44.

72. Short C.L., Bauer M.D. The course of RA in patients receiving simple medical and orthopedic measures. *N Engl J Med*, 1948;**238**:142–8.

73. Short C.L. Long remissions in RA. *Medicine*, 1964;**43**:401–6.

74. Short C.L. RA: types of course and prognosis. *Med Clin North Am*, 1968;**52**:549–57.

75. Ten Wolde S., Dijkmans B.A.C. When to stop second line drugs: risk/benefit ratio of continuation versus cessation in patients with RA in remission. In *Therapy of systemic rheumatic diseases* (van de Putte L.B.A., Furst D., *et al.* eds). New York: Marcel Dekker, 1997; pp. 263–76.

76. Jacoby R.K., Jayson M.I.V., Cosh J.A. Onset, early stages and prognosis of RA: a clinical study of 100 patients with 11 year follow-up *Br Med J*, 1973;2: 96.

77. Aho K., Heliovaara M., Maatela J., Tuomi T., Palosuo T. Rheumatoid factors antedating clinical RA. *J Rheumatol*, 1991;**18**:1282–4.

78. Kerstens P.J.S.M., Boerbooms A.M.T., Jeurissen M.E.C., Fast J.H., Assmann K.J.M., Putte L.B.A. van de. Accelerated nodulosis during low dose methotrexate therapy for RA. *J Rheumatol*, 1992;**19**:867–71.

79. Bonfiglio T., Atwater E.C. Heart disease in patients with seropositive RA. *Arch Int Med*, 1969;**124**:714.

80. Escalente A., Kaufman R.L., Quismoro F.P. jr., *et al.* Cardiac compression in RA. *Semin Arthritis Rheum*, 1990;**20**:148–63.

81. Helmers G.W., Galvin J.R., Hunninghake G.W. Pulmonary involvement in RA. *Sem Arthritis Rheum*, 1995;**24**:242–54.

82. Anaya J.M., Diethelm L., Ortiz L.A., Gutierrez M., Citera G., Welsh R.A., Espinoza L.R. Pulmonary involvement in RA. *Sem Arthriti Rheum*, 1995;**24**:242–54.

83. Saag K.G., Kolluri S., Koehnke R.K., Georgou T.A., Rachow J.W., Hunninghake G.W., *et al.* RA lung disease. *Arthritis Rheum*, 1996;**39**:1711–9.

84. Bacon P.A., Carruthers D.M. Vasculitis associated with connective tissue disorders. *Reum Dis Clin North Am*, 1995;**21**:1077–96.

85. Voskuyl A.E., Zwinderman A.H., Westedt M.L., Vandenbroucke J.P., Breedveld F.C., Hazes J.M.W. Factors associated with the development of vasculitis in RA. *Ann Rheum Dis*, 1996; **55**:190–2.

86. Watts R.A., Carruthers D.M., Symmons D.P., Scott D.G. The incidence of rheumatoid vasculitis in the Norwich health authority. *Br J Rheum*, 1994;**33**:832–33.

87. Vollertsen R.S., Conn D.L., Ilstup D.M., Kamar R.E., Silverfield J.C. Rheumatoid vasculitis: survival and associated risk factors. *Medicine*, 1986;**65**:365–75.

88. Voskuyl A.E., Zwinderman A.H., Westedt M.L., vanden Broucke J.P., Breedveld F.C., Hazes J.M.W. The mortality of rheumatoid vasculitis compared with RA. *Arthritis Rheum*, 1996;**39**:266–71.

89. Lems W.F., Dijkmans B.A.C. Should we look for osteoporosis in patients with RA? *Ann Rheum Dis*, 1998;**57**:325–327.

90. Gough A.K.S., Lilley J., Eyre S., Holder R.L., Emery P. Generalised bone loss in patients with early RA. *Lancet*, 1994;**344**:23–6.

91. Eggelmeijer F., Papapoulos S.E., Paassen H.C. van, Dijkmans B.A.C., Valkema R., Westedt M.L., *et al.* Increased bone mass with pamidronate treatment in RA. *Arthritis Rheum*, 1996;**39**:396–402.

92. Hooyman J.R., Melton L.J., Nelson A.M., O'Fallon W.M., Riggs B.L. Fractures after RA. *Arthritis Rheum*, 1984;**27**:1353–61.

93. Spector T.D., Hall G.M., Mc Closkey E.V., Kanis J.A. Risk of vertebral fracture in women with RA. *Br Med J*, 1993;**306**:58.

94. Felson D.T., Anderson J.J., Boers M., Bombardier C., Chernoff M., Fried B., *et al.* The American College of Rheumatology Core preliminary core set of disease activity measures for RA clinical trials. *Arthritis Rheum*, 1993;**36**:729–40.

95. Leeuwen M.A. van, Rijswijk M.H. van. Acute phase proteins in the monitoring of inflammatory disorders. In: Husby G. (ed). Reactive amyloidosis and the acute phase response. *Balliére's Clinical Rheumatology*, 1994;**8**:531–52.

96. Leeuwen M.A. van, Rijwijk M.H. van, Heijde D.M.F.M. van der, Meermen G.J. te, Riel P.L.C.M. van, Houtman P.M., *et al.* The acute phase response in relation to radiographic progression in early RA: a prospective study during the first three years of the disease. *Br J Rheumatol*, 1993;**32** (suppl 3):9–13.

97. Peeters H.R.M., Jongen-Lavrencic M., Raja A.N., Ramdin H.S., Vreugdenhil G., Breedveld F.C. Course and characteristics of anemia in patients with RA. *Ann Rheum Dis*, 1996;**55**:162–6.

98. Greenwold R.A. Monitoring collagen degradation in patients with arthritis. *Arthritis Rheum*, 1996;**39**:1455–65.

99. Lems W.F., Gerrits M.I., Jacobs J.W.G., Vugt R.M. van, Rijn H.J.M. van, Bijlsma J.W.J. Effect of high dose corticosteroid pulse therapy on (markers of) bone metabolism. *Ann Rheum Dis*, 1996;**55**:288–93.

100. Koopman W.J., Shrohenhofer R.E. A sensitive radioimmunoassay for quantitation of IgM RF. *Arthrtis Rheum*, 1980;**23**:302–8.

101. Wolfe F., Cathey M.A., Roberts F.K. The latex revisited: RFtesting in 8287 rheumatic disease patients. *Arthritis Rheum*, 1991;**34**:951–60.

102. Shmerling R.H., Delbanco T.L. The RF: an analysis of clinical utility. *Am J Med*, 1991;**91**:528–34.

103. Cush J.J., Lipsky P.E., Postlehwaite A.E., Schrohenloher R.E., Saway A., Koopman W.J. Correlation of serologic indicators of inflammation with effectiveness of NSAIDs in RA. *Arthritis Rheum*, 1990;**33**:19–28.

104. Olsen N.J., Callahan L.F., Pincus T. Immunologic studies of RA patients treated with methotrexate. *Arthritis Rheum*, 1987;**30**:481–8.

105. Mc Carthy D.J., O'Duffy J.D., Pearson L., Hunter J.B. Remitting seronegative symmetrical synovitis with pitting edema: RS3PE-syndrome. *JAMA*, 1985;**254**:2763–7.

106. Salvarini C., Macchinoni P., Boiardi L. Polymyalgia rheumatica. *Lancet*, 1997;**350**:43–7.

107. Hench P.S., Rosenberg E.F. Palindromic rheumatism. *Arch Intern Med*, 1994;**73**:293–321.

108. Guerne P.A., Weisman M.H. palindromic rheumatism: part of or apart form the spectrum of RA. *Am J Med*, 1992;**93**:451–60.

109. Ohta A., Yamaguchi M., Kaneoka H., Nagayoshi T., Hida M. Adult Still's disease: review of 228 cases from the literature. *J Rheumatol*, 1987;**14**:1139–46.

110. Gonzalez-Hernandez T., Martin-Mola E., Fernandez-Zamorano A., Balsa Criado A., de Miguel-Medieta E. Serum Ferritin can be useful for diagnosis in Adult Onset Still's disease. *J Rheumatol*, 1989;**16**:412–3.

111. Schaardenburg D van, Breedveld F.C. Elderly-onset RA, a review. *Sem Arthritis Rheum*, 1994;**23**:367–78.

112. Heijde D.M.F.M. van der, Riel P.L.C.M. van, Leeuwen M.A. van, Hof M.A. van 't, Rijswijk M.H. van, Putte LBA van de. Older versus younger onset RA. *J Rheumatol*, 1991;**18**:1285–9.

113. Schaardenburg D. van, Lagaay A.M., Otten H.G., Breedveld F.C. The relation between class-specific serum rheumatoid factors and age in the general population. *Br J Rheumatol*, 1993;**32**:546–9.

114. Heide A. Van der, Jacobs J.W.G., Bijlsma J.W.J., Heurkens A.H., Booma-Frankfort C., *et al*. The effectiveness of early treatment with 'second-line' antirheumatic drugs. *Ann Intern Med*, 1996;**124**:699–707.

115. Fries J.F., Wiliams A., Morfeld D., Singh G., Sibley. Reduction in longterm disability in patients with RA by DMARD-based treatment strategies. *Arthritis Rheum*, 1996;**39**:616–22.

116. Boers M., Verhoeven A.C. van, Markusse H.M., Laar M.A.F.J. van de, Westhovens R., Denderen J.C. van, *et al*. Randomised comparison of combined prednisolone, methotrexate and sulfasalazine with sulfasalazine alone in early RA. *Lancet*, 1997;**350**:309–18.

117. Heijde van der D.M.F.M., Riel P.L.C.M. van, Leeuwen M.A. van, *et al*. Prognostic factors for radiographic damage and physical disability in early RA. *Br J Rheum*, 1992;**31**:519–25.

118. Duguwson C.E., Nelson J.L., Koepsell T.D. Evaluation of the 1987 revised criteria for RA in a cohort of newly diagnosed patients. *Arthritis Rheum*, 1990;**33**:1042–6.

119. Brennan P., Harrison B., Barret E., *et al*. A simple algorithm to predict the development of radiological erosions in patients with early RA. *Br Med J*, 1996;**313**:471–6.

120. Heide A van der, Remme C.A., Hofman D., Jacobs J.W.G., Bijlma J.W.J. Prediction of progression of radiological damage in newly diagnosed RA. *Arthritis Rheum*, 1995;**38**:1466–74.

121. Horst-Bruinsma I.E. van der, Speyer I., Visser H., Breedveld F.C., Hazes J.M.W. Diagnosis and course of early onset arthritis: results of a special early arthritis clinic. *Br J Rheum*, 1998;**37**:1084–8

122. Pinals R.S., Nasi A.T., Larsen R.A., *et al*. Preliminary criteria for clinical remission in RA. *Arthritis Rheum*, 1981;**24**:1308–15.

123. Ten Wolde S., Breedveld F.C., Hermans J., Vandenbroucke J.P., Laar M.A.F.J. van de, Markusse H.M. *et al*. Randomized placebo-controlled study of stopping second-line drugs in RA. *Lancet*, 1996;**347**:347–52.

17 | Extra-articular features of rheumatoid arthritis

D. O'Gradaigh, R.A. Watts, and D.G.I. Scott,

Introduction

Rheumatoid arthritis is characterized by chronic synovial inflammation and pannus formation, involving large and small joints. However, the disease process is not restricted to the joint and its associated structures. Numerous extra-articular manifestations occur particularly in the setting of seropositive disease. These features typically follow years of well-recognized RA, although some may occur early and thereby cause diagnostic confusion. In addition to causing considerable morbidity and interference with quality of life, the excess mortality associated with RA arises largely from its extra-articular organ involvement[1]. Though the psychosocial aspects of RA contribute significantly to illness, they are rarely considered in the context of 'extra-articular disease'.

The study of extra-articular RA has provided some useful clues to the underlying etiology as efforts are made to define common pathways which would account for the protean manifestations of rheumatoid disease. This chapter aims to review the extra-articular features of RA as they present in various organ systems, with emphasis on new insights into pathogenesis, and the resulting therapeutic strategies of value in treating this often complex disease.

Efforts have been made to classify extra-articular disease[2] into those features intrinsic to RA, those which arise as complication of the disease and its treatment, and immunological diseases which may be associated with RA but can occur in isolation (Table 17.1). However, therapeutic interventions do not conform rigidly to these groups, and the appropriate classification of some features is debatable. Table 17.2 highlights the more common extra-articular features of RA. Though well-described, the prevalence and incidence of many extra-articular features is not accurately known. There are inevitable differences between hospital and community-based cohorts, as the former tend to include patients with more severe RA and hence report higher figures than community-based studies. Other factors include the intensity of the search for these extra-articular manifestations and the length of follow-up after diagnosis of RA. Commonly, extra-articular involvement may be asymptomatic, leading to wide variability in figures between clinical and post-mortem studies. The latter introduces a bias towards those with more severe disease. Features common to many autoimmune rheumatic diseases, such as fatigue, weight loss, and fever, are rarely considered in such studies. Weight loss may be quite marked during early, aggressive presentations of RA affecting 67

Table 17.1 Extra-articular features of RA

	Manifestations	Prevalence %* (post-mortem studies)
Intrinsic		
Nodule formation	skin, lung, myocardium	25
Serositis	pleurisy, pericarditis, effusions	10–25 (75)
Vasculitis	ulceration, digital infarcts, mononeuritis	1–10 (14–25)
Felty's syndrome	neutropenia, infection	1 (2)
Complications of chronic inflammation		
Anemia	pallor, dyspnea	75
Lymphadenopathy	axillary nodes	66
Amyloidosis	renal, cardiac, any organ	(21)
Entrapment neuropathy	carpal/tarsal tunnel syndrome	–
Osteoporosis	fracture	–
Associated immunological disease		
Sjögren's syndrome	keratocojunctivitis sicca, dry mouth	35
Interstitial lung disease	dyspnea, dry cough	14 (34)

* Among RA patients; figures are not from a single series (see text).

per cent in one series. This has been related to high levels of TNF-α in both initial presentation of RA and during flare up of disease[3]. Fever is less common, more usually seen in adult Still's disease, but when it occurs during an acute arthritis it may lead to suspicion of joint sepsis. There is a striking tendency for patients to develop more than one extra-articular feature. For example nodules, vasculitis, and pulmonary involvement frequently coexist[4]. Some features, such as nodules and pleuropericardial involvement, usually parallel joint activity while vasculitis typically occurs in the face of quiescent synovitis.

The Norfolk Arthritis Register, a community-based study of inflammatory arthritis, found that 40 per cent of all patients fulfilling ACR criteria for RA had evidence of extra-articular disease at 5-year clinical follow-up[5]. Nodules were the most common feature occurring in isolation in 21 per cent, while 45 per cent had another isolated extra-articular manifestation, and 34 per cent had more than one feature. In other studies, nodules are again the most common feature described, occurring in at least 25 per cent. Pleuropulmonary involvement, clinically evident in perhaps 10 per cent, is detected in over half of patients with early disease when detailed investigations are used[6]. Rarer manifestations include Felty's syndrome seen in 1 per cent. Epidemiological data for rheumatoid vasculitis (RV) are

Table 17.2   Symptoms and associated extra-articular RA features

Skin	nodules	nodulosis, methotrexate therapy
	ulceration	vasculitis, Felty's syndrome
Cardiorespiratory	dyspnea, dry cough	interstitial lung, BOOP[a], methotrexate
		constrictive pericarditis, myocarditis
	hoarse/painful throat	cricoarytenoid arthritis
Neurological	paresthesias	entrapment, mononeuritis, cervical
		myelopathy (AAS)[b]
	muscle weakness	disuse atrophy, neuropathy, steroid use
Eye	dry eye	Sjögren's syndrome
	blurred vision	keratitis/corneal melt, drug therapy
	red eye	scleritis, episcleritis
General	fever	infections, including joint
		flare of arthritis,
		interstitial lung disease, BOOP
	lymphadenopathy	flare of arthritis, joint sepsis,
		lymphoma, methotrexate
Urinalysis	hematuria/proteinuria	amyloidosis, glomerulonephritis, drugs

a BOOP = bronchiolitis obliterans-organizing pneumonia
b AAS = atlanto-axial subluxation

described in more detail later. Post-mortem studies[7,8] demonstrate the importance of extra-articular disease in RA mortality. While the largest series are from non-Caucasian populations, the figures concur with those from smaller series world-wide. Infection is the leading cause of death (25 per cent), followed by cardiac and pulmonary disease (18 per cent), with renal and gastrointestinal disease each identified as cause of death in 10 per cent. Contributory pathology such as vasculitis, amyloidosis, and pulmonary fibrosis are more common than clinically recognized.

Immunogenetic aspects

Etiopathogenesis

In epidemiological studies, it is notable that men are disproportionately affected with extra-articular features; near parity for Felty's syndrome and for vasculitis, and males predominate in lung disease, compared with 1:3 for uncomplicated RA. Patients also tend to be older, though this may simply reflect duration of disease. Ethnic differences exist, largely related to patterns of HLA antigen inheritance. There is a correlation between the severity of RA disease expression and presence of the 'shared epitope' (QKRAA/QRRAA). Westedt *et al.*[9] showed increased frequency of HLA-DR4 in patients with rheumatoid vasculitis (RV) compared with both uncomplicated RA patients and healthy controls. A subsequent study reported a disproportionate increase of the DR4 'subtype' Dw14(DRB1*0404 and *0408) in RV[10], and homozygosity (DRB1 *04,04) is particularly associated (64 per cent), compared with nodular RA without vaculitis (28 per cent) and non-nodular RA (none)[11]. A recently proposed model for the role of HLA molecules in the autoimmune pathogenesis of RA is that an HLA peptide derived from one molecule is presented by another HLA molecule[12]. In

this context, the finding of unusual combinations of DRB1, DQA1, and DQB1 alleles is of particular interest, and observations are consistent with a role for the first and/or second hypervariable region of the DRB1 chain, or for DQA1 *0301 which is in strong linkage disequilibrium with DRB1 *04.

Autoantibody associations

Of note, the 'intrinsic' extra-articular manifestations (see Table 17.1) are rarely seen in those with seronegative disease. IgG isotype rheumatoid factors are strongly associated with extra-articular disease and vasculitis[13] and are associated with disease activity[14]. IgG rheumatoid factor will associate *in vitro* with complement fixing immune complexes. Circulating immune complexes, high serum immunoglobulins, and evidence of complement activation have been observed in extra-articular RA[15]. Histological studies show considerable similarities between many extra-articular manifestations, with high levels of immune complexes, palisading macrophages, and fibrinoid necrosis seen in nodules, serosal involvement, and vasculitis. Adsorption of circulating immune complexes have also been implicated in the peripheral destruction of neutrophils in Felty's syndrome. These suggest that antibody–antigen activation driven by B-cell activity may be involved in these extra-articular manifestations[16]. Antinuclear antibodies (ANA) may be found in up to 60 per cent of patients with uncomplicated RA and do not appear to imply the presence of vasculitis. Antiendothelial cell antibodies (AECA) have been reported to occur in up to 80 per cent of patients with RV. Antineutrophil cytoplasmic antibodies (ANCA) are present in 16 per cent of patients with uncomplicated RA[17], though the presence of ANCA does not appear to correlate with the presence of vasculitis or its severity. ANCA immunoflourescence is typically of the pANCA pattern and is usually directed against antigens other than the classical proteinase 3 or myeloperoxidase, including cathepsin, lactoferrin, elastase, lysozyme, and

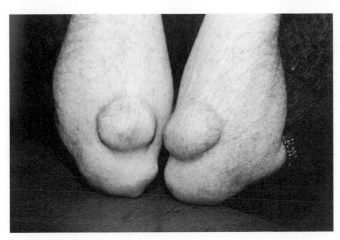

Fig. 17.1 Large rheumatoid nodules at a typical site in the forearm. See also Plate 22.

azuricidin. Lactoferrin is the most commonly-recognized antigen, both in patients with uncomplicated RA[18] And in those with RV[19]. Myeloperoxidase antibodies have been associated with vasculitis in RA[20], but these patients may represent an overlap between RA and microscopic polyangiitis[21]. We too have seen a few patients with positive ANCA who probably represent overlap with MPA or Wegener's granulomatosis.

These findings suggest there are a number of alternative immunopathogenic pathways which might, in part, account for the occurrence of extra-articular disease in the setting of quiescent joint disease.

Clinical features

Nodules

Rheumatoid nodules occur in at least 25 per cent of patients with definite or classical RA[22]. They are typically present over the extensor area of the forearm (Fig. 17.1) and at pressure areas, but can develop in internal organs such as the lungs. There is considerable variability in consistency from small, firm, immobile lumps to large, soft, mobile masses. They may ulcerate and become gangrenous. Rheumatoid factor is almost always present at high titer in the serum of patients with rheumatoid nodules[23]. A rheumatoid nodule is composed of three histological zones: an inner central necrotic zone, a surrounding zone of palisading cells (predominately macrophages), and an outer zone with perivascular infiltration of chronic inflammatory cells[22].

The immunological stimulus that induces formation of nodules and the relation between synovial and nodule-derived lymphocytes is unknown. Expression of HLA-DR is present[24] and collagenase and proteinase production[25] may explain the central necrosis. Lymphocytes in nodules mainly express the CD3 phenotype, with a predominance of CD4 over CD8 T cells. T cells grown from rheumatoid nodules after IL-2 expansion show a significantly oligoclonal pattern reflecting a restricted and clonally biased T cell activation *in situ*[26,27]. Molecular analysis suggests that *in situ* T cell activation is related to classical antigen induced immune activation[28]. Edwards *et al.*[29]

reassessed the immunohistochemical features of the palisading cells and observed that they were a mixture of macrophages and fibroblasts but that the latter did not show evidence of synoviocytic differentiation.

Although the process of formation of rheumatoid nodules is unknown, Ziff has proposed the following sequence of events

(1) trauma to small blood vessels with local pooling of rheumatoid factor immune complexes;

(2) immune complex activation of local monocyte/ macrophages, stimulating the secretion of monocyte chemotactic factors and resulting in mobilization of increased numbers of macrophages;

(3) secretion of procoagulant by activated macrophages, leading to the deposition of fibrinoid;

(4) production of tissue necrosis by cytotoxic agents, proteinases, and collagenases secreted by activated macrophages;

(5) assembly of a palisade of macrophages around the necrotic tissue as a consequence of attraction of macrophages to the necrotic zone by chemotactic factors released by macrophages, and interaction of the macrophage receptors with fibrinoid and fibronectin deposited at the margins of the zone of necrosis[22].

Hematological features

Though a normocytic, normochromic picture is most commonly seen in RA, anemia is multifactorial, sometimes reflected in dimorphic appearances on blood film and wide red-cell differentiation width (RDW). The degree of anemia correlates with disease activity. Ferritin, an acute phase reactant, and lactoferrin are increased and there is increased retention of iron from senescent red cells leading to defects in iron utilization. Inefficient erythropoiesis, reduced response of bone marrow to erythropoietin (EPO), shortened red cell life span, and peripheral destruction of erythrocytes by synovium have all been described[30]. Lower levels of EPO have been found in anemic RA patients than in patients with a similar level of hemoglobin without RA. This has lead to the use of recombinant EPO with good results[31]. Iron deficiency can occur as a consequence of gastrointestinal losses associated with non-steroidal anti-inflammatory drugs (NSAIDs). Methotrexate (MTX) and, to a lesser extent, sulfasalazine are antifolate drugs which may produce megaloblastic anemia, while gold therapy can result in aplastic anemia. Autoimmune hemolytic anemia is an uncommon association with RA.

Platelet numbers are frequently increased as part of an acute phase response. Less commonly, platelets may be depleted, perhaps related to therapeutic drugs or to Felty's syndrome. Intravascular coagulation has been reported, as has hyperviscosity syndrome associated with high titers of IgM rheumatoid factor.

Lymphadenopathy has been reported as a frequent extra-articular manifestation of RA, reflecting chronic immune stimulation. Nodes are almost exclusively axillary[32], and may precede the onset of joint symptoms[33]. Biopsy shows follicular reactive hyperplasia, which recedes as articular disease is controlled.

Lymphoma, however, can occur in the setting of secondary Sjögren's syndrome, with a relative risk for non-Hodgkin's lymphoma of 43.8 compared with the normal population[34]. Lymphadenopathy, reversing on discontinuation of MTX therapy, has also been increasingly recognized[35].

Felty's syndrome

The association of leukopenia, splenomegaly, and RA was first described by Felty in 1924[36]. Splenomegaly is a common feature of both systemic rheumatoid vasculitis and uncomplicated rheumatoid arthritis and may disappear following treatment of the arthritis. Such patients do not necessarily have Felty's syndrome (FS). Patients with and without splenomegaly, who otherwise have FS, are clinically very similar. It effects about 1 per cent of RA patients[37], typically in seropositive disease of long duration, and is strongly associated with HLA-DR4. It is frequently associated with nodule formation. Joint disease is often quiescent when FS occurs[38]. Other features include lower limb ulceration and pigmentation, thrombocytopenia, and positive ANA. Neutropenia predominates and increased susceptibility to infection is the most important consequence of this extra-articular feature of RA. A 12-fold increased risk of non-Hodgkin lymphoma is noted compared with RA patients without FS over a 6-year follow-up[39].

Mechanisms of neutropenia described[40,41] include decreased granulopoiesis, analogous to the anemia and thrombocytopenia described earlier, reduced neutrophil life span, and increased peripheral destruction which may be caused by immune complexes adhering to neutrophils. The risk of infection, which correlates with neutrophil counts below $1.0 \times 10^9/l$, is also thought to be due to defective function of these cells, reduced complement levels, and probably also to steroid therapy.

A chronic T-cell lymphoproliferative disorder with large granular lymphocytes, neutropenia, and splenomegaly has also been described[42]. It has been associated with RA in 25 to 50 per cent of cases, and is considered a variant of FS usually seen earlier in the disease course, typically in older patients and with normal or increased total leukocyte count. However, both forms are clinically very similar and are strongly related to HLA-DR4. Sometimes considered a T-cell clonopathy[43], other workers have found a significant proportion of patients with 'classical' FS have similar clonal expansions, and hypothesize that these T cells may be implicated in impaired granulopoiesis[16].

Although one study[44] found cardiovascular disease to be the commonest cause of death with fatal sepsis occurring no more frequently than in RA controls without FS (10 and 13 per cent respectively), improving neutrophil numbers is the main therapeutic target in FS. While many disease-modifying drugs and others, such as lithium carbonate, have been used, a recent review[45] identified MTX, hemopoietic growth factors, and splenectomy as the most efficacious in increasing granulocyte count and improving clinical outcome. MTX has the advantage of treating both the hematological and joint manifestations of RA. Granulocyte- and granulocyte-macrophage-colony stimulating factors (G-CSF and GM-CSF) have a rapid onset of action but have been increasingly associated with acute flare of arthritis

and with leukocytoclastic vasculitis, which occurs more frequently than when these agents are used in other diseases[46]. Splenectomy produces a rapid and long-term hematological response in 70 to 80 per cent of patients, over half having no further infections. It is a reasonable option perhaps when growth factors have failed. The immunization policy recommended to patients having splenectomy for FS is the same as that for other indications (Turner, personal communication, and Ref. 47). Key points include pneumococcal immunization at least 2 weeks before splenectomy, lifelong prophylactic antibiotics, and urgent admission to hospital in the event of infection. The *Haemophilus influenzae* type b vaccine is recommended. While we do not consider conventional disease-modifying therapy to be immunosuppressive, patients may be immunocompromised by their disease, and influenza immunization is likely to be beneficial.

Vasculitis

Vasculitis complicating rheumatoid arthritis (RA) was first described in 1898 in a patient with involvement of the vasa nervorum[48]. The association was clearly established in the 1940s and 1950s[49,50]. The classical features were peripheral gangrene and mononeuritis multiplex, though a broader spectrum of disease is now recognized.

The annual incidence of systemic rheumatoid vasculitis (SRV) was estimated to be 6/million in the 1970s[4], though recent data using the same diagnostic criteria suggest an annual incidence during 1988–94 of 12.5/million[51]. In this study the lifetime risk for a male with RA developing SRV was estimated to be 1:9 compared with 1:38 for females. Other studies[52] have suggested an occurrence of less than 1 per cent of RA patients, though the occurrence of vascular lesions at post-mortem examination of RA patients is higher, ranging from 14[53] to 25 per cent [54,55]. The median age of onset in one study was 61 years with a median duration of RA before onset of vasculitis of 12 years. However, we and others have seen occasional patients who present with vasculitis, particularly with neuropathies, at the time of or shortly after the diagnosis of RA[55]. Development of rheumatoid vasculitis is associated with male gender, extra-articular features, and a severe disease course as assessed by joint damage and the requirement for disease modifying therapy. The strongest association is with the presence of rheumatoid factor[56].

There are no validated diagnostic criteria for the definition of systemic rheumatoid vasculitis though Scott and Bacon did propose criteria in 1984[58] (Table 17.3). The presence of rheumatoid arthritis is an obligatory criterion. This should prevent confusion with other forms of either primary or secondary vasculitis. The major clinical features of systemic rheumatoid vasculitis are given in Table 17.4, where a series of patients seen in Norwich (UK) between 1988 and 1994 is compared with a series reported from Bath (UK) in the 1970s[56]. The pattern of clinical features has not changed significantly over the past 20 years though the slight decrease in cardiovascular and pulmonary involvement may reflect changes in smoking habits or other factors. Constitutional features are most common with weight loss occurring in up to 80 per cent of patients[4]. This may occur in the absence of active synovitis.

Table 17.3 Classification criteria for systemic rheumatoid vasculitis

The presence in a patient with rheumatoid arthritis of one or more of:

1. Mononeuritis multiplex or acute peripheral neuropathy
2. Peripheral gangrene
3. Biopsy evidence of acute necrotizing arteritis plus systemic illness (e.g. fever, weight loss)
4. Deep cutaneous ulcers or active extra-articular disease (e.g. pleurisy, pericarditis, scleritis) if associated with typical digital infarcts or biopsy evidence of vasculitis

Other causes of such lesions, such as diabetes mellitus and atherosclerosis, should be excluded. Patients with nailfold or digital infarcts alone are excluded. Adapted from Scott and Bacon (1984) Ref 58.

Table 17.4 Clinical features at presentation of patients with systemic rheumatoid vasculitis

	Norwich (%)	Bath* (%)
Number of Patients	47	50
Rheumatoid factor	42 (89)	47 (94)
Erosions	32 (68)	NA
Nodules	16/28 (57)	43/50 (86)
Systemic	23 (49)**	41 (82)
Weight loss	16	41
Malaise	13	NA
Cutaneous	42 (89)	44 (88)
Infarct	33	26
Ulcer	21	12
Purpura	7	28
Gangrene	16	7
Neurological	18 (38)	21 (42)
PN	16	14
MNM	6	7
Stroke	2	2
Pulmonary	13 (28)	17 (34)
Fibrosis	8	9
Pleurisy/Effusion	6	8
Infiltrates	0	NA
Renal	12 (25)	12 (24)
Protein/Hematuria	8	6
Raised creatinine	1	2
Ophthalmic	12 (25)	8 (16)
Scleritis	11	7
CVS	9 (19)	17 (34)
Pericarditis	5	7
Aortic Incomp	2	2
MI	2	3
Gastrointestinal	2 (4)	5 (10)

*from Ref. 4; ** $p < 0.001$ (Norwich vs Bath); PN = peripheral neuropathy, MNM = mononeuritis multiplex, MI = myocardial infarction, NA = data not available.

Three main patterns of rheumatoid vasculitis can be identified;

(1) isolated nailfold vasculitis due to digital endarteritis with intimal proliferation (Fig. 17.2a);

(2) venulitis and small vessel arteritis characterized by rash, skin eruptions, or purpura (Fig. 17.2b);

(3) necrotizing arteritis of small and medium sized arteries with involvement of internal organs and peripheral nerves (Fig. 17.2c).

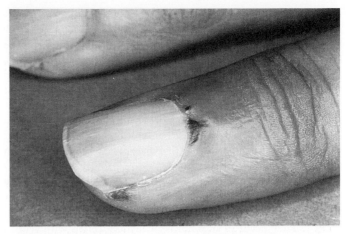

(a)

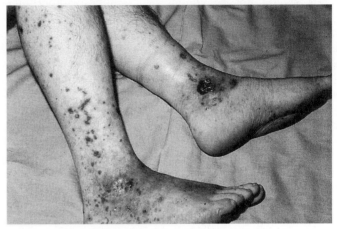

(b)

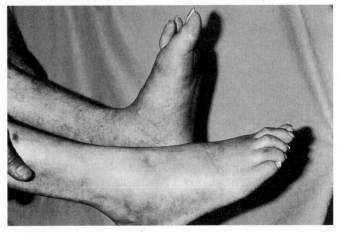

(c)

Fig. 17.2 (a) Isolated nailfold vasculitis; (b) vasculitic rash and ulceration; (c) foot-drop due to mononeurits multiplex. See also Plate 23.

Cutaneous lesions are common, including typical isolated small nail fold or nail edge lesions reflecting mainly small vessel involvement. Nailfold infarcts are evanescent and possibly related to local trauma. The frequency of reported nailfold lesions varies from 15 per cent of males and 5 per cent of females with classical or definite RA[59] to 34 per cent of men and 18 per cent of women with classical RA attending hospital reported by Golding and colleagues[60]. The annual incidence is unknown. Subclinical small vessel vasculitis has been reported in up to 30 per cent of biopsies from clinically uninvolved skin taken from RA patients[61,62]. Isolated nail fold vasculitis is generally believed to be a benign and relatively minor feature of RA[63], though it may herald the onset of major arteritis[49]. However, our own experience has shown that patients developing nailfold vasculitis or systemic rheumatoid vasculitis are of similar age and disease duration supporting the idea, also observed in a cohort study, that there is little progression from localized to systemic disease[64].

Leg ulcers commonly occur in RA patients and are usually multifactorial[65]. Vasculitic ulcers may be clinically recognized as they are typically painful, deep punched out lesions of acute onset[57]. They occur in sites not typically associated with venous stasis ulceration, such as the sacrum or foot. Chronic superficial ulcers should not be considered vasculitic without other evidence of SRV (either histological or clinical). Biopsies are rarely obtained because of fears about poor wound healing. Unusual skin lesions include pyoderma gangrenosum and erythema elevatum diutinum.

Pulmonary involvement (up to 34 per cent) often manifests as fibrozing alvelolitis, though this often occurs in RA uncomplicated by vasculitis. Cardiovascular involvement is uncommon, clinically significant aortitis or valvulitis being rare. Coronary arteritis is rarely diagnosed antemortem. Necropsy series have suggested that coronary arteritis occurs in up to 20 per cent of cases[53,66]. Although pericarditis occurs as a feature of vasculitis, it more typically occurs in rheumatoid disease without SRV.

Scleritis may occur independently of other evidence of vasculitis[67], but occurs in up to 25 per cent of patients with systemic rheumatoid vasculitis. Scleromalacia perforans, a type of nodular vasculitis, is very rare. Retinal vasculitis may occur in up to 18 per cent of patients with RA, but is often asymptomatic and only detectable by fluorescein angiography[68].

Renal vasculitis is a rare complication of RA but has been reported in up to 25 per cent of patients with systemic rheumatoid vasculitis. A post-mortem study by Boers *et al.*[53] of 132 patients with RA showed a large vessel vasculitis in eight out of 18 cases with systemic vasculitis and in four cases there was an extracapillary glomerulonephritis. Harper *et al.*[69] recently reported ten RA patients who developed a focal segmental necrotizing glomerulonephritis with extracapillary proliferation typical of vasculitic glomerulonephritis. Necrotizing and crescentic glomerulonephritis has been ascribed to therapy with D-penicillamine although the typical renal lesion associated with D-penicillamine is membranous nephropathy[21].

Neurological involvement is common with development of acute mononeuritis multiplex or peripheral neuropathy often in association with nailfold lesions. A distal symmetrical sensory or sensori-motor pattern is more common than mononeuritis multiplex (Table 17.4). Peripheral neuropathy is attributable to development of necrotizing vasculitis of the vasa nervorum[70]. Other forms of neurovasculitis are rare though cerebral vasculitis should be considered in any patient who develops central nervous system disturbance in the presence of other features of vasculitis.

As discussed earlier, immune complexes may be important in the pathogenesis of rheumatoid vasculitis. Endothelial and leukocyte adhesion molecules are also important in the pathogenesis of inflammatory injury and might be important in the development of vasculitis by enhancing lymphocyte–endothelial cell molecular interactions and promoting damage to the endothelium. Flipo and colleagues[71] have shown that ICAM-1, E-selectin, and TNF-α expression is significantly increased in endothelial cells and perivascular infiltrates in salivary gland biopsies obtained form patients with rheumatoid vasculitis suggesting that vasculitic lesions may reflect a Th1 response. Levels of von Willebrand factor, a marker of endothelial cell damage, are elevated in patients with vasculitis compared to uncomplicated RA[72].

Isolated nailfold vasculitis does not require specific therapy though the patient should be kept under close observation. Systemic rheumatoid vasculitis, however, is associated with significant mortality and morbidity, which has led to the early use of immunosuppressive regimens. Corticosteroids alone are usually ineffective and rapid changes in dose have been implicated in the pathogenesis and induction of SRV[55,73] and may predispose patients to vascular occlusion. Azathioprine in combination with prednisolone may be effective[74] but no controlled data exist. The only double-blind placebo-controlled trial was abandoned due to a significant number of deaths in both trial groups[75]. A comparison of azathioprine and prednisolone in the treatment of isolated nailfold vasculitis showed no significant advantage over conventional therapy[74]. Cyclophosphamide combined with corticosteroids have now become the standard treatment for SRV. Cyclophosphamide may be given either as pulse intermittent high-dose therapy or as continuous oral therapy. Studies show that intermittent pulse cyclophosphamide combined with prednisolone is more effective than conventional oral regimens in the treatment of SRV[58] and possibly less toxic[76]. Our current regime is shown in Table 17.5.

Other imunosuppressive drugs such as chlorambucil, methotrexate, and cyclosporin have been used in rheumatoid vasculitis. Methotrexate therapy has been associated with development of cutaneous vasculitis though a retrospective study disputes this[77]. MTX has been successfully used in RA patients with vasculitic ulceration to good effect[78] though our own experience does not confirm this. Although used in scleritis, as mentioned earlier, the wider role of cyclosporin in SRV is still to be established; we have found that, like MTX, cyclosporin is only effective in relatively mild rheumatoid vasculitis.

Plasma exchange, used in uncontrolled studies in rheumatoid vasculitis, appears to have little additional benefit over pulse intravenous cyclophosphamide[79]. Intravenous immunoglobulin has also been used in an uncontrolled fashion and we have seen patients with vasculitic leg ulcers who appear to respond effectively to this treatment. It is usually well tolerated and seems to be effective in treating relapses of other types of vasculitis[80].

Patients with isolated nailfold involvement have a much better prognosis than patients with systemic involvement[64], who are generally considered to have a poor prognosis. However, it is important to investigate these patients to ensure there are no other extra-articular features; in our study[64], three patients died who did not have truly 'isolated' nailfold vasculitis. In one study[4], the 1-year mortality was 20 per cent. The 2-year mortal-

Table 17.5 Cyclophosphamide (Cy) protocol for systemic vasculitis

A. Remission induction (0–3 months)

pulses to be given every 2 weeks × 6, each pulse to consist of either:

(1) intravenous Cy 10–15 mg/kg (to max 1 g) over 1 hour, plus Methylprednisolone 1 g over 2 hours

or

(2) Oral Cy 5 mg/kg daily for 3 days plus prednisolone 100 mg/day for 3 days

Continuous oral steroids are not always required. Patients who are systemically unwell with active inflammatory lesions such as scleritis, pleurisy, etc. often do well on 20 mg oral prednisolone which should be reduced to finish within the first 3 months.

Monitoring

White cell count days 7, 10, 14 between first and second pulses; thereafter, WCC on day of treatment only.

If …

(1) lowest WCC < 3 (polymorphs < 2.5) reduce does of next pulse; WCC d 7, 10, 14

(2) WCC d 14 < d10, delay treatment for up to 1 week

(3) WCC satisfactory, look for lymphopenia as indication of immunosuppression.

Caveats

- reduce dose of Cy if renal impairment, e.g. 5–10 mg/kg;
- add H2 receptor antagonist throughout treatment;
- if Cy is required every 10 days, reduce dose by 50–100 mg;
- patients should drink at least 3 litres per 24 h during Cy therapy and the following day; Mesna is optional, but should be considered where there is renal impairment or frequency greater than fortnightly;
- up to 6 pulses intravenously then transfer to oral therapy, though milder cases may transfer sooner, and as some patients tolerate iv therapy better, they may continue iv. Minimum of 6 fortnightly pulses, then maintenance therapy if good response.

B. Maintenance

Increase pulse interval to … 3 weekly × 4 then monthly up to 1 year; if in remission at 1 year, convert to Azathioprine or oral MTX.

C. Relapse

Options include methylprednisolone 1 g iv 3 consecutive days or plasma exchange for severe renal disease or pulmonary hemorrhage

---

ity in this study was 46 per cent, compared with 23 per cent in a later study from a tertiary referral center using actuarial methods[73]. Correction for referral bias reduced calculated 2-year mortality to 10 per cent, and 13 per cent at 5 years, which is similar to patients with RA not complicated by vasculitis. A case-control study showed that, allowing for age and gender, there was only a slight excess mortality in SRV patients compared with RA patients[81].

Pulmonary features

Pulmonary involvement, first described in 1948 and later studied by Cudkowicz[82], includes pleurisy and pleural effusions, nodules, interstitial involvement, and airway disease. According to the classification in Table 17.1, some of the pulmonary features associated with RA are intrinsic to the disease, and others represent immune-mediated processes that can occur independently. It is important to note that chronic bronchitis related to smoking is the most common cause of respiratory symptoms in RA patients[83]. While cricoarytenoid involvement is strictly an articular manifestation, its typical presentations with stridor, dysphagia, or sore throat are clearly extra-articular. Histologically, similarities can be seen between serositis and nodulosis, with palisading macrophages, lymphocytic aggregates, and fibrinoid necrosis, and of course rheumatoid nodules are found in lung parenchyma. The histopathology can be quite varied between and within patients, with lymphocytic infiltrates, bronchiolitis obliterans-organizing pneumonia, lymphoid hyperplasia related to airways (termed follicular bronchiolitis), and interstitial fibrosis. Few of these are specific to RA though useful diagnostic clues can be observed.

Clinically, patients are usually asymptomatic with lesions identified on chest radiographs or physiological tests. Shortness of breath, however, has a wide differential which includes conditions from each of the classifications, and they will be discussed here as clinical diagnoses. The importance of pulmonary disease cannot be over-stressed; studies show it to be one of the leading causes of death in RA patients. We have compared data from three centers (Bath, Birmingham, and Norwich) with respect to systemic RA and have similarly found pulmonary disease as a significant cause of death (unpublished data and Table 17.4). Post-mortem studies in patients with RA of longer duration identify pulmonary, mainly pleural, involvement in as much as 75 per cent of patients[84]. Pleural effusions are the most common manifestation, frequently occurring during periods of active joint disease in men with nodular RA. Nodules are detected incidentally on chest radiographs in less than 1 per cent of patients, though smaller lesions may be detected with high resolution computed tomography (HRCT)[85]. Studies in early RA detected clinically significant interstitial disease in 14 per cent, (compared with largely asymptomatic disease in 44 per cent)[6], and airway involvement is increasingly recognized (16 per cent)[86].

Pleural effusions tend to be small and asymptomatic but may herald the onset of clinically significant extra-articular disease. The effusion has the typical features of an exudate (elevated protein and LDH), with low levels of glucose compared with serum, low levels of complement fractions (particularly CH50), positive rheumatoid factor, and the detection of cholesterol crystals. These features are all helpful in identifying the cause of the effusion[87]. Cytology, usually indicated to rule out associated malignancy, may reveal multinucleated or elongated macrophages and cellular debris[88]. When causing symptoms, the effusion may be drained, but chemical pleurodesis (with povidone iodine or tetracycline) appears only very rarely to be required. Of note, treatment of the underlying arthritis can be effective in resolving the effusion. Surgical decortication can be carried out where marked pleural thickening produces a restrictive lung disease. Pleural involvement rarely causes pneumothorax or empyema, usually in the context of a cavitating rheumatoid nodule.

Pulmonary nodules[89] are histologically identical to those found on the skin and a vasculitic process is similarly implicated in their pathogenesis. They occur more commonly in men but are typically incidental findings, most commonly in the upper lobes or the right middle lobe. Approximately half of these undergo central necrosis and cavitation. Nodules may recede in one part of the lung while new lesions develop elsewhere.

Caplan's syndrome, the association of RA, pulmonary nodules, and pneumoconiosis originally described in coal workers, can arise with other industrial pneumoconioses including silica and asbestos[89]. The clinical prognosis for pulmonary nodules alone is good. The number and size of lesions may reduce with treatment of the underlying joint disease.

Interstitial lung disease (ILD) is clinically and histologically similar to idiopathic pulmonary fibrosis. As diagnostic techniques improve, so the detection of ILD has increased, though the significance of subclinical abnormalities on high resolution computed tomography (HRCT) or pulmonary function tests is unclear. Patients are typically male, 50 to 60 years of age with seropositive nodular RA, complaining of dyspnea and may have clubbing associated with bibasal fine end-inspiratory crepitations. However, in our experience patients with rheumatoid arthritis and interstitial fibrosis are usually not clubbed, compared with patients with cryptogenic fibrozing alveolitis who may show clubbing and have a false-positive rheumatoid factor (i.e. positive test for rheumatoid factor in the absence of rheumatoid disease). In addition to the other risk associations previously outlined for extra-articular manifestations, an increased incidence has been found associated with HLA-B40, in smokers, and in association with particular phenotypes of the α_1-antitrypsin gene. Pulmonary function tests[90] show a restrictive pattern with reduced vital capacity and normal or increased ratio of FEV1 to FVC. Diffusion capacity (DLCO) must be corrected for hemaglobin level, the most common cause of reduced DLCO in RA patients[83]. Chest radiographs and HRCT show reticular, reticulo-nodular, or honeycomb pattern bibasally (Fig. 17.3). Other findings detected on HRCT of patients with clinical signs of ILD include bronchiectasis and emphysema, pleural and pericardial disease. Bronchoalveolar lavage may reveal neutrophilic or lymphocytic infiltrates, though alveolar macrophages producing inflammatory cytokines have been implicated in the pathogenesis of ILD. The treatment of ILD in RA remains somewhat controversial, especially when asymptomatic disease is detected. Immunosuppressive therapy remains the mainstay[91], though trials comparing various regimens are lacking. Prognosis is quite variable, and superimposed infection poses a greater risk than the fibrosis itself[92].

Bronchiolitis obliterans-organizing pneumonia (BOOP) is a specific type of interstitial pneumonia usually presenting acutely or subacutely and running a limited time course. It has also been described in RA[93], and is also recognized as a rare side-effect of D-penicillamine and gold salts. Clinical and radiological manifestations are similar to the idiopathic form, with dyspnea, dry cough, crepitations on auscultation, and linear or acinar shadowing on radiograph. The diagnosis can only be confirmed histologically, where two clinical types are identified. Response to treatment, typically with steroid therapy, is significantly better in 'proliferative' BOOP than in the 'constrictive' type[94]. In many cases, there is an associated fever, and antibiotic therapy is often a first line of management as biopsy will rarely be indicated.

Recent studies with HRCT have found bronchiectasis in 25 to 30 per cent of asymptomatic seropositive patients with normal chest radiograph[95]. A prospective study of patients with bronchiectasis found that this may precede RA, and has indeed been implicated in the antigenic stimulation hypothesis of RA[96].

Treatment of RA may result in pulmonary diseases. 'Methotrexate-lung', an interstitial pneumonitis, occurs in between 2 and 5 per cent of users, presenting with dyspnea, dry cough, and possibly with fever[97]. The condition may be fatal in up to 17 per cent of patients, but differential diagnosis must include infection, BOOP and ILD, and the decision to withdraw this valuable disease-modifying drug can be difficult. Immunosuppression with DMARDs, including methotrexate and cyclosporin, may alter the spectrum of pathogens in respiratory tract infection, and *Pneumocystis carinii*, in particular,

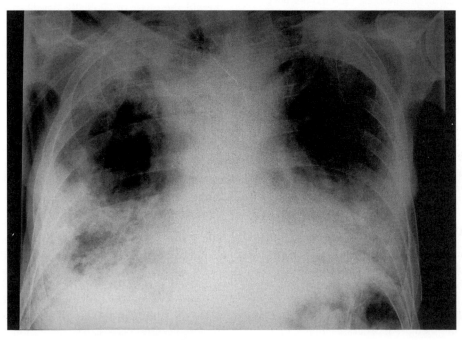

Fig. 17.3 Diffuse, extensive fibrosis extending from both lung bases.

should be considered as definitive diagnosis requires bronchoalveolar lavage[98,99].

Cardiac features

The cardiac manifestations of RA reflect systemic processes which affect many organs including serositis, amyloidosis, vasculitis, and nodule formation. Accelerated atherosclerosis and increased ischaemic heart disease are also seen in RA patients[100] and it is as yet unclear whether this reflects systemic inflammation or the use of corticosteroid therapy in such patients. Post-mortem studies attribute cause of death to heart involvement in 17 per cent. Incidental findings, seen in two-thirds of cases, include pericardial disease, coronary arteritis, myocardial involvement, and valve lesions. Echocardiography, in particular, has led to earlier identification of rheumatoid lesions affecting the heart. Improved therapeutic options from the field of cardiology, such as angiotensin converting enzyme inhibitors and new antiarrhythmic drugs, have led to better prognosis in these patients.

Pericardial disease is similar to pleural involvement with histological features similar to nodules. A 'bread and butter' pericarditis is noted with involvement of both parietal and visceral layers of the pericardium[101]. This may progress to a chronic constrictive pericarditis for which computed tomography is important in diagnosis[102]. Asymptomatic, small effusions are identified on echocardiography in about 25 per cent[103] (Fig. 17.4). Findings on aspiration of these effusions are essentially identical to those described for pleural effusions. Where symptoms occur, typically during increased activity of joint disease, non-steroidal anti-inflammatory drugs are usually sufficient, though the effusion may resolve when the acute flare is controlled. While constrictive pericarditis is rare, it is a serious complication as it may cause heart failure resistant to treatment, and should be treated surgically[104].

Myocardial disease may present with congestive cardiac failure or with isolated diastolic failure[105]. These manifestations may be due to nodular, granulomatous lesions within the myocardium or amyloid involvement which typically produces reduced ventricular compliance and restrictive failure[104]. Coronary artery vasculitis, with consequent myocardial ischaemia and failure, may occur as part of a more generalized SRV, as discussed earlier, though atherosclerotic coronary artery disease is more common. Treatment is as for heart failure in non-RA patients.

Valve lesions, most commonly regurgitation of the aortic and mitral valves, are detected in up to 30 per cent of patients. While these are usually not significant, fulminant heart failure due to aortic valve incompetence is described[101]. Nodular valve lesions infrequently occur, and may mimic endocarditis echocardiographically, impair valve competence, or rarely may embolize producing stroke[106]. Nodular disease may also cause conduction abnormalities detected on electrocardiography, responding to standard antiarrhythmic agents or requiring pacemaker insertion. As with nodules elsewhere, they may reduce in size with improved control of articular disease.

Gastrointestinal features

The gastrointestinal tract (GIT) is relatively spared in RA, though early reports by Tribe and coworkers[107] used rectal mucosal biopsies to identify vasculitis in RA patients. The most common manifestations are a consequence of drug therapy. Peptic ulcer disease may be induced by non-steroidal anti-inflammatory drugs, though the incidence has been reduced by the use of newer, cyclo-oxygenase (COX)-2 selective inhibitors[108]. It is important to note that ulcers may be asymptomatic, and a falling hemoglobin should not be attributed to the anemia of chronic disease without considering

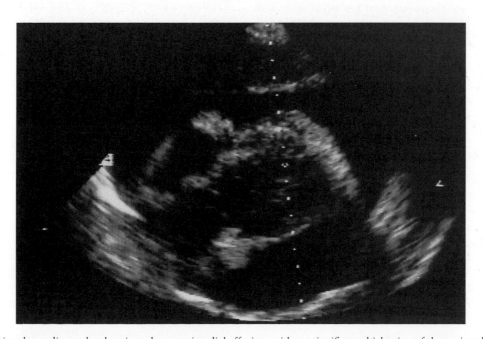

Fig. 17.4 Transthoracic echocardiography showing a large pericardial effusion, without significant thickening of the pericardium in this case.

occult bleeding from the GIT. Less commonly, ulceration may occur due to vasculitic involvement of the GIT (an uncommon feature of SRV), and rare cases of perforation due to CMV infection in the immunocompromised have been described. Aphthous ulcers may accompany any inflammatory disease, particularly during flare-up of joint activity in RA, may be a particular problem in those with sicca syndrome, and can complicate MTX therapy.

Abnormal liver function tests are not unusual in RA. Ultrasound investigation may show diffuse fatty infiltration, consistent with systemic inflammatory disease, or less commonly amyloid may be suspected, confirmed by congo-red staining of rectal or abdominal fat biopsy. However, alkaline phosphatase and gamma-glutamyl transaminase may be elevated as part of an acute phase response with stimulation of hepatocytes by interleukin-6. Methotrexate therapy is routinely monitored for changes in liver transaminases, and NSAIDs may also cause minor changes. The indications for liver biopsy are continually being revised, and it is not currently routinely recommended in patients on MTX unless there are pre-existing risk factors for hepatic cirrhosis before treatment begins, or persisting abnormalities on monitoring[109].

Renal involvement

Clinically significant renal involvement in RA is unusual, though in a clinicopathological study, 10 per cent of patients were felt to have renal failure[8]—however, this could not be attributed to RA with any certainty. Renal involvement in SRV was discussed earlier. Microalbuminuria is the most common manifestation, and may correlate with disease activity[110]. When renal biopsy was carried out in patients thought to have renal disease due to RA[111], the commonest finding (40 per cent) was mesangial glomerulonephritis (GN), especially in those with hematuria; other diagnoses in this group included amyloid and membranous GN. Amyloidosis was the commonest finding in those with nephrotic syndrome. The potential nephrotoxicity of DMARDs is well known, particularly with gold and D-penicillamine (causing proteinuria), and more recently with cyclosporin (hypertension and elevation of serum creatinine)[112,113]. Specific treatment is not usually indicated, and indeed has not been established, though patients do need supportive therapy when peripheral edema is troublesome.

Eye involvement

Keratoconjunctivitis sicca or secondary Sjögren's syndrome is the most common condition to effect the eye in RA, occurring in up to 17 per cent of patients[114]. A dry, gritty or burning sensation is caused by this exocrinopathy which reduces lacrimal gland secretion. The tear becomes hyperosmolar with continued evaporation, and this may result in damage to the cornea and conjunctiva. The condition can be confirmed by a Schirmer tear test and a lack of reflex response to nasal stimulation, and is treated symptomatically with artificial tears. Surgical occlusion of the tear ducts, and other novel therapies such as insertable sponges may be tried in resistant cases.

The differential diagnosis of a patient presenting with a red eye includes episcleritis and scleritis, and prompt evaluation and treatment is essential to avert potential loss of vision. Both these conditions are strongly associated with other systemic manifestations and nodular disease[115]. Episcleritis correlates with joint activity, may be nodular, localized, or diffuse in appearance, occurring in the zone between conjunctiva and sclera. While tender, the eye often is not painful. This form usually does not alter visual acuity, and is typically a mild, self-limiting disease; topical steroid therapy is usually sufficient. Scleritis, however, is a sight-threatening complication and presents with an acutely painful red eye, frequently associated with active vasculitis elsewhere. Both eyes are affected in 70 per cent and involvement may extend to include the optic nerve. Anterior scleritis is the most common, and when aggressive can involve the full thickness of the eye with necrosis and thinning of the scleral wall. Posterior scleritis usually occurs with anterior involvement, but is more difficult to recognize ophthalmoscopically. Isolated scleritis may respond to NSAID therapy. Treatment of severe cases requires immunosuppression[66] with high-dose intravenous methylprednisolone; cyclophosphamide being added in resistant cases or where this is otherwise indicated by active SRV elsewhere. Cyclosporin has also been used in resistant cases with good results[116].

Corneal inflammation (keratitis) may occur in isolation or as part of a generalized sclerokeratitis. The patient may report blurring of vision together with redness and pain, though discomfort may be minimal. Slit-lamp examination may reveal a marginal furrow, typically at the inferior margin of the cornea (the limbus), or more advanced changes with a white, inflammatory infiltrate and adjacent conjunctival or scleral inflammation. The cornea may gradually 'melt' centrally with perforation and subsequent loss of vision, and early treatment is therefore essential. In our experience, this feature is often associated with vasculitis. It is important to rule out infection. Treatment then depends on the extent of corneal thinning, ranging form fitting a bandage contact lens, excision of conjunctiva adjacent to the ulcer, to immunosuppressive therapy, especially if there is coexisting scleritis[67].

It is important to note that RA drug therapy can affect the eye, particularly corticosteroids causing cataracts and glaucoma, and gold compounds deposits in the cornea. The incidence of retinopathy with hydroxychloroquine has been extensively reviewed[117] and guidelines now suggest that patients taking 6.5 mg/kg lean body weight do not require routine ophthalmological assessments[118], though visual acuity should be assessed annually in the rheumatology clinic.

Neurological features

Neurological manifestations of RA occur in several distinct forms. Mononeuritis multiplex and central nervous system features including seizures, aseptic meningitis, and stroke are features of SRV discussed earlier. Diagnosis relies on imaging and examination of cerebrospinal fluid, though the findings are non-specific. Entrapment neuropathies are not uncommon, though nerve impingement by nodules or amyloid deposits is less frequent. Subluxation of the atlantoaxial joint (AAS) is found radiologically in 30 per cent of patients with severe erosive RA[119], and may produce a cervical myelopathy, though involvement at other levels may occur due to synovial hypertrophy in zygoapophyseal joints or discitis.

Carpal tunnel syndrome is the most common of the entrapment neuropathies, producing painful paresthesias in the median nerve distribution, particularly troublesome at night. Phalen's test and Tinel's sign are relatively sensitive and specific in patients with typical distribution of symptoms[120], though nerve conduction studies may be of value in less classical cases to distinguish from a peripheral neuropathy. Entrapment of the ulnar nerve (at the elbow), of the posterior tibial nerve (tarsal tunnel syndrome) or of the posterior interosseus branch of the radial nerve have been described. Treatment options include splinting, injection of the entrapment site with corticosteroid, and surgical release of the involved nerve; the latter is important where muscle atrophy is evident. However, in many cases, symptoms correlate with active synovitis, and improve with treatment directed at the joint disease.

The atlantoaxial joint relies on the integrity of the transverse ligament to prevent subluxation and resultant narrowing of the spinal canal. There is a synovial joint here, and erosive disease may destroy the ligament or effect the odontoid process itself. Cord compression may also occur with upward subluxation and basilar invagination. Radiological indices have been described[119,121] which identify significant subluxation on plain lateral radiographs of the cervical spine. Clinical features include upper motor neuron weakness, hyper-reflexia, and upgoing plantar response (positive Babinski sign). Vertebrobasilar insufficiency can occur on neck flexion, and sudden trauma may cause fatal pressure on the medulla. Management to stabilize the cervical spine includes the use of collars, and surgical fixation is required where there are pyramidal signs or intractable neck pain[122].

Musculoskeletal features

Articular RA often affects nearby structures such as bursas, tenosynovitis may occur and can be complicated by tendon rupture. True extra-articular involvement of the musculoskeletal system include osteoporosis and fractures, and muscular weakness of various etiologies.

Though recognized for over 30 years in both generalized and periarticular forms, osteoporosis secondary to RA has received little attention to date, despite the associated increased fracture risk[123]. Studies have suggested that both immobility and corticosteroid therapy are important, but recent work highlights the importance of osteoclast activation as part of the inflammatory response, and has demonstrated early and substantial loss of bone mineral density in early RA, strongly correlated with measures of disease activity, particularly CRP[124,125]. The most important therapeutic measure would appear to be control of joint disease, though specific antiresorptive treatments have been used in animal models. The importance of corticosteroid therapy in causing osteoporosis is well known and guidelines have been published[126], recommending prophylactic therapy with bisphos-

phonates, or calcium and vitamin D. It is important to note that the rate of bone loss is greatest in the first 6 months of steroid use[124]. Stress fractures can occur as a consequence of osteoporosis, and abnormal biomechanics and muscle weakness are additional risk factors.

Methotrexate osteopathy is an uncommon disorder, causing bone pain, osteoporosis, and fracture, typically in the distal tibia, mimicking ankle arthropathy. Most frequently described in children on high dose MTX, case reports are increasing of this condition in adults treated with the relatively low doses for RA[127,128]. Cyclosporin has also been associated with reduced bone mineral density though patients are frequently also taking corticosteroids[129].

Muscular weakness can be caused in a number of ways. Most commonly, patients develop disuse atrophy as a result of their joint disease, with reduction in isometric and isokinetic strength and in aerobic capacity. Neurological problems such as motor neuropathies described earlier could of course contribute to the problem of weakness and disuse atrophy. True inflammatory myopathy is rare in RA, and there are no specific features to distinguish it from myopathies seen in other systemic inflammatory disorders. Muscle enzymes are usually only slightly elevated and may be normal. Muscle biopsy is also non-specific, and may show evidence of coexisting vasculitis which may be of relevance in the etiology of this extra-articular manifestation. Corticosteroid therapy is the main iatrogenic cause of muscle atrophy, though D-penicillamine and hydroxychloroquine have rarely been implicated.

Amyloidosis

Amyloidosis results from the deposition in various organs of autologous protein in an insoluble fibrillar form. In patients with RA, excess serum amyloid A protein production is stimulated by the cytokines of the inflammatory response. TNF-α in particular has been implicated, which may open new appoaches to treatment of this complication[130]. Our experience in the past decade suggests that amyloidosis is a rare problem in clinical practice. However, post-mortem studies[8] show amyloidosis in 21 per cent and a recent study found evidence of secondary amyloid deposits in abdominal fat in 75 per cent of a selected RA population[131]. Other diagnostic methods include scintigraphy using radiolabeled serum amyloid P componant[132], and labial salivary gland biopsy[133].

In patients with symptomatic amyloidosis, many organ systems may be affected, the main clinical consequences being in restrictive heart failure and in renal involvement causing proteinuria. In these cases, the prognosis is poor, as therapeutic measures are rarely effective. However, colchicine is used in AA amyloidosis in inflammatory bowel disease, and clorambucil has been effective in amyloidosis complicating juvenile RA, where it suppresses the acute phase production of the abnormal protein[134]. Our current clinical practice is to use chlorambucil, in doses sufficient to 'control' the acute phase response, with good effect. If the acute response can be controlled adequately, this may lead to regression of amyloid with improved organ function and survival. In particular, methotrexate[135] in a small group and azathioprine[136] in a single case report have been shown to reduce or resolve proteinuria.

Summary

Systemic or extra-articular manifestations of RA, though clinically quite varied in their presentation, reflect a relatively narrow spectrum of etiopathogenetic mechanisms. The clinician needs to be aware that RA may be directly responsible for a new clinical feature, as tighter control of the active joint disease can improve extra-articular symptoms. However, specific therapies are sometimes necessary.

References

1. Leigh J.P., Fries J.F. Mortality predictors among 263 patients with rheumatoid arthritis. *J Rheumatol*, 1991;**18**:1307–12.
2. Bacon P.A. Extra-articular rheumatoid disease. In: (McCarty D.J., Koopman W.J. eds.) *Arthritis and allied conditions*. Philadelphia: Lee and Febiger, 1993;811–38.
3. Roubenoff R., Roubenoff R., Ward L., Holland S., Hellman D. Rheumatoid cachexia; depletion of lean body mass in rheumatoid arthritis. Possible association with tumor necrosis factor. *J Rheumatol*, 1992;**19**:1505–10.
4. Scott D.G.I., Bacon P.A., Tribe C.R. Systemic rheumatoid vasculitis: a clinical and laboratory study of 50 cases. *Medicine (Baltimore)*, 1981;**60**:288–97.
5. Hailwood S.J., Barrett E.M., Symmons D.P.M., Scott D.G.I., (The Norfolk Arthritis Register). Extra-articular features of early rheumatoid arthritis in a community based population (abstract). *Br J Rheumatol*, 1998;**37** (suppl 1): 102.
6. Gabbay E., Tarala R., Will R., Carroll G., Adler B., Cameron D., Lake F.R. Interstitial lung disease in recent onset rheumatoid arthritis. *Am J Crit Care Med*, 1997;**156**:528–35.
7. Toyosima P., Kusaba T., Yamaguchi T. Cause of death in autopsied rheumatoid arthritis patients. *Ryumachi* 1993;**33**:209–14.
8. Suzuki A., Ohosone Y., Obana M., *et al*. Cause of death in 81 autopsied patients with RA. *J Rheumatol*, 1994;**21**:33–6.
9. Westedt M.L., Breedveld F.C., Schreuder G.M. *et al*. Immunogenetic heterogeneity of rheumatoid arthritis. *Ann Rheum Dis*, 1986;**45**:534–8.
10. Hillarby M.C., Hopkins J., Greenan D.M. A re-analysis of the association between rheumatoid arthritis with and without extra-articular features, HLA-DR4, and DR4 subtypes. *Tissue Antigens*, 1991;**37**:39–41.
11. Weyand C.M., Xie C., Goronzy J.J. Homozygosity for the HLA-DRB1 allele selects for extraarticular manifestations of rheumatoid arthritis. *J Clin Invest*, 1992;**89**:2033–9.
12. Zanelli E., Gonzalez-Gay M.A., David C.S. Could HLA-DRB1 be the protective locus for rheumatoid arthritis? *Immunol Today*, 1995;**16**:274–8.
13. Allen C., Elson C.J., Scott D.G.I., *et al*. IgG antiglobulins in rheumatoid arthritis and other arthritides: relationship with clinical features and other parameters. *Ann Rheum Dis*, 1981;**40**:127–31.
14. Bacon P.A., Carruthers D.M. Vasculitis associated with connective tissue disorders. *Rheum Dis Clin North Am*, 1995;**21**:1077–96.
15. Scott D.G.I., Bacon P.A., Allen C., Elson J., Wallington T. IgG rheumatoid factor, complement and immune complexes in rheumatoid vasculitis; comparative and serial studies during cytotoxic therapy. *Clin Exp Immunol*, 1981;**43**:54–63.
16. Snowdon N., Kay R.A. Immunology of systemic rheumatoid disease. *Br Med Bull*, 1995;**51**:437–48.
17. Braun M.G., Csernok E., Schmitt W.H., Gross W.L. Incidence, target antigens and clinical implications of antineutrophil cytoplasmic antibodies in rheumatoid arthritis. *J Rheumatol*, 1996;**23**:826–30.
18. Brimnes J., Hlaberg P., Jacobsen S., Wiik A., Heegard N.H.H. Specificities of antineutrophil autoantibodies in patients with rheumatoid arthritis. *Clin Exp Immunol*, 1997;**110**:250–6.
19. Coremans I.E.M., Hagen E.C., Daha M.R., *et al*. Antilactoferrin antibodies in patients with rheumatoid arthritis are associated with vasculitis. *Arthritis Rheum*, 1992;**35**:1466–75.
20. Cambridge G., Williams M., Leaker B., *et al*. Anti-MPO antibodies in patients with rheumatoid arthritis: prevalence, clinical correlates and IgG subclass. *Ann Rheum Dis*, 1994;**53**:24–9.
21. Mathieson P.W., Peat D.S., Short A., Watts R.A. Coexistent membranous nephropathy and ANCA-positive crescentic glomerulonephritis in association with penicillamine. *Nephrology Dialysis and Transplantation*, 1996;**11**:863–6.
22. Ziff M. The rheumatoid nodule. *Arthritis Rheum*, 1990;**33**:761–7.
23. Miyasaka N., Sato K., Yamamoto K., Goto M., Nishioka K. Immunological and immunohistochemical analysis of rheumatoid nodules. *Ann Rheum Dis*, 1989;**48**:220–6.
24. Hedfors E., Klareskog L., Lindblad S., Forsum U., Lindahl G. Phenotypic characterisation of cells within subcutaneous rheumatoid nodules. *Arthritis Rheum*, 1983;**26**:1333–9.
25. Palmer D.G., Hogg N., Highton J., Heissian P.A., Denholm I. Macrophage migration and maturation within rheumatoid nodules. *Arthritis Rheum*, 1987;**30**:729–36.
26. De Keyser F., Benoit D., Elewaut D., *et al*. T cell receptor expression in patients with rheumatic diseases. *Progr Histochem Cytochem*, 1992;**26**:218–22.
27. De Keyser F., Verbruggen G., Veys E.M., *et al*. T cell receptor Vβ usage in rheumatoid nodules: marked oligoclonality among IL-2 expanded lymphocytes. *Clin Immunol Immunopathol*, 1993;**68**:29–34.
28. DeKeyser F., Elewaut D., Overmeer-Graus J.P.M., *et al*. Dominant T cell receptor, rearrangements in interleukin 2 expanded lymphocytes from rheumatoid nodules suggest antigen driven T cell activation in situ. *J Rheumatol*, 1997;**24**:1685–9.
29. Edwards J.C.W., Wilkinson L.S., Pitsillides A.A. Palisading cells of rheumatoid nodules: comparison with synovial intimal cells. *Ann Rheum Dis*, 1993;**52**:801–5.
30. Vreugdenhil G., Swaak A.J. Anaemia in rheumatoid arthritis; pathogenesis, diagnosis and treatment. *Rheumatol Int*, 1990;**9**:243–57.
31. Peeters H.R., Jongen-Lavrencic M., Vreugdenhil G., Swaak A.J. Effect of recombinant human erythropoietin on anaemia and disease activity in patients with rheumatoid arthritis and anaemia of chronic disease; a randomised placebo controlled double blind 52 week clinical trial. *Ann Rheum Dis*, 1996;**55**:739–44.
32. Robertson M.D.J., Dudley Hart F., White W.F., Nuki G., Boardman P.L. Rheumatoid lymphadenopathy. *Ann Rheum Dis*, 1968;**27**:253.
33. Kelly C.A., Malcolm A.J., Griffiths I. Lymphadenopathy in rheumatic diseases. *Ann Rheum Dis*, 1987;**46**:224–7.
34. Kassan S.S., Chused T.L., Moutsopoulos H.M., *et al*. Increased risk of lymphoma in sicca syndrome. *Ann Int Med*, 1978;**89**:888–92.
35. Georgescu L., Quinn G.C., Schwartzman S., Paget S.A. Lymphoma in patients with rheumatoid arthritis: association with the disease state or methotrexate treatment. *Sem Arthritis Rheum*, 1997;**26**:794–804.
36. Felty A.R. Chronic arthritis in the adult associated with splenomegaly and leukopoenia. *Bulletins of Johns Hopkins Hospital*, 1924;**35**:16–20.
37. Rosenstein E.D., Kramer N. Felty's syndrome and pseudo-Felty's syndrome. *Sem Arthritis Rheum*, 1991;**21**:129–42.

38. Campion G., Maddison P.J., Goulding N., James I., Ahern M.J., Watt I., Sansom D. The Felty syndrome: a case-matched study of clinical manifestations and outcome, serological features and immunogenetic associations. *Medicine (Baltimore)*, 1990;**69**:69–80.

39. Gridley G., Klippel J.H., Hoover R.N., Fraumeni J.F. Jr. Incidence of cancer among men with the Felty syndrome. *Ann Int Med*, 1994;**120**:35–9.

40. Aboud N.I. Heterogeneity of bone-marrow directed immune mechanisms in the pathogenesis of the neutropoenia of Felty's Syndrome. *Arthritis Rheum*, 1983;**26**:947–53.

41. Breedveld F.C., Lafeber G.J.M., de Vries E., van Krieken J.H.J.M., Cats A. Immune complexes and the pathogenesis of neutropoenia in Felty's Syndrome. *Ann Rheum Dis*, 1986;**45**:696–702.

42. Barton J.C., Prasthofer E.F., Egan M.L. Rheumatoid arthritis associated with expanded populations of granular lymphocytes. *Ann Int Med*, 1986;**104**:314–23.

43. Dhodapkar M.V., Li C.Y., Lust J.A., *et al.* Clinical spectrum of clonal proliferations of t-large granular lymphocytes: a T-cell clonopathy of undetermined significance? *Blood*, 1994;**84**:1620–7.

44. Sibley J.T., Haga M., Visram D.A., Mitchell D.M. The clinical course of Felty's Syndrome compared to matched controls. *J Rheumatol*, 1991;**18**:1163–7.

45. Rashba E.J., Rowe J.M., Packman C.H. Treatment of the neutropoenia of Felty Syndrome *Blood Rev*, 1996;**10**:177–84.

46. Starkebaum G. Use of colony-stimulating factors in the treatment of neutropoenia associated with collagen vascular disease. *Current Opinion Haematol*, 1997;**4**:196–9.

47. Working Party of the British Committee for Standards in Haematology Clinical Task Force. Guidelines for the prevention and treatment of infection in patients with an absent or dysfunctional spleen. *Br Med J*. 1996;**312**:430–4.

48. Bannatyne G.A. In: *Rheumatoid Arthritis*, 2nd Edn. John Wright. Bristol, 1898. p. 73.

49. Bywaters E.G.L. A variant of rheumatoid arthritis characterized by digital pad nodules and palmar fasciitis, closely resembling palidromic rheumatism. *Ann Rheum Dis*, 1949;**8**:2–30.

50. Bywaters E.G.L. Peripheral vascular obstruction in rheumatoid arthritis and its relationships to other vascular lesions. *Ann Rheum Dis*, 1957;**16**:84–103.

51. Watts R.A., Carruthers D.M., Symmons D.P.M., Scott D.G.I. The epidemiology of systemic rheumatoid vasculitis in the United Kingdom. *Br J Rheumatol*, 1994;**33**:832–3.

52. Wilkinson D.S. Rheumatoid vasculitis. In: Wolff K. and Winkelman R.K. eds. *Vasculitis* 1980. London, Lloyd Luke. pp. 188–92.

53. Boers M., Croonen A.M., Dijmans B.A.C., *et al.* Renal biopsy findings in rheumatoid arthritis: Clinical aspects of 132 necropsies. *Ann Rheum Dis*, 1987;**46**:658–63.

54. Cruikshank B. Heart lesions in rheumatoid disease. *J Pathol Bacteriol*, 1957;**76**:223–40.

55. Kemper J.W., Baggenstross A.H., Slocumbe C.H. The relationship of therapy with cortisone to the incidence of vascular lesions in rheumatoid arthritis. *Ann Intern Med*, 1957;**46**:831–35.

56. Luqmani R.A., Watts R.A., Scott D.G.I., Bacon P.A. Treatment of vasculitis in rheumatoid arthritis. *Ann Int Med*, 1994;**145**:566–76.

57. Voskuyl A.E., Zwinderman A.H., Westedt M.L., Vandenbrouke J.P., Breedveld F.C., Hazes J.M.W. Factors associated with the development of vasculitis in rheumatoid arthritis: results of a case-control study. *Ann Rheum Dis*, 1996;**55**:190–2.

58. Scott D.G.I., Bacon P.A. Intravenous cyclophosphamide plus methyl prednisolone in the treatment of systemic rheumatoid vasculitis. *Am J Med*, 1984;**76**:377–84.

59. Dequeker J., Rosberg G. Digital capillaritis in rheumatoid arthritis. *Acta Rheumatol Scand*, 1967;**13**:299–307.

60. Golding J.R., Hamilton M.G., Gill R.S. Arteritis of rheumatoid arthritis. *Brit J Derm*, 1964;**77**:207–210.

61. Westdet M.L., Meijer C.J.L., Vermmer B.L., Cats A., de Vries E. Rheumatoid arthritis – the clinical significance of histo and immunopathological abnormalities in normal skin. *J Rheumatol*, 1984;**11**:448–53.

62. Fitzgerald O.M., Barnes L., Woods R., McHugh L., Barry C., O'Louglin S. Direct immunofluorescence of normal skin in rheumatoid arthritis. *Br J Rheumatol*, 1985;**24**:340–5.

63. Bywaters E.G.L., Scott J.T. The natural history of vascular lesions in rheumatoid arthritis. *J Chron Dis*, 1963;**16**:905–914.

64. Watts R.A., Carruthers D.C., Scott D.G.I. Isolated nailfold vasculitis in RA. *Ann Rheum Dis*, 1995;**54**:927–9.

65. McRorie E.R., Jobanputra P., Ruckley C.V., Nuki G. Leg ulceration in rheumatoid arthritis. *Br J Rheumatol*, 1994;**33**:1078–84.

66. Lebowitz W.B. The heart in rheumatoid disease. *Geriatrics*, 1996;**21**:194–8.

67. Foster C.S., Forstot S.L., Wilson L.A. Mortality rate in rheumatoid arthritis patients developing necrotising scleritis or peripheral ulcerative keratitis. Effects of systemic immunosuppression. *Ophthalmology*, 1984;**91**:1253–62.

68. Giordano N., D'Ettorre M., Giasi G., Fioravanti A., Moretti L., Marcolongon R. Retinal vasculitis in rheumatoid arthritis: an agngiographic study. *Clin Exp Rheumatol*, 1990;**8**:121–5.

69. Harper L., Cockwell P., Howie A.J., *et al.* Focal segmental necrotising glomerulnephritis in rheumatoid arthritis. *Q J Med*, 1997;**90**:125–32.

70. Puéchal X., Said G., Hilliquin P., *et al.* Peripheral neuropathy with necrotising vasculitis in rheumatoid arthritis. *Arthritis Rheum*, 1995;**38**:1618–29.

71. Flipo R.M., Cardon T., Copin M.C., Vandecandelaere M., Duquesnoy B., Janin A. ICAM-1, E-selectin, and TNFα expression in labial salivary glands of patients with rheumatoid vasculitis. *Ann Rheum Dis*, 1997;**56**:41–4.

72. Woolf A.D., Wakerly G., Wallington T.B., Scott D.G.I., Dieppe P.A. Factor VIII related antigen in the assessment of vasculitis. *Ann Rheum Dis*, 1987;**46**:441–7.

73. Vollertsen R.S., Conn D.L., Ballard D.J., Ilstrup D.M., Kazmar R.E., Silverfield J.C. Rheumatoid vasculitis: survival and associated risk factors. *Medicine*, 1986;**65**:365–75.

74. Heurkins A.H.M., Westedt M.L., Breedfeld F.C. Prednisolone plus azathioprine treatment in patients with rheumatoid arthritis complicated by vasculitis. *Arch Intern Med*, 1991;**15**:2249–54.

75. Nicholls A., Snaith M.L., Maini R.N., Scott J.T. Controlled trial of azathioprine in rheumatoid vasculitis. *Ann Rheum Dis*, 197332:589–91.

76. Adu D., Pall A., Luqmani R.A., *et al.* Controlled trial of pulse versus continuous cyclophosphamide in the treatment of systemic vasculitis. *Q J Med*, 199790:401–9.

77. Kaye O, Beckers C.C., Paquet P, Arrese J.E., Piérard G.E., Malaise M.G. The frequency of cutaneous vasculitis is not increased in patients with rheumatoid arthritis treated with methotrexate. *J Rheumatol*, 1996;**23**:253–7.

78. Espinoza L.R., Espinoza C.G., Vasey F.B., Germain B.F. Oral methotrexate therapy for chronic rheumatoid arthritis ulcerations. *J Am Acad Dermatol*, 1986;**15**:508–12.

79. Scott D.G.I., Bacon P.A., Bothamley J.E., Allen C., Elson C.L., Wallington T.B., Plasma exchange in rheumatoid vasculitis. *J Rheumatol*, 1998;**8**:433–9.

80. Jayne D.R.W., Lockwood C.M. Intravenous immunoglobulin as sole therapy for systemic vasculitis. *Br J Rheum*, 1996;**35**:1150–33.

81. Voskuyl A.E., Zwinderman A.H., Westedt Ml., Vandenbrouke J.P., Breedveld F.C., Hazes J.M.W. The mortality of rheumatoid vasculitis compared with rheumatoid arthritis. *Arthritis Rheum*, 1996;**39**:266–71.

82. Cudkowicz L., Madof I.M., Abelmann W.H. Rheumatoid lung disease. *Br J Dis Chest*, 1961;**55**:35–9.

83. Banks, J., Banks, C., Cheong B., An epidemiological and clinical investigation of pulmonary function and respiratory symptoms in patients with rheumatoids arthritis. *Quart J Med*, 1992;**85**:795–806.

84. Shannon T.M., Gale E. Non-cardiac manifestations of rheumatoid arthritis in the thorax: *J Thoracic Imaging*, 1992;**7**:19–29.

85. Mc Donagh J., Concaves M., Wright A.R., *et al.* High resolution computed tomography of the lungs in patients with RA and interstitial lung disease. *Br J Rheumatol*, 1994;32:118–22.

86. Vergnenegre A., Pugnere N., Antonini M.T., Arnaud M., Melloni B., Treves R., Bonnaud F. Airway obstruction and rheumatoid arthritis. *Europ Respir J*, 1997;10:1072–8.

87. Shiel W.C., Prete P.E. Pleuro-pulmonary manifestations of rheumatoid arthritis. *Sem Arthritis Rheum*, 1984;13:235–43.

88. Zufferey P., Ruzicka J., Gerster J.C. Pleural fluid cytology as an indicator of an effusion of rheumatoid origin. *J Rheum*, 1993;20:1449–51.

89. Kelly C.A. Rheumatoid arthritis: classical lung disease. *Bailliere's Clinical Rheumatol*, 1993;7:1–16.

90. Hyland R.H., Duncan A.G., Broder I., *et al.* A systematic study of pulmonary abnormalities in rheumatoid arthritis. *J Rheum*, 1983;10:395–405.

91. McCune W.J., Vallance D.K., Lynch J.P. III. Immunosuppressive drug therapy. *Current Opinion Rheumatol*, 1994;6:262–72.

92. Hakala M. Poor prognosis in patients with rheumatoid arthritis hospitalized for interstitial lung fibrosis. *Chest*, 1988;93:114–8.

93. Geddes D.M., Corrin B., Brewerton D.A., Davies R.J., Turner-Warwick M. Progressive airway obliteration in adults and its association with rheumatoid disease. *Quart J Med*, 1997;66:427–44.

94. Anaya J.M., Diethelm L., Ortiz L.A., Gutierrez M., Citera G., Welsh R.A., Espinoza L.R. Pulmonary involvement in rheumatoid arthritis. *Sem Arthritis Rheum*, 1995;24:242–54.

95. Hassan W.U., Keaney N.P., Kelly C.A. High resolution computed tomography of the lung in lifelong non-smoking patients with rheumatoid arthritis. *Ann Rheum Dis*, 1995;54:308–10.

96. Bamji A., Cooke N. Rheumatoid arthritis and chronic bronchitic suppuration. *Scand J Rheumatol*, 1985;14:15–21.

97. Kremer J.M., Alarcon G.S., Weinblatt M.E., *et al.* Clinical, laboratory, radiographic and histopathologic features of methotrexate-associated lung injury in patients with rheumatoid arthritis. *Arthritis Rheum*, 1997;40:1829–37.

98. Dawson T., Ryan P.F.J., Findeisen J.M., Scheinkestel C.D. Pneumocystis carinii pneumonia following cyclosporin A and methotrexate treated rheumatoid arthritis. *J Rheumatol*, 1992;19:997.

99. Slenger A.A., Houtman P.M., Bruyn G.A., Eggink H.F., Pasma H.R., Pneumocystis carinii pneumonia associated with low dose methotrexate therapy for rheumatoid arthritis. *Scand J Rheumatol*, 1984;23:51–3.

100. Prior P., Symmons D.P.M., Scott D.L., Brown R., Hawkins C.F. Cause of death in rheumatoid arthritis. *Br J Rheumatol*, 1984;23:92–9.

101. Scott D.G.I., Bacon P.A. Cardiac involvement in immunological diseases. *Bailliere's Clinical Immunol Allergy*, 1987;1:537–575.

102. Isner J.M., Carter B.L., Bankoff M.S., Konstan M.A., Salen D.N. Computed tomography in the diagnosis of pericardial heart disease. *Ann Int Med*, 1982;80:453–8.

103. Carrao S., Salli L., Arnone S., Scaglione R., Pinto A., Licata G. Cardiac involvement in RA: evidence of silent heart disease. *Europ Heart J*, 1995;16:253–6.

104. Iveson J.M.I., Pomerance A. Cardiac involvement in rheumatoid disease. *Clinics Rheum Dis*, 1977;3:467–500.

105. Carrao S., Salli L., Arnone S., Scaglione R., Pinto A., Licata G. Echo-Doppler left ventricular filling abnormalities in patients with rheumatoid arthritis without clinically evident cardiovascular disease. *Europ J Clinical Invest*, 1996;26:293–7.

106. Mounet F.S., Soula P., Concina P., Cerene A. A rare case of embolizing cardiac tumor: rheumatoid nodule of the mitral valve. *J Heart Valve Dis*, 1997;6:77–8.

107. Tribe C.R., Scott D.G., Bacon P.A. Rectal biopsy in the diagnosis of systemic vasculitis. *J Clin Pathol*, 1981;34:843–50.

108. Vane J.R. NSAIDs, Cox-2 inhibitors and the gut. *Lancet*, 1995;346:1105–6.

109. Kremer J.M., Alarcon G.S., Lightfoot R.W. Jr., Willkens R.F., Furst D.E., Williams H.J., Dent P.B., Weinblatt M.E. Methotrexate for rheumatoid arthritis. Suggested guidelines for monitoring liver toxicity. The American College of Rheumatology. *Arthritis Rheum*, 1994;37:316–28.

110. Pedersen L.M., Nordin H., Svensson B., Bliddal H. Microalbuminuria in patients with RA. *Ann Rheum Dis*, 1995;54:189–92.

111. Helin H.J., Korpela M.M., Mustonen J.T., Pasternack A.I. Renal biopsy findings and clinicopathologic correlations in RA. *Arthritis Rheum*, 1995;38:242–7.

112. Rodriguez F., Kraenbuhl J.C., Harrison W.B., Forre O., Dijkmans B.A., Tugwell P., Miescher P.A., Mihatsch M.J. Renal biopsy findings and follow-up of renal function in rheumatoid arthritis patients treated with Cyclosporin A. An update from the International Kidney Biopsy Registry. *Arthritis Rheum*, 1996;39:1491–8.

113. Landewe R.B., Dijkmans B.A., van der Woude F.J., Breedveld F.C., Mihatsch M.J., Bruijn J.A. Long-term low dose cyclosporin in patients with rheumatoid arthritis: renal function loss without structural nephropathy. *J Rheumatol*, 1996;23:61–4.

114. Matsuo T., Kono R., Matsuo N., Ezawa K., Natsumeda M., Soda K., Ezawa H. Incidence of ocular complications in rheumatoid arthritis and the relation of keratoconjunctivits sicca to its systemic activity. *Scand J Rheumatol*, 1997;26:113–6.

115. Jayson M.I.V., Jones D.E.P. Scleritis and rheumatoid arthritis. *Ann Rheum Dis*, 1971;30:343–7.

116. McCarthy J.M., Dubord P.J., Chalmers A., Kassen B.O., Rangno K.K. Cyclosporine A for the treatment of necrotizing scleritis and corneal melting in patients with rheumatoid arthritis. *J Rheumatol*, 1992;19:1358–61.

117. Silman A., Shipley M. Ophthalmological monitoring for hydroxychloroquine toxicity: a scientific review of the available data. *Br J Rheumatol*, 1997;36:599–601.

118. Fielder A., Graham E., Jones S., Silman A., Tullo A. *Ocular toxicity and hydroxychloroquine: guidelines for screening*. The Royal College of Ophthalmologists, 1998.

119. Winfield J., Young A., Williams P., *et al.* A prospective study of the radiological changes in the cervical spine in early rheumatoid disease. *Ann Rheum Dis*, 1981;40:109–14.

120. Katz J.N., Larson M.G., Sabra A., Krarup C., Stirrat C.R., Sethi R., Eaton H.M., Fossel A.H., Liang M.H. The carpal tunnel syndrome: diagnostic utility of the history and physical examination findings. *Ann Int Med*, 1990;112:321–7.

121. Redlund-Johnell I. Posterior atlanto-axial dislocation in rheumatoid arthritis. *Scand J Rheumatol*, 1984;13:337–41.

122. Crockard H.A. Surgical management of cervical rheumatoid problems. *Spine*, 1995;20:2584–90.

123. Cooper C., Coupland M., Mitchell M. Rheumatoid arthritis, corticosteroid therapy and hip fracture. *Ann Rheum Dis*, 1995;54:49–52.

124. Gough A.K.S., Lilley J., Eyre S., Holder R.L. Emery P. Generalised bone loss in patients with early rheumatoid arthritis. *Lancet*, 1994;344:23–7.

125. Gough A., Sambrook P., Devlin J., Huissoon A., Njeh C., Robbins S., Nguyen T., Emery P. Osteoclastic activation is the principal mechanism leading to secondary osteoporosis in rheumatoid arthritis. *J Rheumatol*, 1998;25:1282–9.

126. Eastel R. Management of corticosteroid-induced osteoporosis. *J Int Med*, 1995;237:439–47.

127. Preston S.J., Diamond T., Scott A., Laurent M.R. Methotrexate osteopathy in rheumatic disease. *Ann Rheum Dis*, 1993;52:582–5.

128. Zonneveld I.M., Bakker W.K., Dijkstra P.F., Bos J.D., van Soesberg R.M., Dinant H.J. Methotrexate osteopathy in long-term, low-dose methotrexate treatment for psoriasis and rheumatoid arthritis. *Arch Dermatol*, 1996;132:184–7.

129. Thiebaud D., Krieg M.A., Gillard-Berguer D., Jacquet A.F., Goy J.J., Burckhardt P. Cyclosporin induces high bone turnover and may contribute to bone loss after heart transplantation. *Europ Clin Invest*, 1996;26:549–55.

130. Maini R., Brennan F.M., Williams R., Chu C.Q., Cope A.P., Gibbons D., Elliot M., Feldmann M. TNF-alpha in rheumatoid arthritis and prospects of anti-TNF therapy. *Clin Exp Rheumatol*, 1993;11 (Suppl 8):s173–5.

131. Barile L., Ariza R., Muci H., Pizarro S., Fraga H., Lavalle C., Garcia R., Lescano D., Barrios R., Frati A. Tru-cut needle biopsy of subcutaneous fat in the diagnosis of secondary amyloidosis in rheumatoid arthritis. *Arch Med Research*, 1993;**24**:189–92.

132. Hawkins P.N., Richardson S., Viguskin D.M., David J., Kelsey C.R., Gray R.E., Hall M.A., Woo P., Lavener J.P., Pepys M.B. Serum amyloid P componant scintigraphy and turnover studies for diagnosis and quantitative monitoring of AA amyloid in juvenile rheumatoid arthritis. *Arthritis Rheum*, 1993;**36**:842–51.

133. Hachulla E., Janin A., Flipo R.M., Saile R., Facon T., Bataille D., Vanhille P., Hatron P.Y., Devulder B., Duquesnoy B. Labial salivary gland biopsy is a reliable test for the diagnosis of primary and secondary amyloidosis. A prospective clinical and immunohistological study in 59 patients. *Arthritis Rheum*, 1993;**36**:691–7.

134. Gertz M.A., Kyle R.A. Amyloidosis: prognosis and treatment. *Sem Arthritis Rheum*, 1994;**24**:124–38.

135. Fiter J., Nolla J.M., Valverde J., Roig-Escofet D. Methotrexate treatment of amyloidosis secondary to rheumatoid arthritis. *Revue Clinicale Espana*, 1995;**195**:390–2.

136. Shapiro D.L., Spiera H. Regression of the nephrotic syndrome in rheumatoid arthritis and amyloidosis therapy with azothioprine. A case report. *Arthritis Rheum*, 1995;**38**:1851–4.

18 | The neuroendocrine axis in rheumatoid arthritis

Ronald L. Wilder and Ilia J. Elenkov

Introduction

Multiple lines of evidence support the view that the neuroendocrine axis is involved in regulating the expression of rheumatoid arthritis (RA)[1–9]. For example neuroendocrine factors related to age, gender, reproductive status, psychosocioeconomic conditions, and so on have well-recognized associations with both the onset and progression of RA. Animal model data also strongly indicate that neuroendocrine factors play a major role in regulating disease expression[1,3]. Although an understanding of the mechanisms underlying these effects is clearly incomplete, evolving concepts of this important, but controversial, topic will be discussed. A major theme of the discussion is that deficiencies in gonadal and sympathoadrenal hormonal mediator output are important factors in the onset and progression of RA. To provide perspective for the discussion of these concepts, comparisons of RA with other autoimmune diseases, particularly systemic lupus erythematosus (SLE), will also be briefly discussed. A comparison between SLE and RA is of interest because these illnesses appear to be dependent upon different, and apparently antagonistic, cytokines. Current evidence suggests that RA is driven by excessive and sustained production of proinflammatory cytokines, such as tumor necrosis factor alpha (TNF-α) and interleukin-12 (IL-12). Excessive production of these two cytokines is typically accompanied by excessive production of interleukin-1 (IL-1) and interleukin-6 (IL-6). Production of the anti-inflammatory cytokine, interleukin-10 (IL-10), an anti-inflammatory cytokine that antagonizes the effects of TNF-α, IL-1, and IL-12, appears to be deficient in RA patients[10,11]. SLE disease activity, in contrast to RA, is associated with excessive production of IL-10, which appears to drive B-cell-dependent humoral immunopathology. TNF-α and IL-12 production appear deficient in SLE[12–16]. Bidirectional interactions between these cytokines and the neuroendocrine axis appear to play a central role in the modulation of RA and SLE disease activity[1,5]. These concepts will also be briefly discussed.

Age, gender, reproductive status, and RA

RA, like most autoimmune diseases, is much more prevalent and more severe in females than males (3–4.1) overall, but, as shown

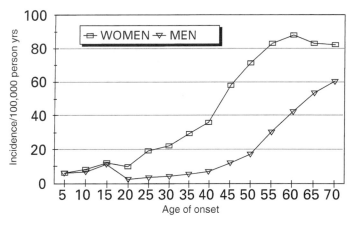

Fig. 18.1 Age of onset of rheumatoid arthritis. Modified from Ref. 17.

in Fig. 18.1, the female:male disparity is much more pronounced in the child-bearing years[17,18]. The risk of RA onset in women increases steadily from about age 5 until it reaches a peak around the perimenopause/menopause. In fact, RA in postmenopausal women is associated with accelerated bone resorption, compared to RA in premenopausal women[19]. RA is, however, uncommon in men under the age of 45, but risk increases markedly in older age groups and approaches female onset incidence rates[17]. In other words, risk of developing RA, for both males and females, increases as a function of age, but risk for females greatly exceeds risk for males during the reproductive years. These data suggest that factors regulating female versus male susceptibility differences are mechanistically linked to aging and reproductive function. As shown in Table 18.1, decreased production of both adrenal and gonadal steroid hormones, including estrogen, progesterone, testosterone,

Table 18.1 Changes in steroid hormone production rates at menopause

	Reproductive age (mg/day)	Postmenopausal (mg/day)
Estrogen	0.35	0.045
Testosterone	0.2–0.25	0.05–0.1
DHEA	6–8	1.5–4
DHEAS	8–16	4–9
Androstenedione	2–3	0.5–1

Data from Rannevik *et al.* Ref. 20.

DHEA, DHEAS, and androstenedione, is well documented at menopause[20]. Each of these adrenal and gonadal hormones warrants consideration for a role in triggering the onset and/or accelerating the progression of RA.

Estrogen deserves attention, particularly in women, because of its well-documented effects on preventing osteoporosis and inhibiting TNF-α, IL-1-, and interleukin-6 (IL-6)-stimulated, osteoclast-mediated bone resorption[21–26]. These processes are important components of the pathogenesis of RA[26,27]. Androgens, such as DHEA, DHEAS, testosterone, may be particularly important, in both men and women with RA, because low androgen levels, inversely correlating with disease severity, have been repeatedly demonstrated[7,17,21]. Moreover, arthritis animal model data, particularly rat models, strongly indicate that androgens influence susceptibility and disease severity. Male rats, in some models, tend to be much more susceptible than females, and castration eliminates the relative resistance to disease in males[3]. In male RA patients, testosterone levels are low in comparison to age-matched controls, and, more striking, in comparison to males less than age 45[28]. Furthermore, a preliminary study indicated that treatment of male RA patients with testosterone supplementation decreased disease activity[29]. One follow-up study in male RA patients, however, failed to demonstrate an effect on disease activity[30]. Another study, in which testosterone was given to postmenopausal women with RA demonstrated modest benefit[31]. More recently, data were published suggesting that the disease-ameliorating effects of cyclosporin A are mediated, in part, by increasing peripheral androgen levels[32]. Thus, the therapeutic value of testosterone replacement therapy in males remains inadequately studied. The available data, however, suggest that the disease-suppressive effects of testosterone therapy alone in established disease are probably modest and 'slow acting'. Since it is unlikely that testosterone mediates its effects through suppressing acute inflammation processes, therapeutic studies on testosterone replacement should probably be focused on the long-term effects on bone and osteoclastic activity.

The subject of DHEA in RA is more controversial than testosterone[1] because it is not clear whether DHEA itself, or a metabolite, is the active androgenic mediator. Nevertheless, DHEA production, a hormone produced predominantly by the adrenal gland, is subject to pronounced age-related variation. In both males and females, DHEA production reaches a peak in the third decade and then progressively declines. At ages of 45–55, its production levels are less than 50 per cent of its peak production[33,34]. Interestingly, plasma levels of DHEA/DHEAS and IL-6 are inversely correlated in both normal and diseased subjects, and DHEA suppresses IL-6 production from peripheral blood mononuclear cells[26,35]. These data suggest that immunosenescence and endocrinosenescence are functionally linked. Thus, the ages of peak onset of RA are associated with precipitous declines in adrenal DHEA and DHEAS production and increasing production of IL-6. Intriguing additional support for the hypothesis that declining DHEA levels are a factor in RA onset is provided by the observation that subnormal plasma DHEA levels were detected in a prospective study of healthy subjects 4–18 years before they developed clinically apparent RA,[17,28,34]. In other words, low DHEA levels may

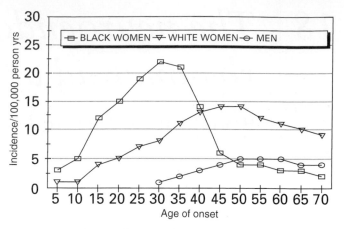

Fig. 18.2   Age of onset of systemic lupus (SLE).

precede the development of disease, rather than being a consequence of disease. There are no reports, however, demonstrating that DHEA replacement therapy affects disease activity. In fact, a recent open study of 13 patients with RA treated for 16 weeks did not show benefit in standard clinical activity measures[36]. If DHEA therapy has disease inhibitory effects, it seems likely that long-term studies focused on osteoclasts and IL-6-mediated bone resorption are required. In summary, the available data are consistent with the view that immune and endocrine functions are linked, but the mechanisms are complex. The putative role of androgens, such as testosterone, DHEA, and DHEAS, to the onset and progression of RA has been reviewed extensively in recent publications[7,34].

Onset of SLE, like RA, varies as a function of age, but similarities and notable differences from RA are apparent (Fig. 18.2). Like RA, males, of all races, are unlikely to develop SLE at ages less than 35, but the onset incidence increases modestly in older age groups. Thus, male gender, or the inheritance of a Y chromosome, reduces SLE risk, but the relative protection provided by male gender declines with advancing age. These data suggest that androgens, at levels produced during the reproductive years, diminish the risk of SLE, as they also appear to do in RA. Risk associated with female gender, in contrast, differs for RA and SLE. Although female:male prevalence disparity in SLE is even greater than in RA (about 9:1), the risk of onset is highest in females, particularly black females, during the child-bearing years. In fact, risk of disease onset in females declines in older age groups (Fig. 18.2). The SLE age–onset risk profile, in contrast to RA, suggests that hormones crucial to female reproductive functions, particularly estrogen, increase risk. Interestingly, abnormalities in estrogen metabolism, which may potentiate their effects, have been described in SLE patients[37–42]. Androgens, in contrast to estrogens, appear to suppress SLE disease activity. In other words, estrogens and androgens, unlike RA, appear to exert opposite effects in determining the onset and activity of SLE. Available data suggest that these differences may, in part, be mediated by estrogenic effects on B cell antibody production. Estrogens appear to enhance humoral immunity, and testosterone appears to have no effect[1,3]. These issues will be discussed further in the following sections.

Pregnancy, the postpartum period and RA risk

Pregnancy and the postpartum period provide compelling indications that RA susceptibility and progression are influenced by neuroendocrine factors[1,5,6,43–50]. It has been recognized for decades that RA frequently goes into remission or substantially improves during pregnancy, particularly in the third trimester. Moreover, the risk of developing new-onset RA during pregnancy, compared to other periods, is decreased by about 70 per cent. In contrast, risk of onset of RA is markedly increased in the postpartum period, particularly in the first 3 months (odds ratio of 5.6). The risk tends to be greatest after the first pregnancy (odds ratio of 10.8). Nulliparity is also associated with increased risk of RA[51–53]. Thus, current pregnancy reduces the risk of RA onset[50], whereas postpartum status is associated with substantially increased risk compared to other periods of time. Breast feeding further increases risk of disease onset or flare[54]. These changing risks of RA onset or flare are notable because they occur in the context of pronounced hormonal changes associated with pregnancy and the postpartum periods. As shown in Fig. 18.3, plasma levels of corticotropin releasing hormone (CRH), adrenocorticotropin (ACTH), cortisol, progesterone, and estradiol increase progressively throughout pregnancy and are maximal around labor and delivery[55,56]. It should be noted that during pregnancy the placenta produces CRH and HCG, and this production terminates at labor and delivery[56]. After labor and delivery, plasma levels of all of these hormones decline. Minimum levels are reached about 2 weeks postpartum (Fig. 18.3). Depressed hormone levels, particularly estradiol, can, however, be detected for up to 1 year postpartum. Furthermore, CRH-induced ACTH responses are severely depressed for up to 3 months postpartum, implying that hypothalamic CRH priming of the pituitary and pituitary–adrenal axis responsiveness is severely deficient[56,57]. Breastfeeding increases plasma prolactin and oxytocin levels, which further attenuates cortisol production in the postpartum period[58,59].

Thus, the postpartum period, in sharp contrast with pregnancy, is characterized by deficient production of both adrenal and gonadal hormones. Interestingly, a substantial fraction (20–30 per cent) of premenopausal onset RA occurs within 1 year of a pregnancy[60] (R. Wilder, unpublished observations). These data suggest that premenopausal onset of RA may be influenced by the same factors that influence perimenopausal/menopausal onset of RA, that is deficient adrenal and gonadal steroid hormone production. A similar situation may apply to multiple sclerosis (MS). Flare rates of MS also decrease during pregnancy, and the highest flare rates are observed in the postpartum period[61–63].

Although some authors have tended to discount the role of hormones in pregnancy-associated remissions of RA and have focused on the role of fetal–maternal MHC disparity[47], it is important to note that hormones and effects of fetal–maternal MHC disparity are not incompatible phenomena. The survival of a histoincompatible fetus is dependent upon diversion/suppression of the maternal cell-mediated immune response to the fetus[64–66]. Similar mechanisms are probably involved in the reported therapeutic effects of allogeneic cell immunization in RA patients[67]. Is appears likely that that pregnancy and allogeneic immunization will involve hormonal mechanisms. As will be discussed in later sections, cortisol is a powerful inhibitor of the production of proinflammatory cytokines such as TNF-α, IL-12, and interferon-γ[1,6,68]. These cytokines play key roles in the rejection of allogeneic tissues. They also play important roles in pathogenesis of RA. Since cortisol is produced during the third trimester of pregnancy at levels similar to those observed in patients with untreated Cushing syndrome, its potential to modify immune responsiveness cannot be ignored[56]. Although not as potent as cortisol, estrogen and progesterone, which, like cortisol, are produced at supraphysiological concentrations during pregnancy, also suppress TNF-α production[23,69–72]. The production of TNF-α, IL-12, and interferon-γ is suppressed during pregnancy[73–75]. In mice, these cytokines impair fetal development and are powerful abortifacients. Survival of the fetus requires that their production is curtailed[75–79] In contrast to TNF-α, IL-12 and interferon-γ, the production of antagonistic, anti-inflammatory cytokines, such as IL-4 and IL-10, is increased during pregnancy, particularly at the maternal–fetal interface[64,80–84]. These anti-inflammatory cytokines suppress cell-mediated immunity but stimulate humoral immunity. Maintained or enhanced humoral immunity is a characteristic of pregnancy. Moreover, cytokines such as IL-10 have been shown to decrease the likelihood of fetal loss or premature spontaneous abortion[6,73,82,85,86]. Cortisol, progesterone, and estrogen, have the capacity to induce this bias in immune response toward humoral immunity[68,74,81,87–91]. The strongest evidence, however, in support of the importance of cortisol and progesterone to fetal survival is the effect of RU486, a cortisol and progesterone receptor antagonist. It is a powerful abortifacient. RU486 is also a potent enhancer of proinflammatory cytokine production and cell-mediated immune function in the setting of an appropriate antigenic challenge[92,93]. Thus, the available evidence is consistent with the hypothesis that hormones, such as cortisol, progesterone, and estrogen, play important roles in regulating the shifts in immune function that occur in pregnancy. These

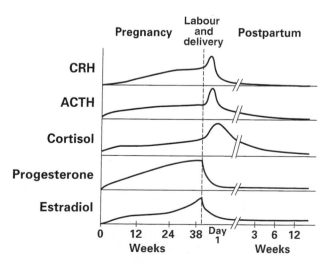

Fig. 18.3 Pregnancy and postpartum plasma hormone levels. Data extracted and modified from Chrousos *et al.*, Ref. 56.

hormonal shifts appear to also suppress RA onset risk and the activity of established disease.

SLE activity during pregnancy and the postpartum periods provides an interesting contrast with RA. Although some investigators have concluded otherwise[94,95], most published data indicate that SLE tends to flare more frequently during pregnancy than in other periods[96-103]. Moreover, there is no dispute that SLE, in contrast to RA, certainly does not improve during pregnancy, and postpartum, SLE activity tends to return to its basal level[103]. In other words, pregnancy-associated increases in cortisol, estrogen, and progesterone do not decrease SLE disease activity, and may, in fact, increase activity. These observations are consistent with the data indicating the maximum risk of SLE onset occurs during the child-bearing years. As will be discussed in more detail in the following sections, one mechanism underlying these clinical data is the capacity of cortisol to suppress macrophage TNF-α and IL-12 production, without affecting IL-10 production, that is during pregnancy the proinflammatory/anti-inflammatory cytokine balance favors humoral immune mechanisms which characterize SLE. Estrogen and progesterone also have suppressive effects on TNF-α and may have similar effects on cytokine balance.

The menstrual cycle, oral contraceptives, and hormone replacement therapy in RA

RA and SLE disease activity, like many other immune diseases such as asthma, irritable bowel syndrome, and diabetes, have been clearly shown to change during the course of the menstrual cycle[104-107]. RA disease activity is measurably worse just before menses, when estrogen and progesterone levels are the lowest. Changes in SLE during the menstrual cycle, on the other hand, have been observed but are more variable. Changes in SLE disease activity have been noted at midcycle through the onset of menses[106,108,109]. Symptoms that exacerbate 2 weeks before menses tend to be more severe than those that occur 10 days before menses[106]. In a case series of three SLE patients, facial rashes, which developed at midcycle, were suppressed with oral contraceptives, presumably by modulating hormonal fluctuations[109]. These observations give further support for the concept that the neuroendocrine axis modulates RA and SLE disease activity.

Oral contraceptive and postmenopausal hormone replacement therapy use provide additional clinical situations to assess the role of gonadal hormones in the pathogenesis of RA and SLE. Oral contraceptives, which produce a hormonal state consistent with pseudopregnancy, are associated with decreased risk of developing RA[1,2,28,51,53,110,111]. Moreover, it is well documented that postmenopausal estrogen replacement therapy decreases RA-Associated bone loss[22,26,112-116]. Effects on other measures of disease activity have not been convincingly shown[115], although the direction of change is clearly towards decreased disease activity. Importantly, there are no data, which are convincing, to suggest that estrogen administration increases the severity of RA.

Oral contraceptive and postmenopausal hormone replacement therapy in SLE patients, because of a perception by many rheumatologists that it increases disease activity, is very controversial[117-120]. The available data suggest that estrogen administration slightly increases the risk of developing SLE or increasing disease activity. Similarly, ovulation-inducing treatment in SLE patients with the antiphospholipid antibody has been noted to increase disease activity[121]. Ovulation-inducing treatment increases plasma estrogen levels. Because of the uncertainty regarding the magnitude of the risk, the relative benefits and risks of estrogen use in SLE patients are currently the subject of a clinical trial. The concern with the use of estrogens in SLE patients definitely contrasts with apparent benefits of the use of estrogens in RA patients.

Interactions between the stress system and the gonadal axis

As illustrated in Fig. 18.4, the hypothalamic–pituitary–adrenal (HPA) axis and the sympathetic nervous system constitute the stress system[1,122,123]. The principal molecular regulators of the stress system are CRH and arginine vasopressin (AVP), both of which are secreted by the parvicellular neurons of the paraventricular nucleus of the hypothalamus. These hormones stimulate pituitary ACTH and, consequently, cortisol production by the adrenal cortex. The brainstem locus ceruleus (LC) and the peripheral sympathetic–adrenomedullary systems are innervated and bidirectionally regulate the activity of the CRH and AVP hypothalamic neurons. The principal mediator produced by the LC is norepinephrine, whereas norepinephrine and epinephrine are produced by the peripheral sympathetic and adrenal medullary systems, respectively. A key point is that the stress system, through a diverse array of hormonal mediators, directly interacts with the innate and acquired immune systems[1,123,124], and vice versa, the immune system, through the production of

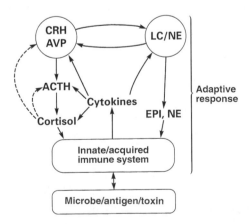

Fig. 18.4 Stress system–immune system interactions. Abbreviations: CRH = corticotropin-releasing hormone, AVP = arginine vasopressin, LC/NE = locus ceruleus/norepinephrine, ACTH = adrenocorticotropin, EPI = epinephrine, NE = norepinephrine. Solid arrows represent stimulatory effects. Dashed arrows represent inhibitory effects.

cytokines such as TNF-α, IL-1, and IL-6[1,26], directly interacts with the stress system.

The bidirectional interactions of these systems facilitate host adaptation to stressful stimuli such as microbes, antigens, and toxins (Fig. 18.4), which threaten physiological homeostasis. Activation of these systems mobilizes adaptive behaviors and peripheral functions that negate the stressor. Stress system activation also suppresses non-adaptive behaviors such as feeding, growth, and gonadal functions related to reproduction.

The suppression of gonadal functions by the stress system occurs through many levels of interaction[56]. Hypothalamic CRH neurons innervate and inhibit the hypothalamic control center of the gonadal axis. In addition, corticosteroids inhibit the gonadal axis at the level of the hypothalamus, the pituitary, gonadal, and end-organ responsiveness. As a consequence, persistent stress-system activation produces functional amenorrhea and secondary hypogonadism[56].

The activity of the stress system is also modulated by the gonadal hormones, particularly estrogen[56,125]. The CRH gene contains a functional estrogen-responsive element[126], which may explain higher levels of CRH in the CRH neurons of female rats, and higher HPA axis responsiveness of women[127,128]. CRH-induced ACTH responses are higher, and the cortisol responses are more prolonged in women compared to men[129]. These data are consistent with observations that pregnant women and women receiving high-dose estrogen treatment have elevated plasma cortisol levels compared to control individuals[130]. Estrogen also increases HPA axis and sympathetic–adrenomedullary catecholamine responsiveness not only in women, but also in normal men[131].

Estradiol also decreases corticosteroid receptor levels in the hypothalamus, the anterior pituitary, and the hippocampus. The net effect, by interfering with corticosteroid feedback, is to increase HPA axis responsiveness and the production of catecholamines by the LC/NE system[56,132]. Conversely, estrogen

deficiency, such as observed in the postpartum period and at menopause, is expected to result in a hyporesponsive HPA axis and suboptimal cortisol and catecholamine production. Thus, the interactions between the stress system and the gonadal axis have the potential to modulate significantly the production of cortisol and catecholamines. These modulatory effects may have profound effects on the activity of innate/acquired immune systems (Fig. 18.4). The potential relevance of these interactions to the onset and progression of RA and SLE will be discussed further in the following sections.

The hypothalamic–pituitary–adrenal axis, corticosteroids, and RA

Corticosteroids and RA are historically intimately linked. The dramatic anti-inflammatory effects of cortisone were first described in RA patients and resulted in the awarding of a Nobel Prize in 1950. Although these observations suggested that RA was possibly a corticosteroid deficiency state, this hypothesis was inadequately evaluated at that time because interest waned with the recognition of the serious side-effects associated with supraphysiological corticosteroid treatment. Renewed interest in this hypothesis has, however, developed in recent years, and Table 18.2 lists many of the observations that support the view that suboptimal production of cortisol is involved in the onset and/or progression of RA[1]. Consistently, low cortisol states, whether primary or acquired, are associated with development or flares of RA, whereas high cortisol states suppress or inhibit disease expression. The dominant observation to date has been that most RA patients have relatively 'normal' plasma cortisol levels in the setting of severe, chronic inflammation. In other words, RA patients appear to have 'inappropriately normal' HPA axis activity in the setting of

Table 18.2 Evidence linking corticosteroid deficiency to the onset and/or progression of RA

Susceptibility to RA-like polyarthritis in some inbred strains of rats (e.g. Lewis) linked to blunted hypothalamic–pituitary–adrenal axis function (1, 92, 141, 142)

Disease activity parallels the daily circadian rhythm of TNF-α, IL-1, and IL-12 production and is inversely related to plasma levels (133, 134, 143–150)

Disease activity, including erosions, is suppressed by low-dose, physiological range corticosteroid therapy (151)

Untreated Cushing disease and RA are probably mutually exclusive illnesses; RA-like symptoms frequently noted after treatment, particularly hypophysectomy, of Cushing disease; classical RA occasionally develops after treatment of Cushing disease (152)

Disease activity increases following periods of severe psychosocial stress (severe stress is initially associated with hypercortisolemia, but may be followed by hypocortisolemia) (8, 9, 153)

Disease activity increases during the week before the onset of menses (plasma cortisol levels decreased) (104, 105)

Disease activity declines during pregnancy in parallel with rising cortisol levels; maximal improvement in third trimester (50)

Disease activity develops or flares in postpartum period, particularly in association with breast feeding (a state associated with increased prolactin and depressed hypothalamic–pituitary–adrenal axis function) (54)

Plasma cortisol levels are frequently subnormal in patients with mild disease (145)

Most patients have 'inappropriately normal', rather than elevated, plasma cortisol levels (inflammation, as a consequence of IL-1 and IL-6 stimulation of the HPA axis, should result in above normal plasma cortisol levels) (134, 145, 154)

Plasma ACTH–cortisol and interleukin-6 (IL-6)–cortisol dose-response relationships are shifted right, indicating defective adrenal responsiveness (134, 155, 156)

Metyrapone exacerbates disease (157, 158)

Blunted plasma cortisol responses noted following surgical stress (133)

High level expression of corticotropin releasing hormone noted in inflamed joints, similar to observations in HPA-axis defective, arthritis-prone Lewis rats (135–137)

markedly enhanced production of proinflammatory cytokines, such as TNF-α, IL-1, and IL-6. Since IL-1 and IL-6 are normally powerful stimulants to the HPA axis and cortisol production, we would have expected significantly elevated cortisol production in RA patients. The available data suggest that this response is blunted in RA patients[133,134]. Whether this abnormality is primary or secondary has not been established, but the data appear analogous to the HPA axis defect noted in autoimmune arthritis-prone Lewis rats. These rats have a globally blunted stress system response and fail, in response to a wide variety of stressors, to activate the hypothalamic CRH neuron appropriately[1,3].

The description of the defect in hypothalamic CRH in Lewis rats has been followed by an explosion of research on CRH and its role in regulating multiple biological processes[56]. Indeed, it is now recognized that CRH production is not limited to the hypothalamus. CRH is also secreted in diverse sites peripherally[56]. Interestingly, it is secreted in the synovial fluids and tissues of RA patients[135]. This observation is provocative because CRH is also expressed at high levels in the inflamed joints of arthritis-prone Lewis rats, but Lewis rats have a defect in expressing CRH in the hypothalamus resulting in blunted HPA axis function and abnormal central stress system responses[136,137]. Although CRH expression in the hypothalamus has not been measured in RA patients, it appears likely that the high-level expression of CRH in the inflamed joints of RA patients may be a reflection of blunted production of hypothalamic CRH. This hypothesis needs investigation. Interestingly, preliminary genetic analysis suggests that a unique polymorphism in the 5' promoter region of the CRH gene may be associated with RA[138]. These observations also need confirmation because of the important implications these data have for understanding the role of the stress system in the pathogenesis of RA. A deficit in hypothalamic production of CRH may have diverse clinical manifestations. As note previously, CRH not only regulates the stress system and immune function, but it also has a role in regulating mood, growth, appetite, and reproductive function[1,56,123]. Since abnormalities of this type are also common in RA, they suggest another dimension to the involvement of the neuroendocrine axis in RA.

Immunoregulatory actions of adrenal and gonadal hormones and RA

The neuroendocrine axis affects the innate and acquired immune systems through an extensive array of mediators and diverse targets[1]. A complete discussion of these neuroendocrine regulatory effects is beyond the scope of this chapter. Nevertheless, a review of the known regulatory actions of cortisol, DHEA/DHEAS, epinephrine, estrogen, progesterone, and testosterone on the production of TNF-α, IL-12, and IL-10 is sufficient to illustrate current concepts. As mentioned in the introduction, excessive and sustained production of TNF-α and IL-12 relative to IL-10 appear to characterize RA, whereas excessive production of IL-10 appears to be a central abnormality in SLE. A summary of the known effects of the major adrenal (cortisol, DHEA/DHEAS, and epinephrine) and gonadal hormones (estrogen, progesterone, and testosterone) hormones on the macrophage production of TNF-α, IL-12, and IL-10 is shown in Table 18.3. A key point is that effects overall of the adrenal and gonadal hormones on TNF-α and IL-12 differs from the effects on IL-10, that is, adrenal and gonadal hormonal deficiency versus excess has potential to shift the proinflammatory/anti-inflammatory cytokine balance in opposite directions.

Cortisol and epinephrine, which are the principal adrenal stress hormones, are clearly the most potent inhibitors of TNF-α, but DHEA/DHEAS, estrogen, and progesterone also have modest direct inhibitory effects on TNF-α production. Cortisol and epinephrine are also the most potent hormonal inhibitors of IL-12 production, which explains their striking effects in suppressing cell-mediated immune mechanisms. IL-12 is a critical bridge between the innate and acquired immune systems, and is particularly important in autoimmune diseases such as RA and MS[139]. Especially noteworthy is that cortisol, in contrast to its potent suppressive effects on TNF-α and IL-12, has negligible suppressive effects on IL-10 production, and epinephrine is even more striking. It strongly stimulates IL-10 production. Thus, disorders driven by IL-10, such as SLE, may flare in high epineph-

Table 18.3 Direct actions of adrenal and gonadal hormones on macrophage production of TNF-α, Interleukin-12, and Interleukin-10

	TNF-α	IL-12	IL-10
Adrenal Hormones			
Cortisol	Potent suppression (150, 159)	Potent suppression (68, 150)	No effects (68)
DHEA/DHEAS	Modest suppression (160, 161) No effects (35)	No published data	Modest suppression (162–164)
Epinephrine	Potent suppression (165–167)	Potent suppression (165, 168)	Potent stimulation (68, 169, 170)
Gonadal Hormones			
Estrogen	Modest suppression (23, 69–71, 171)	No effect (171)	No effect (171)
Progesterone	Modest suppression (72)	No published data	No published data
Testosterone	No effect (69, 172)	No published data	No published data

rine output states, that is acute stress. Conversely, clinical situations associated with relative adrenal insufficiency would be expected to be dominated by excessive TNF-α and IL-12 production relative to IL-10. This situation is suspected to be operative in RA and related diseases.

The direct effects of estrogen on macrophage production of TNF-α are modest. If the enhancing effects of estrogen on the stress system responsiveness are also considered, it is apparent that the combined direct and indirect effects of estrogen on TNF-α and IL-12 production relative to IL-10 production are possibly very large. Most likely, it is this interaction between estrogen and the stress system hormones that underlies the dramatic changes in autoimmune disease in context of changing reproductive status. Declining estrogen levels facilitate the development of cell-mediated autoimmune diseases such as RA, whereas high estrogen levels promote autoimmune diseases associated with humoral immunity such SLE. Progesterone appears to magnify these effects.

The effects of the androgens DHEA/DHEAS and testosterone are difficult to understand. The available data suggest the DHEA modestly suppresses both TNF-α and IL-10, but it is not clear whether this suppression is due to DHEA itself or a metabolic product. Testosterone is even more difficult to understand. No direct suppressive effects of testosterone on TNF-α, IL-12, or IL-10 have been shown. However, testosterone can be converted by aromatase to estrogen, which does have effects as described on TNF-α and so on. Data do exist indicating the some of the immunoregulatory activities of testosterone are modified by conversion to estrogen[140]. Thus, the potential of conversion of DHEA and testosterone to other active products, such as estrogens, makes analysis of their immunoregulatory effects very difficult. Nevertheless, the rudimentary understanding that we now have on the immunoregulatory actions of adrenal and gonadal hormones provides a basis for explaining some aspects of the clinical epidemiology of RA related to age, gender, and reproductive status.

Conclusions

It is now widely recognized that neuroendocrine system interactions with the immune and inflammatory systems are extensive and important. These interactions facilitate bidirectional regulation and co-ordination of systemic adaptive responses to potentially harmful stressful stimuli. This review has focused on a limited array of neuroendocrine mechanisms related to adrenal and gonadal hormones in the context of the immunopathogenesis of RA. A limited comparison with SLE was also presented. The major concept advanced is that RA appears to develop and progress in a setting of both adrenal (cortisol, DHEA, and its metabolites) and gonadal (estrogen, progesterone, testosterone) hormonal deficiency. Data were reviewed suggesting that adrenal and gonadal hormonal deficiencies facilitate the expression of non-specific and cellular immunity mechanisms that characterize RA. Data were reviewed that suggest that the origin of the hormonal deficiencies may include a primary or acquired major central nervous system component (e.g., hypothalamic

CRH deficiency), which may contribute to diverse clinical manifestations of RA such as mood disturbances (fatigue, apathetic depression) and reproductive problems. Most importantly, available data suggest that novel therapeutic approaches may ultimately be developed from continued investigations of the role of the neuroendocrine axis in RA.

References

1. Wilder R.L. Neuroendocrine-immune interactions and autoimmunity. *Ann Rev Immunol*, 1995;**13**:307–38.
2. Da Silva J.A. Sex hormones, glucocorticoids and autoimmunity: facts and hypotheses. *Ann Rheum Dis*, 1995;**54**:6–16.
3. Wilder R.L. Hormones and autoimmunity: Animal models of arthritis. *Baillieres Clin Rheumatol*, 1996;**10**:259–71.
4. Wilder R.L. Adrenal and gonadal steroid hormone deficiency in the pathogenesis of rheumatoid arthritis. *J Rheumatol*, 1996;**44** (Suppl): 10–12.
5. Elenkov I.J., Hoffman J, Wilder R.L. Does differential neuroendocrine control of cytokine production govern the expression of autoimmune diseases in pregnancy and the postpartum period? *Mol Med Today*, 1997;**3**:379–83.
6. Wilder R.L. Hormones, pregnancy, and autoimmune diseases. *Ann N Y Acad Sci*, 1998;**840**:45–50.
7. Cutolo M, Masi A.T. Do androgens influence the pathophysiology of rheumatoid arthritis? Facts and hypotheses. *J Rheumatol*, 1998;**25**:1041–7.
8. Zautra A.J., Burleson M.H., Matt K.S., Roth S, Burrows L. Interpersonal stress, depression, and disease activity in rheumatoid arthritis and osteoarthritis patients. *Health Psychol*, 1994;**13**:139–48.
9. Zautra A.J., Hoffman, J, Potter P, Matt K.S., Yocum D, Castro L. Examination of changes in interpersonal stress as a factor in disease exacerbations among women with rheumatoid arthritis. *Ann Behav Med*, 1997;**19**:279–86.
10. Feldmann M., Brennan F.M., Maini R.N. Role of cytokines in rheumatoid arthritis. *Annu Rev Immunol*, 1996;**14**:397–440.
11. Kotake S., Schumacher H.R. Jr., Yarboro C.H., Arayssi T.K., Pando J.A., Kanik K.S., Gourley M.F., Klippel J.H., Wilder R.L. In vivo gene expression of type 1 and type 2 cytokines in synovial tissues from patients in early stages of rheumatoid, reactive, and undifferentiated arthritis. *Proc Assoc Am Physicians*, 1997;**109**:286–301.
12. Mitamura K., Kang H., Tomita Y., Hashimoto H., Sawada S., Horie T. Impaired tumour necrosis factor-alpha (TNF-alpha) production and abnormal B cell response to TNF-alpha in patients with systemic lupus erythematosus (SLE). *Clin Exp Immunol*, 1991;**85**:386–91.
13. Swaak A.J., van den Brink H.G., Aarden L.A. Cytokine production (IL-6 and TNF alpha) in whole blood cell cultures of patients with systemic lupus erythematosus. *Scand J Rheumatol*, 1996;**25**:233–8.
14. Kroemer G., Hirsch F., Gonzalez-Garcia A., Martinez C. Differential involvement of Th1 and Th2 cytokines in autoimmune diseases. *Autoimmunity*, 1996;**24**:25–33.
15. Horwitz D.A. Gray J.D., Behrendsen S.C. Kubin M., Rengaraju M., Ohtsuka K., Trinchieri G. Decreased production of interleukin-12 and other Th1-type cytokines in patients with recent-onset systemic lupus erythematosus. *Arthritis Rheum*, 1998;**41**:838–44.
16. Del Prete G. The concept of type-1 and type-2 helper T cells and their cytokines in humans. *Int Rev Immunol*, 1998;**16**:427–55.
17. Masi A.T. Incidence of rheumatoid arthritis: do the observed age-sex interaction patterns support a role of androgenic-anabolic steroid deficiency in its pathogenesis? [editorial]. *Br J Rheumatol*, 1994;**33**:697–9.

18. Weyand C.M., Schmidt D., Wagner U., Goronzy J.J. The influence of sex on the phenotype of rheumatoid arthritis. *Arthritis Rheum,* 1998;**41**:817–22.

19. Suzuki M., Takahashi M., Miyamato S., Hoshino H., Kushida K., Miura M., Inoue T. The effects of menopausal status and disease activity on biochemical markers of bone metabolism in female patients with rheumatoid arthritis. *Br J Rheumatol,* 1998;**37**:653–8.

20. Rannevik G., Jeppsson S., Johnell O., Bjerre B., Laurell-Borulf Y., Svanbergy L. A longitudinal study of the perimenopausal transition: altered profiles of steroid and pituitary hormones, SHBG and bone mineral density. *Maturitas,* 1995;**21**:103–13.

21. Sambrook P.N., Eisman J.A., Champion G.D., Pocock N.A. Sex hormone status and osteoporosis in postmenopausal women with rheumatoid arthritis. *Arthritis Rheum,* 1988;**31**:973–8.

22. Sambrook P., Birmingham J., Champion D., Kelly P., Kempler S., Freund J., Eisman J. Postmenopausal bone loss in rheumatoid arthritis: effect of estrogens and androgens. *J Rheumatol,* 1992;**19**:357–61.

23. Cohen-Solal M.E., Graulet A.M., Denne M.A., Gueris J., Baylink D., de Vernejoul M.C. Peripheral monocyte culture supernatants of menopausal women can induce bone resorption: involvement of cytokines. *J Clin Endocrinol Metab,* 1993;**77**:1648–53.

24. Bellido T., Jilka R.L., Boyce B.F., Girasole G., Broxmeyer H., Dalrymple S.A., Murray R., Manolagas S.C. Regulation of interleukin-6, osteoclastogenesis, and bone mass by androgens. The role of the androgen receptor. *J Clin Invest,* 1995;**95**:2886–95.

25. Cutolo M., Sulli A., Seriolo B., Accardo S., Masi A.T. Estrogens, the immune response and autoimmunity. *Clin Exp Rheumatol,* 1995;**13**:217–26.

26. Papanicolaou D.A., Wilder R.L., Manolagas S.C., Chrousos G.P. The pathophysiologic roles of interleukin-6 in human disease. *Ann Intern Med,* 1998;**128**:127–37.

27. Kotake S., Sato K., Kim K.J., Takahashi N., Udagawa N., Nakamura I., Yamaguchi A., Kishimoto T., Suda T., Kashiwazaki S. Interleukin-6 and soluble interleukin-6 receptors in the synovial fluids from rheumatoid arthritis patients are responsible for osteoclast-like cell formation. *J Bone Miner Res,* 1996;**11**:88–95.

28. Masi A.T. Sex hormones and rheumatoid arthritis: cause or effect relationships in a complex pathophysiology? *Clin Exp Rheumatol,* 1995;**13**:227–40.

29. Cutolo M., Balleari E., Giusti M., Intra E., Accardo S. Androgen replacement therapy in male patients with rheumatoid arthritis. *Arthritis Rheum,* 1991;**34**:1–5.

30. Hall G.M., Larbre J.P., Spector T.D., Perry L.A., Da Silva J.A. A randomized trial of testosterone therapy in males with rheumatoid arthritis. *Br J Rheumatol,* 1996;**35**:568–73.

31. Booji A., Biewenga-Booji C.M., Huber-Bruning O., Cornelis C., Jacobs J.W., Bijlsma J.W. Androgens as adjuvant treatment in postmenopausal female patients with rheumatoid arthritis. *Ann Rheum Dis,* 1996;**55**:811–5.

32. Cutolo M., Giusti M., Villaggio B., Barone A., Accardo S., Sulli A., Granata O., Carruba G., Castagnetta L. Testosterone metabolism and cyclosporin A treatment in rheumatoid arthritis. *Br J Rheumatol,* 1997;**36**:433–9.

33. Masi A.T., Feigenbaum S.L., Chatterton R.T., Cutolo M. Integrated hormonal-immunological-vascular (H-I-V triad) systems interactions in the rheumatic diseases. *Clin Exp Rheumatol,* 1995;**13**:203–16.

34. Masi A.T., Da Silva J.A., Cutolo M. Perturbations of hypothalamic-pituitary-gonadal (HPG) axis and adrenal androgen (AA) functions in rheumatoid arthritis. *Baillieres Clin Rheumatol,* 1996;**10**:295–332.

35. Straub R.H., Konecna L., Hrach S. Serum dehydroepiandrosterone (DHEA) and DHEA sulfate are negatively correlated with serum interleukin-6 (IL-6), and DHEA inhibits IL-6 secretion from mononuclear cells in man in vitro: possible link between endocrinosenescence and immunosenescence. *J Clin Endocrinol Metab,* 1998;**83**:2012–7.

36. Giltay E.J., van Schaardenburg D., Gooren L.J., von Blomberg B.M., Fonk J.C., Touw D.J., Dijkmans B.A. Effects of dehy-droepiandrosterone administration on disease activity in patients with rheumatoid arthritis [letter]. *Br J Rheumatol,* 1998;**37**:705–6.

37. Lahita R.G., Bucala R., Bradlow H.L., Fishman J. Determination of 16 alpha-hydroxyestrone by radioimmunoassay in systemic lupus erythematosus. *Arthritis Rheum,* 1985;**28**:1122–7.

38. Lahita R.G. The effects of sex hormones on the immune system in pregnancy. *Am J Reprod Immunol,* 1992;**28**:136–7.

39. Lahita R.G. Sex steroids and SLE: metabolism of androgens to estrogens [editorial]. *Lupus,* 1992;**1**:125–7.

40. Lahita R.G., Cheng C.Y., Monder C., Bardin C.W. Experience with 19-nortestosterone in the therapy of systemic lupus erythematosus: worsened disease after treatment with 19-nortestosterone in men and lack of improvement in women. *J Rheumatol,* 1992;**19**:547–55.

41. Lahita R.G. The importance of estrogens in systemic lupus erythematosus. *Clin Immunol Immunopathol,* 1992;**63**:17–8.

42. Lahita R.G. The basis for gender effects in the connective tissue diseases. *Ann Med Intern,* 1996;**147**:241–7.

43. Wilder R.L. Adrenal and gonadal steroid hormone deficiency in the pathogenesis of rheumatoid arthritis. *J Rheumatol,* 1996;**44**(suppl.):10–2.

44. Hazes J.M., Dijkmans B.A., Vandenbroucke J.P., de Vries R.R., Cats A. Pregnancy and the risk of developing rheumatoid arthritis. *Arthritis Rheum,* 1990;**33**:1770–5.

45. Hazes J.M. Pregnancy and its effect on the risk of developing rheumatoid arthritis. *Ann Rheum Dis,* 1991;**50**:71–4.

46. Spector T.D., Da Silva J.A. Pregnancy and rheumatoid arthritis: an overview. *Am J Reprod Immunol,* 1992;**28**:222–5.

47. Nelson J.L., Hughes K.A., Smith A.G., Nisperos B.B., Branchaud A.M., Hansen J.A. Maternal-fetal disparity in HLA class II alloantigens and the pregnancy-induced amelioration of rheumatoid arthritis [see comments]. *N Engl J Med,* 1993;**329**:466–71.

48. Nelson J.L. Pregnancy immunology and autoimmune disease. *J Reprod Med,* 1998;**43**:335–40.

49. Masi A.T., Feigenbaum S.L., Chatterton R.T. Hormonal and pregnancy relationships to rheumatoid arthritis: convergent effects with immunologic and microvascular systems. *Semin Arthritis Rheum,* 1995;**25**:1–27.

50. Silman A., Kay A., Brennan P. Timing of pregnancy in relation to the onset of rheumatoid arthritis. *Arthritis Rheum,* 1992;**35**:152–155.

51. Spector T.D., Roman E., Silman A.J. The pill, parity, and rheumatoid arthritis. *Arthritis Rheum,* 1990;**33**:782–9.

52. Silman A.J. Parity status and the development of rheumatoid arthritis. *Am J Reprod Immunol,* 1992;**28**:228–30.

53. Silman A.J. Epidemiology of rheumatoid arthritis. *Apmis,* 1994;**102**:721–8.

54. Brennan P., Silman A. Breast-feeding and the onset of rheumatoid arthritis. *Arthritis Rheum,* 1994;**37**:808–13.

55. Magiakou M.A., Mastorakos G., Rabin D., Margioris A.N., Dubbert B., Calogero A.E., Tsigos C., Munson P.J., Chrousos G.P. The maternal hypothalamic-pituitary-adrenal axis in the third trimester of human pregnancy. *Clin Endocrinol (Oxf),* 1996;**44**:419–28.

56. Chrousos G.P., Torpy D.J., Gold P.W. Interactions between the hypothalamic-pituitary-adrenal axis and the female reproductive system: Clinical implications. *Ann Int Med,* 1998;**129**:229–40.

57. Magiakou M.A., Mastorakos G., Rabin D., Dubbert B., Gold P.W., Chrousos G.P. Hypothalamic corticotropin-releasing hormone suppression during the postpartum period: implications for the increase in psychiatric manifestations at this time. *J Clin Endocrinol Metab,* 1996;**81**:1912–7.

58. Amico J.A., Finley B.E. Breast stimulation in cycling women, pregnant women and a woman with induced lactation: pattern of release of oxytocin, prolactin and luteinizing hormone. *Clin Endocrinol (Oxf),* 1986;**25**:97–106.

59. Amico J.A., Johnston J.M., Vagnucci A.H. Suckling-induced attenuation of plasma cortisol concentrations in postpartum lactating women. *Endocr Res,* 1994;**20**:79–87.

60. Pritchard M.H. An examination of the role of female hormones and pregnancy as risk factors for rheumatoid arthritis, using a male population as control group. *Br J Rheumatol*, 1992;31:395–9.

61. Davis R.K., Maslow A.S. Multiple sclerosis in pregnancy: a review. *Obstet Gynecol Surv*, 1992;47:290–6.

62. Damek D.M., Shuster E.A. Pregnancy and multiple sclerosis. *Mayo Clin Proc*, 1997;72:977–89.

63. Confavreux C., Hutchinson M., Hours M.M., Cortinovis-Tourniaire P., Moreau T. Rate of pregnancy-related relapse in multiple sclerosis. *N Engl J Med*, 1998;339:285–91.

64. Formby B. Immunologic response in pregnancy. Its role in endocrine disorders of pregnancy and influence on the course of maternal autoimmune diseases. *Endocrinol Metab Clin North Am*, 1995;24:187–205.

65. Marzi M., Vigano A., Trabattoni D., Villa M.L., Salvaggio A., Clerici E., Clerici M. Characterization of type 1 and type 2 cytokine production profile in physiologic and pathologic human pregnancy. *Clin Exp Immunol*, 1996;106:127–33.

66. Reinhard G., Noll A., Schlebusch H., Mallmann P., Ruecker A.V. Shifts in the Th1/Th2 balance during human pregnancy correlate with apoptotic changes. *Biochem Biophys Res Commun*, 1998;245:933–8.

67. Smith J.B., Fort J.G. Treatment of rheumatoid arthritis by immunization with mononuclear white blood cells: results of a preliminary trial. *J Rheumatol*, 1996;23:220–5.

68. Elenkov I.J. Papanicolaou D.A. Wilder R.L. Chrousos G.P. Modulatory effects of glucocorticoids and catecholamines on human interleukin-12 and interleukin-10 production: clinical implications. *Proc Assoc Am Physicians*, 1996;108:374–81.

69. Ralston S.H., Russell R.G, Gowen M. Estrogen inhibits release of tumor necrosis factor from peripheral blood mononuclear cells in postmenopausal women. *J Bone Miner Res*, 1990;5:983–8.

70. Pacifici R., Brown C., Puscheck E., Friedrich E., Slatopolsky E., Maggio D., McCracken R., Avioli L.V. Effect of surgical menopause and estrogen replacement on cytokine release from human blood mononuclear cells. *Proc Natl Acad Sci U.S.A.*, 1991;88:5134–8.

71. Evans M.J., MacLaughlin S., Marvin R.D., Abdou N.I. Estrogen decreases in vitro apoptosis of peripheral blood mononuclear cells from women with normal menstrual cycles and decreases TNF-alpha production in SLE but not in normal cultures. *Clin Immunol Immunopathol*, 1997;82:258–62.

72. Miller L, Hunt J.S. Regulation of TNF-alpha production in activated mouse macrophages by progesterone. *J Immunol*, 1998;160:5098–104.

73. Delassus S., Coutinho G.C., Saucier C., Darche S., Kourilsky P. Differential cytokine expression in maternal blood and placenta during murine gestation. *J Immunol*, 1994;152:2411–20.

74. Szekeres-Bartho J., Faust Z., Varga P., Szereday L., Kelemen K. The immunological pregnancy protective effect of progesterone is manifested via controlling cytokine production. *Am J Reprod Immunol*, 1996;35:348–51.

75. Lea R.G., McIntyre S., Baird J.D., Clark D.A. Tumor necrosis factor-alpha mRNA-positive cells in spontaneous resorption in rodents. *Am J Reprod Immunol*, 1998;39:50–7.

76. Chaouat G., Menu E., Clark D.A., Dy M., Minkowski M., Wegmann T.G. Control of fetal survival in CBA x DBA/2 mice by lymphokine therapy. *J Reprod Fertil*, 1990;89:447–58.

77. Sacks G.P., Scott D., Tivnann H., Mire-Sluis T., Sargent I.L., Redman C.W. Interleukin-12 and pre-eclampsia. *J Reprod Immunol*, 1997;34:155–8.

78. Dudley D.J. Is pre-eclampsia a Th-1-type immune condition. *J Reprod Immunol*, 1997;34:159–61.

79. Clark D.A., Chaouat G., Arck P.C., Mittruecker H.W., Levy G.A. Cutting edge: cytokine-dependent abortion in CBA x DBA/2 mice is mediated by the procoagulant fg12 prothombinase. *J Immunol*, 1998;160:545–9.

80. Lin H., Mosmann T.R., Guilbert L., Tuntipopipat S., Wegmann T.G. Synthesis of T helper 2-type cytokines at the maternal-fetal interface. *J Immunol*, 1993;151:4562–73.

81. Szereday L., Varga P., Szekeres-Bartho J. Cytokine production by lymphocytes in pregnancy. *Am J Reprod Immunol*, 1997;38:418–22.

82. Rivera D.L., Olister S.M., Liu X., Thompson J.H., Zhang X.J., Pennline K., Azuero R., Clark D.A. Miller M.J. Interleukin-10 attenuates experimental fetal growth restriction and demise. *FASEB J*, 1998;12:189–97.

83. Mattiesen L., Ekerfelt C., Berg G., Ernerudh J. Increased numbers of circulating interferon-gamma- and interleukin-4-secreting cells during normal pregnancy. *Am J Reprod Immunol*, 1998;39:362–7.

84. Lim K.J., Odukoya O.A., Ajjan R.A., Li T.C., Weetman A.P., Cooke I.D. Profile of cytokine mRNA expression in peri-implantation human endometrium. *Mol Hum Reprod*, 1998;4:77–81.

85. Hill J.A. Cytokines considered critical in pregnancy. *Am J Reprod Immunol*, 1992;28:123–6.

86. Gafter U., Sredni B., Segal J., Kalechman Y. Suppressed cell-mediated immunity and monocyte and natural killer cell activity following allogeneic immunization of women with spontaneous recurrent abortion. *J Clin Immunol*, 1997;17:408–19.

87. Piccinni M.P., Giudizi M.G., Biagiotti R., Beloni L., Giannarini L., Sampognaro S., Parronchi P., Manetti R., Annunziato F., Livi C., et al. Progesterone favors the development of human T helper cells producing Th2-type cytokines and promotes both IL-4 production and membrane CD30 expression in established Th1 cell clones. *J Immunol*, 1995;155:128–33.

88. Piccinni M.P. Romagnani S. Regulation of fetal allograft survival by a hormone-controlled Th1- and Th2-type cytokines. *Immunol Res*, 1996;15:141–50.

89. Ramierz F., Fowell D.J., Puklavec M., Simmonds S., Mason D. Glucocorticoids promote a Th2 cytokine response by CD4+ T cells in vitro. *J Immunol*, 1996;156:2406–12.

90. Petrovsky N., McNair P., Harrison L.C. Diurnal rhythms of pro-inflammatory cytokines: regulation by plasma cortisol and therapeutic implications. *Cytokine*, 1998;10:307–12.

91. Szekeres-Bartho J., Par G., Szereday L., Smart C.Y., Achatz I. Progesterone and non-specific immunologic mechanisms in pregnancy. *Am J Reprod Immunol*, 1997;38:176–82.

92. Sternberg E.M., Hill J.M., Chrousos G.P., Kamilaris T., Listwak S.J., Gold P.W., Wilder R.L. Inflammatory mediator-induced hypothalamic-pituitary-adrenal axis activation is defective in streptococcal cell wall arthritis- susceptible Lewis rats. *Proc Natl Acad Sci U.S.A.*, 1989;86:2374–8.

93. Visser J., Methorst D., Brunt T., de Kloet E.R., Nagelkerken L. Differential regulation of interleukin-10 (IL-10) and IL-12 by glucocorticoids in vitro. *Blood*, 1998;91:4255–64.

94. Lockshin M.D. Does lupus flare during pregnancy? [editorial]. *Lupus*, 1993;2:1–2.

95. Derksen R.H., Bruinse H.W., de Groot P.G., Kater L. Pregnancy in systemic lupus erythematosus: a prospective study. *Lupus*, 1994;3:149–55.

96. Petri M., Howard D., Repke J. Frequency of lupus flare in pregnancy. The Hopkins Lupus Pregnancy Center experience [see comments]. *Arthritis Rheum*, 1991;34:1538–45.

97. Urowitz M.B., Gladman D.D., Farewell V.T., Stewart J., McDonald J. Lupus and pregnancy studies. *Arthritis Rheum*, 1993;36:1392–7.

98. Lima F., Buchanan N.M., Khamashta M.A., Kerslake S., Hughes G.R. Obstetric outcome in systemic lupus erythematosus. *Semin Arthritis Rheum*, 1995;25:184–92.

99. Ruiz-Irastorza G., Lima F., Alves J., Khamashta M.A., Simpson J., Hughes G.R., Buchanan N.M. Increased rate of lupus flare during pregnancy and the puerperium: a prospective study of 78 pregnancies. *Br J Rheumatol*, 1996;35:133–8.

100. Khamashta M.A., Ruiz-Irastorza G., Hughes G.R. Systemic lupus erythematosus flares during pregnancy. *Rheum Dis Clin North Am*, 1997;23:15–30.

101. Le Huong D., Wechsler B., Vauthier-Brouzes D., Seebacher J., Lefebvre G., Bletry O., Darbois Y., Godeau P., Piette J.C. Outcome of planned pregnancies in systemic lupus erythematosus: a

prospective study on 62 pregnancies. *Br J Rheumatol*, 1997;**36**:772–7.

102. Buyon J.P. The effects of pregnancy on autoimmune diseases. *J Leukoc Biol*, 1998;**63**:281–7.

103. Petri M. Hopkins Lupus Pregnancy Center: 1987 to 1996. *Rheum Dis Clin North Am*, 1997;**23**:1–13.

104. Latman N.S. Relation of menstrual cycle phase to symptoms of rheumatoid arthritis. *Am J Med*, 1983;**74**:957–60.

105. Rudge S.R., Kowanko I.C., Drury P.L. Menstrual cyclicity of finger joint size and grip strength in patients with rheumatoid arthritis. *Ann Rheum Dis*, 1983;**42**:425–30.

106. Steinberg A.D., Steinberg B.J. Lupus disease activity associated with menstrual cycle [letter]. *J Rheumatol*, 1985;**12**:816–7.

107. Case A.M., Reid R.L. Effects of the menstrual cycle on medical disorders. *Arch Intern Med*, 1998;**158**:1405–12.

108. Yell J.A., Burge S.M. The effect of hormonal changes on cutaneous disease in lupus erythematosus. *Br J Dermatol*, 1993;**129**:18–22.

109. Pando J.A., Gourley M.F., Wilder R.L., Crofford L.J. Hormonal supplementation as treatment for cyclical rashes in patients with systemic lupus erythematosus. *J Rheumatol*, 1995;**22**:2159–62.

110. James W.H. Rheumatoid arthritis, the contraceptive pill, and androgens. *Ann Rheum Dis*, 1993;**52**:470–4.

111. Brennan P., Bankhead C., Silman A., Symmons D. Oral contraceptives and rheumatoid arthritis: results from a primary care-based incident case-control study. *Semin Arthritis Rheum*, 1997;**26**:817–23.

112. van den Brink H.R., Lems, W.F., van Everdingen A.A., Bijlsma J.W. Adjuvant oestrogen treatment increases bone mineral density in postmenopausal women with rheumatoid arthritis. *Ann Rheum Dis*, 1993;**52**:302–5.

113. MacDonald A.G., Murphy E.A., Capell H.A., Bankowska U.Z., Ralston S.H. Effects of hormone replacement therapy in rheumatoid arthritis: a double blind placebo-controlled study. *Ann Rheum Dis*, 1994;**53**:54–7.

114. Hall G.M., Daniels M., Doyle D.V., Spector T.D. Effect of hormone replacement therapy on bone mass in rheumatoid arthritis patients treated with and without steroids. *Arthritis Rheum*, 1994;**37**:1499–505.

115. Hall G.M., Daniels M., Huskisson E.C., Spector T.D. A randomised controlled trial of the effect of hormone replacement therapy on disease activity in postmenopausal rheumatoid arthritis. *Ann Rheum Dis*, 1994;**53**:112–6.

116. Hall G.M., Spector T.D., Delmas P.D. Markers of bone metabolism in postmenopausal women with rheumatoid arthritis. Effects of corticosteroids and hormone replacement therapy. *Arthritis Rheum*, 1995;**38**:902–6.

117. Van Vollenhoven R.F., McGuire J.L. Estrogen, progesterone, and testosterone: can they be used to treat autoimmune diseases? *Cleve Clin J Med*, 1994;**61**:276–84.

118. Sanchez-Guerrero J., Liang M.H., Karlson E.W., Hunter D.J., Colditz G.A. Postmenopausal estrogen therapy and the risk for developing systemic lupus erythematosus [see comments]. *Ann Intern Med*, 1995;**122**:430–3.

119. Liang M.H., Karlson E.W. Female hormone therapy and the risk of developing or exacerbating systemic lupus erythematosus or rheumatoid arthritis. *Proc Assoc Am Physicians*, 1996;**108**:25–8.

120. Buyon J.P. Oral contraceptives in women with systemic lupus erythematosus. *Ann Med Interne*, 1996;**147**:259–64.

121. Huong D.L., Wechsler B., Piette J.C., Arfi S., Gallinari C., Darbois Y., Frances C., Godeau P. Risks of ovulation-induction therapy in systemic lupus erythematosus. *Br J Rheumatol*, 1996;**35**:1184–6.

122. Chrousos G.P., Gold P.W. The concepts of stress and stress system disorders. Overview of physical and behavioral homeostasis [published erratum appears in JAMA, 1992;**268**:200]. *JAMA*, 1992;**267**:1244–52.

123. Chrousos G.P. The hypothalamic-pituitary-adrenal axis and immune-mediated inflammation [see comments]. *N Engl J Med*, 1995;**332**:1351–62.

124. Chikanza I.C., Grossman A.S. Hypothalamic-pituitary-mediated immunomodulation: arginine vasopressin is a neuroendocrine immune mediator. *Br J Rheumatol*, 1998;**37**:131–6.

125. Torpy D.J., Chrousos G.P. The three-way interactions between the hypothalamic-pituitary-adrenal and gonadal axes and the immune system. *Baillieres Clin Rheumatol*, 1996;**10**:181–98.

126. Vamvakopoulos N.C., Chrousos G.P. Evidence of direct estrogenic regulation of human corticotropin- releasing hormone gene expression. Potential implications for the sexual dimophism of the stress response and immune/inflammatory reaction. *J Clin Invest*, 1993;**92**:1896–902.

127. Haas D.A., George S.R. Estradiol or ovariectomy decreases CRF synthesis in hypothalamus. *Brain Res Bull*, 1989;**23**:215–8.

128. Bohler H.C., Jr., Zoeller R.T., King J.C., Rubin B.S., Weber R., Merriam G.R. Corticotropin releasing hormone mRNA is elevated on the afternoon of proestrus in the parvocellular paraventricular nuclei of the female rat. *Brain Res Mol Brain Res*, 1990;**8**:259–62.

129. Galucci W.T., Baum A., Laue L., Rabin D.S., Chrousos G.P., Gold P.W., Kling M.A. Sex differences in sensitivity of the hypothalamic-pituitary-adrenal axis. *Health Psychol*, 1993;**12**:420–5.

130. Lindholm J., Schultz-Moller N. Plasma and urinary cortisol in pregnancy and during estrogen-gestagen treatment. *Scand J Clin Lab Invest*, 1973;**31**:119–22.

131. Kirschbaum C., Schommer N., Federenko I., Gaab J., Neumann O., Oellers M., Rohleder N., Untiedt A., Hanker J., Pirke K.M., Hellhammer D.H. Short-term estradiol treatment enhances pituitary-adrenal axis and sympathetic responses to psychosocial stress in healthy young men [see comments]. *J Clin Endocrinol Metab*, 1996;**81**:3639–43.

132. Peiffer A., Lapointe B., Barden N. Hormonal regulation of type II glucocorticoid receptor messenger ribonucleic acid in rat brain. *Endocrinology*, 1991;**129**:2166–74.

133. Chikanza I.C., Petrou P., Kingsley G., Chrousos G., Panayi G.S. Defective hypothalamic response to immune and inflammatory stimuli in patients with rheumatoid arthritis [see comments]. *Arthritis Rheum*, 1992;**35**:1281–8.

134. Crofford L.J., Kalogeras K.T., Mastorakos G., Magiakou M.A., Wells J., Kanik K.S., Gold P.W., Chrousos G.P., Wilder R.L. Circadian relationships between interleukin (IL)-6 and hypothalamic- pituitary-adrenal axis hormones: failure of IL-6 to cause sustained hypercortisolism in patients with early untreated rheumatoid arthritis. *J Clin Endocrinol Metab*, 1997;**82**:1279–83.

135. Crofford L.J., Sano H., Karalis K., Friedman T.C., Epps H.R., Remmers E.F., Mathern P., Chrousos G.P., Wilder R.L. Corticotropin-releasing hormone in synovial fluids and tissues of patients with rheumatoid arthritis and osteoarthritis. *J Immunol*, 1993;**151**:1587–96.

136. Crofford L.J., Sano H., Karalis K., Webster E.L., Goldmuntz E.A., Chrousos G.P., Wilder R.L. Local secretion of corticotropin-releasing hormone in the joints of Lewis rats with inflammatory arthritis. *J Clin Invest*, 1992;**90**:2555–64.

137. Crofford LJ, Sano H, Karalis K, Webster EA, Friedman TC, Chrousos GP, Wilder RL. Local expression of corticotropin-releasing hormone in inflammatory arthritis. *An NY Acad Sci*, 1995;**771**:459–71.

138. Baerwald C.G., Panayi G.S., Lanchbury J.S. Corticotropin releasing hormone promoter region polymorphisms in rheumatoid arthritis. *J Rheumatol*, 1997;**24**:215–6.

139. Segal B.M., Dwyer B.K., Shevach E.M. An interleukin (IL)-10/IL-12 immunoregulatory circuit controls susceptibility to autoimmune disease. *J Exp Med*, 1998;**187**:537–46.

140. Greenstein B.D., de Bridges E.F., Fitzpatrick F.T. Aromatase inhibitors regenerate the thymus in aging male rats. *Int J Immunopharmcol*, 1992;**14**:541–53.

141. Sternberg E.M., Young W.S.D., Bernardini R., Calogero A.E., Chrousos G.P., Gold P.W., Wilder R.L. A central nervous system defect in biosynthesis of corticotropin-releasing hormone is associated with susceptibility to streptococcal cell wall-induced arthritis in Lewis rats. *Proc Natl Acad Sci USA*, 1989;**86**:4771–5.

142. Wilder R.L. Hormones and autoimmunity: animal models of arthritis. *Baillieres Clin Rheumatol*, 1996;**10**:259–71.

143. Harkness J.A., Richter M.B., Panayi G.S., Van de Pette K., Unger A., Pownall R., Geddawi M. Circadian variation in disease activity in rheumatoid arthritis. *Br Med J (Clin Res Ed)*, 1982;**284**:551–4.

144. Herold M., Gunther R. Circadian rhythm of C-reactive protein in patients with rheumatoid arthritis. *Prog Clin Biol Res*, 1987;**227B**:271–9.

145. Neeck G., Federlin K., Graef V., Rusch D., Schmidt K.L. Adrenal secretion of cortisol in patients with rheumatoid arthritis. *J Rheumatol*, 1990;**17**:24–9.

146. Bellamy N., Sothern R.B., Campbell J., Buchanan W.W. Circadian rhythm in pain, stiffness, and manual dexterity in rheumatoid arthritis: relation between discomfort and disability. *Ann Rheum Dis*, 1991;**50**:243–8.

147. Olsen N.J., Brooks R.H., Furst D. Variability of immunologic and clinical features in patients with rheumatoid arthritis studied over 24 hours. *J Rheumatol*, 1993;**20**:940–3.

148. Masera R.G., Carignola R., Staurenghi A.H., Sartori M.L., Lazzero A., Griot G., Angeli A. Altered circadian rhythms of natural killer (NK) cell activity in patients with autoimmune rheumatic diseases. *Chronobiologia*, 1994;**21**:127–32.

149. Arvidson N.G., Gudbjornsson B., Elfman L., Ryden A.C., Totterman T.H., Hallgren R. Circadian rhythm of serum interleukin-6 in rheumatoid arthritis. *Ann Rheum Dis*, 1994;**53**:521–4.

150. Petrovsky N., Harrison L.C. The chronobiology of human cytokine production. *Int Rev Immunol*, 1998;**16**:635–49.

151. Kirwan J.R. The effect of glucocorticoids on joint destruction in rheumatoid arthritis. The Arthritis and Rheumatism Council Low-Dose Glucocorticoid Study Group [see comments]. *N Engl J Med*, 1995;**333**:142–6.

152. Yakushiji F., Kita M., Hiroi N., Ueshiba H., Monma I., Miyachi Y. Exacerbation of rheumatoid arthritis after removal of adrenal adenoma in Cushing's syndrome. *Endocr J*, 1995;**42**:219–23.

153. Potter P.T., Zautra A.J. Stressful life events' effects on rheumatoid arthritis disease activity. *J Consult Clin Psychol*, 1997;**65**:319–23.

154. Kanik K.S., Chrousos G.P., Yarboro C.H., Schumacher H.R., Wilder R.L. Pituitary-adrenal hormonal abnormalities in patients with new-onset synovitis. *Arthritis Rheum*, 1995;**38**(suppl.):1453.

155. Hall J., Morand E.F., Medbak S., Zaman M., Perry L., Goulding N.J., Maddison P.J., O'Hare J.P. Abnormal hypothalamic-pituitary-adrenal axis function in rheumatoid arthritis. Effects of non-steroidal antiinflammatory drugs and water immersion [see comments]. *Arthritis Rheum*, 1994;**37**:1132–7.

156. Jorgensen C., Bressot N., Bologna C., Sany J.. Dysregulation of the hypothalamo-pituitary axis in rheumatoid arthritis. *J Rheumatol*, 1995;**22**:1829–33.

157. Saldanha C., Tougas G., Grace E. Evidence for anti-inflammatory effect of normal circulating plasma cortisol. *Clin Exp Rheumatol*, 1986;**4**:365–6.

158. Masi A.T., Josipovic D.B., Jefferson W.E. Low adrenal androgenic-anabolic steroids in women with rheumatoid arthritis (RA): gas-liquid chromatographic studies of RA patients and matched normal control women indicating decreased 11-deoxy-17- ketosteroid excretion. *Semin Arthritis Rheum*, 1984;**14**:1–23.

159. Waage A., Bakke O. Glucocorticoids suppress the production of tumour necrosis factor by lipopolysaccharide-stimulated human monocytes. *Immunology*, 1988;**63**:299–302.

160. Padgett D.A., Loria R.M. Endocrine regulation of murine macrophage function: effects of dehydroepiandrosterone, androstenediol, and androstenetriol. *J Neuroimmunol*, 1998;**84**:61–8.

161. Di Santo E., Foddi M.C., Ricciardi-Castagnoli P., Mennini T., Ghezzi P. DHEAS inhibits TNF production in monocytes, astrocytes and microglial cells. *Neuroimmunomodulation*, 1996;**3**:285–8.

162. Inserra P., Zhang Z., Ardestani S.K., Araghi-Niknam M., Liang B., Jiang S., Shaw D., Molitor M., Elliott K., Watson R.R. Modulation of cytokine production by dehydroepiandrosterone (DHEA) plus melatonin (MLT) supplementation of old mice. *Proc Soc Exp Biol Med*, 1998;**218**:76–82.

163. Spencer N.F., Norton S.D., Harrison L.L., Li G.Z., Daynes R.A. Dysregulation of IL-10 production with aging: possible linkage to the age-associated decline in DHEA and its sulfated derivative. *Exp Gerontol*, 1996;**31**:393–408.

164. Norton S.D., Harrison L.L., Yowell R., Araneo B.A. Administration of dehydroepiandrosterone sulfate retards onset but not progression of autoimmune disease in NZB/W mice. *Autoimmunity*, 1997;**26**:161–71.

165. Panina-Bordignon P., Mazzeo D., Lucia P.D., D'Ambrosio D., Lang R., Fabbri L., Self C., Sinigaglia F. Beta2-agonists prevent Th1 development by selective inhibition of interleukin, 12. *J Clin Invest*, 1997;**100**:1513–19.

166. Guirao X., Kumar A., Katz J., Smith M., Lin E., Keogh C., Calvano S.E., Lowry S.F. Catecholamines increase monocyte TNF receptors and inhibit TNF through beta 2-adrenoreceptor activation. *Am J Physiol*, 1997;**273**:E1203–8.

167. Cheng J.B., Watson J.W., Pazoles C.J., Eskra J.D., Griffiths R.J., Cohan V.L., Turner C.R., Showell H.J., Pettipher E.R. The phosphodiesterase type 4 (PDE4) inhibitor CP-80, 633 elevates plasma cyclic AMP levels and decreases tumor necrosis factor-alpha (TNFalpha) production in mice: effect of adrenalectomy. *J Pharmacol Exp Ther*, 1997;**280**:621–6.

168. Elenkov I.J., Hasko G., Kovacs K.J., Vizi E.S. Modulation of lipopolysaccharide-induced tumor necrosis factor-alpha production by selective alpha- and beta-adrenergic drugs in mice. *J Neuroimmunol*, 1995;**61**:123-31.

169. Woiciechowsky C., Asadullah K., Nestler D., Eberhardt B., Platzer C., Schoning B., Glockner F., Lanksch W.R., Volk H.D., Docke W.D. Sympathetic activation triggers systemic interleukin-10 release in immunodepression induced by brain injury. *Nat Med*, 1998;**4**:808–13.

170. Kavelaars A., van de Pol M., Zijlstra J., Heijnen C.J. Beta 2-adrenergic activation enhances interleukin-8 production by human monocytes. *J Neuroimmunol*, 1997;**77**:211–6.

171. Deshpande R., Khalili H., Pergolizzi R.G., Michael S.D., Chang M.D. Estradiol down-regulates LPS-induced cytokine production and NFkB activation in murine macrophages. *Am J Reprod Immunol*, 1997;**38**:46–54.

172. Chao T.C., Van Alten P.J., Greager J.A., Walter R.J. Steroid sex hormones regulate the release of tumor necrosis factor by macrophages. *Cell Immunol*, 1995;**160**:43–9.

19 | *Imaging*

Dolores Kalden-Nemeth and Bernhard Manger

Introduction

The field of radiology has undergone dramatic changes over the past 10 years as a consequence of the rapid technical development of new imaging modalities. It is the aim of this chapter to give an overview of those imaging tools available to the rheumatologist in order to optimize their use in a clinical setting.

Plain film radiography

For the imaging of arthritis, plain film radiography remains the method of choice for the initial examination to evaluate bone and soft tissue changes. Conventional radiography gives an overview of the distribution of joint lesions, reduction of the radiographic joint space, osteopenia, sclerosis, subchondral cyst formation and erosions, osteophytes, periosteal reactions, and soft tissue calcifications to differentiate between degenerative, inflammatory, infectious, and metabolic conditions.

In spite of the availability of numerous technologically sophisticated modalities for the imaging of RA, which offer a high degree of sensitivity and specificity, plain film radiography has maintained its position as the 'work horse' in the evaluation of articular disease. As the method of choice for the initial examination, it accurately evaluates even subtle changes in the bone and, although a definite diagnosis might not immediately be possible, the type of joints affected, the distribution of lesions, and the location and extent of soft tissue involvement usually allow a differential diagnosis. Also, during the course of monitoring therapy, standard radiographic techniques are employed to directly or indirectly visualize disease activity. Depending on the state of the disease, radiographic signs can be subtle or indirect in terms of soft tissue swelling, joint space narrowing, as a consequence of cartilage thinning, or joint space widening as an indication of joint effusion. Juxta-articular osteoporosis is also of the non-specific changes which can confirm the clinical impression of an inflammatory process.

Film–screen combinations

To visualize even discrete abnormalities in conventional radiography it is imperative that among the numerous film–screen combinations available, a perfectly functioning film, intensifying screen, and cassette system are employed. An X-ray film is in principle a photographic film, modified to meet the needs of medical radiography. Today, there are several types of X-ray films available, one being the direct-exposure film, which has a thick emulsion to absorb more efficiently X-rays from the beam and reduce the required exposure level. However, direct-exposure films cannot be processed in automatic film processors. Therefore screen-type films are designed for exposure with light from intensifying screens. Their thinner emulsions are not sensitive to X-rays, but are sensitive to the light emitted by the screens. Among screen-type films there are several different types, most of which have a double emulsion and high speed. Single-emulsion film has a lower speed and, when used with a single screen, it can produce radiographs with precise detail; these are therefore the type of films used in osteoradiology.

In the course of searching for substances which would more efficiently absorb X-rays as a result of their higher specific weight, a group of chemical compounds that all contained what chemists refer to as 'rare earth phosphors', which convert X-rays to light approximately four times more efficiently than calcium tungstate, was discovered. This means that rare earth phosphors have an intrinsic efficiency of 20 per cent, compared with only 5 per cent for calcium tungstate. Their principal advantage over other screens is their speed. Although they are manufactured with different speed levels, each of these is approximately twice as fast as the corresponding calcium tungstate screen.

Therefore, the advantages of using rare earth screens are obvious: they require less exposure to produce the same density on a radiographic film, and consequently the patient exposure dose is reduced. Also, the use of a shorter exposure time reduces the effects of patient movements and therefore increases the detail sharpness.

A given film–screen combination usually has a definite impact on the dose and image quality of a radiograph. The sensitivity of the film-screen combination determines how much radiation is necessary to obtain an image of high quality. The sensitivity of a film–screen combination S (speed) is inversely proportional to the particular exposure level that is necessary to obtain a density D = 1 above fog and background. Fog describes the density that is inherent in the base and emulsion. The base, film tint, and emulsion all produce a small amount of blackening. This dose is called K_S and is defined by the formula $S = (1000 \ \mu Gy/\mu Gy)$. The value S, that is the sensitivity or speed of a given film–screen combination, is stated by the manufacturer, and from this value the required dose can be calculated, using the formula $K_S \ (\mu Gy) = (1000 \ \mu Gy/S)$. The value of the speed (S) in general radiology usually lies between 50 for very insensitive and 1200 for very sensitive film–screen combinations. The sensitivity S for mammography systems lies between 6 and 25. It is obvious that the film speed is inversely proportional to the exposure dose. The lower the exposure dose required to produce a given density on a particular film, the higher the film speed. Conversely, films requiring long exposures to obtain the given density have lower film speeds. The film speed is an important consideration in the selection of radiographic films: higher speed films require less exposure to produce a given density and result in less radiation exposure to the patient, but also give poorer fine-detail resolution. Besides the specification of the S value as the exact measure of the sensitivity for a film–screen combination, for simplified orientation frequently only the sensitivity class is given. In rheumatology the speed used in usually 100 for hands, feet, and shoulders and 200 for shoulder, elbow, hip, and cervical spine.

Digital radiography

The very well known tendency to digitize radiological images in computed tomography (CT), magnetic resonance imaging (MRI), digital subtraction angiology (DSA), and ultrasound (US) is also making inroads in the field of conventional radiology. Imaging considerations are the major reasons but economic advantages are also gradually emerging. Instead of producing a radiological image using the classical film–screen combination method, with digital projection radiography computers develop the image information. The new possibilities for developing and storing digital information can enhance the image quality, reduce the radiation exposure, offer more flexible image documentation, and permit immediate access to radiographs via PACS (Picture Archiving and Communication System).

The main disadvantage of digital radiography is the limited resolution when compared with conventional films. The main advantage, however, is the possibility to produce diagnostic films with lower exposure levels and reduce repeating rates, because of the wide latitude of the system. This wide exposure latitude and the high sensitivity of the system permit excellent images of both bone and soft tissue densities from a single exposure.

Digital intensification fluoroscopy

In the gastrointestinal tract the use of digital intensification fluoroscopy has proven to be of great advantage. Besides offering the possibility of dose reduction, the system offers the possibility of serial imaging with up to eight images per second. Also advantageous is the possibility of last image hold, which makes the last image immediately available. In skeletal diagnostics, however, intensification fluoroscopy has not satisfied the demands placed on a diagnostic system. To depict subperiosteal changes, a very high resolution system is mandatory[1-4].

Digital luminescence radiography

Since 1985, digital luminescence radiography has been in clinical use. Here, the traditional film–screen cassette system is replaced by a reusable phosphor screen together with digital image acquisition and processing. The main advantage is a high-resolution capability of between 2.5 and 5 Lp/mm. The evaluation of the X-ray, however, has to be from the X-ray photograph, since imaging on the monitor with a matrix of 1024 ×1024 pixels, instead of 2000 ×2000 pixels read-out by the laser imager, is not satisfactory in terms of resolution. By contrast, with intensification fluoroscopy, digital luminescence radiography offers sufficient resolution for use in skeletal radiology. Compared to conventional film–screen combinations, additional information can be gained in terms of soft tissue structure[5-7].

Characteristic radiological findings in conventional radiography on routine and special views

General radiographic descriptions of rheumatoid arthritis are:

(1) soft tissue alterations, such as fusiform swelling around joints secondary to effusions and synovitis;

(2) reduced bone density in terms of juxta-articular osteoporosis, which in a later stage can progress to generalized osteoporosis (Fig. 19.1);

(3) discontinuity in the subchondral 'white line' (Fig. 19.2);

(4) loss of joint space—although joint space may initially appear wide due to distension, because of effusion and pannus formation, the subsequent uniform pattern of the destruction of cartilage will result in considerable joint space narrowing;

(5) erosive changes, first depicted as marginal destructions at the bare area; later, when the disease progresses to the point of cartilage destruction, subchondral erosions develop; hypertrophic bone changes, such as osteophyte formation, which may develop in the course of secondary osteoarthritis;

(6) synovial cyst formation—subchondral cysts are common and may communicate with the synovium, especially in the knee and hip, and develop to such a size that the stability of the joint can be endangered or a tumor can be mimicked (Fig. 19.3);

(7) subluxations due to ligamentous laxity and tendon ruptures or contractures leading to deformities and functional alterations;

(8) symmetrical distribution of changes are most frequent in the hands and feet, and the shoulders.

Hands and wrists

The posteroanterior (PA) and Norgaard views of the hand and wrist are the standard views and provide an overview of soft-tissue abnormalities and osseous changes. The Norgaard view, or the so called 'ball catcher', is basically an anterioposterior oblique view to demonstrate the earliest erosive changes which frequently begin at the base of the proximal phalanges and the articulation between the triquetrum and pisiform.

The radiographic features in hands and wrists of RA patients can be separated into early and late changes. Early changes involve periarticular soft-tissue swelling due to edema and synovitis and periarticular osteoporosis in a symmetrical distribution due to hyperemia of the affected joints. For differential diagnosis, the site of the pathological changes is important. In RA patients the joints first involved are the MCP joints. Late changes include erosions, usually beginning at the bare bone areas, those areas of a joint which are not protected by cartilage, for example capsular insertion sides, the ulna styloid and the triquetrum, pan-carpal involvement, MCP ulnar deviation, buttonière, and swan-neck deformity.

Of great importance for the differential diagnosis is the distribution of joint lesions. In RA patients the PIPs and MCPs are involved as well as the carpus while the DIPs are spared. Another differential diagnostic criterion is that there is usually no new bone formation except in the case of postinflammatory arthrosis with osteophyte formation.

Elbows and shoulders

Correct imaging of the shoulders include anterioposterior views in internal and external rotation. In addition, to get a view of the glenohumeral joint without superimposition of images, a 40° posterior oblique special view is necessary.

The radiographic features of shoulder involvement include generalized osteoporosis, uniform narrowing of all compartments (glenohumeral, acromiohumeral, and acromio-clavicular joint) with an upward migration of the humeral head. Associated rotator cuff tears are frequent, resulting from the narrowing between the humerus and acromion. If erosions are present, they are usually found at the rotator cuff attachment. As in all other joints affected by RA, there may be cyst formation. Frequent findings are also lysis of the distal clavicle (Fig. 19.4) and erosions of the proximal end in the sternoclavicular joint.

Elbow involvement is usually symmetrical and begins with uniform joint-space narrowing and the extinction of the subchondral white line. Later in the course of the disease, there may

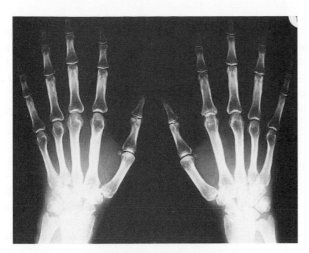

Fig. 19.1   Juxta-articular osteoporosis.

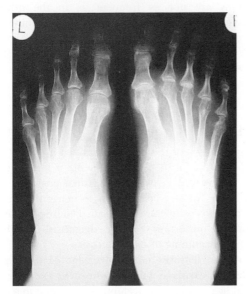

Fig. 19.2   Interruption of subchondral white line; typical distribution of destructions at the medial side of the MTPs beginning from the lateral aspect of the foot.

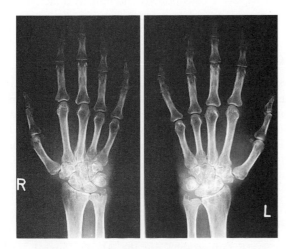

Fig. 19.3   Multiple synovial cysts in the carpal bones.

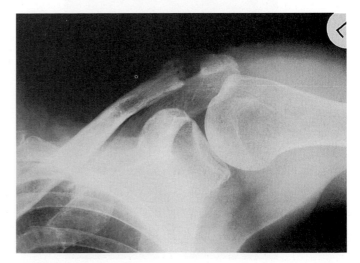

Fig. 19.4   Lysis of distal clavicle.

be a complete destruction of the joint. For differential diagnostic purposes it is helpful to know that there is initially no reparative bone formation (Fig. 19.5a and b).

The feet

The standard views are AP, oblique, and lateral to obtain a radiograph of the calcaneus. Early involvement begins in the MTP joints at the lateral side of the foot and progresses medially, the first sign being discrete interruptions of the continuity of the white cortical line. With disease progression, massive erosive changes around the MTPs and PIPs develop. Additionally, subluxations of the proximal phalanges in the fibular direction occur due to the soft-tissue changes in the capsule with hallux valgus deformity in the big toe. The tarsal bones are uniformly involved with joint-space narrowing ultimately resulting in ankylosis.

The knees

Radiographs of the knees should be taken in an AP and slightly flexed lateral view. The most distinctive initial radiographic feature is soft tissue swelling, juxta-articular osteoporosis, and a symmetrical concentric loss of joint space due to destruction of cartilage that affects all three compartments (medial, lateral, patellofemoral). There is no sign of reparative bone formation, and erosions are not as frequent as in the other joints. Intraosseus cyst formation, however, is a very common feature in knees affected by RA. Cysts develop as a consequence of invasion of pannus into the bone. A different kind of cyst, the Baker's cyst, is a synovial cyst extending into the soft tissue in the posterior compartment of the knee, and is a frequent occurrence in RA.

The hip

Radiographic views of the hip are obtained in an AP and frog-leg lateral position. In the AP view the hip is internally rotated. To image the femoral neck in an optimal position, the hip is abducted in the frog-leg lateral view to image the anterior and posterior portions of the femoral head. The frog-leg lateral view is particularly important for the diagnosis of subchondral lucency in the beginning of osteonecrosis.

Radiographic features of involvement of the hip include uniform loss of cartilage with a consequent axial migration of the femoral head within the acetabulum resulting in a concentric loss of joint space. With progressive migration of the femoral head, protrusion of the acetabulum may occur. It is important to note that affection of the hips is symmetrical. As in other joints, there may be severe osteoporosis and initially a lack of reparative bone formation such as osteophytes.

Sacroiliac joint

Imaging the sacroiliac joint is performed in a supine position with the tube angled to 30° towards the head. SI joint involvement usually leads to uniform narrowing of joint space, possibly resulting in ankylosis around the true synovial part of the SI joint. Erosions usually occur in a discrete way. Involvement of the SI joint in RA patients is not frequent and usually occurs at a very late state of the disease.

Cervical spine

The necessary radiographs are the AP, the lateral, and the lateral-flexed view. The later is the most important view since it

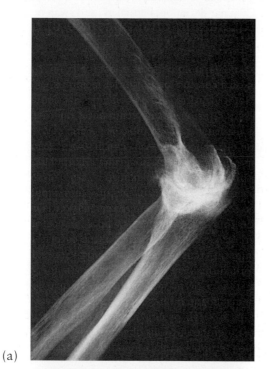

(a)

(b)

Fig. 19.5   Complete destruction of elbow.

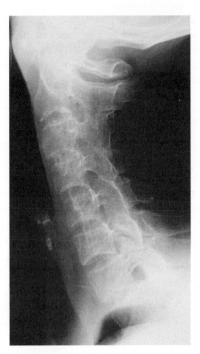

Fig. 19.6 Cervical spine: ankylosis involving only vertebral bodies and small vertebral joints, sparing processus spinosi.

demonstrates the atlantodental joint space, possible erosions of the dens and cervical subluxations. The cervical spine is frequently involved in patients with rheumatoid arthritis. The most common features are abnormalities in the atlantoaxial region. Here, laxity of the transverse ligament, which holds the odontoid to the atlas, is demonstrated in the lateral view resulting in a joint-space widening (gap > 5 mm) which may require surgical intervention. Also frequently found are apophyseal joints leading to disc-space loss and subluxations (Fig. 19.6).

Temporomandibular joint

Involvement of the temporomandibular-joint is frequent. The dominant radiographic features are osteoporosis, erosions, and flattening of the glenoid fossa. Before the age of MRI these changes were demonstrated by conventional tomography. Today, however, MRI is the procedure of choice to evaluate the temporomandibular joint following screening with conventional radiographs.

Conventional tomography

Conventional tomography, or body section radiography, is a technique utilizing geometric principles to produce an image in which the objects in a selected plane remain well defined on the radiograph, while those above and below this plane are blurred. Since there have been enormous technical advances in other such imaging modalities as 3D spiral CT image acquisition and thin-slice spiral CT with multiplanar reconstruction, the indications

for conventional tomography in general, and concerning RA patients in particular, are nowadays very limited.

Computed tomography

Sequential computed tomography

As with conventional tomography, computed tomography (CT) images a section or a slice of a patient. The basis for image acquisition in computed tomography is an X-ray beam, which is summed to a fan beam circulating simultaneously with a detector array around the patient, with the absorption measured at various projections and then fed to a computer. Image reconstruction is performed by a complicated mathematical process, and the various absorption values are then transformed to a numerical matrix. Transforming this numerical matrix to analog gray values then gives an image of differently absorbing structures.

There is a linear relationship between the density and the absorption coefficient, a constant value characterizing the tissue with respect to its capacity for the absorption of radiation. By internal calibration, the density of water is defined as 0 and that of air as −1000. Density values are measured in Hounsfield units (HU). Density units are directly proportional to the linear absorption coefficient.

'Helical' or 'spiral' computed tomography

Whereas in sectional computed tomography each individual slice is exposed, helical computed tomography represents the principle of total volume scanning. Here the patient is moved through the gantry while the X-ray tube revolves a number of times around the patient, so that a data file is acquired for a complete volume. The geometrical path of data acquisition is a spiral, or a helix.

There are various advantages to spiral computed tomography. One is the shortening of the scanning time. For example a distanced of 60 cm can be scanned within 1 minute. Secondly, Spiral CT is a volume scanning method, allowing for considerable variation in the possibilities for reconstruction, so that overlapping slices can be reconstructed at any given location, thus reducing the problems arising due to the partial volume effect. The partial volume effect is a physical phenomenon which occurs during image reconstruction in computed tomography, according to which border lines between different volumes are only partly filled by a structure. As a consequence, there is an averaging of density over the volume, resulting in the blurring of structures at the interface of neighboring volumes. Also, scanning a relatively large volume in a single breath-hold permits gap-free images. In conventional CT, sectional scanning with a new breath-hold for each scan causes gaps between scans because of variations in breathing. This fact is especially important when performing a thorax scan. Finally, contrast medium application can be optimized in the sense that the flow of contrast medium and the scanning speed can be adjusted, which is usually done by computerized automated injection pumps. Because of the timed application of a contrast medium bolus and the shorter scan time, the imaging of vessels can be optimized. With Spiral CT, angiography also becomes possible. By means of MIP (Maximum Intensity Projection) and 3D surface rendering techniques, isolated imaging of vessels becomes possible, so that vessel anatomy and pathology may be evaluated in a three-dimensional technique.

Nevertheless, there are a number of disadvantages, one of these being the limited applicable dose, which consequently results in a worsening of image quality and a higher degree of noise, because the tube is in continuous use up to about 60 seconds and cannot cool down between slices, as in conventional CT. Another disadvantage is that images are not immediately available, since data acquisition and evaluation require a definite time.

High-resolution computed tomography

High-resolution CT means ultra-thin slices with collimation to a width of 1 to 2 mm by a special reconstruction algorithm. In general, the narrower the collimation width the higher the noise. Noise can be reduced by increasing the radiation intensity. This means ultimately that high-resolution computed tomography (HR CT) implies a higher exposure to radiation than standard CT scanning with a collimation width of 5 to 10 mm. High-resolution CT is therefore usually used in addition to, and not instead of, conventional CT, which first covers the entire thoracic space. Afterwards, high-resolution CT is then preformed for three representative levels:

(1) level of the aortic arch;

(2) level of the tracheal bifurcation; and

(3) level of the diaphragm.

HR CT renders the secondary lobuli and the septum of the interlobular space visible. The most frequent indication for HR CT is interstitial lung disease: ground glass opacities, cystic parenchymal defects, reticular or reticular-nodular pattern of interstitial pathology, or thickening of the interlobular septation (Fig. 19.7a–j).

Pulmonary manifestations in RA patients

The major extra-articular manifestations of RA that are found in the thorax are pleural effusion, interstitial fibrosis, pulmonary nodes, and very rare cases of pneumonitis.

Plain film

Plain film radiographs are usually the procedure of choice for screening for pulmonary involvement of RA. Pleural effusions can be easily depicted in the lateral radiograph. Definite interstitial fibrosis should also not be a problem to diagnose on conventional radiographs. The same is the case for pulmonary nodules. Pneumonitis, however, is difficult to view on conventional radiographs, even on a very high quality radiograph.

'Helical' versus 'sequential' CT

Whenever there is a suspicion of pulmonary involvement, which can not be proven in plain film radiographs, computed tomography should be employed. If the patient can co-operate, in the sense that he can hold his breath for approximately 20 seconds, helical computed tomography is to be given preference over sequential CT for reasons mentioned before.

High resolution CT

Especially if there is a clinical suspicion of early interstitial fibrosis but plain film radiographs and computed tomography are not conclusive, high resolution scanning should be used to screen for discrete changes in the interstitium.

Ultrasonography in rheumatoid arthritis

General considerations

Within the last decade, ultrasonograpy (USG) of joints and periarticular tissues has become a well-established imaging technique for the diagnosis and follow-up of patients with RA. Because water is the best ultrasound transducing substance in the body, USG is especially useful for evaluating soft tissue structures, which contain fluid such as effusions, cysts, or edematous synovitic tissue. Because the sound waves used can not penetrate bony surfaces, superficial lesions are more easily examined than deep-seated lesions. Dynamic assessment of joint movements is easily performed and sometimes helps to enhance pathological alterations. USG is a non-invasive method, which is not inconvenient to the patient, does not involve radiation, and can be repeated as often as necessary, which makes it helpful for therapy monitoring.

Technical equipment

The higher the frequency of ultrasound waves, the better is the imaging quality, but the lower is the depth of tissue penetration. For larger joints, linear transducers with 5 to 7.5 MHz are generally used. For smaller joints of hands and feet, technical development of recent years has produced transducers of increasingly higher frequencies from 10 up to 20 MHz. With these high-frequency transducers excellent imaging of finger joints and even minimal lesions of tendons and tendon sheaths of fingers and toes became possible[8].

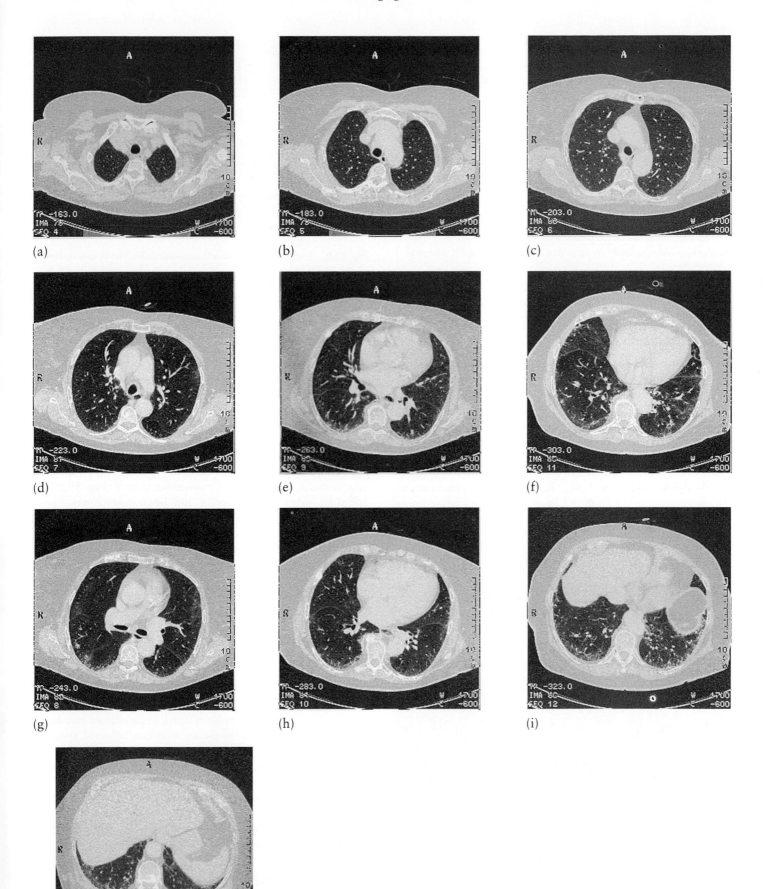

(a)

(b)

(c)

(d)

(e)

(f)

(g)

(h)

(i)

(j)

Fig. 19.7 a–j High resolution CT of RA patient with the beginning of basal and peripheral fibrosis with thickened interlobular septi.

Teaching and training

Of all imaging modalities, ultrasound is the most operator-dependent. Therefore, training and experience of the examiner determine the value of the diagnostic information of USG. While the procedure itself is harmless to the patient, the only harm that can be done is by inexperienced interpretation of obtained images. To ensure the quality of USG education, national societies in various countries hold courses and have established educational criteria for training. This modality is most valuable in a setting in which the clinical rheumatologist, who took the patients history and clinical examination, is trained to perform and interpret the ultrasound examination. Thus, ultrasound waves can become the physicians extended finger. Joint USG can be performed routinely in an office setting, expand a rheumatologist diagnostic potential, save time, and reduce expenses[9,10].

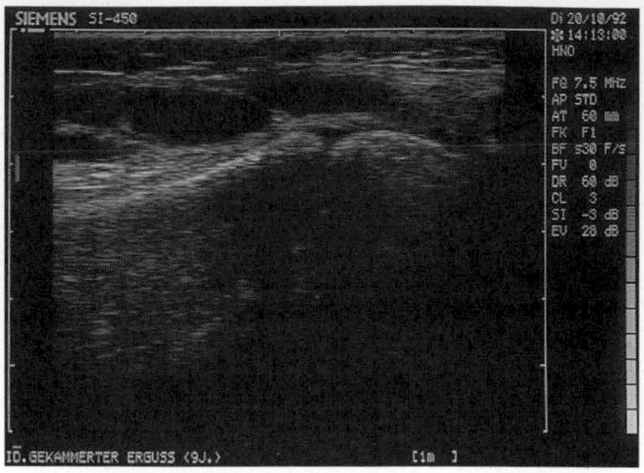

Fig. 19.9 Juvenile arthritis in a 9-year-old child. The epiphyseal plate of the femur is clearly shown beside a large knee joint effusion with septations.

Joint sonography

Bone and cartilage

Bony surfaces are the anatomic landmarks that allow orientation and classification of pathological structures during USG. The intensity of reflection at a bone surface depends on the differences in its sound transducing qualities in comparison to the surrounding tissues. Ultrasound wave frequencies used for USG are not able to penetrate into bone. Therefore, imaging of intra-articular lesions is usually not possible, neither is the differentiation of cortical and trabecular areas of the bone. The detection of erosions in RA is still the domain of conventional roentgenography. USG will not be able to replace conventional radiological diagnosis in this field. However, in specific cases it may be possible to detect bony erosions earlier by USG than by plain X-ray, because ultrasonography is a sectional imaging technique[11] (Figs 19.8). Whether USG with high frequency transducers is able to compete with radiography or MRI in the detection of erosions at small joints of hands and feet in early arthritis is currently under investigation. It is important to confirm any suspected erosion by USG in a second section in a 90° angle because the echogenicity of bone also depends on the angle in which it is met by the ultrasound beam. Those parts of the bone that are met tangentially can fail to produce an echo and mimic a surface defect ('pseudo-erosion') (Fig. 19.9). In addition, other alterations of the bone surface are easily detected by USG such as osteophytes, exostoses, or epiphyseal plates (Fig. 19.9). Hyaline cartilage is generally echo-free when it is met at a 90° angle by the ultrasound beam. The layer of hyaline cartilage can therefore be visualized in various joints using USG[12].

Synovitis

The more inflammatory, exudative, and edematous a connective tissue process is, the easier it is detected by USG. Because of its high water content and few internal structures, which could cause sound reflection, synovial membrane presents as very hypoechoic, sometimes even almost echo-free, tissue (Fig. 19.10). This creates the problem that it is sometimes very hard, if not impossible, to differentiate between inflamed synovial tissue and joint effusion. This can be particularly difficult if the joint effusion contains internal echoes (older effusions, hemarthrosis, pus). One way out of this diagnostic dilemma might be the use of power doppler sonography. This allows the visualization of blood flow in the hyperperfused parts of the inflamed synovial tissue and thus enables a differentiation from exudate[13] (Fig. 19.11).

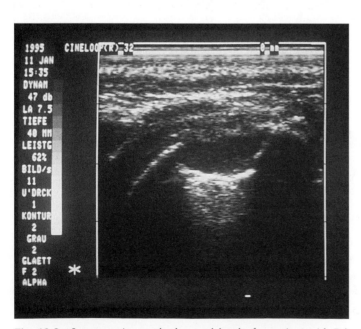

Fig. 19.8 Large erosion at the humeral head of a patient with RA shown in an anterior transverse scan (reproduced with permission from *Rheumatology in Europe* 1997;**26**:89–92).

Joint effusion and synovial cysts

USG is an extremely sensitive method to detect even very small fluid accumulations in joints and is therefore a

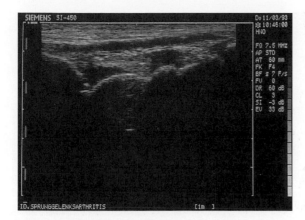

Fig. 19.10 Longitudinal scan of the ankle joint and the proximal dorsum of the foot. Synovitis is shown as dark areas in front of the tibiotarsal and the talotarsal joints in a patient with RA.

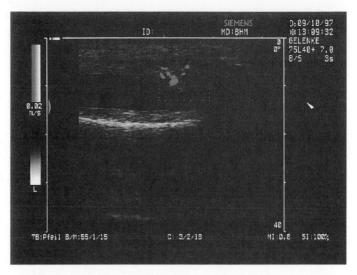

Fig. 19.11 Visualization of perfusion in a hypertrophic, hypoechoic synovium next to an echo-free effusion by power doppler sonography. See also Plate 24.

valuable extension of the clinical examination. In some joints, the diagnostic sensitivity to detect a joint effusion can be enhanced by certain maneuvres such as 30° flexion of the knee or tightening of the extensor muscles of the thigh. In case of the hip joint, it is clinically virtually impossible to assess a joint effusion and USG here is extremely helpful, especially when an arthrocenthesis is planned. In addition, information about internal structures of the inflamed joint space can be obtained (synovial folds, septations, gelatinous or fibrous changes of older effusions). Therefore a routine USG examination is useful before any planned joint puncture[14].

Cystic structures are easily detected by USG, so it is no surprise that large synovial cysts, such as Baker's cysts of the popliteal region, were the first pathological structures examined by joint USG[15]. Again, the extension, shape, and internal structure of a synovial cyst is essential information before any planned therapeutic intervention (Fig. 19.12). USG

is an easy method to distinguish between rupture of a pre-existing Baker's cyst and a deep vein thrombosis, a differential diagnosis that is clinically often difficult. After a recent rupture, fluid accumulation between the calf muscles can be detected (Fig. 19.13). During the same examination, it is possible to visualize and measure the flow in the popliteal vein and thus exclude a deep vein thrombosis with the help of doppler sonography.

Sonography of periarticular tissues

Tendons and tendon sheaths

Chronic tenosynovitis is a frequent complication of RA which can lead to infiltration of tendons and spontaneous tendon ruptures. USG allows the detection of synovitis which is visualized as a dark area around the bright echogenic tendons

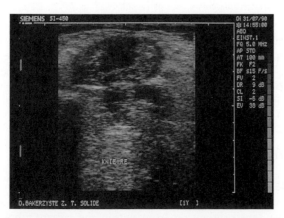

Fig. 19.12 Large Baker's cyst shown in a longitudinal scan of the popliteal region in a patient with RA. Only the innermost part of the cyst is echo free and contains liquid material, the surrounding areas are organized and contain fibrous or gelatinous material.

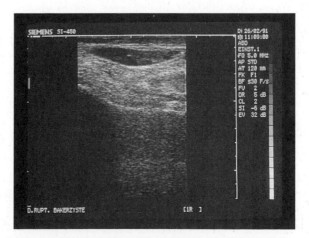

Fig. 19.13 Fluid accumulation between the two heads of M. gastrocnemius after a recent rupture of a popliteal baker cyst. The bone contour below the fluid represents the proximal third of the tibia.

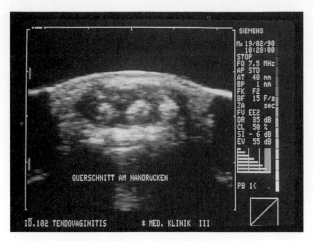

Fig. 19.14 Chronic tenosynovitis shown in a transversal scan of the dorsum of the hand in a patient with RA. The hypoechoic area round the extensor tendons represent synovitis in the common tendon sheath.

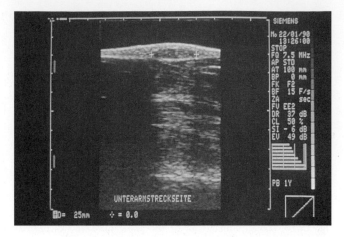

Fig. 19.15 Longitudinal scan at the lower arm of a patient with RA which shows the typical sonographic appearance of a rheumatoid nodule.

(Fig. 19.14). Information can be obtained about the condition of the tendon itself, invasive growth of inflammatory synovial tissue, and partial or complete tears. The most accurate detection and characterization of tenosynovitis of fingers and hands is obtained with high frequency transducers of 10 MHz and more[8]. This may in the future allow a better determination of the exact time point of synovectomy or other surgical procedures.

An important indication for the use of USG is the assessment of a suspected rotator cuff tear. Partial or complete tears of the tendon plate of the rotator cuff are a frequent feature in RA or other causes of shoulder arthritis. In a recent study, it has been demonstrated that the sensitivity of USG to detect a full thickness rotator cuff tear is even higher than that of arthrography using intra-articular contrast media[16].

Rheumatoid nodules

The formation of rheumatoid nodules as an extra-articular manifestation of RA is usually diagnosed clinically. However, in some clinical situations there might be a need to distinguish them from other subcutaneous changes such as gouty tophi, chronic bursitis, tumors, or others. The typical sonographic appearance of a rheumatoid nodule is spindle-shaped, hypoechoic with a distal sound enhancement (Fig. 19.15). Therefore it is easily distinguished from other pathological subcutaneous alterations.

Value of joint sonography in comparison with other imaging technologies

Ultrasonography can not compete with conventional X-rays in the imaging of bony structures. However, it provides valuable additional information with regard to soft tissue processes, which can be assessed only indirectly by conventional radiology. The only other imaging method which provides good images of soft tissue structures is MRI. Compared to MRI, the advantages of USG are the low costs, the easy availability, the possibility of dynamic

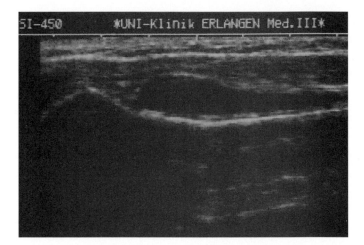

Fig. 19.16 Longitudinal scan over the bicipital groove in a patient with RA before therapy, which shows a hypoechoic area of effusion (reproduced with permission from *Rheumatology in Europe* 1997;26:89–92).

imaging, and the lack of contraindications such as claustrophobia or pacemakers. USG can also be frequently repeated, which makes it a potentially valuable method for monitoring therapy[11] (Figs. 19.16 and 19.17). However, of all imaging technologies, it is the most operator-dependent and skills and experience determine the quality and reproducibility of this technology.

Nuclear medicine

Nuclear imaging in general provides functional data. Following the injection of a radiopharmaceutical agent, gamma rays originating from within the patient's body are then measured and utilized by a gamma camera to produce an image. Bone scans reveal areas with increased blood flow to the bone as foci of increased radiopharmaceutical uptake as

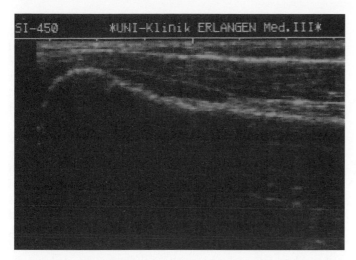

Fig. 19.17 After several months of successful DMARD therapy only a narrow hypoechoic margin can still be visualized along the humerus shaft (reproduced with permission from *Rheumatology in Europe* 1997;26:89–92).

'hot spots'. This technique can detect a wide variety of diseases, including osteomyelitis, primary and secondary bone tumors, arthritis, metabolic bone disease, trauma, and avascular necrosis[17-22].

Technical equipment and radioisotopes

The most widely performed nuclear scan is the bone scan using Tc-99m-DTPA. Tc-99m represents a radioactive isotope and DTPA is a small molecule that is excreted by glomerular filtration. The accumulation of Tc-Phosphate compounds in bone is a function of increased osteoblastic activity in the course of most pathological bone processes.

Depending on the given pathology, either static or dynamic 3-phase scintigraphic procedures are available. In the case of a localized process for differential diagnostic purposes (bone tumor, osteomyelitis, inflammatory or degenerative joint disease) a dynamic 3-phase scintigraphy should be performed consisting of a radionuclid angiography, a blood pooling phase, and the usual static late images.

To perform the radionuclid angiography, the radiopharmaceutical is injected at the site of the camera, which immediately after injection registers the first passage through the arterial vascular system. Simultaneously, the data of the gamma camera are stored at a post processing system for qualitative and semi-quantitative evaluation of perfusion of a the bone process under examination. Also hyperperfused soft tissue and bone tumors can be differentiated.

The early images of the blood pooling phase, which are scanned immediately following radionuclid angiography, demonstrate the arterial as well as the venous perfusion and, within limits, allow for a differential diagnosis, that is inflammatory or degenerative changes. Because of progress in scanner configuration, whole body imaging immediately after injection of the radionuclid is possible and in this way multifocal hyperemia can be demonstrated, a finding that is of great importance in patients with rheumatoid arthritis, especially when radiosynoviothesis is planned (Fig. 19.18).

Three to four hours after injection, static late images are performed, usually as anterior and posterior whole body images. Additionally, special regions of interest can be viewed by a high resolution collimation technique, if necessary with magnification.

SPECT and CNS manifestations of vasculitis

Using a tomographic technique (single-photon-emission-computer tomography, SPECT) reduced perfusion of cortical and subcortical brain areas to a lesser degree of white matter can be visualized. The radiopharmaceutical tracer used is a lipophilic substance which, after intravenous injection, passes the blood–brain barrier and accumulates according to the degree of local perfusion. After accumulation there is nearly no wash-

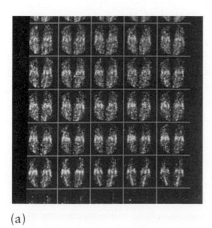

(a)

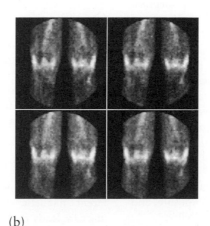

(b)

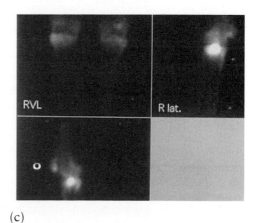

(c)

Fig. 19.18 a–c Three-phase bone scan: (a) dynamic (b) equilibrium (c) delayed.

out effect, so that SPECT images mirror the situation of brain perfusion at the time of injection. Commercially available tracers are technetium-99m-HMPAO (hexamethylen-propylen-amin-oxin) and Technetium-99m-ECD (ethyl-cystein-dimer). Especially in RA patients suspected of having vasculitis with brain involvement, the spectral scan allows a non-invasive evaluation of focal decreased metabolic activity in the brain as a result of reduced blood flow.

Osteodensitometry

Osteodensitometry makes use of the physical principle that there is a nearly linear correlation between tissue density and the absorption of X-radiation. The density of a bone is determined by its mineral content. In computed tomography, by means of calibration phantom which contains defined concentrations of hydroxyl apatite, it is possible to express the HU (Hounsfield Units) in mg hydroxyl apatite/cm^3. The evaluation of bone mineral content in trabecular bone is possible, since trabecular bone has a higher metabolic rate than cortical bone. Osteodensitometry is without doubt the most important radiological tool in the diagnosis of osteoporosis. The synopsis of all results including clinical and laboratory data as well as conventional radiography of the spine together with osteodensitometry should lead to a must reliable diagnosis.

Quantitative computed tomography (QCT)

Quantitative computed tomography can be done by every CT scanner which has the necessary software. The patient is positioned on his back on top of a calibration phantom, this calibration phantom is simultaneously measured with the patient. At least two lumbar spinal bodies between L1 and L4 have to be measured. After the slices are scanned, an automatic evaluation algorithm evaluates osteodensity separately for cortical and trabecular bone. The CT values are then automatically transferred into hydroxylappatite equivalent values. Single-energy-QCT examinations (SIQCT) use high voltage between 120 and 145 KW. As a consequence, the absorption in fat tissue compared to absorption in bone tissue is relatively high, the absorption values are between 10 and 30 per cent lower than the actual values. To avoid this so-called 'fat tissue mistake' usually dual-energy-QCT is applied. Here, two different spectra of energy are applied, usually around 85 and 125 KW. Since bone absorbs more radiation with low energy, those values which are measured with high energy through mathematical calculation are normalized. The price for more precision, however, is higher radiation exposure. Quantitative CT evaluation of the lumbar spine offers the highest degree of information of all osteodensitometric methods. However, fractures, skoliosis, or degenerative changes such as spondylophytes may lead to falsely increased levels because of their higher density. Major disadvantages of quantitative CT evaluations are the high radiation exposure, and the fact that the spine is the only location of applicability.

Peripheral quantitative CT (pQCT)

Special CT scanners for osteodensitometry on the peripheral skeleton such as the lower arm, the tibia, and the calcaneus are especially designed for this application. The major advantage is the very low radiation exposure with less than 1 micro Sv, which is negligible. The major disadvantage, however, is that the values measured on the peripheral skeleton cannot automatically be applied to the general skeleton. Peripheral measuring, especially on the radius, has a number of limitations and can not be used on patients with a radius fracture or patients with RA and degenerative changes in the distal radioulnar and carpal joint. Also reduced perfusion in the arm as well as pathological innervation of the arm which leads to reduced local perfusion, innervation, or mobility have to be excluded, since it is not possible to draw conclusions from the local reduced bone mineral content about the remaining skeleton.

Single energy X-ray absorption (SXA)

SXA examinations being a single energy-method can only be used at the distal arm and the calcaneus. SXA scanners are usually very comfortable for patient and examiner. Radiation exposure is low and scanning time is short. The major disadvantage is the fact that this method does not separate between cortical and trabecular bone. The SXA method is usually employed as a screening method. The method can not be used after radial or calcaneal fractures—here the values achieved would be unjustifiably increased. Also in RA patients who show involvement of the region around the distal radioulna joint and corpus the method can not be used.

Dual X-ray absorptiometry (DXA)

This is the most widely used method today to determine bone mineral content. The method allows the scanning of the whole body, the lumbar spine, the hip, the distal arm, the calcaneus, and the fingers. The DXA evaluation of the calcaneus and the fingers are at present only done for scientific purposes.

Quantitative ultrasound (QUS)

Quantitative ultrasound is not a method to measure osteodensitometry in the true sense of the word, since there is no evaluation of density. What is measured is the reduction of ultrasound waves but what causes the reduction is not clear. It is suspected, however, that different properties of the bone are evaluated compared to the radiological methods.

Quantitative magnetic resonance (QMR)

QMR is based on high resolution ultra-thin MR slices. The different magnetic susceptibility of trabecular bone and bone marrow leads to strong magnetic field inhomogeneities in the tissue, which is expressed by an increased T2(*) DK in the gradient echo. The quantitative evaluation of QMR is done by the relaxation quotient 1:T2(*). In QMR, structure analysis is more pronounced than in the other osteodensitometric procedures. The method is, at present, in an experimental stage and is not yet generally applicable to clinical situations.

In conclusion, it can be said that quantitative computed tomography (QCT) is the method of choice, which offers the highest amount of information, although dual energy X-ray absorption is the most widely used method, which is frequently not applicable to the peripheral skeleton in RA patients.

Osteodensitometric procedures on the peripheral skeleton are to be used only as a screening method and in the case of pathological values, it should be followed by a DXA or QCT examination of the lumbar spine or the femoral neck. Quantitative ultrasound and quantitative MR are at present in an experimental stage, but when standardized in the near future, they might offer an alternative because of the lack of X-ray exposure.

MRI—physical principles

Imaging with clinical MRI is based on the abundant presence of hydrogen atoms in the human body, the nuclei of which consist of only a single particle, the proton, around which a single electron orbits. The proton and electron have opposite electrical charges and the entire atom is therefore electrically neutral. A fundamental property of the proton, in addition to its positive electrical charge, is its 'spin', by virtue of which the proton rotates about its own axis. This property gives rise to two effects: the rotating mass produces an angular momentum, causing the proton to behave similarly to a gyroscope; the electron attempts to maintain the same spatial orientation of its axis of rotation. Simultaneously, however, it also possesses a rotating electrical charge, which can be described as a magnetic moment, and thus it also behaves as a tiny magnet. If the path of the proton is now influenced by the presence of magnetic fields or electromagnetic waves, this induces a voltage in a coil. If an external force is then applied in order to change the position of the axis of rotation of this gyroscope, it is then deflected from its original path. This phenomenon is known as precession. Due to friction, the gyroscope loses energy, is decelerated, and its axis tilts until it finally tips over or otherwise an external magnetic field B and its own intrinsic field B_0 attempt to align the spins along the direction of the field, as indicated by a compass needle. Since the spins also represent tiny gyroscopes, these also react by executing a precessional movement which takes place with a characteristic frequency, the Larmor frequency, and is proportional to the intensity of the magnetic field. Consequently, the spins align themselves parallel to the field by losing energy to the surroundings, just as with a gyroscope.

The Larmor frequency, that is the precessional frequency of the spins, in a magnetic field, is of vital importance, because this is the very basis of the entire MR imaging process. It is exactly proportional to the intensity of the magnetic field B_0;

the spins contributing to this field add vectorially to generate a longitudinal magnetization M_Z in the Z direction. This is similar to that which occurs in the earth's magnetic field, with the difference that the terrestrial magnetic field B_0 is on the order of 60 000 times weaker than the B_0 of an MR scanner, which is therefore able to develop a correspondingly greater longitudinal magnetization. Only a sufficiently strong magnetization makes it possible to measure the—extremely weak—MR signal at all. In the course of time a stable spin system develops, in which energy can be gained through electromagnetic waves. This, in turn, excites the spin system again and in this way generates a signal. With a high-frequency (HF) pulse of suitable power and duration, it is possible to obtain a deflection of exactly 90°: a 90° pulse, with which all spins and, together with these, the entire magnetization M_Z, are flipped into the XY plane. The magnetic field B_0 will then again attempt to flip the spins back to the Z direction, with the result that the spins once again precess about the Z axis. This causes them to rotate in the XY plane, the magnetic sum vector rotating along with them. This vector is now no longer designated as M_Z, but now instead as M_{xy}, because it is aligned in the XY plane. The motion of M_{xy} has the same effect as an electrical generator and induces an alternating voltage in the receiver coil, the frequency of which is equal to the Larmor frequency and which gives the final MR signal. The further processing of this signal by sensitive amplifiers and computers constitutes the imaging process.

Longitudinal (T_1) and transverse (T_2, T_2*) relaxation

Longitudinal (T_1) and transverse (T_2, T_2*) relaxation immediately following excitation cause all spins, and thus the entire magnetization, to execute gyroscopic motion in the XY plane, resulting in the transverse magnetization M_{xy}, which produces the MR signal in the receiver coil. When the transverse magnetization is removed, this MR signal decays over time as a result of two independent processes; the stable ground state prior to excitation is once again attained; the spin–lattice interaction and the spin–spin interaction. These two processes are known as T_1 relaxation and T_2 relaxation.

Fast scans

The spin echo (SE) sequence is the 'working horse' of magnetic resonance imaging. Besides SE sequences, which are composed of 90° HF by the score-pulse and 180° inversion- pulse, there is a group of sequences called gradient-echo sequences (GE). Principally, gradient echo imaging is analogous to SE-sequences in that slice selection and face coding are the same, however the HF pulse is variable with a flip angle smaller than 90°. Also there is no use of a 180° refocusing pulse. A major advantage of GE sequences is the fact that the TR can be drastically reduced down to 20 msec, thus resulting in a far shorter acquisition time. Disadvantageous, however, is the fact that GE sequences are very sensitive to magnetic field in homogenities and therefore susceptibilities are frequent.

Fat suppression methods

Most pathological processes are associated with an increased water content and therefore are bright on T_2 images, also after contrast media uptake in pathological processes these give a bright signal on T_1 images. At the same time the signal of fat tissue is hyperintense on T_1 images and moderately intense on T_2 images. So in both sequences it might be difficult to differentiate between fat and pathological tissue.

Therefore special MR techniques are used to eliminate the bright signal imparted by fat. The most common technique used is the selective saturation of fat protons, such as in bone marrow, since protons associated with the fat behaves slightly differently from the water protons exposed magnetic field. One frequently used sequence is the so called inversion-recovery sequence. The initial magnetization along the Z axis is inverted by 180° pulse which after some time (DI) is followed by a 90° pulse which turns D by now relaxated magnetization into the xy plane where it can be measured. A special variant of this sequence is the short T_1-1R sequence (STIR) which allows suppression of the signal from fat tissue by choosing the inversion time so that fat tissue is exactly at the 0-level when the tissue signal is measured. (Fig. 19.19)

2D imaging versus 3D imaging

Magnetic resonance imaging can be done either in 2D or 3D measuring. In 2-dimensional measuring there are selective excitations for each slice. After the first slice a second slice is excited and the signal received. This procedure continues until all slices are represented by a raw data set. Contrary to 2D-measuring, excitation in 3D technique is not slice but volume selective. The total volume of all slices is excited simultaneously. 3D measurements are used whenever there is a need for a very high resolution in all three planes with excellent contrast, to avoid, for example, partial volume effects or to be able to reconstruct in a different plane. In particular, MR-angiogrames cannot do without a 3D image construction.

Technical equipment

The principal components of an MR tomograph are:

1. Main magnet, i.e. a whole-body magnet. The main magnet produces the magnetic field B0 (0.01–0.4 T) which can be regarded as low field strength (0.5–0.9 T can be regarded as medium field strength, and >1 T implies a high field strength). The correction of local magnetic inhomogeneities is achieved by the use of shim coils.

2. Gradient coils, which provide spatial encoding (10–15 mT/m). These are superimposed on the external magnetic field. There are three gradient coils, providing for 3-dimensional positioning in all planes:
    (i)   slice selection gradient;
    (ii) frequency encoding gradient;
    (iii) phase encoding gradient.

3. The radio-frequency system, which is the equivalent of a radio-frequency sender and receiver. Usually the whole-body

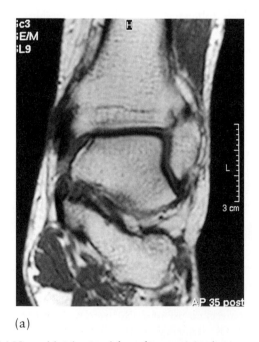

(a)

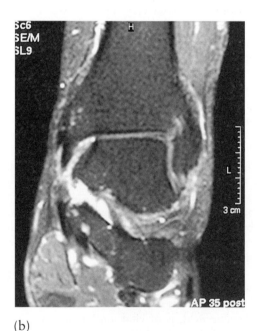

(b)

Fig. 19.19 a, b   (a) Normal bright signal from fat-containing bone marrow, water-containing soft tissue structures are dark. (b) Signal from bone marrow now dark due to fat suppression, after contrast media injection enhancing enflamed ligamentous structures.

coil serves as the sender coil, and for receiving the signal either the whole-body coil is used or special surface coils for various parts of the body (head, knee, axial skeleton).

4. The data processing system, for image acquisition and processing.

While magnetic fields between 0.2 and 0.5 T are produced by a permanent magnet and resistive magnetic systems, for medium and high field techniques superconducting magnets are necessary. These magnets produce the main magnetic field B_0, which should be as homogeneous as possible.

Among the low field MR tomographs there are two which deserve special attention. One is the open MRT, which is useful for claustrophobic patients and also provides image guidance for interventional procedures. Open units image the patient in larger 7-shaped magnets rather than the closed tube in conventional units. Unfortunately, because of their weaker magnets (0.1–0.3 T) these magnets provide only limited anatomic and spatial resolution. High field strength units are to be preferred whenever possible in connection with more diagnostically-oriented images. Open tomographs, however, allow imaging of the whole body. This is not the case with the second group of low field magnets, the so-called dedicated systems. Here, a low field scanner (0.2 T) provides a measuring unit to image individual joints, provided they can be positioned inside the unit; this is usually the case for the feet and knee, as well as the hand, wrist, and elbow.

Of great advantage here is the comfortable patient positioning outside of the scanner. The limitations on image quality are, however, the same or even more than mentioned for open MRI scanners.

Among the different coil types are, as already mentioned, the gradient coils and the radio-frequency-coils. In addition, in MR tomographs of the latest generation there are circularly polarized surface coils, which can be wrapped around a joint for example, and because of the close proximity of the object to be scanned, the coiled produces a better signal-to-noise ratio. Furthermore, there are phased-array coils, which enlarge the anatomical field to be measured and, thanks to their relatively high signal-to-noise ratio, produce a homogeneous image. Anatomical areas of use are the spine, mamma, abdomen, and temperomandibular joint.

Biological effects and safety

There are different forms of exposure of electromagnetic radiation in patients under MR examination:

(1) static magnetic field,

(2) gradient magnetic fields,

(3) radio-frequency (RF), electro magnetic fields.

All three can be harmful to the patient if applied with a sufficiently high intensity. Of particular interest, however, is the specific absorption rate (SAR). The SAR describes the amount of energy which is radiated into a patient by the radio-frequency pulse. Most MR units have a technically fixed SAR limit, above which the sequence will not start.

The SAR is determined by the following factors:

(1) The SAR increases with field strength.

(2) The SAR increases with the flip angle (high SAR with spin-echo sequences, low SAR with gradient-echo sequences).

(3) The SAR increases with increasing frequency of the injected radio-frequency pulse.

(4) The SAR is dependent on the kind of tissue (high SAR in tissue with high liquid content, e.g. brain, blood, liver).

(5) The SAR depends on T_R (the higher the value of T_R, the lower the SAR).

The limit for the SAR is usually < 1 W/kg for whole-body examinations and < 5 W/kg for partial body examinations. Exceeding these limit values makes the control of cardio/pulmonary functions necessary.

There are some absolute contraindications for MRT examinations. These are:

(1) cardiac pacemakers and internal defibrillators;

(2) neurostimulators;

(3) cochlear implants;

(4) ferromagnetic intravascular filters or stents;

(5) Starr-Edward heart valves and old heart valves which have been used before 1970; most other heart valves are not dangerous;

(6) certain ocular implants;

(7) ferro-magnetic vessel clips which have recently been implanted;

(8) ferrometallic bodies, especially in the eye;

(9) implanted infusion pumps;

(10) some penile prostheses.

It is necessary to screen each and every patient for these contraindications before any MRI study. Most manufacturers now produce surgical clips and other devices which are non-ferromagnetic and which are safe for MRI. If there is any question about safety the radiologist or even the manufacturer should be asked. There are also some relative contraindications against an MRT examination. These are non-ferromagnetic clips, which in the course of time can develop ferromagnetic behavior. If metal has been implanted during an operation, there should be no MRI examination for the first six postoperative months. Metallic implants, even when fixed to a bone, can heat up and lead to burns.

During a pregnancy MRT examinations should only be performed in the case of vital indications. A harmful effect on the unborn child has been neither proven or refuted. Gd-DTPA passes the placenta and should not be given during a pregnancy.

Patients with fixed osteosynthetic material can usually undergo an MR examination, an exception being the case when osteosynthetic material is bilateral, this could have the effect of a coil. In general, possible dangers of examining a patient with metal implants are:

(1) heating up of the material;

(2) dislocation of the material;

(3) production of eddy currents;

(4) image artifacts.

Contrast media

In MR images the signal intensity differences between two tissues determine the image contrast. This contrast depends on intrinsic factors of the different tissues and also on extrinsic factors, especially the sequence used.

MR contrast media are pharmaceuticals which improve diagnostic information by enhancing differences in signal intensity. They change the intrinsic properties of a tissue and can usually work either directly, by changing the density of the protons for thinner tissue, or indirectly, by changing the local magnetic field and thus changing the value of T_1 or T_2.

Paramagnetic contrast media are atoms, such as metal ions, which possess a magnetic moment through their unpaired outer electrons. Such a substance is inserted in a magnetic field, after which these atoms move around themselves along the main magnetic field, resulting in a magnetization. Many metal ions show this behavior, for example Co^{2+}, Fe^{2+}, Fe^{3+}, Gd^{3+}, Mn^{2+}. These paramagnetic substances are the most widely used MR contrast media. Thus, gadolinium compounds are frequently used, which primarily shorten the T_1 time by removing energy from the magnetized spins. These spins recover at a faster rate, thus increasing the MR signal. The most widely used gadolinium-based contrast medium is Gd-DTPA. The recommended dose is 0.1 mmole (0.2 ml)/kg body weight. The low molecular Gd-DTPA cannot pass the blood–brain barrier and does not enhance healthy brain tissue. In extracerebral tissue (Gd-DTPA passes the vascular endothelium and accumulates at extracellular, intravascular, and interstitial sites. Individual membranes usually can not be passed by this very hydrophylic substance. Gd-DTPA is not actively transported and is not metabolized, but is excreted unchanged by globular filtration. The speed and quantity of distribution are influenced by the degree of vascularity, capillary permeability, and the extracellular volume of the particular tissue.

Contrast enhanced MRI—static and dynamic

Image acquisition after the injection of contrast media provides information on the vascularization of a lesion. In the valuation of

the musculoskeletal system, usually extracellular paramagnetic or positive enhancers such as Gd-DTPA are used on T_1-weighted images. In obtaining T_1-weighted gadolinium-enhanced images, precontrast T_1-weighted image is produced for comparison before injecting the contrast media and repeating the sequence in the same imaging plane. This means that for each precontrast imaging in a whole volume there is one corresponding postcontrast image. On the other hand, dynamic studies have series of postcontrast images for each precontrast in a defined frame of time and allow evaluation of signal intensity changes over a period of a time (see Figure. 19.20). Since static sequences last 4 minutes, tissues are imaged in a quasi equilibrium state of water-soluble contrast agent between the blood and interstitial space[23-27].

The applicability of dynamic contrast agent enhanced MRI in patients with an inflammatory joint disease has been assessed by a number of authors[28-31]. Several methods for quantitating inflammatory activity by the rate of tissue uptake of paramagnetic contrast agents have been described. All of them are based

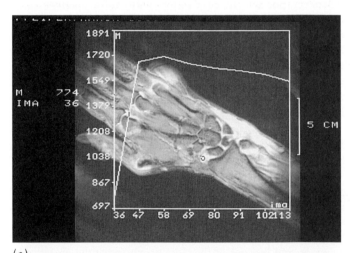

(a)

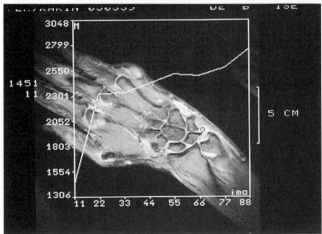

(b)

Fig. 19.20 a–b: a) Time/signal intensity curve prior to therapy with monoclonal antibody shows signal intensity increase of 120%/minute-b) Same patient 4 weeks post therapy with monoclonal antibody shows signal intensity increase reduced to 54%/minute.

on the same signal intensity curve but with variations in the volume of tissue to be evaluated.

The underlying histological features of the signal intensity increased in synovitis seem to be—as has recently been demonstrated by Tamai *et al.*[31]—inflammatory tissue activity. Correlating changes in signal intensity with pathological findings in synovial biopsy specimens obtained during total knee arthroplasty have shown that enhancement is greater in regions with a high degree of fibrin exudation, cellular infiltration, villous hypertrophy, vascular proliferation, and granulation tissue. Likewise, Gaffney *et al.*[32] have identified changes in synovial membrane signal intensity, they have quantified these, and have shown that the rate of synovial membrane enhancement correlates with histological features of acute inflammation. Our group demonstrated a correlation between the slope of the signal intensity curve, inflammatory activity, and the response to therapy[33].

Indications for dynamic MRI

The major indication for dynamic MRI today in rheumatoid arthritis patients is the monitoring of patients under therapy with fast acting immunomodulating drugs.

MRI findings in different joints characteristic for RA patients

The superior soft-tissue discrimination achieved by MR imaging is unrivaled by other imaging modalities, although conventional radiographs have maintained their corner-stone position in screening. Choosing between the multitude of sequences MR-imaging allows for visualization of hyaline articular cartilage, ligaments, tendons, and synovium[34–36].

Wrists and hands

Wrist and hand involvement by rheumatoid arthritis usually involves the carpus and the MCP and PIP joints. Soft tissue swelling can be caused by joint effusion, edema, and tenosynovitis. Frequently subluxations, dislocations, ulnar deviation in the MCP joints, and radial deviation in the radiocarpal articulation are found. Gadolinium-enhanced imaging selectively enhances pannus tissue in synovitis with the involvement of the distal radioulnar joint, the ulnar styloid process, the radiocarpal, intercarpal, and MCP joints as well as the flexor- and extensor-tendons[37, 38].

In the diagnosis of early RA, contrast enhancement of periarticular tissue as a criterion for the presence of disease, was found to have a sensitivity of 100 per cent, specificity of 73 per cent and accuracy of 89 per cent[39]. Making use of fat-suppressed gadolinium-enhanced scanning techniques, periarticular synovial inflammation as well as the subchondral bone marrow edema can be visualized, plus involvement of ligamenteous structures[40]. Subluxations and erosions can be identified both by plain radiographs as well as by MRI; they are, however, overpronounced on MR-images, so that plain radiographs are to be preferred.

Carpal erosions are, on the other hand, delineated better on MR-images. When using fat-suppressed T_2-weighted techniques, changes in articular cartilage can be demonstrated at a very early state.

The elbows

Elbow involvement in RA patients is frequent, usually beginning with painful distension of the joint capsule. In the course of the disease, there is a progressive loss of joint space with erosions developing at the joint surfaces. As a consequence of inflamed synovium herniating into the periarticular soft tissue there may be compression of peripheral nerves[41]. The production of intraosseous synovial cysts is common. All the mentioned features can be clearly visualized on MR. In addition to conventional T_1 and T_2 images, gadolinium enhancement of the inflamed synovia may be necessary to differentiate tissue from joint effusion[42–44]. MR-arthrography with diluted gadolinium or saline solution may also be helpful. The major advantage of MR is its objective evidence of synovitis at an early stage of the disease[45].

The shoulders

Aggressive synovial proliferation in the course of rheumatoid arthritis in the shoulder targets the capsule of the rotator cuff as well as the biceps tendon. Joint space narrowing and cranial subluxation of the humoral head are common features leading to impingement syndromes, especially in the area of the acriomioclavicular joint. Fat-suppressed fast spin-echo sequences combined with an intra-articular contrast agent helps to differentiate humoral head and glenoid-articular cartilage surfaces. Avascular necrosis (AVN) of the humoral head, usually associated with steroid use, can be easily diagnosed and differentiated from osteoarthritis. Especially in stage 1, which is asymptomatic and in which conventional radiographs are not diagnostic, MR imaging results are positive showing alterations in the subchondral marrow.

The hip

The usual imaging plane is coronal. This allows for evaluation of thinning of the hyaline cartilage and evidence of joint space narrowing. Around the hip synovial hypertrophy is not a common finding. RA patients on steroid therapy are, however, at a higher risk for avascular necrosis (AVN) which can be made visible on MR-images on the first signs of pain, long before there are any radiographic changes. Pannus formation around the femoral head is not a very common finding. Erosions, however, are frequently detected and are generally underestimated on conventional radiographs.

The knees

It is beyond the scope of the chapter to describe all MRI-changes associated with RA in the knee. So attention will be paid to the most frequent ones. RA affects all three compartments, the medial, the lateral, and the patellofemoral. Marginal and subchondral erosions and diffuse loss of hyaline articular cartilage is evident on both medial and lateral femoral articular surfaces. Large joint effusions with popliteal cysts are commonly seen and demonstrate uniform high signal intensity on T_2, fat-suppressed T_2-weighted fast spin-echo, and $T_2(*)$-weighted images. Gadolinium-DTPA contrast enhanced images are useful in identifying the pannus or granulation tissue that grows over the surface of articular cartilage in RA. Osteonecrosis and infarction in rheumatoid patients can be identified on MR-scans before corresponding radiographic changes are evident.

Feet and ankles

MR scans demonstrate the presence of an acute or chronic joint effusion as well as concentric joint space narrowing. Pannus formation and inflammatory edema around tendons and ligaments are easily depicted, as well as dislocations.

Cervical spine

Cervical spine represents the site of some of the most significant uses of MR in the evaluation of the arthritides[46–48]. Frequent complications of RA are extradural proliferation of granulation tissue and narrowing of the spinal canal as result of subluxation. These features are delineated easily by MRI. Also the level and degree of cord compression is visualized easily, pannus formation around the odontoid and widening of the joint space of the atlantoaxial joint, due to laxity of the transverse ligament, are easily demonstrated. In general, it can be said that whereas plane radiographs are suitable for assessing the degree of atlantoaxial subluxation, MRI is most valuable for assessing the degree of cord compression. Atlantoaxial subluxation can be diagnosed on T_1-weighted images obtained with the neck in flexion and extension.

MR-findings of the CNS in RA

CNS-manifestations of RA are usually in the form of nonspecific vasculitic changes, such as multifocal areas of increased signal intensity in the subcortical white matter on T_2-weighted images. Some lesions may enhance following contrast administration. Those changes however are highly unspecific and are found in other types of cerebral vascular damage with an identical morphology.

Future perspectives

In conventional radiology, teleradiology and, in this context, digital radiology will gain importance. The medical technical industry is developing imaging systems which offer the extremely high resolution of 5.9 lines per millimeters, necessary for osteoradiology, so that within the next 10 years the classical archiving of X-ray films will become obsolete and radiological information will be stored and transferred electronically.

In computed tomography, a new generation of ultra fast high resolution scanners is entering the market. A highly innovative system of arrayed detectors is increasing scan speed while at the same time reducing radiation exposure dramatically.

Also, in ultrasound, a new generation of high resolution scanners in combination with doppler and color doppler, as well as a special software capable of measuring perfusion and rendering three-dimensional images, is already revolutionizing the method.

In the field of MRI, a number of new developments are on the way. Extremely helpful in increasing patient comfort is the latest generation of superficial coils, which allow for the patient to lie comfortably in a supine position with coils wrapped around various joints at the same time so that two or more joints can be scanned simultaneously or at least sequentially without changing position. Also increasing scan speed is benefiting the image quality of MR angiographies and total volume rendering since motion artifacts can be avoided.

With respect to dynamic studies, three-dimensional volume rendering and special postprocessing computerized techniques to measure signal intensity changes on a pixel by pixel basis, will be progressively developed to allow for an operator-independent objective MRI evaluation of inflammatory activity.

Nevertheless, in spite of all the exciting technical progress it will still be the clinician who, on the basis of his experience and continuing education, has to decide from which of the numerous imaging modalities the patient will profit most at a particular stage of his disease. With respect to cost effectiveness, it should be remembered, however, that frequently what seems the most costly procedure may turn out to be the least expensive since a single high-quality examination may give the diagnostic answer.

References

1. Murphy, M.D. Digital skeletal radiography: spatial resolution requirements for detection of superiosteal resorption. *American Journal of Rheumatology*, 1989;152:541–46.
2. Galanski, M., Prokop, M., Oestmann, J.W., Reichelt, S., von Falkenhausen, U. (1990). Anwendung der digitalen Lumineszenzradiographie in der Skelettdiagnostik: ROC-Studie zur Erkennbarkeit kortikaler Läsionen. In: *Digitale Bildgebung-Interventionelle Radiologie-Integrierte digitale Radiologie.* (ed. Schneider, G.J., Vogeler, E., Kocever, K.), pp. 234–36. Blackwell Ueberreuter Wissenschaft, Berlin.
3. Langer, M., Zwicker, C., Langer, R., Scholz, A., Hinz, A., Eichstädt, E., Mitsch, E., Felix, R. Digitale Bildverstärkerradiographie—Anwendung in der Angiographie. Urographie und Skelettdiagnostik. Rofo *Fortschritte auf dem Gebiet der Röntgenstrahlen und der Neuen Bildgebenden Verfahren,* 1989;**150**(6):723–28.
4. Lehmann, K.J., Busch, H.P., Sommer, A., Georgi, M. Die Wertigkeit digitaler Bildaufnahmeverfahren bei der Skelettdiag

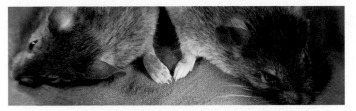

Plate 1 Collagen-induced arthritis in mice expressing an A^q transgene compared with littermate controls (above).

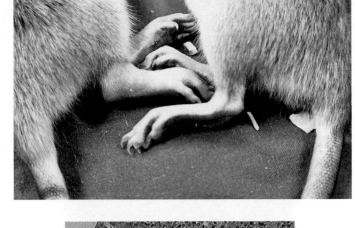

Plate 2 The left paw is from a DA rat injected with 150 μl mineral oil in the back of the skin (opposite). The arthritis is severe but non-erosive and acute, and does not become chronic.

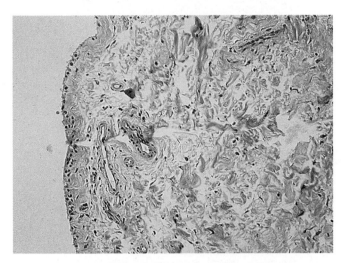

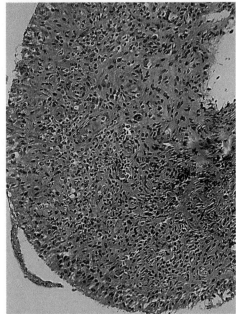

Plate 3 Normal synovial tissue consisting of the intimal lining layer of one to three cell layers and the synovial sublining that contains scattered blood vessels, fat cells, and fibroblasts.

Plate 4 Rheumatoid synovial tissue, showing intimal lining hyperplasia and infiltration of the synovial sublining by mononuclear cells.

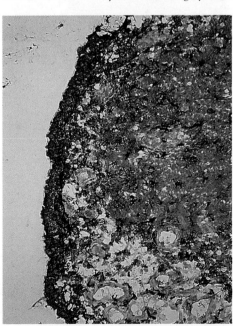

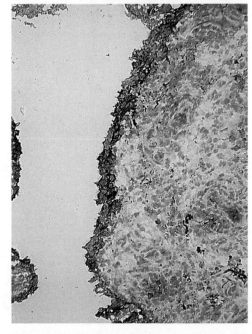

Plate 5 CD68$^+$ macrophages (red-brown) in the intimal lining layer and in the synovial sublining of rheumatoid synovial tissue.

Plate 6 CD55$^+$ fibroblast-like synoviocytes (red-brown) in the intimal lining layer of rheumatoid synovial tissue.

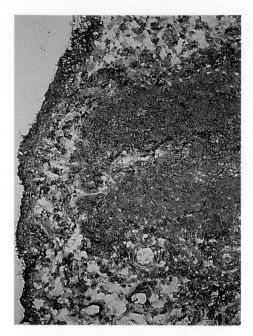

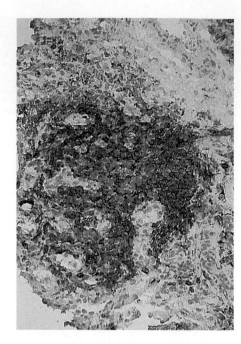

Plate 7 Rheumatoid synovial tissue stained with a monoclonal antibody directed against CD97. Note prominent staining (red-brown) on intimal macrophages and on leukocytes in the synovial sublining.

Plate 9 CD4+ T cells (red-brown) in a lymphocyte aggregate in rheumatoid synovial tissue.

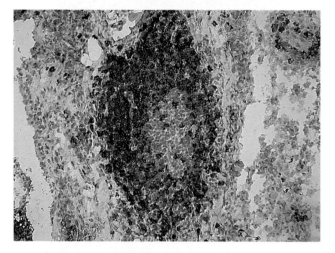

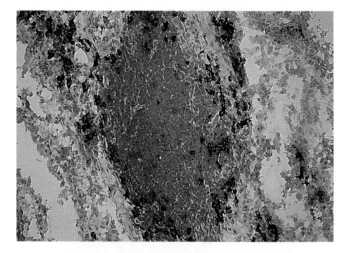

Plate 8 CD22+ B cells (red-brown) in a lymphocyte aggregate in rheumatoid synovial tissue.

Plate 10 CD38+ plasma cells (red-brown) surrounding a lymphocyte aggregate in rheumatoid synovial tissue.

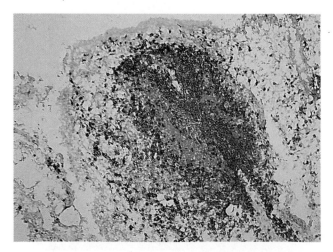

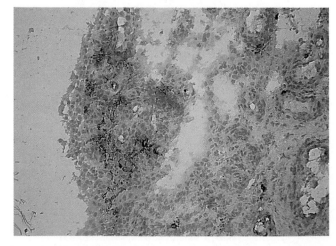

Plate 11 CD3+ T cells (red-brown) in a perivascular lymphocyte aggregate and in the diffuse leukocyte infiltrate in rheumatoid synovial tissue.

Plate 12 Granzyme B+ cytotoxic cells (red-brown) in rheumatoid synovial tissue.

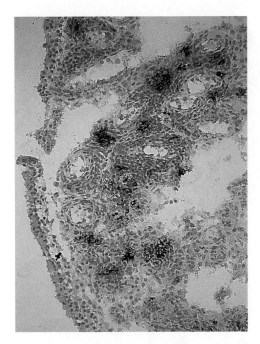

Plate 13   Mast cells (red-brown) in rheumatoid synovial tissue.

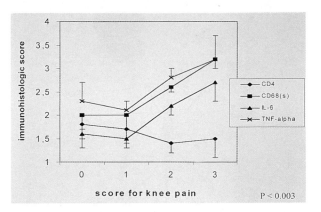

Plate 14   Mean ± SEM semiquantitative scores for the number of CD4+ T cells and CD68+ sublining macrophages and the expression of interleukin-6 and tumor necrosis factor-α in the synovial tisue of 62 patients with rheumatoid arthritis in relation to the scores for knee pain. Reproduced with permission from Lippincott Williams & Wilkins (*Arthritis Rheum*, 1997;40:217–225).

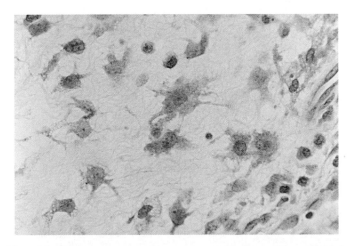

Plate 16   High-power view of a section of fixed, paraffin-embedded synovial tissue, showing T lymphocytes (smaller, rounded cells), in proximity to and interacting with various antigen-presenting cells, including dendritic cells, macrophages, and fibroblasts. (Reprinted with permission from Laboratory Investigation, vol 73, p334, 1995.)

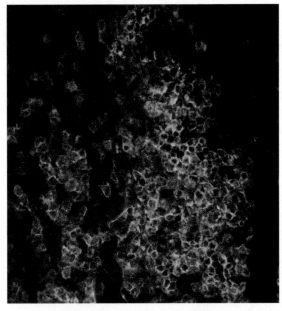

Plate 15   Immunoflourescent micrograph of a frozen section of RA synovial tissue showing a perivascular cluster of T lymphocytes (green fluorescence). The section has been stained with antibody to the CD3 complex, which is associated with the T-cell antigen receptor. (Reprinted with permission from Ref. 7.)

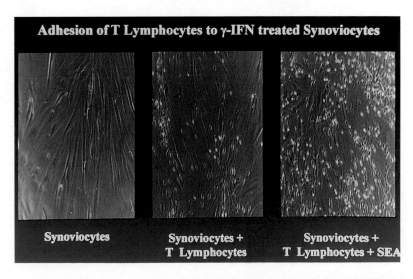

Plate 17   Interaction of T lymphocytes with Type B synoviocytes (synovial fibroblasts) +/− the staphylococcal superantigen SEA (staphylococcal enterotoxin A).

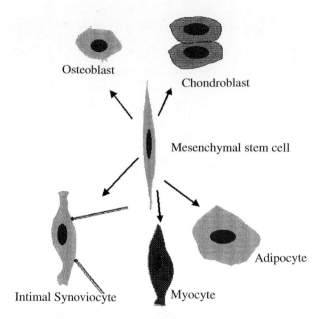

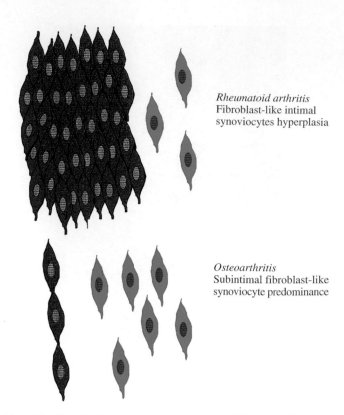

Plate 18 Lineage relationships of cells derived from a mesenchymal stem cell. This cell also givesrise to fibroblasts, including those in the subintima.

Rheumatoid arthritis
Fibroblast-like intimal synoviocytes hyperplasia

Osteoarthritis
Subintimal fibroblast-like synoviocyte predominance

Plate 20 The third interpretation of the basis of the distinctive phenotype of cultured rheumatoid arthritis synoviocytes. This is the lineage model that bases the distinctive phenotype on the fact that the starting point of the culture differs greatly in the proportion of intimal and subintimal synoviocytes in rheumatoid arthritis and osteoarthritis. This model postulates that the intimal and subintimal synoviocytes have different phenotypes based on their differentiation lineages and that the difference in the phenotype of the cultured cells simply reflects the varying starting proportions of the two cell types.

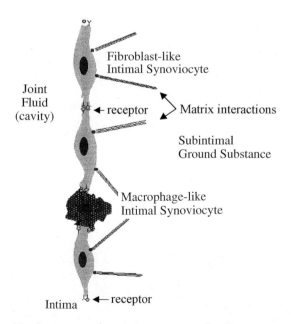

Plate 19 Receptor-mediated homotypic cell–cell interaction of fibroblast-like intimal synoviocytes with each other and their heterotypic interaction with macrophage-like intimal synoviocytes. The polarized state of the intimal cells is indicated by their interaction of one surface, on the right, with the subintimal connective tissue matrix and on the left with the hyaluronate-rich synovial fluid.

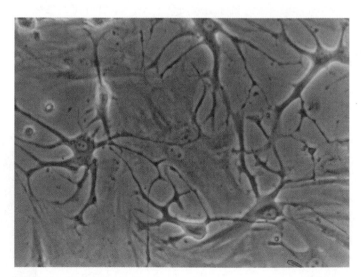

Plate 21 Fibroblast-like intimal synoviocyte exhibiting stellate or 'dendritic' morphology in culture.

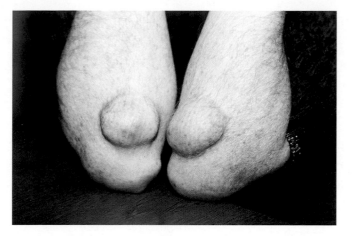

Plate 22   Large rheumatoid nodules at a typical site in the forearm.

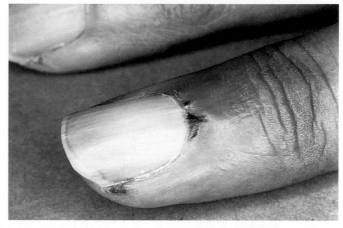

(a)

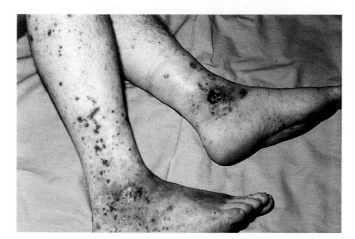

(b)

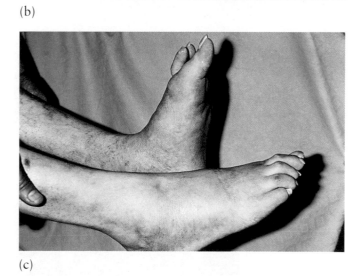

(c)

Plate 24   Visualization of perfusion in a hypertrophic, hypoechoic synovium next to an echo-free effusion by power doppler sonography.

Plate 23   (a) Isolated nailfold vasculitis; (b) vasculitic rash and ulceration; (c) foot-drop due to mononeurits multiplex.

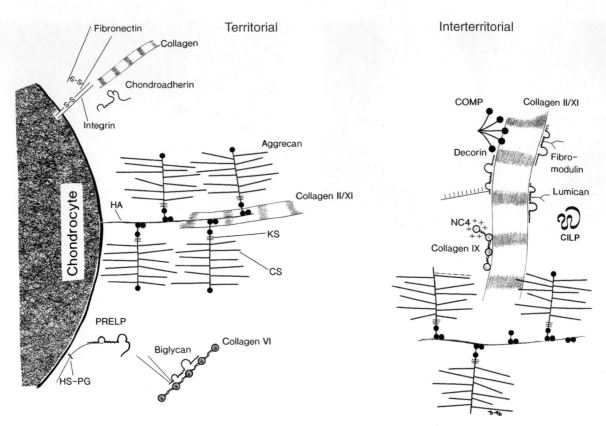

Plate 25 Schematic illustration of the constituents of cartilage matrix. The spatial relationships of the various constituents to the chondrocyte, that is their presence in the territorial (close to the cell) or interterritorial matrix (furthest away from the cell) is shown and the macromolecular organization of matrix molecules is indicated. Adapted from Ref. 10 with permission.

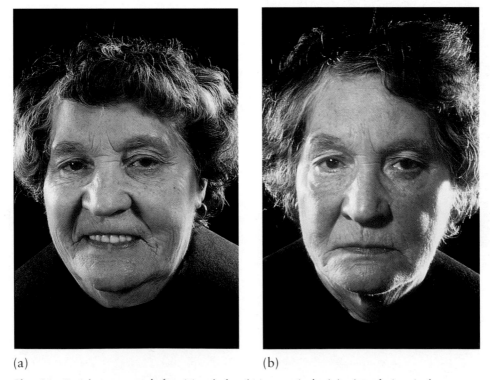

(a)　　　　　　　　　　　　　　　(b)

Plate 26 Facial appearance before (a) and after (b) intra-articular injection of triamcinolone.

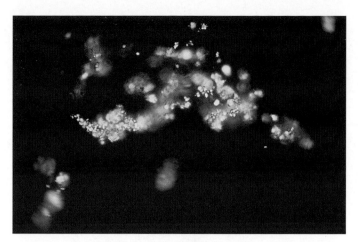

Plate 27 Compensated polarized light microscopy of triamcinolone hexacetonide, aspirated during a steroid flare 72 h postinjection, brightly birefringent material but showing no clear crystalline symmetry.

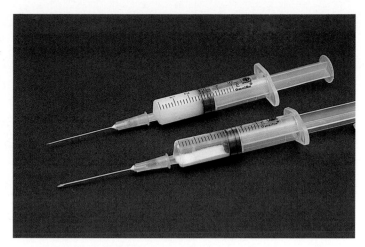

Plate 30 Flocculation and sedimentation occurring after mixing 2 ml 1 per cent lignocaine with methylprednisolone acetate (bottom) but not with triamcinolone hexacetonide (top).

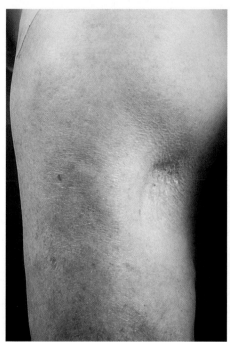

Plate 28 Skin atrophy following fluorinated steroid injection to an anserine bursa.

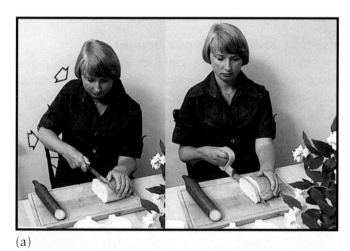

(a)

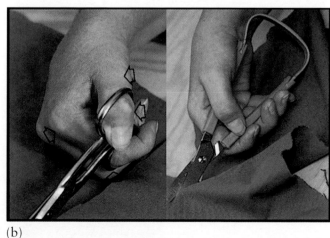

(b)

Plate 31 (a) The ergonomically breadsaw has a handle with a wider gripping area and is specially designed for people with reduced grip force. (b) The specially designed pair of scissors requires low force.

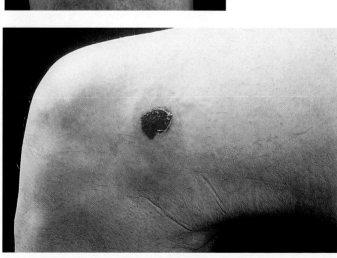

Plate 29 Skin necrosis following over enthusiastic use of a refrigerant spray.

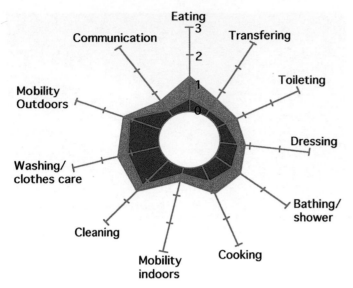

Plate 32 The eleven dimensions in the EDAQ are shown with the scalestep of 0 = no difficulty, 1 = some difficulty, 2 = much difficulty, and 3 unable to do. The upper line marks the difficulty level without assistive devices; the lower line marks the difficulty level with assistive devices. The light field represents the decreased difficulty with devices. The dark field represents the remaining difficulty.

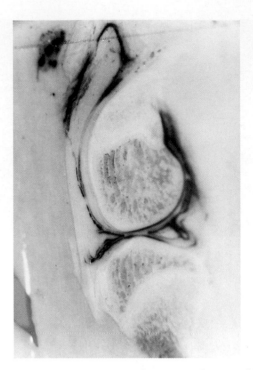

Plate 33 Intra-articular injection of osmic acid in a rabbit joint showing the black coloration of synovium and cartilage.

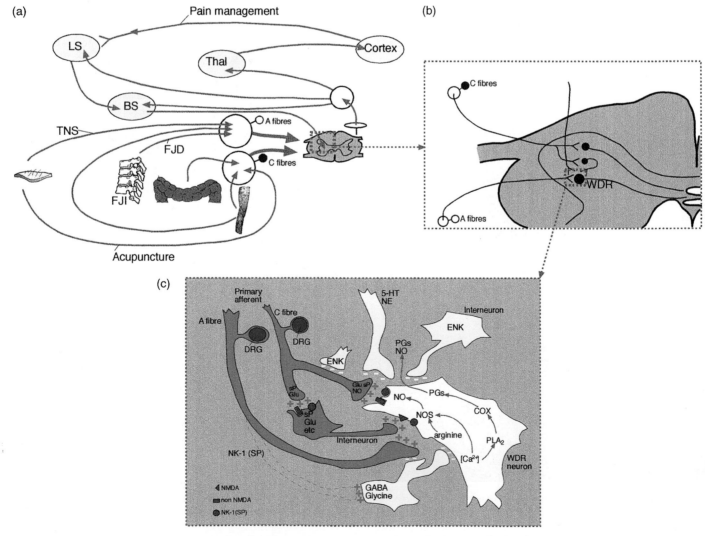

Plate 34 Overview depicting access points of modes of treatment to the pain pathway. See Fig. 33.1 for details.

nostik. Rofo *Fortschritte auf dem Gebiet der Röntgenstrahlen und der Neuen Bildgebenden Verfahren*, 1991;**154**(3):286–91.

5. Zwicker, C., Langer, M., Langer, R., Wasmuth, C., Felix, R. Digitale Bildverstärkerradiographie in der Skelettdiagnostik—Erste klinische Ergebnisse. *Digitale Bilddiagnostik*, 1988;**8**:147–51.

6. Klein, H.M., Wein, B., Langen, J., Glaser, K.H., Stargardt, A., Günther, R.W. Frakturdiagnostik mit der digitalen Lumineszenzradiographie. Rofo *Fortschritte auf dem Gebiet der Röntgenstrahlen und der Neuen Bildgebenden Verfahren*, 1991;**154**(6):582–86.

7. Wiesmann, W., Reiser, M., Pauly, Th., Fiebig, M., Bick, U., Peters, P.E. Darstellung von Metallimplantaten mit der digitalen Lumineszenzradiographie. Rofo *Fortschritte auf dem Gebiet der Röntgenstrahlen und der Neuen Bildgebenden Verfahren*, 1990;**152**(6):687–92.

8. Grassi, W., Tittarelli, E., Blasetti, P., Pirani, 0., Cervini, C. Finger tendon involvement in rheumatoid arthritis. Evaluation with high frequency sonography. *Arthritis & Rheumatism*, 1995;**38**:786–94.

9. Manger, B., Kalden, J.R. Joint and connective tissue ultrasonography—a rheumatological bedside procedure? A German experience. *Arthritis & Rheumatism*, 1995;**38**:736–42.

10. Leeb, B., Stenzel, I., Czembirek, H., Smolen, J.S. Diagnostic use of office based ultrasound. *Arthritis & Rheumatism*, 1995;**38**:859–61.

11. Backhaus, M., Manger, B. The use of ultrasonography in the rheumatological diagnosis of the shoulder. *Rheumatology in Europe*, 1997;**26**:89–92.

12. Sattler, H., Rehart, S. (1997). *Arthrosonographie und klinischer Befund*. Deutscher A[..]rzte-Verlag, Köln.

13. Breisdahl, W.H., Newman, J.S., Taljanovic, M.S., Adler, R.S. Power doppler sonography in the assessment of muskuloskeletal fluid collections. *American Journal of Roentgenology*, 1996;**166**:1443–46.

14. Kern, P., Kalden-Nemeth, D., Kalden, J.R., Manger, B. Ultrasound in the evaluation of an unusual periarticular soft tissue tuberculosis. *Journal of Clinical Rheumatology*, 1998;**4**:32–35.

15. McDonald, D.G., Leopold, G.R. Ultrasound B-scanning in the differentiation of Baker's cyst and thrombophlebitis. *British Journal of Radiology*, 1972;**45**:729–32.

16. Swen, W.A.A., Jacobs, J.W.G., Neve, W.C., Bal, D., Bijlsma, J.W.J. (1998). Is sonography performed by the radiologist as useful as arthrography executed by the radiologist for the assessment of full thickness rotator cuff tears? *Journal of Rheumatology*, in press.

17. Brussatis, F. (1990). Degenerative Skeletterkrankungen. Nuklearmedizinische Diagnostik. In: *Nuklearmedizin in der Orthopädie*. (ed. Brussatis, F., Hahn, K.), pp. 134–48. Springer-Verlag, Berlin.

18. Hahn, K., Hahn, I., Eißner, D., Schaub, T. (1986). Die klinische Wertigkeit der Zweiphasen-Skelettszintigraphie zur Diagnose der Osteomyelitis im Kindesalter. In: *Radioaktive Isotope in Klinik und Forschung*. Bd. 17. (ed. Höfer, R., Bergmann, H.), pp. 115–19. Engermann, Wien.

19. Kraus, W. (1990). Degenerative Skeletterkrankungen. Nuklearmedizinische Diagnostik. In: *Nuklearmedizin in der Orthopädie*. (ed. Brussatis, F., Hahn, K.), pp. 419–28. Springer-Verlag, Berlin.

20. Spitz, J., Lauer, J., Tittel, K. Untersuchungen zur Altersabhängigkeit der traumatisch induzierten ossären Umbaureaktion im Skelettszintigramm. *Nuclear Medicine*, 1991;**30**:155–60.

2l. Steinert, H., Hahn, K. (1989). 3-Phasen-Skelettszintigraphie beim Sudeck-Syndrom. In: *Skelettszintigraphie. Knochendiagnostik mit neuen Verfahren*. (ed. Feine, U., Müller-Schauenburg, W.), pp. 199–203. Wachholz, Nürnberg.

22. Tröger, J., Eißner, D., Otte, D., Weitzel, D. Diagnose und Differentialdiagnose der akuten hämatogenen Osteomyelitis des Säuglings. *Radiologie*, 1979;**19**:99–105.

23. Weber, D.A. (1988) Options in camera technology for the bone scan: role of SPECT. *Seminars in Nuclear Medicine*, 78–9.

24. Brasch, R.C. New directions in the development of MR imaging contrast media. *Radiology*, 1992;**283**:1–11.

25. Dean, P., Kormano, M. Intravenous bolus of 1251 labeled meglumine diatrizoate: early extravascular distribution. *Acta Radiologica: Diagnosis*, 1977;**18**:293–304.

26. Kormano, M., Dean, P.B. Extravascular contrast material: the major component of contrast enhancement. *Radiology*, 1976;**121**:379–82.

27. Verstraete, K.L., De Deene, Y., Roels, H., Dierick, A., Uyttendaele, D., Kunnen, M. Benign and malignant musculoskeletal lesions: dynamic contrast-enhanced MR imaging—parametric 'first-pass' images depict tissue vascularization and perfusion. *Radiology*, 1994;**192**:835–43.

28. Braun, J., Bollow, M., Eggens, U., Konig, H., Distler, A., Sieper, J. Use of dynamic magnetic resonance imaging with fast imaging in the detection of early and advanced sacroiliitis in spondylarthropathy patients. *Arthritis & Rheumatism*, 1994;**37**:1039–45.

29. Nagele, M., Kunze, V., Koch, W., Bruning, R., Seelos, K., Strohmann, I., Wall, B., Reiser, M. Rheumatoid arthritis of the wrist. Dynamic Gd-DTPA enhanced MRT. Rofo *Fortschritte auf dem Gebiet der Röntgenstrahlen und der Neuen Bildgebenden Verfahren*, 1993;**185**:141–6.

30. Ostergaard, M., Lorenzen, I., Henrikson, O. (1994). Dynamic gadolinium-enhanced MR imaging in active and inactive immuno-inflammatory gonarthritis. *Acta Radiologica: Diagnosis*, 35–275.

31. Tamai, K., Yamato, M., Yamaguchi, T., Ohno, W. Dynamic magnetic resonance imaging for the evaluation of synovitis in patients with rheumatoid arthritis. *Arthritis & Rheumatism*, 1994;**37**:1151–7.

32. Gaffney, K., Cookson, J., Blake, D., Coumbe, A., Blades, S. Quantification of rheumatoid synovitis by magnetic resonance. *Arthritis & Rheumatism*, 1995;**38**:610–17.

33. Kalden-Nemeth, D., Grebmeier, J., Antoni, C., Manger, B., Wolf, F., Kalden, J.R. NMR monitoring of rheumatoid arthritis patients receiving anti–TNF–alpha monoclonal antibody therapy. *Rheumatology International*, 1997;**16**:249–55.

34. Yulish, B. S., *et al*. Juvenile rheumatoid arthritis: assessment with MR imaging. *Radiology*, 1987;**165**:149.

35. Baker, L.L., *et al*. (1987). High resolution magnetic resonsnace imaging of the wrist: normal anatomy. *Skeletal Radiology*, 16–128.

36. Meske, S., *et al*. (1990). Rheumatoid arthritis lesions of the wrist examined by rapid gradient echo magnetic resonance imaging. *Scandinavian Journal of Rheumatology*, 19–235.

37. Watson, K.H. (1988). Degenerative disorders of the carpus. In: *The wrist and its disorders*. (ed. D. Lichtman). Philadelphia: W.B. Saunders, p. 286.

38. Renner, W.R., *et al*. Early changes of rheumatoid arthritis in the hand and wrist. *Radiologic Clinics of North America*, 1988;**26**:1185.

39. Rominger, M.B., Bernreuter, W.K., Kenney, P.J., *et al*. MR imaging of the hands in early rheumatoid arthritis: preliminary results. *Radiographics*, 1993;**13**:47.

40. Sugimoto, H., Takeda, A., Masuyama, J., Furuse, M. Early-stage rheumatoid arthritis: diagnostic accuracy of MR imaging. *Radiology*, 1996;**198**:185.

41. Inglis, A.E., Figgle, M.P. (1993). Rheumatoid arthritis. In: *The elbow and its disorders* (ed. Morrey, B.F.). 2nd edn. Philadelphia, WB Saunders, p. 751.

42. Singson, R.D., Zalduondo, F.M. Value of unenhanced spin-echo MR imaging in distinguishing between synovitis and effusion of the knee. *American Journal of Rheumatology*, 1992;**159**:569.

43. Adam, G., Dammer, M., Bohndorf, K., Christoph, R., Fenke, F., Gunther, R.W. Rheumatoid arthritis of the knee: value of gadopentetate dimenglumine-enhanced MR imaging. *American Journal of Rheumatology*, 1991;**156**:125.

44. Bjorkengren, A.G., Geborek, P., Rydholm, U., Holtas, S., Petterson, H. MR imaging of the knee in acute rheumatoid arthritis: synovial uptake of gadolinium-DOTA. *American Journal of Rheumatology*, 1990;**155**:329.

45. Sugimoto, H., Takeda, A., Masuyama, J., Furuse, M. Early-stage rheumatoid arthritis: diagnostic accuracy of MR imaging. *Radiology*, 1996;**176**:831.

46. Breedveld, F.C., Algra, P.R., Vielvoye, C.J., Cats, A. Magnetic resonance imaging in the evaluation of patients with rheumatoid arthritis and subluxations of the cervical spine. *Arthritis & Rheumatism*, 1987;30:624.

47. Aisen, A.M., Martel, W., Ellis, J.H., McCune, W.J. Cervical spine involvement in rheumatoid arthritis: MR imaging. *Radiology*, 1987;**165**:159.

48. Larsson, E.M. Holtås, S., Zygmunt, S. Pre- and postoperative MR imaging of the craniocervical junction in rheumatoid arthritis. *American Journal of Roentgenology*, 1989;**152**:561.

20 | *Outcome and mortality*

Marjatta Leirisalo-Repo

Introduction

The determination of long-term outcome of patients with rheumatoid arthritis depends on the patient populations studied, on the follow-up time, and on the therapeutic interventions applied during the follow-up period. The natural outcome can not be determined, because all the patients have been treated by some medications and/or other means.

In previous population studies on patients fulfilling the ARA criteria for suspected, possible, or definite rheumatoid arthritis[1], many of the subjects had no evidence of chronic disease when studied a few years later[2]. These studies cannot easily be applied to the present situation because diagnostic criteria for rheumatoid arthritis were less strict. In particular, patients with possible rheumatoid arthritis might have had other more benign forms of arthritis such as reactive arthritis, psoriasis arthritis, arthritis in association with viral infections such as parvovirus, or other self-limiting arthritides of unknown etiology. However, recent studies have also shown that population cohorts with rheumatoid arthritis have a less severe course of disease compared with patients collected from specialist clinics[3,4].

Reports from many countries have also shown that a considerable proportion of patients with rheumatoid arthritis are only treated in primary health care and do not seek or are not referred to specialist care. As high as 50 per cent of patients with rheumatoid arthritis have been reported to be treated only by primary care in Sweden[5,6]. In Hannover, Germany, only 16 per cent of rheumatoid arthritis patients had consulted a rheumatologist or internist during the previous 12 months[7]. In a primary-care-based register of incident cases of inflammatory polyarthritis with duration of disease less than 12 weeks, 80 per cent of whom fulfilled the ACR diagnostic criteria[8] during the first year, 35 per cent of the patients were solely treated by the general practitioner[9].

Unselected patients with inflammatory polyarthritis studied prospectively have a benign disease with a majority recovering within the first 2 years[10,11]. By contrast, the subgroup of patients with early rheumatoid arthritis, mostly seropositive, have progressive arthritis, with the rate of remission during the first 3 years of disease of 6.5 to 19 per cent[12,13,14].

This review will discuss the outcome and mortality of patients with rheumatoid arthritis addressing the question from information available from population and hospital studies and from prospective cohort studies. In addition, the contributing effect of treatment modalities on the outcome and mortality will be discussed. As all these end points are highly dependent on the time course, only studies on patients with disease duration of at least 5 years will be included.

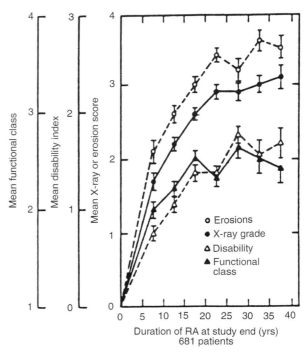

Fig. 20.1 Cross-sectional analysis of erosion score, radiological grade, disability index, and functional class in 681 rheumatoid arthritis patients. Reproduced from Ref. 15: Sherrer Y.S., Bloch D.A., Mitchell D.M., Young D.Y., and Fries J.F. (1986). The development of disability in rheumatoid arthritis. *Arthritis and Rheumatism*, 29:494–500, with permission of Lippincott Williams and Wilkins.

Population and hospital studies

Functional disability

Most of the reports are on patients with chronic rheumatoid arthritis, either cross-sectional or with varying information on the course of the disease (either retrospective or prospective). Of patients with rheumatoid arthritis treated at specialist clinics, 36 to 80 per cent have functional disability of Steinbrocker class III–IV after 9 to 20 years from onset of the disease (Table 20.1). Only 10 per cent do not develop significant disability[15]. Deterioration of functional capacity seems to be progressive and starts within the first years of the disease (Fig. 20.1). The figures are for patients surviving at least 12 years[15]. The slopes would be even steeper, if all patients presenting with early disease were included prospectively because the most severely handicapped are probably excluded due to increased mortality[18,19]. Measured by a Health Assessment Questionnaire (HAQ), patients with chronic rheumatoid arthritis who attended a private practice

Table 20.1 Development of disability in patients with rheumatoid arthritis

Reference	Entry years	Number of patients	Disease duration at entry (years)	Follow-up time (years)	Cohort	Intervention[1]	Steinbrocker I/II/III/IV (%)	% with III/IV	HAQ
91	NG	500 403 387 246 176	233: ≤2 127: 2–5 140: ≥6	...[4] 1–5 6–10 11–15 ≥16	Hospital out-patients, retrospective	NG	NG	18 26 42 50 55	NG
27	1948–1951	307	6–7	9	Hospital patients, active/poor function at entry, prospective	NG	20/40/27/13	40	NG
72, 74	NG	100	<1	20	Early consecutive hospital admissions, prospective	NG	NG	45	NG
37	1973	75	11	25	Hospital patients, drug trial, Retrospective	NG In 1973 intra-articular thiotepa Later therapy NG	31/43/17/9 16/42/34/8	26 42	NG 0.96 (MHAQ)[3]
15	1966–1974	681	10	12	Out-patient clinic, cross-sectional	NG	17/47/20/16	36	NG
21	1965–1967	239	NG[2]	17	Population survey, prospective	NG	16/62/15/6	21	NG
69	1964–1986	112	64% < 5	20	Clinical patients, prospective	DMARD/steroids 100%	Modified: I/II 28 III 43 IV/V 29	72	NG
31	1966–1974	292	9	6	Multicenter prospective	NG	NG	NG	1.20
113	1983–1988	574	10	5	Rheumatology practices, prospective, observational	100% im. Gold	NG	NG	1.00
90	1981	209	12	8	Population study	NG	NG	NG	1.16
68	1988–1989	129	Newly diagnosed	6	Multiple centers, elderly, retrospective	DMARD 77%	4/63/27/6	33	NG
16, 19	1966–1971	102	<1	15	Hospital referrals, prospective	During first three years: 64% DMARD 15% steroids	0/58/28/14	42	0.95
94	NG	127	5	7	Hospital referrals, prospective	100% DMARD	20/50/27/3	30	1.63
106	1982–1986	132	1.6	6	Clinical patients, female, 20–50 years, prospective	75%DMARD	45/45/10/0	10	0.82
22	1989	103	30: ≤10 44: 11–20 28: >20	...	Population survey, cross-sectional	DMARD 97%	0/67/33/0 0/45/55/0 0/28/61/4	33 55 65	} 0.85
4	1985	128	<1	6–7	Inception cohort, retrospective	DMARD 85%	NG	NG	0.49 (MHAQ)
117	NG	2888	8–11	10	Multicenter prospective	DMARD 84% Steroids 64%	NG	NG	1.18–1.60
67	1983–1989	142	0.7	6	Hospital inception cohort, prospective	100% DMARD 35% steroids	49/29/21/3	24	0.64
17	NG	200	11	...	Out-patient clinic, cross-sectional	70% DMARD 10% Steroids	NG	NG	1.30
66	1985–1987	106	1	7	Hospital inception cohort, prospective	65% DMARD	8/90/2/0	2	1.3
112	1986–1990	440	106: 0–2 93: > 2–5 235: >5	5	Clinical patients, prospective	100% im. Gold 0% steroids	NG	NG	1.25 1.81 2.13

1 Treatment received some time during follow-up; 2 not given; 3 modified HAQ; 4 not applicable.

rheumatic disease clinic in 1977–1988, were estimated to reach the disability score of 1 (difficulty in activities of daily living) at a median time of 10 years, score 2 (great difficulty in activities of daily living/need of assistance) at 21 years, and score 2.5 (severe disability) at 35 years after the onset of the disease[20].

Cases selected from the general population do best: about 20 per cent of patients selected from the general population are moderately or severely incapacitated after 20 years[21]. With increasing duration of disease, a high proportion of patients has developed at least moderate disability but severe functional handicap is rare[22].

Work disability

Rheumatoid arthritis has a major impact on the work capacity of patients. Most of the studies on work disability have been performed on patients in gainful employment while the work disability in homemakers has been analysed less frequently.

Mäkisara and Mäkisara[23] analyzed the work disability of patients treated at the Heinola Rheumatism Foundation Hospital in the 1970s. They observed a steady decrease in work capacity of patients with increasing duration of the disease. Thus, work disability was 40 per cent in patients with duration of disease of 5 years, 50 per cent in those with disease duration of 10 years, and 67 per cent in those with disease duration of 15 years. The figure reported 20 years later for patients during the

first 4 years of the disease in the Netherlands, 42 per cent, is not remarkably different from the Finnish report[24].

A long-term study of a cohort of patients with chronic rheumatoid arthritis collected in 1948–1951 and prospectively followed up for 9 years ended up with lower figures 12 to 20 per cent for work disability during 2 to 9 years of follow-up (Table 20.2). These figures are not representative of the whole patient population because they were based only on the available subgroup of patients in gainful employment at various periods[25,26,27].

The risk of losing work capacity has been prospectively analyzed by two groups. Out of 75 patients fully employed during the first year of the disease, 37 per cent were disabled at the end of 6-year follow-up[28]. The figure is similar in another group of patients treated for chronic rheumatoid arthritis by rheumatologists in the United States. Of those fully employed at the start of the study, 34 per cent were not able to work after 5 years[29]. The work ability decreased most rapidly during the first 3 years of the disease (Fig. 20.2).

Radiological destruction

Inflammation in the synovium leads to pannus formation adjacent to cartilage. Prolonged inflammation causes destruction in the cartilage and bone, ending with erosions. Joint destruction is a hallmark of rheumatoid arthritis and few patients escape from it. In cross-sectional studies of patients with chronic

Table 20.2 Work disability of patients with rheumatoid arthritis

Reference	Number of patients	Disease duration (years)	Follow-up time (years)	Cohort	Work disability at entry (%)	Work disability at outcome (%)
25	307	6–7	...	Hospital patients, active disease/poor function	8	...
			2			12
26			6			18
27			9			20
91	500	233: ≤2	...	Hospital outpatients, retrospective	28	...
	403	127: 2–5	1–5			24
	387	140: ≥6	6–10			27
	246		11–15			29
	176		≥16			32
23	405	144: 5	...	Hospital patients, cross-sectional	40	...
		131: 10			50	
		130: 15			67	
37	75	11	9	Hospital patients, drug trial	60	85
75	84	1	2	Hospital inception cohort, prospective	32	47
66	106	1	7	"	42	37
24	119	≤4	...	Early rheumatoid arthritis, interview	42	...
29	392	61% > 5	5	Rheumatologists' patients, prospective interview	0	34
28	75	≤1	6	Early rheumatoid arthritis, all gainfully employed, prospective	0	37

Abbreviations as in Table 20.1.

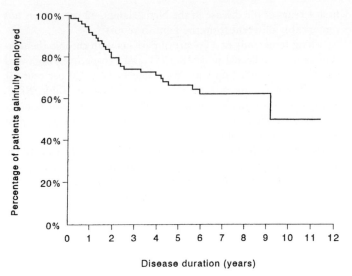

Fig. 20.2 Loss of work capacity during the first years of disease. Reproduced from Ref. 28: Mau W., Bornmann M., Weber H., Weidemann H.F., Hecker H., and Raspe H.H. (1996). Prediction of permanent work disability in a follow-up study of early rheumatoid arthritis: results of a tree structured analysis using RECPAM. *British Journal of Rheumatology*, **35**:652–9, with permission of the British Society for Rheumatology.

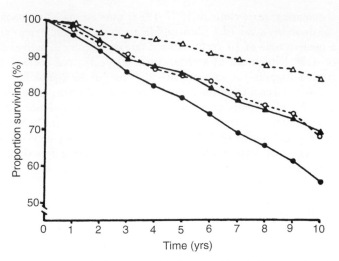

Fig. 20.3 Survival of patients with rheumatoid arthritis treated at the Rheumatism Foundation Hospital, Finland in 1959–1968 and control population. Circles, men; triangles, women; closed symbols, patients; open symbols, controls. Reproduced from Ref. 48: Mutru O., Laakso M., Isomäki H. and Koota K. (1985). Ten year mortality and causes of death in patients with rheumatoid arthritis. *British Medical Journal*, **290**:1979–9, with permission of the British Medical Journal.

rheumatoid arthritis, more than 90 per cent of the patients had erosive changes[30]. The progression of the changes is considered to be more rapid during the first years (Fig. 20.1) but the destruction usually continues with increased duration of the disease[15,31]. About 5 to 6 per cent of the joints show new erosions annually during the first years of the disease[30].

Most of the studies on long-term radiological outcome of patients with rheumatoid arthritis are cross-sectional. Therefore, it is hard to determine whether there are any changes in the

outcome in patients acquiring the disease in different decades. However, Heikkilä and Isomäki[32] addressed this question by analyzing hand and feet radiographs of four cohorts of female patients aged 45 to 64 years, seropositive, and with disease duration between 10 and 15 years but admitted to hospital in 1962, 1972, 1982 and 1992. Interestingly, during the 30-year span, the proportion of intact joints in fingers rose from 53.5 to 70.4 per cent, in wrists from 14.0 to 29.0 per cent, and in feet from 29.8 to 40.0 per cent. The most evident explanation for this good result, reasoned by the authors, is that the disease has

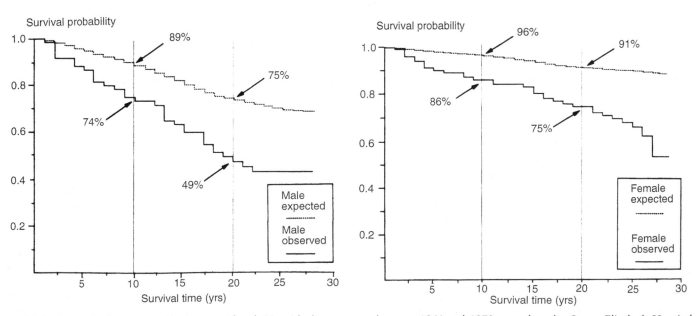

Fig. 20.4 Survival of patients with rheumatoid arthritis with disease onset between 1964 and 1978 treated at the Queen Elizabeth Hospital, Birmingham, England compared with population figures. Reproduced from Ref. 52: Symmons D.P.M., Jones M.A., Scott D.L., and Prior P. (1998). Long-term outcome in patients with rheumatoid arthritis: early presenters continue to do well. *Journal of Rheumatology*, **25**:1072–7, with permission of the Journal of Rheumatology.

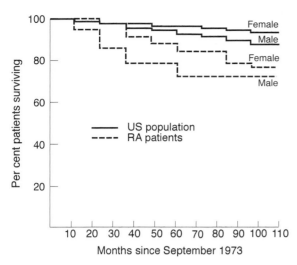

Fig. 20.5 Survival of patients with rheumatoid arthritis participating in a drug trial in 1973 at Vanderbilt University, United States, compared with population figures. Reproduced from Ref. 38, Pincus T., Callahan L.F., and Vaughn W.K. (1987). Questionnaire, walking time and button test measures of functional capacity as predictive markers for mortality in rheumatoid arthritis. *Journal of Rheumatology*, 14:240–51, with permission of the Journal of Rheumatology.

become either more benign or that there has been a change during the study period to start drug treatments more vigorously and in an earlier phase of the disease.

Mortality

A vast majority of studies have reported that patients with rheumatoid arthritis have an increased risk for mortality compared with populations without rheumatoid arthritis (Figs 20.3–20.7). This can be estimated by the standardized mortality ration (SMR) (Table 20.3). The median life expectancy is 4 to 7 years shorter for male, and 3 to 10 years shorter for female, patients[33,34,35]. The mortality figures depend on the age of the cohorts, follow-up time, entry selection criteria, and also on the criteria for diagnosis for rheumatoid arthritis. Some studies have included only patients with seropositive rheumatoid arthritis[36], with or without a definite laboratory abnormality[33], previously participating in a drug trial[37,38], or those of a cohort collected by previous mail survey[39]. The comparison of the results collected from these heterogeneous studies cannot be done reliably. Earlier studies also included patients with a low number of classification criteria for rheumatoid arthritis. Such patients have a low risk for the development of chronic rheumatoid arthritis[2,21].

There have been three population studies, two of which showed increased risk for mortality[41,42], while the third study observed no increased mortality rates compared with the background population[40]. This was a population study of incidence and prevalence of rheumatoid arthritis in Rochester, Minnesota, which also included patients with probable rheumatoid arthritis. In an extensive analysis of long-term prognosis of different patient cohorts by Wolfe *et al.*[43], patients belonging to a community-based cohort also had increased mortality risk (SMR 2.18).

Because of the heterogeneity of the studies, it is hard to analyze the contribution of the duration of the disease to the increased risk of mortality. However, there seems to be no major

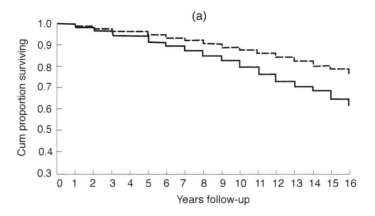

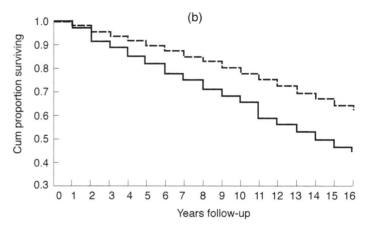

Fig. 20.6 Survival of patients with seropositive rheumatoid arthritis (solid lines); (a) shows figures for females treated at the Department of Rheumatology, University of Umeå, Sweden, in 1979 compared with population figures (dashed lines), (b) shows figures for males. Reproduced from Ref. 36: Wållberg-Jonsson S., Öhman M.-L., and Rantapää Dahlqvist S. (1997). Cardiovascular morbidity and mortality in patients with seropositive rheumatoid arthritis in Northern Sweden. *Journal of Rheumatology*, 24:445–51, with permission of the Journal of Rheumatology.

trend for an increase in the SMR with the duration of the disease (Table 20.3).

The causes for increased mortality can be divided into three categories: (1) mortality due to rheumatoid arthritis; (2) mortality due to intervening illness; and (3) mortality caused by the treatment. Rheumatoid arthritis has been reported as a primary or underlying cause of mortality in 0 to 11 per cent[35,39,42,44]. This is, however, not reliable, because in most studies which are based on analysis of death certificates, rheumatoid arthritis is underreported as a cause or as a contributing factor[45,46].

The shortening of life expectancy is evident after 5 years of the disease[47], and is mainly due to increased frequency of infections and cardiovascular, renal, and pulmonary diseases[11,46]. Amyloidosis has contributed to excess renal mortality, especially in Finland[35,48]. Mortality figures due to cancer are not higher than that of the general population, but there is an increased frequency of hematological malignancies[36,43,49,50,51,52]. The hematological malignancies are usually lymphomas, but myeloma patients have increased frequency of rheumatoid arthritis compared with matched population controls[53,54]. Risk for mortality due to lymphoma increases with the duration[51] and high inflammatory activity of the disease[55].

complications[62]. In many studies, the mortality of patients treated with glucocorticoids was higher compared with those who had not received such a treatment[19,38,43]. The impact on the mortality, however, is hard to estimate because the studies have not been randomized, with a bias to more severe disease in those treated with glucocorticoids. However, there is increasing evidence that glucocorticoids are an independent risk factor for cardiovascular mortality[63,64]. In addition to arteriosclerosis, glucocorticoids can increase the risk for infections and osteoporotic fractures, both of which can contribute to increased mortality. In the nation-wide analysis of mortality of patients with rheumatoid arthritis, 0.7 per cent of deaths were associated with glucocorticoids[57].

In conclusion, the mortality of patients with rheumatoid arthritis treated at hospitals is increased. Rheumatoid arthritis as a contributing factor is usually underestimated. Cardiovascular, hematological, nephrological, and gastrointestinal causes are increased. Part of the excess mortality is related to the NSAID treatment.

Early rheumatoid arthritis cohorts

Functional disability

Ideally, the best information would be achieved on an unselected patient cohort attending a prospective study at an early phase of disease followed up by the same team with structured questionnaires for 20 to 30 years. However, most of the studies available have some limitations and have been running less than 10 years. In five prospective studies on patients with early rheumatoid arthritis (entry into the trial within the first 2 years of symptoms), functional disability analyzed either by Steinbrocker or HAQ seems to vary greatly (Table 20.1). Part of this variation depends on the follow-up time but other factors such as age and functional stage of the patients at entry, treatment with DMARDs and glucocorticoids, and orthopedic surgery, cannot be ruled out.

Contrary to cross-sectional studies, in prospective studies on patients with early rheumatoid arthritis a decrease in the functional capacity with time is less obvious. There are some prospective studies on patients with early disease followed up for 5 to 6 years. In a study from Sweden, median HAQ changed during 5 years non-significantly from 0.8 to 0.9[65], but increased to 1.3 during the next 3 years[66]. A study from Finland showed a change in mean HAQ from 0.28 to 0.64 within the first 6 years[67]. After 15 years of disease, patients followed from early disease still had a mean HAQ of 0.95[19]. A non-significant progression from Steinbrocker class II toward class III was observed in a cohort of patients with late-onset, seropositive, erosive disease[68]. Patients with early rheumatoid arthritis seem to get better or stay at least stable during the first 10 years of the disease, but start to lose functional capacity during the second decade of the disease[69].

Results from one early cohort with reports on the functional outcome at various intervals[70,71,72,73,74] show that there seems to be a decrease in the severity of disability with time. However, this may be explained by the report of functional outcome being made only for patients who attended follow-up—with increasing time, the numbers of patients dying between follow-up visits increases. Patients with high functional disability have an

Table 20.4 Functional capacity (%) of patients in a prospective study of early rheumatoid arthritis, functional capacity measured at 20 and 25 years in survivors and at latest review in deceased

Functional capacity (Steinbrocker)	Survivors		Dead
	at 20 years	at 25 years	at latest visit
I	24	35	26
II	31	40	15
III	39	16	24
IV	6	8	35

Reproduced from Ref. 18: *Bailliereé's Clinical Rheumatology*, Vol. 6 (1), Rasker, J.J., Cosh, J.A.: Long-term effects of treating rheumatoid arthritis, pp. 141–160, 1992, by permission of the publisher WB Saunders Company Limited.

increased risk for mortality[69,41]. Rasker and Cosh[18] have also shown that the functional capacity of patients who died during a prospective study of long-term outcome was lower at last review than in those who survived for 20 to 25 years (Table 20.4).

Work disability

Work disability is observed early in the disease course: in the Swedish cohort of early rheumatoid arthritis, during the first 2 years after entry 47 per cent of 84 patients, and, during seven years, 37 per cent of 106 patients were unable to work[66,75]. Importantly, 70 per cent of those who had stopped working had done so during the first year of the disease, that is often before having been referred to specialist care[75].

Radiological destruction

In prospective studies on cohorts of early rheumatoid arthritis, erosive changes at entry (mean duration of symptoms less than 12 months) have been detected in about 8[76], 4[77], and 47 per cent[67,68] of the patients. During the next few years, most of the patients non-erosive at entry developed erosions. Plant *et al.*[79] have followed up prospectively a selected cohort of patients with early (symptoms less that 3 years) rheumatoid arthritis without erosions at entry: 70 per cent of the patients developed erosions during the next 8 years. Erosions developed in 73 per cent of patients with early (symptoms less than 1 year) rheumatoid arthritis followed prospectively for a mean of 9 years at the Middlesex Hospital[80]. Initial studies showed that the progression was most advanced during the first 2 years of follow-up[30,76,78,79]. However, an extensive, prospective study of the early arthritis cohort in Heinola revealed that destruction is continuing up to 20 years[81]. While individual progression during the first 8 years varies[79,82] (Fig. 20.8), the average radiological destruction shows continuing progression (Fig. 20.9).

Mortality

Of patients with early rheumatoid arthritis in 1966–1971, followed up at the Middlesex Hospital, 28 per cent (SMR 1.13) died during a mean of 13 years of follow-up[19]. A patient cohort with very early rheumatoid arthritis (duration of symptoms less than 6 months at entry) recruited from the pop-

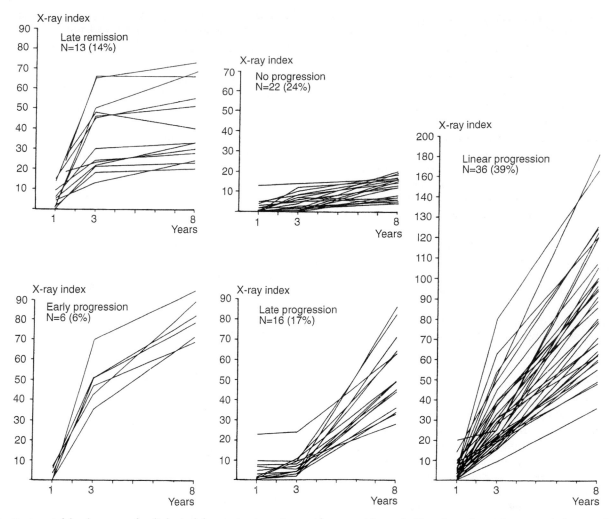

Fig. 20.8 Patterns of development of radiological destruction in patients with seropositive early (duration < 6 months at entry) rheumatoid arthritis. Joint destruction analyzed by Larsen score 0–200 (Ref. 83). Reproduced from Ref. 82, Isomäki H. (1992). Long-term outcome of rheumatoid arthritis. *Scandinavian Journal of Rheumatology*. **21** (**Suppl. 95**):3–8, with permission of the Scandinavian Journal of Rheumatology.

ulation in 1973–1975 and followed up prospectively at the Rheumatism Foundation Hospital in Heinola, had no increased risk for mortality during the next 20 years (SMR 1.09)[84]. The figures are comparable to the population study by

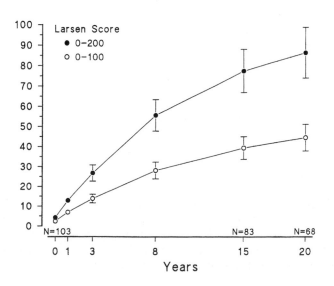

Linos *et al.*[40] in the United States (Table 20.3), but they are lower compared with other reports on patient cohorts with chronic rheumatoid arthritis in prospective or cross-sectional studies (Table 20.3). The recruitment of patients from the community might be one explanation for the low mortality risk in these two studies with the lowest mortality ratios since patients not referred routinely to specialist care have a milder disease[85]. In a population study from Sweden, the mortality was not increased in those patients who had not been hospitalized during the observation period[41]. The role of early treatment, medical, vocational, orthopedic, cannot be ruled out as patients referred for treatment within the next 5 years of the disease seem to have a better prognosis than those with a longer duration of disease before referral[52].

◀ **Fig. 20.9** Development of radiological destruction (means and 95% confidence limits) in patients with seropositive early (duration < 6 months at entry) rheumatoid arthritis analyzed by Larsen score (score 0–200; Ref. 83), and a modification by Kaarela (score 0–100; Ref. 81). Reproduced from Ref. 81: Kaarela K. and Kautiainen H. (1997). Continuous progression of radiological destruction in seropositive rheumatoid arthritis. *Journal of Rheumatology*, **24**:1285–7, with permission of the Journal of Rheumatology.

Can we predict the outcome in rheumatoid arthritis?

Clinical features of the disease

Clinical features early in the disease seem to have predictive value: early loss of function, female sex, low education level, and persistent active disease with clinical and laboratory evidence of continuous inflammation are all associated with poor functional outcome and progressive joint destruction[58,86]. Most of the information is, however, based on studies on patients with chronic rheumatoid arthritis with varying disease duration and follow-up time. Information on such patient cohorts can be biased, only the most severe ones and those surviving to the evaluation time point, being analyzed. The most reliable information is that obtained on early arthritis cohorts followed up prospectively from the start. The results of two such studies are conflicting. In a study from Sweden, none of the conventional variables had predictive value on radiological progression during the first 5 years of follow-up[78] while another study from Finland observed that initially active disease predicted disability and radiological progression during the next 6 years[87].

Risk factors for work disability are remarkably similar in various reports from different countries. Active disease, seropositivity, erosive disease, poor functional status at entry, duration of the disease, low educational level, and older age predict the loss of work capacity[23,24,28,29,66,74,88]. Social and work-related factors also have a substantial effect on work disability[29,85,89,90].

Risk factors for increased mortality are increasing age[36,38,42,43,44], male sex[36,42,43], poor function at study entry[18,19,38,41,43,91], and poor level of general health by self-reported questionnaire[39]. Poor function evaluated by HAQ predicted mortality during the next 8 years in a community cohort[90].

Variables directly related to the activity of the disease, such as high number of involved joints[38,43], high inflammatory activity[43], extra-articular features[43,92], and seropositivity[41,42,43,44], are also predictors of mortality. In some studies, the increased risk is observed only in seropositive patients[42,44]. The presence of joint destruction and extra-articular features is also reflected in the increased mortality of patients with classical versus definite rheumatoid arthritis[18]. Other factors, less directly associated with the rheumatoid disease, have also been associated with decreased life span, such as low level of education[38,43], hypertension, and previous cardiovascular event[36].

Laboratory markers

There is an increasing interest in the search for laboratory markers which would predict the functional and radiological outcome of patients. Of the conventional markers, high sedimentation rate, high C-reactive protein, low hemoglobin level, and high platelet counts are all markers of active disease[93]. Low hemoglobin and high sedimentation rate present at entry predict the 6-year radiological outcome of patients with early rheumatoid arthritis[87]. Also, persistent elevation of erythrocyte sedimentation rate or C-reactive protein levels associate with more severe joint destruction[79,94,95]. Rheumatoid factor is a hallmark for rheumatoid arthritis. Nearly all studies available agree that it is also a marker for more severe disease and predicts both joint destruction and functional disability. The level, as well as a persistently positive value, of rheumatoid factor during the early years of the disease is also associated with progressive radiological destruction (Fig. 20.10). Other autoantibodies, such as antinuclear, antikeratin, antiperinuclear factor, and anti-RA 33, have been analyzed in the context of predicting joint destruction. Only the presence of antikeratin antibodies was associated with

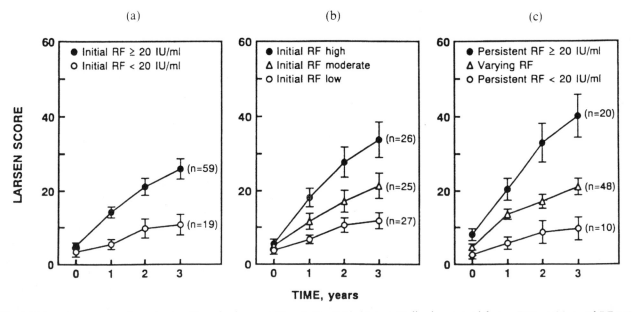

Fig. 20.10 (a) Mean Larsen score in patients with early rheumatoid arthritis divided into initially rheumatoid factor (RF) positive and RF negative patients. (b) Mean Larsen score in patients divided into subgroups according to the initial RF levels by tertile distribution. (c) mean Larsen score in patients divided into persistently positive, persistently negative, and variably positive and negative patients. Reproduced from Ref. 96: Paimela L., Palosuo T., Leirisalo-Repo M., Helve T., and Aho K. (1995). Prognostic value of quantitative measurement of rheumatoid factor in early rheumatoid arthritis. *British Journal of Rheumatology*, 34:1146–50, with permission of the British Society for Rheumatology.

an increased the risk for severe radiological damage during the first 8 years of the disease[97].

In addition to markers measuring or associated with inflammation, much interest has been recently focused on the search for biochemical markers reflecting inflammation in the synovium, or changes in the metabolism of cartilage or underlying bone, as predictors of joint destruction. Persistently high serum level of hyaluronan, produced in increased amounts by the inflamed synovium, is associated with increased radiological destruction during early rheumatoid arthritis[98]. It has a similar predictive value as a high sedimentation rate or C-reactive protein[99]. Interestingly, serum levels of a cartilage derived protein, cartilage oligomeric protein (COMP), were elevated in a subgroup of patients with early rheumatoid arthritis who subsequently developed rapid destruction of hip joints[100] but the serum levels of COMP did not predict the radiological destruction of the small joints[99]. A marker of collagen I breakdown, carboxyterminal telopeptide (ICTP), in serum, is associated with active disease and radiological erosions in early rheumatoid arthritis[101]. Serum levels of ICTP correlate both with inflammation[102], destruction of knee joints[103], and predict radiological destruction during the first 3 years of the disease[102]. The markers of synovium, cartilage, and bone predict radiological destruction when analyzed in patient cohorts but they cannot be used in clinical practice to predict the radiological destruction in the small joints of a single patient. Their value in monitoring destruction of large joints has to be studied further.

Genetic markers

While the frequency of HLA-DR4 (in some populations of HLA-DR1) is higher in RA patients compared with the population as a whole, the role of genetic factors, HLA-DR4 or the shared epitope, as determining the course of the disease is controversial. The presence of the shared epitope has been shown to predict the development of erosive arthritis in a population attending an early arthritis clinic[104]. Patients with established, chronic rheumatoid arthritis with severe articular damage also had higher frequency of HLA-Dw4, -Dw14 or–DR1 compared with control patients with limited destruction[95]. However, the groups were not comparable. The patients with more extensive joint destruction also more often had systemic and extra-articular manifestations, positive rheumatoid factor, and had more active disease compared with the rest of the patients. Prospective studies on early rheumatoid arthritis have found no significant contribution of HLA-DR4, HLA-Dw4, or the shared epitope on the radiological destruction or functional outcome of the patients during the following 5 to 9 years[67, 80,105].

Interestingly, however, patients homozygous for the shared epitope had about three times greater risk of undergoing joint replacement[105]. In a prospective study of patients followed up since the first 5 years of the disease, the number of swollen joints, rheumatoid factor, and erosion score worked well as predictors of the number of inflamed joints, radiological destruction, and functional outcome of the patients. HLA-DR4 contributed little or no additional information[106]. Genetic analysis might be most useful for patients with chronic, compli-

cated rheumatoid arthritis treated at specialist centers. Genetic analysis in the determination of late prognosis in the early arthritis patient does not seem to have a major role.

Can we modify the outcome and mortality in rheumatoid arthritis?

Long-term effects of pharmacological therapy

There are many controlled studies showing that patients treated with DMARDs have decreased joint inflammation. Some of the studies have also shown an effect on the radiological progression[107]. As discussed by Pincus[108], most of the studies are of short duration, extending only up to 2 to 3 years. These studies are too short to tell whether the long-term outcome of the patients would be influenced by such a treatment.

The effect of DMARDs with respect to functional outcome, work disability, or mortality is hard to estimate in the many observational studies reported. Many such studies include either no information of the drug therapies or only give information on the numbers of patients receiving DMARDs for some time during the study. In addition, the treatment has been empirical and mostly limited to patients with more active disease (see Table 20.1).

However, there is some uncontrolled evidence in favor of the role of early treatment. Radiological destruction was less frequent if gold treatment was started within the first 3 years of the disease[109]. Early treatment, if it resulted in decrease of C-reactive protein, has been shown to result in a fall in functional disability measured by HAQ during the subsequent 2 years[110]. DMARD therapy, if started within the initial 2 years of the disease, resulted in improved functional outcome[111, 112]. Such an effect is not reached if the treatment is delayed beyond that time[112]. Individually tailored, continuous DMARD therapy started within the initial 2 years of symptoms cannot prevent radiological progression but most of the patients preserve their functional capacity. During the next 6 years, 77 per cent of patients have normal or only slightly decreased functional capacity, but 3 per cent end up with severe handicap[67].

The duration of DMARD therapy might be important in determining long-term outcome. The functional disability and number of painful joints were unchanged during the 10-year course of disease of patients with chronic rheumatoid arthritis treated with parenteral gold for at least 2 consecutive years[113]. This was true both for patients with chronic disease as well as those in whom the treatment was started within the initial 2 years of the disease. However, the survival of patients first treated at the Rheumatism Foundation Hospital in Heinola in 1961–1966 was best in those who had been treated with parenteral gold for at least 10 years and lowest in those who had never received gold[114]. Results from England on patients followed-up for a period of 10 years from the time of prescription of the initial DMARD favor the conclusion by the Heinola group since patients remaining on DMARD showed significant improvement while those not on treatment at the final analysis had deteriorated in function[115]. During follow-up, patients were also treated with multidisciplinary care, with 71 per cent of the patients having had joint surgery as part of the treatment. Only 20 per cent of the patients had died and 3 per cent had become wheelchair-bound. The outcome can be compared to the results of a community-based survey by Hakala *et al.*[22], who explain the good functional outcome by early and active treatment with DMARDs, prescribed to 97 per cent of the patients, multi disciplinary care, and by the high number of orthopedic operations[116]. Use of DMARD also predicted survival in a community survey[90] and reduction of long-term disability in a large, multicenter databank analysis[117]. The results suggest up to 30 per cent reduction in the long-term disability with consistent use of DMARDs.

Patients treated with corticosteroids seem to be at increased risk for mortality[36,38,43]. The significance of this information is biased by the indications used for the treatment. A case-controlled study on the use of prednisone showed no increased mortality but the outcome by 10 years was slightly worse with more complications due to prednisone treatment[118]. An extensive review on the use of low-dose corticosteroids in rheumatoid arthritis concluded that corticosteroids are equivalent or slightly better than placebo and active controls in improving disease activity[119]. The side-effects in long-term use of the treatment were also evident in this analysis.

The effect of treatment on work disability is hard to evaluate because in addition to physical handicap, social and work-related factors and support available by the community contribute to the subjective disability. Yelin *et al.*[89] showed that work disability was effected by stage and duration of the disease but not by therapies received by the patient.

Role of orthopedic surgery

Despite active medical treatment and rehabilitation procedures, joint destruction proceeds in most patients. The figures for joint arthroplasties seem to vary between different prospective studies. The lowest figure is from the Heinola study: during the first 8 years of disease, 20 per cent of patients with rheumatoid arthritis had radiological evidence of hip involvement, mostly asymptomatic; 1 per cent had been operated on[120]. In another prospective study of early rheumatoid arthritis from Sweden, 13 per cent of the patients had undergone hip arthroplasty during the first 7 years of disease[121]. The third prospective cohort study, from Finland, reported a figure of 7 per cent for all major joint prosthesis during a mean of 7 years of disease[67]. Different populations and varying access to orthopedic surgery can contribute to the number of operations. A large database on 1600 patients with chronic rheumatoid arthritis in the United States showed that, within the first 20 years, about 25 per cent of the patients will undergo total joint arthroplasty[122]. The figure is astonishingly similar to that reported by Scott *et al.*[69] from England. Laboratory markers of inflammation and poor function increase the risk for orthopedic intervention. While it is an indicator of failure of conservative treatment, the availability of prosthetic surgery is an important contribution to the well-being of the patients. Operation improves, often dramatically, the quality of life of the patient and prevents the patient entering a lower functional class.

Conclusion

Rheumatoid arthritis is a chronic disease, which usually leads to decreasing function and contributes to increased mortality. Patients treated at specialist centers usually have more advanced and severe disease and the prognosis of such patients is usually worse compared with population cohorts or with patients belonging to early arthritis cohorts. Early destruction, early functional handicap, and persistent inflammation are the best predictors of poor outcome and increased mortality. Early multidisciplinary intervention with DMARDs, rehabilitation, and orthopedic surgery can postpone the functional deterioration in most of the patients.

References

1. Ropes M.V., Bennett G.A., Cobb S., Jacos R., Jessar R.A. 1958 revision of diagnostic criteria for rheumatoid arthritis. *Bull Rheum Dis*, 1958; 9:175–6.
2. Mikkelsen W.M. and Dodge H. A four year follow-up of suspected rheumatoid arthritis: the Tecumseh, Michigan, community health study. *Arthur Rheum*, 1969; 12:87–91.
3. Hochberg M.C. Predicting the prognosis of patients with rheumatoid arthritis: is there a crystal ball? *J Rheumatol*, 1993: 20:1265–7.
4. Suarez-Almazor M.E., Soskolne C.L., Saunders D., Russell A.S. Outcome in rheumatoid arthritis. A 1985 inception cohort study. *J Rheumatol*, 1994; 21:1438–46.
5. Allebeck P. and Lindberg G. Rheumatic diseases in a health interview survey and in in-patient care. *Scand J Soc Med*, 1984; 12:147–54.
6. Recht L, Brattström M., Lithman T. Chronic arthritis. Prevalence, severity and distribution between primary care and referral centres in a defined rural population. *Scand J Rheumatol*, 1989; 18:205–12.
7. Wasmus A., Kindel P., Raspe H.H. Epidemiologie der Behandlung bei an chronischer Polyarthritis Erkrankten in Hannover. *Z Rheumatol*, 1989;48:236–42.
8. Arnett F.C., Edworthy S.M., Bloch D.A., McShane D.J., Fries J.F., Cooper N.S., Healey L.A., *et al*. The American Rheumatism Association 1987 revised criteria for the classification of rheumatoid arthritis. *Arthritis Rheum*, 1988;31:315–24.
9. Harrison B.J., Symmons D.P.M., Brennan P., Barrett E.M., Silman A.J. Natural remission in inflammatory polyarthritis: issues of definition and prediction. *Br J Rheumatol*, 1996; 35:1096–100.
10. Wolfe F., Ross K., Hawley D.J., Roberts F.K., Cathey M.A. The prognosis of rheumatoid arthritis and undifferentiated polyarthritis syndrome in the clinic: a study of 1141 patients. *J Rheumatol*, 1993;20:2005–9.
11. Wolfe F. The natural history of rheumatoid arthritis. *J Rheumatol*, 1996;23 (suppl. 44):13–22.
12. Nissilä M., Isomäki H., Kaarela K., Kiviniemi P., Martio J., Sarna S. Prognosis of inflammatory joint diseases. A three-year follow-up study. *Scand J Rheumatol*, 1983;21:33–8.
13. Young A. Short-term outcomes in recent-onset rheumatoid arthritis. *Br J Rheumatol*, 1995;34 (suppl. 2): 79–86.
14. Harrison B.J., Symmons D.P.M., Brennan P., Bankhead C.R., Baret E.M., Scott D.G.I., Silman A.J. Inflammatory polyarthritis in the

community is not a benign disease: predicting functional disability one year after presentation. *J Rheumatol*, 1996; 23:1326–31.

15. Sherrer Y.S., Bloch D.A., Mitchell D.M., Young D.Y., Fries J.F. The development of disability in rheumatoid arthritis. *Arthritis Rheum*, 1986; 29:494–500.

16. Young A., Corbett M., Winfield J., Jaqueremada D., Williams P., Papasavvas G, *et al*. A prognostic index for erosive changes in the hands, feet, and cervical spine in early rheumatoid arthritis. *Br J Rheumatol*, 1988; 27:94–101.

17. Houssein D.A., McKenna S.P., Scott D.L. The Nottingham Health Profile as a measure of disease activity and outcome in rheumatoid arthritis. *Br J Rheumatol*, 1997; 36:69–73.

18. Rasker J.J., Cosh J.A. Long-term effects of treating rheumatoid arthritis. *Baillière's Clin Rheumatol*, 1992; 6:141–60.

19. Corbett M., Dalton S., Young A., Silman S., Shipley M. Factors predicting death, survival, and functional outcome in a prospective study of early rheumatoid disease over fifteen years. *Br J Rheumatol*, 1993; 32:717–23.

20. Wolfe F., Cathey M.A. The assessment and prediction of functional disability in rheumatoid arthritis. *J Rheumatol*, 1991; 18:1298–306.

21. Isacson J., Allander E., Broström H. L-Å. A seventeen-year follow-up of a population survey of rheumatoid arthritis. *Scand J Rheumatol*, 1987; 16:145–52.

22. Hakala M., Nieminen P, Koivisto O. More evidence from a community based series of better outcome in rheumatoid arthritis. Data on the effect of multi-disciplinary care on the retention of functional ability. *J Rheumatol*, 1994; 21:1432–7.

23. Mäkisara G.L., Mäkisara P. Prognosis of functional capacity and work capacity in rheumatoid arthritis. *Clin Rheumatol*, 1982; 1:117–25.

24. Doeglas D., Suurmeijer T., Krol B., Sanderman R., van Leeuwen M, Rijswijk M. Work disability in early rheumatoid arthritis. *Ann Rheum Dis*, 1995; 54:455–60.

25. Duthie J.J.R., Thompson M., Weir M.M., Fletcher W.B. Medical and social aspects of the treatment of rheumatoid arthritis with special reference to factors affecting prognosis. *Ann Rheum Dis*, 1955; 14:133–49.

26. Duthie J.J.R., Brown P.E., Know J.D.E., Thompson M. Course and prognosis in rheumatoid arthritis. *Ann Rheum Dis*, 1957; 16:411–24.

27. Duthie J.J.R., Brown P.E., Truelove L.H., Baragar F.D., Lawrie A.J. Course and prognosis in rheumatoid arthritis. A further report. *Ann Rheum Dis*, 1964; 23:193–204.

28. Mau W., Bornmann M., Weber H., Weidemann H.F., Hecker H., Raspe H.H. Prediction of permanent work disability in a follow-up study of early rheumatoid arthritis: results of a tree structured analysis using RECPAM. *Br J Rheumatol*, 1996; 35:652–9.

29. Reisine S., McQuillan J., Fifield J. Predictors of work disability in rheumatoid arthritis patients. A five-year follow-up. *Arthritis Rheum*, 1995; 38:1630–7.

30. van der Heijde D.M.F.M. Joint erosions and patients with early rheumatoid arthritis. *J Rheumatol*, 1993;34(suppl 2):74–8.

31. Sharp J.T., Wolfe F., Mitchell D.M., Bloch D.A. The progression of erosion and joint space narrowing scores in rheumatoid arthritis during the first twenty-five years of disease. *Arthritis Rheum*, 1991;34:660–8.

32. Heikkilä S., Isomäki H. Long-term outcome of rheumatoid arthritis has improved. *Scand J Rheumatol*, 1989;23:13–15.

33. Vandenbroucke J.P., Hazevoet H.M., Cats A. Survival and cause of death in rheumatoid arthritis: A 25-year prospective follow-up. *J. Rheumatol*, 1984;11:158–61.

34. Mitchel D.M., Spitz P.W., Young D.Y., Bloch D.A., McShane D.J., Fries J.F. Survival, prognosis, and causes of death in rheumatoid arthritis. *Arthritis Rheum*, 1986;29:706–14.

35 Myllykangas-Luosujärvi R., Aho K., Kautiainen H., Isomäki H. Shortening of life span and causes of excess mortality in a population-based series of subjects with rheumatoid arthritis. *Clin Exp Rheumatol*, 1995;13:149–53.

36. Wållberg-Jonsson S., Öhman M-L., Rantapää Dahlqvist S. Cardiovascular morbidity and mortality in patients with seropositive rheumatoid arthritis in northern Sweden. *J Rheumatol*, 1997;24:445–51.

37. Pincus T., Callahan L.F., Sale W.G., Brooks A.L., Payne L.E., Vaughn W.K. Severe functional declines, work disability, and increased mortality in seventy-five rheumatoid arthritis patients studied over nine years. *Arthritis Rheum*, 1984;27:864–72.

38. Pincus T., Callahan L.F., Vaughn W.K. Questionnaire, walking time and button test measurers of functional capacity as predictive markers for mortality in rheumatoid arthritis. *J Rheumatol*, 1987;14:240–51.

39. Kazis L.E., Anderson J.J., Meenan R.F. Health status as a predictor of mortality in rheumatoid arthritis: a five year study. *J Rheumatol*, 1990;17:609–13.

40. Linos A., Worthington J.W., O'Fallon W.M., Kurland L.T. The epidemiology of rheumatoid arthritis in Rochester, Minnesota: A study of incidence, prevalence, and mortality. *Am J Epidemiol*, 1980;111:87–98.

41. Allebeck P., Ahlbom A., Allander E. Increased mortality among persons with rheumatoid arthritis, but where RA does not appear on death certificate. *Scand J Rheumatol*, 1981;10:301–6.

42. Jacobsson L.T.H., Knowler W.C., Pillemer S., Hanson R.L., Pettitt D.J., Nelson R.G., *et al*. Rheumatoid arthritis and mortality. A longitudinal study in Pima Indians. *Arthritis Rheum*, 1993;36:1045–53.

43. Wolfe F., Mitchell D.M., Sibley J.T., Fries J.F., Bloch D.A., Williams C.A., *et al*. The mortality of rheumatoid arthritis. *Arthritis Rheum*, 1994;37:481–94.

44. van Schaardenburg D., Hazes J.W., de Boer A., Zwinderman A.H., Meijers K.A.E., Breedveld F.C. Outcome of rheumatoid arthritis in relation to age and rheumatoid factor at diagnosis. *J Rheumatol*, 1993;20:45–52.

45. Pincus T. The paradox of effective therapies but poor long-term outcomes in rheumatoid arthritis. *Seminars Arthritis Rheum*, 1992;21 (suppl.3):2–15.

46. Myllykangas-Luosujärvi R.A., Aho K., Isomäki H. Mortality in rheumatoid arthritis. *Seminars Arthritis Rheum*, 1995;25:193–202.

47. Young A., van der Heijde D.M.F.M. Can we predict aggressive disease? *Baillière's Clin Rheumatol*, 1997;11:27-48.

48. Mutru O., Laakso M., Isomäki H., Koota K. Ten year mortality and causes of death in patients with rheumatoid arthritis. *Br Med J*, 1985;290:1797–9.

49. Laakso M., Mutru O., Isomäki H., Koota K. Cancer mortality in patients with rheumatoid arthritis. *J Rheumatol*, 1986;13:522–6.

50. Matteson E.L., Hickey A.R., Maquire L., Tilson H.H., Urowitz MB. Occurrence of neoplasia in patients with rheumatoid arthritis enrolled in DMARD registry. Rheumatoid arthritis azathioprine registry steering committee. *J Rheumatol*, 1991;18:809–14.

51. Myllykangas-Luosujärvi R., Aho K., Isomäki H. Mortality from cancer in patients with rheumatoid arthritis. *Scand J Rheumatol*, 1995;24:76–8.

52. Symmons D.P.M., Jones M.A., Scott D.L., Prior P. Long-term mortality outcome in patients with rheumatoid arthritis: early presenters continue to do well. *J Rheumatol*, 1998;25:1072–7.

53. Isomäki H.A., Hakulinen T., Joutsenlahti U. Excess risk of lymphomas, leukemia and myeloma in patients with rheumatoid arthritis. *J Chron Dis*, 1978;31:691–6.

54. Eriksson M. Rheumatoid arthritis as a risk factor for multiple myeloma: a case-control study. *Eur J Cancer*, 1993;29A:259–63.

55. Bäcklund E., Ekbom A., Sparén P., Feltelius N., Klareskog L. Disease activity and risk of lymphoma in patients with rheumatoid arthritis: nested case-control study. *Br Med J*, 1998;317:180–1.

56. Symmons D. Excess mortality in rheumatoid arthritis—is it the disease or the drugs? *J Rheumatol*, 1995;22:2200–2.

57. Myllykangas-Luosujärvi R., Aho K., Isomäki H. Death attributed to antirheumatic medication in a nation-wide series of 1666 patients with rheumatoid arthritis who have died. *J Rheumatol*, 1995;22:1121–7.

58. Pincus T., Callahan L.F. The 'side effects' of rheumatoid arthritis: joint destruction, disability, and early mortality. *Br J Rheumatol*, 1993;**32** (suppl. 1):28–37.

59. Silman A.J., Petrie J., Haxleman B., Evans S.J. Lymphoproliferative cancer and other malignancy in patients with rheumatoid arthritis treated with azathioprine: a 20 year follow up study. *Ann Rheum Dis*, 1988;**47**:988–92.

60. Jones M., Symmons D., Finn J., Wolfe F. Does exposure to immuno-suppressive therapy increase the 10 year malignancy and mortality risks in rheumatoid arthritis? A matched cohort study. *Br J Rheumatol*, 1996;**35**:738–45.

61. Alarcón G.S., Tracy I.C., Strand G.M., Singh K., Macaluso M. Survival and drug discontinuation analyses in a large cohort of methotrexate treated rheumatoid arthritis patients. *Ann Rheum Dis*, 1995;**54**:708–12.

62. Fries J.F., Williams C.A., Bloch D.A., Michel B.A. Nonsteroidal anti-inflammatory drug-associated gastropathy: incidence and risk factor models. *Am J Med*, 1991;**91**:213–22.

63. Maxwell S.R.J., Moots R.J., Kendall M.J. Corticosteroids: do they damage the cardiovascular system? *Postgrad Med J*, 1994;**70**:863–70.

64. Raynaud J.P. Cardiovascular mortality in rheumatoid arthritis. How harmful are corticosteroids? *J Rheumatol*, 1997;**24**:415–6.

65. Eberhardt K.B., Fex E. Functional impairment and disability in early rheumatoid arthritis—development over 5 years. *J Rheumatol*, 1995;**22**:1037–42.

66. Fex E., Larsson B-M., Nived K., Eberhardt K. Effect of rheumatoid arthritis on work status and social and leisure time activities in patients followed 8 years from onset. *J Rheumatol*, 1998;**25**:44–50.

67. Möttönen T., Paimela L., Ahonen J., Helve T., Hannonen P., Leirisalo-Repo M. Outcome in patients with early rheumatoid arthritis treated according to the 'sawtooth' strategy. *Arthritis Rheum*, 1996;**39**:996–1005.

68. Lance N.J., Curran J.J. Late-onset, seropositive, erosive rheumatoid arthritis. *Seminars Arthritis Rheum*, 1993;**23**:177–182.

69. Scott D.L., Symmons D.P.M., Coulton B.L., Popert A.J. Long-term outcome of treating rheumatoid arthritis: results after 20 years. *Lancet*, 1987;**i**:1108–11.

70. Jacoby R.K., Jayson M.I.V., Cosh J.A. Onset, early stages, and prognosis of rheumatoid arthritis. A clinical study of 100 patients with 11-year follow-up. *Br Med J*, 1973;**2**:96–100.

71. Rasker J.J., Cosh J.A. Cause and age of death in a prospective study of 100 patients with rheumatoid arthritis. *Ann Rheum Dis*, 1981;**40**:115–20.

72. Cosh J.A., Rasker J.J. A 20-year follow-up of 100 patients with rheumatoid arthritis (RA). *Ann Rheum Dis*, 1982;**41**:317.

73. Rasker J.J., Cosh J.A. The natural history of rheumatoid arthritis over 20 years. Clinical symptoms, radiological signs, treatment, mortality, and prognostic significance of early features. *Clin Rheumatol*, 1987;**6** (suppl. 2):5–11.

74. Reilly P.A., Cosh J.A., Maddison P.J., Rasker J.J., Silman A. Mortality and survival in rheumatoid arthritis: a 24-year prospective study of 100 patients. *Ann Rheum Dis*, 1990;**49**:363–9.

75. Eberhardt K., Larsson B-M., Nived K. Early rheumatoid arthritis—some social, economical, and psychological aspects. *Scand J Rheumatol*, 1993;**22**:119–23.

76. van der Heijde D.M.F.M., van Leeuwen M.A., van Riel P.L.C.M., Koster A.M., van't Hof M.A., van Rijswijk M., van de Putte L.B.A. Biannual radiographic assessment of hands and feet in a three-year prospective follow-up of patients with early rheumatoid arthritis. *Arthritis Rheum*, 1992;**35**:26–34.

77. Kaarela K., Kauppi M.J., Lehtinen K.E.S. The value of the ACR 1987 criteria in a very early rheumatoid arthritis. *Scand J Rheumatol*, 1995;**24**:279–81.

78. Fex E., Jonsson K., Johnson U., Eberhardt K. Development of radiologic damage during the first 5–6 yr of rheumatoid arthritis. A prospective follow-up study of a Swedish cohort. *Br J Rheumatol*, 1996;**35**:1106–15.

79. Plant M.J., Jones P.W., Saklatvala J., Ollier W.E.R., Dawes P.T. Patterns of radiological progression in early rheumatoid arthritis: results of an 8 year prospective study. *J Rheumatol*, 1998;**25**:17–26.

80. Young A., Jaraquemada D., Awad J., Festenstein H., Corbett M., Hay F.C., Roitt I. Association of HLA-DR4/Dw4 and DR2/DW2 with radiologic changes in a prospective study of patients with rheumatoid arthritis. Preferential relationship with HLA-Dw rather than HLA-DR specificities. *Arthritis Rheum*, 1984;**27**:20–25.

81. Kaarela K., Kautiainen H. Continuous progression of radiological destruction in seropositive rheumatoid arthritis. *J Rheumatol*, 1997;**24**:1285–7.

82. Isomäki H. Long-term outcome of rheumatoid arthritis. *Scand J Rheumatol*, 1992;**21** (suppl 95):3–8.

83. Larsen A., Dale K., Eek M. Radiographic evaluation of rheumatoid arthritis and related conditions by standard reference films. *Acta Radiol Diagn*, 1977;**18**:481–91.

84. Isomäki H., Kautiainen H., Kaarela K., Nieminen M. Low 20-year mortality in RA patients with early hospitalisation. *Scand J Rheumatol*, 1995;**24**:189.

85. Weisman M.H. Natural history and treatment decisions in rheumatoid arthritis revisited. *Arthritis Care Res*, 1989;**2** (suppl.):S75–S83.

86. Alarcón G.S. Predictive factors in rheumatoid arthritis. *Amer J Med*, 1997;**103** (suppl. 6A):19S–24S.

87. Möttönen T., Paimela L., Leinsalo-Repo M., Kautiainen H., Ilonen J., Hannonen P. Only high disease activity and positive RF indicate poor prognosis in patients with early rheumatoid arthritis treated with 'sawtooth' strategy. *Ann Rheum Dis*, 1998;**57**:533–9.

88. Sherrer Y.S., Bloch D.A., Mitchell D.M., Roth S.H., Wolfe F., Fries J.F. Disability in rheumatoid arthritis: comparison of prognostic factors across three populations. *J Rheumatol*, 1987;**14**:705–9.

89. Yelin E., Meenan R., Nevitt M., Epstein W. Work disability in rheumatoid arthritis: effects of disease, social, and work factors. *Ann Int Med*, 1980;**93**:551–6.

90. Leigh J.P., Fries J.F. Mortality predictors among 263 patients with rheumatoid arthritis. *J Rheumatol*, 1991;**18**:1307–12.

91. Ragan C., Farrington E. The clinical features of rheumatoid arthritis. *JAMA*, 1962;**181**:663–7.

92. Erhardt C.C., Mumford P.A., Venables P.J.W., Maini R.N. Factors predicting a poor life prognosis in rheumatoid arthritis: an eight year prospective study. *Ann Rheum Dis*, 1989;**48**:7–13.

93. van der Heijde D.M.F.M., van Riel P.L.C.M., van Rijswijk M.H., van de Putte L.B.A. Influence of prognostic features on the final outcome in rheumatoid arthritis: review of the literature. *Seminars Arthritis Rheum*, 1988;**17**:284–92.

94. Hassell A.B., Davis M.J., Fowler P.D., Clarke S., Fisher J., Shadforth M.F., Jones P.W., Dawes P.T. The relationship between serial measures of disease activity and outcome in rheumatoid arthritis. *Quart J Med*, 1993;**86**:601–7.

95. Combe B., Eliaou J.F., Daurès J.P., Meyer O., Clot J., Sany J. Prognostic factors in rheumatoid arthritis. Comparative study of two subsets of patients according to severity of articular damage. *Br J Rheumatol*, 1995;**34**:529–34.

96. Paimela L., Palosuo T., Leirisalo-Repo M., Helve T., Aho K. Prognostic value of quantitative measurement of rheumatoid factor in early rheumatoid arthritis. *Br J Rheumatol*, 1995;**34**:1146–50.

97. Meyer O., Combe B., Elias A., Benali K., Clot J., Sany J., Elianou JF. Autoantibodies predicting the outcome of rheumatoid arthritis: evaluation in two subsets of patients according to severity of radiographic damage. *Ann Rheum Dis*, 1997;**56**:682–5.

98. Paimela L., Heiskanen A., Kurki P., Helve T., Leirisalo-Repo M. Serum hyaluronate level as a predictor of radiologic progression in early rheumatoid arthritis. *Arthritis Rheum*, 1991;**34**:815–21.

99. Fex E., Eberhardt K., Saxne T. Tissue-derived macromolecules and markers of inflammation in serum in early rheumatoid arthritis: relationship to development of joint destruction in hands and feet. *Br J Rheumatol*, 1997;**36**:1161–5.

100. Forslind K., Eberhardt K., Jonsson A., Saxne T. Increased serum concentrations of cartilage oligomeric matrix protein. A prognos-

tic marker in early rheumatoid arthritis. *Br J Rheumatol*, 1992;31:593–8.

101. Kotaniemi A., Isomäki H., Hakala M., Risteli L., Risteli J. Increased type I collagen degradation in early rheumatoid arthritis. *J Rheumatol*, 1994;21:1593–6.

102. Paimela L., Leirisalo-Repo M., Risteli L., Hakala M., Helve T., Risteli J. Type I collagen degradation product in serum of patients with early rheumatoid arthritis: relationship to disease activity and radiological progression in a 3-year follow-up. *Br J Rheumatol*, 1994;33:1012–6.

103. Hakala M., Åhman S., Luukkainen R., Risteli H.L., Kauppi M., Nieminen P., Risteli J. Application of markers of collagen metabolism in serum and synovial fluid for assessment of disease process in patients with rheumatoid arthritis. *Ann Rheum Dis*, 1995;54:886–90.

104. Emery P., Salmon M., Bradley H., Wordsworth P., Tunn E., Bacon P., Waring R. Genetically determined factors as predictors of radiological change in patients with early symmetrical arthritis. *Br Med J*, 1992;305:1387–9.

105. Eberhardt K., Fex E., Johnson U., Wollheim F.A. Associations of HLA-DRB and -DQB genes with two and five year outcome in rheumatoid arthritis. *Ann Rheum Dis*, 1996;55:34–9.

106. van Zeben D., Hazes J.M.W., Zwinderman A.H., Vandenbroucke JP, Breedveld FC. Factors predicting outcome of rheumatoid arthritis: results of a follow-up study. *J Rheumatol*, 1993;20:1288–96.

107. Iannuzzi L., Dawson N., Zein N., Kushner I. Does drug therapy slow radiographic deterioration in rheumatoid arthritis. *New Engl J Med*, 1983;309:1023–8.

108. Pincus T. Long-term outcomes in rheumatoid arthritis. *J Rheumatol*, 1995;34 (suppl. 2):59–73.

109. Luukkainen R. Chrysotherapy in rheumatoid arthritis with particular emphasis on the effect of chrysotherapy on radiological changes and on the optimal time of initiation of therapy. *Scand J Rheumatol*, 1980;(suppl. 34):1–56.

110. Devlin J., Gough A., Huissoon A., Perkins P., Holder R., Reece R., *et al*. The acute phase and function in early rheumatoid arthritis. C–reactive protein levels correlate with functional outcome. *J Rheumatol*, 1997;24:9–13.

111. Egsmose C. Lund B., Borg G., Pettersson H., Berg E., Brodin U., Trang L. Patients with rheumatoid arthritis benefit from early 2nd line therapy: 5 year follow-up of a prospective double blind placebo controlled study. *J Rheumatol*, 1995;22:2208–13.

112. Munro R., Hampson R., McEntegard A., Thomson E.A., Madhok R., Capell H. Improved functional outcome in patients with early rheumatoid arthritis treated with intramuscular gold: results of a five year prospective study. *Ann Rheum Dis*, 1998;57:88–93.

113. Epstein W.V., Henke C.J., Yelin E.H., Katz P.P. Effect of parenterally administered gold therapy on the course of adult rheumatoid arthritis. *Ann Int Med*, 1991;114:437–44.

114. Lehtinen K., Isomäki H. Intramuscular gold therapy is associated with long survival in patients with rheumatoid arthritis. *J Rheumatol*, 1991;18:524–9.

115. Capell H.A., Murphy E.A., Hunter J.A. Rheumatoid arthritis: workload and outcome over 10 years. *Quart J Med* (new series), 1991;290:461–76.

116. Hakala M., Nieminen P. Functional status assessment of physical impairment in a community based population with rheumatoid arthritis: severely incapacitated patients are rare. *J Rheumatol*, 1996;23:617–23.

117. Fries J.F., Williams C.A., Morfeld D., Singh G., Sibley J. Reduction in long-term disability in patients with rheumatoid arthritis by disease-modified antirheumatic drug-based treatment strategies. *Arthritis Rheum*, 1996;39:606–22.

118. McDougall R., Sibley J., Haga M., Russell A. Outcome in patients with rheumatoid arthritis receiving prednisone compared to matched controls. *J Rheumatol*, 1994;21:1207–13.

119. Saag K.G. Low-dose corticosteroid therapy in rheumatoid arthritis: balancing the evidence. *Am J Med*, 1997;103 (suppl. 4):31S–39S.

120. Lehtimaki M.Y., Kaarela K., Hämäläinen M. Incidence of hip involvement and need for total hip replacement in rheumatoid arthritis. An eight-year follow-up study. *Scand J Rheumatol*, 1986;15:387–91.

121. Eberhardt K., Fex E., Johnsson K., Geborek P. Hip involvement in early rheumatoid arthritis. *Ann Rheum Dis*, 1995;54:45–8.

122. Wolfe F., Zwillich S.H. The long-term outcomes of rheumatoid arthritis. A 23-year prospective, longitudinal study of total joint replacement and its predictors in 1,600 patients with rheumatoid arthritis. *Arthritis Rheum*, 1998;41:1072–82.

21 | Molecular markers for assessment of cartilage damage in rheumatoid arthritis

Tore Saxne and Bengt Månsson

Introduction

Cartilage, like other connective tissues, continuously remodels in a finely tuned balance between matrix synthesis and degradation[1]. In common diseases such as osteoarthritis (OA) and rheumatoid arthritis (RA), the normal balance is disturbed and shifted towards degradation in established disease. This eventually leads to disruption of the structural and functional integrity of the joint. As a consequence of the disturbed matrix turnover, increased amounts of macromolecules or fragments thereof are released into synovial fluid and may subsequently reach the blood stream. Some fragments may also be found in the urine[2-4]. This sequence of events, schematically depicted in Fig. 21.1, forms the rationale for efforts to identify alterations in the tissue by quantifying matrix macromolecules, 'molecular markers', in body fluids by immunoassay with the purpose of defining non-invasive methods to monitor pathological tissue processes[5,6].

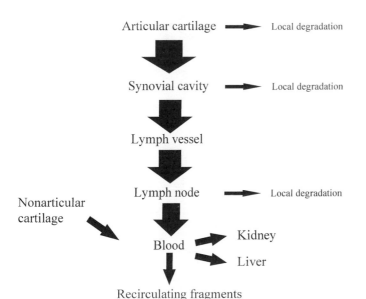

Fig. 21.1 Pathways for release and catabolism of articular cartilage macromolecules. Macromolecules are fragmented by proteases and released into synovial fluid. Fragments are eliminated by lymphatic drainage to the blood and are then removed by hepatic degradation or renal clearance. Note influx of fragments from extra-articular cartilage.

Table 21.1 Examples of potential applications of molecular markers for cartilage involvement in rheumatoid arthritis

1. Diagnostic test
2. Monitor and quantify tissue damage
3. Monitor and predict progression of tissue damage
4. Monitor response to therapy/provide proof of concept in clinical trials
5. Predict response to therapy
6. Elucidate pathophysiological mechanisms for cartilage destruction
   - Define cleavage patterns of macromolecules which will reveal the enzymatic mechanisms for cleavage and thereby facilitate development of inhibitors
   - By monitoring effects of therapy molecular markers will aid in understanding how mediators, e.g. cytokines, drive the destructive process

In this review, the basic principles of the molecular marker technology for assessment of pathological processes in cartilage will be highlighted, focusing on its potentials both for elucidation of pathophysiological mechanisms for tissue destruction and for clinical purposes Table 21.1. The limitations and pitfalls of this novel approach to the study of tissue involvement in arthritis will be discussed. Most of the points raised apply not only to markers for cartilage but also for bone markers and some reference to the use of such markers in RA will be given when appropriate. The current status, as well as future perspectives of the field, will be discussed in the light of key findings pertaining to the different applications of the technology.

Structure and function of cartilage

Cartilage is a mesenchymal tissue, and forms the precursor of long bone. Joint cartilage is devoid of blood vessels and is thus dependent on synovial fluid for nutrition and drainage of waste products. The main function of articular cartilage in diarthrodial joints is to provide smooth, low resistance surfaces that can withstand compression when loaded. To accomplish this, the tissue has an abundant, resilient extracellular matrix. In this matrix relatively few cells, chondrocytes, are embedded. For review see Ref. 7.

The cartilage matrix contains several matrix molecules specific for the tissue, but also includes many molecules with a ubiquitous distribution among connective tissues. The major components are collagen type II and the large aggregating proteoglycan, aggrecan, both essentially cartilage specific. The collagen fibers with their other constituent molecules form a network in the tissue with major functions to provide tensile stiffness and in distributing load. The interactions between collagen fibrils, essential for the properties of the collagen network, as well as those between collagen fibers, largely rely on a number of other matrix proteins which are often of proteoglycan nature, for example decorin and fibromodulin, but also on integral, minor collagens. These proteins apparently also have the potential to regulate collagen fibril formation and thus to modulate matrix assembly.

Aggrecan represents some 5 per cent of the cartilage wet weight but the abundance varies between different types of cartilage and between different parts of a given cartilage. Thus, in articular cartilage the concentration is much lower in the superficial than in the deep layers. Aggrecan contains anionic glycosaminoglycan side chains with high fixed negative charge density which creates high osmotic pressure. This results in a pronounced capacity to imbibe water and creates a very high swelling pressure, which is resisted by the network of collagen fibers. A consequence of this organization is that even high loads on the tissue will result in only minor volume changes. The cartilage matrix can thus be viewed as a composite, with fibers embedded in and reinforcing a charged matrix.

The structure of the cells and matrix is not homogenous throughout the articular cartilage (Fig. 21.2.) In the superficial

layers the cells are relatively scarce, have a somewhat flattened shape and are oriented in parallel with the surface. Deeper in the cartilage the cells are somewhat more abundant and have a rounded shape. The extracellular matrix also differs in different depths of the cartilage. Collagen type II fibers exemplifies this. In the superficial layers, collagen fibers run in parallel to the surface but deeper in the cartilage they run more perpendicular to the surface to meet varying types of load.

In each layer there is also a heterogeneity in the composition of the matrix depending on the distance from the cells. Light and/or electron microscopy reveals thin, less dense collagen fibers around the cells and an abundance of metachromatically stained (negatively charged) material. This zone is called the territorial matrix. In the periphery of the territorial matrix, the collagen fibers become more dense forming the so called basket. The matrix localized outside the basket is called interterritorial matrix. For review see Refs. 7–9.

The only cell type in cartilage, the chondrocyte, is capable of both synthesizing and degrading all matrix components. Normally the cartilage matrix turnover is a highly controlled, finely tuned process. This becomes dysregulated in disease. Newly synthesized molecules are secreted into the pericellular zone where some of them remain. The cells receive information from the matrix enabling them to maintain tissue homeostasis. It is reasonable to speculate that molecules responsible for matrix to cell signaling are enriched in the pericellular zone. Other molecules are transported further away to become incorporated in

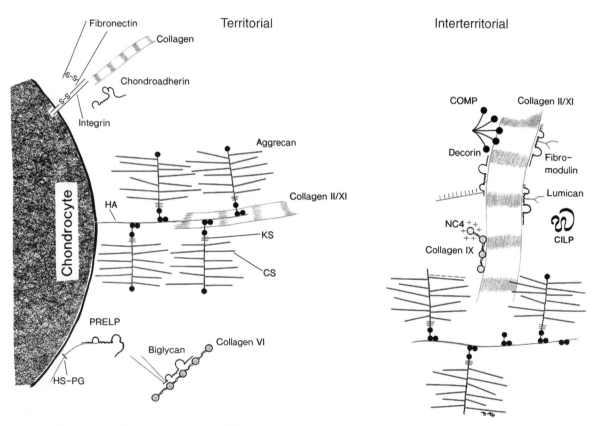

Fig. 21.2   Schematic illustration of the constituents of cartilage matrix. The spatial relationships of the various constituents to the chondrocyte, that is their presence in the territorial (close to the cell) or interterritorial matrix (furthest away from the cell) is shown and the macromolecular organization of matrix molecules is indicated. Adapted from Ref. 10 with permission. See also Plate 25.

the territorial matrix and in the interterritorial matrix, providing the structural properties of the matrix.

The different distribution of matrix constituents may indicate different functional roles which may be studied using the molecular marker technology. Another consequence of the variable distribution is that molecules or fragments thereof detected in body fluids may be used to localize disease process to a certain zone or compartment at a certain stage of, for example rheumatoid arthritis.

Macromolecular constituents

Cartilage consists of approximately 75 per cent water. The organic material consists of collagens, proteoglycans, and other non-collagenous matrix proteins[10]. Some of the most important features of these constituents will be discussed.

Collagens

Collagen type II is the dominating collagen in articular cartilage comprising 70 per cent of the tissue dry weight. Collagen type II is a triple helix composed of three α 1 (II)-chains. It is synthesized as a procollagen containing non-helical ends. After cleavage of the N- and C-terminal propeptides, fibrils are formed. However, in both the N- and C-terminal parts of the triple helix, non-helical telopeptides remain. The fibrils are held together, amongst other bonds, by cross links between the telopeptides. These cross links retain their structure when collagen is broken down[11].

Articular cartilage also contains other collagens such as types V, VI, IX, X, and XI collagen[12]. Type VI collagen, which has a wide tissue distribution, consists of a short helical domain and a large globular domain. In the tissue it forms a network of microfilaments. Collagen type IX is a so called FACIT-collagen (Fibril Associated Collagen with Interrupted triple-helices). It consists of three triple helical domains (C1–C3) and four globular domains (NC1–NC4). It is sometimes substituted with one glycosaminoglycan chain and is thus, in these cases, also a proteoglycan. It interacts with collagen type II in such a way that the NC4 domain, which is positively charged, sticks out from the complex[13,14]. Collagen IX thus provides the collagen II fibril with properties that might facilitate interaction with other fibrils or other matrix constituents. Type X collagen is a short-chained collagen synthesized by hypertrophic chondrocytes and it is also present in the superficial layers of articular cartilage. It might form fine filaments[15] and be associated with collagen type II fibers[16]. Type XI collagen is an integral part of the collagen II fibers and seems to have a role in regulating fiber diameter[17].

Proteoglycans

The large aggregating proteoglycan, aggrecan, is the second most dominant component of articular cartilage. Aggrecan consists of a protein core of molecular weight 220–250 kD, which is heavily substituted with glycosaminoglycans, mainly chondroitin sulfate and, to a lesser extent, keratan sulfate. The glycosaminoglycan side chains confer a high negative charge density and water binding. The protein core consists of three globular domains, G1–G3, separated by stretched areas. Via the G1 domain aggrecan interacts with hyaluronan to form extensive complexes which are fixed in the collagen network and provide the tissue pressure through water binding[18].

Cartilage also contains different small proteoglycans such as decorin[19,20], biglycan, and fibromodulin[21]. These proteins belong to a family of leucine-rich repeat (LRR) proteins[22]. They have a protein core of molecular weight 37–41 kD and are often substituted with glycosaminoglycan side chains (dermatan-/chondroitin-sulfate in decorin and biglycan, keratan sulfate in fibromodulin). Decorin and fibromodulin on one hand and biglycan on the other hand are present at different locations in articular cartilage. All of them are more prominent in superficial layers as compared to deep layers but decorin and fibromodulin are most prominent in the interterritorial matrix while biglycan is more abundant in the pericellular matrix[23–24]. The immunolocalization corroborates the observation that fibromodulin and decorin, on different sites, interacts with collagen, thereby modulating fibrillogenesis. Synthesis of small proteoglycans is regulated by transforming growth factor β (TGF-β), a protein to which they also bind[25,26]. The functional implication of this interaction is not fully understood but it may be involved in TGF-β mediated cartilage repair.

Other non-collagenous extracellular matrix proteins

Cartilage oligomeric matrix protein, COMP, deserves special attention as a promising marker of cartilage metabolism. COMP belongs to the thrombospondin family of proteins[27]. It consists of five identical subunits, each with a molecular weight of 83 kD, held together in an α-helical bundle which is stabilized by disulfide bridges close to the N-terminal end[28]. It has globular domains in the C-terminal end. In this way a bouquet-like structure is formed[29] Fig. 21.3. Each subunit contains eight Ca-binding domains and four epidermal growth factor- (EGF-) like domains[30]. COMP isolated from fetal and adult cartilage differs with regard to glycosylation[31]. COMP is located pericellularly and territorially in developing cartilage but mainly interterritorially in mature cartilage[32]. Its true function is not fully elucidated but it has been shown to interact with collagen of type I and type II at very specific sites on the collagen molecule[33]. This feature, and its interterritorial localization in mature cartilage, indicates a structural role in cartilage. The different glycosylation and localization in fetal cartilage suggests yet another function. Point mutations in COMP result in severe chondrodysplasias or epiphyseal dysplasias indicating its critical role in cartilage formation and/or function[34–36].

COMP is most prominent in cartilage but the protein is also present in other pressure loaded tissues, for example tendon and meniscus. More recently, the protein has also been found in synovial membrane[37–39]. The relative abundance of the protein differs considerably, being significantly higher in cartilage as

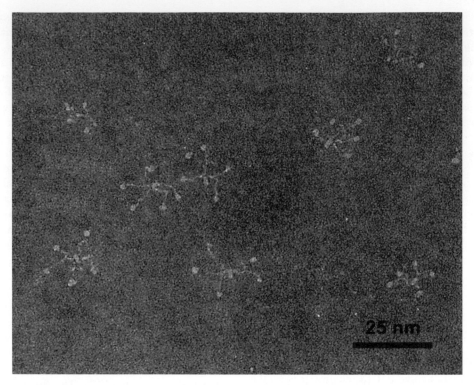

Fig. 21.3 Structure of COMP as revealed by rotary shadowing electron microscopy. Note the five-armed, bouquet-like structure. Picture provided by Mathias Mörgelin.

compared to synovial membrane (Heinegård D, Saxne T, Månsson B, unpublished observations).

The link protein is a globular protein with molecular weight of 40–48 kD which has sequence homologies to the G1 domain of aggrecan[40–41]. It has a widespread tissue distribution. The link protein interacts with hyaluronan and the G1 domain in aggrecan, thereby stabilizing the interaction between aggrecan and hyaluronan and forming large complexes of aggrecan, hyaluronan, and link protein.

Chondroadherin, like the small proteoglycans, belongs to the leucine-rich repeat (LRR) protein family[42]. It has a molecular weight of 38 kD with minor carbohydrate substitutions. The protein is extractable from cartilage in two different forms, differing in 9 C-terminal amino acids[42]. The two forms have different tissue distribution. The protein was primarily isolated from cartilage but has also been found in tendons. Chondroadherin has been showed to bind to cells via the $\alpha_2\beta_1$ integrin. It may thus have a signaling function between chondrocytes and the extracellular matrix[43]. Chondroadherin is mainly localized in the deeper portion of articular cartilage[44].

Cartilage matrix protein (CMP) was the first-described member of a family of proteins called matrilins. It has an intriguing tissue distribution in that it is present in extra-articular cartilage but not in normal articular cartilage[45]. The protein consists of three identical subunits[46]. Each subunit consists of two von Willebrand factor A-like domains separated by an EGF-like domain[47]. The subunits are assembled in the C-terminal end by a coiled-coil α-helical structure stabilized by disulfide bridges. The function of CMP is basically unknown, but it can interact with both type II collagen and proteoglycans[48].

Cartilage intermediate layer protein, CILP, is a recently-characterized cartilage protein with a molecular weight of 91.5 kD. It is distributed mainly to the middle layer of articular cartilage and has thereby a unique localization in the tissue[49]. It is synthesized as a part of a precursor protein which is cleaved to CILP and a homologue to a porcine nucleotide pyrophosphohydrolase, NTPPHase[50]. Its function is unknown but the cartilage content of the protein increases with age and the synthesis is upregulated in early phases of osteoarthritis.

Understanding and monitoring RA based on biochemical assays of cartilage macromolecules in body fluids

The disease process in the joint in RA is characterized by inflammation of the synovium and progressive damage to cartilage and bone[51]. Although it is clear that in many patients persistent inflammation predisposes to accelerated tissue destruction, the mechanisms responsible are not fully elucidated. Some patients with only low grade inflammation, as determined by various measures of the acute-phase response, may develop extensive joint damage whereas other patients with a pronounced systemic inflammatory response will develop little joint damage[52]. Also, therapeutic intervention which suppresses inflammation may be very effective in reducing symptoms directly related to inflammation but may have little influence on the process leading to irreversible joint damage. Thus, it may be reasonable to use different approaches when addressing the inflammatory and the destructive process, respectively. It is also likely that different measures for evaluation of therapy are required, depending on the target of therapy.

The inflammatory process is currently assessed by well-established clinical and biochemical measures, although the degree of generalized inflammation as measured by, for example, C-reactive protein, may not fully reflect the local inflammatory process[53,54]. In contrast, assessment of the tissue destructive process is much more difficult. Established imaging techniques are insensitive for detection of early destructive events, and radiography represents a record of anatomical changes resulting from processes that may have occurred long ago. Therefore, sensitive procedures for the assessment of ongoing processes in cartilage and bone would represent a major advantage in investigative and clinical studies aimed to elucidate and modify the processes leading to permanent joint damage[55–57].

Quantification and characterization of tissue-derived macromolecules or fragments thereof in synovial fluid and serum represents a novel, promising approach for monitoring pathological processes in cartilage and bone[5,6]. Although still in an early stage of development, this approach has already yielded informative results in several settings. It is important to realize that this technology enables studies of processes that until now were not possible to monitor with non-invasive techniques suitable for clinical use. Furthermore, since there is no immediate connection between clinical symptoms and destructive processes in cartilage and bone, there is no reason to expect close correlations between measures of inflammation or symptoms and circulating levels of a tissue marker.

Cartilage markers applied in studies of RA

In Table 21.2 the cartilage markers that have been assayed by immunochemical techniques in synovial fluid and serum in studies of RA are listed. Key findings showing the utility of these markers are discussed in the sections below. A number of other potential cartilage markers are under study but at present no data pertaining to their use in RA is available.

Diagnostic test

A diagnostic test may be defined as a test that discriminates between affected and non-affected individuals, for example an RA patient from a healthy individual[58]. Such tests are rarely available in rheumatological practice, and this also applies to

Table 21.2 Molecular markers of cartilage in synovial fluid and serum applied in studies of rheumatoid arthritis (for reference, see text)

Aggrecan	Core protein (intact or fragmented)
	Core protein (cleavage site specific epitopes)
	Keratan sulfate epitopes
	Chondroitin sulfate epitopes
Collagen	Type II collagen C-propeptide
Matrix proteins	Cartilage oligomeric matrix protein (COMP)
	Cartilage matrix protein (matrilin-1)

tissue-derived molecular markers. In part, this is due to disease-heterogeneity[59]. Furthermore, it is often difficult to identify the onset of disease. For practical reasons a diagnostic test should preferably work with serum or possibly urine since normal synovial fluid is hard to come by. As expected, a number of studies show group average differences for serum levels between patients with different forms of arthritides and 'normal' individuals but the overlap of individual specimens is marked which precludes diagnostic utility[60, 61]. At present, it seems unrealistic to expect that a tissue-derived molecule that is released also during normal turnover would be diagnostic for RA. The situation is quite different in other specialities, for example cardiology, where leakage of enzymes from the cardiac muscle occurs in relation to a very dramatic event, a myocardial infarction. Thus a prerequisite for a useful tissue marker is not that serum levels discriminate between healthy individuals and those afflicted by disease. The diagnostic value of tissue markers instead lies in their ability to elucidate pathophysiological and prognostic differences between patients with various forms and stages of arthritis. For example we were able to distinguish patients with effusion having acute onset oligoarthritis, including knee joint arthritis with a benign disease course, from those who develop a chronic joint disorder including RA, by distinctly different synovial fluid patterns of aggrecan and COMP[62].

Monitoring and quantification of the tissue process and elucidation of cleavage patterns of matrix macromolecules

The cartilage structure is, as described above, very different in various layers and compartments. The consequences of a disease process may vary considerably with tissue location. Different parts of the tissue may be involved at different time points in a progressive process, with ensuing different functional and structural consequences. Thus it is likely that structural disturbances close to the chondrocyte are easier to correct than those occurring in the interterritorial matrix, where the distance to the cell is larger and the assembly of the structural elements will be more complex to regulate. In a given compartment, the organization of the matrix is finely regulated and the cells may be able to repair damaged structures. Aggrecan fragments may be lost and replaced without influencing the long-term function or structure. This is amply demonstrated by the marked synovial release of aggrecan in patients with reactive arthritis[63]. If more widespread structural derangement occurs, including impaired function of the collagen network, progressive joint destruction is likely. Thus in early stages of disease, we may find one pattern of fragmentation of macromolecules and in later stages another pattern may emerge due to involvement of different compartments of the tissue.

The concept of assessing the damage at the molecular level has been substantiated in both cross-sectional and longitudinal studies of patients with RA[64–69]. In early stages, high synovial fluid content of aggrecan is found, even before any radiographic changes are apparent. Subsequently, as the tissue damage increases the levels gradually decrease, most likely reflecting the reduced cartilage mass. The synovial fluid COMP levels vary less

Table 21.3 Effects of glucocorticoid treatment in rheumatoid arthritis on synovial fluid (SF) and serum (S) concentrations of aggrecan and COMP (data derived from both cross-sectional and longitudinal studies, see text), N.d. = not determined

Preparation and route of administration	Aggrecan SF	S	COMP SF	S
Triamcimolone hexacetonide intra-articularly	⇓	N.d.	⇑	⇔
Methylprednisolone intramuscularly	N.d.	⇓	N.d.	⇓
Prednisolone (<10 mg daily) orally	⇑	N.d.	⇔	⇔

low-dose oral glucocorticoid treatment did not influence serum concentrations of glycosaminoglycans[79]. These preliminary observations also focused on some of the difficulties of this approach that need to be clarified. The effects of glucocorticoids seemed to vary in relation to the administered dose and possibly the route of administration. Tissue sampling was not possible in these studies so the response of the serum/synovial fluid marker could not be correlated to the tissue response. Consequently, the decreasing aggrecan levels and increasing COMP levels in synovial fluid in arthritis after glucocorticoid injections, could suggest both beneficial and detrimental effects on the cartilage turnover[77] (Fig. 21.7), (Saxne T, Heinegård D, unpublished observations). For serum results, effects on the extra-articular processing of the fragments or effects on the cartilage turnover could not be distinguished.

Studies in experimental arthritis have been initiated to explore further tissue-derived macromolecule measurements for the monitoring of the cartilage turnover in arthritis, especially for evaluation of therapy. Initially, serum concentrations of COMP were monitored. In studies of collagen II-induced arthritis in rats and mice and pristane-induced arthritis in rats, serial observations indicate that serum COMP increases during development of arthritis to reach a maximum coinciding with developing cartilage changes, as confirmed by histopathological observations[80–82]. The increase in COMP correlates with the number of involved joints, determined by clinical joint scoring. The increases in serum fibrinogen or serum hyaluronan occur considerably earlier during arthritis development than that of COMP and peak at a time when the serum COMP levels are only slightly increased (Larrson E, Saxne T, unpublished observations). Furthermore, the levels of the inflammatory markers in most cases returned to normal at a stage when the COMP levels are most markedly elevated. These results are in line with findings in collagen-induced arthritis in rhesus monkeys where a dissociation between changes in plasma C-reactive protein levels and urinary hydroxylysylpyridinoline levels during arthritis development was observed[83]. Cytokine modulating treatment which reduced cartilage pathology also reduced serum COMP, whereas treatment which only reduced inflammation without influencing cartilage pathology did not influence the serum levels of COMP[84,85] (Joosten LAB, Saxne T unpublished observations). Taken together, these observations show that changes in serum COMP reflect cartilage involvement in these models. Thus, COMP should be a suitable marker for monitoring cartilage response to therapy. The results also demonstrate that a matrix macromolecule that is not completely tissue-specific, as well as its fragments, may be useful for evaluating changes in a partic-

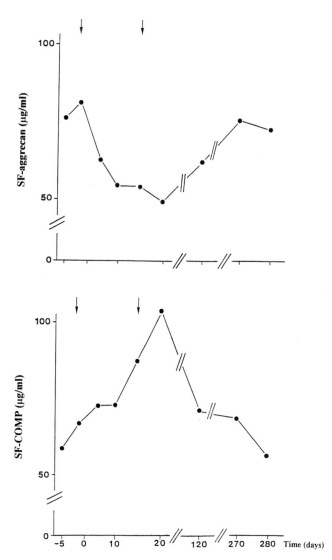

Fig. 21.7 Knee joint synovial fluid aggrecan and COMP concentrations in a patient with seronegative polyarthritis given intra-articular glucocorticoid injections. The arrows denote the times of injections of 10 and 20 mg triamcinolone hexacetonide, respectively.

ular tissue (see below). A therapeutic principle aimed at retarding cartilage damage may, in initial phases, be tested in such experimental models using serum COMP as a marker for effects on cartilage. In future experiments, it will be possible to measure certain fragments of COMP which potentially could allow new insight into the pathophysiological mechanisms operating in different stages or types of arthritides and in cytokine pathophysiology.

Predict response to therapy

Another application of molecular marker measurements would be to identify subsets of RA patients who are most likely to respond to chondroprotective measures[86]. In other words, can we distinguish potential responders by selecting patients with, for example, high serum COMP levels or high concentrations of a certain COMP fragment early in disease. This relates to the discussion about prognostic utility of markers but broadens the question since it is not self-evident that patients with the worst prognosis will benefit from a given therapy. For example if we were to test a drug which selectively blocks a crucial enzymatic cleavage step we would anticipate that patients exhibiting high serum or synovial fluid content of the cleavage products will respond more favorably than patients releasing small amounts of the cleavage product.

Potential difficulties and factors to consider in molecular marker measurements

The molecular marker approach, although very promising, has some inherent difficulties that need to be sorted out for each marker and should be considered when interpreting results. However, none of the difficulties impose severe limitations to the exploration of molecular marker measurements as instruments for monitoring tissue involvement in disease. Some principal aspects of the potential confounding factors regarding molecular marker measurements are reviewed below.

Formation and clearance of fragments

It is important to understand the generation and clearance of molecular fragments (Fig. 21.1)[87,88]. Macromolecules that are enzymatically cleaved in articular cartilage will be released into synovial fluid and/or taken up by the chondrocytes and degraded further. One fraction of the molecules are phagocytosed and further degraded by cells in the synovial lining or in the joint fluid, but the bulk of fragments leaves the joint cavity via lymphatic drainage. The half-life in synovial fluid of the fragments varies with the permeability of the synovial interstitium to different macromolecules. Thus, accelerated clearance has been observed in conditions with inflammation in the synovial lining cells[89,90]. Differences in marker concentrations between inflamed and non-inflamed joints may therefore underestimate the corresponding differences between release rates. As mentioned above, the joint fluid content of cartilage-derived molecules may also be influenced by the amount of cartilage remaining in the joint[67]. This correlation outweighs the influence of synovial inflammation and has proved useful in the monitoring of tissue damage.

The concentration of a protein in synovial fluid is highly dependent on the amount of fluid present. Reliable assessment of the synovial fluid volume is problematic. However, we have generally found a close correlation between concentration and total amount (concentration corrected for fluid volume) of individual fragments in most samples[65,77,91]. The use of ratios of concentrations of two markers instead of absolute concentrations is an attractive way to overcome this problem. This approach has proven most useful particularly in longitudinal studies of patients and when lavage procedures are used[92]. The turnover rate of the different compounds may vary but this appears to be of little practical significance. Thus, increased aggrecan/COMP ratios in synovial fluid early in disease indicated rapid progression of cartilage damage in a longitudinal study of RA patients[64].

Factors affecting the interpretation of serum analyses

A substantial portion of released fragments are entrapped, further degraded, or eliminated in the regional lymph nodes. The remainder reaches the blood stream. Preliminary observations indicate that up to 80 per cent of aggrecan core protein antigenic fragments are removed in the lymph node[87]. In contrast, the majority of antigenic fragments of COMP passes the lymph node, suggesting that COMP may be a more sensitive serum marker of the tissue turnover than aggrecan. This is corroborated by clinical studies, particularly in OA, where serum COMP correlated with progressive disease both in very early phases of the disorder and in more advanced stages[93,94]. Also, in a group of patients with hip OA, those patients who had the highest serum concentrations of COMP showed the most marked progression at follow-up 1 year later[95]. In RA, as discussed above, serum COMP is prognostic for the development of large joint destruction[74].

The macromolecules in the circulation are rapidly eliminated by uptake in the liver or by renal clearance. The hepatic or renal elimination is dependent on the function of these organs, which may be altered by disease processes or drug treatment. Clearly, the recirculating pool of any tissue marker represents only a fraction of all fragments released from the tissue[96]. Furthermore, serum will also contain molecules released from extra-articular cartilage or bone. This indicates that the contribution from single joints must be extensive to show up against a background of fragments released during normal turnover of extra-articular tissues. Nevertheless, numerous examples indicate that increased release from single or multiple joints can be recognized against the background of circulating molecules[97]. The proportion of fragments from the extra-articular source may vary depending on the condition and the type of molecule. Involvement of extra-articular cartilage is indicated by elevated serum levels, both in RA and relapsing polychondritis, of CMP, matrilin-1, which is not found in articular cartilage[98]. Furthermore, serum levels of BSP are increased in RA, presumably reflecting generalized bone involvement[68].

Release of structural and newly synthesized molecules

It should be realized that molecules released from cartilage into synovial fluid will be a mixture of fragments of macromolecules that have been part of the matrix and fragments of newly practice. Each marker will evidently have its own advantages and weaknesses, but by combining a number of well-characterized and validated markers, which need not be the same for research and clinical purposes, the non-invasive monitoring of disease processes in cartilage will be greatly facilitated.

References

1. Poole A.R., Alini M., Hollander A.P. Cellular biology of cartilage degradation. In: Henderson B., Edwards J.C.W., Pettipher E.R., eds. *Mechanisms in Rheumatoid Arthritis*. London: Academic Press, 1995; p. 163–204.

2. Heinegård D., Saxne T. Macromolecular markers in joint disease. *J Rheumatol*, 1991;**27** (suppl.):27–9.

3. Poole A.R., Dieppe P.A. Biological markers in rheumatoid arthritis. *Semin Arthritis Rheum*, 1994;**23**:17–31.

4. Thonar E.J., Shinmei M., Lohmander L.S. Body fluid markers of cartilage changes in osteoarthritis. *Rheum Dis Clin North Am*, 1993;**19**:635–57.

5. Lohmander L.S., Saxne T., Heinegård D.. Molecular markers for joint and skeletal diseases. *Acta Orthop Scand*, 1995;**66** (suppl. 266):1–212.

6. Saxne T., Heinegård D. Matrix proteins: potentials as body fluid markers of changes in the metabolism of cartilage and bone in arthritis. *J Rheumatol*, 1995;**43**(suppl.):71–4.

7. Ratcliffe A., Mow V.C., Comper W.D., eds. *Extracellular matrix*. Vol 1. Tissue function. 1st edn. Amsterdam: Harwood Academic Publishers; 1996;**9**, Articular cartilage. p. 234–302.

8. Horton W.A. Morphology of connective tissue: cartilage. In: Royce P.M., Steinmann B., eds. *Connective tissue and its heritable disorders. Molecular, genetic, and medical aspects*. New York: Wiley-Liss; 1993;**2**, part II, p. 73–84.

9. Hunziker E.B. Articular cartilage structure in humans and experimental animals. In: Kuettner K.E., Schleyerbach R., Peyron J.G, Hascall V.C., eds. *Articular cartilage and osteoarthritis*. New York: Raven Press, 1992;**13**, p. 183–99.

10. Heinegård D., Bayliss M.T., Lorenzo P. Biochemistry and metabolism of normal and osteoarthritic cartilage. In: Brandt K.D., Doherty M., Lohmander L.S., eds. *Osteoarthritis*. 1st edn. Oxford University Press, 1998; p. 74–84.

11. Bateman J.F., Lamandé S.R., Ramshaw J.A.M. Collagen superfamily. In: Comper W.D., ed. *Extracellular matrix*. Vol 2. Molecular components and interactions. 1st edn. Amsterdam: Harwood Academic Publishers, 1996; p. 22–67.

12. Eyre D.R., Wu J.J., Woods P. Cartilage-specific collagens. Structural studies. In: Kuettner K.E., Schleyerbach R., Peyron J.G., Hascall V.C., eds. *Articular cartilage and osteoarthritis*. New York: Raven Press, 1992; 119–31.

13. Eyre D.R., Apon S., Wu J.J., Ericsson L.H., Walsh K.A. Collagen type IX: evidence for covalent linkages to type II collagen in cartilage. *FEBS Lett*, 1987;**220**:337–41.

14. Wu J.J., Woods P.E., Eyre D.R. Identification of cross-linking sites in bovine cartilage type IX collagen reveals an antiparallel type II-type IX molecular relationship and type IX to type IX binding. *J Biol Chem*, 1992;**267**:23007–14.

15. Kwan A.P., Cummings C.E., Chapman J.A., Grant M.E. Macromolecular organization of chicken type X collagen in vitro. *J Cell Biol*, 1991;**114**:597–604.

16. Schmid T.M., Linsenmayer T.F. Immunoelectron microscopy of type X collagen: supramolecular forms within embryonic chick cartilage *Dev Biol*, 1990;**138**:53–62.

17. Mendler M., Eich-Bender S.G., Vaughan L., Winterhalter K.H., Bruckner P. Cartilage contains mixed fibrils of collagen types II, IX, and XI. *J Cell Biol*, 1989;**108**:191–7.

18. Heinegård D., Oldberg Å. Glycosylated matrix proteins. In: Royce P.M., Steinmann B., eds. *Connective tissue and its heritable disor-*

ders. *Molecular, genetic, and medical aspects*. 1st edn. New York: Wiley-Liss, 1993; p. 189–209.

19. Heinegård D., Paulsson M., Inerot S., Carlström C.A. novel low-molecular weight chondroitin sulfate proteoglycan isolated from cartilage. *Biochem J*, 1981;**197**:355–66.

20. Rosenberg L.C., Choi H.U., Tang L.H., Johnson T.L., Pal S., Webber C., Reiner A., Poole A.R. Isolation of dermatan sulfate proteoglycans from mature bovine articular cartilages. *J Biol Chem*, 1985;**260**:6304–13.

21. Heinegård D., Larsson T., Sommarin Y., Franzen A., Paulsson M., Hedbom E. Two novel matrix proteins isolated from articular cartilage show wide distributions among connective tissues. *J Biol Chem*, 1986;**261**:13866–72.

22. Patthy L. Detecting homology of distantly related proteins with consensus sequences. *J Mol Biol*, 1987;**198**:567–77.

23. Hedlund H., Mengarelli W.S., Heinegård D., Reinholt F.P., Svensson O. Fibromodulin distribution and association with collagen. *Matrix Biol*, 1994;**14**:227–32.

24. Miosge N., Flachsbart K., Goetz W., Schultz W., Kresse H., Herken R. Light and electron microscopical immunohistochemical localization of the small proteoglycan core proteins decorin and biglycan in human knee joint cartilage. *Histochem J*, 1994;**26**: 939–45.

25. Hildebrand A., Romaris M., Rasmussen L.M., Heinegård D., Twardzik D.R., Border W.A., Ruoslahti E. Interaction of the small interstitial proteoglycans biglycan, decorin and fibromodulin with transforming growth factor beta. *Biochem J*, 1994;**302**:527–34.

26. Westergen T.G., Antonsson P., Malmström A., Heinegård D., Oldberg Å. The synthesis of a family of structurally related proteoglycans in fibroblasts is differently regulated by TFG-beta. *Matrix*, 1991;**11**:177–83.

27. Oldberg Å., Antonsson P., Lindblom K., Heinegård D. COMP (cartilage oligomeric matrix protein) is structurally related to the thrombospondins. *J Biol Chem*, 1992;**267**:22346–50.

28. Efimov V.P., Lustig A., Engel J.. The thrombospondin-like chains of cartilage oligomeric matrix protein are assembled by a five-stranded alpha-helical bundle between residues 20 and 83. *FEBS Lett*, 1994;**341**:54–8.

29. Mörgelin M., Heinegård D., Engel J., Paulsson M. Electron microscopy of native cartilage oligomeric matrix protein purified from the Swarm rat chondrosarcoma reveals a five-armed structure. *J Biol Chem*, 1992;**267**:6137–41.

30. Newton G., Weremowicz S., Morton C.C., Copeland N.G., Gilbert D.J., Jenkins N.A., Lawler J. Characterization of human and mouse cartilage oligomeric matrix protein. *Genomics*, 1994;**24**:435–9.

31. Zaia J., Boyton R.E., McIntosh A., Marshak D.R., Ollson H., Heinegård D., Barry F.P. Post-translational modifications in cartilage oligomeric matrix protein. Characterization of the N-linked oligosaccharides by matrix-assisted laser desorption ionization time-of flight mass spectrometry. *J Biol Chem*, 1997;**272**:14120–6.

32. DiCesare P.E., Mörgelin M., Carlson C.S., Pasumarti S., Paulsson M. Cartilage oligomeric matrix protein: isolation and characterization from human articular cartilage. *J Orthop Res*, 1995;**13**:422–8.

33. Rosenberg K., Olsson H., Mörgelin M., Heinegård D. Cartilage oligomeric matrix protein shows high affinity zinc-dependent interaction with triple helical collagen. *J Biol Chem*, 1998;**273**: 20397–403.

34. Ballo R., Briggs M.D., Cohn D.H., Knowlton R.G., Beighton P.H., Ramesar R.S. Multiple epipyseal dysplasia, ribbing type: a novel point mutation in the COMP gene in a South African family. *Am J Med Genet*, 1997;**68**:396–400.

35. Briggs M.D., Mortier G.R., Cole W.G., King L.M., Golik S.S., Bonaventure J., Nuytinck L., De-Paepe A., Leroy J.G., Biesecker L., et al. Diverse mutations in the gene for cartilage oligomeric matrix protein in the pseudoachondroplasia-multiple epiphyseal dysplasia disease spectrum. *Am J Hum Genet*, 1998;**62**:311–9.

36. Susic S., McGrory J., Ahier J., Cole W.G. Multiple epiphyseal dysplasia and pseudoachondroplasia due to novel mutations in the

calmodulin-like repeats of cartilage oligomeric matrix protein. *Clin Genet*, 1997;**51**:219–24.

37. Hedbom E., Antonsson P., Hjerpe A., Aeschlimann D., Paulsson M., Rosa P.E., Sommarin Y., Wendel M., Oldberg Å., Heinegård D. Cartilage matrix proteins. An acidic oligomeric protein (COMP) detected only in cartilage. *J Biol Chem*, 1992;**267**:6132–6.

38. DiCesare P., Hauser N., Lehman D., Pasumarti S., Paulsson M. Cartilage oligomeric matrix protein (COMP) is an abundant component of tendon. *FEBS Lett*, 1994;**354**:237–40.

39. Di-Cesare P.E., Carlson C.S., Stollerman E.S., Chen F.S., Leslie M., Perris R. Expression of cartilage oligomeric matrix protein by human synovium. *FEBS Lett*, 1997;**412**:249–52.

40. Neame P.J., Perin J.P., Bonnet F., Christner J.E., Jolles P., Baker J.R. An amino acid sequence common to both cartilage proteoglycan and link protein. *J Biol Chem*, 1985;**260**:12402–4.

41. Neame P.J., Christner J.E., Baker J.R. The primary structure of link protein from rat chondrosarcoma proteoglycan aggregate. *J Biol Chem*, 1986;**261**:3519–35.

42. Neame P.J., Sommarin Y., Boynton R.E., Heinegård D. The structure of a 38-kDa leucine-rich protein (chondroadherin) isolated from bovine cartilage. *J Biol Chem*, 1994;**269**:21547–54.

43. Camper L., Heinegård D., Lundgren A.E. Integrin alpha2beta1 is a receptor for the cartilage matrix protein chondroadherin. *J Cell Biol*, 1997;**138**:1159–67.

44. Shen Z., Gantcheva S., Månsson B., Heinegård D., Sommarin Y. Chondroadherin expression changes in skeletal development. *Biochem J*, 1998;**330**:549–57.

45. Paulsson M., Heinegård D. Radioimmunoassay of the 148-kilodalton cartilage protein. Distribution of the protein among bovine tissues. *Biochem J*, 1982;**207**:207–13.

46. Paulsson M., Heinegård D. Purification and structural characterization of a cartilage matrix protein. *Biochem J*, 1981;**197**:367–75.

47. Kiss I., Deak F., Holloway-RG J., Delius H., Mebust K.A., Frimberger E., Argraves W.S., Tsonis P.A., Winterbottom N., Goetnick P.F. Structure of the gene for cartilage matrix protein, a modular protein of the extracellular matrix. Exon/intron organization, unusual splice sites, and relation to alpha chains of beta 2 integrins, von Willebrand factor, complement factors B and C2, and epidermal growth factor. *J Biol Chem*, 1989;**264**:8126–34.

48. Hauser N., Paulsson M., Heinegård D., Mörgelin M. Interaction of cartilage matrix protein with aggrecan. Increased covalent cross-linking with tissue maturation. *J Biol Chem*, 1996;**271**:32247–52.

49. Lorenzo P., Bayliss M.T., Heinegård D. A novel cartilage protein (CILP) present in the mid-zone of human articular cartilage increases with age. *J Biol Chem*, 1998;**273**:23463–8.

50. Lorenzo P., Neame P.J., Sommarin Y., Heinegård D. Cloning and deduced amino acid sequence of a novel cartilage protein (CILP) identifies a proform including a nucleotide pyrophosphohydrolase. *J Biol Chem*, 1998;**273**:23469–75.

51. Harris-ED J. Rheumatoid arthritis. Pathophysiology and implications for therapy. *N Engl J Med*, 1990;**322**:1277–89.

52. Mulherin D., Fitzgerald O., Bresnihan B. Clinical improvement and radiological deterioration in rheumatoid arthritis: evidence that the pathogenesis of synovial inflammation and articular erosion may differ. *Br J Rheumatol*, 1996;**35**:1263–8.

53. Wollheim F.A., Eberhardt K.B. The search for laboratory measures of outcome in rheumatoid arthritis. *Baillieres Clin Rheumatol*, 1992;**6**:69–93.

54. Otterness I.G. The value C-reactive protein measurement in rheumatoid arthritis. *Semin Arthritis Rheum*, 1994;**24**:91–104.

55. Breedveld F.C., Dijkmans B.A. Differential therapy in early and late stages of rheumatoid arthritis. *Curr Opin Rheumatol*, 1996;**8**:226–9.

56. Cawtson T.E., Rowan A. Prevention of cartilage breakdown by matrix metalloproteinase inhibition—a realistic therapeutic target? *Br J Rheumatol*, 1998;**37**:353–6.

57. Bresnihan B., Alvar-Garcia J.M., Cobby M.D.M., Doherty M., Domljan Z., Emery P., Nuki G., Pavelka K., Rau R., Rozman B., Watt I., Williams B., Aitchison R., McCabe D., Musikic P. Treatment of rheumatoid arthritis with recombinant human interleukin-1 receptor antagonist. *Arthritis Rheum*, 1998; in press.

58. Ward M.M. Evaluative laboratory testing. Assessing tests that assess disease activity. *Arthritis Rheum*, 1995;**38**:1555–63.

59. Arnett F.C., Edworthy S.M., Bloch D.A., McShane D.J., Fries J.F., Cooper N.S., Healey L.A., Kaplan S.R., Liang M.H., Luthra H.S., et al. The American Rheumatism Association 1987 revised criteria for the classification of rheumatoid arthritis. *Arthritis Rheum*, 1998;**31**:315–24.

60. Spector T.D., Woodward L., Hall G.M., Hammond A., Williams A., Butler M.G., James I.T., Hart D.J., Thompson P.W., Scott D.L. Keratan sulfate in rheumatoid arthritis, osteoarthritis, and inflammatory diseases. *Ann Rheum Dis*, 1992;**51**:1134–7.

61. Saxne T., Heinegård D. Cartilage oligomeric matrix protein: a novel marker of cartilage turnover detectable in synovial fluid and blood [published erratum appears in Br J Rheumatol 1993 Mar; 32 (3):247]. *Br J Rheumatol*, 1992;**31**:583–91.

62. Lindqvist E., Saxne T. Cartilage macromolecules in knee joint synovial fluid. Markers of the disease course in patients with acute oligoarthritis. *Ann Rheum Dis*, 1997;**56**:751–3.

63. Saxne T., Glennås A., Kvien T.K., Melby K., Heinegård D. Release of cartilage macromolecules into the synovial fluid in patients with acute and prolonged phases of reactive arthritis. *Arthritis Rheum*, 1993;**36**:20–5.

64. Månsson B., Geborek P., Saxne T. Cartilage and bone macromolecules in knee joint synovial fluid in rheumatoid arthritis: relation to development of knee or hip joint destruction. *Ann Rheum Dis*, 1997;**56**:91–6.

65. Saxne T., Heinegård D, Wollheim F.A., Pettersson H. Difference in cartilage proteoglycan level synovial fluid in early rheumatoid arthritis and reactive arthritis. *Lancet*, 1985;**2**:127–8.

66. Saxne T., Heinegård D. Synovial fluid analysis of two groups of proteoglycan epitopes distinguishes early and late cartilage lesions. *Arthritis Rheum*, 1992;**35**:385–90.

67. Saxne T. Differential release of molecular markers in joint disease. *Acta Orthop Scand*, 1995;**266**(suppl.):80–3.

68. Saxne T., Zunino L., Heinegård D. Increased release of bone sioloprotein into synovial fluid reflects tissue destruction in rheumatoid arthritis. *Arthritis Rheum*, 1995;**38**:82–90.

69. Haraoui B., Thonar E.J., Martel P.J., Goulet J.R, Raynauld J.P., Ouellet M., Pelletier J.P. Serum keratan sulfate levels in rheumatoid arthritis: inverse correlation with radiographic staging. *J Rheumatol*, 1994;**21**:813–7.

70. Flannery C.R., Lark M.W., Sandy J.D. Identification of a stromelysin cleavage site within the interglobular domain of human aggrecan. Evidence for proteolysis at this site in vivo in human articular cartilage. *J Biol Chem*, 1992;**267**:1008–14.

71. Lohmander L.S., Neame P.J., Sandy J.D. The structure of aggrecan fragments in human synovial fluid. Evidence that aggrecanase mediates cartilage degradation in inflammatory joint disease, joint injury, and osteoarthritis. *Arthritis Rheum*, 1993;**36**:1214–22.

72. Sandy J.D., Plaas A.H., Koob T.J. Pathways of aggrecan processing in joint tissues. Implications for disease mechanism and monitoring. *Acta Orthop Scand Suppl*, 1995;**266**:26–32.

73. Hughes C.E., Caterson B., Fosang A.J., Roughley P.J., Mort J.S. Monoclonal antibodies that specifically recognize neoepitope sequences by 'aggrecanase' and matrix metalloproteinase cleavage of aggrecan: application to catabolism in situ and in vitro. *Biochem J*, 1995;**305**:799–804.

74. Månsson B., Carey D., Alini M., Ionescu M., Rosenberg L.C., Poole A.R., Heinegård D., Saxne T. Cartilage and bone metabolism in rheumatoid arthritis. Differences between rapid and slow progression of disease identified by serum markers of cartilage metabolism. *J Clin Invest*, 1995;**95**:1071–7.

75. Fex E., Eberhardt K., Saxne T. Tissue-derived macromolecules and markers of inflammation in serum in early rheumatoid arthritis: relationship to development of joint destruction in hands and feet. *Br J Rheumatol*, 1997;**36**:1161–5.

76. Saxne T., Wollheim F.A., Petterson H., Heinegård D. Proteoglycan concentration in synovial fluid: predictor of future cartilage destruction in rheumatoid arthritis? *Br Med J Clin Res Ed*, 1987;**295**:1447–8.

77. Saxne T., Heinegård D., Wollheim F.A. Therapeutic effects on cartilage metabolism in arthritis as measured by release of proteoglycan structures into the synovial fluid. *Ann Rheum Dis*, 1986;45:491–7.

78. Saxne T., Heinegård D., Wollheim F.A. Cartilage proteoglycans in synovial fluid and serum in patients with inflammatory joint disease. Relation to systemic treatment. *Arthritis Rheum*, 1987;30:972–9.

79. Sharif M., Salisbury C., Taylor D.J., Kirwan J.R. Changes in biochemical markers of joint tissue metabolism in a randomized controlled trial of glucocorticoid in early rheumatoid arthritis. *Arthritis Rheum*, 1998;41:1203–9.

80. Larsson E., Müssener A., Heinegård D., Klareskog L., Saxne T. Increased serum levels of cartilage oligomeric matrix protein and bone sialoprotein in rats collagen arthritis. *Br J Rheumatol*, 1997;36:1258–61.

81. Vingsbo C., Sahlstrand P., Brun J.G., Jonsson R., Saxne T., Holmdahl R. Pristane-induced arthritis in rats: a new model for rheumatoid arthritis with a chronic disease course influenced by both major histocompatibility complex and non-major histocompability complex genes. *Am J Pathol*, 1996;149:1675–83.

82. Vingsbo C., Saxne T., Olsson H., Holmdahl R. Increased serum levels of cartilage oligomeric matrix protein in chronic erosive arthritis in rats. *Arthritis Rheum*, 1998;41:544–50.

83. 'T Hart B.A., Bank R.A., De-Roos J.A., Brok H., Jonker M., Theuns H.M., Hakimi J., Te Koppele J.M. Collagen-induced arthritis in rhesus monkeys: evaluation of markers for inflammation and joint degradation. *Br J Rheumatol*, 1998;37:314–23.

84. Joosten L.A.B., Helsen M.M.A., Saxne T., van de Loo F.A.J., Heinegård D., van den Berg W.B. IL-1α,β blockade prevents cartilage and bone destruction in murine type II collagen-induced arthritis, whereas TNFα blockade only ameliorates joint inflammation. *J Immunol*, 1999;163:5049–55.

85. Joosten L.A.B., Helsen M.M.A., Saxne T., Heinegård D., van de Putte L.A.B., van den Berg W.B. Synergistic protection against cartilage destruction by low dose prednisolone and interleukin-10 in established murine collagen arthritis. *Inflammation Research*, 1999;48:48–55.

86. Lohmander L.S., Felson D.T. Defining and validating the clinical role of molecular markers in osteoarthritis. In: Brandt K.D., Doherty M., Lohmander L.S., eds. *Osteoarthritis* Oxford: Oxford University Press, 1998; p. 519–30.

87. Saxne T., Heingård D., Wollheim F.A. Cartilage macromolecules and the development of new molecules and the development of new methods for the assessment of joint disease. *Rheumatol Europe*, 1997; 26:108–10.

88. Levick J.R. In: The 'clearance' of macromolecular substances such as cartilage markers from synovial fluid and serum. In: Maroudas A, Kuettner K, eds. *Methods in Cartilage Research*. London: Academic Press, 1990; p. 352–7.

89. Myers S.L., Brandt K.D., Eilam O. Even low-grade synovitis significantly accelerates the clearance of protein from the canine knee. Implications for measurement of synovial fluid 'markers' of osteoarthritis. *Arthritis Rheum*, 1995;38:1085–91.

90. Myers S.L., O'Connor B.L., Brandt K.D. Accelerated clearance of albumin from the osteoarthritis knee: implications for interpretation of concentrations of "cartilage markers" in synovial fluid. *J Rheumatol*, 1996;23:1744–8.

91. Lohmander L.S., Saxne T., Heinegård D.K. Release of cartilage oligomeric matrix protein (COMP) into joint fluid after knee injury and in osteoarthritis. *Ann Rheum Dis*, 1994;53:8–13.

92. Flygare L., Wendel M., Saxne T., Ericson S., Eriksson L., Petersson A., Rohlin M. Cartilage matrix macromolecules in lavage fluid of temporomandibular joints before and 6 months after diskectomy. *Eur J Oral Sci*, 1997;105:369–72.

93. Petersson I.F., Boegård T., Svensson B., Heinegård D., Saxne T. Changes in cartilage and bone metabolism identified by serum markers in early osteoarthritis of the knee joint. *Br J Rheumatol*, 1998;37:46–50.

94. Sharif M., Saxne T., Shepstone L., Kirwan J.R., Elson C.J., Heinegård D., Dieppe P.A. Relationship between serum cartilage oligomeric matrix protein levels and disease progression in osteoarthritis of the knee joint. *Br J Rheumatol*, 1995;34:306–10.

95. Conrozier T., Saxne T., Shan Sei Fan C., Mathieu P., Tron Am, Piperno M., Heinegård D., Vignon E. Serum levels of cartilage oligomeric matrix protein and bone siloprotein in hip osteoarthritis: A one-year prospective study. *Ann Rheum Dis*, 1998;57:527–32.

96. Laurent T.C. Hyaluronan as a clinical marker of pathological processes. In: Laurent TS, ed. *The Chemistry, Biology and Medical Applications of Hyaluronan and its Derivatives*. London: Portland Press Limited, 1998; p. 305–13.

97. Wollheim F.A. Serum markers of articular cartilage damage and repair. *Rheum Dis Clin N Am*, 1999;25:417–32.

98. Saxne T., Heinegård D. Involvement of nonarticular cartilage, as demonstrated by release of a cartilage-specific protein, in rheumatoid arthritis. *Arthritis Rheum*, 1989;32:1080–6.

99. Hummel K.M., Neidhart M., Vilim V., Hauser N., Aicher W.K., Gay R.E., Gay S., Haüselmann H.J. Analysis of cartilage oligomeric matrix protein (COMP) in synovial fibroblasts and synovial fluids. *Br J Rheumatol*, 1998;37:721–8.

100. Neidhart M., Hauser N., Paulsson M., DiCesare P.E., Michel B.A., Haüselmann H.J. Small fragments of cartilage oligomeric matrix protein in synovial fluids and serum as markers for cartilage degradation. *Br J Rheumatol*, 1997;36:1151–60.

101. Recklies A.D., Baillargeon L., White C. Regulation of cartilage oligomeric matrix protein synthesis in human synovial cells and articular chondrocytes. *Arthritis Rheum*, 1998;41:997–1006.

102. Smith R.K., Zunino L, Webbon P.M., Heinegård D. The distribution of cartilage oligomeric matrix protein (COMP) in tendon and its variation with tendon site, age and load. *Matrix Biol*, 1997;16:255–71.

103. Lohmander L.S., Dahlberg L., Eyre D., Lark M.W., Thonar E., Ryd L. Longitudinal and cross-sectional variability in markers of joint metabolism in patients with knee pain and articular cartilage abnormalities. *Osteoarthritis Cartilage*, 1998;6:351–61.

104. Lohmander L.S., Roos H., Dahlberg L., Lark M.W. The role of molecular markers to monitor disease, intervention and cartilage breakdown in osteoarthritis. *Acta Orthop Scand*, 1995;266(suppl.):84–7.

105. Thonar E.J., Pachman L.M., Lenz M.E., Hayford J., Lynch P., Kuettner K.E.. Age related changes in the concentration of serum keratan sulfate in children. *J Clin Chem Clin Biochem*, 1988;26:57–63.

106. Saxne T., Castro F., Rydholm U., Svantesson H.. Cartilage derived proetoglycans in body fluids of children. Inverse correlation with age. *J Rheumatol*, 1989;16:1341–4.

107. Carey D.E., Alini M., Ionescu M., Hyams J.S., Rowe J.C., Rosenberg L.C., Poole A.R.. Serum content of the C-propeptide of the cartilage molecule type II collagen in children. *Clin Exp Rheumatol*, 1997;15:325–8.

108. Tortorella M.D., Burn T.C., Pratta M.A, et al. Purification and cloning of aggrecanase-1: a member of the ADAMTS family of proteins. *Science* 1999;284:1664–6.

109. Abbaszade I., Liu R.Q., Yang F., et al. Cloning and characterization of ADAMTS11, an aggrecanase from the ADANTS family. *J Biol Chem* 1999;274:23443–50.

SECTION
4 | *Drug therapy*

22 | NSAIDs and analgesics

Richard Day, David Quinn, Lynnette March, Garry Graham, and Kenneth Williams

Non-steroidal anti-inflammatory drugs (NSAIDs) are pre-scribed more than any other class of drugs. This reflects the prevalence of musculoskeletal disorders and the need for pain relief in these conditions. The most common of these painful conditions, such as osteoarthritis (OA) and spinal pain, are pri-marily not inflammatory conditions. However, the NSAIDs are also effective analgesics as well as having anti-inflammatory and antipyretic properties. The anti-inflammatory properties of NSAIDs are obviously useful in the inflammatory rheumatic conditions such as rheumatoid arthritis (RA) and the spondy-larthropathies such as ankylosing spondylitis, reducing joint swelling and pain. NSAIDs are associated with important adverse effects, particularly on the upper gastrointestinal tract. As our populations age, increasingly older cohorts of patients are exposed to NSAIDs. This has important consequences with respect to adverse effects, particularly those affecting the upper gastrointestinal tract and the cardiovascular system. There has been considerable debate about the proper drug management of rheumatic conditions and the place of NSAIDs, with increased advocacy of analgesics such as paracetamol (aceta-minophen) as the first pharmacological step in the management of the non-inflammatory rheumatic conditions. The place of opioids, such as codeine, in the management of chronic painful rheumatic disorders has also been the subject of reassessment recently. The advent of a new class of NSAIDs, namely the COX (cyclooxygenase)-2-specific inhibitors, has further increased interest in the pharmacological management of the rheumatic disorders. This chapter reviews the important prop-erties of analgesics, the traditional NSAIDs, and the COX-2 specific inhibitors.

Analgesics

Paracetamol (acetominophen)

Paracetamol is an effective analgesic and antipyretic when given in appropriate doses. The important contrast with NSAIDs is that acetominophen has no anti-inflammatory action in man. In fact, the drug has been considered a very weak inhibitor of the enzyme cyclooxygenase but it is a potent inhibitor in several cellular systems, with EC50 values within the range of therapeutic plasma concentrations[1-4]. However, acetominophen will not inhibit cyclooxygenase if peroxides are present in high concentrations, as found in association with inflammation[5]. The widely employed antipyretic actions of acetominophen result from inhibition of the synthesis of prostaglandins in the hypothalamus. Surprisingly, the mechanism of the analgesic action of acetominophen remains unknown but effects on prostaglandin synthesis in non-inflamed areas such as the nervous system are possible[6].

Paracetamol is about as effective as NSAIDs in patients with OA even when 'anti-inflammatory' doses of the NSAIDs are administered[7]. Surprisingly, this finding is not influenced by the presence of signs of inflammation in these OA patients[8,9]. However, there is substantial resistance to using acetominophen in non-inflammatory rheumatic conditions. Patients commonly have taken one to two acetominophen tablets or capsules occa-sionally and experience an inadequate response. This, combined with easy access to the drug through supermarkets, suggests to patients and perhaps physicians that the drug cannot be very efficacious. Thus, most patients and many physicians need re-assurance that the drug is indeed efficacious as an analgesic when an adequate dosing regimen is instituted.

Peak analgesic actions are observed about 2.5 h post oral dose[6]. The plasma half-life is 1 to 3 h. Dosing is usually 6 hourly, with a maximum daily dose of 4 g in otherwise healthy adults. This dose produces peak plasma concentrations of about 15 mg/l. Formulations that consist of fast and slow release com-ponents are now available which allow less frequent dosing (e.g. 8 hourly) and an improvement in the convenience associated with taking the drug. Paracetamol is not protein bound. Daily doses of not much greater have been associated with serious hepatotoxicity but are sometimes used for short periods in pal-liative medicine.

The metabolism of acetominophen is of major importance. At low doses, it is primarily metabolized to inactive glucuronide and sulfate conjugates. The conversion of acetominophen to the glucuronide conjugate is inhibited at the enzymatic level by probenecid and, consequently, the half-life is increased from about 2 h to about 4 h. Consequently, the long-term dosage of acetominophen should be reduced during treatment with probenecid. At high doses, the amount of oxidative metabolism to the reactive compound, N-acetylbenzoquinoneimine, becomes significant and this explains the hepatotoxicity of large, usually intentional, overdoses of acetominophen. Paracetamol is also metabolized by the neutrophil enzyme, myeloperoxidase, the result being decreased production of the normal product, hypochlorous acid, by both intact neutrophils and isolated myeloperoxidase[6]. Recently it has been discovered that about 1 to 2 per cent of a dose of acetominophen is deacetylated to p-aminophenol and then reacetylated to form acetaminophen again[10]. The intermediate, p-aminophenol, is a renal toxin but it is not known where the process occurs or if toxic concentrations are achieved *in vivo*. The percentage of the dose undergoing this futile deacetylation pathway is low but, considering the high dose of acetaminophen, up to 40 mg of p-aminophenol is formed daily.

A major advantage for acetaminophen in comparison with conventional NSAIDs is the absence of gastrointestinal toxicity, notably upper gastrointestinal ulceration, perforation, and bleeding. Serious hepatotoxicity occurs with acetaminophen overdose and is a considerable problem. Hepatotoxicity can occur rarely in patients with liver disease and those who have taken the drug at a high dose rate. Therefore the daily dose should be carefully monitored in all patients, particularly in those with possible liver disease (e.g. alcoholism) or when more than one acetaminophen-containing formulation is being ingested. For example acetaminophen tablets may be taken along with a combination codeine–acetaminophen formulation.

Regular, high-dose acetaminophen has been recorded as enhancing the anticoagulant effects of warfarin. However, the increase in prothrombin time reported is small and the strength of the evidence for a significant drug interaction is low[11].

Although little studied, it is apparent also from clinical practice that the use of acetaminophen along with NSAIDs can reduce the daily dose of NSAIDs in patients with rheumatic problems. This does not lead to loss of overall analgesic efficacy but the risk for upper gastrointestinal toxicity is reduced[12,13].

Opioid analgesics in rheumatic disorders

Opioids such as codeine and dextropropoxyphene are used extensively in the acute and chronic management of rheumatic disorders. However, the appropriate use of opioids in these disorders has received inadequate attention and remains contentious[14]. There is little debate that short-term, oral use of opioids for problems such as acute mechanical back pain is appropriate. Once pain becomes chronic the use of opioids becomes problematic. Many of the patients with chronic rheumatic problems are elderly and the adverse effects of opioids become critically important. Constipation, cognitive impairment, drowsiness, increased risk of falls and fractures, and opioid dependence are well recognized problems with these drugs. Also, the quality of pain relief in chronic pain states often is unsatisfactory and opioids in themselves are not adequate therapy.

Codeine and dextropropoxyphene are usually used in formulations that include aspirin or acetaminophen. Oxycodone, methadone, slow release formulations of morphine, and other opioids such as fentanyl delivered topically via patch formulations are being used increasingly in patients with chronic pain problems. Studies indicate that a minimum of 20 mg of codeine added to acetaminophen 500 mg in a regular dosing regimen is needed to show any increment in pain relief over full dose acetaminophen alone, that is 4 g daily. Thus, a daily dose of 120–240 mg codeine might be needed when treating a patient with a chronic painful, musculoskeletal condition. This dosage

of codeine can be achieved by formulations that combine codeine 15–30 mg with acetaminophen 500 mg[15,16].

Codeine

First pass metabolism of codeine is about 60 per cent. The half-life of the parent drug is 2–4 h. Codeine is only an extremely weak ligand for opioid receptors. However, about 10 per cent of codeine is metabolized to morphine by the hepatic cytochrome P450 metabolic system. The 2D6 isoenzyme is employed in the transformation. Approximately, 8–10 per cent of Caucasians will be unable to transform codeine to morphine and the drug will be much less effective as a result of genetic polymorphisms of the 2D6 isoenzyme rendering it inoperative. It is now well established that morphine is metabolized by glucuronidation largely in the liver to morphine 6-glucuronide and morphine 3-glucuronide. Morphine 6-glucuronide is an agonist at the mu opioid receptor producing analgesia. It has a longer half-life than morphine and is retained in renal impairment. Morphine 3-glucuronide may antagonize the analgesic effects of morphine. Therefore it high dose codeine or morphine are used in the management of rheumatic disorders, analgesic efficacy and careful monitoring for adverse effects is needed, especially in the elderly.

Dextropropoxyphene

Dextropropoxyphene has been shown in a limited number of studies in patients with rheumatic disorders to increment the analgesic efficacy achieved with acetaminophen. However, the use of this drug is controversial and not generally recommended in the chronic musculoskeletal disorders. This is because the drug has been associated with a number of sudden cardiac deaths especially in overdose. There is some suspicion that elderly patients with coronary artery disease and renal impairment may be at greater risk for sudden cardiac death if taking dextropropoxyphene. This risk may be further increased by alcohol. The mechanism of increased cardiac risk is considered to be via the formation of an oxidative metabolite of dextropropoxyphene, namely nor-dextropropoxyphene[17].

Non-steroidal anti-inflammatory drugs (NSAIDs)

NSAIDs are used extensively for their anti-inflammatory and analgesic properties. They account for about 10 per cent of all prescribing and are increasingly available 'over-the-counter'. In most developed countries, around 20 per cent of individuals older than 65 years take these drugs regularly, establishing NSAIDs as an important community risk factor for upper gastrointestinal bleeding and perforation, hypertension, and possibly cardiac failure[18]. There has been a decline in usage of NSAIDs around the world in the last decade, partly as a result of concerns regarding adverse effects. For example in Australia a 25 per cent drop in NSAID usage has been recorded with most decline occurring in elderly patients suffering with osteoarthritis. The fall in NSAID use has been promoted by educational programs directed to prescribers and copayments for NSAIDs prescriptions by patients[19].

Of great interest has been the expanding indications for NSAIDs beyond the rheumatic diseases. Aspirin, the index NSAID, is very widely used now for the prevention of cardiovascular and cerebrovascular diseases. Analgesic indications have widened to include cancer pain and pain associated with biliary and renal colic. Inflammatory states ranging from eye inflammations, coronary artery disease, and post-operative inflammation are being treated with NSAIDs. Possibly Alzheimer's disease and colon cancer prevention will become major new indications for NSAIDs and particularly for the COX-2-specific inhibitors. Increasingly, NSAIDs are applied topically. There is good evidence for reasonable efficacy via this route of delivery in acute and chronically painful musculoskeletal conditions, although there are very few comparative studies or comparisons with simple liniments. There is good evidence for the enhanced safety of NSAIDs by this route[20].

NSAID chemistry

The common chemical structure of most of the classical NSAIDs makes several aspects of the their pharmacokinetics very similar. NSAIDs are weak acids, that are highly lipid soluble in the unionized forms. Typically, they have pKa values in the range 4 to 5. The atypical NSAIDs, aspirin and salicylate, are somewhat different with pKa values of 3.7 and 3, respectively. The chemistry of the simple analgesic, acetominophen, differs to a greater extent. It is a very weak acid (pKa 9.7) and, consequently, is almost totally unionized at physiological pH values. The new COX-2-specific inhibitors, such as celecoxib and rofecoxib, are also very weak acids or neutral and are almost totally unionized at physiological pH values.

Mechanism of action of NSAIDs

As classical NSAIDs are typically weak acids, they partition into and are trapped in cells found in relatively acidic environments. These areas are the stomach, kidney, and inflamed joints, namely sites of action and toxicity of NSAIDs[21]. Inhibition of the ubiquitous enzyme cyclooxygenase, and therefore the synthesis of prostaglandins, explains most of the therapeutic and toxic actions of NSAIDs[22]. The discovery of two isoforms of cyclooxygenase, COX-1 and COX-2, has opened up an exciting opportunity to separate the desired from the toxic effects of NSAIDs in the treatment of the rheumatic diseases[23-26]. The COX-1 isoenzyme is constitutively expressed and is responsible for the synthesis of prostaglandins involved in normal physiological functions in platelets, the gastrointestinal tract, and the kidney. COX-2 is an inducible isoform of cyclooxygenase with massive expression occurring in sites of inflammation thereby providing substantial amounts of prostaglandins to contribute to the inflammatory process. COX-2 interestingly has a very limited distribution otherwise, namely in brain, spinal cord, kidney, and testes (Fig. 22.1).

The genes for COX-1 and COX-2 reside on chromosomes 9 and 1 respectively, *COX-1* being a 22.5 kilobase gene and *COX-*

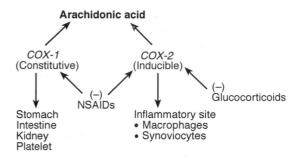

Fig. 22.1 Metabolism of arachidonic acid either by the largely constitutively expressed cyclooxygenase, COX-1, or the largely inducible form, COX-2. From Needleman and Isakson[167] with the permission of the publishers.

2, 2.8 kilobases[27-29]. The *COX-2* gene is one of a number of 'primary response' or 'immediate early' genes which include inducible nitric oxide synthase. These genes are heavily induced by inflammatory stimuli and mediators including NF-KB, IL-1, and TNFα[30,31]. The *COX-2* promoter is notable for the presence of a TATA box with sites for NF-kB whereas the *COX-1* promoter does not have a TATA box, reflecting the inducible nature of the former gene and the constitutive nature of the latter [32]. There is about 60 per cent homology of the amino acid sequences of the COX-1 and -2 proteins although very few differences in the amino acid sequences in the active sites of the enzymes[33]. The tertiary structures of COX-1 and COX-2 have been determined, an important contrast being a side pocket as part of the inhibitor binding site in the COX-2 molecule. This results in a substantially larger inhibitor binding site in the COX-2 molecule[34]. Specific COX-2 inhibitors have been designed to fit closely into the side pocket. The Vmax and Km for arachidonic acid are similar for the two isoforms. COX-1 is found on the endoplasmic reticulum only whereas COX-2 is found on the nuclear envelope as well as the endoplasmic reticulum.

NSAIDs vary in their inhibitory potency against the two isoforms of cyclooxygenase[33]. Our present knowledge strongly suggests that the optimal NSAID for the treatment of the inflammation and pain of the rheumatic diseases should be a potent inhibitor of COX-2 but a weak or non-inhibitor of COX-1 at clinically relevant doses. Recent studies with a highly specific COX-1 inhibitor, SC-560, at doses that inhibited COX-1 activity substantially *in vivo*, revealed no evidence of therapeutic efficacy against the inflammation or hyperalgesia associated with the rat paw carrageenan inflammation assay[35]. This contrasted with the significant anti-inflammatory activity seen with celecoxib, the COX-2-specific inhibitor. Of great interest was the finding that prostaglandin levels were reduced equally in the inflamed rat paw by SC-560 and celecoxib. Elevated cerebrospinal fluid concentrations of prostaglandins were reduced by celecoxib but not SC-560 suggesting an important central nervous system component to inflammatory pain by way of COX-2-derived prostaglandins[35]. There are a number of COX-2 'specific' inhibitors in the clinical phase of development or recently registered. MK 966 or rofecoxib (Vioxx) and celecoxib (Celebrex) are the first two of this new class of drugs now known as COX-2-specific inhibitors to be registered widely[36]. These drugs are efficacious as reversibly acting anti-inflammatory and analgesic drugs in RA and OA and do not contrast notably in this respect with conventional NSAIDs. However, they appear to be substantially safer as suggested in endoscopic studies of the upper gastrointestinal tract and large-scale clinical trials of up to 3 months elicited ulcer rates indistinguishable from placebo and significantly less than conventional NSAIDs given in usual doses.

Much has been made of the ratio of inhibitory concentrations against COX-1 and COX-2 of particular, currently available NSAIDs. This information has been related to epidemiological studies ranking NSAIDs for the risk of causing serious upper gastrointestinal bleeding or perforation. There seems to be a very rough relationship between the COX-2/-1 inhibitory concentration ratio and the relative risk for serious upper gastrointestinal bleeding or perforation[36]. It is expected that the relationship suggested between COX-2/-1 selectivity and relative risk for serious upper gastrointestinal adverse events will be much stronger for the COX-2-specific drugs. In the meantime, intensive marketing of some conventional NSAIDs has been based on a 'good' or 'low' ratio for COX-2/-1 inhibitory potency and an apparent relatively lower risk for serious gastrointestinal toxicity. There are many technical issues in establishing a meaningful COX-2/-1 inhibitory potency ratio before comparisons can be contemplated and there has been much appropriate criticism of the establishment and use of these ratios in this way[37]. Thus, ratios derived from *in vitro* assay systems differ widely relating to the species from which COX enzymes are obtained, whether microsomes or whole cells are employed, incubation times, whether exogenous or endogenous arachidonate substrate is used, the concentration of arachidonate employed, and the concentration of plasma proteins in the assay, amongst other variables.

A useful guide has recently been promulgated in response to confusion concerning categories of COX-2 inhibitors[38]. It is suggested that a COX-2 'specific' inhibitor is a drug that when given in usual clinically-relevant dose rates to humans will inhibit COX-2 as assessed by a validated, *ex vivo* assay, while at the same time showing no inhibitory activity against COX-1 in human blood or other tissues[38–40]. Systematic study of the relationship between the *ex vivo* assays for COX-1 and COX-2 and *in vivo* production of prostaglandins are awaited with interest. None of the conventional NSAIDs currently marketed meet this standard set for a COX-2-specific drug. Meloxicam, nimuleside, and nabumetone show some 'selectivity' for COX-2 inhibition but COX-1 activity is inhibited in whole blood assays *ex vivo* during routine, chronic oral dosing[38].

Rofecoxib, a specific COX-2 inhibitor, is potent at blocking COX-2 activity in the human blood assay *ex vivo* with single doses of drug from 5 to 1000 mg but has no effect on COX-1 at these doses. By contrast, indometacin 5 to 75 mg in single doses inhibits both COX-1 and COX-2[41]. Efficacy of rofecoxib has been demonstrated in OA, RA and post surgical dental pain in doses up to 50 mg daily indicating specificity for COX-2. Similarly, celecoxib at clinically effective doses, and also at substantially higher doses, that are associated with substantial COX-2 inhibition, is inactive in inhibiting the synthesis of thromboxane B2 production from whole blood *ex vivo*, a

measure of COX-1 activity. Thus celecoxib also qualifies as a COX-2 'specific' inhibitor[42].

NSAIDs have also been reported to block a number of other processes important in the inflammatory response, such as the production of the superoxide anion and intracellular transduction mechanisms in polymorphs. These have been suggested as possible reasons for the observed variations in response between NSAIDs. However, this remains hypothetical and the subject of ongoing studies[18,43].

Pharmacokinetics of NSAIDs: critical features

The physicochemical properties of conventional, acidic NSAIDs are responsible for the common pharmacokinetic features of these drugs (and indeed other weakly acidic drugs), namely good absorption from the gastrointestinal tract, low to negligible first-pass metabolism, and extensive binding to albumin leading to a small volume of distribution.

Dose and plasma concentration response relationships

Relationships between plasma NSAID concentrations and anti-inflammatory response have been demonstrated in patients with RA (Fig. 22.2) and also in patients with postoperative pain[44–46]. However, much variation in patient response remains unaccounted for by plasma NSAID concentration differences. Overall, the data do not suggest that plasma NSAID concentration monitoring would substantially improve clinical outcomes although plasma salicylate concentrations have been found useful in monitoring anti-inflammatory therapy with high-dose aspirin. Salicylate plasma concentrations need to be maintained between 1.1 and 2.2 mmol/l (150–300 mg/l) for anti-inflammatory effect. These concentrations are associated with doses of the order of 4–6 gm aspirin daily in adults[47]. It has also been observed that aspirin dose and plasma concentrations of salicylates predict

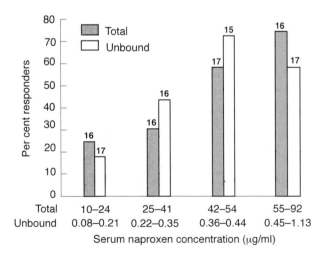

Fig. 22.2 Relationship between total and unbound plasma naproxen concentrations and response to the drug in patients with RA using a 'summed' efficacy score. From Day *et al.*[44] with permission of the publishers.

ototoxicity. A linear relationship between plasma salicylate concentrations and the degree of hearing loss and the loudness of salicylate-induced tinnitus respectively has been demonstrated[48]. Plasma indomethacin concentration measurement in neonates with patent ductus arteriosus has been helpful in dose adjustment[49]. Large epidemiological studies have revealed an important relationship between the daily dose of NSAID and serious upper gastrointestinal bleeding or perforation[50-52].

Responders and non-responders to NSAIDs: relevance of pharmacokinetics

A proportion of patients with RA can be designated as responders or non-responders to individual NSAIDs and this 'label' has been applied to some patients with RA[53]. Also, a subset of RA and ankylosing spondylitis patients sustain preferences for particular NSAIDs over considerable periods of time[54] and in clinical trials involving blinded, re-exposure to drug[55,56]. No pharmacokinetic contrasts for these NSAIDs, comparing responders to non-responders, have been discovered[57,58]. For example a proportion of RA patients dosed with naproxen 1500 mg/day did not respond irrespective also of their plasma naproxen concentration whereas the majority of subjects in this study had increasing anti-inflammatory effect with increasing dose of naproxen[44]. It is difficult to conceive that prostaglandin synthesis is not suppressed in all patients taking reasonable doses of NSAIDs. An hypothesis for an individual's lack of response to even a maximal dose of NSAID is that the pathophysiological processes involved in that person are less responsive to that drug's range of mechanisms additional to prostaglandin synthesis. An alternate NSAID may work in that individual because it has some different mechanisms of action. More recently, studies have indicated that RA patients who respond to particular NSAIDs contrast with non-responders in alterations in plasma concentrations of markers of inflammation such as the acute phase reactants, effects not usually associated with NSAID action[55,59]. These effects on other components of the inflammatory response may hold the key to NSAID variability but much work remains to be done.

Absorption and bioavailability of NSAIDs

The bioavailability of NSAIDs is essentially complete. The NSAIDs have high oral bioavailabilities because of:

(1) high lipid/water partition coefficients;

(2) sufficient aqueous solubilities within the gastrointestinal tract—some NSAIDs are administered as their sodium salts which gives them high aqueous solubilities but they are converted to their less soluble unionized forms in the stomach, e.g. naproxen sodium;

(3) resistance to hydrolytic enzymes;

(4) hepatic clearance which is small in relation to hepatic plasma flow rates (about 800 m/min).

However, diclofenac with a bioavailability of about 54 per cent[60] and aspirin with 50–70 per cent[61] are exceptions.

Virtually all of a dose of aspirin is metabolized to salicylate eventually. The absorption rate of NSAIDs is slowed when taken with food but bioavailability is generally unaffected. Despite the effect on absorption rate, NSAIDs should be taken with food to decrease the symptoms of gastric irritation. No decrement in anti-inflammatory or analgesic efficacy in the treatment of rheumatic diseases is expected. Antacids taken with NSAIDs usually improve gastric tolerance but there is no reduction in the risk of serious upper gastrointestinal bleeding. Again, as with concurrent food intake, the extent of absorption or bioavailability is not affected by antacids[62].

Much effort has been invested in developing aspirin formulations that are less irritating to the gastrointestinal tract, especially when the drug is used in anti-inflammatory doses. The advent of newer NSAIDs has reduced the demand for anti-inflammatory treatment with aspirin. However, when aspirin is used to treat chronic rheumatic conditions, it is usually administered as slow release or enteric formulations because plain or soluble forms are associated with considerable gastric irritation. It was observed that there could be a substantial delay before enteric-coated tablets reached the small intestine and release and absorption could begin as a result of delays in gastric emptying. Such variation in the onset of absorption is unlikely to be a problem in the treatment of inflammatory conditions because the half-life of salicylate is about 15 h when full anti-inflammatory doses of aspirin are administered chronically. In this situation, steady-state salicylate concentrations are likely to be maintained satisfactorily. Interestingly, although upper gastrointestinal symptoms such as reflux and indigestion are reduced, the risk of serious upper gastrointestinal complications remains[63]. There has been a vogue for the development of sustained release formulations of NSAIDs, with short to medium half-lives, in order to increase the duration of action of the drugs. However, no improvement in symptom control has been documented except that administration can be less frequent. Thus, ketoprofen SR is given once daily as compared to twice to three times daily for the conventional release formulation. Interestingly, studies with short half-life NSAIDs such as ibuprofen revealed that 8 or 12 hourly administration produced symptom control indistinguishable from a 6-hourly regimen of the same total daily dose. This result may be explained from the observation that synovial fluid NSAID concentration time profiles remain essentially unchanged for short half-life NSAIDs when comparing 6-hourly to 12-hourly regimens or conventional release with immediate-release formulations[64].

There is the suggestion that sustained release NSAIDs may be more damaging to the gastrointestinal tract. Collins *et al.*[65] did not demonstrated any difference in peptic ulcer rate on endoscopic examination between immediate and slow release preparations of ketoprofen. There is an increased risk for serious upper gastrointestinal toxicity associated with ketoprofen compared to ibuprofen despite their similar, short half-lives. It has been suggested that the increased risk could be a function of the slow release formulation of ketoprofen and, thus, the apparent long half-life[66].

Distribution and protein binding

NSAIDs are extensively bound to plasma albumin thereby explaining the small volumes of distribution of the NSAIDs. Binding of NSAIDs to plasma albumin is a reversible reaction. An important equilibrium between albumin bound NSAID, known as the 'bound' drug, and unbound NSAID in the plasma, also known as 'free' drug, exists. Free drug is able to diffuse across cell membranes and bind to COX-1 and 2 intracellularly. The fraction of NSAID unbound is defined as the free drug/free plus bound drug. This ratio is altered by a number of factors such as the plasma albumin concentration, age, gender, renal and hepatic impairment, other albumin bound drugs, and pregnancy. The fraction unbound for NSAIDs increases when plasma albumin is low from any cause and in states of renal impairment. It is important to remember that it is the free concentration which is critical to a change in performance of a drug, for example changes in efficacy or toxicity. Free concentrations are proportional to the dose rate and inversely proportional to the clearance of free drug. Free drug concentrations of naproxen are found to be higher in the elderly and also in individuals whose RA activity has increased. These changes in free drug concentration must be due to a decrease in the clearance of free drug in the elderly and active RA[67].

As dosages of phenylbutazone, salicylate, and naproxen increase, a less than proportional increment in total NSAID plasma concentrations (bound plus free concentrations) occurs. This phenomenon is due to the saturation of the available binding sites for NSAIDs on plasma albumin. More importantly, the unbound naproxen concentrations still increase linearly with dose. Thus the free fraction increases whereas in the 'unsaturated' state it would remain unchanged as the dose was increased. As an example, total plasma concentrations of naproxen fail to increase linearly with dose and approach a

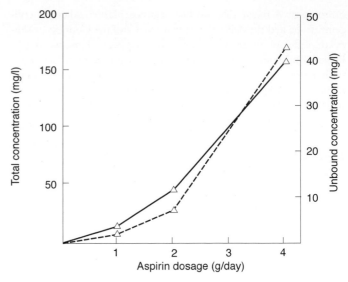

Fig. 22.4 Relationships between total (continuous line) and unbound (broken line) concentrations of salicylate and increasing daily dosage with aspirin. Note the more than proportional increase in total and unbound concentrations related to saturable metabolism and the relatively greater increase in unbound drug concentration. Adapted from Bochner *et al.*[69].

plateau with increasing doses above 750 mg/day. However, the unbound concentrations of naproxen increase proportionally with the dose increase (Fig. 22.3). An exception is seen with salicylate. Not only is albumin binding saturated with high dose rates with aspirin but also the metabolism of salicylate is saturable. In this case, unbound or free concentrations of salicylate as well as total concentrations of the drug increase more than proportionally as the dose increases[68,69] (Fig. 22.4).

Half-life of NSAIDs

NSAIDs can be divided usefully into those with short initial half-lives (< 6 h) and those with long half-lives (> 12 h) (Table 22.1)[53]. As noted, NSAIDs have small volumes of distribution (about 10 l) and the variation in the half-lives is mostly due to differences in clearance. The major practical difference is that NSAIDs with long half-lives can usually be given once or twice daily. This is helpful for compliance and patient convenience. Plasma concentrations of long half-life drugs will not fluctuate substantially during a dosing interval but this conveys no substantive clinical advantage (Fig. 22.5). NSAIDs with long half-lives will accumulate in the body significantly after chronic dosing is commenced. Steady-state or plateau concentrations are reached in four to five half-lives. Maximal effects of NSAIDs are expected when plasma concentrations are at steady-state. This is within a few days for NSAID with short half-lives[70,71] and longer for NSAID with long half-lives. Pain seems to respond faster than joint swelling[70]. Piroxicam with a half-life of approximately 60 h, will reach 90 per cent of its ultimate steady-state plasma concentration in about 7.5 days. Naproxen has a half-life of about 14 h (Table 22.1) and will therefore accumulate for about 2 days following the onset of dosing. Loading doses may be employed to achieve steady-state concentrations of long half-

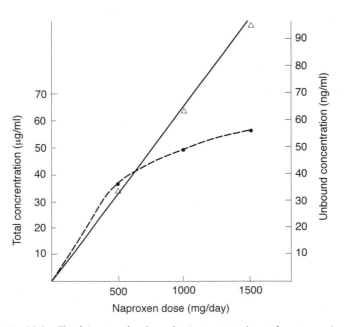

Fig. 22.3 Total (●---) and unbound (Δ) concentrations of naproxen in plasma versus daily dose of naproxen illustrating the linear increase in unbound concentrations with increasing dose. From Dunagan *et al.*[45] with permission of the publishers.

Table 22.1 Pharmacokinetic features of NSAIDs, adapted from Day *et al.* (168)

NSAID	Total daily dose range (mg); (dose divisions/day)	Half-life (hours)	Notes (Decrease dose in renal and hepatic impairment and in the elderly for all NSAID)
Aspirin	4800; (bid, tid)	0.25	
Azapropazone	1200; (bid, tid, qds)	15	Renal excretion unchanged drug 60 per cent; reduce dose in renal impairment
Carprofen	300; (bid)	12	Given as R and S isomers
Diclofenac	50–150; (od, bid, tid)	1–2	
Diflunisal	500–1000; (bid)	7–15	Decrease dose 50 per cent in renal failure (creatinine clearance < 10 ml/min)
Etodolac	400–600; (bid)	7	Given as R and S isomers
Fenbufen	900; (bid)	11	Given as R and S isomers
Fenoprofen	1200–2400; (bid	1–2	R converted virtually completely to active S enantiomer
Flurbiprofen	150–300; (bid)	3–4	R and S enantiomers; no inversion in man
Ibuprofen	1200–2400; (bid; tid)	2–3	About 60 per cent R converted to active S enantiomer; safest NSAID for GI tract in low dose
Indometacin	25–200; (od, bid, tid)	5	Enterohepatic circulation; headaches, depersonalization reactions; suppositories for night pain
Ketoprofen	100–300; (od; bid)	1–4	Commonly prescribed as slow release formulation; given as R and S isomers
Ketorolac	60 (elderly)- 90 (IMI and IVI); 30(elderly)- 40 (oral; (4–6 hourly for pain)	4–6	i.m/i.v and oral routes; 60 per cent excreted unchanged in urine; used as an analgesic; great caution needed in post operative situation and renal impairment
Meclofenamate	200–400; (bid)	2.5	Caution needed as it can prolong the bleeding time
Nabumetone	1000–2000; (od)	26	Active metabolite is 6-methoxy-2-naphthylacetic acid
Naproxen	500–1000; (bid)	12–15	Administered as S isomer
Oxaprozin	1200–1800; (od)	49–60	Hepatic metabolism
Piroxicam	10–20; (od)	30–86	Decrease dose in liver disease
Salicylate	2000–4000; (tid; qds)	4–15	Half life increases with increasing dose; choline magnesium trisalicylate or salsalicylate well tolerated
Sulindac	200–600; (bid)	16–18 (sulfide)	Reduced to active 'sulfide'; enterohepatic circulation
Tenoxicam	10–20; (od)	60	Hepatic metabolism
Tiaprofenic acid	600; (bid; tid)	3	Given as R and S isomers; be alert for cystitis
Tolmetin	1200–2000; (bid, tid, qds)	1–1.5	Renal excretion unchanged drug 17 per cent
COX-2 specific drugs			No COX-1 inhibition in clinical dose ranges
Celecoxib	100–200; (bd)		Platelet function not affected; gastric ulcer rate indistinguishable from placebo
Rofecoxib	12.5–25; (od)		Platelet function not affected; gastric ulcer rate indistinguishable from placebo

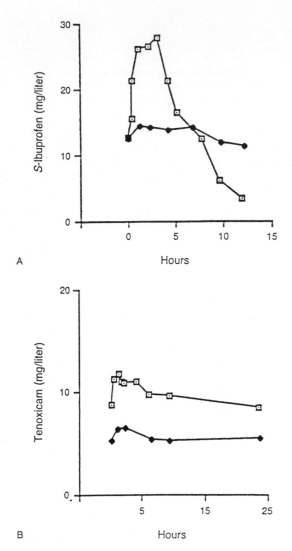

Fig. 22.5 Total concentrations of drug in plasma (□) and synovial fluid (♦) after the administration of an NSAID with a short half-life (ibuprofen) and a long half-life (tenoxicam). Note the greater fluctation in the plasma concentrations in the short half life ibuprofen and the 'cross-over' in plasma and synovial fluid concentrations for that drug. Adapted from Day *et al.* (1988)[74] and Day *et al.* (1991)[77], respectively.

life NSAIDs quickly. Thus it is recommended that naproxen 500 to 750 mg is given as a loading dose to be followed by 250 mg every 8 h as treatment for the pain of acute gout[72].

NSAIDs with short elimination half-lives of the order of 1–3 h are administered every 6 to 8 h and occasionally 12 hourly. This interval is substantially greater than their half-lives. As expected, there are substantial fluctuations in plasma concentrations, from zero or close to it prior to the next dose. However, analgesic and anti-inflammatory activity is well maintained throughout the dosing interval[73]. One possible reason for their long duration of effect may be their more sustained concentrations in synovial fluid. Data from large epidemiological studies and meta-analyses reveal that NSAIDs with short half-lives such as ibuprofen and diclofenac exhibit a lower risk for serious upper gastrointestinal bleeding when used in usual doses[66].

Synovial fluid concentrations of NSAIDs

The major site of action of the NSAIDs is probably within the synovium of joints but there is little information on the distribution of the NSAIDs into this tissue. There is considerably more knowledge on the distribution in synovial fluid although practically all information has been obtained on the distribution in synovial fluid of the knee because of the relatively easy access to this large joint. NSAIDs are distributed slowly into and out of synovial fluid. The predictable result is that the pattern of distribution in synovial fluid depends on the half-life of the NSAID. NSAIDs with short half-lives, such as ibuprofen, show a crossover pattern during long-term dosage and the concentrations in synovial fluid are more sustained at a lower mean range than in plasma. Concentrations are lower in synovial fluid than in plasma for approximately the first 6 h post dose, then higher than plasma concentrations subsequently (Fig. 22.5). By contrast, the synovial concentrations of tenoxicam, a NSAID with a long half life of elimination, are lower than in plasma and are variable but generally follow the pattern of concentrations in plasma. The unbound concentrations of naproxen, an intermediate half-life NSAID, show the crossover pattern seen with the short half-life NSAIDs although the total plasma concentrations are higher than in synovial fluid because of the higher binding to the higher concentrations of albumin in plasma.

Mean total concentrations (bound plus unbound) of NSAIDs in synovial fluid over a dosage interval are approximately 60 per cent of the mean total concentration in plasma[74–76] due to the lower levels of albumin and consequent lesser protein binding of NSAIDs in synovial fluid. By contrast, the mean unbound concentrations of NSAIDs in synovial fluid and plasma are very similar across a dosage interval[74,77].

Clearance of NSAIDs

Active metabolites

A notable feature of NSAID pharmacokinetics is that interpatient differences in the metabolic clearances of individual NSAIDs are quite marked. Therefore, there is substantial variation in the steady-state concentrations of NSAIDs. The predominant clearance mechanism for NSAIDs is hepatic metabolism. The metabolites are generally inactive. However, there are several NSAIDs that are themselves inactive but have active metabolites (Table 22.1). Nabumetone is a widely used NSAID with apparent relative safety for the upper gastrointestinal tract. It has no intrinsic activity until metabolized to 6-methoxy-2-naphthylacetic acid (6-MNA), which has an elimination half-life of about 24 h. The apparent gastrointestinal safety may be more related to the dose of drug generally employed and possibly a favourable COX-2/1 inhibitory ratio for 6-MNA than to the inactive parent drug. Sulindac is metabolized by a reduction reaction to a sulfide metabolite, sulindac sulfide, by microflora in the large intestine[78]. This metabolite has a long half-life (16–18 h) and is responsible for the anti-inflammatory activity of sulindac. The conversion of sulindac to its sulfide is a reversible metabolic reaction and the sulfide is metabolized back to sulindac in the kidney. The conversion of the sulfide back to inactive sulindac may explain the apparent diminished effect of sulindac on renal function compared to other NSAIDs. The significance of this contrast with other NSAIDs is debated[79].

Aspirin irreversibly inhibits prostaglandin synthesis as seen in its inhibition of platelet aggregation. Aspirin is rapidly cleared by hydrolysis to salicylate. Salicylate is an effective anti-inflammatory agent when steady-state, trough plasma concentrations fall between 100 and 300 mg/l (1.1–2.2 mmol/l). Additionally, it has a much longer half-life than its parent, of the order of 15 h when concentrations approach 300 mg/l. Salsalate is a dimer of salicylic acid (salicylsalicylic acid) and is inactive but is metabolized to salicylate. The absence of aspirin from this salicylate formulation eliminates platelet inhibition and probably reduces the risk of serious upper gastrointestinal bleeding.

Glucuronides

Glucuronide conjugates of drugs and their oxidative metabolites generally increase solubility and detoxify the drug or metabolite. An exception is the formation of the active metabolite of morphine, namely morphine-6-glucuronide. Some glucuronide metabolites of NSAIDs have been demonstrated to be active metabolic intermediates with the ability to acylate proteins and transfer NSAID residues from the glucuronide conjugate to the protein. This phenomenon may be significant for the serious allergic reactions to NSAIDs that occur rarely.

Chirality of NSAIDs

Some NSAIDs are asymmetric and therefore exist as two optical isomers or enantiomers[80] (Table 22.1). Sulindac has two enantiomers that have equal anti-inflammatory effect. The members of the 2-arylpropionic acid class of NSAIDs that include ibuprofen, fenoprofen, ketoprofen, naproxen, flurbiprofen, and tiaprofenic acid are asymmetric and are generally administered as the racemate, that is an equal mixture of the R and S enantiomers. The S-configured enantiomer inhibits COX-1 and COX-2 and therefore prostaglandin production. Naproxen was the first of this group to be marketed as the pure S-enantiomer. The remainder are available as racemic mixtures. The inactive R-enantiomers of ibuprofen and fenoprofen are metabolized to the active S-enantiomers *in vivo*. The R-enantiomers can thus be considered prodrugs for the active S-enantiomers. Approximately, 60 per cent of the R-enantiomer of ibuprofen is converted to the active S-enantiomer, however this proportion is variable[81]. Inversion of R to S-fenoprofen is extensive[82]. The initial step in R to S inversion involves the stereoselective formation of a coenzyme A thioester. This intermediate metabolite can also participate in fatty acid metabolism such that the NSAID is incorporated into triglycerides ('hybrid' lipids; k1, k2). Recent studies have further demonstrated that clofibrate, by activating COA ligases, can shunt an increased proportion of R-ibuprofen into lipids in rats (k3) and that a similar process probably occurs in humans (k4). The therapeutic and/or toxicological consequences of these novel metabolic effects have yet to be elucidated.

Saturable metabolism

Steady-state plasma concentrations of NSAIDs increase or decrease in proportion to alterations in dosage rate. An exception to this general rule is salicylate. Its major two metabolic pathways, namely glycine conjugation and phenolic glucuronidation, are saturable at clinically relevant dose rates[83,84]. The result is that steady-state plasma concentrations of salicylate increase more than proportionally with increases in dosage (Fig. 22.4). The half-life of elimination of salicylate increases from a few hours at low doses such as 300 mg to about 15 h when plasma levels approach the upper end of the therapeutic range for anti-inflammatory effect, namely 300 mg/l. Also the drug induces its own metabolism. Steady-state plasma salicylate concentrations decline significantly from about 5 to 20 days after commencement of dosing[85–87]. Diflunisal, like salicylate, exhibits saturable metabolism and there is a disproportionate increase in plasma concentrations with increasing dosage[88]. The drug is marketed as an analgesic and is a salicylate derivative but interestingly is it is not metabolized to salicylate (Table 22.1).

Biliary clearance of NSAIDs

Sulindac and its metabolites and indomethacin undergo enterohepatic cycling such that the effective half-life of elimination of indomethacin and sulindac sulfide is prolonged[89]. Hepatic impairment has not been identified as a particular problem with NSAID metabolic clearance. Thus, the clearance of ibuprofen[90], diclofenac[91], and salicylate[92] is unaffected by liver failure. However, plasma sulindac sulfide concentrations are increased about four-fold in patients with alcoholic hepatic disease[90]. It is of interest that the clearance of azapropazone decreases as hepatic function deteriorates as the drug is largely renally excreted.

Renal clearance

Only small proportions of the doses of most NSAIDs are excreted unchanged in urine, the only exception being salicylate and azapropazone. Renal clearance of salicylate is substantially greater when urinary pH is above 6.5, leading to significant decreases in plasma concentrations[93]. The clearance of a number of NSAIDs, including ketoprofen, naproxen, diflunisal, fenoprofen, and indomethacin decreases with renal impairment and when probenecid is also prescribed. This is a surprising fact as a fraction only of these drugs is excreted unchanged in the urine. Acyl glucuronide metabolites of these drugs are retained in renal failure and in patients on probenecid. The acylglucuronides are hydrolyzed to release their parent NSAIDs thereby prolonging their presence and establishing a so-called 'futile-cycle'[94]. In renal impairment, the R and S acylglucuronides are retained and both are hydrolyzed to the R and S parent NSAID but only the R-enantiomer is inverted to the S-enantiomer. Thus, there are two additional sources of active S-enantiomer, namely S-glucuronide and R-enantiomer released from R-glucuronide[95]. This mechanism is identified as contributing toward the deaths associated with the release of the NSAID benoxaprofen. Over 60, generally elderly, patients with varying degrees of renal impairment died of benoxaprofen-induced hepatic and renal failure. Renal impairment increases the risk of further NSAID-induced renal impairment as a result of inhibition of renal prostaglandin synthesis. Thus, these drugs must be used with great care in the elderly and renally impaired[96].

Age and NSAID clearance

NSAIDs are used extensively in the elderly and this group are most at risk for adverse reactions to NSAIDs. There is good evidence that higher dose rates of NSAIDs are associated with greater risk for serious adverse effects, notably gastrointestinal bleeding. Some of the increased risk most likely relates to reduced clearance of some NSAIDs with age. Thus, naproxen[97,98], azapropazone[99], ketoprofen[100], benoxaprofen (withdrawn), and salicylate[92,101,102] exhibit reduced clearance in the elderly. The most plausible mechanism is the reduced renal function associated with age. Age-related decrease in hepatic clearance mechanisms does not seem to be a significant effect with most NSAIDs. In the case of naproxen, benoxaprofen, and ketoprofen the retention of their labile acyl glucuronide metabolites in renal impairment that hydrolyze to their parent NSAIDs is a possible mechanism. Plasma concentrations of piroxicam have been found to vary widely in elderly patients and although toxicity has not been related formally to high plasma concentrations of the drug[103] the possibility should be borne in mind. NSAID toxicity has not been correlated directly with impaired NSAID clearance in individual elderly patients, although it has with dose, so it is sound practice to start with lower than usual doses of NSAIDs. Dose can be increased if required and if side-effects are not problematic.

Adverse reactions to NSAIDs

The commonest drug class associated with reports to adverse drug reaction reporting agencies is the NSAIDs. About, 25 per cent of all reports to these agencies relate to NSAIDs. The elderly patient has a greater risk for gastrointestinal, renal, central nervous system, and hematological adverse effects from NSAIDs and this is most likely due to a combination of reduced clearance of drug from the body and increased tissue sensitivity commonly observed in the elderly. As a result of greater risk in the elderly, a more cautious approach to the use of NSAIDs in this age group is warranted.

Gastrointestinal adverse reactions

NSAID-induced upper gastrointestinal symptoms are common, occurring in 20–30 per cent of individuals taking NSAIDs regularly, and include dyspepsia or indigestion, epigastric pain (heartburn), and, less commonly, nausea. Lesions found upon upper gastrointestinal endoscopy encompass mucosal erythema, erosions, and peptic ulceration. Endoscopic lesions are found in 20–30 per cent of subjects taking NSAIDs chronically but not necessarily those with upper gastrointestinal symptoms. In fact, no correlation has been demonstrated between upper gastrointestinal symptoms and endoscopic abnormalities. NSAID-induced gastric ulcers are located on the antral or prepyloric areas of the stomach. Duodenal injury is much less common on endoscopy than gastric injury. However, studies have shown considerable loss of protein and blood across the mucosa and into the upper small intestine in subjects taking NSAIDs[104]. The presence or absence of upper gastrointestinal symptoms also has been unsatisfactory as a predictor of serious bleeding from the upper gastrointestinal tracts, especially in the elderly. However,

an interesting recent study demonstrated that patients who knew least about the risk of NSAIDs were more likely to continue NSAID therapy when upper GI symptoms occurred and were significantly more likely to bleed[105].

An individual's relative risk for serious complications of peptic ulcer disease, namely hemorrhage and perforation, as a result of taking NSAIDs ranges from 2 to 6. The absolute risk has been estimated to be about 3–6/1000 patient years of NSAID therapy. A substantially higher estimate of 2–4/100 patient years of therapy comes from a large data base of patients which contains a high proportion of inflammatory rheumatic disease patients[106,107]. It is increasingly likely that the risk is closer to the 1–2/100 patient years of therapy, particularly in the elderly. It is estimated that 7600 deaths and 76 000 admissions in the United States per annum are due to NSAID gastric adverse effects[106,107]. It is also estimated that 15–30 per cent of all peptic ulcer complications are due to NSAIDs[108]. There are estimated to be 1200 deaths due to NSAID gastropathy per year in the United Kingdom[109].

The risk is known to increase in the elderly, patients with a history of peptic ulcer or bleeding, patients concomitantly dosed with glucocorticosteroids, and patients given higher doses of NSAIDs. Two large meta-analyses have revealed that the risk for serious upper gastrointestinal bleeding or perforation varies between NSAIDs when they are used at their most common dose rates[50,66]. Ibuprofen and diclofenac are ranked the safest with piroxicam and azapropazone at the least safe end of the spectrum. It is apparent that the longer half-life NSAIDs are also clustered at the less safe end of the distribution. It is important to re-emphasize that risk alters with the dose of NSAID being used so that an anti-inflammatory dose of ibuprofen of 2400 mg daily has a substantially higher risk than apparent from the meta-analyses presented[66]. Indeed, the reason for the difference in risk between NSAIDs may be in part related to the relative potency of usual doses of individual NSAIDs, for example ibuprofen having a lower anti-inflammatory potency than piroxicam at usually used dose. The contribution of *Helicobacter pylori* to the risk of NSAID-induced gastrointestinal complications remains uncertain and controversial[110]. One study has suggested that identification of *Helicobacter pylori* before NSAID therapy was useful in reducing the incidence of GI complications[111]. Other work suggests that the bacterium might protect against NSAID GI damage[112]. The proton-pump inhibitor, omeprazole, might be more effective as a prophylaxis against NSAID-induced gastric ulcer in patients infected with *H. pylori*[113]. Finally, the high prevalence of usage of NSAIDs in the elderly is consistent with 20–30 per cent of all serious ulcer complications of bleeding and perforation being attributable to these drugs. This fact presents a major, but addressable, public health challenge. This is particularly the case given that many of these elderly patients have OA or soft tissue rheumatic complaints and may not need NSAIDs in the first instance[114].

Antacids, the surface-active agent sucralfate, histamine 2-antagonists (H2 antagonists) such as cimetidine and ranitidine, the prostaglandin analogue misoprostol, and proton pump inhibitors including omeprazole are used extensively to treat NSAID-induced upper gastrointestinal symptoms, and to treat and prevent NSAID-induced peptic ulcers and their complications[115]. Upper gastrointestinal symptoms, notably indigestion and dyspepsia, are reduced by taking NSAIDs with food and/or antacids. Histamine 2 antagonists are heavily used for treating dyspepsia induced by NSAIDs. However, there is virtually no robust evidence of efficacy available but anecdotal evidence for benefit against dyspeptic symptoms is widely accepted.

Histamine-2-antagonists, proton pump inhibitors, and misoprostol are effective in healing NSAID-induced mucosal damage even if the NSAID is continued, although healing is slower if NSAIDs are continued. Despite the widely held perception that H2 antagonists protect against NSAID-induced gastric ulcers, only misoprostol the prostaglandin analogue or the proton pump inhibitor omeprazole have proven efficacy in reducing the incidence of NSAID-induced gastroduodenal lesions as observed endoscopically[76,110,113,116,117]. High-dose famotidine, a newer histamine-2-antagonist, has also shown efficacy but the cost makes this an unattractive option[118]. Misoprostol has been shown to reduce the incidence of NSAID-induced gastric ulcers by 50–90 per cent and the incidence of serious bleeding and perforation is reduced significantly by this drug[119]. Omeprazole is as effective as misoprostol in treating NSAID-induced gastric lesions, but there is a less relapse and better tolerance in comparison to misoprostol[113]. Misoprostol causes diarrhea in a small percentage of patients and this could be more of a problem in the elderly sick. However, studies of the cost-effectiveness of misoprostol and omeprazole in this setting have produced conflicting results. Cost effectiveness studies of prophylactic therapy with misoprostol or omeprazole are required in patients who have a compelling indication for NSAID therapy, are using an NSAID designated as 'safer' from epidemiological studies at the lowest effective dose and for the shortest appropriate time and also have an increased risk for serious upper gastrointestinal adverse effects form NSAIDs.

The availability of selective COX-2 inhibitors may have a profound effect on the need for prophylactic therapy but, again, economic analysis will be critical. Endoscopic studies on substantial numbers of normal volunteers with rofecoxib and celecoxib, in repeated dose studies at the upper limit for clinical use or substantially higher, has revealed gastrointestinal damage values indistinguishable from those seen with placebo and substantially and significantly less than ibuprofen and naproxen. Thus, gastrointestinal damage defined as a Lanza score of ≥ 2 was 12.2 per cent for rofecoxib 250 mg daily, 8 per cent for placebo, and 71 per cent for ibuprofen 2400 mg daily[120]. Similar results were obtained for celecoxib[121] (Fig. 22.6). The gastrointestinal symptoms associated with NSAIDs such as heartburn, dyspepsia, and acid reflux are also described with COX-2-specific drugs but the rate of these relative to conventional NSAIDs and placebo remains undetermined—the rate may be either slightly greater than placebo and less that conventional NSAIDs or the same as placebo. Interestingly, hemoglobin concentrations do not decline over time with chronic COX-2-specific therapy in contrast to conventional NSAIDs; presumably a result of gastric microbleeding in the case of the NSAIDs.

Three NSAIDs that were available prior to the discovery of the COX-2 enzyme, namely meloxicam, nabumetone, and nimuleside, have been identified as having some selectivity for

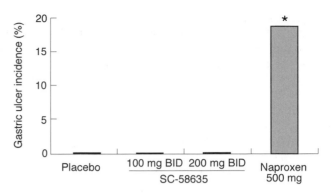

Fig. 22.6 Gastric ulcer incidence comparing celecoxib with naproxen and placebo. Adapted from Simon *et al.*[121].

the inhibition of COX-2 versus COX-1 using *in vitro* test systems. As noted previously, the *in vitro* findings do not reflect the fact that oral therapy with usual therapeutic dose rates of these drugs is associated with COX-1 inhibitory activity. Thus, although it had been strongly suggested that these drugs should have reduced adverse effects, especially gastrointestinal, on the basis of their selectivity for COX-2, studies with meloxicam and nimuleside at least are not convincing. Nimuleside had a relative risk for serious upper gastrointestinal bleeding of 4.4, similar to naproxen[122] while very large, short-term studies with meloxicam showed similar rates of upper gastrointestinal bleeds, perforations, and ulcers to diclofenac and piroxicam respectively[123,124]. Although gastric perforations and bleeds appear to be lower with nabumetone, studies are limited to date.

Renal adverse effects

NSAIDs can affect the kidney in two ways—impairing kidney function and causing damage to kidney tissue[96] (Table 22.2). The functional effects are prevalent in comparison to the tissue damaging effects.

Renal prostaglandin synthesis is vital for the maintenance of renal function when renal perfusion is reduced in hypovolemic states (cirrhosis with ascites; nephrotic syndrome), ineffective circulatory volume (congestive heart failure), or primary renal disorders. In these conditions vasoconstrictor hormones, such as noradrenaline and vasopressin, are secreted in the kidney to maintain renal perfusion pressure. Compensatory secretion of prostaglandins by the kidney is essential to prevent unopposed vasoconstriction of renal blood vessels and thus damaging decreases in glomerular perfusion pressure. NSAIDs will jeopardize this protective response by inhibiting the synthesis of the vasodilatory prostaglandins. This can lead to a decrease of glomerular filtration rate and renal blood flow that can progress to irreversible renal failure if prolonged. Concurrent diuretic therapy which leads to prostaglandin secretion in the kidney is another risk factor for NSAID impairment of renal function. NSAID-induced renal functional impairment results in a rise in plasma creatinine within days of commencing the NSAID. Serum potassium also rises in more severe cases and weight gain is noted along with decreasing urine output. Cessation of the NSAID usually leads to rapid improvement. Careful monitoring of renal function is important especially in the elderly or renally

Table 22.2   Renal adverse drug reactions to NSAIDs (Day *et al.* (168))

Type	Adverse reaction	Features
Functional adverse effects	Decreased GFR Sodium and water retention Hyperkalemia	Commonest; elderly and renally impaired at greatest risk; regular monitoring in at risk patients with plasma creatinine and electrolytes, weight and blood pressure
Pathological adverse effects		Rare; can happen with any NSAID
	Acute interstitial nephritis	With or without nephrotic syndrome; can happen with any NSAID; immunological origin; ? T-cell mediated
	Papillary necrosis	Incidence declining since removal of phenacetin containing combination analgesics from the market
	Chronic renal failure	Mechanisms uncertain

impaired and early recognition of functional impairment can prevent acute renal failure[125,126].

NSAID-induced sodium and water retention with dependent edema has been reported in up to 25 per cent of patients given NSAIDs depending on the general health, renal function, and age of the patient[127]. Hyperkalemia can be marked but is uncommon. Risk factors identified are the patient's age, the presence of renal impairment, diabetes, and concurrent therapy with angiotensin-converting enzyme inhibitors, potassium-sparing diuretics, or cyclosporin-A.

Kidney tissue damage is uncommon with NSAIDs. Acute interstitial nephritis with and without proteinuria in the nephrotic range, minimal change of glomerulonephritis with nephrotic syndrome, papillary necrosis, acute tubular necrosis, and vasculitis are reported adverse reactions to NSAIDs. NSAID-induced interstitial nephritis is unusual and there are case reports linking this effect to most NSAIDs. Most commonly this adverse reaction occurs 2 weeks–18 months after starting NSAIDs, often proteinuria and renal failure occur and the abnormality recovers slowly over a year following the cessation of the NSAIDs. An important adverse renal effect of NSAIDs is associated with tiaprofenic acid. This drug is rarely associated with intense interstitial cystitis. Unfortunately, quite a few patients have undergone investigation and multiple surgical interventions for this drug-induced problem[128,129].

Disappointingly, the new, specific COX-2 inhibitors appear to induce the physiological impairment of renal functional typical of conventional NSAIDs. This may relate to constitutive expression of COX-2 enzyme in the macula densa of the kidney[130]. Thus, peripheral edema up to 3 per cent has been reported in clinical studies of the COX-2 specific inhibitors.

Hematological adverse effects

Chronic NSAID therapy can be associated with anemia resulting from blood loss from the gastrointestinal tract that is often unsuspected. An occasional full blood count for any patient taking NSAIDs regularly is warranted. This effect is not a feature of COX-2-specific drugs to-date. Anemia related to chronic inflammatory disease and vitamin and nutritional deficiencies also contribute to anemia in patients with rheumatic disease.

Serious NSAID-induced bone marrow toxicity is rare, an exception being phenylbutazone which has been withdrawn from routine availability in many countries because of the risk of aplastic anemia. It appears that the risk factors for aplastic anemia are age, female gender, and excessive dose rates. A relationship with high blood concentrations is indicative of the importance of high dosage rates and/or low body clearance rates in the genesis of this adverse effect. A rate of phenylbutazone-induced aplastic anemia of about 1/30 000 monthly prescriptions has been estimated.

NSAIDs inhibit platelet COX-1 enzyme thereby inhibiting platelet adhesiveness and prolonging the bleeding time. Low doses of aspirin irreversibly acetylate the COX-1 enzyme. Bleeding time is prolonged significantly for 10–12 days, return to basal bleeding time being dependent upon the generation of new platelets. Other NSAIDs inhibit COX-1 reversibly so bleeding time normalizes in concert with the elimination of the NSAID. For the majority of NSAIDs, bleeding time has normalized within 24 h of the last dose. Platelet function may take longer to return to normal with NSAIDs with long half-lives such as tenoxicam and piroxicam. Thus it may be about 70 h after piroxicam is ceased until platelet function is normal. COX-2-specific inhibitors celecoxib and rofecoxib do not inhibit platelet function or prolong bleeding time at clinically used or even supra-therapeutic doses[24,41,42,121,131].

NSAID-induced thrombocytopenia is a rare, idiosyncratic adverse reaction that occurs with all NSAIDs. However, because of the widespread use of NSAIDs in the community the total number of cases reported to adverse reaction reporting agencies is substantial. NSAID-induced thrombocytopenia is usually mild and reversible. However serious bleeding and death do occur and have been reported more often with phenylbutazone and indometacin.

Neurological adverse effects

NSAID-induced central nervous system adverse effects are often overlooked in elderly patients. Confusion, cognitive dysfunction, somnolence, disturbances of behavior, and dizziness are some of the central nervous system adverse effects described[132]. The problem is that these symptoms are not unusual in the elderly. Therefore the link to NSAIDs is often unsuspected. Most reports implicate indometacin, ibuprofen, and naproxen. Psychotic reactions have been reported with indometacin and sulindac[133–136]. Given that the antipyretic and at least a component of the analgesic effects of NSAIDs depend on central nervous system actions, it is to be expected that there will be other central nervous system effects[137].

Aseptic meningitis is an uncommon adverse reaction reported with ibuprofen and sulindac and occurs particularly in individuals with systemic lupus erythematosus or juvenile rheumatoid arthritis. Migraine type headaches are commonly noted in patients taking indometacin, particularly if they are known sufferers of migraine.

Hepatic adverse effects

NSAID-related hepatotoxicity leading to fibrosis or cirrhosis is quite rare and idiosyncratic when it does occur. Reversible liver function abnormalities are more common. Thus, anti-inflammatory doses of aspirin are associated with mild, usually asymptomatic elevations of hepatic enzymes in serum in 50 per cent of patients, occurring within the first few weeks of therapy. Sulindac and diclofenac appear to be associated with a higher incidence of reversible hepatotoxicity in comparison to other NSAIDs. Hepatotoxicity is more common in juvenile rheumatoid arthritis and patients with systemic lupus erythematosus. There is no consistent liver function or histopathological abnormality in NSAID-induced hepatotoxicity. NSAID-hepatotoxicity is a contraindication to further use in an affected patient.

Rarely, severe liver toxicity occurs with aspirin even at low doses. Reyes syndrome, characterized by severe hepatic damage, occurs in children and for this reason aspirin is no longer recommended for use as an antipyretic in children less than 12 years of age. Phenylbutazone has also been associated with rare cases of severe hepatotoxicity with a high fatality rate. This drug should only be contemplated for second-line use in patients with significant and problematic inflammatory disease.

Cardiovascular adverse effects

Variable and sometimes very significant increases in blood pressure can occur in patients commenced on NSAIDs, particularly if they are already hypertensive[138]. Therefore, blood pressure should be more intensively monitored in hypertensive patients commencing NSAIDs. This effect is most commonly observed with indomethacin. This drug dosed chronically will oppose the effects of antihypertensive drugs and has also been demonstrated to increase blood pressure in healthy elderly individuals significantly[139–142].

NSAIDs inhibit the synthesis of vasodilatory prostaglandins in renal and vascular tissue. These important counter-regulatory hormones are secreted in response to various diuretics and antihypertensive drugs contributing to their effects. Removal of prostaglandins by NSAID inhibition of synthesis promotes an increase in blood pressure.

An important, but unresolved, matter is whether NSAIDs precipitate or worsen cardiac failure. Unconfirmed case control data suggests this might be a very significant cause of morbidity and mortality, especially in the elderly who would be most susceptible[143,144]. Elevation of systemic blood pressure would be likely to increase the demands on the left ventricle but further work needs to be undertaken to determine the contribution of NSAIDs to cardiac failure.

Pulmonary adverse effects

Prescribers and patients need to be aware that aspirin and NSAIDs can precipitate or exacerbate asthma. Aspirin or NSAID-induced bronchospasm is often acute and can be lethal. Those most at risk have a history of 'aspirin-allergy' and frequently complain of symptoms from nasal polyps. All NSAIDs are contraindicated in this extreme form of aspirin allergy. Many tragedies from NSAID-bronchospasm occur when a new 'pain-relieving' drug is not known to be an NSAID by the prescriber or patient. Interestingly some individuals with aspirin allergy are able to tolerate salicylate derivatives. Salicylate is an extremely weak inhibitor of prostaglandin synthesis whereas aspirin is potent. It has long been suspected that this contrast may be related to the differing potential for 'allergy'. The propensity for COX-2-specific inhibitors to cause bronchospasm remains unknown and data is eagerly awaited. Exciting recent work promises to, at last, shed some light on the mechanism for this important and dangerous adverse event. Accumulation of leukotriene C4 to an excessive degree in association with NSAID-induced prostaglandin synthesis inhibition may be the explanation for this adverse effect[145].

Dermatological adverse effects

Skin rashes are uncommon with NSAIDs although serious, idiosyncratic reactions such as erythema multiforme and blistering skin reactions are reported. Photosensitivity reactions are also well known although uncommon.

Cartilage and NSAIDs

Chronic NSAID therapy has long been suspected of inducing cartilage damage although this remains an unproven hypothesis in man and is also contentious. *In vitro* studies have suggested that NSAIDs might have a deleterious effect upon chondrocyte function but these have been marred by often employing excessive concentrations of aspirin and NSAIDs. Confirmation that this is an important clinical effect has been difficult to demonstrate. One clinical study[146] has suggested that cartilage deterioration was more rapid in patients taking diclofenac, a potent prostaglandin synthetase inhibitor, than those taking azapropazone, a relatively mild prostaglandin inhibitor. One NSAID, tiaprofenic acid, even has reference to

Table 22.3   Drug interactions involving NSAIDs (Day *et al.*[168])

Drug affected	NSAID implicated	Effect of interaction	Management considerations
Pharmacodynamic interactions			
Antihypertensive drugs Beta-blockers Diuretics ACE inhibitors Calcium channel blockers	Indomethacin; others less problematic; sulindac possbily least problematic	Blunting of antihypertensive effect	Avoid NSAID if possible; increased monitoring; adjust dose of antihypertensive
Diuretics	Indomethacin (reversible renal failure has occurred with triamterene); others less problematic; sulindac possibly least problematic	Blunting of natriuretic and diuretic effects; cardiac failure worsened; increased risk of renal impairment; increased risk of hyperkalemia with potassium sparing diuretics	Avoid NSAIDs; indometacin and triamterine contraindicated; increased clinical and laboratory monitoring; adjust dose of diuretic; particular care with potassium sparing diuretics
Anticoagulants	All	Inhibition of platelets; GI lesions a bleeding risk	Avoid NSAIDs; low dose, intermittent NSAID such as ibuprofen if needed
Hypoglycemic agents	Anti-inflammatory dose salicylate	Potentiates hypoglycemia; mechanism unknown	Avoid high dose salicylate; monitor BSL
Pharmacokinetic interactions	*NSAIDs affecting other drugs*		
Warfarin	Phenylbutazone; azapropazone	Inhibits metabolism of S warfarin (more potent isomer)	Avoid combination; use another NSAID
Oral hypoglycemics e.g. tolbutamide, glipizide	Phenylbutazone, azapropazone	Inhibits metabolism of oral hypoglycemic drugs	Avoid combination; use another NSAID
Phenytoin	Phenylbutazone; azapropazone	Inhibits metabolism of phenytoin and displaces phenytoin off albumin	Avoid combination; phenytoin requirements decreased; beware toxicity; monitor unbound phenytoin
Phenytoin	Other NSAIDs e.g. ibuprofen and salicylates (high dose)	Displace phenytoin from albumin but unbound concentrations only rise if phenytoin metabolism is saturated or if folate depletion occurs	Monitor for phenytoin toxicity; unbound phenytoin concentrations may be helpful; may need phenytoin dose reduction
Methotrexate	All	Risk of methotrexate toxicity; inhibition of renal excretion of methotrexate; not usually a problem; beware elderly, renally impaired; folate depleted	Be careful not to dose too heavily with methotrexate in the elderly and those with renal impairment; careful regular monitoring of blood count

Table 22.3   *cont.*

Drug affected	NSAID implicated	Effect of interaction	Management considerations
Digoxin	All	NSAID-induced decrease in renal function leads to reduced clearance	Beware possible digoxin toxicity; monitor digoxin more closely
Aminoglycosides	All	Decreased renal function by NSAID increases aminoglycoside concentration and risk of nephrotoxicity	Close monitoring of aminoglycoside concentrations and renal function
Lithium	All	Decreased renal function increases risk of lithium toxicity	Closer monitoring of lithium concentrations; beware dehydration and concomitant illness
Valproic acid	Aspirin	Inhibition of valproate metabolism increasing valproate concentrations	Avoid aspirin; monitor valproate concentrations more closely
Antacids	Salicylates	Alkalinization of urine increases renal clearance of salicylate and plasma concentrations fall	Monitor plasma salicylate concentrations more closely
Cholestyramine	All	Reduce absorption of NSAID	Avoid combination
Metoclopramide	Aspirin; all	Increases absorption rate	Useful in migraine attacks

'cartilage-sparing' properties incorporated into its label in some countries but clinical data indicating superiority in this domain is not available. Recently, *in vitro* work suggests that COX-2 is expressed in cartilage. Thus, the COX-2-specific inhibitors potentially may be more deleterious than the conventional NSAIDs[147].

NSAID drug interactions

The most clinically important drug interactions of NSAIDs are pharmacodynamic in nature. Perhaps the best example is the decreased activity of diuretics and antihypertensives in patients taking NSAIDs, especially indometacin[148,149] (Table 22.3). Those most at risk are the elderly and patients with diabetes, cardiovascular, or renal diseases. Thus, these categories of patient require increased surveillance when potentially interacting drugs are prescribed.

Pharmacokinetic interactions involving NSAIDs are less important as the NSAIDs most involved are infrequently prescribed. NSAIDs as a class are not expected to interfere with the hepatic clearance of other drugs. Exceptions include the inhibition of the metabolism of warfarin, phenytoin, and tolbutamide,

by the chemically-related pyrazole NSAIDs, phenylbutazone and azapropazone.

As NSAIDS bind extensively to plasma albumin, it is to be expected that this class will displace other drugs from plasma albumin. However, the possibility of clinically important potentiation of pharmacological effects of the displaced drug has been exaggerated[150,151]. An important case in point is that of the widely used anticoagulant warfarin. This drug is displaced from its binding site on albumin by many NSAIDs but increased anticoagulant activity has never been demonstrated. This relates to the fact that steady-state, unbound concentrations of warfarin are unchanged. This is to be expected as the only pharmacokinetic parameter that can influence steady-state concentrations of unbound drug is the clearance of unbound drug. NSAIDs do not affect the clearance of unbound warfarin. However, caution is still warranted when contemplating the use of warfarin with NSAID because of inhibition of platelet function by NSAIDs and the propensity to bleed more from the upper gastrointestinal tract with the combination. Another example is that of phenytoin. Its binding to plasma albumin is reduced by high dose salicylate but, again, the effect of phenytoin is not potentiated[152]. However, as expected with all these protein-binding interactions, the total plasma concentrations of phenytoin will be lower. The free concentrations of phenytoin at steady-state will be no different after the introduction of NSAID explaining why there is not the risk of phenytoin toxicity when NSAID is added. Because total (free plus bound) concentrations of phenytoin are monitored, and these will be lower in the face of concurrent NSAID therapy, the therapeutic range should be adjusted accordingly. The new range should be reduced by approximately 25 per cent to 30–60 mmol/l (7.5–15 mg/l). By an identical mechanism, high dose aspirin leads to the fall in steady-state total concentrations of a number of other NSAIDs but there is no advantage for such combinations being used as adverse effects will increase as a function of a higher dose of NSAIDs[153].

An important interaction occurs between lithium and NSAIDs. The clearance of lithium, which is largely renal, is reduced by diclofenac[154], ketorolac[155], and flurbiprofen[156]. It is likely that most other NSAIDs will have a similar effect as the mechanism is NSAID-induced inhibition of renal prostaglandin synthesis. It is possible that sulindac may be less likely to cause this interaction because of lower exposure of kidney tissue to the active sulindac sulfide metabolite[157]. As plasma lithium concentrations need to be kept in a narrow therapeutic range, concentrations need to be monitored more frequently when NSAIDs are introduced or ceased.

An interaction between methotrexate and NSAIDs is described, however serious interactions between these drugs prescribed at doses appropriate for inflammatory rheumatic diseases are uncommonly reported. The mechanism is thought to be inhibition of the renal secretion of methotrexate[158,159]. Increased concentrations of the potentially toxic 7-hydroxy-metabolite of methotrexate have also been described[160]. The risk for an interaction leading to dangerous methotrexate toxicity increases as renal impairment increases because methotrexate is retained in these circumstances. Therefore great caution is needed in the elderly and those with renal impairment even with low methotrexate doses as the addition of an NSAID to the treatment could tip the balance leading to methotrexate toxicity[161]. This situation is increasingly likely as older patients with inflammatory rheumatic diseases are treated with higher doses of methotrexate. Also, caution in the combined use of NSAIDs and methotrexate has also been recommended on the basis of studies in children with arthritis[162]. Drugs that deplete folic acid, such as the antibiotics, trimethoprim, and various sulfonamides including sulfamethoxasole contribute to increased risk for methotrexate toxicity.

Finally, the availability of diclofenac is markedly enhanced by cyclosporin leading to the recommendation that lower doses of diclofenac be administered initially when coadministered with cyclosporin. The mechanism is probably inhibition of the first pass metabolism of diclofenac by cyclosporin[163]. Other NSAIDs are not susceptible to this interaction.

Practical guidance for safe and effective NSAIDs usage

Firstly, it should be clear that NSAID therapy is indicated in a rheumatic disorder and physical and other 'non-drug' therapies and simple analgesic therapy have been carefully considered and, if appropriate, prescribed. If NSAID treatment is indicated, most prescribers commence with one of the newer NSAIDs rather than aspirin or indometacin. Anti-inflammatory doses of aspirin are associated with troubling deafness and tinnitus. Indometacin is associated with a substantial incidence of headaches and other CNS effects. However, indometacin retains popularity for the short-term, high-dose treatment of acute gout. Phenylbutazone is no longer recommended for initial therapy rheumatic disorders because of the risk of marrow aplasia. It is still preferred by many patients with ankylosing spondylitis and is a good second-line choice in this condition if the patient is young, the dose is not excessive, and regular monitoring is undertaken.

Generally, the choice of an NSAID is a matter of personal preference of the physician and patient. Selection might reasonably be based on the patient's previous experience with NSAIDs, the dosing frequency preferred, and perhaps influenced by the information regarding relative gastrointestinal safety of NSAIDs[66,161]. Appropriately, the cost of prescriptions is an increasing influence and more recently the estimated costs of NSAID-induced adverse events is being factored into the selection criteria[164]. Logically, combining data on the relative safety of NSAIDs and their relative costs should provide a rational approach to NSAID selection and indeed such an approach has been associated with substantial savings without decrement in outcomes in United States studies[165,166]. Ibuprofen in lowest effective dose emerges as an appropriate first choice from these sorts of analyses. In respect of dosing regimens, once daily dosing with piroxicam, tenoxicam, or slow release formulations of ketoprofen or naproxen may be preferred to a twice or three times daily dosage with other NSAIDs such as ibuprofen and diclofenac. Many patients with inflammatory rheumatic diseases find that an NSAID suppository at night helps to control morning symptoms of pain and stiffness.

NSAID doses ought to be the minimum to produce symptom relief. They should also be appropriate for the rheumatic condition and the age and general health of the patient. Larger doses are indicated for inflammatory arthritis such as acute gout and rheumatoid arthritis while smaller does are appropriate for osteoarthritis. The value of concurrent acetominophen in maintaining analgesia with lower exposure to NSAIDs should be explored. Special care with dosing and monitoring is needed for the elderly, particularly those with low body weight, and patients with hypertension or cardiac, renal, or liver impairment.

NSAID dose needs to be altered according to clinical response, the goal being to use the minimal effective dose especially in the elderly with increased risk of serious adverse effects. If NSAID dosage increases, do not deliver a satisfactory response, or dyspepsia or other adverse effect occurs, then substitution with another NSAID is indicated. Concurrent acetominophen may also be helpful. Why swapping one NSAID for another sometimes is successful is not understood.

An important problem is that NSAIDs are too often prescribed indefinitely without careful, regular, re-evaluation of need. This is especially the case in the elderly with osteoarthritis or non-specific rheumatic symptoms[114]. Any patient taking NSAIDs chronically needs a clinical review regularly as to ongoing need for NSAIDs and with particular note of gastrointestinal risk factors, blood pressure, cardiac status, blood count, and renal function. The advent of specific COX-2 inhibitors heralds an exciting period of change in analgesic anti-inflammatory therapy of the rheumatic disorders and will undoubtedly lead to reconsideration of the most appropriate drug therapy for the various rheumatic conditions.

References

1. Malmberg A.B., Yaksh T.L. Capsaicin-evoked prostaglandin E2 release in spinal cord slices: relative effect of cyclooxygenase inhibitors. *European Journal of Pharmacology*, 1994;**271**(2–3):293–9.

2. Lanz R., Polster P., Brune K. Antipyretic analgesics inhibit prostaglandin release from astrocytes and macrophages similarly. *European Journal of Pharmacology*, 1986;**130**(1–2):105–9.

3. Brune K., Rainsford K.D., Wagner K., Peskar B.A. Inhibition of anti-inflammatory drugs of prostaglandin production in cultured macrophages. *Naunyn-Schmiedebergs Archives of Pharmacology*, 1981;**315**(3):269–76.

4. Yaksh T.L., Malmberg A.B. Spinal actions of NSAIDs in blocking spinally mediated hyperalgesia: the role of cyclooxygenase products. *Agents Actions*, 1993;**41**(Suppl.):89–100.

5. Marshall P.J., Kulmacz R.J., Lands W.E. Constraints on prostaglandin biosynthesis in tissues. *Journal of Biological Chemistry*, 1987;**262**(8):3510–7.

6. Graham G.G., Milligan M.K., Day R.O., Williams K.M., Ziegler J.B. Therapeutic considerations from pharmacokinetics and metabolism: ibuprofen and paracetamol. In: Rainsford K.D., Powanda M.C., eds. *Safety and efficacy of non-prescription (OTC) analgesics and NSAIDs*. London: Kluwer Academic Publishers,, 1998:77–92.

7. Bradley J.D., Brandt K.D., Katz B.P., Kalasinski L.A., Ryan S.I. Comparison of an anti-inflammatory dose of ibuprofen, an analgesic dose of ibuprofen, and acetaminophen in the treatment of patients with osteoarthritis of the knee. *New England Journal of Medicine*, 1992;**325**(2):87–91.

8. Bradley J.D., Brandt K.D., Katz B.P., Kalasinski L.A., Ryan S.I. Treatment of knee osteoarthritis: relationship of clinical features of joint inflammation to the response to a nonsteroidal antiinflammatory drug or pure analgesic. *Journal of Rheumatology*, 1992;**19**(12):1950–4.

9. Williams H.J., Ward J.R., Egger M.J., *et al.* Comparison of naproxen and acetaminophen in a two-year study of treatment of osteoarthritis of the knee [see comments]. *Arthritis Rheum*, 1993;**36**(9):1196–206.

10. Nicholls A.W., Farrant R.D., Shockcor J.P., *et al.* NMR and HPLC-NMR spectroscopic studies of futile deacetylation in paracetamol metabolites in rat and man. *Journal of Pharmaceutical and Biomedical Analysis*, 1997;**15**(7):901–10.

11. Bartle W.R., Blakely J.A. Potentiation of warfarin anticoagulation by acetaminophen. *Journal of the American Medical Association*, 1991;**265**(10):1260.

12. Seideman P., Samuelson P., Neander G. Naproxen and paracetamol compared with naproxen only in coxarthrosis. Increased effect of the combination in,18 patients. *Acta Orthopaedica Scandinavica*, 1993;**64**(3):285–8.

13. Seideman P., Melander A. Equianalgesic effects of paracetamol and indometacin in rheumatoid arthritis. *British Journal of Rheumatology*, 1988;**27**(2):117–22.

14. Graziotti P.J., Goucke C.R. The use of oral opioids in patients with chronic non-cancer pain. Management strategies. *Medical Journal of Australia*, 1997;**167**(1):30–4.

15. de Craen A.J., Roos P.J., Leonard de Vries A., Kleijnen J. Effect of colour of drugs: systematic review of perceived effect of drugs and of their effectiveness. *British Medical Journal*, 1996;**313**(7072):1624–6.

16. Kjaersgaard-Andersen P., Nafei A., Skov O., *et al.* Codeine plus paracetamol versus paracetamol in longer-term treatment of chronic pain due to osteoarthritis of the hip. A randomised, double-blind, multi-centre study. *Pain*, 1990;**43**(3):309–18.

17. Chan G.L., Matzke G.R. Effects of renal insufficiency on the pharmacokinetics and pharmacodynamics of opioid analgesics. *Drug Intelligence and Clinical Pharmacy*, 1987;**21**(10):773–83.

18. Brooks P.M., Day R.O. Nonsteroidal antiinflammatory drugs—differences and similarities. *New England Journal of Medicine*, 1991;**324**(24):1716–25.

19. McManus P., Primrose J.G., Henry D.A., Birkett D.J., Lindner J., Day R.O. Pattern of non-steroidal anti-inflammatory drug use in Australia, 1990–1994. A report from the Drug Utilization Sub-Committee of the Pharmaceutical Benefits Advisory Committee. *Medical Journal of Australia*, 1996;**164**(10):589–92.

20. Moore R.A., Tramer M.R., Carroll D., Wiffen P.J., McQuay H.J. Quantitative systematic review of topically applied non-steroidal anti-inflammatory drugs. *British Medical Journal*, 1998;**316**(7128):333–8.

21. Brune K., Graff P. Non-steroid anti-inflammatory drugs: influence of extra-cellular pH on biodistribution and pharmacological effects. *Biochemical Pharmacology*, 1978;**27**(4):525–30.

22. Vane J.R. Inhibition of prostaglandin synthesis as a mechanism of action for aspirin-like drugs. *Nature—New Biology*, 1971;**231**(25):232–5.

23. Vane J.R., Bakhle Y.S., Botting R.M. Cyclooxygenases 1 and 2. *Annual Review of Pharmacology and Toxicology*, 1998;**38**:97–120.

24. Lipsky P.E., Isakson P.C. Outcome of specific COX-2 inhibition in rheumatoid arthritis. *Journal of Rheumatology*, 1997;**24**(Suppl.49):9–14.

25. Frolich J.C. Prostaglandin endoperoxide synthetase isoenzymes: the clinical relevance of selective inhibition. *Annals of the Rheumatic Diseases*, 1995;**54**(12):942–3.

26. Bahkle Y.S., Botting R.M. Cyclooxygenase-2 and its regulation in inflammation. *Mediators of Inflammation*, 1996;**6**:765–768.

27. Crofford L.J. COX-1 and COX-2 tissue expression: implications and predictions. *Journal of Rheumatology*, 1997;**24**(Suppl.49):15–9.

28. Herschman H.R. Prostaglandin synthase 2. *Biochimica et Biophysica Acta*, 1996;**1299**(1):125–40.

29. Otto J.C., Smith W.L. Prostaglandin endoperoxide synthases-1 and -2. *J Lipid Mediat Cell Signal*, 1995;**12**(2–3):139–56.

30. Smith W.L., DeWitt D.L. Biochemistry of prostaglandin endoperoxide H synthase-1 and synthase-2 and their differential susceptibility to nonsteroidal anti-inflammatory drugs. *Seminars in Nephrology*, 1995;**15**(3):179–94.

31. Appleby S.B., Ristimaki A., Neilson K., Narko K., Hla T. Structure of the human cyclo-oxogenase-2 gene. *Biochemical Journal*, 1994;**302**(3):723–7.

32. Sirois J., Richards J.S. Transcriptional regulation of the rat prostaglandin endoperoxide synthase 2 gene in granulosa cells. Evidence for the role of a cis-acting C/EBP beta promoter element. *Journal of Biological Chemistry*, 1993;**268**(29):21931–8.

33. Luong C., Miller A., Barnett J., Chow J., Ramesha C., Browner M.F. Flexibility of the NSAID binding site in the structure of human cyclooxygenase-2. *Nature Structural Biology*, 1996;**3**(11):927–33.

34. Kurumbail R.G., Stevens A.M., Gierse J.K., *et al.* Structural basis for selective inhibition of cyclooxygenase-2 by anti-inflammatory agents [published erratum appears in *Nature*, 1997 Feb 6;**385**(6616):555]. *Nature*, 1996;**384**(6610):644–8.

35. Smith C.J., Zhang Y., Koboldt C.M., *et al.* Pharmacological analysis of cyclooxygenase-1 in inflammation. *Proceedings of the National Academy of Science USA*, 1998;**95**(22):13313–8.

36. Vane J.R. NSAIDs, Cox-2 inhibitors, and the gut. *Lancet*, 1995;**346**(8982):1105–6.

37. Frolich J.C. A classification of NSAIDs according to the relative inhibition of cyclooxygenase isoenzymes [see comments]. *Trends in Pharmacological Sciences*, 1997;**18**(1):30–4.

23 | Systemic glucocorticoids in rheumatoid arthritis

Roger Hällgren

The discovery of the dramatic anti-inflammatory effects of glucocorticoids in rheumatoid arthritis (RA) half a decade ago revolutionized the treatment of rheumatic diseases and other immunologically mediated diseases. The demonstration that glucocorticoids could induce reversibility of RA marks the beginning of modern rheumatology. However, the substantial and often catastrophic complications which appeared during extended use of high doses of glucocorticoids tempered the enthusiasm for the use of glucocorticoids in RA. The role and value of systemic glucocorticoids still remain under debate and many pertinent questions have to be answered regarding both basic and clinical aspects of glucocorticoid therapy. Among available drugs, glucocorticoids offer the most powerful and predictable symptomatic relief in RA but their long-term effect is a most controversial issue. Patients with RA easily become addicted to oral glucocorticoids and the long-term adverse effects are definitely present. Minimizing the incidence and severity of glucocorticoid-related side-effects is an urgent task since glucocorticoids remain widely used. New approaches to the management of osteoporosis, better definition of the therapeutically relevant effect of glucocorticoid, optimal dosage and timing of glucocorticoid intake, and molecular alterations of the glucocorticoid molecule, may hopefully decrease its complications in the treatment of rheumatoid arthritis.

Mechanisms of glucocorticoid action in inflammation

The principal endogenous adrenal glucocorticoid hormone is cortisol (hydrocortisone), derived from cortisone. In common with other steroid hormones, cortisol has a basic structure of four carbon rings. The two hydroxyl groups, 11β and 17α, are important for the glucocorticoid anti-inflammatory activity. Glucocorticoids circulating in blood are either in the free form or in association with cortisol-binding protein. Free cortisol and its analogues being lipophilic substances pass very easily through the cell membrane into the cell where they bind to specific phosphorylated cytosolic receptors (GR). This receptor protein exists in two isoforms, $GR\alpha$ and $GR\beta$. $GR\alpha$ mediates the classical hormonal effects, and it in its unligated state is bound to a complex of heat-shock proteins (HSP). Binding of glucocorticoid to the carboxyterminal region of GR induces a dissociation of the glucocorticoid–$GR\alpha$ complex from the HSP.

The glucocorticoid–receptor complex leaves the cytoplasm, moves to the nucleus and there binds reversibly to specific sequences of DNA in the regulatory regions of glucocorticoid-responsive genes[1-2]. This initiates the transcription of genes which results in increased production of enzymes and other proteins, of which lipocortin 1 is of great importance for the anti-inflammatory action of glucocorticoids[3]. Lipocortin inhibits phospholipase A2 and thereby blocks the arachidonic cascade[4]. Cyclooxygenase (COX) catalyses the first committed step in arachidonic acid metabolism. Two isoforms of the membrane protein COX are known; COX-1 and COX-2. COX-1 is constitutively expressed and is responsible for the physiological production of prostaglandins. The enhanced prostaglandin synthesis seen after an inflammatory stimulus results from the induction and activity of COX-2. Glucocorticoids selectively and directly inhibit the expression of COX-2[5]. Glucocorticoids can also interfere with the transcription of certain other genes, and thereby reduce the synthesis of various cytokines such as interleukin 1 (IL-1), IL-2, IL-6, interferon-α, and tumor necrosis factor-α[6,7]. Glucocorticoids also inhibit the expression of an inducible nitric oxide synthase in vascular endothelial cells and the synthesis of a variety of proinflammatory enzymes including collagenase, elastase, and plasminogen activator[8]. As a result, glucocorticoids affect the synthesis of most major immunological and inflammatory mechanisms contributing to the pathogenesis of rheumatoid arthritis.

Administration of 7.5 mg and 15 mg prednisolone results in 42 per cent and 63 per cent binding of the classical cytosolic steroid receptors, respectively[9]. These binding figures are impressive and have raised the question of whether the clinical results of high-dose prednisolone (500 mg–1 g) in certain inflammatory situations are mediated by mechanisms other than classical genomic effects. High glucocorticoid dosage might affect the receptor synthesis and expression as well as receptor off-loading and reoccupance. It has also been proposed that glucocorticoids may mediate effects by membrane-bound receptors or by physicochemical interactions with cellular membranes.[10]

Glucocorticoids influence the traffic of circulating leukocytes and inhibit many of their functions. Glucocorticoids increase the number of circulating neutrophils by reduced margination of cells due to inhibition of neutrophil adhesion to endothelial cells, increased cell circulating time, and increased release of immature cells from the bone marrow. The anti-inflammatory glucocorticoid effect on neutrophils in RA is mainly attributed to an inhibition of neutrophil ingress into inflamed joints partly due to effect on neutrophil adhesion to endothelial cells[11]. Pharmacological doses of glucocorticoids have marginal effects on neutrophil function but more clinical relevant doses do not seem to influence neutrophil phagocytosis and intracellular killing, chemotaxis, lysosomal enzyme release, and respiratory burst[12].

Glucocorticoids induce reduced numbers of eosinophils in blood as well as in inflammatory lesions by unknown mechanisms. Circulating basophils are slightly reduced in number by glucocorticoids, which also reduce basophil and mast cell degranulation[11]. The glucocorticoid action on monocytes/macrophages includes reduction of circulating number, inhibition of cell arrival at reactive sites, and depression of chemotaxis and intracellular killing[10]. Glucocorticoids also antagonize macrophage differentiation and inhibit expression of class II major histocompatibility antigens induced by interferon-γ. Furthermore, these agents block the macrophage release of proinflammatory cytokines, prostaglandins, and leukotrienes and depress the macrophage microbiocidal activity.

The therapeutically relevant actions of glucocorticoids are also directed at the traffic and function of lymphocytes. These agents induce lymphopenia involving all subpopulations not primarily due to cell death but mainly due to changes in the T cell circulation pattern and redistribution of circulating lymphocytes[12]. Changes in the adhesion molecular expression and their ligands may be responsible for the altered distribution[13]. *In vitro* studies have demonstrated that glucocorticoids depress activation and proliferation of T cells induced by antigens and non-specific mitogens[14] and also suppress T-cell cytotoxicity[15]. Cytokines are essential for T-cell function. Since glucocorticoids inhibit the synthesis and also the action of several cytokines, the functional effects on T cells mediated by these agents may be primarily because of blockade of cytokine expression[16,17].

Glucocorticoids inhibit the proliferation of B cells when present in culture during cell stimulation but have only minimal effect on differentiated B cells. *In vivo*, high doses are needed to decrease antigen-induced humoral immune response while low doses of glucocorticoids have no effect on specific antibody production[18,19].

Glucocorticoid receptors and the hypothalamo–pituitary–adrenal axis in inflammation and rheumatoid arthritis

The potency of endogenous glucocorticoids is influenced by its bioavailability, that is its concentration in free form, its affinity to the specific receptor, and the ability of the cell to respond to the glucocorticoid-mediated signal. The plasma and tissue concentrations of corticosteroid-binding globulin are determined by a complex regulatory system. The glucocorticoid receptor can be subject to a number of modulating influences but glucocorticoids themselves appear to be the most potent down regulator of the receptor expression[20]. The hormone-binding affinity of

the glucocorticoid receptor is also influenced by a number of factors including the cellular ATP levels of the cell[21] and point mutations of receptor ligand-binding domain[22]. The combined treatment with IL-2 and IL-4 may reduce glucocorticoid receptor affinity in lymphocytes[23].

Most, but not all, cells respond to glucocorticoids. The distal tubule cells are examples of unresponsive cells. Furthermore, glucocorticoid-responding cells have varying degree of glucocorticoid sensitivity, partly due to different expression level of the glucocorticoid receptor. From a clinical point of view, it is important that impaired glucocorticoid sensitivity has been described in association with various human diseases. Generalized impaired glucocorticoid sensitivity has been reported to be familial due to mutation of the glucocorticoid-binding domain of the receptor[22,25]. Acquired reduced hormone binding of the receptor is seen in a subgroup of patients with AIDS[26]. This generalized form of resistance can be compensated for by increased synthesis of cortisol. Tissue-specific glucocorticoid resistance may be present in certain lymphoid tumors[27] and ACTH-producing tumors[28]. A tissue-specific glucocorticoid resistance seems to be present in a subgroup of patients with asthma[29]. In RA, the concentration of glucocorticoid receptors in leukocytes is reduced by approximately 50 per cent, a finding which cannot be explained by endogenous or exogenous hypercortisolism[30]. A selected tissue or cell-specific resistance should not easily be detected by the HPA-axis and thus not be compensated for by increased synthesis of cortisol. Since an increased propensity for immune-mediated inflammation may be mediated by glucocorticoid resistance in target tissues or immune cells, future therapeutic perspective should be to sensitize hyporesponsive cells/organs to glucocorticoids or to target the administration of these agents.

During recent years, attention has been paid to the importance of the endogenous production of glucocorticoids for the development of RA and other immune-mediated inflammatory reactions[31]. The endogenous cortisol production is dependent on the hypothalamic release of corticotropin-releasing hormone (CRH), which stimulates the pituitary to release corticotropin (adrenocorticotropic hormone, ACTH), which in turn, stimulates the adrenal cortex to release cortisol. When CRH is absent, very little corticotropin is secreted. CRH and noradrenergic neurons of the central stress system stimulate each other and both are in turn stimulated by serotonergic and cholinergic systems and inhibited by opioid-peptide systems of the brain. Every hour a secretory pulse of CRH occurs, and early in the morning these pulses increase with associated increase of the cortitropin and cortisol pulses. CRH-neutralizing antibodies, glucocorticoids, and prostanoid-synthesis inhibitors depress CRH secretion while proinflammatory cytokines, TNF-α, IL-1, and IL-6, enhance CRH secretion independently but also synergistically. These cytokines also stimulate the hypothalamic arginine vasopressin secretion and may thereby activate the HPA-axis through a neural–spinal route. However, the net result, that is the cortisol synthesis, may also be influenced by the inhibitory effect of IL-6 and TNF-α on CRH-mediated corticotropin secretion and the inhibitory effect of TNF-α on corticotropin-mediated cortisol production. Nociceptive and motorsensory afferent neurons involved in a local inflammatory process also stimulate the CRH and noradrenergic stress systems and a number of other inflammatory mediators may also participate in the regulation of the HPA axis. Thus, the short and long-term influences of the inflammatory processes on the complex systems involved in the HPA axis regulation are hard to predict in RA, since not only inflammatory signals but also the influence of a chronic, painful, and stressing illness must be considered.

Cortisol has been demonstrated in animal experimental studies to be a potent endogenous anti-inflammatory regulatory system. A chronic, proliferative erosive arthritis is seen in the female Lewis rat after injections of the streptococcal cell wall peptidoglycan but not in the histocompatible female Fischer rat[32]. A deficient corticotropin hormone release with an associated inability of the adrenals to release adequate amounts of glucocorticoids is congenitally present in the Lewis rats and could explain their susceptibility to arthritis, in particular since replacement doses with glucocorticoids reverse this susceptibility[33]. The HPA axis studies that have been performed in RA suggest that these patients have a relatively hypofunctional axis with defective central and peripheral components[34]. We reported impairment of the cortisol response to constitutive and CRH-induced corticotropin in a study of HPA axis function in untreated RA subjects. The findings suggest impaired cortisol secretion in RA despite intact ACTH secretion, and are consistent with a relative adrenal glucocorticoid insufficiency[35]. These findings are, however, at odds with earlier findings which implied a hypothalamic defect in RA[36].

The combined findings in RA of low glucocorticoid receptor concentration in leukocytes and impaired cortisol secretion are intriguing. Whether these findings originate in a pre-existing genetic and/or constitutional disturbance or whether they are the result of a chronic inflammatory process, is unknown. The concept that altered HPA axis function and leukocyte glucocorticoid receptor expression may contribute to the expression and outcome of RA is exciting but needs further research.

Synthetic glucocorticoids

Synthetic glucocorticoids are cortisol derivatives designed to increase glucocorticoid and reduce mineralocorticoid activity. The most frequently prescribed compounds with limited mineralcorticoid potency are prednisone, prednisolone, methylprednisolone, betamethasone, dexamethasone, and triamcinolone. Their actions are similar and the relative differences in anti-inflammatory potency are due to differences in circulating half-life and plasma protein binding, different affinity for the glucocorticoid receptor, and different ability to cross membranes. It is clearly desirable to modify future analogs so as to maintain the anti-inflammatory potency but reduce the harmful actions on bone and other tissues or alternatively to identify substances that may be protective against therapeutically irrelevant actions of glucocorticoids. The synthetic glucocorticoids are metabolized in the liver, conjugated, and excreted in the urine. Glucocorticoids may interact with other drugs with effect on hepatic microsomal glucocorticoid-metabolizing enzymes resulting in enhancement or depression of the glucocorticoid metabolism.

Therapeutic use of glucocorticoids

The value and optimal role of glucocorticoids in the management of RA is still under debate. Nevertheless they are widely used. Suppression of rheumatoid activity by glucocorticoids is most complex and not well defined. A number of challenging questions remain to be definitely addressed, such as issues of dosage and timing of glucocorticoids, benefits versus adverse effect of low dosage glucocorticoid treatment, and whether or not glucocorticoids have disease-modifying properties.

Glucocorticoids are effective and reliable anti-inflammatory agents, that rapidly suppress synovitis in rheumatoid arthritis. Short and long-term studies of glucocorticoids in RA have clearly demonstrated that they are superior to non-steroidal anti-inflammatory drugs in reducing pain and morning stiffness[37].

Most physicians define low dose glucocorticoid treatment as prednisolone dosages up to 5 mg daily for women and up to 7.5 mg for men in their active years. However, even these doses are not quite safe during long-term treatment and may predispose patients with RA to fractures. Elderly females develop more adverse effects, particularly osteoporosis, from chronic low dosage glucocorticoid treatment than young males. Patients with impaired responsiveness of the HPA glucocorticoid axis are presumed to benefit relatively more from low dosages of glucocorticoids. The severity of the disease may, during certain periods, dictate higher prednisolone dosages. High daily or split dose therapy may be indicated the early phases of a particular aggressive RA. The use of adjunctive immunosuppressive drug therapy as a means to decrease glucocorticoid intake should definitely be considered. Several agents including methotrexate, antimalarial agents, azathioprine, and cyclosporin A have been used. Moderate doses of glucocorticoids in the region of 15 mg prednisolone per day are also commonly used to induce a rapid remission while other drugs are taking effect. Patient education is an important factor in optimal glucocorticoid therapy and the patient should be aware of the consequences of adrenal insufficiency and informed about symptoms suggesting serious adverse events[38].

Several studies appear to suggest that corticosteroids may possess disease-modifying properties. A study that has created a stir was published by Kirwan *et al.*[39], who reported a reduction in joint erosions in glucocorticoid-treated patients with early, active RA. Prednisolone, 7.5 mg daily, given for 2 years in addition to other treatments, substantially reduced the rate of radiologically-detected progression of disease. The addition of prednisolone accelerated the clinical improvement initially but this symptomatic benefit did not persist into the second year of treatment. A major conclusion of the study, that the progression of erosions and clinical and laboratory evidence of inflammation may be uncoupled in RA, is intriguing. However, some concerns about unintentional skewing of the patient sample in the study have been raised. Confirmatory studies have to be awaited before low-dose corticosteroids in RA can be accepted as routine[40,41].

A single, daily morning dose of low dosage glucocorticoid is conventional and the rationale is to match the circadian rhythm of endogenous cortisol secretion. The issue of timing of glucocorticoid administration in RA was recently raised in a short-term study of the anti-inflammatory effect of 5 or 7.5 mg prednisolone given as a single dose either at 2.00 am or 7.30 am[42]. The rationale for the study design was the circadian rhythm in patients with RA of increased stiffness, joint pain at rest, and indices of joint activity in the mornings and the diurnal rhythm of circulating levels of IL-6[43]. In patients with RA, this cytokine peaks early in the morning and declines towards normal concentrations during the afternoon and evening. Assuming that the variation in circulating IL-6 mirrors its production and is associated with a flare in inflammatory activity early in the morning, the timing of glucocorticoid administration might be important for its effect on the rheumatoid inflammatory process. After oral administration of prednisolone tablets, peak plasma concentrations are attained after 1–3 h and the plasma half-life is 2–3.5 h. The biological half-life is estimated to be 6 h. These pharmacokinetic and biological actions of prednisolone are essential for the understanding of the dramatic improvement observed in morning clinical symptoms and the decrease of serum IL-6 concentrations following a short term period of low dose glucocorticoids given at 2 am. This exploratory study suggests that timed dosing of prednisolone may substantially improve treatment outcome but needs to be confirmed in a properly controlled, long-term trial[44]. Attention should also be directed to the suppression of morning ACTH/cortisol secretion and bone toxicity exerted by night time administration of prednisolone.

In an attempt to reduce the side-effects of long-term oral glucocorticoid therapy and increase the efficacy, the intermittent intravenous administration of high doses of glucocorticoids was introduced. Stimulated by the results obtained in renal allograft rejection and glomerulonephritis associated with systemic lupus erythematosus, corticosteroid pulse therapy (CPT) has been used to treat RA. Intravenous infusion of large doses of glucocorticoids are given, usually 1 g methylprednisolone over a short time period (30–60 min). A variety of regimens have been used, but mostly CPT is given on three consecutive or alternate days followed by a resting phase of about 6 weeks. The initial reports in RA were very promising with long-lasting effects after the last glucocorticoid infusion[45,46], but have not been confirmed in later publications reporting improvement of clinical variables for only 4 to 10 weeks and improvement of biochemical inflammatory variables, such as CRP protein, for only 2 weeks[47,48]. Several investigators have studied the effects of reduced doses of methylprednisolone and the results have been conflicting, partly due to small clinical trials with limited statistical power. In one study, the outcome of a regimen of 1000 mg methylprednisolone on 3 consecutive days was not significantly different from a regimen of three intravenous doses of 100 mg[49]. Other investigators concluded that using only 500 mg results in a substantial loss of efficacy[50]. Comparisons of intravenous high-dose methylprednisolone with equivalent oral prednisolone have been performed in a double-blind cross-over study. No statistical differences were seen during the 6 weeks of follow up[51,52].

The adverse effects of high-dose intravenous methylprednisolone after renal transplantation and in lupus nephritis have been severe and include sudden death due to cardiovascular collapse, myocardial infarction, or severe infections, osteonecrosis of the femoral head, and several other complications. A retrospective study in RA patients demonstrated frequent side-effects after CPT, but in most cases they were mild[53]. Some investigators have stressed the favorable risk/benefit ratio of pulsed methylprednisolone in this disease[54]. Nevertheless, the utility of CPT for extended maintenance treatment in RA appears to be limited.

Complications of glucocorticoid therapy

The side-effects of systemic glucocorticoids are numerous and are determined by dosage, duration of treatment, and probably also by genetic factors. The negative consequences in the early days of aggressive, extended glucocorticoid therapy were quite severe, and included mortality in infection and cardiovascular complications. Such complications are now unusual. However, a number of expected to rare medical complications are present during treatment with the more moderate dosages of glucocorticoids used today. Some of the widely believed glucocorticoid adverse effects have to be questioned while others still await improved regimens. Patients treated with moderate or low doses of corticosteroid frequently develop symptoms such as fatigue, myalgia, and nausea during rapid reduction or withdrawal of glucocorticoid therapy. These symptoms may be part of the HPA axis insufficiency but generally there appears to be no correlation between the withdrawal reaction and adrenal function. In an attempt to avoid the withdrawal reaction, slow reduction and alternate day administration of prednisolone may be recommended.

Osteoporosis

The bony complications to glucocorticoid therapy are insidious and perplexing and are today the chief concern relating to the long-term use of glucocorticoids. In RA, glucocorticoid-induced bone loss is superimposed on bone loss which is already increased in this disease because of immobilization and chronic inflammation. Risk factors for steroid-induced osteoporosis include documented low bone mineral density, history of osteoporotic fracture, or premature menopause.

Glucocorticoid-induced osteoporosis is the result of multiple factors that affect calcium homeostasis and bone formation. Pharmacological doses of glucocorticoids inhibit intestinal absorption of calcium, an effect which is at least partially independent of vitamin D. Glucocorticoid administration also induces fasting hypercalciuria due to increased resorption and decreased renal tubular calcium reabsorption. This negative calcium balance has been one possible explanation for the mild hyperparathyroidism seen in patients taking long-term glucocorticoids[55]. Glucocorticoids suppress secretion of gonadotropins and thereby the synthesis by ovary and testis of estradiol and precursors of testosterone[56,57]. The adrenal synthesis of DHEA, androstenedione, and estrogens is also reduced due to adrenal atrophy induced by glucocorticoid suppression of ACTH. Estrogen deficiency and glucocorticoids are additive in increasing the bone loss in experimental studies, and estrogen replacement therapy reduces bone loss in women taking glucocorticoids. Gonadal hormone deficiency makes a bone more susceptible to PTH induced bone resorption. Glucocorticoids also exert potent direct inhibitory effects on bone formation by suppressing osteoblastic recruitment, shortening of the life span of active osteoblasts, and depression of their function[58].

The glucocorticoid-induced bone loss is most prominent in trabecular bone and the cortical rim of the vertebral body. Compression fractures of the spine are therefore the most common sign of glucocorticoid-induced osteoporosis but increased fragility of the proximal femur and long bones is also seen. A relative risk of 6.2 of vertebral fractures is reported in glucocorticoid-treated RA patients compared with a healthy population and the current use of glucocorticoids doubles the risk of hip fracture[59,60]. The rate of bone loss seems to be most marked during the early glucocorticoid treatment period and slows down after about 6–12 months of therapy[61].

Studies of bone loss in patients treated with corticosteroids do not clearly suggest a threshold dose below which osteoporosis can be avoided. Bone loss has been reported with prednisolone doses as low as 2.5–5 mg daily, while other investigators have suggested that prednisolone doses up to 7.5 mg daily have no significant impact on bone mass. However, a single dose of 2.5 mg prednisone given in the evening will prevent the normal nocturnal rise in osteocalcin, a marker of bone synthesis[62]. Neither is the relationship between severity of bone loss and cumulative dose of glucocorticoid definitely settled. At higher doses (greater than 10 mg/day of prednisolone) all patients lose significant amounts of bone. Changes of markers of bone turnover suggest that intra-articular corticosteroid injections have minimal effect on bone resorption, and that high-dose intravenous pulse corticosteroid administration in RA may hold advantages over continuous therapy. However, these markers may be inappropriate guides to long-term bone loss in RA and many investigators believe that the total glucocorticoid dose is closely related to the degree of bone loss.

It is important to identify those patients who are at greater risk for bone loss during long-term glucocorticoid therapy. Postmenopausal women receiving steroids are more at risk for fractures, presumably because they also have age- and menopause-related bone loss. Patients with low bone mineral density due to, for example, defective calcium balance or secondary hyperparathyroidism are also at greater risk. Bone mineral density measurement should be considered in such patients. The possible predictive value of measurement of calcium absorption, urinary levels of calcium, serum levels of gonadal hormones, and markers of bone turnover are unproven.

The guidelines for prevention of steroid-induced osteoporosis include physical exercise and an active life-style, and adequate intakes of calcium and vitamin D. Food intake should also be well balanced with adequate intake of calories. Dietary calcium should be 1500 mg/day, a level that usually requires supplementation. Treatment with elemental calcium and vitamin D has, in prospec-tive studies, been shown to prevent steroid-induced bone loss, predominantly in the lumbar spine[63]. The use of large doses of vitamin D to prevent or treat glucocorticoid-induced osteoporosis is of questionable benefit, and may be hazardous. It is of greatest value to implement a muscle training program in RA patients.

Sex hormones should be replaced if gonadal failure is present. Inhibition of testosterone secretion is not uncommon in men taking steroids. Although deficiencies of male and female sex hormones enhance osteoporosis, pharmacological doses of these hormones are not indicated, because of potential adverse conse-quences on prostate and breast tumors. Postmenopausal women and premenopausal women with low estrogen levels, benefit from estrogen therapy[64]. Intramuscular testosterone injections have been tested in male patients on chronic glucocorticoids, resulting in improvement of bone mineral density, but the definite value of testosterone in primary prevention in glucocor-ticoid bone loss has to be addressed by prospective long-term studies. Whether or not anabolic steroids in female RA may prevent glucocorticoid-induced bone loss is unknown.

Bisphosphonates and calcitonin have been tested in an attempt to increase bone formation during glucocorticoid treat-ment. Etidronate given cyclically and with calcium supplementa-tion has a significant protective effect on the loss of vertebral and trochanteric bone[65,66]. In one study, treatment with etidronate was associated with an 85 per cent reduction in verte-bral fractures[65]. Alendronate therapy together with calcium and vitamin supplementation also significantly increases lumbar-spine and hip bone density in patients receiving glucocorticoid therapy but has no influence on the incidence of new vertebral fractures[67]. Cacitonin may also have a favorable effect on bone density and bone pain[68].

The treatment and prevention of bone loss in patients with RA and other diseases treated with glucocorticoids is an urgent and previously neglected problem. The current principles used may have significant effects on bone loss, but the optimal regimen for prevention of glucocorticoid-induced osteoporosis has not yet been found. Attempts to stimulate the local produc-tion of growth factors, for example IGF-1 and TNF-β, in bone which are altered by glucocorticoids may be useful. Hopefully, we shall in the future have new glucocorticoid molecules which retain anti-inflammatory properties but have less effect on calcium metabolism and bone remodeling.

Infections

The risk of infection is dependent on the dose and duration of glucocorticoid therapy[69]. In a meta-analysis involving more than 2000 glucocorticoid-treated patients in various clinical settings, the relative risk for infection was calculated to be two times that of controls[70]. The risk for infection seems, in part, to depend on the underlying disease, due to disease-associated deficits in host-defense mechanisms. Also, concomitant treatment with immunosuppressive agents may contribute. Furthermore, patients may be exposed to atypical organisms in a hospital environment[71]. Certain viral and fungal infections often occur. Staphylococcal, Gram-negative, and Listeria infections, and tuberculosis have been claimed to be frequently associated with glucocorticoid treatment. However, the risk for reactivation of tuberculosis during treatment with low doses of corticosteroids over long periods of time seems to be much lower than previously suspected[72]. The ability of glucocorticoids to mask infectious symptoms such as fever and malaise may lead to underestimation of clinical problems related to infection.

Peptic ulceration

Peptic ulceration has been considered a complication of glucocorticoid therapy. A large prospective study of patients receiving glucocorticoid therapy reported a two-fold risk for peptic ulceration. Multivariate analysis, however, showed that concomitant use of non-steroidal anti-inflammatory drugs could account for most or all of this risk[73].

Glucose and lipid metabolism

Glucocorticoids exert diabetogenic effects by stimulation of gluconeogenesis and inhibition of glucose metabolism in peripheral tissue. Thus, glucocorticoid therapy may uncover a genetic impairment of glucose handling. However, glucose handling is also influenced by inflammation. Thus, abnormal carbohydrate metabolism may occur in non-diabetic subjects during acute infections of bacterial and viral origin[74,75]. Patients with untreated but inflammatory active RA have also abnormal carbohydrate metabolism characterized by glucose intolerance, hyperinsulinemia, and peripheral insulin resistance[76,77,78]. These abnormalities in RA can be related to the inflammatory activity of the disease as measured by the acute-phase reaction. A seemingly paradoxical restoration of normal glucose handling is seen in the rheumatoid patients after short-term treatment with glucocorticoids[77]. This glucocorticoid effect may be mediated by a reduction of the synthesis of inflammatory products which influence the peripheral insulin sensitivity. Successful long-term treatment with chloroquine, penicillamine, and immunosuppressive drugs also improve or normalize the glucose handling in patients with RA[77]. When patients with very active RA have uncontrolled diabetes, the addition of low-dose glucocorticoids may improve the efficacy of insulin treatment.

The lipoprotein metabolism is altered in untreated, inflammatory active RA. Thus, serum cholesterol and cholesterol in very low density lipoprotein (VLDL), low density lipoprotein (LDL), and high density lipoprotein (HDL) fractions are reduced by 20–30 per cent and triglycerides in VLDL and HDL are reduced to a similar extent[79]. The fractional elimination rate at an intravenous fat tolerance test is about 30 per cent higher in the patients[79]. The degree of inflammatory activity governs the altered lipoprotein metabolism. Corticosteroids normalize the lipoprotein pattern in RA patients[80] and do not substantially affect total cholesterol or LDL in healthy volunteers but increase the HDL fraction[81].

Atherosclerosis

An increased cardiovascular mortality, partly due to ischemic heart disease, is documented in RA. An accelerated atherosclerosis has been claimed to be associated with glucocorticoid treatment[82,83]. Whether or not this is true can be debated, but available clinical data clearly merit future controlled studies of factors leading to atherosclerosis in RA. If glucocorticoids themselves are atherogenic, the process would involve mechanisms other than a change in lipoprotein profiles. Glucocorticoid-mediated weight gain, fluid retention, and hypertension may enhance an atherosclerotic process. It also seems important to normalize the glucose handling by reduction of the inflammatory activity. Patients should be advised regarding smoking cessation and reduction of cholesterol intake to minimize cardiovascular risk factors. Even though glucocorticoids do not induce lipoprotein abnormalities associated with cardiovascular risk, initial assessment of cholesterol levels with high-density and low-density lipoproteins may be included in patients with a family history of ischemic heart disease.

Glaucoma and cataract formation

Pre-existing cataracts and glaucoma are definitely risk factors for ophthalmic adverse effects. The incidence of cataracts is high in elderly patients but only if the prednisolone dose is > 12.5 mg/day. The adjusted odds ratio of ocular hypertension for elderly users of oral glucocorticoids compared with non-users has been calculated at 1.41[84]. The odds ratios were dependent on the glucocorticoid dose and the duration of treatment. The incidence of glaucoma is normally low in a dose range of prednisolone < 12.5 mg/day. Baseline eye examination and tonometry should be considered in patients over the age of 65 or with a family history of glaucoma. Monitoring of intraocular pressure may be justified in elderly patients on long-term treatment with higher doses of glucocorticoids.

References

1. Baxter H.D., Forssham P.H. Tissue effects of glucocorticoids. *Am J Med*, 1972;**53**:573–589.
2. Bamberger C.M., Schulte H., Chrousos G.P. Molecular determinants of glucocorticoid receptor function and tissue sensitivity to glucocorticoids. *Endocrine Reviews*, 1996;**17**:245–261.
3. Barnes P.J., Adcock I. Anti-inflammatory actions of steroids; molecular and mechanisms. *Trends Pharmacol Sci*, 1993;**14**:436–441.
4. Goulding N.J., Guyre P.M. Glucocorticoids, lipocortins and the immune response. *Curr Opin Immunol*, 1993;**5**:108–113.
5. Kurumbail R.G., Stevens A.M., Gierse J.K., *et al*. Structural basis for selective inhibition of cyclooxygenase-2 by anti-inflammatory agents. *Nature*, 1996;**384**:644–8.
6. Grabstein K., Dower S., Gillis S., *et al*. Expression of interleukin-2, interferon-gamma and the IL-2 receptor by human peripheral blood lymphocytes. *J Immunol*, 1986;**15**:136:4503–4508.
7. Buttgereit F., Brink I., Thiele B., *et al*. Effects of methylprednisolone and 21-aminosteroids on mitogen-induced IL-6 and TNF-α production in human peripheral blood mononuclear cells. *J Pharmacol Exp Ther*, 1995;**275**:850–853.
8. Werb Z. Biochemical actions of glucocorticoids on macrophages in culture-specific inhibition of elastase, collagenase and plasminogen activator secretion and the effects on other metabolic functions. *J Exp Med*, 1978;**147**:1695–1712.
9. Tyrell J.B. Glucocorticoid therapy. In: Felig P., Baxter J.D., Frohman L.A., eds. *Endocrinology and metabolism*. 3rd edn. New York: McGraw-Hill, 1995;855–882.

10. Buttgereit F., Wehling M., Burmester G-R. A new hypothesis of modular glucocorticoid actions. Steroid treatment of rheumatic diseases revisited. *Arthritis Rheum*, 1998;**41**:761–767.

11. Sternberg E.M., Chrousos G.P., Wilder R.L., Gold P.W. The stress response and the regulation of inflammatory disease. *Ann Intern Med*, 1992;**117**:854–866.

12. Sternberg E.M., Wilder R.L. Corticosteroids. In: McCarty D.J., Koopman W.J., eds. *Arthritis and Allied Conditions*. Philadelphia: Lea and Febiger, 1993:p.665–682.

13. Fauci A.S., Dale D.C. The effects of in vivo hydrocortisone on subpopulations of human lymphocytes. *J Clin Invest*, 1974;**53**:240–246.

14. Fauci A.S., Dale D.C., Balow J.E. Glucocorticosteroid therapy: mechanisms of action and clinical consideration. *Ann Intern Med*, 1976;**84**:304–315.

15. Boumpas D.T., Paliogianni F., Anastassiou E.D., Balow J.E. Glucocorticosteroid action on the immune system. Molecular and cellular aspects. *Clin Exp Rheumatol*, 1991;**9**:413–423.

16. Almawi W.Y., Lipman M.L., Stevens A.C., *et al.* Abrogation of glucocorticoid-mediated inhibition of T cell proliferation by the synergistic action of IL-1, IL-6, and INF-gamma. *J Immunol*, 1991;**146**:3523–3527.

17. Arya S.K., Wong-Staal F., Gallo R.C. Dexamethasone-mediated inhibition of human T cell growth factor and gamma-interferon messenger RNA. *J Immunol*, 1984;**133**:273–276.

18. Wu C.Y., Fargeas C., Nakajima T., Delespesse G. Glucocorticoids suppress the production of interleukin 4 by human lymphocytes. *Eur J Immunol*, 1991;**21**:2645–2647.

19. Butler W.T., Rossen R.D. Effects of corticosteroids on immunity in man. 1. Decreased serum IgG concentrations caused by 3 or 5 days of high doses of methylprednisolone. *J Clin Invest*, 1973;**52**:2629–2640.

20. Tuchinda M., Newcomb R.W., Devald B.L. Effect of prednisone treatment on the human immune response to keyhole limpet haemocyanin. *Int Arch Allergy Appl Immunol*, 1972;**42**:533–544.

21. Silva C.M., Powell-Oliver F.E., Jewell C.M., *et al.* Regulation of the human glucocorticoid receptor by long-term and chronic treatment with glucocorticoid. *Steroids*, 1994;**59**:436–442.

22. Hu L-M., Bodwell J., Hu J-M., Orti E., Munck A. Glucocorticoid receptors in ATP-depleted cells. *J Biol Chem*, 1994;**269**:6571–6577.

23. Hurley D.M., Accili D., Stratakis C.A., *et al.* Point mutation causing a single amino aid substitution in the hormone binding domain of the glucocorticoid receptor in familial glucocorticoid resistance. *J Clin Invest*, 1991;**87**:680–686.

24. Kam J.C., Szefler S.J., Surs W., *et al.* Combination IL-2 and IL-4 reduces glucocorticoid receptor-binding affinity and T-cell response to glucocorticoids. *J Immunol*, 1993;**151**:3460–3466.

25. Karl M., Lamberts S.W., Detera-Wadleigh S.D., *et al.* Familial glucocorticoid resistance caused by a splice site deletion in the human glucocorticoid receptor gene. *J Clin Endocrinol Metab*, 1993;**76**:683–689.

26. Norbiato G., Bevilacqua M., Vago T., *et al.* Cortisol resistance in acquired immunodeficiency syndrome. *J Clin Endocrinol Metab*, 1992;**74**:608–613.

27. Strasser-Wozak E.M., Hattmannstorfer R., Hala M., *et al.* Splice site mutation in the glucocorticoid receptor gene causes resistance to glucocorticoid-induced apoptosis in a human acute leukemic cell line. *Cancer Res*, 1995;**55**:348–353.

28. Karl M., von Wichert G., Kempter E., *et al.* Nelsons's syndrome associated with a somatic frame shift mutation in the glucocorticoid receptor gene. *J Clin Endocrinol Metab*, 1996;**81**:124–129.

29. Sher E.R., Leung D.Y., Surs W., *et al.* Steroid-resistant asthma. Cellular mechanisms contributing to inadequate response to glucocorticoid therapy. *J Clin Invest*, 1994;**93**:33–39.

30. Schlaghecke R., Kornely E., Wollenhaupt J., Specker C. Glucocorticoid receptors in rheumatoid arthritis. *Arthritis Rheum*, 1992;**35**:740–744.

31. Chrousos G.P. The hypothalamic-pituitary-adrenal axis and immune-mediated inflammation. *N Engl J Med*, 1995;**332**:1351–1362.

32. Wilder R.L., Calandra G.B., Garvin A.J., *et al.* Strain and sex variation in the susceptibility to streptococcal cell wall-induced polyarthritis in the rat. *Arthritis Rheum*, 1982;**25**:1064–1072.

33. Sternberg E.M., Hill J.M., Chrousos G.P., *et al.* Inflammatory mediator induced arthritis is defective in streptococcal cell arthritis susceptible Lewis rats. *Proc Natl Acad Sci USA*, 1989;**86**:2374–2378.

34. Masi A.T., Chrousos G.P. Hypothalamic-pituitary-adrenal-glucocorticoid axis function in rheumatoid arthritis. *J Rheumatol*, 1996;**23**:577–581.

35. Gudbjörnsson B., Skogseid B., Öberg K., *et al.* Intact adrenocorticotropic hormone secretion but impaired cortisol response in patients with active rheumatoid arthritis. *J Rheumatol*, 1996;**23**:596–602.

36. Chikanza I.C., Petrou P., Kingsley G., *et al.* Defective hypothalamic response to immune and inflammatory stimuli in patients with rheumatoid arthritis. *Arthritis Rheum*, 1992;**35**:1281–1288.

37. George E., Kirwan J.R. Corticosteroid therapy in rheumatoid arthritis. *Bailliere's Clin Rheumatol*, 1990;**4**:621–647.

38. American College of Rheumatology ad Hoc Committee on Clinical Guidelines. Guidelines for the management of rheumatoid arthritis. *Arthritis Rheum*, 1996;**39**:713–722.

39. Kirwan J.R. Arthritis and Rheumatism Council Low-dose Glucocorticoid Study Group. The effect of glucocorticosteroids on joint destruction in rheumatoid arthritis. *New Engl J Med*, 1995;**333**:142–146.

40. Cohen M.D., Conn D.L. Benefits of low dose corticosteroids in rheumatoid arthritis. *Bull Rheum Dis*, 1997;**46**:4–7.

41. Ramos-Remus C., Russel A.S. Dangers of low dose corticosteroid therapy in rheumatoid arthritis. *Bull Rheum Dis*, 1997;**46**:1–4.

42. Arvidson N.G., Gudbjörnsson B., Larsson A., Hällgren R. The timing of glucocorticoid administration in rheumatoid arthritis. *Ann Rheum Dis*, 1997;**56**:27–31.

43. Arvidson N.G., Gudbjörnsson B., Elfman L., *et al.* Circadian rhythm of serum interleukin-6 in rheumatoid arthritis. *Ann Rheum Dis*, 1994;**53**:521–524.

44. Masi A.T., Chrousos G.P. Dilemmas of low dosage glucocorticoid treatment in rheumatoid arthritis: considerations of timing. *Ann Rheum Dis*, 1997;**56**:1–4.

45. Liebling M.R., Leib E., McLaughlin K., *et al.* Pulse methylprednisolone in rheumatoid arthritis: a double-blind cross-over trial. *Ann Intern Med*, 1981;**94**:21–26.

46. Forster P.J., Grindulis K.A., Neumann V., *et al.* High-dose intravenous methylprednisolone in rheumatoid arthritis. *Ann Rheum Dis*, 1982;**41**:444–446.

47. Smith M.D., Bertouch J.V., Smith A.M. The clinical and immunological effects of pulse methylprednisolone therapy in rheumatoid arthritis. I. Clinical effects. *J Rheumatol*, 1988;**15**:229–232.

48. Radia M., Furst D.E. Comparison of three pulse methylprednisolone regimens in the treatment of rheumatoid arthritis. *J Rheumatol*, 1988;**15**:242–246.

49. Iglehart I.W., Sutton J.D., Bender H., *et al.* Intravenous pulsed steroids in rheumatoid arthritis: a comparative dose study. *J Rheumatol*, 1990;**17**:159–162.

50. Shipley M.E., Bacon P.A., Berry H., *et al.* Pulsed methylprednisolone in active early rheumatoid disease: A close ranging study. *Br J Rheumatol*, 1988;**15**:242–246.

51. Smith M.D., Ahern M.J., Roberts-Thomson P.J. Pulse steroid therapy in rheumatoid arthritis: can equivalent doses of oral prednisolone give similar clinical results to intravenous methylprednisolone? *Ann Rheum Dis*, 1988;**47**:28–33.

52. Needs C.J., Smith M., Boutagy J., *et al.* Comparison of methylprednisolone (1 g i.v.) with prednisolone (1 g orally) in rheumatoid arthritis. A pharmacokinetic and clinical study. *J Rheumatol*, 1988;**15**:224–228.

53. Weusten B., Jacobs J.W.G., Bijlsma J.W.J. Corticosteroid pulse therapy in active rheumatoid arthritis. *Seminar Arthritis Rheum*, 1993;**23**:183–192.

54. Smith M.D., Ahern M.J., Roberts-Thompson P.J. Pulse methylprednisolone therapy in rheumatoid arthritis: unproved therapy,

unjustified therapy or effective adjunctive treatment? *Ann Rheum Dis*, 1990;49:265–267.

55. Fucik R.F., Kukreja S.C., Hurgis G.K., *et al*. Effect of glucocorticoids on function of the parathyroid glands in man. *J Clin Endocrinol Metabol*, 1975;40:150–155.

56. Hsueh A.J., Erickson G.F. Glucocorticoid inhibition of FSH-induced estrogen production in cultured rat granulosa cells. *Steroids*, 1976;32:639–648.

57. Mac Adams M.R., White R.H., Chipps B.E. Reduction of serum testosterone levels during chronic glucocorticoid therapy. *Ann Intern Med*, 1986;104:648–651.

58. Lukert B.P., Johnson B.E., Robinson R.G. Estrogen and progesterone replacement therapy reduces glucocorticoid-induced bone loss. *J Bone Miner Res*, 1992;7:1063–69.

59. Cooper C., Kirwan J.R. The risk of local and systemic corticosteroid administration. *Bailliere's Clin Rheumatol*, 1990;4:305–332.

60. Cooper C., Barker D.J.P., Wickham C. Physical activity, muscle strength and calcium intake in fracture of the proximal femur in Britain. *Br Med J*, 1988;297:1443–1446.

61. Reid I.R., Evans M.C., Stapleton J. Lateral spine densitometry is a more sensitive indicator of glucocorticoid-induced bone loss. *J Bone Miner Res*, 1992;7:1221–25.

62. Nielsen H.K., Thomsen K., Eriksen E.F., *et al*. The effect of high-dose glucocorticoid administration on serum bone gamma carboxyglutamic acid-containing protein, serum alkaline phosphatase and vitamin D metabolites in normal subjects. *Bone Miner*, 1988;4:105–113.

63. Sambrook P., Birmingham J., Kelly P., *et al*. Prevention of corticosteroid osteoporosis: a comparison of calcium, calcitriol, and calcitonin. *N Engl J Med*, 1993;328:1747–52.

64. Lukert B.P., Johnsson B.C., Robinson R.G. Estrogen and progesterone replacement therapy reduces glucocorticoid-induced bone loss. *J Bone Miner Res*, 1992;7:1063–1069.

65. Adachi J.D., Bensen W.G., Brown J., *et al*. Intermittent etidronate therapy to prevent corticosteroid-induced osteoporosis. *N Engl J Med*, 1997;337:382–387.

66. Roux C., Oriente P., Laan R., *et al*. Randomized trial of effect of cyclical etidronate in the prevention of corticosteroid-induced bone loss. *J Clin Endocrinol Metab*, 1998;83:1128–1133.

67. Saag K.G., Emkey R., Schnitzer T.J., *et al*. Alendronate for the prevention and treatment of glucocorticoid-induced osteoporosis. *N Engl J Med*, 1998;339:292–299.

68. Healey J.H., Paget S.A., Williams-Russo P., *et al*. A randomized controlled trial of salmon calcitonin to prevent bone loss in corticosteroid-treated temporal arthritis and polymyalgia rheumatica. *Calcif Tissue Int*, 1996;56:73–80.

69. Dale D.C., Petersdorf R.G. Corticosteroids and infectious diseases. *Med Clin North Am*, 1973;57:1277–1287.

70. Stuck A.E., Minder C.E., Frey F.J. Risk of infectious complications in patients taking glucocorticoids. *Rev Infect Dis*, 1989;11:954–963.

71. Grieco M.H. The role of corticosteroid therapy in infection. *Hospital Practice*, 1984;18:131–143.

72. Haanaes Q.C., Bergman A. Tuberculosis in patients treated with corticosteroids. *Eur J Respir Dis*, 1983;64:294–297.

73. Piper J.M., Ray W.A., Daugherty J.R., Griffin M.R. Corticosteroid use and peptic ulcer disease: role of nonsteroidal anti-inflammatory drugs. *Ann Intern Med*, 1991;114:735–740.

74. Rayfield E.J., Curnow R.T., George D.T., Beisel W.R. Impaired carbohydrate metabolism during a mild viral illness. *N Engl J Med*, 1973;289:618–621.

75. Drobny E.C., Abramsson E.C., Baumann G. Insulin receptors in acute infection: A study of factors conferring insulin resistance. *J Clin Endocrinol Metab*, 1984;58:710–716.

76. Svenson K.L., Lundquist G., Wide L., Hällgren R. Impaired glucose handling in active rheumatoid arthritis: relationship to the secretion of insulin and counter-regulatory hormones. *Metabolism*, 1987;36:940–943.

77. Svenson K.L., Lundquist G., Wide L., Hällgren R. Impaired glucose handling in active rheumatoid arthritis: effects of corticosteroids and antirheumatic treatment. *Metabolism*, 1987;36:944–948.

78. Svenson K.L., Pollare T., Lithell H., Hällgren R. Impaired glucose handling in active rheumatoid arthritis: relationship to peripheral insulin resistance. *Metabolism*, 1988;37:125–130.

79. Svenson K.L., Lithell H., Hällgren R., *et al*. Serum lipoprotein in rheumatoid arthritis and other chronic inflammatory arthritides. I. Relativity to inflammatory activity. *Arch Intern Med*, 1987;147:1912–1916.

80. Svenson K.L., Lithell H., Hällgren R., Vessby B. Serum lipoproteins in rheumatoid arthritis and other inflammatory arthritides. II. Effects of anti-inflammatory and disease-modifying drug treatment. *Arch Intern Med*, 1987;147:1917–1920.

81. Ettinger W.H., Hazzard W.R. Prednisone increases very low density lipoprotein and high density lipoprotein in healthy men. *Metabolism*, 1988;37:1055–1058.

82. Million R., Poole P., Kellgren J.H., *et al*. Long term study of management of rheumatoid arthritis. *Lancet*, 1984;1:812–816.

83. Nashel D.J. Is atherosclerosis a complication of long-term corticosteroid treatment? *Am J Med*, 1986;80:925–929.

84. Garbe E., LeLorier J., Boivin J.F., Suissa S. Risk of ocular hypertension or open-angle glaucoma in elderly patients on oral glucocorticoids. *Lancet*, 1997;350:979–82.

24 | Methotrexate

Rolf Rau

Introduction

In 1947, aminopterin was synthesized as an antifolate for the treatment of tumors. Four years later, Gubner[1] reported the successful treatment of seven patients with rheumatoid arthritis (RA) with aminopterin and dramatic improvement of skin lesions in two patients additionally suffering from psoriasis. Following this observation, aminopterin was extensively used by American dermatologists in patients with refractory psoriasis[2]. Methotrexate (amethopterin), synthesized in 1948[3], proved to be less toxic than aminopterin and could be applied in higher doses. However, because of the dramatic effects of corticosteroids in the treatment of RA, it took many years before the use of methotrexate (MTX) became widespread. Only very few reports were published on the effectiveness of MTX in rheumatic diseases: psoriatic arthritis in 1964[4], SLE in 1965[5], RA with weekly i.v. doses of 50 mg[6], and RA with oral weekly doses of 10–15 mg[7]. It was not until the early 1980s that the first pilot studies appeared and encouraged a systematic evaluation of low-dose MTX treatment in RA. The introduction of MTX is one of the major achievements in the pharmacotherapy of RA. Because of its superior efficacy and tolerability, today it is the most widely used DMARD worldwide.

Pharmakokinetics

Bioavailability

Bioavailability of MTX decreases with increasing dose. Low doses between 10 and 25 mg result in a mean absorption rate of 70 per cent, ranging between 25 and 100 per cent[8–11] (Table 24.1). In the same individual, absorption remains constant with doses of 7.5 mg[12] but decreases by 13.5 per cent at the maintenance dose of 17 mg[13]. There is no difference in the bioavailability between intravenous and intramuscular administration[14]. When taken after meals, absorption was delayed[15], slightly reduced[10], or unchanged[16].

Plasma kinetics

After low oral dosage (7.5–15 mg/week) peak plasma concentrations ranged between 0.31 and 0.72 μM[17]. MTX concen-

Table 24.1 Absorption of MTX

Author		Dose	Range (%)	Mean (%)
Hermann[8]	1989	10 mg p.o.	25–100	73
Auvinet[9]	1992	15 mg p.o.	45–80	60
Oguey[10]	1992	15 mg p.o.	28–94	67
Krober[11]	1973	25 mg p.o.		73

Absorption rate is constant between 7.5 g and 25 mg (Kremer[68]).
No change in absorption after long-term therapy (Anaya[12]).
Decrease in the absorption rate with increasing dose (Hamilton[13]).
After food intake, absorption is delayed (Kozloski[15]), slightly reduced (Oguey[10]), or unchanged (Hamilton[16]).

trations in synovial fluid are usually comparable to those of plasma. Elimination of MTX after low doses is generally biphasic[8] or triphasic[14]. After peak plasma concentrations are reached during the initial disposition phase the drug is distributed in the body fluids with a half life of 1 h leading to a rapid decline of plasma concentration. The second phase predominantly reflects renal elimination: 50–80 per cent of the drug are eliminated unchanged through glomerular filtration with a half-life of 2–4 h. Renal clearance ranges between 40 and 190 ml/min/m^2 with a mean of 110 ml/min/m^2 [8]. Nine to 26 per cent of MTX are eliminated through the bile[18]. The terminal phase of MTX excretion refers to enterohepatic circulation[18] and release from tissues and third spaces resulting in a terminal half-life of 15–21 h[8]. Total half-life ranges between 6 and 7 h[19]. Impaired renal function[20] and older age[21] may lead to decreased clearance and increased toxicity. However, a meta-analysis revealed no higher toxicity in elderly patients[20].

Metabolism

Less than 50 per cent of MTX[22,23] is bound to plasma proteins. Approximately 10 per cent is oxidized to 7-hydroxy-MTX, a less potent inhibitor of dihydrofolate reductase. Both remain within cells in polyglutamated forms maintaining constant concentrations over 1 week as demonstrated in RA patients treated with low-dose weekly MTX[24]; they are responsible for the prolonged inhibition of dihydrofolate reductase.

Drug interactions

MTX can be partly displaced from its binding to plasma proteins by aspirin and NSAIDs[22], but this mechanism has only minor impact since less than 50 per cent of MTX is bound to plasma proteins. NSAIDs can interfere with the renal excretion of MTX, exemplified by a significant reduction of creatinine and MTX clearance in patients additionally treated with ibuprofen, naproxen, ketoprofen, or salicylates. An 80 per cent reduction of 7-hydroxy-methotrexate clearance through aspirin has also been reported[25]. No significant interactions have been reported with etodolac and piroxicam. Pharmacokinetic variables were not affected by NSAIDs or salicylates at weekly doses of 7.5 mg MTX; however, when patients received their usual maintenance dose (mean 17 mg) NSAIDs reduced the renal clearance of both MTX and creatinine by 20 per cent[26]. Meloxicam had no overall effect on pharmacokinetics during treatment with 15 mg MTX weekly, but resulted in a significant reduction of MTX clearance in two elderly patients[27]. This indicates substantial individual variations regarding drug interactions, and single cases with severe side-effects have been reported[22,28]. MTX clearance was reduced by approximately 20 per cent in patients receiving long-term steroid therapy, while short-term administration of 15 mg prednisone did not affect MTX pharmacokinetics[29]. Probenecid increases 24-h MTX plasma levels up to 400 per cent by decreasing its clearance[30]. Trimetoprim-sulfamethoxazol also belongs to the group of folic acid antagonists and may cause severe bone marrow depression if combined with MTX.

Mechanism of action

MTX (Figure 24.1) is an antifolate and inhibits dihydrofolate reductase (DHFR), thus impairing the conversion of dihydrofolate to tetrahydrofolate. This decreases the intracellular supply of reduced folates which are needed for the synthesis of pyrimidin and purines[31,32]. Both, MTX and 7-hydroxy-methotrexate are intracellularly polyglutamated and are then even stronger inhibitors of DHFR. They can also inhibit other folate-dependent enzymes in the purine biosynthesis pathway. This effect may be even more important in RA than the inhibition of DHFR. The rapid onset of clinical effect in rheumatoid arthritis, including changes in acute phase response and the rebound after discontinuation, indicate a strong anti-inflammatory effect of MTX. The occurrence of opportunistic infections indicates additional immunosuppressive properties of MTX.

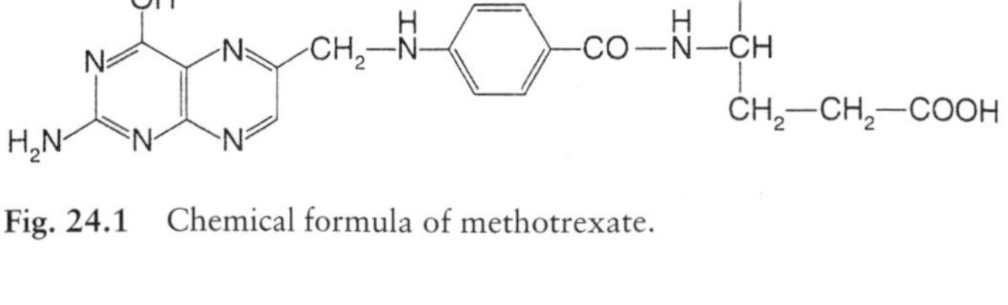

Fig. 24.1   Chemical formula of methotrexate.

Immune system

While in most clinical studies there was no change in rheumatoid factor[33,34], two studies demonstrated a decrease in serum level of IgM, IgG, and IgA rheumatoid factor[35,36]. Peripheral blood mononuclear cells from patients treated with MTX produce less IgM rheumatoid factor than cells from patients without MTX treatment[37].

No reduction of lymphocyte proliferation after antigen stimulation, measuring tritiated thymidine uptake, could be demonstrated[33,34]; however, when using deoxyuridine uptake to measure proliferation a reduction in lymphocyte proliferation by 85 per cent[37] and fibroblast proliferation by 90 per cent[38] was observed. The discrepancy between results with thymidine and deoxyuridine assays may be explained by the inhibition of thymidilate synthetase with MTX resulting in a thymidine depletion of cells[39]. Primary delayed hypersensitivity can be suppressed by MTX[40], while secondary reaction is not affected[41]. The clonal growth of T and B cells and of rapidly proliferating fibroblasts can be inhibited by therapeutic MTX concentrations[42]

Cytokines

Several studies examined the influence of MTX on different cytokines. MTX significantly decreased the production of IL-1 in experimental arthritis[43]. In RA patients, MTX treatment induced a reduction of IL-1 production by mononuclear cells *ex vivo*[44] and biological activity of IL-1[45], while IL-1 serum concentrations remained unchanged[44]. MTX has little effect on TNF-α production, although liposome preparations of MTX dramatically inhibit TNF-α production *in vitro*, most likely because of improved uptake of liposomal MTX by target cells[46]. In the adjuvant arthritis model, MTX treatment results in a profound decrease of TNF-α in the synovial fluid[47]. In patients with RA, however, MTX did not demonstrate any substantial effect on TNF-α concentrations[48,49]. Soluble IL-2 receptors (sIL2R) are elevated in RA in relation to disease activity and decline with MTX treatment[50]. The proinflammatory cytokine IL-6 was also found to decline during MTX therapy[45]. The production of IL-8, a potent chemoattractant for neutrophils, can be inhibited by MTX[51].

Anti-inflammatory effects

An anti-inflammatory effect is indicated by a significant decrease of CRP and ESR within days after a single MTX injection[52]. The antiphlogistic effect is also documented in animal models of arthritis[53,54]. MTX decreases chemotaxis of polymorphonuclear cells, activation and migration of neutrophils through capillar membranes, and leucotriene-B4 induced infiltration of the psoriatic skin. In other studies, an inhibition of macrophage activation, granuloma formation, and lymphatic cell infiltration could be demonstrated in animal models of chronic inflammation. The anti-inflammatory effect of MTX has been explained by an inhibition of methylation reactions and/or increased adenosine release into the extracellular space[55].

Clinical efficacy

Pilot and placebo-controlled studies

In the early 1980s, open pilot studies indicated effectiveness of 7.5–15 mg MTX weekly in RA patients not responding to conventional DMARDs[56–58,59]. Randomized placebo-controlled trials over 6–26 weeks with weekly MTX doses between 7.5 mg and 25 mg demonstrated a significant improvement in several clinical parameters[33,60–62]. A meta-analysis of four studies[63] revealed a reduction of tender joints by 39 per cent and of swollen joints by 26 per cent when compared to placebo. Furst[64] documented a significant dose–effect relationship of MTX. Dose dependency has also been indicated by a rapid and excellent response to weekly i.v. doses of 25 mg[65] and 50 mg[66].

Long-term observational studies

Clinical efficacy accompanied by good tolerability and low discontinuation rates have been demonstrated in several long-term observational trials[67–79]. These studies had follow-up periods up to 11 years and included between 26 and 453 patients, in general suffering from long-lasting disease unresponsive to conventional DMARD therapy. MTX resulted in a significant improvement of all relevant clinical parameters, including acute phase reactants, with a peak effect after 6 months. Moreover, the effect was sustained during the entire follow-up period. Marked improvement (> 50 per cent decrease) in the number of swollen joints occurred in more than 50 per cent[78] and 69 per cent[72] of patients. Clinical remissions according to the definition of Pinals[80], however, are infrequent and are difficult to achieve in patients with severe destructive disease.

Good tolerability and effectiveness has been demonstrated with 'drug survival rates' of more than 5 years in over 50 per cent of patients (Table 24.2). This compares favorably with other DMARDs[81–84]. Pincus[85] estimated a treatment continuation rate of 57 per cent for MTX after 5 years and between 20 and 25 per cent for other DMARDs (p < 0.01). However, in two other studies, the continuation rate after 4 years did not differ between MTX and other DMARDs[86,87]. The potential for large dosage variations makes it easier for patients to stay on MTX compared to other compounds. In patients older than 65 years, MTX was equally effective[88,89], but withdrawal rates were higher[79,83].

Effect on radiograph progression

Long-term studies measuring radiographic outcome usually demonstrated continued progression[68,70,78,90,91]. However, most patients in these studies still had clinically active disease, as indicated by the number of swollen joints and the ESR. In contrast, patients who achieved an abrogation of disease activity, displayed an arrest of progression[68,70,78,91]. Nordstroem[92] found no difference in radiological progression when comparing a period of 33 months of clinically insufficient pretreatment with 30 months of effective MTX-treatment in 18 RA patients. In another study, the progression rate during MTX therapy was significantly reduced when compared to a pretreatment period[93]. In 31 patients who switched to MTX because of rapid radiograph progression, the mean radiographic progression was significantly reduced during 3.9 years of MTX treatment when compared with a mean observation period of 2.2 years while on treatment with other DMARDs[94]. A comparative trial in patients with early erosive RA showed no significant difference in the radiographic progression between patients treated with parenteral gold or intramuscular MTX; however, progression was clearly delayed during the second half year when compared with the first half year in both groups[95,96]. Other studies comparing MTX to other DMARDs also demonstrated a flattening of the progression curve over time[97]. Progression was compara-

Table 24.2 Long-term observational studies

Author	Year	n	Type of study	Disease duration (years)	Treatment duration in months (range)	Dose (mg/week)	Efficacy	Treatment continued (%)	After years
Kremer[68]	1992	29	prospective	11.7	90 (79–107)	11.7	Good	62	71/2
Weinblatt[70]	1992	26	prospective	8.9	84	10.2	Good	46	7
Sany[73]	1991	191	prospective	8.5	19 (3–58)	10.2	Good	46	5
Hanrahan[74]	1989	128	prospective	12	22 (1–60)	12.8	Moderate	50	5
Alarcon[75]	1989	152	prospective	9.1			Good		
Mielants[76]	1991	92	prospective	11	appr. 16	7.5	Moderate		
Rau[78]	1988	271	prospective	8.5	31.4 (1–108)	12.1	Good	60	5
Krause[210]	1995	271	prospective	8.5	120 (12–198)	11.7	Good	60	10
Bologna[79]	1997	453	retrospective		35 (3–106)		Good	73	5

Qualification: MTX is often the last-resort DMARD; a wider dosage range is possible.

Table 24.3　Comparative studies with other DMARDs

Author	Year	Drugs	Centers	n	Disease duration	Treatment duration	MTX dose	MTX efficacy	MTX tolerability
Weinblatt[100]	1990	MTX/Auran	Multi	281	6 yrs	36 wks	7.5–15	superior	superior
Williams[101]	1992	MTX/Auran	Multi	229	5 yrs	48 wks	7.5–15	equal	superior
Morassut[102]	1989	MTX/Au	1	35	6 yrs	26 wks	12.5	equal	superior
Suarez-Almasor[103]	1988	MTX/Au	1	40	6 yrs	26 wks	10	equal	superior
Rau[104]	1991	MTX/Au	1	57	13 mths	26 wks	15 i.m.	equal	superior
Rau[105]	1992	MTX/Au	2	174	11 mths	2 yrs	15 i.m.	equal	superior
Hamdy[107]	1987	MTX/AZA	1	42	8.7 yrs	24 wks	10	equal/ superior	equal
Jeurissen[97]	1991	MTX/AZA	1	64	10 yrs	48 wks	7,5–15	superior	superior

MTX = methotrexate; Auran = auranofin; Au = parenteral gold; AZA = azathioprine.

ble to that seen with parenteral gold[95,96,98] but slower than with other DMARDs[97–99] (Table 24.3). On the basis of these observations, it is reasonable to assume that MTX delays radiological progression, provided a good clinical response is achieved.

Comparison with other DMARDs

In a double-blind multicenter study including 281 patients over 36 weeks, 7.5–15 mg MTX weekly was superior to 6–9 mg auranofin/day in terms of improving disease activity with fewer side-effects and a lower withdrawal rate[100]. In contrast, a multicenter comparison between 7.5 mg MTX weekly (n=114) and 6 mg auranofin/day (n=115) showed no significant differences[101].

A significant improvement in all clinical parameters was documented in three trials comparing parenteral gold and MTX with no intergroup differences, but there was slightly less toxicity with MTX[102–104]. In a two-center double-blind comparison between parenteral gold (50 mg per week) and parenteral MTX (15 mg per week) in 174 patients with early erosive RA (median disease duration 11 months) all clinical parameters and acute phase reactants improved significantly (> 50 per cent) after 1 and 3 years without significant intergroup differences. Marked improvement (> 50 per cent reduction) occurred in 68 per cent of MTX patients and 76 per cent of patients treated with gold, but tolerability was significantly better with MTX[105,106].

In 42 patients treated over 24 weeks, there was no significant difference between 100 mg azathioprin/day and 10 mg MTX/week with a trend towards earlier and larger improvement with MTX[107]; 7.5–15 mg MTX/week (n = 33) was significantly better than 100–150 mg AZA/day (n = 31) over a period of 48 weeks[97]; after 48 weeks, just 36 per cent of patients remained on AZA, while 91 per cent continued on MTX.

A meta-analysis of clinical trials in 3957 patients found MTX to be more effective than auranofin and comparable to D-penicillamine and parenteral gold[108].

Combination of MTX with other DMARDs

MTX has emerged as the ideal compound for combination with other DMARDs. A combination of MTX and auranofin was not more effective than the individual drug; however, fewer patients withdrew from the combination because of lack of efficacy[101]. A combination MTX/azathioprine was not more effective than MTX alone, however, in the combination group, the study protocol allowed an increase of 5 to 7.5 mg MTX/week and of 50 to 100 mg azathioprine/day, while in the individual drug arms, doses could be increased up to 15 mg/week (MTX) and up to 150 mg (AZA). Yet, fewer patients in the combination required a dose increase compared to the single drug arms[109,110]. The combination MTX/chloroquine was more effective than MTX alone[111], but in a pharmacokinetic study, chloroquine was found to reduce the bioavailability of MTX substantially[112] In two studies, there was only a marginally superior effect of the combination MTX/sulfasalazine (SAS) compared to the individual compounds[113,114]. Triple combination including MTX, SAS, and chloroquin demonstrated high effectiveness in one study[115].

In RA patients responding partially to the 'maximal tolerated dose' (approximately 10–12.5 mg/week), the combination with 2.5–5.0 mg cyclosporin/day improved efficacy significantly, while creatinine levels increased only marginally[116]. The treatment effect could be maintained in an open-label extension study during additional 24 weeks of follow-up[117].

Recently it could be shown that the addition of TNF-α inhibitors to ongoing MTX treatment with only partial response is well tolerated and enhances efficacy when compared with single treatment[214–217].

Effect on extra-articular manifestations of RA

Two case reports[118,119] and two case series of four[120] and seven patients[121] with Felty's syndrome, observed an increase in the number of neutrophils accompanied by an improvement of ESR and the number of swollen joints as well as a reduction of the steroid dose when treated with MTX. Rheumatic vasculitis may respond favorably to MTX, resulting in the healing of vasculitic ulcerations and digital infarctions[122,123]. On the other hand, MTX therapy can also induce vasculitic lesions, which can disappear even when treatment is continued[124].

An accelerated nodulosis has been estimated to occur in approximately 8 per cent of RA patients treated with MTX[125]. Histologically, these nodules are not different from rheumatoid nodules. They heal with discontinuation of MTX and reappear with reintroduction. They also may develop in the heart or in the lungs[126].

Side-effects of low-dose methotrexate treatment

Most adverse events relate to the antifolate activity of MTX and mimic symptoms of folate deficiency. Clinically relevant side-effects are fortunately rare, however. In prospective, long-term studies with frequent visits[68,70,73–76,78,127] as well as in studies with i.v. application of high MTX doses[66], 60–85 per cent of patients reported adverse events and 10–30 per cent discontinued MTX due to toxicity. Elevated creatinine serum levels, older age[83,128], and low folic acid levels predispose to adverse events. When MTX is discontinued, adverse reactions are generally reversible. A post-dosing reaction, occurring in approximately 10 per cent of patients within hours after dosing, is characterized by arthralgias/myalgias, or fatigue/malaise, or both[129].

Gastrointestinal side-effects

The accumulation of MTX polyglutamate in the cells of the intestinal mucosa[130] may explain the frequency of gastrointestinal side-effects. Nausea, malaise, and vomiting, observed in prospective studies among 10–50 per cent of patients, may begin 1–8 h after medication and last for a few hours up to 1 week. Healing of peptic ulcers, caused by concomitant NSAID medication, can be delayed in patients treated with MTX[131]. Hence, an active peptic ulcer should be regarded as relative contraindication for MTX.

Skin and mucous membranes

Stomatitis has been observed in long-term studies in 12–37 per cent of patients[69,75,128,132] and was the reason for discontinuation in 6 per cent[78]. Mild alopecia occurs in up to 27 per cent of cases[67,75,128,132] but prompted discontinuation in only 4 per cent[78]. Urticaria[133], small vessel vasculitis[124], and granulomatous vasculitis are usually rare.

Hematopoetic system

MTX-related bone marrow suppression is a rare but potentially fatal complication. In short-term studies hematological adverse events were observed in 2–3 per cent[65,66,131], and in 11 per cent according to one report[134], while long-term studies encounter bone marrow side-effects in up to 24 per cent[69,75,132], frequently induced through interactions of MTX with NSAIDs. The most frequent abnormality is mild to moderate leucopenia[68]. In a long-term follow-up of 271 RA patients mild leucopenia ($< 4000/mm^3$) was observed in only eight and mild thrombocytopenia ($< 100\,000/mm^3$) in seven patients[78]. After conclusion of the study, we observed two cases of agranulocytosis during comedication with NSAIDs, analgetics and antibiotics. The number of withdrawals due to cytopenia ranges between 0 and 5.9 per cent[69,75,132]. Five of six patients with pancytopenia had creatinine levels far exceeding 2.0 mg/dl and all had multiple comedication[135]. Seventy cases of pancytopenia were published in the medical literature between 1980 and 1995; 63 were case reports and seven were reported from 511 patients included in five prospective long-term studies; 12 of the 70 patients (17 per cent) died[136]. The majority of patients with pancytopenia had impaired renal function, concurrent infection, and/or concomitant comedication with more than five drugs. All 26 patients in whom a bone marrow biopsy had been performed exhibited megaloblastosis and hypocellularity[136]. Other risk factors include folic acid depletion[137], older age, and treatment with trimetoprim-sulfamethoxazol. In cases of mild to moderate abnormalities, blood count normalizes within 2 weeks after withdrawal of MTX, but patients with severe bone marrow suppression may require supplementation of folinic acid[31,137] or even colony stimulating factors[138]. Recovery from pancytopenia can be accompanied by eosinophilia in up to 56 per cent[139].

Central nervous system

Central nervous disturbances including headache, dizziness, vertigo, light-headedness, and mood alterations were reported in up to 36 per cent in long-term studies[68,75,127]. Older age and elevated serum creatinine are predisposing factors[140]. In two of our patients with a history of epilepsy, seizures reappeared within 6 weeks of starting MTX treatment and disappeared only when MTX was discontinued.

Respiratory system

MTX-induced lung disease is a rare but potentially life threatening complication. The rapid evaluation of newly developed pulmonary symptoms in patients receiving MTX is crucial[141]. MTX pneumonitis is predominantly characterized by shortness of breath, a dry non-productive cough, and fever[142], accompanied by headache, malaise, cyanosis, hypoxemia, and restrictive pulmonary function changes. Rales can be present, and chest radiographs may demonstrate interstitial infiltrates. Lung biopsy reveals hypersensitivity pneumonitis with massive interstitial and alveolar infiltrations with inflammatory cells (predominantly lymphocytes) with granuloma formation and giant cells[143]. Other causes of pulmonary disease, for example nosocomial infections[144–146], have to be excluded before a diagnosis of MTX-induced pneumonitis can be established. Whether pre-existing lung disease predisposes for MTX-induced adverse events[147,148] is still a matter of controversy. There is much discussion about the frequency of pulmonary complications with MTX treatment. Many clinical studies did not encounter any pulmonary complications[109,149,150], while in others adverse pulmonary events occurred in between 2.1 and 6.8 per cent of patients[148,151,152]. Six clinical centers identified 27 patients with MTX pneumonitis between 1981 and 1993 in addition to 68 patients that had been reported in the medical literature[142]. The mortality in these patients was approximately 17.5 per cent[142]. Pulmonary complications can develop after cumulative doses as low as 12.5 mg and up to 4 weeks after discontinuation of MTX. The vast majority of patients with pulmonary symptoms during MTX treatment, however, suffer from airway infections[152,146] related to the immunosuppressive effect of MTX.

Table 24.4 Roenigk graduation[160]

Grade I	Normal fatty infiltration, mild nuclear variability, mild portal inflammation, mild
Grade II	Fatty infiltration, moderate to severe nuclear variability, moderate to severe portal tract expansion, portal tract inflammation, necrosis, moderate to severe
Grade IIIa	Fibrosis, mild formation of fibrotic septa extending into the lobules Connective tissue stain required
Grade IIIb	Fibrosis, moderate to severe
Grade IV	Cirrhosis

Liver toxicity

Hepatotoxicity is a potentially serious, long-term problem in the treatment of rheumatoid arthritis with MTX. Transient slight elevations of liver enzymes are among the most frequent side-effects of MTX treatment and have been observed in up to 48 per cent of patients during long-term studies, generally in the initial phase of treatment[153]. Liver function tests (LFT) usually returned to normal after dose reduction, change of concurrent NSAID therapy, or folic acid supplementation, and even in patients where MTX treatment is continued unchanged[78,154]. In one study, AST increased significantly up to 53 months of follow-up and subsequently decreased when patients were followed for 90 months[68]. Frequent elevations of aminotransferases indicate structural liver abnormalities[155–158], and correlate significantly with liver biopsy grades[159,160] (Table 24.4). Galactose elimination capacity and aminopyrine breath test declined significantly with MTX treatment during a mean follow-up period of 3.8 years[161].

In patients with psoriasis treated with MTX, liver fibroses and cirrhoses developed with increasing cumulative doses[162] and

were reported in 24 and 21 per cent of patients[163]. In 1990, three additional cases with liver cirrhosis were published in patients treated with cumulative MTX doses between 9.5 and 26 g[164]. Daily administration of MTX, unlimited alcohol consumption, prior vitamin-E-therapy, obesity, and diabetes are considered potential risk factors for the development of MTX-induced liver fibrosis and cirrhosis among patients with psoriasis.

In RA, there is a high prevalence of minor histological changes[165,166], which can be classified as mild reactive hepatitis in 1/3 of patients[166] even without any drug treatment. Moreover, RA patients are treated with hepatotoxic drugs other than MTX. Comparative liver biopsy studies (Table 24.5) showed no differences in a number of histological parameters between biopsies taken before and during MTX treatment, even up to cumulative MTX doses of 8400 mg[167]. Minor fibrosis was present in approximately 25 per cent of cases before and during MTX treatment[168]; scores for 'necrosis', 'inflammation' and 'fibrosis' were not different between the groups[78,169].

Table 24.5 Liver biopsy studies

Author		MTX treatment		No of Controls (RA before MTX)	Result
		No. of biopsies	Cumulative dose		
Mackenzie[167]	1986	60	4400 mg	25	No difference
Mackenzie	1985	30	2500–8400 mg	42	No difference
Rau[168]	1989	40	200–3000 mg	60	No difference (25% minor fibrosis)
Rau[169]a	1991	131	1500 ± 1000 mg	135	Fibrosis score 1.7/2.1 (n.s.)[a] Inflammation score 1.0/1.3 (n.s)[b]
Frenzel	1991	25c	1660 ± 900 mg	25	Fibrosis score 1.0/2.2 (n.s.)[a] Inflammation score 1.0/1.3 (n.s)[b]
Aponte[170]	1988	23	4700–10200 mg		5 cases of mild fibrosis
Kremer[171]	1989	29	Monitored every 1–2 years, total 4.5 years		Slight increase of fibrosis Collagen deposition/lysosomal changes
Kremer[172]	1995	27	Follow-up 8.2 years	0	Roenigk score 1.8 → 2.3 → 2.4 (p = 0.05) No sign of progression in electronmicroscopy

a Fibrosis score (1 = mild, 2 = moderate, 3 = severe).
b Inflammation score (1 = mild, 2 = moderate, 3 = severe).
c same patients before and during MTX therapy.

In patients who received MTX for more than 10 years (4700–10 200 mg) only five of 25 liver biopsies demonstrated minor fibrosis which had not deteriorated in subsequently performed control biopsies[170]. Kremer observed a significant increase of fibrosis in 29 patients with baseline and yearly follow-up biopsies over 4 years[171] and a significant increase of the Roenigk-score after 6 years[172] (Table 24.4). Electron microscopic evaluation showed collagen depositions in the space of Disse and lysosomal changes not seen in controls[173]; however, these changes had not increased after a mean follow-up period of 8.2 years[172]. In several overviews, the frequency of fibrosis was estimated to be between 3 and 11 per cent. In one review, the number of RA patients treated with MTX for more than 5 years was estimated at 16 600. Among these, 17 patients with clinically serious liver diseases were identified; of these seven had histologically proven cirrhosis, giving a 5 year incidence of 1:1000[174]. Regular alcohol consumption has been identified as an important risk factor for the development of MTX-induced liver disease.

Infections

Infections occur more often with MTX than with other DMARDs[175,176], especially in patients with severe RA[177] and during the first years of treatment. In prospective studies, infections were observed in 25 per cent of patients[69]. A series of opportunistic infections[144,145,178] and serious fungal infections[87,179] have been reported. Herpes zoster also occurs more frequently[176,180,181]. Some patients have to discontinue MTX permanently because of recurrent infections, predominantly affecting the small airways or the urinary tract.

There is no consensus whether the rate of perioperative complications increases among patients with MTX therapy. In some studies, wound infections and and wound healing disturbances were increased after orthopedic surgery, in other studies they were not. Although there are at present no definite studies, withholding MTX for 2 weeks prior to surgery is a prudent approach[141].

Kidneys

The excretion of MTX and its metabolites is delayed in patients with impaired renal function leading to increased toxicity[20]. MTX treatment may impair renal function, at least in elderly patients: among 13 RA patients with a mean age of 64 years glomerular filtration rate and tubular excretion was reduced by 10 per cent during oral MTX treatment with 15 mg weekly without any comedication[182]. Renal MTX clearance and creatinine clearance decreased significantly during stable MTX treatment with 7.5 mg/week[183]. These observations underline the importance of creatinine tests during MTX treatment. In patients developing proteinuria after gold treatment, this side-effect could be prevented when gold was combined with MTX[184].

Reproductive system

Oligospermia, impotence, and gynecomastia have been reported. In 11 cases malformations have been documented after the use of methotrexate to induce abortion[180]. Although malformations were not detected among 10 pregnancies during MTX treatment of RA patients[185], multiple congenital anomalies have been described after weekly low dose MTX treatment for RA during the first trimester of pregnancy[186].

Oncogenicity

Large studies of cancer and psoriasis did not establish an association between MTX and malignancies[162,187]. In RA patients, the risk of developing malignancy is increased even without any treatment. RA patients treated with MTX developed non-Hodgkin lymphoma[135,172,188–192], Hodgkin's disease[193], and leukemia[194]. Many of these cases demonstrate the features of immunosuppression-associated lymphoma[191]. Risk factors for RA patients to develop lymphoma while on MTX include severe disease, intense immunosuppression, genetic predisposition, and an increased frequency of latent infections with pro-oncogenic viruses such as Epstein-Barr virus[191,195]. Many of the lymphomas associated with EBV infection come into remission after discontinuation of MTX[191,195].

Bone

Active rheumatoid arthritis is associated with osteoporosis, especially in patients taking corticosteroids[196]. It has not yet been clarified whether MTX treatment can aggravate this osteoporosis. In rats, low-dose MTX treatment decreased osteoid volume specifically, reduced bone formation markedly[197], and induced a significant osteopenia through suppression of osteoblast activity[198,199]. In RA patients, a prospective study with 3 years follow-up revealed no difference in the change of bone mineral density with or without MTX treatment; however, patients treated with MTX + prednisone ($\geq$ 5 mg/day) had significantly greater bone loss in the lumbar spine compared to patients treated with a similar dose of prednisone without MTX ($p = 0.004$)[200].

Supplementation with folates

The mode of MTX action is characterized by its antifolate activity, hence, MTX toxicity mimics clinical manifestations of folate deficiency. MTX toxicity can be reduced with folate supplementation[201–205], although two studies revealed no change in toxicity[206,207]. While in most studies, folic acid supplementation seemed not to interfere with clinical efficacy, two studies demonstrated an exacerbation of arthritis when high-dose folinic acid was supplemented 2 hours after oral and 4–6 hours after i.v. administration of MTX[205,207]. In one double-blind study, the group treated with MTX and folic acid required higher MTX doses than patients treated with MTX and placebo[208]. In another study with 23 RA patients, red cell folate levels decreased during treatment, and side-effects were inversely related to red cell folate values; when side-effects were reported, folic acid values were below 800 nmol/l[27]. Unfortunately, in all other studies mentioned above the folate status has not been documented and the doses of folic acid supplementation varied greatly. American authorities recommend routine folic acid supplementation with 1 mg/day. Recently, it was demonstrated that with folic acid supplementation a decline in folate serum and red blood cell levels as well as an increase in homocystein concentrations in serum could be prevented[209]. Hyperhomocysteinemia is considered an independent risk factor for cardiovascular disease. However, there are no reports of increased cardiovascular mortality in RA patients treated with MTX; in contrast, effective MTX therapy may reduce mortality[210]. The possibility that beneficial effects of folic acid supplementation regarding toxicity reflect a relative dose reduction of MTX resulting in decreased efficacy has not yet been excluded[211]. Recently, Kremer[212] demonstrated that patients responding best to MTX treatment have a significant decrease in their red blood cell folate levels during treatment compared to those who respond minimally or not at all. This supports the recommendation to supply folic acid only in patients with established folate deficiency.

A recent and elegant trial in 434 patients with active RA over 48 weeks demonstraed that folic acid (1 mg/day) and folinic acid (2.5 mg/week), respectively, reduced hepatotoxicity-related withdrawals of MTX significantly while there was no difference regarding other side effects. To obtain similar efficacy the mean doses of MTZ was higher (18.0, 16.4 and 14.5 mg/week) in the groups with folic or folinic acid supplementation[218].

Personal recommendations for administration and drug monitoring

Today, MTX treatment can be recommended as single or combination therapy not only after failure of other DMARDs but as initial treatment in patients with active disease. MTX can be administered orally or by intramuscular, intravenous, or subcutaneous injection with doses ranging from 7.5–25 mg once a week. The dose depends on body weight, gender, renal function, concomitant disease, general health status, and disease activity.

We usually start treatment with a relatively high dose of 15–25 mg given parenterally to exclude the individual differences in bioavailability of oral medication and to achieve a rapid response; after 6–12 weeks, we switch to oral medication in most patients and adjust the dose according to efficacy and tolerability. Most rheumatologists prefer to start with lower oral doses and to increase dosage subsequently. In the case of adverse events, tolerability can be improved by administering the drug in the evening or in two equal doses in the morning and evening of the same day, by changing the route of administration (parenteral versus oral), reducing the dose, or supplementation of folic acid. Nausea and vomiting frequently indicate the presence of a peptic ulcer. We consider folate supplementation when side-effects occur in the presence of concomitant folate deficiency. With 5 mg of folic acid 2 days after MTX application folate levels usually normalize after several weeks and supplementation can be stopped. Possible interactions with NSAIDs have to be considered.

Relative or absolute contraindications to MTX treatment are listed in Table 24.6. We avoid starting MTX in patients with

Table 24.6   Contraindications to MTX therapy

1. Renal insufficiency (serum creatinine > upper limit)
2. Inadequate contraception
3. Active liver disease
4. Regular alcohol intake
5. Acute or chronic infection
6. Leucopenia or thrombocytopenia (exception: Felty's syndrome)
7. Serious underlying systemic disease
8. Non-compliance

renal impairment defined as a serum creatinine outside the normal range. If there is no alternative, we start with lower doses (5 mg/week) and check the MTX serum level after 24 h to ensure it is below 0.05 mM/l. Regular monitoring of serum creatinine is most important since the majority of patients reported with bone marrow toxicity had elevated serum creatinine levels. As MTX is contraindicated during pregnancy, women with childbearing potential have to practice adequate contraception. Because the probability of liver toxicity is significantly increased with alcohol intake we always urge the patients to avoid alcohol when treated with MTX. We allow a maximum of one or two glasses of wine or beer per week. However, the safe amount of alcohol consumption while taking MTX is not known and may differ from patient to patient.

During MTX treatment full blood counts including differential white blood count and platelets, serum creatinine, and aminotransferases should be monitored weekly in the first month, fortnightly in month 2 and 3, and monthly thereafter.

MTX should be discontinued temporarily in the following conditions: serum creatinine exceeding normal values; aminotransferases exceeding threefold normal values; leucopenia or thrombocytopenia; stomatitis; acute infections; severe concurrent illness; 1 week before and 2 weeks after surgery; concomitant treatment with sulfonamides or acute pulmonary symptoms. Pretreatment liver biopsies are recommended only in patients with significant alcohol consumption or a history of liver disease. Biopsies during MTX treatment are recommended only if over 50 per cent of the ALT (alanine aminotransferase) determinations within 1 year—measured every 4–8 weeks— are elevated or the serum albumin concentration falls below the normal. Treatment can be continued if liver biopsies reveal a Roenigk-class I, II or IIIa (see Table 24.4). In patients with moderate to severe fibrosis or cirrhosis (class IIIb or IV) MTX should be permanently discontinued[158,213].

Parameters of disease activity, radiographic progression, development of deformities, and functional capacity should be monitored regularly. In the case of unsatisfactory response we increase the dose or, if this is impossible, combine MTX with an other DMARD. A new option will be the combination of MTX with a 'biological' agent, that is an antibody or receptor to TNFα.

References

1. Gubner R., August S., Ginsberg V. Therapeutic suppression of tissue reactivity. II. Effect of aminopterin in rheumatoid arthritis and psoriasis. *Am J Med Sci*, 1951;**221**:176–182.
2. Rees R.B., Bennett j.H., Bostick W.L. Aminopterin for psoriasis. *Arch Dermatol*, 1955;**72**:133–143.

3. Smith J.M. Jr, Cosulich D.B., Hultquist M.E., Seeger D.R. The chemistry of certain pteroylglutamic acid antagonists. *Trans NY Acad Sci*, 1948;**10**:82–83.

4. Black R.L., O'Brien W.M., van Scott E.J., *et al.* Methotrexate therapy in psoriatic arthritis. Double-blind study on 21 patients. *JAMA*, 1964;**180**:141–145.

5. Miescher P.A., Riethmüller D Diagnosis and treatment of systemic lupus erythematosus. *Semin Hematol*, 1965;**2**:1.

6. Gross D., Enderlin M., Fehr K. Die immunsuppressive Behandlung der progredient chronischen Polyarthritis mit Antimetabolica und Cytostatika. *Schweiz Med Wschr*, 1967;**97**:1301.

7. Hoffmeister R.T. (1972) Methotrexate in rheumatoid arthritis (abstract). *Arthritis Rheum*, **15**:114.

8. Herman R.A., van Pedersen P., Hoffman J., Furst D.E. Pharmacokinetics of low dose methotrexate in rheumatoid arthritis patients. *J Pharm Sci*, 1989;**78**:165–171.

9. Auvinet B., Jarrier I., Le-Levier F., *et al.* Comparative bioavailability of methotrexate given orally or intramuscularly in rheumatoid arthritis. *Presse Med*, 1992;**21**:822.

10. Oguey D., Kölliker F., Gerber N.J., Reichen J. Effect of food on the bioavailability of low-dose methotrexate in patients with rheumatoid arthritis. *Arthritis Rheum*, 1992;**35**:611–614.

11. Korber H., Iven H., Gross W.L. Bioavailability and pharmacokinetics of methotrexate and its metabolite 7-hydroxy-MTX after low-dose MTX (25 mg) in patients with chronic rheumatoid diseases. *Arthritis Rheum*, 1992;**35**:S142 (abstract).

12. Anaya JM., Fabre D., Bressolle F., *et al.* Unchanged methotrexate pharmacokinetics upon initial therapy compared with prolonged therapy in rheumatoid arthritis. *Arthritis Rheum*, 1992;**35**:142.

13. Hamilton R.A., Kremer J.M. Why intramuscular methotrexate may be more efficacious than oral dosing in patients with rheumatoid arthritis. *Br J Rheumatol*, 1997;**36**:86–90.

14. Edelman J., Biggo D.F., Tandy N., Russel A.S. Low dose methotrexate kinetics in arthritis. *Clin Pharm Ther*, 1984;**35**:382–386.

15. Kozloski G.D., Devito J.M., Kisitzki J.C., Johnson J.B. The effect of food on the absorption of methotrexate sodium tablets in healthy voluntiers. *Arthritis Rheum*, 1992;**35**:761–764.

16. Hamilton R.A., Kremer J.M. The effects of food on methotrexate absorption. *J Rheumatol*, 1995;**22**:630–632.

17. Sinnett M.J., Groff G.D., Raddatz D.A., *et al.* Methotrexate pharmacokinetics in patients with rheumatoid arthritis. *J Rheumatol*, 1989;**16**:745–748.

18. Nuernberg B., Kunkl R., Hoffmann J., Furst D.E. Biliary elimination of low dose methotrexate in humans. *Arthritis Rheum*, 1990;**33**:898–902.

19. Furst D.E. (1986) Pharmacocinetics of very low dose methotrexate. In: Rau R (ed) *Low dose methotrexate therapy in rheumatoid diseases*. Karger, Basel.

20. Rheumatoid Arthritis Clinical Trial Archive Group The effect of age and renal function on the efficacy and toxicity of methotrexate in rheumatoid arthritis. *J Rheumatol*, 1990;**22**:218–223.

21. Bresolle F., Bologna C., Kinowski J.M., *et al.* Total and free methotrexate pharmacokinetics in elderly patients with rheumatoid arthritis. A comparison with young patients. *J Rheumatol*, 1997;**24**:1903–1909.

22. Evans W.E., Christensen M.L. Drug interactions with methotrexate. *J Rheumatol*, (Suppl) 1985;**12**:15–20.

23. Edno L., Bressolle F., Gomeni R., *et al.* Total and free methotrexate pharmakokinetics in rheumatoid arthritis patients. *Ther Drug Monit*, 1966;**18**:128–134.

24. Kremer J.M., Galivan J., Strelkfuss A., Kamen B. Methotrexate metabolism analysis in blood and liver of rheumatoid arthritis patients. Association with hepatic folate deficiency and formation of polyglutamates. *Arthritis Rheum*, 1986;**29**:832–835.

25. Furst D.E., Herman R.A., Koshnike R. The effect of aspirin and sulindac on methotrexate clearance. *J Pharm Sci*, 1990;**79**:782–786.

26. Kremer J.M., Hamilton R.A. The effects of nonsteroidal antiinflammatory drugs on methotrexate (MTX) pharmacokinetics: impairment of renal clearance of MTX at weekly maintenance doses but not at 7.5 mg. *J Rheumatol*, 1995;**22**: 2072–2077.

27. Hübner G., Sander O., Degner F.L., Turck D., Rau R. Lack of pharmacokinetic interaction of meloxicam with methotrexate in patients with rheumatoid arthritis. *J Rheumatol*, 1997;**24**:845–851.

28. Rooney T., Furst D.E. Methotrexate. In: McCarty DJ, ed. *Arthritis and allied conditions*, 12th edn. Philadelphia: Lea & Febiger, 1992;621–636.

29. Lafforgue P., Monjanel-Mouterde S., Durand A., *et al.* Is there an interaction between low doses of corticosteroids and methotrexate in patients with rheumatoid arthritis. *J Rheumatol*, 1993;**20**: 263–267.

30. Ahern G.W., Piall E., Marks V. Prolongation and enhancement of serum methotrexate concentrations by probenecid. *Br Med J*, 1978;**1**:1097–1099.

31. Buckley L.M., Vacek P.M., Cooper S.M. Administration of folinic acid after low-dose methotrexate in patients with rheumatoid arthritis. *J Rheumatol*, 1990;**17**:1158–1161.

32. Bruce-Gregorios J.H., Agarwal R.P., Oracion A., *et al.* Effects of methotrexate on RNA and purine synthesis of astrocytes in primary culture. *J Exp Neurol*, 1991;**50**:770–778.

33. Andersen P.A., West S.G., O'Dell J.R. *et al.* Weekly pulse methotrexate in rheumatoid arthritis. *Ann Intern Med*, 1985;**103**: 489–496.

34. Olsen N.J., Callahan L.F., Pincus T. Immunologic studies of rheumatoid arthritis patients treated with methotrexate. *Arthritis Rheum*, 1987;**30**:481–488.

35. Alarcon G.S., Schrohenloher R.E., Bartolucci A.A., *et al.* Suppression of rheumatoid factor production by methotrexate in patients with rheumatoid arthritis. Evidence for differential influences of therapy and clinical status on IgM and IgA rheumatoid factor expression. *Arthritis Rheum*, 1990;**33**:1156–1161.

36. Spadaro A., Taccari E., Riccieri V. *et al.* Relationship of soluble interleukin-2-receptor and interleukin-6 with class-specific rheumatoid factors during low-dose methotrexate treatment in rheumatoid arthritis. *Rev Rhum* Engl Ed, 1997;**64**:89–94.

37. Olsen N.J., Murray L. Antiproliferative effects of methotrexate on peripheral blood mononuclear cells. *Arthritis Rheum*, 1989;**32**:378–385.

38. Rosenblatt D.S., Whitehead V.M., Vera N. *et al.* Prolonged inhibition of DANN synthesis associated with the accumulation of methotrexate polyglutamates by cultured human cells. *Mol Pharmacol*, 1978;**14**:1143–1147.

39. Martinez-Osuna P., Zwolinska J.B., Sikes D.H., *et al.* Lack of immunosuppressive effect of low-dose oral methotrexate on lymphocytes in rheumatoid arthritis. *Clin Exp Rheumatol*, 1993;**11**:249–253.

40. Mitchell M.S., Wade M.E., DeConti R.C. *et al.* Immunosuppressive effects of cytosine arabinoside and methotrexate in man. *Ann Intern Med*, 1969;**70**:535–546.

41. O'Callaghan J.W., Bretscher P., Russell A.S. The effect of low dose chronic intermittent parenteral methotrexate on delayed type hypersensitivity and acute inflammation in a mouse model. *J Rheumatol*, 1968;**13**:710–714.

42. Nakajiama A., Hakoda M., Yamanaka H. *et al.* Divergent effects of methotrexate on the clonal growth of T and B lymphocytes and synovial adherent cells from patients with rheumatoid arthritis. *Ann Rheum Dis*, 1996;**55**:237–242.

43. Connolly K.M., Stecher V.J., Danis E. *et al.* Alteration of interleukin-1 production and the acute phase response following medication of adjuvant arthritis rats with cyclosporin-A or methotrexate. *Int J Immunopharmacol*, 1988;**10**:717–728.

44. Chang D.M., Weinblatt M.E., Schur P.H. The effects of methotrexate on interleukin 1 in patients with rheumatoid arthritis. *J Rheumatol*, 1992;**19**:1678–1682.

45. Segal R., Mozes E., Yaron M., Tartakovsky B. The effects of methotrexate on the proliferation and activitiy of interleukin 1. *Arthritis Rheum*, 1989;**32**:370–377.

46. Williams A.S., Punn Y.L., Amos N. *et al.* The effect of liposomally conjugated methotrexate upon mediator release from human peripheral blood monocytes. *Br J Rheumatol*, 1965;**34**:241–245.

47. Smith-Oliver T., Noel L.S., Stimpson S.S. *et al.* Elevated levels on TNF in the joints of adjuvant arthritic rats. *Cytokine*, 1993;**5**: 298–304.

48. Seitz M, Loetscher P, Dewald B *et al.* Methotrexate action in rheumatoid arthritis: Stimulation of cytokine inhibitor and inhibition of chemokine production by peripheral blood mononuclear cells. *Br J Rheumatol*, 1995;**34**:602–609.

49. Barrera P., Haagsma C.J., Boerbooms A.M.T. *et al.* Effect of methotrexate alone or in combination with sulfasalazine on the production and circulating concentrations of cytokines and their antagonists: longitudinal evaluation in patients with rheumatoid arthritis. *Br J Rheumatol*, 1995;**34**:747–755.

50. Barrera P., Boerbooms AMTh, Janssen E.M., *et al.* Circulating soluble tumor necrosis factor receptors, interleukin-2 receptors, tumor necrosis factor α, and interleukin-6 levels in rheumatoid arthritis. Longitudinal evaluation during methotrexate and azathioprine therapy. *Arthritis Rheum*, 1993;**36**:1070–1079.

51. Seitz M., Dewald B., Ceska M., *et al.* Interleukin-8 in inflammatory rheumatic diseases: synovial fluid levels, relation to rheumatoid factors, production by mononuclear cells, and effects of gold sodium thiomalate and methotrexate. *Rheumat Int*, 1992;**12**:159–164.

52. Segal R., Caspi D., Tishler M. *et al.* Short term effects of low dose methotrexate on the acute phase reaction in patients with rheumatoid arthritis. *J Rheumatol*, 1989; **16**:914–917.

53. Welles W.L., Sikworth J., Oronsky A.L. *et al.* Studies on the effect of low dose methotrexate in adjuvant arthritis. *J Rheumatol*, 1985;**12**:904–906.

54. Ridge S.C., Rath N., Galivan J. *et al.* Studies on the effect of D-penicillamine, gold thioglucose and methotrexate on streptococcal cell wall arthritis. *J Rheumatol*, 1986;**13**:895–898.

55. Cronstein B.N.: Molecular therapeutics—Methotrexate and its mechanism of action. *Arthritis Rheum*, 1996;**39**:1951–1960.

56. Willkens R.F. *et al.* Low-dose pulse methotrexate in rheumatoid arthritis. *J Rheumatol*, 1980;**7**:501–505.

57. Wilke W.S., Calabrese L.H., Scherbel A.L. Methotrexate in the treatment of rheumatoid arthritis. Pilot study. *Cleve Clin Q*, 1980;**47**: 305–309.

58. Hoffmeister R.T. Methotrexate therapy in rheumatoid arthritis: 15 years experience. *Am J Med*, 1983;**75**:69–73.

59. Karger T., Rau R. Treatment of rheumatoid arthritis with methotrexate. *Z Rheumatol*, 1982;**41**:164.

60. Thompson R.N., Watts C., Edelman J., Russell A.S. A controlled two-centre trial of parenteral methotrexate therapy for refractory rheumatoid arthritis. *J Rheumatol*, 1984;**11**:760–762.

61. Weinblatt M.E., Coblyn J.S., Fox D.A. *et al.* Efficacy of low-dose methotrexate in rheumatoid arthritis. *N Engl J Med*, 1985;**312**:818–822.

62. Williams H.J., Willkens R.F., Samuelson C.O. *et al.* Comparison of low-dose oral pulse methotrexate and placebo in the treatment of rheumatoid arthritis—A controlled clinical trial. *Arthritis Rheum*, 1985;**28**:721–729.

63. Tugwell P., Bennett K., Gent M. Methotrexate in rheumatoid arthritis. *Ann Intern Med*, 1987;**107**:358–366.

64. Furst D.E., Koehnke R., Burmeister L.F. *et al.* Increasing methotrexate effect with increasing dose in the treatment of resistant rheumatoid arthritis. *J Rheumatol*, 1989;**16**:313–320.

65. Rau R., Herborn G. (1986) Intravenous treatment of highly active rheumatoid arthritis with methotrexate. In: Rau R (ed) *Low dose methotrexate therapy in rheumatic diseases*. Karger, Basel.

66. Michaels R.M., Nashel D.J., Leonard A., Sliwinski J., Derbes S.J. Weekly intravenous methotrexate in the treatment of rheumatoid arthritis. *Arthritis Rheum*, 1982;**25**:339–341.

67. Kremer J.M., Lee J.K. The safety and efficacy of the use of methotrexate in long-term therapy for rheumatoid arthritis. *Arthritis Rheum*, 1986;**29**:822–831.

68. Kremer J.M., Phelps C.T. Long-term prospective study of the use of methotrexate in the treatment of rheumatoid arthritis. *Arthritis Rheum*, 1992;**35**:138–145.

69. Weinblatt M.E., Trentham D.E., Fraser P.A. Longterm prospective trial of low-dose methotrexate in rheumatoid arthritis *Arthritis Rheum*, 1988;**31**:167–175.

70. Weinblatt M.E., Weissman B.N., Holdsworth D.E., *et al.* Long-term prospective study of methotrexate in the treatment of rheumatoid arthritis. 84-month Update. *Arthritis Rheum*, 1992;**35**:129–137.

71. Weinblatt M.E., Maier A.L., Fraser P.A., Coblyn J.S. Longterm prospective study of methotrexate in rheumatoid arthritis: Conclusion after 132 months of therapy. *J Rheumatol* 1998;**25**:238–242.

72. Weinblatt M.E., Kaplan H., Germain B.F., *et al.* Methotrexate in rheumatoid arthritis. A five-year prospective multicenter study. *Arthritis Rheum*, 1994;**37**;1492–1498.

73. Sany J., Anaya J.M., Lussiez V., *et al.* Treatment of rheumatoid arthritis with methotrexate: a prospective open longterm study of 191 cases. *J Rheumatol*, 1991;**18**:1323–1327.

74. Hanrahan P.S., Scrivens G.A., Russell A.S. Prospective long term follow-up of methotrexate therapy in rheumatoid arthritis: Toxicity, efficacy and radiological progression. *Brit J Rheum*, 1989;**28**:147–153.

75. Alarcon G.S., Tracy I.C., Blackburn W.D. Jr Methotrexate in rheumatoid arthritis: toxic effects as the major factor in limiting long-term treatment. *Arthritis Rheum*, 1989;**32**:671–676.

76. Mielants H.., Veys E.M., van der Straeten C., Ackerman C., Goemaere S. The efficacy and toxicity of a constant low dose of methotrexate as a treatment for intractable rheumatoid arthritis: An open prospective stud. *J Rheumatol*, 1991;**18**:978–983.

77. Rau R., Karger T. Clinical experience with methotrexate in the treatment of rheumatoid arthritis. *Internistische Welt*, 1987;**12**: 335–348.

78. Rau R., Schleusser B., Herborn G., Karger T. Long-term treatment of destructive rheumatoid arthritis with methotrexate. *J Rheumatol*, 1997;**24**:1881–1889.

79. Bologna C., Viu P., Picot M.C., *et al.* Long-term follow-up of 453 rheumatoid arthritis patients treated with methotrexate: an open, retrospective, observational study. *Br J Rheumatol*, 1997;**36**: 535–540.

80. Pinals R.S., Masi A.T., Larsen R.A., Subcommittee for Criteria of Remission in Rheumatoid Arthritis of the American Rheumatism Association Diagnostic and Therapeutic Criteria Committee Preliminary criteria for clinical remission in rheumatoid arthritis. *Arthritis Rheum*, 1981;**24**:1308–1315.

81. Wolfe F., Hawley D.J., Cathey M.A. Termination of slow acting antirheumatic therapy in rheumatoid arthritis. A 14-year prospective evaluation of 1017 consecutive starts. *J Rheumatol*, 1990;**17**:994–1002.

82. Morand E.F., McCloud P.I., Littlejohn G.O. Life table analysis of 879 treatment episodes with slow acting antirheumatic drugs in community rheumatology practice. *J Rheumatol*, 1990;**1**:704–708.

83. Buchbinder R., Hall S., Sambrook P.N., Champion G.D., Harkness A. *et al.* Methotrexate therapy in rheumatoid arthritis: a life table review of 587 patients treated in community practice. *J Rheumatol*, 1993;**20**:639–644.

84. Hawley D.J., Wolfe F. Are there results of controlled clinical trials and observational studies of second line therapy in rheumatoid arthritis valid and generalisable as measures of outcome: analysis of 122 studies. *J Rheumatol*, 1991;**18**:1008–1014.

85. Pincus T., Callahan L.F. Methotrexate is significantly more likely to be continued over two years than gold salts, penicillamine or hydroxycholoroquine in rheumatoid arthritis. *Arthritis Rheum* 1989;**32**:128.

86. Mc Kendry R.J.R., Dale P. Advers effects of low-dose methotrexate therapy in rheumatoid arthritis. *J Rheumatol*, 1993;**20**:1850–1856.

87. Furst D.E. Proposition: Methotrexate should not be the first second-line agent to be used in rheumatoid arthritis if NSAIDs fail. *Arthritis Rheum*, 1990;**20**:69–75.

88. Wolfe F., Cathey M.A. The effect of age on methotrexate efficacy and toxicity. *J Rheumatol*, 1991;**18**:973–977.

89. Poole P., Yeoman S., Caughey D. Methotrexate in older patients with rheumatoid arthritis. *Br J Rheum*, 1992;**31**:860.

90. Sany J., Kaliski S., Couret M., *et al.* Radiologic progression during intramuscular methotrexate treatment of rheumatoid arthritis. *J Rheumatol*, 1990;17:1636–1641.

91. Drosos A.A., Karantanas A.H., Psychos D., *et al.* Can treatment with methotrexate influence the radiological progression of rheumatoid arthritis? *Clin Rheumatol*, 1990;9:342–345.

92. Nordstrom D.M., West S.G., Andersen P.A., Sharp J.T. Pulse methotrexate therapy in rheumatoid arthritis. A controlled prospective roentgenographic study. *Ann Intern Med*, 1987;107: 797–801.

93. Reykdal S., Steinsson K., Sigurjonsson K., Brekkan A. Methotrexate treatment of rheumatoid arthritis: effects on radiological progression. *Scand J Rheumatology*, 1989;18:221–226.

94. Rau R., Herborn G., Karger T., Werdier D. Retardation of radiologic progression in rheumatoid arthritis with methotrexate therapy. *Arthritis Rheum*, 1991;10:1236–1244.

95. Rau R., Herborn G., Menninger H., Sangha O. (1998) Progression in early erosive rheumatoid arthritis: 12 month results from a randomised controlled trial comparing methotrexate and gold sodium thiomalate. *Br J Rheumatol*–in press.

96. Rau R., Herborn G., Menninger H., Elhardt D. Radiologic outcome after two years of treatment with parenteral MTX and gold sodium thiomalate in early erosive arthritis. *Rivista Espanola de Rheumatologia*, 1993;20 (suppl 1):440 (abstract).

97. Jeurissen M.E.C., Boerbooms AMTh, van de Putte L.B.A. *et al.* Methotrexate versus azathioprine in the treatment of rheumatoid arthritis. A forty-eight-week randomised, double blind trial. *Arthritis Rheum*, 1991;34:951–960.

98. Alarcon G.S., Lopez-Mendez A., Walter J., *et al.* Radiographic evidence of disease progression in methotrexate-treated and non-methotrexate disease modifying antirheumatic drug treated rheumatoid arthritis patients. A meta-analysis. *J Rheumatol*, 1992;19:1868–1873.

99. Weinblatt M.E., Polisson R., Blotner S.D., *et al.* The effects of drug therapy on radiographic progression of rheumatoid arthritis. *Arthritis Rheum*, 1993;5:613–619.

100. Weinblatt M.E., Kaplan H., Germain B.F. Low dose methotrexate compared with auranofin in adult rheumatoid arthritis. *Arthritis Rheum*, 1990;33:330–338.

101. Williams H.J., Ward J.R., Reading J.C., *et al.* Comparison of auranofin, methotrexate, and the combination of both in the treatment of rheumatoid arthritis. *Arthritis Rheum*, 1992;3:259–269.

102. Morrasut T., Goldstein R., Cyr M., *et al.* Goldsodiumthiomalat compared to low-dose methotrexate in the treatment of rheumatoid arthritis—a randomised double-blind 26-week trial. *J Rheumatol*, 1989;16:302–306.

103. Suarez-Almazor M.E., Fitzgerald A., Grace M., Russell A.S. A randomised controlled trial of parenteral methotrexate compared with sodium aurothiomalate. *J Rheumatol*, 1988;15:753–756.

104. Rau R., HerbornG., Karger T., *et al.* A double blind randomised parallel trial of intramuscular methotrexate and goldsodiumthiomalate in early erosive rheumatoid arthritis. *J Rheumatol*, 1991;18:328–333.

105. Rau R., Herborn G., Menninger H., Blechschmidt J. Comparison of intramuscular methotrexate and gold sodium thiomalate in the treatment of early erosive rheumatoid arthritis: 12 month data of a double-blind parallel study of 174 patients. *Brit J Rheum* 1997;36:345–352.

106. Menninger H., Herborn G., Blechschmidt J., Rau R. A 36-month comparative trial of methotrexate and gold sodium thiomalate in the treatment of early active and erosive rheumatoid arthritis. *Brit J Rheum*, 1998;37:1060–1068.

107. Hamdy H., McKendry R.J.R., Mierins E., Liver J.A. Low-dose methotrexate compared with azathioprine in the treatment of rheumatoid arthritis. *Arthritis Rheum*, 1987;30:361–368.

108. Felson D.T., Anderson J.J., Meenan R.F. The comparative efficacy and toxicity of second-line drugs in rheumatoid arthritis. *Arthritis Rheum*, 1990;33:1449–1460.

109. Willkens R.F., Urowitz M.B., Stablein D.M. *et al.* Comparison of azathioprine, methotrexate, and the combination of both in the treatment of rheumatoid arthritis: A controlled clinical trial. *Arthritis Rheum*, 1992;35:849–856.

110. Willkens R.F., Stablein D. Combination treatment of rheumatoid arthritis using azathioprine and methotrexate: a 48 week controlled clinical trial. *J Rheumatol*, 1996;44:64–68.

111. Ferraz M.B., Pinheiro G.R., Helfenstein M., *et al.* Combination therapy with methotrexate and chloroquine in rheumatoid arthritis. A multicenter randomised placebo-controlled trial. *Scand J Rheumatol*, 1994;23:231–236.

112. Seideman P., Albertioni F., Beck O., *et al.* Chloroquine reduces the bioavailability of methotrexate in patients with rheumatoid arthritis. A possible mechanism of reduced hepatotoxicity. *Arthritis Rheum*, 1994;37:830–833.

113. Dougados M., Combe B., Cantagrel A., *et al.* Combination therapy in early rheumatoid arthritis: A randomized, controlled, double-blind 52 week clinical trial of sulfasalazine and methotrexate versus the single components. *Ann Rheum Dis*, 1999;58: 220–225.

114. Haagsma C.J., van Riel P.L., de Jong A.J., van de Putte L.B. Combination of sulfasalazine and methotrexate versus the single components in early rheumatoid arthritis: a randomised, controlled, double-blind, 52 week clinical trial. *Brit J Rheum*, 1997; 36:1082–1088.

115. O'Dell J.R., Haire C., Erikson N. *et al.* Efficacy of triple DMARD therapy in patients with RA with suboptimal response to methotrexate. *J Rheumatol*, 1996;44:72–74.

116. Tugwell P., Pincus T., Yocum D., Stein M., *et al.* Combination therapy with cyclosporin and methotrexate in severe rheumatoid arthritis. *N Engl J Med*, 1995;333:137–141.

117. Stein C.M., Pincus T., Yocum D., *et al.* Combination treatment of severe rheumatoid arthritis with cyclosporin and methotrexate for forty-eight weeks: an open-label extension study. *Arthritis Rheum*, 1997;40:1843–1851.

118. Allen L.S., Groff G. Treatment of Felty's syndrome with low-dose oral methotrexate. *Arthritis Rheum*, 1986;29:902–905.

119. Isasy C., Lopez-Martin J.A., Trujillo M.A., Andreu J.L., Palacio S., Mulero J. Felty's syndrome: Response to low dose oral methotrexate. *J Rheumatol*, 1989;16:983–985.

120. Fiechtner J.J., Miller D.R., Starkebaum GA. Methotrexate use in Felty's syndrome: Correlation of clinical response with neutrophil reactive IgG. *Arthritis Rheum*, 1987;30:28.

121. Wassenberg S., Herborn G., Rau R. Methotrexate treatment in Felty's syndrome. *Brit J Rheumatol*, 1998;37:908–911.

122. Bacher D.E., Wilke W.S. (1989) Methotrexate in extraarticular rheumatoid disease. In: Wilke W.S. (ed) *Methotrexate therapy in rheumatic disease*. Marcel Dekker, New York.

123. Espinoza L.R., Espinoza C.G., Vasey F.B., Germain B.F. Oral methotrexate therapy for chronic rheumatoid arthritis ulcerations. *J Am Acad Dermatol*, 1986;15:508–512.

124. Marks C.R., Willkens R.F., Wilskek R., Brown P.B. Small vessel vasculitis and methotrexate. *Ann Intern Med*, 1984;100:916.

125. Kerstens P.J.S.M., Boerbooms A.M.T., Jeurissen M.E.C., *et al.* Accelerated nodulosis during low dose methotrexate therapy for rheumatoid arthritis. An analysis of ten cases. *J Rheumatol*, 1992;19:867–871.

126. Alarcon G.S., Koopman W.J., McCarty M.J. Nonperipheral accelerated nodulosis in a methotrexate-treated rheumatoid arthritis patient. *Arthritis Rheum*, 1993;36:132–133.

127. Weinblatt M.E., Kaplan H., Germain B.F. Methotrexate in rheumatoid arthritis: Effects on disease activity in a multicenter prospective study. *J Rheumatol*, 1991;18:334–338.

128. Fehlauer C.S., Carson C.W., Cannon G.W. Methotrexate therapy in rheumatoid arthritis: 2-year retrospective follow up study. *J Rheumatol*, 1989;16:307–312.

129. Halla J.T., Hardin J.G. Underrecognized postdosing reactions to methotrexate in patients with rheumatoid arthritis. *J Rheumatol*, 1994;21:1224–1226.

130. Bertino J. The mechanism of action of the folate antagonists in man. *Cancer Res*, 1963;23:1286–1306.
131. Karger T., Rau R. (1986) Methotrexate therapy of highly active polyarthritis. In: Rau R (ed) *Low dose methotrexate therapy in rheumatic diseases*. Karger, Basel.
132. Kremer J.M., Lee J.K. A long-term prospective study of the use of methotrexate in rheumatoid arthritis: update after a mean of fifty-three months. *Arthritis Rheum*, 1988;31:477–584.
133. Willkens R.F., Watson M.A. Methotrexate: A perspective of its use in the treatment of rheumatic disease. *J Lab Clin Med*, 1982;100:314–321.
134. Groff G.D., Shenberger K.N., Wilke W.S., Taylor T.H. Low dose oral methotrexate in rheumatoid arthritis: an uncontrolled trial and review of the literature. *Semin Arthritis Rheum*, 1983;12:333–347.
135. Mackinnon S.K., Starkebaum G., Willkens R.F. Pancytopenia associated with low-dose pulse methotrexate in the treatment of rheumatoid arthritis. *Semin Arthritis Rheum*, 1985;15:119–126.
136. Gutierrez-Urena S., Molina J.F., Garcia C.O., et al. Pancytopenia secondary to methotrexate therapy in rheumatoid arthritis. *Arthritis Rheum*, 1996;39:272–276.
137. Weinblatt M.E., Fraser P. Elevated mean corpuscular volume as a predictor of hematologic toxicity due to methotrexate therapy. *Arthritis Rheum*, 1989;32:1592–1596.
138. Tanaka Y., Shiozawa K., Nishibayashi Y., Imura S. Methotrexate induced early onset pancytopenia in rheumatoid arthritis: Drug allergy? Idiosyncrasy? *J Rheumatol*, 1992;19:1320–1321.
139. Bruyn G.A., Velthuysen E., Joosten P., Houtman P.M. Pancytopenia related eosinophilia in rheumatoid arthritis: a specific methotrexate phenomen? *J Rhematol*, 1995;22:1373–1376.
140. Wernick R., Smith D.L. Central nervous system toxicity associated with weekly low-dose methotrexate therapy. *Arthritis Rheum*, 1989;32:770–775.
141. Cannon G.W. Methotrexate pulmonary toxicity. *Rheum Dis Clin North Am*, 1997;23:917–937.
142. Kremer J.M., Alarcon G.S., Weinblatt M.E., et al. Clinical, laboratory, radiographic, and histopathologic features of methotrexate-assocaited lung injury in patients with rheumatoid arthritis: a multicenter study with literature review. *Arthritis Rheum*, 1997;40:1829–1837.
143. Williams H.J., Cannon G.W., Ward J.R. (1986) Methotrexate induced pulmonary toxicity in patients with rheumatoid arthritis. In: Rau R (ed) *Low dose methotrexate therapy in rheumatic diseases*. Karger, Basel.
144. Dawson T., Ryan P.F.J., Findeisen J.M., Scheinkestel C.D. Pneumocystis carinii pneumonia following cyclosporin A and methotrexate treated rheumatoid arthritis. *J Rheumatol*, 1992;19:997.
145. Lang B., Riegel W., Peters T., Peter H.H. Low dose methotrexate therapy for rheumatoid arthritis complicated by pancytopenia and pneumocystis carinii pneumonia. *J Rheumatol*, 1991;18:1257–1259.
146. Hilliquin P., Renoux M., Perrot S., et al. Occurrence of pulmonary complications during methotrexate therapy in rheumatoid arthritis. *Br J Rheumatol*, 1996;35:441–445.
147. Golden M.R., Katz R.S., Balk R.A., Golden H.E. The relationship of preexisting lung disease to the development of methotrexate pneumonitis in patients with rheumatoid arthritis. *J Rheumatol*, 1995;22:1043–1047.
148. Ohosone Y., Okano Y., Kameda H., et al. Clinical characteristics of patients with rheumatoid arthritis and methotrexate induced pneumonitis. *J Rheumatol*, 1997;24:2299–2303.
149. Weinblatt M.E. (1985) Toxicity of methotrexate in rheumatoid arthritis. 16. *International Congress of Rheumatology*, Sydney, p 28: abstract R78.
150. Wilke W.S., Calabrese L.H., Krall P.L., Segal A.M. (1986) Incidence of toxicity in patients with rheumatoid arthritis treated with methotrexate. In: Rau R (ed) *Low dose methotrexate therapy in rheumatic disease*. Karger, Basel.
151. Salaffi F., Mangenelli P., Carotti M., et al. Methotrexate-induced pneumonitis in patients with rheumatoid arthritis and psoriatic arthritis: report of five cases and review of the literature. *Clin Rheumatol*, 1997;16:296–304.
152. Carson C.W., Cannon G.W., Egger M.J. et al. Pulmonary disease during the treatment of rheumatoid arthritis with low-dose pulse methotrexate. *Semin Arthritis Rheum*, 1987;16:186–195.
153. Weinblatt M.E. Toxicity of low dose methotrexate in rheumatoid arthritis. *J Rheumatol*, (Suppl 12), 1985;12:35–39.
154. Rau R. Toxicity of methotrexate in rheumatoid arthritis. In: Weinblatt M.E. (ed) *A comprehensive guide to new therapeutic approaches of methotrexate in rheumatoid arthritis*. Chicago, Pharma Libri, 1987;63–77.
155. Phillips C., Cera P.J., Mangan T.F., Newman E.D. Clinical liver disease in rheumatoid arthritis patients on methotrexate. *J Rheumatol*, 1992;19:229–233.
156. Kremer J.M., Lee R.G., Tolman K.G. Liver histology in rheumatoid arthritis patients receiving long-term methotrexate therapy. A prospective study with baseline and sequential biopsy samples. *Arthritis Rheum*, 1989;32:121–127.
157. Bjorkman D.J., Hammond E.H., Lee R.G., et al. Hepatic ultrastructure after methotrexate therapy for rheumatoid arthritis. *Arthritis Rheum*, 1988;31:1465–1472.
158. Kremer J.M. Liver biopsies in patients with rheumatoid arthritis receiving methotrexate: Where are we going? *J Rheumatol*, 1992;19:189–191.
159. Kremer J.M., Furst D.E., Weinblatt M.E., Blotner S.D. Significant changes in serum AST across hepatic histological biopsy grades: prospective analysis of 3 cohorts receiving methotrexate therapy for rheumatoid arthritis. *J Rheumatol*, 1996;23: 459–461.
160. Roenigk H.H., Maibach H.I., Weinstein G. Guidelines on methotrexate therapy for psoriasis. *Arch Dermatol*, 1972;105:363–365.
161. Beyeler C., Reichen J., Thomann S.R. et al. Quantitative liver function in patients with rheumatoid arthritis treated with low-dose methotrexate: a longitudinal study. *Br J Rheumatol*, 1997;36:338–344.
162. Nyfors A. (1986) Methotrexate hepatotoxicity in psoriasis and psoriatic arthritis. A review. In: Rau R. (ed) *Low dose methotrexate therapy in rheumatic diseases*. Karger, Basel.
163. Nyfors A. Liver biopsies from psoriatics related to methotrexate therapy. *Acta pathol Microbiol*, 1977;85:511–518.
164. Gilbert S.C., Klintamalm G., Menter A., Silverman A. Methotrexate-induced cirrhosis requiring liver transplantation in three patients with psoriasis. *Arch Intern Med*, 1990;150:889–891.
165. Lefkowitz A.M.; Farrow I.J. The liver in rheumatoid disease. *Ann Rheum Dis*, 1955;14:162–168.
166. Rau R. (1978) *Die Leber bei entzündlich-rheumatischen Erkrankungen* (The liver in inflammatory rheumatic diseases). Steinkopff, Darmstadt.
167. Mackenzie A.H. (1986) Liver biopsy findings after prolonged methotrexate therapy for rheumatoid arthritis. In: Rau R (ed) *Low dose methotrexate therapy in rheumatic diseases*. Karger, Basel.
168. Rau R., Karger T., Herborn G., Frenzel H. Liver biopsy findings in patients with rheumatoid arthritis undergoing longterm treatment with methotrexate. *J Rheumatol*, 1989;16:489–493.
169. Rau R., Frenzel H., Cepin A., Herborn G. 131 liver biopsies of MTX treated RA patients compared with 135 pretreatment biopsies (abstract) *Arthritis Rheum*, 1992;35:S147.
170. Aponte J., Petrelli M. Histopathologic findings in the liver of rheumatoid arthritis patients treated with longterm bolus methotrexate. *Arthritis Rheum*, 1988;31:1457–1464.
171. Kremer J.M., Lee R.G., Tolman K.G. Liver histology in rheumatoid arthritis patients receiving longterm methotrexate therapy. *Arthritis Rheum*, 1989;32:121–127.
172. Kramer J.M., Kaye G.I., Kaye N.W. et al. Light and electron microscopic analysis of sequential liver biopsy samples from rheumatoid arthritis patients receiving long-term methotrexate therapy. Follow-up over longterm treatment intervals and correlation with clinical and laboratory variables. *Arthritis Rheum*, 1995;38:1194–1203.

173. Kremer JM, Kaye GI Electron-microscopic analysis of sequential liver biopsy samples from patients with rheumatoid arthritis: Correlation with light microscopic findings. *Arthritis Rheum*, 1989;**32**:1202–1213.

174. Walker A.M., Funch D., Dreyer N.A. *et al*. Determinants of serious liver disease among patients receiving low-dose methotrexate for rheumatoid arthritis. *Arthritis Rheum*, 1993;**36**:329–335.

175. Singh G., Fries J.F., Williams C.A. *et al*. Toxicity profiles of disease modifying antirheumatic drugs in rheumatoid arthritis. *J Rheumatol*, 1994;**18**:188–194.

176. van der Veen M.J., van der Heijde A., Kruize A.A., Bijlsma J.W. Infection rate and use of antibiotics in patients with rheumatoid arthritis treated with methotrexate. *Ann Rheum Dis*, 1994;**53**: 224–228.

177. Boerbooms A.M., Kerstens P.J., van Loenhout J.W., *et al*. Infections during low-dose methotrexate treatment in rheumatoid arthritis. *Semin Arthritis Rheum*, 1995;**24**:411–421.

178. Kerstens P.J., van Loenhout J.W., Boerbooms AM, van de Putte LB (1992) Methotrexate, pneumonitis, and infection. *Ann Rheum Dis*, **51**:1179.

179. Altz-Smith M., Kendall L.G., Stamm A.M. Cryptococcosis associated with low-dose methotrexate for arthritis. *Am J Med*, 1987;**83**: 179–181.

180. Segal A.M., Wilke S (1989) Toxicity of low-dose methotrexate in rheumatoid arthritis. In: Wilke WS (ed) *Methotrexate therapy and rheumatic diseases*. Marcel Dekker New York/Basel.

181. Antonelli M.A.S., Moreland L.W., Bruck J.L. Herpes zoster in patients with rheumatoid arthritis treated with weekly, low-dose methotrexate. *Am J Med*, 1991;**90**:295–298.

182. Seideman P., Müller-Suur R., Ekman E. Renal effects of low dose methotrexate in rheumatoid arthritis. *J Rheumatol*, 1993;**20**:1126–1128.

183. Kremer J.M., Petrillo G.F., Hamilton R.A. Pharmacokinetics and renal function in patients with rheumatoid arthritis receiving a standard dose of oral weekly methotrexate: association with significant decreases in creatinine clearance and renal clearance of the drug after 6 months of therapy. *J Rheumatol*, 1995;**22**:38–40.

184. Rau R., Wassenberg S., Herbon G. Can methotrexate reduce the renal toxicity of parenteral gold? *J Rheumatol*, 1993;**20**: 759–761 (letter).

185. Segal A.M., Kozlowski R.D., Steinbrunner J.V., *et al*. Outcome to first trimester exposure to low-dose methotrexate (MTX) in eight pregnant rheumatoid arthritis (RA) patients. *Arthritis Rheum*, 1987;**30**:59.

186. Buckley L.M., Bullaboy C.A., Leichtman L., Marquez M. Multiple congenital anomalies associated with weekly low-dose methotrexate treatment of the mother. *Arthritis Rheum*, 1997;**40**:971–973.

187. Rustin G.J.S., Rustin F., Dent J. *et al*. No increase in second tumors after cytotoxic chemotherapy for gestational trophoblastic tumors. *N Engl J Med*, 1983;**308**:473–476.

188. Ellman M.H., Hurwitz H., Thomas C. Lymphoma developing in a patient with rheumatoid arthritis taking weekly low dose methotrexate. *J Rheumatol*, 1991;**18**;1741–1743.

189. Kingsmore S.F., Hall B.D., Allen N.B., *et al*. Association of methotrexate, rheumatoid arthritis and lymphoma: report of two cases and literature review. *J Rheumatol*, 1992;**19**:1462–1465.

190. Taillon B., Garnier G., Ferrari E., *et al*. Lymphoma developing in a patient with rheumatoid arthritis taking methotrexate. *Clin Rheumatol*, 1993;**12**:93–94.

191. Georgescu L., Quinn G.C., Schwartzman S., Paget S.A. Lymphoma in patients with rheumatoid arthritis: associatoin with the disease state or methotrexate treatment. *Semin Arthritis Rheum*, 1997;**26**: 794–804.

192. Usman A.R., Yunus M.B. Non-Hodgkin's lymphoma in patients with rheumatoid arthritis treated with low dose methotrexate. *J Rheumatol*, 1996;**23**:1095–1097.

193. Padeh S., Sharon N., Schiby., *et al*. Hodgkin's lymphoma in sytemic onset juvenile rheumatoid arthritis after treatment with low dose methotrexate. *J Rheumatol*, 1997;**24**;2035–2037.

194. Dubin-Kerr L., Troy K., Isola L. Temporal association between the use of methotrexate and development of leukemia in 2 patients with rheumatoid arthritis. *J Rheumatol*, 1995;**22**: 2356–2358.

195. Salloum E., Cooper D.L., Howe G., *et al*. Spontaneous regression of lymphoproliferate disorders in patients treated with methotrexate for rheumatoid arthritis and other rheumatic diseases. *J Clin Oncol*, 1996;**14**:1943–1949.

196. Verstraeten A., Dequeker J. Vertebral and peripheral bone mineral content and fracture incidence in postmenopausal patients with rheumatoid arthritis: Effects of low-dose corticosteroids. *Ann Rheum Dis*, 1986;**45**:852–857.

197. Friedlander G.E., Tross R.B., Dopganis A.C. *et al*. Effects of chemotherapeutic agents on bone. *J Bone Joint Surg*, 1984;**66**: 602–607.

198. May K.P., West S.G., McDermott M.T., Huffer W.E. The effect of low dose methotrexate on bone metabolism and histomorphometry in rats. *Arthritis Rheum*, 1994;**37**:201–206.

199. van der Veen M.J., Scheven B.A., van Roy J.L., *et al*. In vitro effects of methotrexate on human articular cartilage and bone-derived osteoblasts. *Br J Rheumatol*, 1996;**35**:342–349.

200. Buckley L.M., Leib E.S., Cartularo K.S., *et al*. Effects of low dose methotrexate on the bone mineral density of patients with rheumatoid arthritis. *J Rheumatol*, 1997;**24**:1489–1494.

201. Morgan S.L., Daggott J.E., Vaugh W.H. *et al*. The effect of folic acid supplementation on the toxicity of low-dose methotrexate in patients with rheumatoid arthritis. *Arthritis Rheum*, 1990;**33**: 9–18.

202. Weinblatt M.E., Maier A.L., Coblyn J.S. Low dose leucovorin does not interfere with the efficacy of methotrexate in rheumatoid arthritis: an 8 week randomised placebo controlled trial. *Arthritis Rheum*, 1993;**20**;950–952.

203. Shiroky J.B., Neville C., Esdaile J.M., *et al*. Low-dose methotrexate with leucovorin (folinic acid) in the management of rheumatoid arthritis. *Arthritis Rheum*, 1993;**36**:795–803.

204. Buckley L.M., Vacek P.M., Cooper S.M. Administration of folinic acid after low dose methotrexate in patients with rheumatoid arthritis. *J Rheumatol*, 1990;**17**:1158–1161.

205. Tishler M., Caspi D., Fishel B., Yaron M. The effects of leucovorin (folinic acid) on methotrexate therapy in rheumatoid arthritis patients. *Arthritis Rheum*, 1988;**31**:906–908.

206. Hanrahan P.S., Russell A.S. Concurrent use of folinic acid and methotrexate in rheumatoid arthritis. *J Rheumatol*, 1988;**15**: 1078–1080.

207. Joyce D.A., Will R.K., Hoffmann D.M., *et al*. Exacerbation of rheumatoid arthritis in patients treated with methotrexate after administration of folinic acid. *Ann Rheum Dis*, 1991;**59**:913–914.

208. Morgan S.L., Baggot J.E., Altz-Smith M. Folate status of rheumatoid arthritis patients receiving long-term, low-dose methotrexate therapy. *Arthritis Rheum*, 1987;**30**:1348–1356.

209. Morgan S.L., Baggott J.E., Lee J.Y., *et al*. Folic acid supplementation prevents deficient blood folate levels and hyperhomocyteinemia during longterm, low dose methotrexate therapy for rheumatoid arthritis: implications for cardiovascular disease prevention. *J Rheumatol*, 1988;**25**:441–446.

210. Krause D., Schleusser B., Herborn G., Rau R. Response to methotrexate treatment is associated with reduced mortality in patients with severe rheumatoid arthritis. *Arthritis Rheum* (in press).

211. Stenger A.A.M.E., Houtman P.M., Bruyn G.A.W. Does folate supplementation make sense in patients with rheumatoid arthritis treated with methotrexate (review). *Ann Rheum Dis*, 1992;**51**: 1019–1020.

212. Kremer J.M., Davey B.T., Hall M.J., Lawrence D.A. Significant differences in red blood cell folate levels between best and worst responders to methotrexate in patients with rheumatoid arthritis. *Arthritis Rheum*, 1998;**41**:S158 (abstract).

213. Kremer J.M., Alarcon G.S., Lightfood R.W. Jr., *et al*. Methotrexate for rheumatoid arthritis. Suggested guidelines for monitoring liver toxicity. *Arthritis Rheum*, 1994;**37**:316–328.

214. Weinblatt M.E., Kremer J.M., Bankhurst A.D., *et al*. A trial of etanercept, a recombinant tumor necrosis factor receptor: Fc fusion protein, in patients with rheumatoid arthritis receiving methotrexate. *N Engl J Med* 1999;**340**:253–59.

215. Weinblatt M.E., Kremer J.M., Lange M., Burge D.J. Longterm safety and efficacy of combination therapy with methotrexate (MTX) and etanercept (Enbrel®). *Arthritis Rheum* 1999;**42**:S401.

216. Lipsky P. St. Clair W., Furst D., et al. 54-week clinical and radiographic results from the attract trial: a phase III study of infliximab (RemicadeTM) in patients with active RA despite methotrexate. *Arthritis Rheum*, 1999;**42**:S401.

217. Rau R., Simianer S., Weier R., et al. Effective combination of the fully human anti-TNF antibody D2E7 and methotreate in active rheumatoid arthritis. *Ann Rheum Dis-Eular Congress 1999*;217.

218. van Ede A., Laan R., Rood M., et al. Effect of folic and folinic acid suppletion on toxicity efficacy of methotrexate in rheumatoid arthritis: a randomised, double-blind, 48 week, clinical trial. *Arthritis Rheum*, 1999;**42**:S380.

25 | Gold, antimalarials, sulfasalazine, and other DMARDs

Piet LCM van Riel and Eric-Jan JA Kroot

Introduction

Although many treatment modalities are now involved, pharmacotherapy is still considered as the cornerstone in the management of rheumatoid arthritis (RA). Due to insights into the course of RA and the availability of an increasing number of antirheumatic therapies, the strategy of the treatment of rheumatoid arthritis has changed dramatically in the past decades.

Changes in the pharmacotherapeutic management

Until half a century ago, only a few disease modifying antirheumatic drugs (DMARDs) were available for the treatment of rheumatoid arthritis: antimalarials, sulfasalazine, and injectable gold salts. The management of rheumatoid arthritis at that time was mainly based on a 'wait and see' policy. This was on the assumption that prognosis could be benign, on the fear for adverse reactions of the gold salts, and on the lack of alternative treatments. It was common to treat the patient with active RA as long as possible with (bed)rest and salicylates, in the mean time the patient was reassured that the disease was not severe enough to 'dig up the gold'. From 1950 onwards, gradually more first- and second-line agents became available. Almost all the DMARDs were primarily developed for the treatment of other diseases and were found to be useful in the treatment of RA by coincidence. Only sulfasalazine was developed for the treatment of RA and inflammatory bowel disease (IBD), assuming that RA as well as IBD were caused by an infectious agent. As it was not directly clear in which order these drugs had to be used—it was proposed to follow the 'pyramid' treatment approach. This strategy was mainly toxicity driven, which meant that it was proposed to start with the less toxic drug and keep the more toxic drugs, which frequently appeared to be also the most effective, in reserve. In the 1980s the pyramid approach was abandoned, as it became clear that RA had a significant morbidity and mortality with major consequences both for the individual and for society. In addition, it was shown that joint destruction already started in the first years of disease and that it was possible to slow down this process both early and late in the disease course[1]. As a consequence, DMARDs are used earlier in the disease course as monotherapy. Additionally, combinations of different DMARDs are given. It is to be foreseen that in the coming years this strategy will have to be adjusted due to the use of biological agents targeting the important mediators in the pathogenesis of RA such as TNFα, IL-1 or certain adhesion molecules (see Chapters 4 and 7).

Antimalarials

History

Hydroxychloroquine and chloroquine, two drugs used for the treatment and prophylaxis of malaria, have been widely used for the treatment of rheumatoid arthritis and systemic lupus erythematosus. In the early 1950s, Page first suggested remission of associated RA in his series of patients using antimalarials for other reasons. Since that time, several double-blind, placebo-controlled trials have been conducted testing antimalarials in RA[2,3]. The efficacy has been proven to be somewhat weaker than that of most other DMARDs. However, one major advantage of antimalarials is their lack of life-threatening toxicity compared to other DMARDs. Therefore, antimalarials are frequently used in the moderate active RA and in combination with other DMARDs for more severe disease[5,7].

Pharmacology

Both hydroxychloroquine and chloroquine are efficiently absorbed in the gastrointestinal tract and rapidly cleared from the plasma unchanged, after which their disposition is characterized by distribution in the tissues, including liver, spleen, kidney, and red and white blood cells[4]. Their extended half-lives of almost 40 days are caused by their unusually large volumes of distribution[5]. Thus steady state concentrations are still achieved after 3 or 4 months. This tissue accumulation can be explained by the avid intracellular uptake of antimalarials by acidic cytoplasmic vesicles, particularly by the lysosomes. This explains the high concentrations in the liver, containing an abundance of lysosomes. Both drugs are metabolized by dealkylation. However excretion is different; chloroquine is predominantly excreted in the urine, whereas hydroxychloroquine is predominantly excreted in the feces. Two studies showed correlation between a better clinical response and higher serum hydroxychloroquine levels[6,7]. However, there is a great interindividual variability in serum levels of both drugs and a dose–response relationship needs further support[8].

Mechanism of action

The mechanism of action of chloroquine and hydroxychloroquine remains controversial. The most likely explanation is the inhibition of the antigen processing ability of macrophages and monocytes, including inhibition of lymphocyte transformation, chemotaxis, and IL-1 secretion by monocytes. Through decrease of the intracytoplasmic pH, the acid hydrolases, and molecular assembly required for processing antigenic peptides are altered. As a result of the inhibition of the antigen processing, a decreased stimulation of autoimmune CD4+ T cells occurs, leading to a down-regulation of autoimmune responses[9].

Therapeutic efficacy

Several double-blind, placebo-controlled clinical trials and randomized comparative studies in patients with RA have demonstrated the efficacy[2,10,11]. Improved functional class, joint count, pain, grip strength, patient and observer's assessments, ESR, and hemoglobin have been reported. Studies comparing sulfasalazine and hydroxychloroquine showed no statistically significant differences in disease activity variables, including pain, general health, and number of tender and swollen joints. In one study, hydroxychloroquine had a slower onset of antirheumatic effect in comparison with sulfasalazine, but no difference was seen at 48 weeks[10]. However, sulfasalazine seemed to be effective in reducing radiological progression[1]. Improvements or slowing of joint destruction have not yet been demonstrated for antimalarials. A meta-analysis comparing the therapeutic efficacy of hydroxychloroquine and chloroquine, by using the generally accepted doses for both drugs (200–400 mg for hydroxychloroquine and 250 mg for chloroquine), showed that chloroquine was more effective than hydroxychloroquine, a finding which requires confirmation[12]. In a double-blind trial in which patients with juvenile RA were treated with hydroxychloroquine, no therapeutic effect was reported[13]. In conclusion, both hydroxychloroquine and chloroquine have been proven to be effective in the treatment of up to 60–80 per cent of patients with RA or SLE. Maximum antirheumatic effect is usually achieved after 4–6 months of treatment.

Toxicity

The range of adverse effects is similar for hydroxychloroquine and chloroquine. However hydroxychloroquine has been reported to have an incidence of adverse effects about half of that chloroquine in the usual doses. Both drugs have been shown to have the mildest toxicity profile in comparison with other DMARDs. Gastrointestinal side-effects are the most common and include epigastric discomfort and nausea. Headache and dermatological side-effects, such as urticaria, lichenoid changes, and erythema multiforme, have also been reported in a number of studies[5,14]. The most serious side-effect reported so far is retinopathy. However, most case reports of retinopathy date from the 1960s when patients were prescribed higher doses than are now recommended. In these reports irreversible retinal damage (bull's eye retinopathy) involving blurred vision, accommodation problems, scotoma or night blindness, and loss of central vision have been reported. Retinal damage is not related to duration of therapy or to total cumulative dose, but rather to daily dose of the drug. Although severe toxicity is rare, baseline and 6-monthly eye examination, including funduscopy and visual field charting, are recommended[15,16]. However, simple testing of visual activity combined with testing of color vision is as sensitive in early detection of occular toxicity.

Daily clinical practice

Dosage limits of 6 mg/kg/day for hydroxychloroquine and 4 mg/kg/day for chloroquine are recommended. This drug should only be used in patients under the age of 65 and with a normal liver function. Increases or decreases in dosing should be instituted when the body weight is outside the range of 60–70 kg[17]. Patients should be instructed to report any visual symptoms as soon as possible. Complete blood counts and urine analysis should be performed at the same intervals as the ophthalmological examinations. The drug should be used with caution in patients with renal disease or epilepsy. Use of antimalarials in pregnancy should be avoided[18].

Cyclosporin

History

Cyclosporin has first been used in the management of rejection in solid organ transplantation. Its immunosuppressive properties were discovered in 1972 by Borel. At that time several studies started in patients undergoing renal transplantation. Shortly thereafter, cyclosporin was introduced in the treatment of several autoimmune diseases, including psoriasis and inflammatory bowel disease[19]. In 1979, Hermann and Muller introduced cyclosporin in the treatment of RA[20]. Since then, several studies have confirmed the modest efficacy of cyclosporin in the treatment of RA[21,22].

Pharmacology

The cyclosporins, a family of nine distinct polypeptides (termed A to I), each composed of 11 amino acid residues, have been isolated from mycelia of two fungi, *Cyclocarpon leucidum* and *Trichoderma polysporum*. These fungi were found in the search for newer antimicrobial agents in Norway. Only cyclosporin A (cyclosporin) is immunologically active[19,23]. Cyclosporin, lipophilic by nature, is efficiently absorbed in the gastrointestinal tract and metabolized by the liver cytochrome P450-dependent mixed function oxidase system and eliminated in the bile. So the metabolism of cyclosporin may be affected by enzyme inhibitors and inducers. The elimination half-life is about 15 h in RA patients. Only 6 per cent is eliminated through the urine[24]. Recently a microemulsion-based formulation of cyclosporin has been developed, which possesses more predictable and improved absorption with a consequent increased peak concentration and systemic bioavailability[25]. This finding leads to an improved efficacy and short term safety profile.

Mechanism of action

Cyclosporin forms a complex with specific intracellular proteins known as cyclophillins. This cyclosporin/cyclophillin complex binds to calcineurin, thereby inhibiting its intracellular phosphatase activity[20]. As a result, there is inhibition of IL-2 production, which suppresses T-cell activation. Also, release from macrophages of IL-1, IL-3, granulocyte-macrophage colony-stimulating factor, tumor and TNF-α is inhibited. As cyclosporin also inhibits the expression of the CD40 ligand, needed for proliferation and differentiation of B cells, after which calcineurin activity is inhibited. In conclusion cyclosporin inhibits T-cell initiation of humoral immunity[25,26].

Therapeutic efficacy

Most studies investigating the efficacy of cyclosporin have been performed in RA patients refractory to other DMARDs. At the moment, only a small number prospective, randomized, double-blind clinical trials on the efficacy of cyclosporin, at doses of 2.5 to 5 mg/kg per day, have been reported. Improvements in several clinical parameters and a 40 per cent improvements in CRP were noted compared with placebo[27]. Clinical benefit was evident after 3 to 6 months. No effect of cyclosporin on ESR has been reported in almost all studies evaluating the efficacy of cyclosporin. No long-term comparative trials have been performed to compare the efficacy of cyclosporin with that of methotrexate and azathioprine. In comparative trials in which cyclosporin was compared with d-penicillamine (2 years) and azathioprine (6 months), comparable efficacy, but a higher number of adverse events for cyclosporin-treated patients was reported[28,29]. Retardation of radiological progression in patients with active RA has been found in a controlled clinical trial in which patients were treated with cyclosporin or placebo[30]. However another study showed no difference between cyclosporin and parenteral gold[31]. There has only been one study combining cyclosporin with another DMARD, methotrexate in particular. This combination appeared to be a promising option as clinical improvements without a substantial increase in adverse events were found[32].

Toxicity

The most important side-effects leading to discontinuation of cyclosporin treatment include gastrointestinal intolerance and renal dysfunction. This renal toxicity is predictable and dose dependent but urinary protein and 24 h creatinine are recommended at the start of cyclosporin treatment. When, during the treatment, the creatinine levels are persistently increased up to 30 per cent of pretreatment levels, the dose should be reduced. Initial concern that cyclosporin treatment is associated with an increased incidence of malignancies has been proven unfounded. Another common, but less serious, side-effect is hypertension, which is usually reversible by stopping the treatment or reducing the dose. Other frequently occurring side-effects include parasthesias, hyperthrichosis, headaches, and gingival hyperplasia[33]. There is concern with regard to the occurrence of slowly progressive renal fibrosis, which has been convincingly documented in patients with psoriasis[34].

Daily clinical practice

The starting dosage for cyclosporin should be 2.5 mg/kg daily to 3.5 mg/kg daily as a twice-daily regimen, but in daily clinical practice the starting dose is often lower, 1–2 mg/kg daily. After 4–8 weeks the dose can be increased by increments of 0.5 to 1.0 mg/kg daily, up to a maximum of 5 mg/kg daily, at monthly or bimonthly intervals. Clinical response might be expected after 8 to 12 weeks. Cyclosporin should be stopped if no, or only partially, clinical response is achieved after 3 months, at maximal dosing of the drug. A complete blood count and liver function tests should be performed at baseline and periodically thereafter. The blood pressure and serum creatinine should be measured at baseline and biweekly for at least 3 months and monthly thereafter if at stable dose. When creatinine increases to 30 per cent above the baseline value, the dose has to be reduced. If the creatinine remains elevated the drug has to be discontinued. The drug has to be used with caution in patients with: age above 65 years, controlled hypertension, use of drugs with known cyclosporin interactions, use of NSAIDs, previous or concurrent use of alkylating agents, premalignant conditions, active infections, and pregnancy or breastfeeding. The drug is contraindicated in patients with known renal dysfunction, uncontrolled hypertension, current or past malignancy except for basal cell carcinoma, leukopenia or thrombocytopenia, abnormal liver enzymes defined as twice baseline values, or patients with an immunodeficiency disorder[35].

Gold salts

History

At the end of last century the antimocrobial activity of gold salts *in vitro* was demonstrated. However, in patients with tuberculosis treatment with intramuscular administered gold salts appeared not to be successful. As it was thought at that time that RA and tuberculosis had some similarities, gold salts were subsequently successfully tried in patients with RA. Most studies with gold salts have been performed in the 1970s and 1980s due to the introduction of an oral gold compound, auranofin, as that time the intramuscular gold salts were viewed as the 'gold standard' disease modifying agent. Although gold salts are no longer considered as the first choice in the treatment of RA, since the introduction of sulfasalazine and methotrexate, they still have a place in the treatment of RA.

The orally administered gold compound, auranofin, has a different efficacy and toxicity profile than the parenteral gold compounds and will be dealt with separately.

Parenteral gold compounds

Mechanism of action

Many effects of gold compounds on cellular and humoral immunoresponses have been demonstrated. However, the exact mechanism of action is still unknown. Worldwide, different gold compounds are used. The two most frequently used are sodium aurothiomalate and aurothioglucose. Both are water-soluble and administered intramuscularly; sodium aurothiomalate is an aqueous solution while aurothioglucose is an oily suspension. Other preparations used intramuscularly include sodium aurothiopropanol sulfonate, aurothiopolypeptide, and sodium aurothiosulfate.

Therapeutic efficacy

The efficacy of the parenteral gold compounds has been clearly demonstrated in many controlled clinical trials. In addition to effects on clinical and laboratory features of rheumatoid arthritis, which are usually observed after a period of 8–12 weeks, it has been shown that treatment with parenteral gold compounds improves functional status and may slow down radiographic progression. Treatment with parenteral gold compounds resulted in similar efficacy percentages as treatment with sulfasalazine, d-penicillamine, azathioprine (2.5 mg/kg/day), cyclophosphamide (1.5 mg/kg/day), or methotrexate (15 mg/week). However, the withdrawal rate due to adverse reactions during gold treatment is significantly higher than during treatment with most other second-line agents[36]. Furthermore, a randomized 18-month open trial showed equivalence with cyclosporin A[31].

A recent study investigated whether the effect of intramuscular gold salts on functional status (Health Assessment Questionnaire, HAQ) was dependent on disease duration[37]. Significant reductions in disease activity variables were seen in all disease duration groups although the HAQ only improved in the patient population with a disease duration below 2 years.

In an another study, the efficacy and safety of intramuscular gold compounds was compared with methotrexate in 174 patients with a rather early, erosive, rheumatoid arthritis[38]. Patients were treated with weekly doses of either 50 mg aurothiomalate or 15 mg methotrexate. A significant response (more than 50 per cent improvement in swollen and tender joints and erythrocyte sedimentation rate) was observed more frequently in the methotrexate treated patients than in the gold treated patients (76 versus 68 per cent) while a complete remission was more frequently observed in the gold treated patients (24 versus 11 per cent). As expected, significantly more gold-treated patients were withdrawn due to adverse reactions (6/87 versus 32/87).

However, as has been observed earlier, those patients who were withdrawn due to adverse reactions on the gold compound experienced a marked improvement or even a clinical remission which sustained for months after stopping the treatent which is never the case in methotrexate withdrawals.

For many years it was not clear whether or not patients who were treated for the second time with a parenteral gold compound experienced the same response as during the first course. In a study in which the data from 45 patients who had received more than one gold course were reviewed it was shown that more than 95 per cent of the patients who responded to the first course also responded to the second course[39]. The patients who had to discontinue the first course due to adverse reactions also developed an adverse reaction to the second course in 65 per cent of the cases. Patients who did not respond to the first course also did not respond to the second one.

Toxicity

Sodium aurothiomalate is an aqueous gold salt that is rapidly absorbed from the injection site in contrast to the lipid aurothioglucose which is more slowly absorbed. The adverse reactions for both gold compounds are similar with one exception: 'nitritoid' cardiovascular reactions such as flushing, hypotension, tachycardia, and palpitations are unique to sodium aurothiomalate, probably due to the rapid absorption from the injection site.

Treatment with gold salts is characterized by a high number of adverse reactions, the incidence varying from 25–40 per cent. In particular, mucocutaneous reactions are frequently observed followed by proteinuria and hematological adverse reactions such as leukopenia and thrombocytopenia; aplastic anemia is rarely observed.

Some of the adverse reactions are at least partly dose dependent while others are fully idiosyncratic in nature. The drop-out rate due to adverse reactions is 20–30 per cent.

Daily clinical practice

Although several different dosing regimes are in use, most frequently one starts with a weekly dose of 50 mg for a period of 20 weeks. When a response occurs the dose can be gradually tapered by increasing the dosing interval. If no response is observed after 20 weeks, the dose can be increased up to 100 mg for a period of 6–8 weeks. Complete blood counts, urinalysis, renal and liver function tests, and chest radiograph should be performed before starting treatment. During the first 8 weeks complete blood counts, liver function tests, and urinalysis should be performed every week, thereafter tests should be performed following every second injection. In the case of a mild adverse reaction it has to be decided whether to lower the dose or to temporarily withdraw the gold treatment until the adverse reaction has disappeared.

Oral gold

Mechanism of action

The orally absorbable gold compound, auranofin is a lipid-soluble triethylphosphine monomeric gold compound. About 25 per cent of auranofin is absorbed from the gastrointestinal tract, the blood levels of gold are one-quarter to one-sixth of those achieved with the parenteral administered gold compounds. Auranofin is more effective than the parenteral gold compounds in models of acute inflammation and is a potent inhibitor of lysosomal enzyme release and superoxide production. Like the parenteral gold compounds it affects cellular and humoral immune reactions.

Efficacy

Auranofin has a slow onset of response—first results on inflammatory symptoms are seen after 4 to 6 months, the plateau being reached after 6 months. Auranofin is less effective than aurothioglucose and aurothiomalate but better tolerated. Auranofin has been found to be less effective than most of the other second-line agents but also less toxic except for hydroxychloroquine[40]. However, early therapy with auranofin has been found to retard radiographic progression after 2 and 5 years[41]. A recent publication reported 5 years follow-up data of a randomized study in which sulfasalazine was compared to auranofin[42]. Significantly more patients were still on sulfasalazine after 5 years follow-up. In this study it was also shown that those patients who did not respond, or had adverse reactions, to previous parenteral gold treatment had the most unfavorable results: only 4 per cent of those patients were still on auranofin after 5 years.

Toxicity

The nature of the adverse reactions with auranofin appears to be similar to that with parenteral gold compounds, but generally are less severe with auranofin. Adverse reactions affecting the lower gastrointestinal tract (loose stools and diarrhea) are the most common complaints. Most adverse reactions occur during the first months of treatment, in less than 10 per cent of the patients this is reason to discontinue the treatment.

Daily clinical practice

Auranofin is effective in doses of 6–9 mg daily, the usual starting dose is 6 mg, which in case of inefficacy can be increased up to 9 mg. Complete blood counts, urinalysis, and renal and liver function tests should be performed before starting treatment. During the first 12 weeks complete blood counts, liver function tests, and urinalysis should be performed biweekly, thereafter every month. In the event of adverse reactions, it will depend on the severity whether one should only lower the dose or withdraw the treatment temporarily or definitely.

Leflunomide

Mechanism of action

Leflunomide is a novel isoxazole drug with immunosuppressive and antiproliferative properties. Leflunomide causes cell arrest of autoimmune lymphocytes at doses that are not associated with leukopenia, thrombocytopenia, or the occurrence of opportunistic infections. Two mechanisms of action have been proposed: inhibition of the enzyme dihydroorotate dehydrogenase, a critical step for uridine monophosphate production, and inhibition of tyrosine kinases[43]. Leflunomide is rapidly metabolized to its active form which has a plasma half-life of 15 days.

By oral administration of cholestyramine 8 g three times daily it is possible to lower the plasma half-life to 1–2 days.

Efficacy

A multicenter, phase II, placebo-controlled study evaluating 5, 10, and 25 mg daily showed that the 10 and 25 mg group were significantly superior compared to placebo, the highest dose being the most effective one[44]. In two recently-presented 12-month, placebo-controlled studies leflunomide (20 mg daily after a loading dose) was compared to respectively methotrexate (maximum dose 15 mg weekly) and sulfasalazine (2000 mg daily)[45,46]. Leflunomide was statistically superior to placebo and as efficacious as the comparators. The onset of response was significantly earlier with leflunomide compared to methotrexate. Already after 4 weeks a significant response was observed in the leflunomide patients. Radiographic analysis showed a retardation in radiographic progression in the leflunomide patients after 12 months compared to the placebo-treated patients.

Toxicity

Not only the efficacy of leflunomide but also the adverse reactions are dose related. In decreasing order the most frequently reported adverse reactions are gastrointestinal symptoms (anorexia, diarrhea, nausea, gastritis), elevated liver function tests, rash/allergic reactions, weight loss, hypertension, and reversible alopecia. The frequency of adverse reactions during leflunomide treatment in these studies was not different from those during sulfasalazine or methotrexate.

Immunosuppressive agents

The two most frequently used immunosuppressive at present, the 'anticancer' agents cyclophosphamide and azathioprine, were introduced in the treatment of RA in the 1960s. Their efficacy in the treatment of RA has been clearly demonstrated in many studies. However, especially for cyclophosphamide, the indications for use in RA have become restricted due to the severe adverse reactions.

Cyclophosphamide

Cyclophosphamide has been thought to be the most effective antirheumatic drug in the treatment of RA. Unfortunately it is also the most toxic agent with potential severe adverse reactions including bone marrow suppression, infections, gonadal failure, hemorrhagic cystitis, alopecia, and the risk of developing secondary malignancies, especially of the skin and bladder cancer[47]. Cyclophosphamide and its metabolites are mainly excreted by the kidney. Hemorrhagic cystitis results from contact of the bladder with the metabolite and its occurrence can be reduced by ingestions of large amounts of fluid and administration of cyclophosphamide in a single morning dose.

with D-penicillamine, parental gold, or azathioprine has also been successful in several clinical studies, but was generally less well tolerated than monotherapy[65,66].

Toxicity

The adverse reaction profile of sulfasalazine is extensively known since it has been used in the treatment of inflammatory bowel diseases for more than 40 years. Gastrointestinal and central nervous system reactions are the most frequently reported adverse reactions[63]. Up to half of the patients may suffer from these reactions at some time. Nausea, vomiting, anorexia, dyspepsia, headache, and dizziness are the most common side-effects[67]. The gastrointestinal side-effects, in particular, are dose related and probably also relate to sulfapyridine level and acetylatorship. Dose reduction with or without interruption of the medication for a couple of days is often effective in reducing these adverse effects[60]. The majority of these side-effects occur in the first 2–3 months of treatment and are less likely if dosage is increased gradually or when enteric-coated tablets are used[58]. Most of these effects disappear spontaneously after withdrawal of sulfasalazine. As most side-effects occur early in the treatment, biweekly monitoring of full blood counts and liver function tests during the first 3 months and once every 4–12 weeks thereafter have been recommended. Other less frequent adverse reactions include: skin rash, leukopenia and mild hemolysis, hepatitis, eosinophilic pneumonia, agranulocytosis, and hypogammaglobulinemia. The most severe hematological adverse reaction, agranulocytosis, is most likely to occur in the first 6 months of treatment. It is reversible in most cases after dose cessation or reduction[58].

No teratogenic effect or perinatal morbidity or mortality in the progeny of male or female patients taking sulfasalazine at conception or during pregnancy have been reported, but the use of this drug should be avoided in these circumstances, if possible. Also fertility is often reduced in male patients treated with sulfasalazine due to a reversible effect on sperm motility and absolute sperm count[59].

Withdrawal rates for adverse reactions in sulfasalazine recipients varied from 10 to 36 per cent in large comparative studies[12,40]. No differences in withdrawals due to adverse reactions have been reported between sulfasalazine, auranofin, and D-penicillamine[58].

Daily clinical practice

Sulfasalazine is administered orally as enteric coated tablets in the treatment of RA. Patients usually start with 0.5 g daily, whereafter the daily dose may be incremented by 0.5 g at 4-day intervals. The usual maintenance dose is 2.0 to 3.0 g daily given in two divided doses. Complete blood counts and liver function tests should be performed before starting treatment and at least every 4 weeks during the first 6 months of treatment and every 3 months thereafter. As there is always a possibility of serious hematological side-effects, patients should be instructed to learn to recognize clinical signs such as rash, fever, or significant malaise.

As the drug is extensively metabolized by the liver and excreted by the kidney, it should be used with caution in patients with hepatic or renal disease. By incrementing the dose at 4-day intervals, gastrointestinal side-effects are usually avoided. In patients with an ileostomy the drug is contraindicated[68].

Conclusion

In the last decade an increasing number of DMARDs have become available which has influenced the pharmacotherapeutic management of RA. The old pyramid approach has been abandoned definitely and is being replaced by a more aggressive treatment early in the disease course with effective, fast-acting DMARDs[69]. Due to new insights (change in dosages or route of administration, different ways of combining therapies, etc) and the development of new promising therapies the current pharmacotherapeutic approach changes all the time. It is therefore not possible to present a fixed treatment outline. In general, one should try to suppress the disease activity rapidly and as completely as possible with the least toxic agent(s).

References

1. Heijde van der D.M., Riel van P.L., Nuver-Zwart H.H., Gribnau F.W., Putte van de L.B. Effects of hydroxychloroquine and sulfasalazine on progression of joint damage in rheumatoid arthritis. *Lancet*, 1989;I:1036–38.
2. Clark P., Casas E., Tugwell P., Medina C., Gheno C., Tenorio G., Orozco J.A. Hydroxychloroquine compared with placebo in rheumatoid arthritis. A randomized controlled trial. *Annals of Internal Medicine*, 1993;**119**(11):1067–71.
3. A randomized trial of hydroxychloroquine in early rheumatoid arthritis: the HERA Study [see comments] *American Journal of Medicine*, 1995;**98**(2):156–68.
4. Cutler D.J., MacIntyre A.C., Tett S.E. Pharmacokinetics and cellular uptake of 4-aminoquinoline antimalarials. *Agents Actions Supplement*, 1988;**24**:142–57.
5. Tett S., Culter D., Day R. Antimalarials in rheumatic diseases. *Baillieres Clinical Rheumatology*, 1990;**4**(3):467–89.
6. Miller D.R., Fiechtner J.J., Carpenter J.R., Brown R.R., Stroshane R.M., Stecher V.J. Plasma hydroxychloroquine concentrations and efficacy in rheumatoid arthritis. *Arthritis & Rheumatism*, 1987;**30**(5):567–71.
7. Tett S.E., Day R.O., Cutler D.J. Concentration-effect relationship of hydroxychloroquine in rheumatoid arthritis- a cross sectional study. *Journal of Rheumatology*. 1993;**20**:1874–79.
8. McLachlan A.J., Tett E., Cutler D.J., Day R.O. Bioavailability of hydrochloroquine tablets in patients with rheumatoid arthritis. *British Journal of Rheumatology*, 1994;**33**(3):235–9.
9. Fox R. Mechanism of action of hydroxychloroquine as an antirheumatic drug. *Seminars in Arthritis in Rheumatism*, 1993;**23**(2)(suppl. 1):82–91.
10. Nuver-Zwart I.H., van-Riel P.L., van-de-Putte L.B., Gribnau F.W. A double blind comparative study of sulfasalazine and hydrochloroquine in rheumatoid arthritis: evidence of an earlier effect of sulfasalazine. *Annals of the Rheumatic Diseases*, 1989;**48**(5):389–95.
11. Faarvang K.L., Egsmose C., Kryger P., Podenphant J., Ingeman-Nielsen M., Hansen T.M. Hydroxychloroquine and sulfasalazine alone and in combination in rheumatoid arthritis: a randomised

double blind trial. *Annals of the Rheumatic Diseases*, 1993;**52**(10):711–5.

12. Felson D.T., Anderson J.J., Meenan R.F. The comparative efficacy and toxicity of second-line drugs in rheumatoid arthritis. Results of two metaanalyses [see comments]. *Arthritis & Rheumatism*, 1990;**33**(10):1449–61.

13. Brewer E., Giannini E., Kuzmina N., Alekseev L. Penicillamine and hydroxychloroquine in the treatment of severe juvenile rheumaroid arthritis. *New England Journal of Medicine*, 1986;**314**:1269–76.

14. Rynes R.I. Toxicity of antimalarial drugs in rheumatoid arthritis. *Agents Actions Supplement*, 1993;**44**:151–7.

15. Bernstein H.N. Ocular safety of hydroxychloroquine. *Annals of Ophthalmology*, 1991;**23** (8):292–6.

16. Easterbrook M. The ocular safety of hydroxychloroquine. *Seminars in Arthritis & Rheumatism*, 1993;**23**(2 Suppl. 1):62–7.

17. Paulus H. Antimalarial agents compared with or in combination with other disease modifying antirheumatic drugs. *American Journal of Medicine*, 1988;**85**:45–52.

18. American College of Rheumatology Ad Hoc Committee on Clinical Guidelines Guidelines for monitoring drug therapy in rheumatoid arthritis. *Arthritis & Rheumatism*, 1996;**39**(5):723–31.

19. Yocum D. Immunological actions of cyclosporin A in rheumatoid arthritis. *British Journal of Rheumatology*, 1993;**32**(Suppl 1):38–41.

20. Chaudhuri K., Torley H., Madhok R. Disease-modifying antirheumatic drugs. Cyclosporin. *British Journal Rheumatology*, 1997;**36**(9):1016–21.

21. Dougados M., Torley H. Efficacy of cyclosporin A in rheumatoid arthritis: worldwide experience. *British Journal of Rheumatology*, 1993;**32**(Suppl 1):57–9.

22. Wells G., Tugwell P. Cyclosporin A in rheumatoid arthritis: overview of efficacy. *British Journal of Rheumatology*, 1993;**32**(Suppl 1):51–6.

23. Rainsford K.D. Disease-modifying antirheumatic and immunoregulatory agents. *Baillieres Clinical Rheumatology* 1990;**4**(3):405–32.

24. Faulds D., Goa K.L., Benfield P. Cyclosporin. A review of its pharmacodynamic and pharmacokinetic properties, and therapeutic use in immunoregulatory disorders. *Drugs*, 1993;**45**:953–1040.

25. Richardson C., Emery P. Clinical use of cyclosporin in rheumatoid arthritis [published erratum appears in Drugs 1996 Apr;51(4): 570]. *Drugs*, 1995;**50**(Suppl. 1):26–36.

26. Bentin J. Mechanism of action of cyclosporin in rheumatoid arthritis. *Clinical Rheumatology*, 1995;**14**(Suppl 2):22–5.

27. Tugwell P., Bombardier C., Gent M., Bennett K.J., Bensen W.G., Carette S., et al. Low-dose cyclosporin versus placebo in patients with rheumatoid arthritis. *Lancet*, 1990;**335**(8697):1051–5.

28. Tugwell P., Bombadier C., Gent M. et al. Low dose cyclosporin in rheumatoid arthritis: a pilot study. *Journal of Rheumatology*, 1987;**14**:1108–14.

29. Van Rijthoven A.W., Dijkmans B.A., Goeithe H.S., et al. Comparison of cyclosporin and D-penicillamine for rheumatoid arthritis: a randomized, double blind, multicenter study. *Journal of Rheumatology*, 1991;**18**:815–20.

30. Pasero G., Priolo F., Marubini E., Fantini F., Ferraccioli G., Magaro M. et al. Slow progression of joint damage in early rheumatoid arthritis treated with cyclosporin A. *Arthritis & Rheumatism*, 1996;**39**(6):1006–15.

31. Zeidler H., Kvien T., Hannonen P., Wollheim F., Forre O., Geidel H. et al. Progression of joint damage in early active severe rheumatoid arthritis during 18 months of treatment: comparison of low-dose cyclosporin and parenteral gold. *British Journal Rheumatology*, 1998;**37**(8):874–82.

32. Tugwell P., Pincus T., Yocum D., Stein M et al. Combination therapy with cyclosporin and methotrexate in severe rheumatoid arthritis. *New England Journal of Medicine*, 1995;**333**:137–41.

33. Dijkmans B.A. Safety aspects of cyclosporin in rheumatoid arthritis. *Drugs*, 1995;**50**(Suppl.1):41–7.

34. Zachariae H., Kragballe K., Hansen H., Marcussen N., Olsen S Renal biopsy findings in long-term cyclosporin treatment of psoriasis. *British Journal Dermatology*, 1997;**136**(4):531–35.

35. Panayi G.S., Tugwell P. The use of cyclosporin A in rheumatoid arthritis: conclusions of an international review. *British Journal of Rheumatology*, 1994;**33**:967–69.

36. Gestel van A.M., Haagsma C.J., Furst D.E., Riel van P.L.C.M. Treatment of early rheumatoid arthritis patients with slow-acting anti-rheumatic drugs (SAARDs). *Balliere's Clinical Rheumatology*, 1997;**11**:65–82.

37. Munro R., Hampson R., McEntegart A., Thomson E.A., Madhok R., Capell H. Improved functional outcome in patients with early rheumatoid arthritis treated with intramuscular gold: results of a five year prospective study. *Annals of the Rheumatic Diseases*, 1998;**57**:88–93.

38. Rau R., Herborn G., Menninger H., Blechschmidt J. Comparison of intramuscular methotrexate and gold sodium thiomalate in the treatment of early erosive rheumatoid arthritis: 12 month data of a double-blind parallel study of 174 patients. *British Journal of Rheumatology*, 1997;**36**:345–352.

39. Klinkhoff A.V., Teufel A. The second course of gold. *Journal of Rheumatology*, 1995;**22**:1655–1666.

40. Felson D.T., Anderson J.J., Meenan R.F. Use of short-term efficacy/toxicity tradeoffs to select second-line drugs in rheumatoid arthritis. A metaanalysis of published clinical trials. *Arthritis & Rheumatism*, 1992;**35**(10):1117–25.

41. Egsmose C., Lund B., Borg G., Petterson H., Berg E., Brodin U., Trang L. Patients with rheumatoid arthritis benefit from early 2nd line therapy: 5 year followup f a prospective double blind placebo controlled study. *Journal of Rheumatology*, 1995;**22**(12):2208–13.

42. McEntegart A., Porter D., Capell H.A., Thomson E.A. Sulfasalazine has a better efficacy/toxicity profile than auranofin-evidence from a 5 year prospective, randomized trial. *Journal of Rheumatology*, 1996;**23**:1887–90.

43. Fox R.I. Mechanism of action of leflunomide in rheumatoid arthritis. *Journal of Rheumatology*, 1998;**25**(Suppl, 53):20–26.

44. Mladenovic V., Domljan Z., Rozman B., Jajjic I., Mihajlovic D., Dordevic J. et al. Safety and effectiveness of leflunomide in the treatment of patients with active rheumatoid arthritis. Results of a randomized, placebo-controlled, phase II study. *Arthritis & Rheumatism*, 1995;**38**:1595–1603.

45. Weaver A., Caldwell J., Olsen N., Cohen S. for the Leflunomide Investigators group, Strand V. (1998). Treatment of active rheumatoid arthritis with leflunomide compared to placebo or methotrexate. *Arthritis & Rheumatism*, **41**(suppl), S131.

46. Smolen J.S., Kalden J.R., Scott D.L., Rozman B., Kvien T.K., Larsen A. et al. and the European Leflunomide Study Group. Efficacy and safety of leflunomide compared with placebo and sulfasalazine in active rheumatoid arthritis: a double blind, randomised, multicentre trial. *Lancet*, 1999;**353**:259–266.

47. Radis C.D., Kahl, L.E., Baker G.L., Morgan Wasko M.C., Cash J.M., Gallatin A. et al. Effects of cyclophosphamide on the development of malignancy and on long-term survival of patients with rheumatoid arthritis. A 20 year followup study. *Arthritis & Rheumatism*, 1995;**38**:1120–1127.

48. Jeurissen M.E.C., Boerbooms A.M.Th., Putte van de L.B.A., Doseburg W.H., Lemmens A.M. Influence of methotrexate and azathioprine on radiologic progression in rheumatoid arthritis. *Annals of Internal Medicine*, 1991;**114**:999–1004.

49. Jeurissen M.E.C., Boerbooms A.M.Th., Putte van de L.B.A., Doesburg W.H., Mulder J., Rasker J.J. et al. Methotrexate versus azathioprine in the treatment of rheumatoid arthritis. A forty-eight-week randomized, double-blind trial. *Arthritis & Rheumatism*, 1991;**34**:961–972.

50. Durez P., Desager J.P., Appelboom T. (1998) Intravenous loading dose of azathioprine in active rheumatoid arthritis. *Arthritis & Rheumatism*, **41** (Suppl):Abstract 726, S153.

51. Munro R., Capell H.A. Penicillamine. *British Journal of Rheumatology*, 1997;**36**(1):104–9.

52. Joyce D.A. D-penicillamine. *Baillieres Clinical Rheumatology*, 1990;4(3):553–74.
53. Bird (1998).
54. Eberhardt K., Rydgren L., Fex E., Svensson B., Wollheim F.A. D-penicillamine in early rheumatoid arthritis: experience from a 2-year double blind placebo controlled study. *Clinical Experimental Rheumatology*, 1996;14(6):625–31.
55. Joyce D.A. Variability in response to D-penicillamine: pharmacokinetic insights. *Agents Actions Supplement*, 1993;44:203–7.
56. Situnayacke R.D., Gurindulis K.A., Mcconkey B. Longterm treatment of rheumatoid arthritis with sulfasalazine, gold or penicillamine: A comparison using life table methods. *Annals of the Rheumatic Diseases*,1987; 46:177–183.
57. Barrera P., den Broeder A., van der Hoogen F., van Engelen B.G., van de Putte L.B. Postural changes, dysphagia, and systemic sclerosis. *Annals of the Rheumatoid Diseases*, 1998;57:331–38.
58. Rains C.P., Noble S., Faulds D Sulfasalazine. A review of its pharmacological properties and therapeutic efficacy in the treatment of rheumatoid arthritis [published erratum appears in Drugs 1995 Oct;50(4): 625]. *Drugs*, 1995;50(1):137–56.
59. Porter D.R., Capell H.A. The use of sulfasalazine as a disease modifying antirheumatic drug. *Baillieres Clinical Rheumatology*, 1990;4(3):535–51.
60. Bird H.A. Sulphasalazine, sulfapyridine or 5-aminosalicylic acid—which is the active moiety in rheumatoid arthritis? *British Journal of Rheumatology*, 1995;34 (Suppl. 2), 16–9.
61. Wahl C., Liptay S., Adler G., Schmid R. Sulfasalazine: a potent and specific inhibitor of nuclear factor kappa B. *Journal of Clinical Investigations*, 1998;101(5):1163–74.
62. van der Heijde D.M., van Riel P.L., Nuver-Zwart I.H., van de Putte L.B. Sulphasalazine versus hydroxychloroquine in rheumatoid arthritis: 3-year follow-up [letter]. *Lancet*, 1990;3, 335(8688):539.
63. van Riel P.L., van Gestel A.M., van de Putte L.B. Longterm usage and side-effect profile of sulfasalazine in rheumatoid arthritis. *British Journal of Rheumatology*,1995; 34(Suppl. 2):40–2.
64. Haagsma C.J., van Riel P.L., de Rooij D.J., Vree T.B., Russel F.J., van't Hof M.A., van de Putte L.B. Combination of methotrexate and sulfasalazine vs methotrexate alone: a randomized open clinical trial in rheumatoid arthritis patients resistant to sulfasalazine therapy. *British Journal of Rheumatology*, 1994;33(11):1049–55.
65. Conaghan P.G., Brooks P. Disease-modifying antirheumatic drugs, including methotrexate gold, antimalarials, and D-penicillamine. *Current Opinion Rheumatology*, 1995;7(3):167–73.
66. McEntegart A., Porter D., Capell H.A., Thomson E.A. Sulfasalazine has a better efficacy/toxicity profile than auranofin-evidence from a 5 year prospective, randomized trial. *Journal of Rheumatology*, 1996;23(11):1887–90.
67. The Australian Multicentre Clinical Trial Group Sulfasalazine in early rheumatoid arthritis. *Journal of Rheumatology*, 1992;19(11):1672–7.
68. Dougados M. (1998) Sulfasalazine. In: *Therapy of Systemic Rheumatic Disorders* (ed. Van de Putte L.B.), pp. 165–83. Marcel Dekker, New York.
69. van de Putte L., van Gestel A., van Riel P. Early treatment of rheumatoid arthritis: rationale, evidence, and implications. *Annals of the Rheumatic Diseases*, 1998;57:511–12.

26 | *Intra-articular therapy*

Peter Lanyon and Michael Doherty

Introduction

This chapter primarily focuses on intra-articular steroid therapy, although other experimental intra-articular agents will be briefly discussed. Intra-articular steroids are used widely in the management of rheumatoid arthritis (RA). The main objectives of intra-articular injection are to:

- provide temporary pain relief;
- reduce joint inflammation;
- retard tissue damage.

Historical perspective

Many attempts have been made at intra-articular injection of a variety of substances to try and provide pain relief or lubrication for the RA joint. On finding chronic inflammatory synovial fluid to have an alkaline pH, Grant Waugh in 1938 advocated the intra-articular injection of lactic acid and novocain, reporting good results in individual cases[1]. In 1944, a study of the effects of a longer acting acid solution, potassium phosphate, injected into 284 rheumatoid joints reported a lasting improvement in 60 per cent of patients[2]. This approach, however, did not gain widespread acceptance into medical practice. Shortly, after the introduction of cortisone by Hench in 1950[3], numerous reports documented the antirheumatic effects of this compound when administered orally or parentally. However, the first results from utilizing direct intra-articular injection of cortisone were disappointing; the effect was reported as inconsistent, mild and too transient to be of any practical value[4]. However, the future of intra-articular therapy changed dramatically with the introduction of hydrocortisone in 1951. This was reported by Hollander to produce significant improvement in RA synovial joint swelling, tenderness, and motion within 24 h, with improvement

lasting an average of 8 days[4,5]. Over the last 40 years intra-articular injection of steroids has become an important means of obtaining rapid control of synovitis and pain in the inflamed RA joint.

Intra-articular steroids

There are many potential benefits of intra-articular steroid therapy in RA. It clearly targets anti-inflammatory therapy to the site of disease. Treatment response occurs rapidly, often with pain relief and restoration of function within just a few days. In isolated synovitis of one or two joints, it may be the only definitive treatment that is required, thus avoiding exposure to the potential side-effects of systemic drugs. Where there is more widespread disease, selective joint injection may be effective in 'debulking' synovitis, prior to the onset of DMARD action[6]. However, there are a number of important practical considerations to this therapy since both local and systemic complications may occur. Moreover, frequently repeated injections may insidiously equate with continuous oral steroid therapy and may defer attention from the fundamental fact that the patient's DMARD therapy needs to be reviewed. Table 26.1 shows the benefits and drawbacks of intra-articular steroids.

Efficacy

In 1953, Hollander reported the results of injection in a large, open, personal series of 850 patients, most of whom had RA; 20 per cent of his patients had obtained relief from symptoms and signs for at least a year following a single injection, and a further 50 per cent obtained temporary relief which was maintained throughout a year by repeated injections[5]. By 1969, in reporting nearly 250 000 injections to over 8000 patients,

Table 26.1 Benefits and drawbacks of intra-articular steroid injections

Benefits	Drawbacks
Effective, rapid reduction of inflammation	Suitable for use in limited number of
Good patient tolerability	joints at any one time
Simple	Low prevalence, definite side-effects
Cheap	(local and systemic)

Table 26.2   Preparations and dosage of intra-articular steroids

Preparation	Concentration/ml	Dose
Hydrocortisone acetate	25 mg	5–50 mg
Methylprednisolone acetate	40 mg	20–80 mg
Prednisolone acetate	25 mg	5–25 mg
Dexamethasone phosphate	4 mg	0.8–4 mg
Triamcinolone acetonide	10 mg	2.5–15 mg
Triamcinolone acetonide	40 mg	5–40 mg
Triamcinolone hexacetonide	20 mg	2–40 mg

Hollander concluded that 'no other form of treatment for arthritis has given such consistent local relief from pain to so many for so long with so few harmful effects[7]. Numerous subsequent studies have confirmed the efficacy of intra-articular steroids.

Some of the most commonly used preparations and their recommended doses are listed in Table 26.2. As there are no available intrasynovial dose response curves, conventional practice is to arbitrarily inject 1–2 ml into large joints and less into smaller joints. Compared to hydrocortisone acetate, the synthetic preparations, by virtue of esterified side chains, have a reduced water solubility and hence slower systemic absorption from the joint. The duration of action is generally shortest for hydrocortisone acetate and increases as the solubility of the preparation decreases. However, there are only a few comparative studies of efficacy. Triamcinolone hexacetonide has generally been reported to have a longer duration of action than any other preparation[7]. In an open study of 12 patients who received 124 hand and wrist injection followed by 3 weeks of splinting, McCarty reported an 87 per cent remission rate over an average 21 month follow-up[8]. A reduction in the development of hand erosions in the injected joints was also observed. While a subsequent study of similar unilateral 'total hand' injection reported a significant reduction in joint swelling and tenderness at 1 year in the injected compared to control hand, no significant improvement in hand function or retardation of radiographic change was observed[9]. One suggested explanation for these differing results is that the later study used less rigorous postinjection splinting. In double-blind studies in rheumatoid knee synovitis, a longer duration of benefit has been observed with triamcinolone hexacetonide than methylprednisolone acetate[10,11]. In a single blind comparison of hydrocortisone, triamcinolone acetonide, and triamcinolone hexacetonide in 300 patients with knee synovitis, a significantly greater number of patients were pain free for longer with triamcinolone hexacetonide[12].

Mode of action

The precise mode of action of intra-articular steroids is unknown[13] and may not be analogous to the mechanism of systemically-administered steroids. The mechanism of rapid pain relief, in particular, remains unclear and may be independent for the concomitant reduction in synovitis and intra-articular hypertension. Pain relief, of course, occurs following intra-articular injection of steroid into an OA knee in which synovitis and intra-articular hypertension is less evident or even absent. Steroids modulate multiple aspects of cell metabolism by binding to specific cytoplasmic receptors, forming complexes which influence gene expression. Steroid receptors are present in human articular cartilage.

Contrast MRI studies have demonstrated reduced GdDTPA (gadopentetate dimeglumine) enhancement after intra-articular steroid, reflecting decreased synovial inflammation[13,14]. Intra-articular steroids decrease synovial permeability[15] and reduce both the total leukocyte count and the percentage of polymorphonuclear leukocytes[16,17]. The percentage PMN leucocytosis preinjection has been reported to correlate with reduction in knee joint circumference at 2 and 6 months post injection; however, this result may simply reflect a higher grade of pretreatment inflammatory activity[17].

Systemic effects

Systemic absorption clearly does occur after an intra-articular steroid injection. Most clinicians are aware that injection into one joint may produce beneficial effects on inflamed joints distal to the injection site. This may be paralleled by a significant fall in the acute phase response at 1 week, lasting for 1–6 months[18].

The amount of systemic absorption has a stronger relationship to the number of joints injected at one sitting rather than the total steroid dose given[19], presumably reflecting drug exposure to a greater volume of synovium from which absorption can take place.

Depression of endogenous cortisol after intra-articular injection, of duration ranging from 14–28 days has been observed in some studies[10,19–21] but not in others[22,23]. The clinical significance of this effect is not known. There are no reports of adrenal crisis after isolated injection, although some authors have recommended supplemental steroids if patients undergo a significant stress within 1 week of intra-articular injection[24].

Potential complications

Flushing

Marked flushing of the face and neck occurs in up to 15 per cent of subjects (see Table 26.3), with onset within a few hours and lasting up to 3–4 days (Fig. 26.1)[25]. It is more common in women,

Table 26.3   Potential complications of intra-articular steroids

Complication	Estimated frequency(%)
facial flushing	1–15
postinjection flare	2–6
skin/fat atrophy	1–24
septic arthritis	0.01–0.07
anaphylaxis	< 1
tendon rupture	< 1

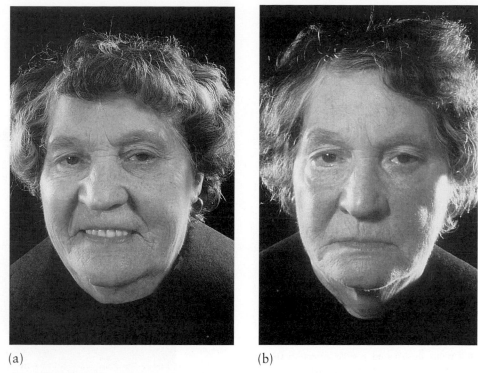

(a)   (b)

Fig. 26.1 Facial appearance before (a) and after (b) intra-articular injection of triamcinolone. See also Plate 26.

and is likely to recur if the procedure is repeated with the same preparation[25,26].

Postinjection flare

A localized inflammatory reaction, clinically evident 4 to 24 h after the injection, occurs in 2–6 per cent of subjects. It is more common with the earlier steroid formulations (e.g. hydrocortisone acetate) than triamcinolone, and may be associated with the presence of intracellular steroid crystals. Triamcinolone hexacetonide 'crystals' may be observed in

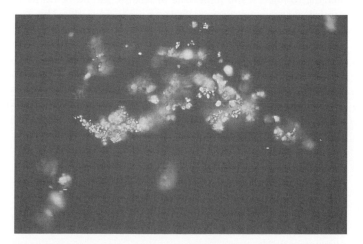

Fig. 26.2 Compensated polarized light microscopy of triamcinolone hexacetonide, aspirated during a steroid flare 72 h postinjection, brightly birefringent material but showing no clear crystalline symmetry. See also Plate 27.

aspirated synovial fluid several days following injection; they can show similar morphology and birefringence to urate, but are larger in length[27]. Commonly however, brightly birefringent material with no clear crystalline structure is seen (Fig. 26.2). If post injection pain lasts for longer than 48 h, or clearly if it is associated with skin erythema, reaspiration to exclude iatrogenic infection is mandatory. The peripheral leukocyte count is not a reliable guide to the presence of infection, as intra-articular steroids have been shown to induce a peripheral leukocytosis[28].

Skin

Fat and skin atrophy may occur after injection, due to leakage of steroid back along the needle track. These complications are more likely to occur with the fluorinated triamcinolone preparations[29] which, for this reason, are not recommended for superficial injection (Fig. 26.3). Where small finger joints are injected under pressure with triamcinolone, skin atrophy has been reported to occur in up to a quarter of cases[8]. Local skin rashes due to delayed type hypersensitivity may also occur[30].

Infection

In several large series, post injection infection rates of 1 in 14 to 85 000 have been reported[7,27,31]. The usual causative organism is *Staphylococcus aureus*, although infection with other organisms including *Clostridia* and *Serratia marscescans* (from contamination of the drug preparation) has been

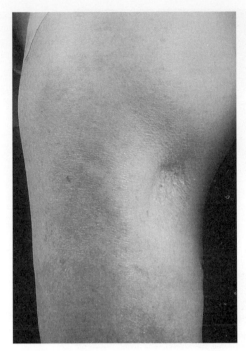

Fig. 26.3 Skin atrophy following fluorinated steroid injection to an anserine bursa. See also Plate 28.

reported[32]. The most common route of joint sepsis is through skin penetration[32], resulting in inoculation of the patient's own flora or organisms from the operator's skin or nose[33]. Intra-articular injection may also allow preferential hematogenous seeding from other sites of occult (usually skin) infection by interrupting the normal capillary integrity of the joint[34]. Clearly, some of the reported cases may reflect injection into an already infected joint, which may have lacked the typical features of sepsis due to the immunosuppressive effects of the disease or drugs.

Rare side-effects

Other reported adverse effects include anaphylaxis to the steroid preparation or coadministered local anesthetic, sickle cell crisis[35], joint capsule calcification[8], and needle fracture[26]. Tendon rupture has been very rarely reported after intra-articular injection, most commonly the extensor tendons of the wrist, although it is often impossible to distinguish the role of injection from the underlying disease process[36].

Contraindications

Contraindications to injections are listed in Table 26.4. Most of these relate to sepsis. Anticoagulant therapy is not a contraindication to cautious aspiration and injections; as with venepuncture, more prolonged pressure on the puncture site is advised following the procedure.

Table 26.4   Contraindications to intra-articular injection

Septic arthritis
Periarticular cellulitis
Bacteremia
Joint prosthesis
Osteochondral fracture

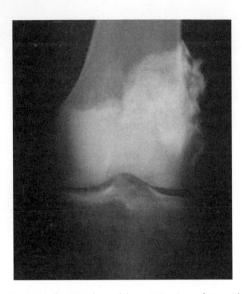

Fig. 26.4   Attempted superolateral knee injection of steroid plus radiographic contrast. Although the operator withdrew synovial fluid and thought the injection went in under low resistance, it was clearly extra-articular.

Practical issues

Accessibility

Before any injection is undertaken, the patient should be comfortable, co-operative, and the joint accessible. All non-axial joints affected by RA are readily accessible. Many would use imaging to inject a hip joint. The procedure should be no more painful than venepuncture if performed correctly. The one common exception is the temporomandibular joint which is commonly a more painful experience.

Accessibility is an important issue, because failure to enter the joint space and hence extra-articular injection may explain some of the variability in the response to steroid injection[37] and in the frequency of local tissue damage. A radiographic study after injection of steroid and contrast medium reported that intra-articular injections are often inaccurate, even if undertaken by experienced operators[38]. In the case of readily-accessible joints, such as the knee, 28 per cent of injections were extra-articular (Fig. 26.4). In this study, the clinical response, as judged by a reduction in joint inflammation, was much more likely to occur with intra-articular than extra-articular injection. As expected, accurate injection strongly associates with successful aspiration of synovial fluid.

Paradoxically, attempting to aspirate a joint to complete dryness may lead to extra-articular injection; with increasing retraction on the syringe the needle tip may be pulled out of the joint capsule.

Other indicators that the injection is being misplaced include immediate discomfort and any resistance to injection.

Preinjection counselling

Prior to injection, the patient should be fully counselled. This should include an explanation of, and opportunity to ask questions, about the following:

- nature of the procedure and drugs used;
- expected likelihood and duration of benefit;
- the frequency and nature of any potential complications;
- what the patient should do if these occur, including how and when to seek medical advice;
- the duration and type of postinjection rest.

A record should be made in the patients' notes that these issues have been discussed.

The procedure

Each doctor will develop his/her own routine to maximize patient comfort and the accuracy of injection and to minimize potential risks. In a questionnaire survey of 172 United Kingdom consultant rheumatologists, there was very little consensus regarding technique[39]. The following procedure is suggested as a minimum guide:

- use only single-use sterilized needles and syringes and single dose drug ampoules;
- hands should be domestically washed and adequately dried to avoid droplet contamination;
- the appropriate site for injection should be identified, and, if required, marked with either a thumbnail or the retracted tip of a ballpoint pen;
- the skin should be cleaned with isopropyl alcohol swabs or chlorhexidine and allowed to dry completely;
- all drugs should be checked after drawing up for correct preparation and expiry date;
- the operator should don gloves;
- a no-touch technique should be used to enter the joint and any fluid aspirated to confirm correct location prior to injection;
- all needles should be disposed of safely.

What to do if things go wrong

Inadvertent intra-articular injection of the wrong substance obviously occurs (e.g. medroxyprogesterone acetate instead of methylprednisolone acetate, 50 per cent dextrose instead of radiographic contrast medium) and is probably under reported[40]. This complication is probably more likely to occur where different preparations have similar packaging ('trade dress') and where office suites and drug cabinets are shared with other spe-

cialities. It is vital for all operators to personally check all drugs prior to administration. If such an error does occur, the following procedure should be followed:

- the patient needs to be informed of the error and counselled regarding potential short and long-term consequences;
- the joint should be immediately reaspirated to try and reduce systemic drug absorption;
- if the drug is potentially irritant, the joint should be treated with immediate lavage (arthroscopic or needle).

Areas of continued debate

Method of skin preparation

There is no consensus as to whether a single isopropyl alcohol swab is sufficient, or a fuller sterile aseptic technique using chlorhexidine in spirit-soaked cotton wool balls should be used[39]. In a study of 64 patients where bacteriological examination of the needles was performed post joint injection, no significant difference in needle contamination rates was found between these two methods[41]. Whichever method is employed, skin drying should be complete; this takes longer for chlorhexidine, which is also more expensive.

Should the operator wear gloves?

Many rheumatologists do not wear gloves[39]. Although these are not necessary for the patient's safety, their use is recommended to prevent the contamination of the operator and any assistant by potentially infectious blood or synovial fluid[42].

Should the joint be rested and for how long?

Whether to rest joints postinjection, and for how long, is controversial and also subject to practical constraints, since most injections are given in an out-patient rather than in-patient setting. The rationale for instituting postinjection rest is to try and delay the systemic absorption of steroid suspension from the joint and reduce any leakage of crystalline steroid along the needle track. In addition, it may avoid the hazard of the patient immediately 'overworking' an inflamed joint which may lead to further hypoxia–reperfusion damage. Some authorities recommend three days' bed rest after lower extremity injection followed by 3–6 weeks modified weight bearing, and 3–5 days' use of a sling for the upper extremity[43,44]. However, in a randomized controlled study of 28 subjects, no benefit from postinjection rest could be ascertained at 2 days and 10 months postinjection, although the methodology of this study has been criticized[45,46]. A more recent study of 91 knees demonstrated that 24 hours hospital bed rest compared to standard out-patient injection was associated with greater clinical and serological improvement for up to 6 months, though of course bed rest itself may help control of synovitis[47].

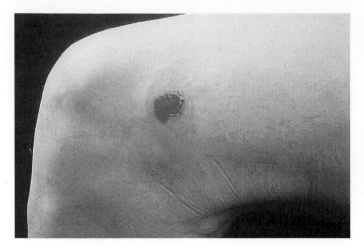

Fig. 26.5 Skin necrosis following over enthusiastic use of a refrigerant spray. See also Plate 29.

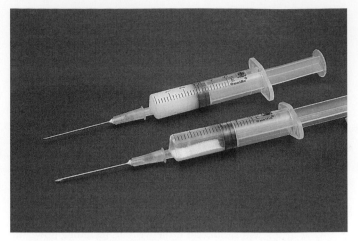

Fig. 26.6 Flocculation and sedimentation occurring after mixing 2 ml 1 per cent lignocaine with methylprednisolone acetate (bottom) but not with triamcinolone hexacetonide (top). See also Plate 30.

Clearly, hospital bed rest is not practical and economically feasible for the majority of patients. However, it should be considered particularly where rheumatoid synovitis responds poorly to several injections. In practice, all patients should be advised to reduce weight bearing as much as possible for 48 hours postinjection.

Use of local anesthetic

There is no consensus on the use of local anesthesia either to skin alone or down to the joint capsule prior to injection. In practice, it's use will depend on the joint to be injected, patients' preference, and their previous experiences of the procedure and the skill of the operator. Arguments against the use of local anesthetic are that it may actually be more painful than a single injection needle. Some practitioners use refrigerant sprays, though these must be used with caution since overenthusiastic spraying may lead to cold injury and painful blistering (Fig. 26.5).

More controversial is whether local anesthetic should be mixed with steroid prior to injection. The theoretical advantage of this approach is that it might result in more rapid pain relief and reduce the incidence of postinjection flares, although there is no evidence to support the latter. For large joints such as the knee, a volume of anesthetic may help to disperse the steroid within the joint. However, there are potential drug compatibility

problems with this approach. The data sheet recommendations for some intraarticular steroid is shown in Table 26.5.

For only one preparation, triamcinolone hexacetonide, is there specific advocacy for the addition of lignocaine. For methylprednisolone acetate it is specifically stated that no other fluid should be added; the addition of lignocaine results in flocculation of the steroid shortly after mixing (Fig. 26.6). Whether there are any adverse therapeutic implications of this flocculation is not known, but it is good practice not to depart from datasheet recommendations.

Is routine culture of synovial fluid necessary?

Some authors suggest that steroid should never be injected into a rheumatoid joint unless the synovial fluid is being sent for culture[48]. The arguments in favor of this approach are that in rheumatoid patients the signs of sepsis may be subtle and unrecognized. Additionally, a 'baseline' may be useful in the event of subsequent iatrogenic sepsis, although the overall risk of this occurring postinjection is very low (1 in 14 to 85 000). Conversely, it has been argued that routine culture is unnecessary[31]. Two studies of over 600 joint aspirates reported that no positive synovial fluid culture results were obtained where sepsis had not been suspected clinically[49,50].

Avoiding routine culture would result in significant cost savings (e.g. estimated United Kingdom savings £2million per year)[50]. It is therefore recommended that fluid only be cultured if the patient has symptoms of infection, non-specific malaise, tachycardia, or if purulent fluid is obtained.

Do intra-articular steroids have adverse effects on the joint?

Whether intra-articular steroids have an adverse effect on the joint ('steroid arthropathy') has been debated for many years. Early reports suggested that radiological deterioration occurred

Table 26.5 Manufacturers datasheet recommendations for addition of diluents to steroid preparations

Preparation	Acceptable diluents
Hydrocortisone acetate	no comments in datasheet
Methylprednisolone acetate	do not mix with any other fluid
Prednisolone acetate	no comments in datasheet
Dexamethasone phosphate	sodium chloride BP
Triamcinolone acetonide	no comments in datasheet
Triamcinolone acetonide	no comments in datasheet
Triamcinolone hexacetonide	sodium chloride BP, lignocaine hydrochloride BP

after repeated steroid injection, with articular damage being attributed to 'joint abuse' as a consequence of the increased movement and analgesia obtained after injection[51]. Conversely, Keagy reported no evidence of steroid arthropathy in a group of 123 patients treated with over 800 injections of triamcinolone acetonide and, in some patients, the joint space actually increased[52]. Most of the reports of 'steroid arthropathy' have been isolated cases[53,54] where subsequent joint destruction may well have been attributable to pre-existing primary joint disease, for example erosive OA. McCarty has reported only one case of local osteonecrosis after 25 years of using triamcinolone[55].

In a small study of 13 patients where one joint had been injected at least 25 per cent more often than the contralateral joint, no increased risk of joint replacement was observed over a 5-year period in the more heavily injected joint[56]. Intra-articular steroids have not been shown to have a significant effect on bone resorption markers and only a transient (14 day) effect on bone formation[57].

Experimental animal studies have also given conflicting results. Some studies of injection of hydrocortisone[58] or triamcinolone hexacetonide[59] into rabbit knees reported the development of cartilage lesions such as thinning, fibrillation, and cyst formation. However, other studies have suggested that triamincolone hexacetonide may have a protective effect following cartilage damage induced by meniscectomy[60] or chemicals[61]. Methylprednisolone acetate has been reported to have a protective effect on the development of radiological change in immobilized rabbit knees[62] and after cruciate injury in dogs[63]. This proposed chondroprotective effect may be due to reduced intra-articular metalloproteinase activity following steroid injection[64]. IGF-1 signaling is important in proteoglycan synthesis in cartilage and is down-regulated in arthritic cartilage. In tissue culture models, triamcinolone acetonide resulted in repaired IGF-1 responsiveness, probably through down-regulation of proinflammatory IL-1 synthesis[65].

It is therefore likely that in routine clinical practice intra-articular steroids do not carry any significant risk of joint damage.

How many joints should be injected at one time, and how often repeated?

To minimize systemic steroid effects, most clinicians recommend a maximum of two to three large joints should be injected at any one sitting[27], less often than monthly. Current convention has been to limit their use to no more than three injections to a single site per year.

Other intra-articular agents

Methotrexate

Intra-articular administration of methotrexate has been advocated in order to avoid the toxicity of oral therapy, although in fact it is rapidly absorbed from the joint. However, no advantage has been demonstrated for this agent either alone or in combination with steroid injection[66,67].

Rifampicin

This broad-spectrum antibiotic is a potent inhibitor of RNA and DNA polymerases and has been reported to possess anti-inflammatory effects when injected intra-articularly at weekly intervals[68]. In a double-blind study of subjects with rheumatoid knee synovitis, median duration of improved pain scores was longer after injection of rifampicin plus triamcinolone (19 weeks) than with trimacinolone alone (13.5.weeks)[67]. However, 40 per cent of subjects suffered from postinjection pain, which is likely to limit the future of this therapy.

Rimexolone

In a small dose-ranging study of rimexolone, a novel antiinflammatory steroid, in 20 patients with rheumatoid knee synovitis, an improvement in joint pain and tenderness was sustained for up to 94 days[69].

Somastatin

Somastatin has an analgesic effect through inhibition of the release of substance P, and may also have an effect in inhibiting neurogenic inflammation. Elevated levels of substance P are found in rheumatoid synovial fluid. In an open study of 16 patients who received six intra-articular injections of somastatin at 15-day intervals, a reduction in synovial membrane thickness was observed by ultrasound[70].

Hyaluronans

Hyaluronate, a major component of synovial fluid, is decreased in concentration and in molecular weight in rheumatoid synovial fluid as a result of increased enzymatic degradation. Intra-articular injection of high molecular weight hyaluronate reduces inflammatory synovial exudate and cell proliferation. In an open study of eight patients who received injections of hyaluronate biweekly for 12 weeks, pain in 50 metre walking was significantly reduced compared to baseline from week 2. No improvement in spontaneous pain at rest or in systemic inflammatory parameters was observed[71]. Several preparations of different molecular weight hyaluronan are currently available; Hyalgan® is licensed in several countries for pain relief of OA knees and most studies relate to OA not RA.

Summary

Intra-articular steroid injection is a simple, safe way of obtaining rapid control of pain and local joint inflammation and should be commonly considered as part of an overall management strategy.

References

1. Waugh W.G. Treatment of certain joint lesions by injection of lactic acid. *Lancet*, 1938;487–9.
2. Crowe H.W. Treatment of arthritis with acid potassium phosphate. *Lancet*, 1944;563–4.
3. Hench P.S., Slocumb C.H., Polley H.F., Kendall E.C. Effect of cortisone and pituitary adrenocorticotrophic hormone (ACTH) on rheumatic diseases. *JAMA*, 1950;144:1327–35.
4. Hollander J.L., Brown E.M., Jessar R.A., Brown C.Y. Hydrocortisone and cortisone injected into arthritic joints. *JAMA*, 1951;147:1629–35.
5. Hollander J.L. Intra-articular hydrocortisone in the treatment of arthritis. *Ann Intern Med*, 1953;39:735–46.
6. McCarty D.J., Harman J.G., Grassanovich J.L., Qian C. Treatment of rheumatoid joint inflammation with intrasynovial triamcinolone hexacetonide. *J Rheumatol*, 1995;22:1631–5.
7. Hollander J.L. Intrasynovial corticosteroid therapy in arthritis. *Md State Med J*, 1970;19:62–6.
8. McCarty D.J. Treatment of rheumatoid joint inflammation with triamcinolone hexacetonide. *Arthritis Rheum*, 1972;15:157–73.
9. Hardin J.G. Controlled study of the long term effects of 'total hand' injection. *Arthritis Rheum*, 1979;22:619.
10. Bird H.A., Ring E.F.J., Bacon P.A. A thermographic and clinical comparison of three intra-articular steroid preparations in rheumatoid arthritis. *Ann Rheum Dis*, 1979;38:36–9.
11. Bain L.S., Balch H.W., Wetherly J.M.R. Intraarticular triamcinolone hexacetonide: double-blind comparison with methylprednisolone. *Br J Clin Practice*, 1972;26:559–61.
12. Blyth T., Hunter J.A., Stirling A. Pain relief in the rheumatoid knee after steroid injection. A single-blind comparison of hydrocortisone succinate, and triamcinolone acetonide or hexacetonide. *Br J Rheumatol*, 1994;33:461–3.
13. Creamer P., Keen M., Zananiri F., Waterton J.C., Maciewicz R.A., Oliver C., et al.. Quantitative magnetic resonance imaging of the knee: a method of measuring response to intra-articular treatments. *Ann Rheum Dis*, 1997;56:378–81.
14. Leitch R., Walker S.E., Hillard A.E. The rheumatoid knee before and after arthrocentesis and prednisolone injection: evaluation by Gd-Enhanced MRI. *Clin Rheumatol*, 1996;15:358–66.
15. Eymontt M.J., Gordon G.V., Schumacher H.R., Hansell J.R. The effects on synovial permeability and synovial fluid leukocyte counts in symptomatic osteoarthritis after intraarticular corticosteroid administration. *J. Rheumatol*, 1982;9:198–203.
16. Goetzl E.J., Bianco N.E., Alpert J.S., Sledge C.B., Schur P.H. Effects of intra-articular corticosteroids *in vivo* on synovial fluid variables in rheumatoid synovitis. *Ann Rheum Dis*, 1974;33:62–6.
17. Luukkainen R., Hakala M., Sajanti E., Huhtala H., Yli-Kerttula U., Hameenkorpi R. Predictive value of synovial fluid analysis in estimating the efficacy of intra-articular corticosteroid injections in patients with rheumatoid arthritis. *Ann Rheum Dis*, 1992;51:874–6.
18. Taylor H.G., Fowler P.D., David M.J., Dawes P.T. Intra-articular steroids: confounder of clinical trials. *Clin Rheumatol*, 1991;10:38–42.
19. Armstrong R., English J., Gibson T., Chakraborty J., Marks V. Serum methylprednisolone levels following intra-articular injection of methylprednisolone acetate. *Ann Rheum Dis*, 1981;40:571–4.
20. Weiss S., Fischel B., Kisch E. Systemic effects of intra-articular steroid preparations. *Ann Rheum Dis*, 1980;39:413–6.
21. Shuster S., Williams I.A. Adrenal suppression due to intra-articular corticosteroid therapy. *Lancet*, 1961;2:171–2.
22. Weiss S., Kisch E.S., Fischel B. Systemic effects of intraarticular administration of triamcinolone hexacetonide. *Isr J Med Sci*, 1983;19:83–4.
23. Esselinckx W., Kolanowski J., Nagant de Deuxchaisness C.H. Adrenocortical function and responsiveness to tetracosactrin infusions after intra-articular treatment with triamcinolone acetonide and hydrocortisone acetate. *Clin Rheumatol*, 1982;1:176–7.
24. Koehler B.E., Urowitz M., Killinger D.W. The systemic effects of intra-articular corticosteroid. *J Rheumatol*, 1974;1:117–25.
25. Pattrick M., Doherty M. Facial flushing after intra-articular injection of steroid. *Br Med J*, 1987;295:1380.
26. Gottlieb N.L., Riskin W.G. Complications associated with locally injected microcrystalline corticosteroid esters. *JAMA*, 1980;243:1547.
27. Gray R.G., Tenenbaum J., Gottlieb N.L. Local corticosteroid injection treatment in rheumatic disorders. *Semin Arthritis Rheum*, 1981;10:231–54.
28. Salomon F., Levy L., Pinkhas J., Weinberger A., Gelber M. Intra-articular corticosteroid-induced peripheral leukocytosis. *Isr J Med Sci*, 1986;22:408–9.
29. Price R., Sinclair H., Heinrich I., Gibson T. Local injection treatment of tennis elbow—hydrocrotisone, triamcinolone and lignocaine compared. *Br J Rheumatol*, 1991;30:39–44.
30. Konttinen Y.T., Friman C., Tolvanen E., Reitamo S., Johansson E. Local skin rash after intraarticular methyl prednisolone acetate injection in a patient with rheumatoid arthritis. *Arthritis Rheum*, 1983;26:231–3.
31. Gray R.G., Poppp M. Comment on the article by Goldenberg. *Arthritis Rheum*, 1989;32:1487.
32. McCarty D.J. Joint sepsis: A choice for cure. *JAMA*, 1982;247:835.
33. Grayson M. Three infected injections from the same organism. *Br J Rheumatol*, 1998;37:592–3.
34. Von Essen R., Savolainen H.A. Bacterial infection following intra-articular injection. A brief review. *Scand J Rheumatol*, 1989;18:7–12.
35. Gladman D.D., Bombardier C. Sickle crisis following intraarticular steroid therapy for rheumatoid arthritis. *Arthritis Rheum*, 1987;30:1065–8.
36. Gray R.G., Gottlieb N.L. Intra-articular corticosteroids—an updated assessment. *Clin Orthop Rel Res*, 1983;177:235–63.
37. Hollander J.L. Intrasynovial corticosteroid therapy. In: *Arthritis and Allied conditions*. 7th edn. Philadelphia: Lea and Feibiger; 1966; pp. 381–98.
38. Jones A., Regan M., Ledingham J., Pattrick M., Manhire A., Doherty M. Importance of placement of intra-articular steroid injections. *Br Med J*, 1993;307:1329–30.
39. Haslock I., MacFarlane D, Speed C. Intra-articular and soft tissue injections: a survey of current practice. *Br J Rheumatol*, 1995;34:449–52.
40. Lanyon P., Regan M., Jones A., Doherty M. Inadvertent intra-articular injection of the wrong substance. *Br J Rheumatol*, 1997;36:812–3.
41. Cawley P.J., Morris I.M. A study to compare the efficacy of two methods of skin preparation prior to joint injection. *Br J Rheumatol*, 1992;31:847–8.
42. American College of Rheumatology Council on Rheumatological Care. *Safety Guidelines for Performing Arthrocentesis*, 1992.
43. Neustadt D.H. Treatment of rheumatoid joint inflammation with intrasynovial triamcinolone (letter). *J Rheumatol*, 1996;23:1666–7.
44. McCarty D.J., Dr McCarty replies. *J Rheumatol*, 1997;24:1850.
45. Chatham W., Williams G., Moreland L. Intraarticular corticosteroid injections: Should we rest the joints? *Arthritis Care Res*, 1989;2:70–4.
46. Neustadt D.H. Treatment of rheumatoid joint inflammation with intrasynovial triamcinolone (letter). Neustadt D.H.: (reply). *J Rheumatol*, 1997;24:1849–50.
47. Chakravarty K., Pharoah P.D.P., Scott D.G.I. A randomized controlled study of post-injection rest following intra-articular steroid therapy for knee synovitis. *Br J Rheumatol*, 1994;33:464–8.
48. Goldenberg D.L. Infectious arthritis complicating rheumatoid arthritis and other chronic rheumatic disorders. *Arthritis Rheum*, 1989;32:496–502.
49. Gupta M.N., Gemmell C., Kelly B., Sturrock R.D. Can the routine culture of synovial fluid be justified? *Br J Rheumatol*, 1998;37:798–9.

50. Pal B., Nash E.J., Oppenheim B., Maxwell S., McFarlane L. Routine synovial fluid (SF) culture: Is it necessary? Lessons from an audit. *Br J Rheumatol*, 1996;**35**:(suppl. 2):34.

51. Chandler G.N., Wright V. Deleterious effect of intra-articular hydrocortisone. *Lancet*, 1958;ii:661–3.

52. Keagy R.D., Keim H.A. Intra-articular steroid therapy: repeated use in patients with chronic arthritis. *Am J Med Sci*, 1967;**253**:45–51.

53. Bentley G., Goodfellow J.W. Disorganisation of the knees following intraarticular Hydrocortisone injection. *J Bone Jt Surg*, 1969;**51B**:498–502.

54. Steinberg C., Duthie R.B., Piva A.E. Charcot-like arthropthy following intraarticular hydrocortisone. *JAMA*, 1962;**181**:851–4.

55. McCarty D.J., McCarthy G., Carrera G. Intraarticular corticosteroids possibly leading to local osteonecrosis and marrow fat induced synovitis. *J Rheumatol*, 1991;**18**:1091–4.

56. Roberts W.N., Babcock E., Breitbach S., Owen D.S., Irby W.R. Corticosteroid injection in rheumatoid arthritis does not increase rate of total joint arthroplasty. *J Rheumatol*, 1996;**23**:1000–4.

57. Emkey R.D., Lindsay R., Lyssy J., Weisberg J.S., Dempster D.W., Shen V. The systemic effect of intraarticular administration of corticosteroid on markers of bone formation and bone resorption in patients with rheumatoid arthritis. *Arthritis Rheum*, 1996;**39**:277–82.

58. Salter R.B., Gross A., Hall J.H. Hydrocortisone arthropathy—an experimental investigation. *Canad Med Ass J*, 1967;**97**:374–7.

59. Moksowitz R.W., Davis W., Sommarco J., Mast W., Chase S.W. Experimentally induced corticosteroid arthropathy. *Arthritis Rheum*, 1970;**13**:236–43.

60. Butler M., Colombo C., Hickman L., O'Byrne E., Steele R., Steinetz B., *et al.* A new model of osteoarthritis in rabbits. *Arthritis Rheum*, 1983;**26**:1380–6.

61. Williams J.M., Brandt K.D. Triamcinolone Hexacetonide protects against fibrillation and osteophyte formation following chemically induced articular cartilage damage. *Arthritis Rheum*, 1985;**28**:1267–74.

62. Michelsson J.E., Juntunen S., Valtakari T. Methylprednisolone has a preventive effect on the development of radiological changes, thickening and stiffening of the rabbit knee following immobilization. *Clin Exp Rheumatol*, 1990;**8**:439–43.

63. Pelletier J., Mineau F., Raynauld J., Woessner J.F., Gunja-Smith Z., Martel-Pelletier J. Intraarticular injections with methylprednisolone acetate reduce osteoarthritic lesions in parallel with chondrocyte stromelysin synthesis in experimental osteoarthritis. *Arthritis Rheum*, 1994;**37**:414–23.

64. Pelletier J.P., Martel-Pelletier J., Cloutier J.M., Woessner J.F. Proteoglycan-degrading acid metalloprotease activity in human osteoarthritic cartilage, and the effect of intraarticular steroid injections. *Arthritis Rheum*, 1987;**30**:541–8.

65. Verschure P.J., van der Kraan P.M., Vitters E.L., van den Berg W.B. Stimulation of proteoglycan synthesis by triamcinolone acetonide and insulin-like growth factor 1 in normal and arthritic murine articular cartilage. *J Rheumatol*, 1994;**21**:920–6.

66. Hall G.H., Jones B.J.M., Head A.C., Jones V.E. Intra-articular methotrexate: Clinical and laboratory study in rheumatoid and psoriatic arthritis. *Am Rheum Dis*, 1978;**37**:351–6.

67. Blyth T., Stirling A., Coote J., Land D., Hunter J.A. Injection of the rheumatoid knee: Does intra-articular methotrexate or rifampicin add to the benefits of triamcinolone hexacetonide? *Br J Rheumatol*, 1998;**37**:770–2.

68. Caruso I., Montrone F., Fumagalli M., Patrono C., Santandrea S., Gandini M.C. Rheumatoid knee synovitis successfully treated with intra-articular rifamycin SV. *Ann Rheum Dis*, 1982;**41**:232–6.

69. Gevers G., Dequeker J., Van Holsbeeck M., Van vliet-Daskalopoulou E. A high dose (up to 200 mg) tolerance and efficacy study of intra-articular rimexolone (Org 6216) in rheumatoid synovitis of the knee. *Clin Rheumatol*, 1994;**13**:103–9.

70. Coari G., Franco D.I., Iagnocco A., DiNovi M.R., Mauceri M.T., Ciocci A. Intra-articular somatostatin 14 reduces synovial thickness in rheumatoid arthritis: an ultrasonographic study. *Int J Clin Pharm*, 1995;**15**:27–32.

71. Goto M., Hosoko Y., Katayama M., Yamada T. Biochemical analysis of rheumatoid synovial fluid after serial intra-articular injection of high molecular weight sodium hyaluronate. *Int J Clin Pharm*, 1993;**13**:161–6.

27 | *Combination therapy for rheumatoid arthritis*

Philip G. Conaghan and Peter M. Brooks

Introduction

It is now well recognized that rheumatoid arthritis (RA) causes significant morbidity and mortality, with 50 per cent of RA patients having significant impairment of work capacity 10 years after diagnosis[1,2,3]. It is also clear from early arthritis clinics that, once the disease has been established with persisting synovitis of over 3 months duration, it is unusual for remission to occur spontaneously or with drug therapy[4,5]. Recent magnetic resonance imaging data in early RA has demonstrated more extensive bony damage than has been appreciated with conventional radiography[6].

These facts have given rise to the concept that the management of RA should be approached as a medical emergency and that aggressive therapy needs to be commenced at the earliest possible stage[7]. The prescribing practices of rheumatologists vary considerably but over the last few years there has been a significant shift to early use of disease modifying antirheumatic drugs (DMARDs)[8] although the majority of rheumatologists would commence with single agents rather than using these drugs in combination[9].

Over the last decade the strategy for management of rheumatoid arthritis has also changed with suggestions for the 'step-down' approach[10], where more potent drugs are used initially to dampen down inflammation and synovitis and then withdrawn, or the 'sawtooth' approach[11] where goals are set *a priori* in terms of inflammation control and the patient is reviewed at frequent intervals from the perspective of achieving those goals.

An increasing number of DMARDs have now been shown to retard the progression of erosions in RA and can reduce progression of disability[12]. These drugs and their proposed mechanisms of action are shown in Table 27.1. However the poor results obtained in terms of remission for individual agents, and the lessons learned from oncological therapies, have led to the search for effective combination therapies in RA.

The rationale for combination therapy

Research on the etiopathogenesis of joint destruction in RA has defined, to a very large extent, the multiplicity of interacting cells and mediators that result in joint destruction (Fig. 27.1) and with these interacting pathways it is unlikely that one single agent, unless directed specifically at the triggering mechanism

Table 27.1 Mechanism of action

Drug	Mechanism of action
Antimalarials	Inhibitis lysosomal enzymes
	Inhibits PMNs and lymphocytes (*in vitro*)
	Inhibits IL-1 release (*in vivo*)
	Inhibits T cell proliferation
Sulfasalazine	Inhibits PMN migration
	Reduces lymphocyte responses
	Inhibits angiogenesis
	Inhibits synovial cell proliferation
Gold	Inhibits PMN function
	Inhibitis of T and B cell activity
	Inhibits macrophage activation (*in vitro*)
D-penicillamine	Inhibits neovascularization (*in vitro*)
	Inhibits PMN myeloperoxidase
	Scavenges free radicals
	Inhibits T cell function
	Impairs antigen presentation
	Inhibits protease
Corticosteroids	Increases lipocortin levels leading to inhibition of phosphilipase A$_2$
	Reduces cytokine production
	Inhibits Fc receptor expression
	Suppresses lymphocyte function
	Redistributes circulating leukocytes
	Inhibits transcription factors
Methotrexate	Decreases thymidilate synthetase activity and subsequent DNA synthesis
	Diminishes PMN chemotaxis
Azathioprine	Interferes with DNA synthesis
	Inhibits lymphocyte proliferation
Cyclophosphamide	Crosslinks DNA leading to cell death
	Decreases circulating T and B cells
Chlorambucil	Similar to cyclophosphamide
Cyclosporin	Blocks synthesis/release of IL-1 and IL-2

PMN = polymorphonuclear leukocyte

for the disease, will significantly dampen down the pathological process. The rationale for using combinations of DMARDs is that, by using drugs which have a different mechanism of action and, in particular, a different side-effect profile, it might be possible to have additive or synergistic effects on efficacy without an increase in adverse events.

Another reason for using combination therapy is that it might slow the development of so-called drug resistance. It is clear from long-term drug studies that a significant number of patients with RA, who are initially controlled on a DMARD or combination of DMARDs, will then have a flare of their disease despite initial control[13]. Studies from the cancer literature have demonstrated the

Cytokine Network

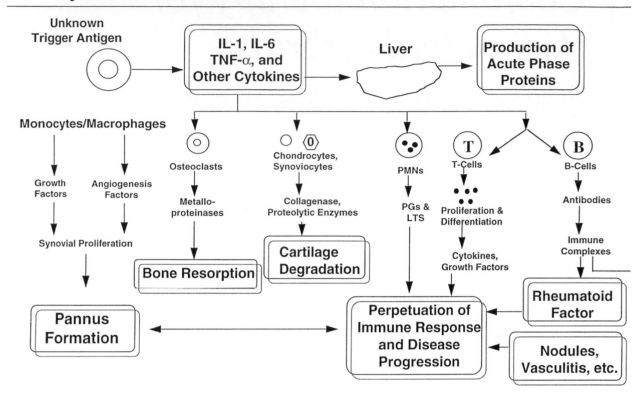

Fig. 27.1 The pathogenetic mechanisms of joint destruction in rheumatoid arthritis (RA).

development of drug resistance to anticancer agents as being associated with the generation of the P-glycoprotein, a cell membrane pump which rapidly transports anticancer drugs out of tumor cells thus reducing their effect[14]. Whether 'drug resistance' in RA is associated with an increase in P-glycoprotein is not known but a number of antirheumatic drugs including cyclosporin and chloroquine have been shown to competitively inhibit the efflux function of P-glycoproteins[15]. This inhibition blocks tumor necrosis factor α (TNFα) release by macrophages, TNFα activation of natural killer (NK) cells, and NK cell secretion of cytotoxins within the rheumatoid joint[15,16]. Corticosteroids also induced an increase in P-glycoprotein expression in a cell line suggesting that corticosteroid resistance may be explained by P-glycoprotein efflux function[17]. Salmon and Dalton[16] have hypothesized that the use of a DMARD which has an effect on the P-glycoprotein function (such as cyclosporin and antimalarials) together with drugs that are not subject to P-glycoprotein efflux (such as methotrexate) might provide added benefit in RA and this may be reflected in clinical trials using these agents (see below).

Designing rational combination therapies

Our limited knowledge on the mechanism of action of most DMARDs hampers rational combination design. The toxicities of all agents are well described and should be taken into account, although again the mechanism for many of these adverse reactions is not known. Potential pharmacokinetic interactions between DMARD drug combinations should also be considered in trial design. Investigation should be carried out at an early stage to ensure that there is no significant increase in the concentration of any drug in a given combination. If so, this needs to be incorporated into the study design as it may be more appropriate to test two dosages of a single drug against the combination. These interactions are particularly important for drugs that might interfere with renal function. The rationale for combinations in terms of mechanism, pharmacokinetics, and toxicity has recently been summarized[18] and pharmacokinetic data for the commonly used DMARDs is shown in Table 27.2.

Cost effective issues need to be considered since use of combination therapy may be associated with an increase in the frequency or type of safety monitoring that is required. These cost issues need to be considered particularly if only small gains are obtained with a combination treatment over single agents. For example cyclosporin and methotrexate combination therapy (reviewed below) may provide benefits; but the cost of increased monitoring, potential for adverse drug reactions (due to renal dysfunction[19]), and potential for cardiovascular complications (due to hypertension) in a group with higher cardiovascular mortality[20] may be significant.

The data from *in vitro* and animal model studies should also be considered in combination therapy design, and these will be briefly discussed before looking at combination therapies reported in clinical trials.

Table 27.2 Kinetics of antirheumatic drugs

	AZA[a]	CSA	DPA	GST	HCQ	MTX
Bioavailability (%)		20–50	50–70	> 95	74	70
Tissue binding (%)			3+*		4+	3+
Serum protein building (%)	70	90		> 90	40–60	50
Renal clearance (%)			47	30–60	20	30–80
Biliary clearance (%)		94	35			3–23
Hepatic clearance	2+*		3+		4+	3+(H)

a AZA – azathioprine; CSA – cyclosporin A; DPA – D-penicillamine; GST – gold sodium thiomalate; HCQ – hydroxychloroquine; MTX – methotrexate; SSZ = sulfasalazine.
* on a qualitative scale of 04+, where '0' = none, 4+ is 'major effect'.
H = hydroxylation.
Adapted from Furst[18].

Table 27.3 Drug combinations in animal models

		Efficacy	
Drug or combination	Animal model	Single agent	Combination
Cyclosporin			
+ Methotrexate	CIA	–	
+ Calcitriol	AA	–	+
+ AGM-1470	CIA	+	
AGM-1470			
+ Anti CD5 Mono	CIA	–	
+ Taxol	CIA	–	

AA = Adjuvant Arthritis; CIA = Collagen-induced Arthritis. From: Oliver and Brahne[24].

Using drug combinations in vitro

A number of *in vitro* systems have been used to study the effect of drug combinations. Danis *et al.*[21] examined the effects of a variety of DMARD combinations on the production of interleukin-1 (IL-1) and TNFα by purified human monocytes stimulated with the cytokines granulocyte-macrophage colony stimulating factor and IFN-γ. In this system the inhibition of IL-1 and TNFα production was seen with many DMARDs although there were individual differences. Interestingly, combinations of gold sodium thiomalate plus auranofin, and hydroxychloroquine plus sulfasalazine were extremely effective at suppressing cytokine production although other combinations were not so effective. In another study by this group[22], chloroquine was shown to decrease the inhibition of pokeweed mitrogen stimulated blast formation of monocytes that was induced by D-penicillamine—suggesting that this particular combination would not be useful. In a recent study of IFN-γ-production by CD4+ and CD8+ T cell clones, the combination of chloroquine and cyclosporin were found to synergistically inhibit production[23].

These data would suggest that certain combinations of DMARDs might be particularly useful in inhibiting the inflammatory responses in RA but further work needs to be done to establish whether *in vitro* assays can predict subsequent clinical response.

Using drug combinations in animal models

Despite the fact that animal models of inflammation have significantly influenced the development of DMARDs for use in man, few studies have been carried out using combinations of these drugs[24]. The combinations of antirheumatic and other drugs used in animal models are shown in Table 27.3. In the collagen-induced arthritis rodent model, low doses of cyclosporin A do not significantly affect the disease process although when combined with low doses of methotrexate significant reduction in inflammation and joint damage is seen[25]. A combination of cyclosporin and calcitriol has again been shown to be suppressive of inflammation in the adjuvant arthritis model when both drugs used singly have little effect (and in fact may promote inflammation)[26]. Studies with novel agents such as a potent angiogenesis inhibitor in combination with an anti-CD5 (pan-T cell) monoclonal antibody or taxol (a microtubule-stabilizing drug that has potential effects on cell mitosis and migration) have also demonstrated that combinations are more effective than single agents in a collagen-induced arthritis model[27–29].

Although it is often difficult to extrapolate the results of treatment of animal models to man, they may provide a useful screening milieu in which single drugs and combinations can be tested to see whether drug synergy is obtained.

Evaluating combination therapies in clinical trials

Rheumatologists have been using combinations of antirheumatic drugs since 1963[30]. Subsequent randomized studies have failed to produce the impressive evidence seen in uncontrolled studies and the continuing publication of underpowered, non-randomized, and non-blinded studies has only confused the data base. Trials of combination therapy have usually been either poorly designed or underpowered[31,32]. Felson *et al.*[32] found only five studies up to the time of their review in 1994 that fulfilled strict criteria for study size, appropriate drug doses, and outcome measurements.

Trial design issues in the use of combination therapy in RA have been summarized[33] and include the problems of:

(1) the choice of controls, trial design, and sufficient patients to ensure a fair comparison between therapies;

(2) the issue of safety assessment as well as efficacy;

(3) the problems of maintaining blinding over a significant period of time.

One of the major difficulties in evaluating combination therapies has been that the differences between DMARDs in their ability to slow erosions may not be very great. Although the issues of outcome assessment in RA have now been addressed to a large extent with the development of the OMERACT core

Table 27.4 Combination therapy in rheumatoid arthritis: randomized, double-blind trials

Reference	Combination	No. of patients	Results
Trnavsky et al. (1993)[40]	Methotrexate and hydroxycholroquine	40	Combination more effective for some outcomes
Ferraz et al. (1994)[41]	Methotrexate and chloroquine	82	Combination more effective for some outcomes
Clegg et al. (1997)[42]	Methotrexate and hydroxychloroquine	121	Combination more effective, using flare of RA as the outcome measure
Tugwell et al. (1995)[45]	Methotrexate and cyclosporin	148	Combination more effective
Haasgsma et al. (1997)[51]	Methotrexate and sulfasalazine	105	No advantage to combination in early RA
Williams et al. (1992)[52]	Methotrexate and auranofin	335	No advantage to combination. More withdrawals with combination due to side-effects
Willkens et al. (1992)[54]	Methotrexate and azathioprine	209	Combination and methotrexate alone superior to azathioprine alone
O'Dell et al. (1996)[58]	Methotrexate, hydroxychloroquine and sulfasalazine	102	Triple combination more effective than sulfasalazine plus hydroxychloroquine or methotrexate alone
Boers et al. (1997)[60]	Methotrexate, sulfasalazine and prednisolone	155	Combination more effective
Scott et al. (1989)[61]	Gold and hydroxychloroquine	101	Combination more effective than gold alone
Porter et al. (1993)[63]	Gold and hydroxychloroquine	142	No advantage to combination
Corkill et al. (1990)[65]	Gold and methylprednisolone	59	No advantage after cessation of corticosteroids
Van Gestel et al. (1990)[66]	Gold and prednisolone	40	No advantage after cessation of corticosteroids
Ciconelli et al. (1996)[67]	Sulfasalazine and methylprednisolone	38	No advantage after cessation of corticosteroids
Faarvang et al. (1993)[70]	Sulfasalazine and hydroxychloroquine	91	No advantage to combination over sulfasalazine alone
Bunch et al. (1984)[71]	D-penicillamine and hydroxychloroquine	56	Combination not as effective as D-penicillamine
Moreland et al. (1995)[74]	Methotrexate and anti-CD4 monoclonal	64	No advantage to combination over methotrexate alone

set[34], careful definition and detection of erosions at an early stage remains difficult. The duration of the study is also important since small differences in the slowing of erosion rates may only be detectable over a 1 to 2-year period.

The published trials of combination therapy have also been critically reviewed by a number of authors[35–39].

Published trials of combination therapies in rheumatoid arthritis

For the purposes of this review we have selected published reports of clinical trials of drug combinations in RA, based on a MEDLINE database review. Reports in abstract form only and articles where an English translation were not available have not been included. Some reports with small patient numbers and open design have also been omitted. The randomized, controlled trials and their outcomes are summarized in Table 27.4. This list of trials is similar to that selected by Verhoeven et al.[39] in their recent combination therapy analysis, further indicative of the relatively small number of good combination studies.

Many of the more recent trials have used DMARD combinations that include methotrexate, reflecting the increased popularity of this agent in the last decade.

Drug combinations that include methotrexate therapy

Methotrexate has been studied in combination with antimalarials, cyclosporin, sulfasalazine, oral gold, azathioprine, and in multiple drug combinations.

Methotrexate and antimalarials

Trnavsky et al.[40] studied 40 patients on hydroxychloroquine 200 mg and either methotrexate 7.5 mg or placebo. This 6 months, double-blind study demonstrated significant improvement in patient global assessment and erythrocyte sedimentation rate (ESR) in the combination group. In a double-blind study of 82 RA patients, Ferraz et al.[41] randomized subjects to either methotrexate 7.5 mg or methotrexate and chloroquine 250 mg. Again there was no dose escalation for methotrexate. At 6 months of combination group had significant reduction in tender joint counts and significant improvement in grip strength and functional assessment as measured by the Health Assessment Questionnaire. Early morning stiffness, patient pain, and ESR were not significantly different. Clegg et al.[42] reported an interesting study where 121 patients who had responded to a combination of methotrexate and hydroxychloroquine in an open label study were then randomized blindly to one of three treatments. Forty patients continued on hydroxychloroquine with pulse methotrexate for a flare(Group 1), 41 patients continued on hydroxychloroquine with placebo pulse for a flare (Group 2), and 40 patients were randomized to placebo with pulse methotrexate for a flare (Group 3). Half of the patients in Groups 1 and 3 flared within 8 weeks of randomization. Of those not flaring in the first 8 weeks, 61 per cent of Group 1, 72 per cent of Group 2, but only 21 per cent of Group 3 remained 'flare free' for the duration of the study (36 weeks). 'Flares' seen in Group 2 were also much longer lasting than those seen in Groups 1 and 3. In summary, patients improved on a combination of methotrexate and hydroxychloroquine while maintenance of hydroxychloroquine delayed the onset and seemed to shorten the duration of flares when methotrexate was discontinued.

Seideman et al.[43] demonstrated a reduced bioavailability of methotrexate in RA patients using methotrexate and chloroquine which might explain the observation that patients on this combination have a lower incidence of liver function abnormalities[44].

Methotrexate and cyclosporin

Tugwell *et al.*[45] conducted a 6-month, randomized trial of cyclosporin (2.5–5 mg/kg body weight/day) and methotrexate (at maximal tolerated dose) in patients who were partial responders to methotrexate. Patients were randomized to receive cyclosporin or placebo and continue their methotrexate. A high proportion of each treatment group had received multiple DMARDs previously and approximately 80 per cent in each group were on prednisone. At the end of the 6-month period the combination group had a net improvement in tender joint count of 25 per cent and three times the number (36 patients) on the combined regimen fulfilled ACR 20 per cent improvement criteria than on placebo (12 patients). Of note, serum creatinine concentrations increased significantly in those patients on cyclosporin. A later report from this study[46] demonstrated no increase in the frequency of abnormal liver function tests in the 6 months of the trial. The same group recently reported an open, extension study[47] That found the improvement rates in the original combination group were maintained, while adding cyclosporin to the original methotrexate and placebo group resulted in similar clinical improvement rates. Given the known renal excretion of N-methotrexate it is likely that cyclosporin influences methotrexate kinetics, possibly increasing methotrexate concentrations. If this is so then the relatively small improvement with cyclosporin should be weighed against the significant potential for increased cardiovascular morbidity of this combination.

Methotrexate and sulfasalazine

There was some concern that this combination of two agents with antifolate activity may lead to increased toxicity. In a retrospective review of 32 patients treated with a combination of methotrexate and salazopyrin, Nisar *et al.*[48] showed that the combination of methotrexate and salazopyrin was well tolerated in comparison to methotrexate alone. Other small studies demonstrated similar safety with the combination[49].

A Dutch group has published interesting and conflicting results using the combination, reflecting different study designs and perhaps the different RA patient groups. Haasgsma *et al.*[50] studied the addition of methotrexate (7.5 to 15 mg/week) to patients not responding to 3 g of sulfasalazine. In a 24-week, unblinded study, patients continued on 2 g daily of sulfasalazine alone or in combination with 7.5–15 mg weekly of methotrexate. At study completion the combination appeared superior to methotrexate in terms of efficacy and had comparable toxicity. This study did address pharmacokinetic issues and demonstrated no change in methotrexate kinetics in a small subset of patients. However, this group of researchers subsequently studied early (less than 12 months symptom duration) RA patients randomized to methotrexate, sulfasalazine, or the combination in a parallel design using similar dose ranges to the previous study[51]. This 12-month, double-blind study failed to demonstrate an advantage for the combination over single agents, using the Disease Activity Score as outcome measure.

Methotrexate and auranofin

The effect of combining auranofin and methotrexate was investigated in a well conducted, double-blind, randomized study comparing 6 mg per day auranofin, 7.5 mg per week methotrexate, and a third group given the combination[52]. The study duration was 48 weeks and there was no dose escalation for either agent. There were no statistical differences in response for clinical and laboratory variables between the groups. Withdrawals because of lack of efficacy were less frequent in the combination group who also, however, had more terminations due to adverse events. A later report from this study[53] found progression of erosions and joint space narrowing in hand/wrist radiographs in all three groups, although this reached significance only in the auranofin treated group.

Methotrexate and azathioprine

Willkens *et al.*[54] compared azathioprine, methotrexate and a lower dose combination of each in 209 patients followed for 24 weeks. Combination therapy and methotrexate alone were slightly better than azathioprine alone although the differences were not large. The same group reported the 48 week follow-up of this study and again there was no advantage with the combination, but more withdrawals due to adverse events in the combination and azathioprine groups[55]. There was also no significant difference between groups in radiological progression reported at 48 weeks.

Methotrexate and multiple drug combinations

McCarty[56] was one of the first to report treatment of rheumatoid arthritis patients with multiple therapies, in a small-number report using a combination of azathioprine, hydroxychloroquine, and cyclophosphamide. This report represented the experience of a single rheumatologist, and methotrexate was substituted for cyclophosphamide in this combination during the 1980s. Recent uncontrolled follow-up[57] of a large group of patients treated with this combination demonstrated an impressive response with complete remission being achieved in 43 per cent of patients and a low incidence of side-effects.

In an important 2-year, double-blind, randomized study. compared methotrexate alone (7.5 to 17.5 mg/week), sulfasalazine (1 g daily) plus hydroxychloroquine (400 mg/daily), or all three drugs.[58] The primary endpoints of the study were 50 per cent improvement in composite symptoms of arthritis and no evidence of drug toxicity. Fifty of 102 patients had a 50 per cent improvement at 9 months and maintained at least that degree of improvement for the 2-year period. Of these 'responders', 24 of 31 were treated with the three drug combination, 12 of 36 treated with methotrexate alone, and 14 of 35 were treated with sulfasalazine and hydroxychloroquine. A slightly higher number of patients (seven) in the methotrexate group discontinued treatment because of drug toxicity. A later report from this study group[59] looked at all the patients who had suboptimal response to single drug therapy in the previous protocol and treated them with the triple combination. This open-label study demonstrated a significant improvement in all patients, with greater improvement in the sulfasalazine–hydroxychloroquine suboptimal responders.

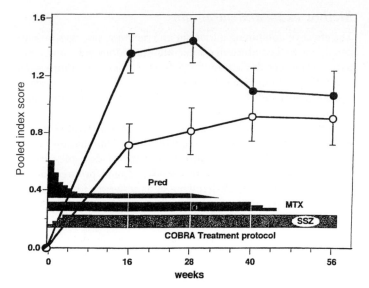

Fig. 27.2 Methotrexate, prednisolone, and sulfasalazine combination and sulfasalazine alone in rheumatoid arthritis (Boers *et al.*, 1997). Open circles—sulfasalazine alone; close circles—combination.

Boers *et al.*[60] recently conducted an interesting multicenter study using an initial high-dose prednisolone combination regimen in early RA. This double-blind, randomized controlled trial compared a combination of sulfasalazine (2 g daily), methotrexate (7.5 mg weekly) and prednisolone reducing from an initial dose of 60 mg daily to 7.5 mg daily after 6 weeks, with sulfasalazine alone. The study enrolled 155 patients with early rheumatoid arthritis, with median duration of 4 months. The primary outcome measure was a pooled index derived by weighting the change scores of five variables: tender joint count, independent observer assessment, grip strength, ESR, and the McMaster Toronto arthritis questionnaire. The drug regimen is shown in Fig. 27.2 along with the clinical outcomes; note that prednisolone and methotrexate were tapered and stopped at 28 and 40 weeks respectively. At week 28 the mean pooled index in the combined treatment group was significantly higher than in the sulfasalazine group, with 72 per cent of the combined group improving according to ACR criteria in contrast to 49 per cent in the sulfasalazine group. However, the difference between the groups was only maintained while prednisolone was given. At 28 weeks the radiographic damage score had increased by a median of one in the combined therapy group and four in the sulfasalazine group—again this was a statistically significant difference. These differences in radiographic scores remained throughout the duration of the trial (80 weeks).

Drug combinations that include parenteral gold therapy

In a recent, parenteral gold therapy (sodium aurothiomalate) was compared with a combination of gold plus hydroxychloroquine[61]. Patients with an average disease duration of 2 years were randomized to receive hydroxychloroquine or placebo in addition to their gold treatment. Hydroxychloroquine dosage was 400 mg daily for 6 months followed by 200 mg for the following 6 months as well as background NSAIDs and analgesics. Significantly more patients in the combined group developed side-effects (particularly rash) but more patients withdrew from gold therapy than from the combination therapy because of lack of benefit. There were statistically significant benefits in overall disease activity and C-reactive protein levels in those patients completing the 12 months of combination therapy.

A number of studies have added a combination agent to patients having inadequate response to parenteral gold therapy. In a small open study, D-penicillamine, chlorambucil, or levamisole was added to patients with inadequate response to 12 months of gold therapy and found the best response rate in the gold–penicillamine combination.[62,63] studied the combination of hydroxychloroquine and intramuscular gold in 142 patients who had a suboptimal response to 6 months of intramuscular gold therapy. Patients continued gold and were randomized to receive either hydroxychloroquine 400 mg daily or placebo, and followed for a 6-month period. No significant differences between treatments were seen in terms of either efficacy or toxicity. Another study looked at patients with inadequate response after at least 6 months of aurothiomalate therapy and randomized them to the addition of cyclosporin or placebo[64]. This 6-month, double-blind study of 40 patients demonstrated a statistical improvement in the patients overall health assessment score in the combination group, but no other between-group differences for clinical and laboratory variables.

Two groups used step-down protocols in looking at the combination of corticosteroids at induction of parenteral gold therapy in patients with established disease. One randomized 59 patients to three doses of intramuscular methylprednisolone 120 mg or placebo at monthly intervals while starting sodium aurothiomalate therapy and followed the groups for 24 weeks[65]. Van Gestel *et al.* looked at 40 patients starting aurothioglucose and randomized to oral prednisolone (starting at 10 mg/day and dose reduced until ceased at week 19 to 20) or placebo and followed for 44 weeks[66]. Both studies found significant improvement in outcome markers in the combination groups while corticosteroids were used, but at the end of both studies there was no difference between the combination and single agent groups. In the latter study, there was also no difference in radiological progression.

Other drug combinations

Corticosteroids have also been used as additive therapy at commencement of sulfasalazine treatment. 38 refractory RA patients were treated with standard doses of sulfasalazine and randomized to intravenous methylprenisolone (5 mg/kg each month for 3 months) or placebo.[67] After 6 months this double-blind study failed to demonstrate any difference between treatment groups.

Trials involving sulfasalazine and D-penicillamine have been small-number, open studies. Taggart *et al.*[68] assessed the combination versus sulfasalazine alone in 30 patients. Their data suggested a small benefit of combination treatment over sulfasalazine alone, with nine responders in the combination group and six in the single agent group. However there were twice as many withdrawals in the combination group. Farr et al.[69] demonstrated that D-penicillamine in a dose of 125–1000 mg/day or aurothiomalate produced a favorable response in over 70 per cent of patients when added to established sulfasalazine treatment (1.5–3.0 g daily). A third of patients discontinued gold and d-penicillamine because of side-effects.

Faarvang et al.[70] conducted a 6-month, randomized, double-blind study comparing sulfasalazine and hydroxychloroquine alone and in combination in 91 patients. Although the combination resulted in more rapid response and was significantly better than hydroxychloroquine alone for some clinical variables, there was no difference between the combination and sulfasalazine alone. Radiographic progression was similar for all groups.

Combinations of antimalarials and D-penicillamine have also been studied. Bunch et al.[71] reported a 2-year, randomized, double-blind, comparison of hydroxychloroquine, D-penicillamine, and a combination of both in 56 RA patients with an average duration of disease of over 6 years. The combination group did not improve as much as the penicillamine-alone group, although toxic events were less frequent in the combination group than in the penicillamine-alone group. Another group compared chloroquine, D-penicillamine, and a combination of both in a randomized, non-blinded study with 72 patients.[72] At the end of 12 months no significant differences were seen between the patient groups in terms of efficacy although adverse events and withdrawals due to side-effects were significantly more frequent in the combination therapy group. Radiological progression was more marked in the chloroquine-alone group.

Drug combinations involving biological agents

The role of biological agents in the treatment of RA is as yet unclear, but a number of therapies look promising[73]. Combination therapies involving DMARDs and biologics remain preliminary. Moreland et al. added three different doses of a T-cell depleting anti-CD4 monoclonal antibody to RA patients using methotrexate.[74] Sixty-four patients with refractory disease were randomized in this double-blind study but there were no differences in outcome measures after 3 months. There has been a promising report of methotrexate in combination with an anti-TNF monoclonal antibody (cA2) that suggested not only a benefit in clinical outcome measures for the combination, but a methotrexate-related reduction in antiglobulin response[75]. As well, there is potential for biological combination therapies, although these too remain experimental at present[76].

Conclusions

Felson et al.[77] have reported the patient numbers required to detect differences in efficacy between antirheumatic drugs used to treat RA (Table 27.5). Obviously the trial size in excess of 3000 patients needed to achieve the appropriate statistical power to detect a clinically important difference between single

Table 27.5   Numbers required in trials to detect differences in efficacy between antirheumatic drugs used to treat rheumatoid arthritis

	Actual differences in efficacy (Standardized effect units)				
	0.1	0.2	0.3	0.4	0.5
2 Drug comparison					
No. per drug	1500	400	170	96	62
No. per trial	3000	800	340	192	124
3 Drug comparison					
No. per drug	1300	325	143	80	52
No. per trial	3900	975	429	240	156

Power = 80% α = 0.05 (2 tailed). From: Felson et al.[77].

drugs and combination therapy is impractical[78]. Careful attention to trial design, however, could improve the data base on these combinations considerably. Editors of medical journals should adopt clear principles for the publication of all clinical trials but particularly those on combination therapy in rheumatoid arthritis[79]. These should include:

(1)   adequate numbers;

(2)   appropriate design including randomization;

(3)   an indication of consideration of pharmacokinetic interactions; and

(4)   an indication of cost benefit of the combined therapy.

Many important questions remain unanswered concerning combination therapy, despite the studies presented. Which are the best combinations and how early should they be commenced? Should all patients with early RA receive combination therapy, or should we target those with poor prognostic markers? After an excellent response, should drugs be tapered or discontinued?

It is time for rheumatologists to establish large multicenter trials with appropriate numbers of patients to clearly demonstrate one way or the other the benefits of combination therapies.

References

1.   Wolfe F., Mitchell D.M., Sibley J.T., Fries J.F., Bloch D.A., Williams C.A., et al. The mortality of rheumatoid arthritis. *Arthritis Rheum*, 1994;**37**:481–94.

2.   Yelin E., Henke C., Epstein W.V. The work dynamics of the person with rheumatoid arthritis. *Arthritis Rheum*, 1987;**30**:507–12.

3.   Yelin E., Callahan L. The economic cost and social and psychological impact of musculoskeletal conditions. *Arthritis Rheum*, 1995;**38**:1351–62.

4.   Eberhardt K.B., Rydgen L.C., Petterson H., Wollheim F.A. Early rheumatoid arthritis: onset, course and outcome over two years. *Rheumatol Int*, 1990;**10**:135–42.

5.   Mottonen T., Paimela L., Ahonen J., Helve T., Hannonen P., Leirisalo-Repo M. Outcome in patients with early rheumatoid arthritis treated according to the 'sawtooth' strategy. *Arthritis Rheum*, 1996;**39**:996–1005.

6.   McGonagle D., Gibbon W., Green M., Proudman S., O'Connor P., Emery P. A longitudinal MR study of bone changes of the MCP joints in early rheumatoid arthritis [abstract]. *Arthritis Rheum*, 1997;**40**:S246.

7. Emery P. The optimal management of early rheumatoid disease: the key to preventing disability. *Br J Rheumatol*, 1994;**33**:765–8.

8. Conaghan P.G., Crotty M., Oh E.S., Day R.O., Brooks P.M. Antirheumatic drug prescribing behaviour of Australasian Rheumatologists 1984–1994. *Br J Rheumatol*, 1997;**36**:487–90.

9. Galindo-Rodriguez G., Avina-Zubieta J.A., Fitzgerald A., LeClerq S.A., Russell A.S., Suarez-Almazor M.E. Variations and trends in the prescription of initial second-line therapy for patients with rheumatoid arthritis. *J Rheumatol*, 1997;**24**:633–8.

10. Wilske K.R., Healey L.A. Challenging the therapeutic pyramid: a new look at treatment strategies for rheumatoid arthritis. *J Rheumatol*, 1990;**17**(Suppl 25):4–7.

11. Fries J.F. Evaluating the therapeutic approach to rheumatoid arthritis: the 'sawtooth' strategy. *J Rheumatol*, 1990;**22**(Suppl):12–5.

12. Fries J.F., Williams C.A., Morefeld D., Singh G., Sibley J. Reduction in long-term disability in patients with rheumatoid arthritis by disease modifying antirheumatic drug-based treatment strategies. *Arthritis Rheum*, 1996;**36**:616–22.

13. Wolfe F. The epidemiology of drug treatment failure in rheumatoid arthritis. *Baillière's Clin Rheumatol*, 1995;**9**:619–32.

14. Shulstik C., Dalton W., Gros P. P-glycoprotein-mediated multidrug resistance in tumour cells: biochemistry, clinical relevance and modulation. *Molec Aspects Med*, 1995;**16**:1–78.

15. Klimecki W.T., Taylor C.W., Dalton W.S. Inhibition of cell-mediated cytolysis and P-glycoprotein function in natural killer cells by verapamil isomers and cyclosporin A analogs. *J Clin Immunol*, 1995;**15**:152–8.

16. Salmon S.E., Dalton W.S. Relevance of multidrug resistance to rheumatoid arthritis: development of a new therapeutic hypothesis. *J Rheumatol*, 1996;**23**(Suppl 44):97–101.

17. Bourgeoi S., Gruol D.J., Newby B.R.F., Rajah F.M. Expression of an MDR gene is associated with a new form of resistance to dexamethasone-induced apoptosis. *Mol Endocrinol*, 1993;**7**:840–51.

18. Furst D.E. Clinical pharmacology of combination DMARD therapy in rheumatoid arthritis. *J Rheumatol*, 1996;**23**(Suppl 44):86–90.

19. Chaudhuri K., Torley H., Madhok R. Cyclosporin. *Br J Rheumatol*, 1997;**36**:1016–21.

20. Wålleberg-Johnson S., Öhman M., Dahlquest S.R. Cardiovascular morbidity and mortality in patients with seropositive rheumatoid arthritis in Northern Sweden. *J Rheumatol*, 1997;**24**:445–51.

21. Danis V.A., Franic G.M., Brooks P.M. The effect of slow acting antirheumatic drugs (SAARDs) and combinations of SAARDs on monokine production in vitro. *Drugs Exptl Clin Res*, 1991;**17**:549–54.

22. Danis V.A., Kulesz A.J., Nelson D.S., Brooks P.M. Cytokine regulation of human monocyte interleukin-1 production in vitro. Enhancement of IL-1 production by interferon-γ, tumour necrosis factor γ, IL-2 and IL-1 and inhibition by interferon-alpha. *Clin Exp Immunol*, 1990;**8**:435–43.

23. Landewe R.B.M., Miltenburg A.M.M., Breedfeld F.C., Daha M.R., Dijkmans B.A.C. Cyclosporin and chloroquine synergistically inhibit the interferon-gamma production by CD4 positive and CD8 positive synovial T cell clones derived form a patient with rheumatoid arthritis. *J Rheumatol*, 1992;**19**:1353–7.

24. Oliver S.J., Brahn E. Combination therapy in rheumatoid arthritis. The animal model perspective. *J Rheumatology*, 1996;**23**(Suppl 44):56–60.

25. Brahn E., Peacock D.J., Banquerigo M.L. Suppression of collagen-induced arthritis by combination cyclosporin A and methotrexate therapy. *Arthritis Rheum*, 1991;**34**:1282–8.

26. Boissier M.C., Chioccha G., Fournier C. Combination of cyclosporin A and calcitriol in the treatment of adjuvant arthritis. *J Rheumatol*, 1992;**19**:754–7.

27. Oliver S.J., Cheng T.P., Banquerigo M.L., Brahn E. Suppression of collagen-induced arthritis by an angiogenesis inhibitor, AGM-1470, in combination with cyclosporin reduction of vascular endothelial growth factor (VEGF). *Cell Immunol*, 1995;**166**:196–206.

28. Peacock D.J., Banquerigo M.L., Brahn E. An angiogenesis inhibitor in combination with anti-CD5 Mab suppresses estab-lished collagen-induced arthritis significantly more than single agent therapy [abstract]. *Arthritis Rheum*, 1992;**35**:S140.

29. Oliver S.J., Banquerigo M.L., Brahn E. Suppression of collagen-induced arthritis using an angiogenesis inhibitor AGM 1470, and a microtubule stabilizer, Taxol. *Cell Immunol*, 1994;**57**:291–9.

30. Sievers K., Hurri L. Combined therapy of rheumatoid arthritis with gold and chloroquine. I. Evaluation of the therapeutic effect. *Acta Rheumatol Scand*, 1963;**9**:48–55.

31. Bombardier C., Tugwell P. Controversies in the analysis of long term clinical trials of slow acting drugs. *J Rheumatol*, 1998;**12**:403–5.

32. Felson D., Anderson J., Meenan R. The efficacy and toxicity of combination therapy in rheumatoid arthritis: a meta-analysis. *Arthritis Rheum*, 1994;**37**:1487–91.

33. Johnson K. Efficacy assessment in trials of combination therapy for rheumatoid arthritis. *J Rheumatol*, 1996;**23** (Suppl 44):107–9.

34. Tugwell P., Boers M. Developing consensus and preliminary core efficacy endpoints for rheumatoid arthritis clinical trials. The OMERACT Committee. *J Rheumatol*, 1993;**20**:555–61.

35. Boers M., Ramsden M. Long-acting drug combinations in rheumatoid arthritis: a formal review. *J Rheumatol*, 1991;**18**:316–24.

36. Tugwell P., Boers M. Long-acting drug combinations in rheumatoid arthritis. Updated overview. In: Wolfe F., Pincus T., eds. *Rheumatoid arthritis pathogenesis, assessment, outcome and treatment*. New York: Marcel Dekker; 1994; p. 357–371.

37. Borgini M., Paulus H.E. Combination therapy. *Baillière's Clin Rheumatol*, 1995;**9**:689–710.

38. Williams H.J. Overview of combination second-line or disease-modifying antirheumatic drug therapy in rheumatoid arthritis. *Br J Rheumatol*, 1995;**34**(Suppl 2):96–9.

39. Verhoeven A.C., Boers M., Tugwell P. Combination therapy in rheumatoid arthritis: updated systematic review. *Br J Rheumatol*, 1998;**37**:612–9.

40. Trnavsky K., Gatterova J., Linduskova M., Peliskova Z. Combination therapy with hydroxychloroquine and methotrexate in rheumatoid arthritis. *Z Rheumatol*, 1993;**52**:292–6.

41. Ferraz M.B., Pinheiro G.R.C., Helfenstein M., Albuquerque E., Rezende C., Roimicher L., *et al*. Combination therapy with methotrexate and chloroquine in rheumatoid arthritis: a multicentre randomised placebo controlled trial. *Scand J Rheumatol*, 1994;**23**:231–6.

42. Clegg D.O., Dietz F., Duffy J., Willkens R.F., Hurd E., Germain B.F., *et al*. Safety and efficacy of hydroxycholoroquine as maintenance therapy for rheumatoid arthritis after combination therapy with methotrexate and hydroxychloroquine. *J Rheumatology*, 1997;**24**:1896–902.

43. Seideman P., Albertoni F., Beck O., Eksborg S., Peterson C. Chloroquine reduces the bioavailability of methotrexate in patients with rheumatoid arthritis. *Arthritis Rheum*, 1994;**37**:880–3.

44. Fries J.F., Singh G., Lenert L., Furst D. Aspirin, hydroxychloroquine and hepatic abnormalities with methotrexate in rheumatoid arthritis. *Arthritis Rheum*, 1990;**33**:1611–9.

45. Tugwell P., Pincus T., Yocum D., Stein M., Gluck O., Kragg G., *et al*. Combination therapy with cyclosporin A and methotrexate in severe rheumatoid arthritis. *N Engl J Med*, 1995;**333**:137–41.

46. Stein C.M., Brooks R.H., Pincus T. Effect of combination therapy with cyclosporin and methotrexate on liver function test results in rheumatoid arthritis. *Arthritis Rheum*, 1997;**40**:1721–3.

47. Stein C.M., Pincus T., Yocum D., Tugwell P., Wells G., Gluck O., *et al*. Combination treatment of severe rheumatoid arthritis with cyclosporin and methotrexate for forty-eight weeks. An open-label extension study. *Arthritis Rheum*, 1997;**40**:1843–51.

48. Nisar M., Carlisle L., Amos R.S. Methotrexate and sulfasalazine in combination therapy in rheumatoid arthritis. *Br J Rheumatol*, 1994;**33**:651–4.

49. Shiroky J.B. Combination sulfasalazine and methotrexate in the management of rheumatoid arthritis. *J Rheumatol*, 1996;**23**(Suppl 44):69–71.

50. Haagsma C.J., van Reil P.L.C.M., de Rooij D.J.R.A.M., Vree T.B., Russel F.J.M., van't Hof M.A., *et al*. Combination of

methotrexate and sulfasalazine vs methotrexate alone: a randomised open clinical trial in rheumatoid arthritis patients resistant to sulfasalazine therapy. *Br J Rheumatol*, 1994;**33**:1049–55.

51. Haagsma C.J., van Reil P.L.C.M., de Jong A.J.L., van de Putte L.B.A. Combination of sulfasalazine and methotrexate versus the single components in early rheumatoid arthritis: a randomised, controlled, double-blind, 52 week clinical. *Br J Rheumatol*, 1997;**36**:1082–8.

52. Williams H.J., Ward J.R., Reading J.C., Brooks R.H., Clegg D.O., Skosey J.L., *et al*. Comparison of auranofin, methotrexate and the combination of both in the treatment of rheumatoid arthritis: a controlled trial. *Arthritis Rheum*, 1992;**35**:259–69.

53. Lopez-Mendez A., Daniel W.W., Reading J.C., Ward J.R., Alarcon G.S. Radiographic assessment of disease progression in rheumatoid arthritis patients enrolled in the cooperative systematic studies of the rheumatic diseases program randomised clinical trial of methotrexate, auranofin, or a combination of the two. *Arthritis Rheum*, 1993;**36**:1364–9.

54. Willkens R.F., Urowitz M.B., Stablein D.M., McKendry R.J.R., Berger R.G., Box J.H., *et al*. Comparison of azathioprine, methotrexate, and a combination of both in the treatment of rheumatoid arthritis: a controlled clinical trial. *Arthritis Rheum*, 1992;**35**:849–56.

55. Willkens R.F., Sharp J.T., Stablein D., Marks C., Wortmann R. Comparison of azathioprine, methotrexate, and the combination of the two in the treatment of rheumatoid arthritis. A forty-eight week controlled clinical trial with radiologic outcome assessment. *Arthritis Rheum*, 1995;**38**:1799–806.

56. McCarty D.J., Carrera G.F. Treatment of intractable rheumatoid arthritis with combined cyclophosphamide, azathioprine and hydroxychloroquine. *JAMA*, 1982;**248**:1718–23.

57. McCarty D.J., Harman J.G., Grassanovich J.L., Qian C., Klein J.P. Combination drug therapy of seropositive rheumatoid arthritis. *J Rheumatol*, 1995;**22**:1636–45.

58. O'Dell J.R., Haire C.E., Erikson N., Drymalski W., Palmer W., Eckhoff P.J., *et al*. Treatment of rheumatoid arthritis with methotrexate alone, sulfasalazine and hydroxychloroquine, or a combination of all three medications. *N Engl J Med*, 1996;**334**:1287–91.

59. O'Dell J.R., Haire C., Erikson N., Drymalski W., Palmer W., Maloley P., *et al*. Efficacy of triple DMARD therapy in patients with RA with suboptimal response to methotrexate. *J Rheumatol*, 1996;**23**(Suppl 44):72–4.

60. Boers M., Verhoeven A.C., Markusse H.M., van de Laar M.A.F., Westhovens R., van Denderen J.C., *et al*. Randomised comparison of combined step-down prednisolone, methotrexate and sulfasalazine with sulfasalazine alone in early rheumatoid arthritis. *Lancet*, 1997;**350**:309–18.

61. Scott D.L., Dawes P.T., Tunn E., Fowler P.D., Shadforth M.F., Fisher J., *et al*. Combination therapy with gold and hydroxychloroquine in rheumatoid arthritis: a prospective, randomised, placebo-controlled study. *Br J Rheumatol*, 1989;**28**:128–33.

62. Bitter T. Combined disease modifying chemotherapy for intractable rheumatoid arthritis. *Rheum Dis Clin N Am*, 1984;**10**:417–28.

63. Porter D., Capell H., Hunter J. Combination therapy in rheumatoid arthritis: no benefit of addition of hydroxychloroquine to

patients with a sub-optimal response to intra-muscular gold therapy. *J Rheumatol*, 1993;**20**:645–9.

64. Bendix G., Bjelle A. Adding low-dose cyclosporin A to parenteral gold therapy in rheumatoid arthritis: a double-blind placebo-controlled study. *Br J Rheumatol*, 1996;**35**:1142–9.

65. Corkill M.M., Kirkham B.W., Chikanza I.C., Gibson T., Panayi G.S. Intramuscular depot methylprednisolone induction of chrysotherapy in rheumatoid arthritis: a 24-week randomised controlled trial. *Br J Rheumatol*, 1990;**29**:274–9.

66. Van Gestel A.M., Laan R.F.J.M., Haagsma C.J., van de Putte L.B.A., van Riel P.L.C.M. Oral steroids as bridge therapy in rheumatoid arthritis patients starting with parenteral gold. A randomised double-blind placebo-controlled trial. *Br J Rheumatol*, 1995;**34**:347–51.

67. Ciconelli R.M., Ferraz M.B., Visioni R.A., Oliviera L.M., Atra E. A randomised double-blind controlled trial of sulfasalazine combined with pulses of methylprednisolone or placebo in the treatment of rheumatoid arthritis. *Br J Rheumatol*, 1996;**35**:150–4.

68. Taggart A.J., Hill J., Astbury C., Dixon J.S., Bird H.A., Wright V. Sulphasalazine alone or in combination with d-penicillamine in rheumatoid arthritis. *Br J Rheumatol*, 1987;**26**:32–6.

69. Farr M., Kitas G., Bacon P.A. Sulphasalazine in rheumatoid arthritis, combination therapy with d-penicillamine or sodium aurothiomalate. *Clin Rheumatol*, 1988;**7**:242–8.

70. Faarvang K.L., Egmose C., Krygar P., Podenphant J., Ingeman-Nielsen M., Hansen T.M. Hydroxychloroquine and sulfasalazine alone and in combination in rheumatoid arthritis: a randomised double blind trial. *Ann Rheum Dis*, 1993;**52**:711–5.

71. Bunch T.W., O'Duffy J.D., Tompkins R.B., O'Fallon W.M. Controlled trial of hydroxychloroquine and d-penicillamine singly or in combination in the treatment of rheumatoid arthritis. *Arthritis Rheum*, 1984;**27**:267–76.

72. Gibson T., Emery P., Armstrong R.D., Crisp A.J., Panayi G.S. Combined d-penicillamine and chloroquine treatment of rheumatoid arthritis: a comparative study. *Br J Rheumatol*, 1987;**26**:279–84.

73. Choy E.H.S., Kingsley G.H., Panayi G.S. Monoclonal antibody therapy in rheumatoid arthritis. *Br J Rheumatol*, 1998;**37**:484–90.

74. Moreland L.W., Pratt P.W., Mayes M.D., Postlethwaite A., Weisman M.H., Schnitzer T., *et al*. Double-blind, placebo controlled multicenter trial using chimeric monoclonal anti-CD4 antibody, cM-T412, in rheumatoid arthritis patients receiving concomitant methotrexate. *Arthritis Rheum*, 1995;**38**:1581–8.

75. Maini R.N., Breedveld F.C., Kalden J.R., Smolen J.S., Davis D., MacFarlane J.D., *et al*. Low dose methotrexate (MTX) suppresses anti-globulin responses and potentiates efficacy of a chimeric monoclonal anti-TNFα antibody (cA2) given repeatedly in rheumatoid arthritis. *Arthritis Rheum*, 1997;**40**(Suppl):S126.

76. Strand V. The future use of biologic therapies in combination for the treatment of rheumatoid arthritis. *J Rheumatol*, 1996;**23**(Suppl 44):91–6.

77. Felson D.T., Anderson J.J., Meenan R.F. The comparative efficacy and toxicity of second-line drugs in rheumatoid arthritis: results of two meta-analyses. *Arthritis Rheum*, 1990;**30**:1449–61.

78. Tugwell P. Combination therapy in rheumatoid arthritis: meta-analysis. *J Rheumatol*, 1996;**23**(Suppl 44):43–6.

79. Brooks P.M. Should disease modifying drugs be used alone or in combination? In: *Questions and uncertainties in rheumatoid arthritis*, (ed.) H. Bird and M. Snaith. Blackwell Science, Oxford, 1999; in press.

SECTION 5 | *Non-drug therapy*

28 | *The impact of physiotherapy*

Ulrich Moritz

Decline of function over time is found in most patients with rheumatoid arthritis. About 50 per cent of patients show evidence of articular damage with radiographic joint space narrowing and/or erosions within the first 2 years of disease[1]. Early retirement, within 3 years, has been found in 37 per cent of early cases of rheumatoid arthritis[2]. The main functional limitations pertain to pain, decreased joint motion, muscle weakness, reduced endurance, and limitations in aerobic capacity. The unpredictable course of the disease often causes anxiety and depression and reduces self-efficacy.

Physiotherapy is an essential part of comprehensive management for patients with rheumatoid arthritis, and there is a growing body of knowledge concerning the efficacy of physiotherapeutic interventions. Most of the research during recent years has been performed in the field of exercise therapy. The aim of physiotherapy is to prevent or reduce functional consequences of the disease. The basis of intervention are needs experienced by the patient and relevant findings of functional impairment. In addition, cognitive and behavioral factors have to be taken into account[3,4].

Exercise therapy

Range of motion (ROM) exercises

Decreased range of passive motion may be due to capsular swelling and increased intra-articular fluid volume. In more advanced stages, contracture and articular structural changes contribute. Adhesions sometimes add to the restriction. The increased frictional force, due to cartilage destruction, on ROM becomes apparent when the joint is loaded. In the unloaded joint, cartilage destruction and joint space narrowing appear to play a minor role among factors contributing to stiffness. Elastic, as well as viscous, joint stiffness are more closely related to local, active inflammatory changes such as capsular swelling[5]. External restrictions of flexibility are pain-induced muscle tension or increased stiffness of muscle tissue. Inflammatory changes in flexor and extensor tendons cause increased viscous stiffness of, for example, finger joints[5]. Destruction of stabilizing tissues impairs mobility because of incongruency of the joint.

There are three types of ROM exercises: passive, assisted, and active. In order to increase extensibility, terminal stretching is applied. It is a general rule that the stretch should be held at the maximally achieved range for 5–20 s, with at least three repetitions. However, the implications of different tissue changes limiting joint motion have not been tested. ROM exercises are usually combined with strength training. Muscle function is necessary to preserve mobility.

Only a few randomized controlled studies have tested the effect of joint-specific ROM exercise programs in RA patients. A home training program for patients with arthritic shoulder dysfunction has been evaluated by Mannerkorpi and Bjelle[6]. Twenty-eight consecutive female out-patients with shoulder pain, functional class I and II, were randomly assigned to two groups. One group (n = 14) received instructions for shoulder training to be performed three times a week, comprising (1) warming up and relaxation exercises, (2) retraction exercises of the shoulder blades, (3) pulley-assisted movements in flexion and abduction, (4) light stretching of shoulder muscles (6–10 s), and (5) endurance training of the outward rotator muscles with an elastic rubber band. The number of repetitions was individually adapted depending on pain, limitation of ROM, and endurance. No instructions were given to the control group. After 8 weeks, the training group reported decreased pain on active motion. Abduction of the left arm and hand-to-neck mobility of the right arm were improved compared with the controls. Muscle endurance in both arms was increased. There was a trend towards improvement of the arm activites of daily living (ADL)-index in the training group, however, the difference was not significant. The long-term effect was not studied. No adverse effects were observed.

The role of exercise with particular reference to the RA hand has been highly controversial[7]. It has been suspected that resistive exercises accelerate the development of hand deformities. The effect of daily, simple hand exercises has been tested in a randomized, controlled, 48-month trial in 44 female patients with seropositive, active RA for at least 1 year and erosions in the metacarpophalangeal joint (MCP) and/or proximal interphalangeal joint (PIP) joints[7]. All patients were classified as functional class I. None had severe deformities. The exercise program comprised warm-up exercises, stretching, dexterity training, grip strengthening exercises, and flexion and extension training of the MCP and PIP joints, with five to ten repetitions each. The patients were strongly encouraged to perform the exercises on a regular basis. The control group was given no exercise instructions. Parameters recorded were grip strength, pincer grip strength, and flexion and extension ROM of individual MCP and PIP joints. The examiner was blinded. About 80 per cent of the patients completed the study. At the end of the 48 months, grip strength and pincer grip strength were significantly improved in the training group, while there was a significant deterioration in the control group. There was a significant loss of MCP joint extension in both groups, somewhat less in the training group. Flexion in the MCP joints deteriorated in the control group but this did not reach statistical significance; nor was the improvement of flexion in the training group significant. Changes in the flexion and extension of the PIP joints did not reach statistical significance. It can be concluded that this type of simple exercise regimen improves muscle strength but is less efficacious with regard to joint motion. No adverse effects were observed.

The effect of 12 weeks of home hand exercises performed for 10–20 min twice a day has been studied in 44 patients, functional class II and III[8]. The patients were randomly assigned to one of three exercise groups or a control group. The exercise groups were ROM exercises, resistive (RES), and RES + ROM exercises. Immediate and short term effects at 3 months follow-up were studied. The exercises were well tolerated and only caused transient, mild to moderate discomfort. Examinations were performed by a blinded observer. There were no significant changes in range of motion of the PIP and MCP joints over the study period, with the exception of increased left PIP extension in the RES group. There were no significant changes in deformities, ulnar deviation, or joint circumference. Compared with the control group, there was a significant decrease in right hand joint count in the ROM group and an increase in left hand dexterity in the RES + ROM group. The combined intervention groups gained significant strength in the left hand after 3 months of exercise (RES 22 per cent, ROM 6 per cent). Follow-up evaluation 3 months after the exercise period revealed no statistically significant changes in any of the intervention groups.

The effect of active exercises and warm wax bath treatment was evaluated in 52 rheumatoid arthritis patients, functional class I and II, with a mean age of 53 years and an average duration of the disease of 7.6 years[9]. The patients were randomized into four groups: (1) both exercise and wax bath, (2) exercise only, (3) wax bath only, and (4) controls. Treatment was given three times a week for 4 weeks. Twenty min of wax bath treatment was followed by hand exercises including eight different movements with slight resistance (soft exercise dough) for 20 min. Active exercise was found to significantly reduce pain with non-resistent motion, stiffness, and flexion deficits. Total grip function and pinch test improved significantly in group (1) compared to all other groups. No significant effect was observed with wax bath except that pain relief was registered immediately after treatment in groups (1) and (3). Stiffness was reduced in all treatment groups immediately after treatment.

Dynamic exercise programs intended to improve muscle function and aerobic capacity may have a short-term effect on joint mobility (Tables 28.1–28.3). During a 12-week, high-intensity exercise program joint flexibility improved significantly in the high-intensity group only, and in particular in the joints of the lower extremities[10]. Range of motion was not changed significantly in the control groups which had programs including ROM exercises. There was no significant difference between the groups at 24 weeks follow-up, except knee extension with high-intensity training.

A 12-week, home exercise program including exercises for strength and mobility in upper and lower extremities, stretching, and walking has been found to improve total joint mobility (joint mobility index) significantly in both the upper and the lower extremities[11]. The study included no control group without training. The long-term effect was not evaluated. A long-term (2-year) program comprising different training modalities was not found to prevent deterioration of joint function measured as the functional score of 26 joints[12]. The decrease in joint function was not associated with any increase in pain experience or disease activity. Radiographic examination revealed progression of joint destruction in both the experimental and the control group.

To summarize, capsular and muscular stiffness are temporarily reduced by regular motion exercises. However, in the long run, reduced mobility associated with progressive joint destruction can not be significantly prevented by ROM exercises.

Training of muscle strength, endurance, and aerobic capacity

Pain or inhibition caused by pressure-induced joint capsular distension can result in muscular weakness[13]. Changes in muscle

Table 28.1 Randomized controlled trials of exercise interventions in RA

Study	Patients (n)	Functional class	Age	Duration (years)	Inclusion criteria	Exclusion criteria
Harkcom[24]	20	II	52	9	NR	NR
Minor[20]	40	NR	54	11	Symptomatic weight-bearing joints Age: > 20 y	Not on stable medication Currently exercising
Ekdahl[21]	67	II	53	11	Functional class II Age: 20–65 y	Other disease states that might influence the results
Hansen[12]	75	I–II	52	7	Age: 20–60 y Functional class I and II	Training 3 × per week Comorbidity
Lyngberg[25]	24	I–III	67	9	Corticosteroid treatment > 6 month	Heart disease Unable to train
Hakkinen[22,31]	43	NR	44	1	Recent-onset arthritis	NR
Stenström[26,32]	54	I–II	54	14	Functional class I and II Age: < 65 y	NR
Van den Ende[10]	100	NR	52	10	Age: 20–70 y Able to bicycle	Arthroplastics of weight-bearing joints, comorbidity
Komatireddy[23]	49	II–III	61	11	NR	Chest pain, abnormal ECG Pulmonary function abnormalities

NR, not reported

Table 28.2 Type of exercise, frequency, and duration of intervention and follow-up after intervention

Study	Type of exercise		Frequency	Duration of intervention	Follow-up
Harkcom[24]	EG:	Bicycle exercise 70% max heart rate	3 × per week	12 weeks	0
	CG:	No exercise			
Minor[20]	EG:	Aerobic walking or aquatics 60–80% max heart rate	1 h 3 × per week	12 weeks	9 months
	CG:	Non-aerobic ROM exercises			
Ekdahl[21]	EG:	Dynamic exercises + ROM Bicycle exercise > 50% heart rate	Supervised 1–2 × per week + 45 min daily home exercise	6 weeks	3 months
	CG:	Low intensity static training + ROM exercises			
Hansen[12]	EG:				
	A.	Self training after instruction	15 + 30 min 3 × per week	2 years	0
	B.	As A + training with PT in private practice once a week			
	C.	As A + weekly group training in the hospital			
	D.	As C but including training in hot water pool			
	CG:	No instruction			
Lyngberg[25]	EG:	Bicycle training heel lifts, step-climbing	45 min 2 × per week	3 months	0
	CG:	No training			
Häkkinen[22,31]	EG:	Strength training trunk, upper, and lower extremity			36 months
		40% RM	2 × per week	2 months	
		50–60% RM	2–3 × per week	2 months	
		70–80% RM	2–3 × per week	2 months	
		Walking, biking, swimming	2 × per week		
	CG:	Habitual physical activities	3–4 × per week	6 months	
Stenström[26,32]	EG:	Strength and mobility, stretching, walking	30 min 5 × per week	3 months	9 months
	CG:	Progressive muscle relaxation	15 min 5 × per week + 15 min rest	3 months	
Van den Ende[10]	EG:	Cycling 70–85% max. heart rate Intensive dynamic group exercises	1 h 3 × per week	3 months	3 months
	CG 1:	ROM exercises. Low intensity isometric group exercises	1 h 2 × per week	3 months	3 months
	CG 2:	Individual ROM and low intensity isometric exercises	1 h 2 × per week	3 months	3 months
	CG 3:	Home instructions for ROM and isometric exercises	15 min 2 × per week	3 months	3 months
Komatireddy[23]	EG:	Home instructions (video tape) Low load resistive exercise, high repetitions with moderate exertion	20–27 min 3 × per week	3 months	0
	CG:	No training			

RM = repetition maximum; ROM = range of motion; EG = exercise group; CG = control group; PT = physiotherapist.

Table 28.3 Effects of therapeutic exercises

Study	Muscle strength	Aerobic capacity	Joint mobility	Physical capacity	Self-reported pain	Disease activity	Radiograph
Harkcom[24]	=	+	NR	=	NR	+[a]	NR
Minor[20]	NR	+	+*	+	=	+	NR
Ekdahl[21]	+	+	=	+	=	+	NR
Hansen[12]	+*	=	–*	NR	=	=	–*
Lyngberg[25]	=	=	NR	+	NR	=	NR
Häkkinen[22]	+	NR	NR	NR	NR	+*	=
Stenström[26]	=	NR	=	=	=	=	NR
Van den Ende[10]	+	+	+	+*	=	+[a]	NR
Komatireddy[23]	+*	=	NR	+	+	+*	NR

=, no change within exercise group; +, significant improvement; –, significant deterioration; *, no significant difference between groups;
anumber of swollen joints;
NR, not reported.

strength have been found to be closely correlated with changes in systemic disease activity[5]. An additional factor is atrophy of type I and Type II muscle fibers. Except for intrinsic muscles of the hand, electromyographic signs of myopathy or neuropathy are an unusual finding in patients with RA[14]. Rheumatoid arthritis patients also experience impaired control of balance and an increased body-sway in standing position has been found[15].

Training of muscle strength introduces a considerable load on the joint on which the muscles act. Compressive forces in the knee joint in the extented position are about ten times higher than the load applied at the ankle during training of the quadriceps muscle. During maximal contraction of the knee extensor muscles, an increased intra-articular hydrostatic pressure varying between 15 and > 380 mm Hg has been observed in RA patients, depending on the volume of joint effusion and capsular stiffness[13]. An increase in the intra-articular pressure of as little as 20 mm Hg decreases synovial blood flow significantly, inducing a risk of anoxic joint destruction. Because of possible risks induced by intensive muscle training, articular rest and static training with low loads have been recommended[16]. Rest is therefore indicated in patients with acute and very active arthritis[17], but the majority of patients need physical activity to preserve joint and muscle function and to overcome the effect of inactivation. During the recent two decades it has become apparent that short-term, high-intensity static or dynamic training of patients with non-acute RA can improve strength, aerobic capacity, and physical performance without increasing disease activity or accelerating joint destruction (reviewed in Ref. 3, 18). However, previous reviews included, to a varying extent, trials that were not randomized; also outcome evaluations confined to subgroups have low power and introduce a risk of bias[19].

The following review is based on randomized, controlled trials with a duration of at least 6 weeks (Table 28.1). As a rule, only patients with stable medication and low to moderate disease activity were included, except in one of the trials where patients were included without regard to the extent or severity of arthritis[20]. The disability level was usually low to moderate and the patients were not hospitalized. The compliance in the different intervention studies was satisfactory; around 85 per cent (70–91) completed the program. A considerable variety in study design, with regard to types of training, intensity, frequency, and duration, was found (Table 28.2), which, in part, was due to the different aims of the studies.

Out-come measures (Table 28.3) were according to the following methods. Muscle strength, mostly of the lower extremities, was tested isometrically[10,12,21–23], isokinetically[10,21,24,25], or with a dynamometer for isotonic contraction[22]. Evaluation of muscle training in one study was based on an index of muscle function including endurance, and balance/co-ordination[26]. Aerobic capacity was measured with a cycle ergometer[10,12,21,22,24,25] or treadmill test[20,23]. Goniometer[10,21,22] and/or flexibility scores[12,20,26] were used to assess joint mobility. Assessment of physical capacity included a stair climbing test[12,21,25], walk test[10,20,21,24–26], grip test[20,23–25], step test[25], and/or sit-to-stand time[23]. Conventional methods were used to assess disease activity, such as the Ritchie index[10,21,22,26], tenderness, number of swollen joints, morning stiffness, and pain rating. Evaluations were performed by examiners who were blinded to the experimental condition, in all but three studies[10,20,24].

The results confirm previous non-randomized trials[27–29]. Dynamic training improves muscle strength and physical capacity significantly. Measurement of the cross-sectional area of the femoral quadriceps muscle by means of computerized tomography in one of the experimental groups with high intensity training revealed a significant increase after 6 months[22]. Low-intensity static training, however, did not improve strength[10,21]. In a group of elderly subjects, dynamic training did not improve muscle strength[25]. On the other hand, muscle strength decreased more than 20 per cent in the control group during the same time. The effect of exercise therapy on impairment of balance was tested in one study only[21]. No significant differences in standing balance were found during the training period of 18 weeks despite intensive, dynamic training of the lower extremities.

Weight-bearing exercises were used in several studies. This type of closed chain-training instead of open chain-training (isokinetic training or quadriceps table) has become popular in sports medicine rehabilitation. During this type of strength training, the extremity is loaded as a functional unit with activation of all stabilizing muscles of the extremity. If load tolerance is reduced in one of the joints of the extremity, open-chain training may be used. Isokinetic training has been shown to be safe and effective[30], but the equipment is expensive. Isometric training is equally effective and strength training can be performed with the joint in a pain-free position.

High intensity training three times a week increased aerobic capacity significantly. No improvement was found in groups with aerobic training once a week only[12] or with repetitive resistive exercises with moderate exertion[23].

Follow-up studies

Increases in muscle strength in patients with early RA were lost to a great extent during the follow-up period of 3 years, during which the patients had resumed their habitual physical activities[31]. If training activities are continued, improvements in muscle strength and endurance can be maintained. This has been shown for a follow-up time of 3 months after 6 weeks of supervised high-intensity training[21]. In this study, patients' diary records indicated good compliance. Similar results have been reported by Minor[20]. Re-examination 9 months after physical conditioning showed persistent improvement of aerobic capacity, 50-foot walking time, and grip strength. The patients had been encouraged to continue exercising but the compliance was not studied. Aerobic capacity and joint mobility appear to be more sensitive to detraining than muscle strength and physical capacity[10].

In order to maintain the improved physical fitness, continued exercise is required. The outcome depends on the compliance of the patient. Compliance with a 1-year home exercise program was found to be predicted by habitual, regular ROM exercises before the intervention and by high self-efficacy for exercises[32]. Interestingly, health status, initial disease activity, or treatment priorities had no influence.

The impact on functional ability and well being

Different performance tests such as walking test and stair climbing test showed significant improvement in the majority of the studies reviewed (Table 28.3), confirming previous reports (reviewed in Ref. 3). To assess functional capacity for activities of daily living the Health Assessment Questionnaire (HAQ)[33] was used in five of the studies[10,12,21–23]. This instrument showed that the majority of patients were only mildly disabled before training; the median HAQ score varied between 0.53 and 0.83. A significant improvement in the score of the experimental groups was reported in only two of the studies[22,23]. The HAQ score seems insensitive to measure outcome in short-term exercise trials, at least in patients with a low degree of disability. After 12 weeks of exercise therapy, changes in the HAQ score were found to be significantly correlated with changes in pain, depression, and quadriceps strength, but not with changes in joint mobility or physical condition[34]. It is not apparent whether the training really focused on problems in activities of daily living experienced by the patients in this study.

Significant improvement in AIMS scores of physical activity and depression[35] was reported after 12 weeks of physical conditioning exercises[20]. However, the effect on depression was not maintained at the follow-up 3 months later. Another exercise trial with high or low-intensity training during 12 weeks did not change the AIMS score of depression[10]. The Nottingham Health Profile was used in one of the studies[26]. Strength and mobility training as a home exercise resulted in only minor physical improvements and had no effect on the total score or the sub-scores. Progressive relaxation training of the control group was found to reduce lack of energy. Cognitive and behavioral effects of exercise therapy have been described in previous studies (reviewed in Ref. 3).

The heterogeneity of outcome measures makes it difficult to compare the different studies. It is apparent that more long-term studies are needed to clarify the effect of physiotherapeutic interventions on activities of daily living and well being.

Adverse effects

The dynamic training did not increase the progression of joint destruction. However, no protective effect, as described by Nordemar and coworkers[28], was found. No negative effect on the experience of pain or disease activity was observed. Indeed, in six of the studies, reduced signs of activity were found. It has been suggested that an increase of circulating neuropeptides after exercise training might reduce pain caused by physical loading of inflamed joints. A study of neuropeptide levels in RA patients and in healthy subjects after high-intensity training for 6 weeks showed a significant increase in the corticotropin releasing hormone levels in RA patients but not in the healthy training group. In addition, significantly higher levels of β-endorphin were found in arthritis patients compared to healthy controls after high-intensity training and after low-intensity training for another 6 months[36]. It is suggested that the results indicate a higher activity level during training for the RA patients as compared to the healthy subjects.

Aerobic training has been shown to have an effect on immune parameters in healthy subjects with increase in natural killer cytotoxicity, monocyte concentration, and interleukin-1 levels in plasma[37]. Eight weeks of bicycle training increased aerobic capacity significantly in patients with RA but did not induce changes in blood mononuclear cell subpopulations, proliferative response, or natural killer cell activity[37]. Furthermore, there was no change in plasma concentrations of IL-1α, IL-1β, and IL-6. Thus, the decrease in the disease activity observed in arthritis patients after intensive physical training is not explained by changes in these proinflammatory cytokines.

As a rule, the patients were instructed to reduce the training load and/or the number of repetitions for some days if the training caused pain lasting for more than 2 h. To influence pain behavior in other chronic musculoskeletal disorders, the training intensity has been based on goal-setting and not on pain attention. This approach has been found to be effective in, for example, chronic low back pain. A comparative study has therefore been performed, with RA patients in a home training program, to investigate whether additional cognitive training with goal-setting and reinterpretation of pain versus a recommendation to avoid overload and increased pain, would influence the exercise results[11]. After 12 weeks no significant difference was noted between the groups with regard to functional capacity or joint mobility. However, the goal-setting group had a significantly larger decrease in the Ritchie's index and pain rating during one of the lifting tasks. In addition, self-efficacy for mood and fatigue had increased. To avoid negative effects during intensive training, attention has to be paid to the coping strategies of the patients. Some patients have been found to be caught in a vicious cycle of avoidance and low self-appraisal when exposed to this type of training[38]. This study also showed that avoidance coping in these patients resulted in an increase in pain during intensive dynamic training.

Hydrotherapy

Water exercise

Exercises in heated swimming pools have a long tradition. The weight-relieving effect of water immersion allows easier movement with less pain. Increased water resistance during rapid movements can be used to train muscle strength[39] and aerobic capacity[20].

Despite its popularity, the efficacy of this therapy has not been adequately evaluated in the treatment of RA[40]. In a randomized, controlled trial comprising 130 patients with RA involving at least six joints, exercise hydrotherapy was compared with seated immersion in a pool with a water temperature of about 36°C, land exercise, or progressive relaxation[40]. All interventions were limited to two sessions per week for four consecutive weeks. The outcome was evaluated immediately after the intervention and 3 months later. The overall effect was a significant reduction in joint tenderness after intervention, but between groups the difference was significant for the hydrotherapy only. At follow-up the reduction was no longer significant. Grip strength, range of motion, and duration of morning stiffness did not change significantly. There

29 | *Occupational therapy and assistive technology*

Ulla Nordenskiöld

Introduction

Historically, occupational therapy arose in recognition of the universal human need for activity[1] and the belief that activity organizes and integrates human beings into the normal routines of their cultures. Subsequently, occupational therapy practice, based on this belief, developed in different configurations in most countries of the world[2]. Activity is a central concept in occupational therapy and comprises all situations in which the individual takes an active part, assuming that the individual is an active person with his or her own resources. The importance of activity to health is central. The patient is seen as an active definer rather than a passive recipient of rehabilitative goals[3].

Pörn[4] has given an explanation of the concept of health which does not rely on the concept of disease. He presented three basic factors that can be distinguished in the dynamic of the actor subject: the repertoire, the environment, and the goals of the subject. By repertoire he means the individual's skills, which are not static. New skills can be developed and skills deteriorate when they are not used. Occupational therapy, based on a holistic view of the person, emphasizes that individuals must be actively involved in their own treatment. Activity encompasses all such situations as personal care, living conditions, work, leisure and relations to other people, typically referred to as activities of daily living (ADLs). Occupational therapy seeks to prevent disabilities while re-establishing and maintaining abilities so that the individual may function optimally in the environment.

Individuals with rheumatoid arthritis (RA) have problems conducting their daily, lives because of joint pain, muscle weakness, stiffness, fatigue, reduced grip force, and hand deformities. They are often unable to perform daily activities in what is considered a normal manner. Pincus *et al.*[5] also noted that difficulties in daily activities were among the predictors of a higher mortality rate in RA patients.

Consequences of rheumatoid arthritis for daily living

In order to understand different levels of function and how to distinguish among pathology, impairment, disability, and handicap, many rehabilitation teams use the concepts developed by the World Health Organization (WHO) in 1980[6]. However, the way in which a person reacts to difficulties and hardship is not only due to impairments and disabilities but to a great extent on the individual's personality and social situation[7,8]. Some patients feel threatened or guilty, while others may see a challenge in learning cope with their situation. When analyzing the situation of patients with RA, the occupational therapist may, however, find this International Classification of Impairment, Disability, and Handicap (ICIDH) model helpful, since it clarifies the different levels of consequences.

Impairment — body functions and structures

Impairment describes the consequences at the organic level; for example in RA this applies to joint motion, pain, and reduced grip force. Most patients with rheumatoid arthritis experience chronic pain.

Pain relief and assistive devices

Pain creates fatigue and impairs the ability to concentrate. For that reason the struggle against pain is one of the main tasks in clinical care. Pain relief is an important reason for seeking medical care in the form of occupational therapy. Frustration over the inability to perform tasks, dependence upon others, limitation due to the disease in daily life, and difficulties in adjusting routines have been identified in RA.

The purpose of ergonomically-designed assistive devices such as an upright-handled breadknife and cheese slicer is to decrease or eliminate the consequences of reduced joint function and pain. One study[9] has shown that using assistive devices such as a spring-assisted scissors, a cheese slicer, a broad-handled potato peeler, and designed breadknife, resulted in significant pain reduction compared with using ordinary household tools (Fig. 29.1a and b). The hand and finger joints were positioned in an ergonomically natural grip, since the handles of hand devices are designed with a wider gripping area[10].

Grip force, hand function, and orthoses

The hand has a very complex structure and, when inflamed, the possibilities of reduced mobility and muscle function, as well as instability, are manifold. As early as 1940, Lansbury[11] showed that grip strength can be used as a measure of disease activity in RA. Gripping power is dependent on pain and deformity. Reduced strength in the wrist and fingers, which often occurs at an early stage of the disease, has a strong impact on the person's

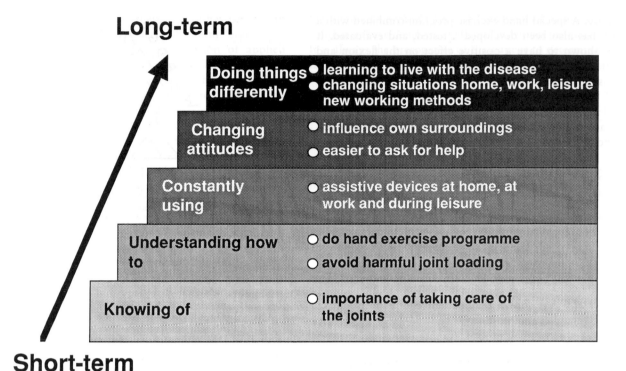

Long-term

Doing things differently
- learning to live with the disease
- changing situations home, work, leisure new working methods

Changing attitudes
- influence own surroundings
- easier to ask for help

Constantly using
- assistive devices at home, at work and during leisure

Understanding how to
- do hand exercise programme
- avoid harmful joint loading

Knowing of
- importance of taking care of the joints

Short-term

Fig. 29.5 The 'educational staircase' illustrates the process for achievement of established needs and goals and adaptation to the disease. Changing work methods and attitudes requires more engagement than just 'knowing about' something.

force increased significantly when patients used an elastic wrist orthosis.

Reduced grip force and pain are highly correlated to difficulties in daily activities. To what extent patients' ADL problems can be explained by reduced grip force has been analyzed in one daily task—vacuuming[34]. Eight of the 41 women avoided the activity vacuuming, the mean grip force in these women was 42 Newton (N) (confidence interval 25–58). The women who were still doing the vacuuming had a mean grip force value of 80 N (confidence interval 63–100) (Fig. 29.6). Thus the threshold value of grip force for performing vacuum-cleaning would be 60 N. Such information could be used for designing technical adaptations, since the results showed the relationship between grip force, pain, and difficulty in daily activities. Another study[35] has suggested that the grip force level below 88 N was the threshold level for performing daily activities.

Outcome measures reflect the noticeable consequences of the disease process. As the goals of assistive technologies are to decrease disability and to help reduce the problems for the individuals, the outcome measures should reflect these factors. Instruments which are specifically developed for people with arthritis should highlight typical problems expressed by arthritics, such as buttoning clothes, turning faucets, opening cans, lifting frying pans, and shopping on a large scale. These may not be included in other generic functional assessments. Outcomes in RA should be viewed as multidimensional, and no single measure can account for all aspects. When analyzing the effect of an intervention such as the use of assistive devices, a large number of items may be required.

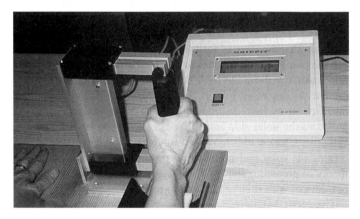

Fig. 29.6 The Grippit®: an electronic handpower instrument developed to measure peak grip force and mean force over a set period of time[33].

The Stanford Health Assessment Questionnaire (HAQ)[36] has been widely used as an outcome index. The problem with the HAQ model is that it mixes two different aspects of disability: dependence in terms of use of assistive devices and perceived difficulty. The score number 2 on the ordinal scale, in the HAQ, is described as; with much difficulty, with the use of assistive devices or other person. Information on performance in daily activities is also lost when using scores from the eight subscales as recommended instead of using all 20 questions[34,37].

By using the Rasch model[38] to transform ordinal scores from an instrument to obtain unidimensional linear measures, we can analyse whether items change in difficulty and follow changes in the subjects' degree of ability. The Rasch analysis has been widely used for functional assessment tests in rehabilitation medicine and for performance tests in occupational therapy.

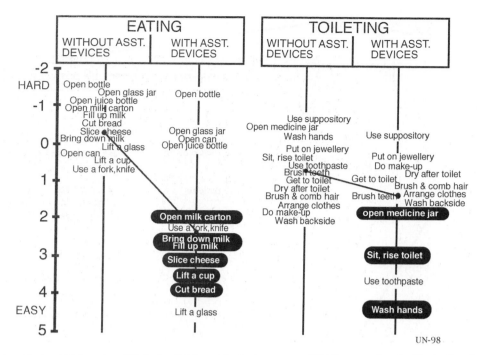

Fig. 29.7 The dimensions Eating (12 items) and Toileting (13 items) in the instrument EDAQ are analyzed with the Rasch analysis. The items have been marked on the scale, which ranges from 'hard' to 'easy' both without assistive devices/altered working methods and with devices/altered methods. ASST = assistance.

In a report[17] using the Rasch analysis to transform the patients' ratings on the ordinal scale (using the instrument EDAQ) to a linear measure, it was possible to construct a hierarchical model ranging from hard items to easy ones and with the patients' overall difficulties ranging from less able to more able. The variation in difficulty in the items was clearly shown and it was possible to demonstrate a reduction in overall difficulty thanks to assistive devices in most of the women. All subjects were helped in some way by devices and or altered method (Figs 29.3 and 29.7). The use of devices or altered methods led to a reduction in perceived difficulty in 42 per cent of the ratings. The results from this study clearly show the importance of providing assistive devices for patients with RA. This was further emphasized by the fact that there was reduction in difficulty in many aspects of daily living, and that the women were able to do things they had not done before.

As outcome assessments are being used in routine clinical practice, occupational therapists, like other health professionals, will feel obliged to use more evidence-based methods and instruments. The assessments must include the patients' own experience as well as the sensitivity of the instruments and choosing which instrument is most efficient at describing important changes within an individual. In order to understand why a person is more, or less, able to do the activities, it is important to consider both the person's physical capacity and the person's mental ability to perform in relevant situations. The occupational therapist should always remember that the home for the patient is a place of activities. Other types of evaluation, such as the quality of life[39], may help the occupational therapist to understand the patient's total situation and avoid the label 'someone with a chronic disease'.

Cost-effectiveness/utility analysis

Economy in health care implies using the resources in the most effective way. Consequently, the occupational therapists should describe their aims, measurements, and treatments and establish the effects to the patients of the interventions. The 'direct' cost could comprise costs for the selection process, the devices, and the domestic services. The 'indirect' costs reflect resource use in other areas not directly concerned with the provision of services[40]. The aim is to link outcome to costs in studies of technologies or health care. The methods for economic evaluation could be used in assessments of occupational therapy. A model (Fig. 29.8) is presented in an attempt to illustrate the costs for the personnel and the devices as well as the effects from the perspective of the patient. When analyzing and describing effectiveness (utility) in the health-care system one must identify the effect on the subject, otherwise the system can only be described as showing the productivity. The cost of the joint protection program, including provision of assistive devices, could be judged to be low in relation to its effectiveness—the utility to the patient[9].

In occupational therapy for individuals with rheumatoid arthritis a combination of assessments and treatments of grip force, pain, and the subjects' perceived ability/difficulty and needs in performing daily activities is to be recommended. The use of adaptive occupation with assistive devices, introducing alternative methods and strategies, or modifying social environments are other aspects of the occupational therapists intervention process. Both the benefit of assistive technology in relation to the individual's goals and their own solutions should be identified and described.

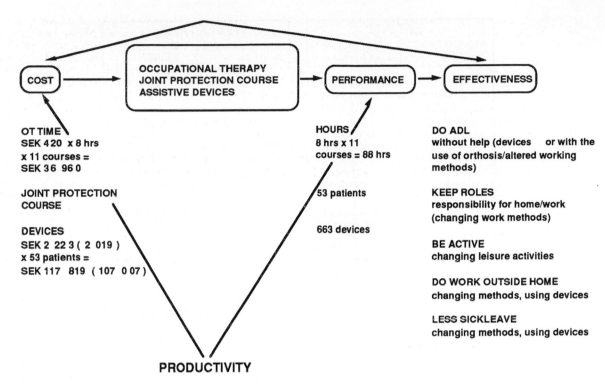

Fig. 29.8   A cost-effectiveness analysis of the joint protection course, the assistive devices, and the utility to the patient. SEK = Swedish krona; OT time = occupational therapist's time.

The role of an occupational therapist entails great responsibility: to develop the ability to switch between the role of 'efficient professional' and that of a caring fellow human being and have the ability to see the person/patient with rheumatoid arthritis as both healthy and sick. The most important goal is to build a basis for the individual's creative thinking that will enable them to find their own solutions to their problems.

The words of a women with RA after a joint protection course:

'I'm not alone with my problems, I can—I have important experiences and knowledge, I want and know how to influence around me'.

References

1. Meyer A. The philosophy of occupational therapy. *Archives Occup Ther*, 1992;1:1–10.
2. Yerxa E. In search of good ideas for occupational therapy. *Scand J Occup Ther*, 1994;1:7–15.
3. Robinson I. The rehabilitation of patients with long-term physical impairments: the social context of professional roles. *Clin Rehabil*, 1988;2:339–47.
4. Pörn I. Health and adaptedness. *Theor Med*, 1993;14:295–303.
5. Pincus T., Callahan L.F., Vaughn W.K. Questionnaire, walking time and button test measures of functional capacity as predictive markers for mortality in rheumatoid arthritis. *J Rheumatol*, 1987;14:240–51.
6. WHO, *World Health Organization: International classification of impairment, disabilities and handicaps. A manual of classification relating to consequences of disease (ICIDH).* Geneva, Switzerland: WHO, 1980. Revised.
7. Berglund K., Persson L.O., Brattström M. Effects of group councelling for rheumatoid arthritis patients on measures of psycho-
logical adjustment to illness. In: Balint G. ed. *Rheumatology state of the art*. Elsevier Science Publishers, Amsterdam, 1992:432–5.
7a. WHO, *ICIDH-2*. Geneva, Switzerland: WHO, 1999.
8. Nordenfelt L. On the notion of disability and handicap. *Scand J Soc Welfare*, 1993;2:17–24.
9. Nordenskiöld U. Evaluation of assistive devices after a course in joint protection. *Intl J of Technology Assessment in Health Care*, 1994;10:294–304.
10. Althoff B., Nordenskiöld U. *Joint protection—for active living*, Course booklet. The Swedish Rheumatism Association, Stockholm, 1994.
11. Lansbury J. Report of a three year study on the systemic and articular indices in rheumatoid arthritis: theoretic and clinical considerations. *Arthritis Rheum*, 1958;1:505–22.
12. Kjeken I., Möller G., Kvien T. Use of commercially produced elastic wrist orthoses in cronoc arthritis: a controlled study. *Arthritis Care Res*, 1995;8:108–13.
13. Nordenskiöld U. Elastic wrist orthoses—Reduction of pain and increase in grip force for women with rheumatoid arthritis. *Arthritis Care Res*, 1990;3:158–62.
14. Verbrugge L.M., Jette A.M. The disablement process. *Soc Sci Med*, 1994;38:1–14.
15. Törnquist K., Sonn U. Towards on ADL taxonomy for occupational therapists. *Scand J Occup Ther*, 1994;1,2:69–76.
16. Nordenskiöld U., Grimby G., Dahlin-Ivanoff S. Questionnaire to evaluate the effects of assistive devices and altered working methods in women with rheumatoid arthritis. *Clin Rheumatol*, 1998;17:6–16.
17. Nordenskiöld U., Grimby G., Hedberg M., Wright B., Linacre J.M. The structure of an instrument for assessing the effect of assistive devices and altered working methods in women with rheumatoid arthritis. *Arthritis Care Res*, 1996;9:21–30.
18. Mann M. Assistive technology for persons with arthritis. In: Melvin J., Jensen G. (eds). *Rheumatologic rehabilitation*, The American Occupational Therapy Association Inc, Bethesda, 1998:369–92.
19. Abraham B., Clamp S. Aids and adaptations: A new practice model. *Br J Occup Ther*, 1991;54:341–5.

20. Benktzon, M. Designing for our future selves: The Swedish experience. *Appl Ergonomics*, 1993;**24**:19–27.

21. Rogers J.C., Holm M.B. Assistive technology device use in patients with rheumatic disease: A literature review. *Am J Occup Ther*, 1992;**46**:120–7.

22. Hass U., Brodin H., Andersson A., Persson J. Assistive technology selection: a study of participation of users with rheumatoid arthritis. *IEEE Trans Rehabil Eng*, 1997;**5**:263–75.

23. Nordenskiöld U., Althoff B., Hansen A.M. *Joint Protection for Active Living Guide*. Stockholm: The Swedish Rheumatism Association, 1994.

24. Dellhag B., Wollersjö I., Bjelle A. Effect of active hand exercise and waxbath treatment in rheumatoid arthritis patients. *Arthritis Care Res*, 1992;**5**:287–92.

25. Fitinghoff H., Söderback I., Nordemar R. An activity analysis of hand grips used in housework by female rheumatoid arthritics. *Work*, 1994;**4**:128–36.

26. Dellhag B., Bjelle A. A grip ability test use in rheumatology practice. *J Rheumatol*, 1995;**22**:1559–65.

27. Lindroth Y., Nilsson J.Å., Wollheim F.A. Demographic variables and knowledge, behaviour and health outcome among patients with rheumatoid arthritis. Correlation before and seven years after a patient education program, 1997; personal communication.

28. Cordery J. Joint protection: A responsibility of the occupational therapist. *Am J Occup Ther*, 1965;**19**:285–94.

29. Cordery J., Rocchi M. Joint protection and fatigue management. In: Melvin J., Jensen G. (eds). *Rheumatologic rehabilitation*. The American Occupational Therapy Association, Bethesda, 1998:279–322.

30. Smith E., Juvinal R., Bender L., Pearson R. Role of the finger flexors in rheumatoid deformities of the metacarpophalangeal joints. *Arthritis Rheum*, 1964;**7**:467–80.

31. Chao E.Y., Opgrande J.D., Axmear F.E. Three dimensional force analysis of finger joints in selected isometric hand functions. *J Biomechanics*, 1976;**9**:387–96.

32. Hammond A. Joint protection behaviour assessment. *Arthritis Care Res*, 1994;**7**:abstracts, S9, S15.

33. Nordenskiöld U., Grimby G. Grip force in patients with rheumatoid arthritis and fibromyalgia and in healthy subjects. A study with the Grippit instrument. *Scand J Rheumatol*, 1993;**22**:14–9.

34. Nordenskiöld U. Daily activities in women with rheumatoid arthritis. Aspects of patient education, assistive devices and methods for disability and impairment assessment. *Scand J Rehab Med*, 1997;**37** (Suppl).

35. Philips C. Rehabilitation of the patient with rheumatoid hand involvement. *Phys Ther*, 1989;**69**:1091–9.

36. Fries J.F., Spitz P., Krainer G., Holman H. Measurement of patient outcome in arthritis. *Arthritis Rheum*, 1980;**23**:137–45.

37. Tennant A., Hillman M., Fear J., Pickering A., Chamberlain M.A. Are we making the most of Stanford Health Assessment Questionnaire? *Br J Rheumatol*, 1996;**35**:574–8.

38. Wright B.D., Masters G. *Rating Scale analysis: Rasch measurement*. Chicago:MESA, 1982.

39. Burckhardt C., Archenholtz B., Bjelle A. Measuring of the quality of life in women with rheumatoid arthritis or systemic lupus erythematosus. *Scand J Rheumatol*, 1992;**21**:190–5.

40. Andrich R., Ferrario M., Moi M. A model of cost-outcome analysis for assistive technology. *Disabil Rehabil*, 1998;**20**;1–24.

30 | Diets

Lars Sköldstam

Is diet important in rheumatoid arthritis?

In a recent editorial article on quackery Ames and Gold wrote[1]: 'We must not be seduced into accepting, or even tolerating, reasoned nonsense based on junk science premises'. Their statement is not contradictive to the more humble writing of CK Wasner, who in his article on *The art of unproven remedies* wrote[2]: 'The effort of traditional medicine to look at areas that are important to patients will help the work with patients go easier'. In addition, Wasner honored what he called 'open minded contemporary investigators who are willing to trudge through the murky waters of nutritional science'.

In their review article on diet and RA, Buchanan *et al.*[3] Stated: 'There can be no more commonly asked question by patients with RA than whether diet has any role in their disease'. According to Nenonen[4] 'the idea of a positive and therapeutic potential of dietary manipulation is probably as old as the written history of mankind', and to quote Darlington: 'such ideas are part of the folklore of RA'[5].

In fact, patients even in prehistoric times adjusted their diets, trying to reduce symptoms, until recently with little scientific support for their actions.

Does diet affect rheumatoid inflammation?

More recent research fostered by the application of molecular and cellular biological techniques has revealed that many nutrients and vitamins seem to act essentially in the same way as hormones, that is by binding to soluble intranuclear receptors[6]. This novel approach, known as molecular nutrition, has raised new, fascinating perspectives, and will eventually give us better knowledge about the functional significance of many nutrients.

It is evident from a number of studies that modulation of diet composition and caloric intake can have marked effect on the establishment and progression of autoimmune disease in murine models[7,8].

Twin studies in rheumatoid arthritis have shown a concordance rate of 12–21 per cent for RA among monozygotic twins[9]. These data indicate that less than one-third of the cause of RA within a given population can be attributed to genetics. The rest remains to be explained by environmental factors. With this in mind, data from epidemiological studies on RA should be of significant interest.

A hospital-based, case-control study of self-reported diet in Greece, indicated that increased consumption of fish and olive oil was associated with a reduced prevalence of RA[10]. In a district of northwestern Greece, Drosos *et al.* identified 428 cases of RA, which suggested a low prevalence of RA in the area. The course of RA was reported to be mild, and extra-articular manifestations, such as rheumatoid nodules and vasculitis, were rare[11]. The investigators assumed that genetic and environmental factors could explain their findings, and that one possible contributing factor could have been the relatively high consumption of olive oil in the area.

Faroe Islanders, who eat a diet high in fish and whale meat, have been reported to experience a milder clinical course of RA than patients in Denmark[12].

Shapiro *et al.*[13] analyzed data from a population-based, case-control study from Washington state in United States to assess the association between diet and the incidence of RA. Cases were 324 women who were first diagnosed during a 4.5-year long period. These were compared with 1245 matched controls. Self-administered semi quantitative food frequency questionnaires were used to ascertain subjects usual diet during a 1-year period before the patients were affected with RA. The primary purpose of the study was to investigate the hypothesis that n-3 fatty acids, as measured by fish consumption, were protective against RA. The results showed that a high consumption of broiled or baked fish was associated with a decreased risk of RA, and the relation was stronger for cases positive for rheumatoid factor.

Guillemin *et al.*[14] measured the incidence of RA in the Lorraine district, eastern France, restricted to people aged 20–70 years, over the period 1986–1989. In a population of 530 000 people, 205 cases were identified giving an incidence rate of 9.0/100 000, which is a low figure compared to other incidence studies conducted in Caucasian populations[15].

Epidemiological studies conducted in Third World countries are perhaps even more difficult to evaluate with respect to the importance of environmental factors for the development of RA. Somewhat surprisingly, several studies suggest a high prevalence of RA among Eskimo populations[16,17], that is results that do not support the hypothesis of anti-inflammatory effects of n-3 PUFA from fish oil.

The prevalence of RA seems to be low in rural and urban areas in China and in the Philippines[18]. Early reports suggested that in Africans RA was a mild disease[19]. More recent experience shows that severe disease with deformities, radiographic changes, and extra-articular features as seen although they may be less common than in Caucasians[19]. The prevalence in African urban populations seems to be similar to that in Western communities.

Of course, the results from these epidemiological studies in Third World countries should be interpreted very cautiously. The diets of most Third World populations differ significantly from that of Western societies, and with the cited epidemiological information in mind, the data could indicate that Western dietary habits may be less favorable with respect to RA.

Methodological problems in investigating diet and RA

By definition, a *nutraceutical* is any food, food ingredient, or food supplement which is considered to provide medical or health benefits, including the prevention and treatment of disease. The effects of nutraceuticals are difficult to evaluate for many reasons. People eat foods, not single nutrients. Among factors that effect eating habits are age, body fat distribution, physical activity, alcohol consumption, tobacco use, psychological stress, etc.

Investigations of micro nutrients may appear to be less complex. A particular micro nutrient can be encapsulated like a drug and tested against placebo in randomized, double-blinded clinical trials. Ethical constraints normally preclude withholding proven effective therapy. Johnson[20] has recommended the rheumatology community to work toward therapy comparisons of one strategy versus another, rather than one drug versus another. This approach would be suitable for therapeutic trials of nutrients when tested as supplements to other known effective therapy. The endpoints of clinical trials should be different if the trial concerns a 'remitting', 'bridging', or a 'background sparing' agent. Based on present knowledge, nutraceuticals and different dietary regimes fall under the last category mentioned.

As with all therapy trials[21] diet intervention studies should be randomized and double-blinded. Panush *et al.*[22] applied this criterion on their 10-week study of the Dong diet[23] for treatment of patients with RA. The Dong diet, which is a Chinese poor man's diet, contains little meat except fish and occasional fowl, no dairy products, no fruit, and no herbs. A placebo diet was designed to resemble the experimental diet, while including those foods eliminated from the experimental diet. No demonstrable benefit emerged.

However, the double-blinded design may not always be possible. For example trials of extraordinary tasty nutrients, and of diets that exclude common food components, or of very involved regimes such as vegetarianism, are not easy to control. Obviously, a single, open diet interventional study offers little scientific evidence. In addition, we also tend to underestimate the ability of patients to discover which treatment arm they are receiving. This fact is distressing as single blinded observational studies also control placebo effects rather poorly. Treatment with placebo can induce up to 40 per cent response rates, as has been documented in many pharmacological, surgical, or non-pharmacological trials.

Preferably we need large observational studies as in cancer[24] and cardiovascular research[25]. In order to detect putative effects of 20 per cent or more with a power of 80 per cent or more, large patient groups are required. With nutrients, no such large studies have been published so far. In the future, meta-analysis of multiple, well-performed, blinded, as well as open studies could be one instrument for scientists to reach valid consensus on issues of diets and RA.

The inference of dietary intervention studies is often impaired by the existence of inclusion difficulties and of substantial numbers of drop-out patients. Thus, it is difficult to recruit non-biased subjects that are willing to participate in diet intervention studies. In addition, patients need to understand the trial design, and especially the randomized procedure. This is not the least important for those who become allocated to the control group, as exemplified by the recent study by Hansen *et al.*[26]. These researchers met with the problem that the patients in the control diet group tended to adopt features of the experimental diet.

Nutritional status and body composition of patients with RA

Chronic disease may affect nutritional status and body composition of patients[27]. Anthropometric evaluation of the upper limb is a simple, inexpensive and non-invasive bedside method used in the assessment of nutritional status of individuals. It is assumed that the triceps skin fold thickness indicates the energy reserves stored in the form of fat, and the upper arm circumference reflects the reserves of muscle protein. Both measures are associated with a systematic bias. They underestimate any change in body composition. In addition, in older patients, the compressibility of fat increases disproportionately, which results in an overestimation of muscle and an underestimation of fat component.

Plasma albumin is similarly assumed to represent the visceral protein status. However, RA by itself has an affect on anthropometric data and plasma protein concentrations. Active inflammation is accompanied by muscle wasting, partly due to physical inactivity, and decrease in plasma albumin is a well known acute phase protein reaction to inflammation.

Cachexia has been used to denote the loss of body cell mass (BCM) which regularly accompanies severe illness[27]. Approximately 99 per cent of potassium in the human body is located within cells. With the help of the naturally-occurring radioactive isotope ^{40}K, and an expensive whole body counter equipment, total body potassium, and indirectly BCM, can be calculated. Decrease of BCM requires a catabolic process of such magnitude that it induces prolonged negative energy, protein, and micro nutrient balances. Losses accelerate during times of increases disease activity. Loss of BCM is a powerful predictor of outcome in various clinical situations. Decrease of > 40 per cent from baseline BCM is associated with death[28]. It is unlikely that nutritional intervention alone will reverse inflammatory-driven catabolism[29]. Roubenoff *et al.*[28] found that a low BCM correlated with the summation of the disease activity status over many years, and not with the actual disease activity on the day of study.

Collins *et al.*[30] Studied a cohort of 38 patient with active, severe RA. The patients were middle aged, in functional class II–III, and with an average disease duration of 9 years. Upper arm anthropometrics, body weight, and height were measured and a food intake history was obtained by a dietitian. Malnutrition was found in 27 of the 38 RA patients. There was no difference with respect to adequate social and financial support between the malnourished and non-malnourished patients. A high degree of malnutrition was associated with a poor outcome in over 80 per cent of the patients. Malnourished patients tended to have significantly higher erythrocyte sedimentation rates, higher C-reactive protein levels, larger functional impairments, and worse medical outcomes than well-nourished patients.

Based on clinical observations, others have found lower prevalence of malnutrition in RA patients. Roubenoff *et al.*[28] Reported close correlation between ARA functional class of patients and their amount of BCM. In addition, most patients had a reduced BCM (cachexia) even during periods of low disease activity[28]. Their patients with clinically well controlled RA had 13 per cent lower body cell mass, higher resting energy expenditures, and lower levels of vigorous physical activity compared to healthy controls matched for age, sex, race, and weight. Yet these patients consumed similar amounts of protein and energy and their fat mass and total body weight were not significantly different from that of controls. These data suggest that the hypermetabolism of chronic inflammation smolders even when clinical control of RA is achieved. The hypermetabolism is thought to be an effect of increased release of proinflammatory cytokines.

Of course, several other factors may have negative effects on nutritional status. These include: anti nutrient effects of drug therapy, inability to perform grocery and food preparation, and oral dysfunction due to Sjögren's syndrome or temporo-mandibular joint involvement.

Macronutrient intake patterns in patients with RA

Measurement of nutritional adequacy is essential in the evaluation of an individuals nutritional status. Commonly, a structured dietary history is obtained, for example a 24-hour dietary recall[27]. Patients can also be instructed to record measured quantities of foods and beverages immediately after ingestion and to do so prospectively over a certain time period. However, most current methods to assess food intake tend to over-report small intakes and under-report large intakes. In particular, total energy intake measurements systematically tend to be under-estimated. There is also a 'respondent bias', which means over-reporting of the consumption of 'good foods', such as fruits and vegetables, and under-reporting of 'bad foods', with high energy

content, such as fatty foods and alcohol. Nowadays, it is recommended that biological markers of food intake should regularly be used to complement the various forms of food intake records[31].

Cross-sectional studies have confirmed that many patients with RA have a poor dietary intake pattern. Morgan *et al.*[32] recently reported that 40 per cent of a cohort of patients with RA in an urban area of southern United States, had varying degrees of obesity, while only 14 per cent were underweight. The patients had active disease and no serious concomitant medical illness. They were predominantly female Caucasians, in their early 50s, and had a mean disease duration of 9 years, and were all under the care of rheumatologists and on disease modifying medication. Patients who were on prednisone, used doses of less than 10 mg/day. Their mean intake of fat and sweets was estimated to be 50 per cent higher than that of the average United States population. In contrast, their mean intake of all other food groups was below the officially recommended levels. Only 46 per cent of their total energy intake was from carbohydrate. In comparison, FAO/WHO experts[33] recently advocated, that ideally more than 55 per cent of the energy intake should come from carbohydrate. This relative shift from carbohydrate to fat as source of the dietary energy content is not unique for this particular cohort of RA patients. The average citizen in any developed society world wide follows this trend[34], and it is more pronounced among smokers[35].

Kremer *et al.*[36] performed dietary assessments with a 3-day detailed food diary in 41 patients with active RA, and found that they consumed more than recommended of total fat, and too little of polyunsaturated fatty acids and fibers.

It may appear strange that many patients with RA are obese, considering that most RA patients are cachectic[28] even during periods of inactive disease. The likely explanation is that over many years the BCM, that is the lean body mass and especially the content of muscle declines, while the total body weight remains unchanged or goes up, due to absolute increase in body fat. Consequently, the body weight tends to remain constant and does not usually to relate to measures of disease activity[28].

A high fat intake with a high percentage of saturated fatty acids is associated with elevated levels of total cholesterol and low-density lipoprotein in otherwise healthy people. However, in patients with active RA lower serum levels of total cholesterol and total triglycerides are observed, and these levels are reduced in all lipoprotein classes[37]. With active inflammation, triglycerides seemed to be cleared more rapidly from the circulation, as demonstrated with intravenous fat tolerance tests[37]. The likely explanation was considered to be increased elimination of intermediate forms of lipoproteins via the reticular endothelial system and the scavenger receptors of macrophages. However, despite reduced serum lipid levels, patients with RA are at an increased risk of developing atherosclerotic cardiovascular disease[38], as discussed elsewhere in this volume.

The carbohydrate metabolism is also impaired in patients with RA. Glucose handling, as tested by an intravenous glucose tolerance test, was shown to be impaired[39] and related to the intensity of the inflammatory process was defined by the acute phase reaction. It was proposed that the altered glucose metabolism was due to increased peripheral insulin resistance mediated by the inflammatory process[39].

Micronutrient intake of patients with RA

Vitamins and essential trace elements are micronutrients that are vital to cell function. Some are denominated 'antioxidants' because of their defensive functions in tissues against free radical damage. Free oxygen radicals originate from normal metabolism and are formed at sites that encompass all cellular constituents. Free radicals are also generated from exogenous sources such as tobacco smoke, chemicals, and radiation. Large amounts of oxygen radicals are liberated within inflamed rheumatoid joints from activated synovial macrophages and granulocytes, from the up-regulated prostaglandin pathway, and from xanthine oxidase-mediated ischemic repurfusion injury.

Vitamin C and B-carotenes are present in high concentrations in serum and tissue fluids, where they directly interact with emerging free radicals[40]. Vitamin E is lipid soluble and is enriched in cellular membranes, where it is protective against lipid peroxidation. Other essential antioxidative nutrients are selenium, copper, zinc, and manganese. These minerals participate as cofactors to enzymes. Together vitamins, minerals, and enzymes interact in a complicated network. The nutritional intake of each vitamin and mineral has to be adequate in order to maintain optimal protective capacity.

'Optimal' antioxidant plasma levels are for vitamin C in the order of: ≥ 50 μmol/l, for vitamin E: ≥ 30 μmol/l, for vitamin A:≥ 2.2 μmol/l, and for β-carotene: ≥ 0.4 μmol/l[25]. Data from cross-cultural epidemilogical surveys[25] indicate that levels below these threshold predict an increased risk of developing important health hazards. Suboptimal levels of any single antioxidant may increase the relative risk independently. Accordingly, 'suboptimal' levels of several antioxidants predict an additive increase in risk.

Studies on the dose response of plasma levels to oral intake of vitamins indicate that healthy, middle-aged subjects in westernized societies can achieve an 'optimal' plasma status by intake amounts close to or moderately above recommended daily allowances (RDA)[25]. At present, these are for vitamin C:60–80 mg, for vitamin E:15–30 mg, and for β-carotene:2–3 mg[25].

Recent studies performed in Germany, Sweden, and United Kingdom on representative samples of the general population, indicate that the average intake of antioxidative vitamins are close to RDA[41]. A survey from 1985 of United States women showed a mean intake that was below the RDA for pyridoxine, folacin, vitamin E, calcium, iron, magnesium, and zinc.[42]. In fact, the scientific basis for stating the optimum intake of vitamins is under debate. A growing body of knowledge indicates a need for higher intake of antioxidants to protect against sudden and unforeseen oxidative stress. Recently two independent American authorities, the United States Department of Agriculture and the United States Department of Health and Human Services, have suggested figures that are between 50–100 per cent higher for several vitamins compared with present RDA figures[25].

In normal health individuals, the level of dietary intake of micronutrients directly affects the serum levels of these nutrients, and the activity of antioxidant metalloenzymes. In patients with manifest RA, the relationship between nutritional intake and serum levels of antioxidative micronutrients is more complex. Measurements of sera from patients with RA have indicated an ongoing and increased antioxidant activity, and have shown evidence of a redox stress probably imposed by chronic inflammation[43]. Honkanen et al.[44] studied plasma zinc and copper concentrations in 40 Finnish patients with RA. The patients had decreased levels of zinc and increased levels of copper as compared to controls. The patients diets were assessed by using a 1-week food diary. Their average daily intakes of zinc and copper were at the lower end of the recommended dietary allowances. However, the authors concluded that the observed plasma concentrations of zinc and copper were abnormal due to the extent of the inflammation and not due to dietary factors[44].

Plasma levels of vitamins A, C, and E, as well as plasma levels of iron, selenium, and zinc are regularly decreased in patients with active RA in direct relation to the degree of inflammatory activity[44–48]. The plasma level of copper tends to move in the other direction, and shows increase with inflammation[44].

Cross-sectional studies have confirmed that many patients with RA have poor dietary intake patterns and have deficient levels of several vitamins. Data from Morgans cohort of middle-aged patients with RA in Alabama, United States[32] Indicated that these patients consumed less than 67 per cent of the recommended daily intake for the nutrients: folate, vitamin B_{12}, vitamin E, calcium, iron, magnesium, copper, and zinc. Blood vitamin levels of these patients were also assessed. Greater than 15 per cent of the patients had low values with regards to vitamin B_{12}, pyridoxine, vitamin C, carotene, plasma folate, and vitamin E.

Kremer et al.[36] performed dietary assessments with a 3-day detailed food diary on 41 patients from the state of New York, United States with active RA. For both men and women a deficient dietary intake of pyridoxine was observed. Deficiencies in trace element intake were seen for zinc, magnesium, copper, and potassium.

Two recent case control studies[49,50] suggest a link between low serum concentrations of common antioxidants and the relative risk of individuals to develop RA. In a case control study of food intake and recent onset of RA, no association was found between low intake of antioxidants prior to diagnosis and the subsequent development of RA[13].

Supplementation with vitamins and/or minerals

With the intension to suppress RA, megadoses of any antioxidant micro nutrients is not justified by the available observational data. There appears to be an upper limit above which increase in intake of antioxidant micronutrients does not lead to further increase in endogenous capacity of health control. In addition and in theory, there still remains the possibility, that nutritional supplementation actually may enhance the underlying immunologic aberration, thus exacerbating disease activity.

For vitamins C and E, the risks of health hazard by high doses of supplemental dietary therapy seem to be negligible. The safety of β-carotene preparations remains still to be settled. It has to be explored whether the increase of cancer mortality in notorious Finnish smokers in response to a daily intake of a preparation of 20 mg of β-carotene was not a chance finding in spite of its statistical significance[24]. The liposoluble vitamins A and D have very high biological potency and hormone-like actions, and excess intake of these vitamins can provoke adverse, toxic effects.

A small number of double-blinded clinical trials of substitution with "supraoptimal" daily doses of antioxidant vitamins or minerals have been done in patients with RA, involving vitamin C[48], vitamin E[51], zinc[45], and selenium[46].

These trials were all of short duration and comprised limited numbers of patients. Therefore power to detect eventual effects was low. No anti-inflammatory effects on RA were documented. However, in a recent observational investigation[52] On 640 patients, over 10 years, knee osteoarthritis progression and the development of knee pain was reduced in people with high intakes of vitamin C and possibly other antioxidants. Still another recent investigation[51] provides preliminary evidence that vitamin E may exert a small but significant analgesic action from influence on nociceptive transmission within central nervous pathways.

However, as stated before, substitution with one, two, or more preparations of antioxidants seems to be suboptimal strategy. Antioxidant-related health benefits seem to depend on an adequacy of all antioxidants, and possibly of non-antioxidative nutrients as well. Evidence from epidemiological surveys indicates that under steady-state conditions, diets rich in antioxidants (from vegetables/fruits and suitable vegetable oils) can reduce the relative risk of premature death from cardiovascular disease and cancer[25].

Intriguing 'new' conutrients of antioxidants have been isolated from health promoting fruits and vegetables. Such substances are phenols/bioflavonoids, anthocyanins, caretenoids other than β-carotene, folate, riboflavin, oleic acid, and potentially carcinostatic compounds in garlic, broccoli, and others[25].

Polyunsaturated fatty acids (PUFA)

Polyunsaturated fatty acids (PUFA) are dominant and manifold compounds in cell membranes. In competition with each other, they are readily incorporated into cell membrane phospholipids, where they support structure and participate in vital functions. Examples of their functions are production, regulation, and release of eicosanoids, as well as signal transduction through the phospholipid-dependent pathways. Other effects of PUFA include regulation of ion channels[53] and suppression of smooth muscle cell proliferation[54]. It has recently been shown that dietary fatty acids as well as vitamins can react like steroidal hormones with nuclear receptors and influence gene transcription[6]. As stated by Zurier *et al.*[55]: 'The potential regulation of cell activation, immune responses, and inflammation by certain

fatty acids is exciting to consider at clinical, cellular, and molecular levels'.

PUFA of the n-6 family and especially arachidonic acid (20:4 n-6) are dominating in human cell membranes. Linoleic acid (18:2 n-6) is the obligate precursor for longer n-6 PUFA, and is an essential micro nutrient for humans. It is abundant in dairy products, meat, and in many vegetable seed oils. Gamma-linolenic acid (GLA; 18:3 n-6) is an essential n-6 PUFA found in certain plant seed oils and is precursor of prostaglandin E_I, an eicosanoid with known anti-inflammatory and immunoregulatory properties[55].

Human cell membranes contain considerably less PUFA of the n-3 family, and Western diets are usually low on these acids. In practice only fish, and especially pink salmon, tuna, herring, mackerel, and pitchard are rich in longer n-3 PUFA.

Eicosapentaenoic (20:5 n-3) and docosahexaenoic acids (22:6 n-3) are the most well known. Alfa linolenic acid (18:3 n-3) is a shorter n-3 PUFA found in flax, rape, and soy oils. It can be elongated endogenously and further desaturated into longer n-3 PUFA, and this probably explains why vegetarians still have longer n-3 PUFA in their phospholipids, even though the levels are low compared to those of omnivores. A new PUFA of interest is conjugated dienoic linoleate (CLA), which is another linoleic acid derivative. It has recently received considerable attention for chemoprotective qualities[56], and possibly modulatory effects on carcinogenesis in humans[56]. The highest food source of CLA is ruminant meat and dairy products. The pattern of fatty acids in blood is widely used as a biomarker to assess differences in fatty acid intake between populations. Human blood contains a number of discrete fatty acid pools. These are triglycerides, cholesteryl esters, phospholipids, and fats that are cellularly bound to erythrocytes and platelets. PUFA have been measured preferentially in the plasma phosphatidylcholine and erythrocyte lipid pools. Patients with RA, and juvenile chronic arthritis (JCA) seemed to have increased proportions of saturated acids, while linoleic acid (18:2 n-6) was reduced in these pools. Also eicosapentaenoic acid and other fatty acids of the n-3 series seemed to be proportionally decreased[57,58]. These abnormalities increased with disease duration and correlated with the acute phase protein response. It was assumed that inflammation and not altered dietary habits could explain the abnormal lipid profile seen in patients with RA.

Supplementation with specific PUFA

Certain PUFA of the n-6, as well as the n-3 families are especially recognized for their potential modulatory effects on inflammation and immune reactions[55,56,59]. Gamma-linolenic acid (GLA; 18:3 n-6) and longer n-3 PUFA have been tested in clinical trials on patients with RA. For the present, no formal trials of conjugated dienoic linoleate (CLA) on patients with RA have been presented.

Zurier *et al.*[55] performed a randomized double blind trial of GLA versus sunflower seed oil (placebo) in patients with RA over a period of 6 months. The daily dose was 2.8 gm of GLA provided in eight gelatin capsule. 22 patients on GLA completed the trial and achieved statistically significantly improvement in swollen joint count, tender joint count, pain (by VAS), and

HAQ score compared to 19 patients in the placebo group. Differentiation from the placebo response as measured in number of tender joints did not occur until after 3 months of therapy. Twenty per cent of patients experienced some adverse reactions from belching and/or diarrhea.

Several trials have studied the effect of supplementation with longer n-3 PUFA in patients with RA[60-66]. The results have been fairly consistent and have shown moderate improvements in selected subjective symptoms, with little effect on objective measurements of disease activity. A modest NSAID-sparing was documented in some of the studies. Somewhat surprisingly, a recent Mexican study reported no effect[67].

The range of doses of n-3 PUFA tested were 2.6–6g or 7–20 gelatin capsules daily. Very high daily doses of n-3 PUFA (20 g) have been associated with gastrointestinal intolerance including eructions, nausea, abdominal bloating, flatulence, diarrhea, and an bad taste[68]. In clinical trials on RA patients the doses have been considerably lower but still many patients recognized an aftertaste, although acceptable[63]. Twelve months was the longest treatment period[66,68]. All studies had rather limited numbers of patients in the treatment arms, and most probably each of them had suboptimal power to verify potential effects of therapy. Thus supplementation with GLA or n-3 PUFA seem to provide only modest improvement and it may not be worth while to prescribe these substances[55,59]. However, for patients, with a perspective of a persistent disease process prevailing for decades even a modest anti-inflammatory effect could be of interest, provided that it is safe, well tolerated, and affordable. A normal diet enriched in fish (700 g per week) can induce similar changes in the fatty acid composition of membrane and serum lipids as substitution with a daily intake of 15 capsules with fish oil concentrates (3.1 g n-3 PUFA per day)[69]. These findings indicate that some fish meals per week could have similar anti-inflammatory effect for patients with RA as do fish oil concentrates.

Rheumatologists have paid much less attention to alfa-linolenic acid (18:3, n-3) which is a precursor for longer n-3 PUFA in humans. Flax seed oil is rich in this fatty acid, and it has been shown that use of flax seed oil in domestic food preparation may inhibit production of TNF-α and IL-1β by mononuclear cells[70]. No formal trial of domestic foods enriched in alfa-linolenic acid on patients with RA have been presented so far. However, it is of interest that French investigators on atherosclerotic vascular disease[71] have shown results which indicate that a diet enriched with alpha-linolenic acid and fish oils may have anti-inflammatory effects, and that this kind of diet seemed to have induced secondary prevention against coronary heart disease.

Elimination of nutrients from the diet

The anti-inflammatory effect of fasting

Fasting had a reputation among laymen to improve RA. The idea was tested and found valid[72] and has been repeatedly confirmed[73-77]. At the end of a 7–10-day long fasting period the Ritchie index of joint tenderness showed a decrease and the plasma concentrations of acute phase proteins were reduced[72,78]. However, the most striking effect was reduced pain and stiffness, experienced by most patients, and a reduction in their daily intake of NSAID[72].

The improvement was usually present on the 4th or 5th day of fasting and lasted throughout the rest of the fast. Many patients felt a return of pain and stiffness already on the day after the fast was concluded, and most of the benefit was lost within a week or two of return to normal diet. The effect wained irrespectively of which diet the patients returned to. This could be a ordinary Western diet[74], lactovegetarian[72], or vegan diet[79].

Although fasting is not a feasible approach for long-term treatment, it may serve as a model for studying pathogenic mechanisms. The way by which fasting exerts its anti-inflammatory effect are largely unknown, as discussed by Palmblad *et al.*[80]. Fasting promptly imposes a shortage of exogenous energy, internal metabolism has to be reorganized, and priority given to vital functions[81]. Tissue concentrations of metabolic hormones have to be readjusted[82,83], and endogenous energy sources are mobilized from liver glykogen, fat tissue, and muscular proteins.

Considerable data support effects of fasting on inflammatory and immunlogical processes. The exposure of healthy subjects to 10 days of fasting was accompanied by lower levels of acute phase proteins[78,84], reduced DNA synthesis in circulating mononuclear leukocytes after *in vitro* stimulation with bacterial antigens[85], and decreased ability of PMNs to kill bacteria[86].

In patients with RA, a period of 3–6 days of total fast induced a significant increase in antigen-specific mucosa-driven B-lymphocyte response[87], and at the end of a fast for 7 days patients with RA showed normalization in impaired con A suppressor cell activity[88]. In other patients with RA, fasting reduced the ability of serum to generate cytotaxins, reduced the release of LTB 4 from neutrophils, and altered the fatty acid composition in neutropil phospholipids[77].

Fasting very dramatically reduced the amounts of nutrients and foreign antigens that gain access to the gastrointestinal (GI) canal, which has effects on intestinal bacterial colonisation, and possibly on GI-immune function. Recent data of Trollmo *et al.*[89] support the occurrence of gut-derived lymphocytes in synovial tissues.

Gastrointestinal conditions and functions with implications for RA

The enterocytes of the intestinal mucosa and the overlying mucus 'glycolax' are, under most conditions, an effective barrier[90]. The intestinal mucosa selectively absorbs nutrients after enzymatic digestion down to dipeptides, triglycerides, fatty acids, and disaccharides[90]. Besides these, only small molecules penetrate the gut wall freely, while macromolecules with antigenic properties are not readily absorbed. However, there are special mechanisms through which antigenic material might penetrate to the interior body[91]. A specialized epithelial cell, the M-cell, covers agglomerates of intestinal lymphoid tissue, Peyer's patches. The M-cell is in direct contact with the liquid content of the intestinal lumen, where, by active pinocytosis, it randomly picks up foreign antigenic material and presents it to closely underlying macrophages and lymphocytes for immunological surveillance and processing.

Non-self macromolecules penetrate the intestinal mucosa through other less controlled and ill-defined routes[92], presumedly through injuries to the epithelium caused by toxic[93,94], infectious[95], or allergic[96] processes. NSAID caused an increase of intestinal permeability in healthy volunteers[94] and in patients with RA[97]. Another factor that can augment permeability is local intestinal anaphylaxis to food-derived antigens[96].

Coeliac disease is accompanied by altered intestinal permeability[98,99], elevated levels of circulating immune complexes, and lesions outside the gastrointestinal tract, most commonly dermatitis herpitiforms. The disease characteristics are strictly correlated to the dietary intake of gluten[100]. Although coeliac disease has been reported in association with RA, this is not common[101]. O'Farrely et al.[102] reported on a surprisingly large subgroup of RA patients with raised levels of IgG antibodies to gliadin, which is a component of gluten. These patients showed intestinal villious atrophy compared to a control group of RA patients lacking such antibodies. These findings need confirmation.

Recently Trollmo et al.[89] have shown that antigen-specific B cells, triggered by oral immunization with influenza virus vaccine, displayed a strong propensity to home to synovium, indicating an immunological communication between the gut and the synovial tissue in patients with RA. They also demonstrated that patients with RA showed normal responsiveness in their gastrointestinal mucosal immune system, and that these functions were not significantly altered by medication with NSAID. Trollmo et al. hoped that their findings would stimulate researchers to look for induction of tolerance/vaccination procedures in RA patients[89].

Food hypersensitivity and RA

Food antigens do cross the gastrointestinal barrier and can be detected in the circulation as food antigens and as immune complexes[91]. Already in 1941, Hench and colleagues[103] concluded: 'allergy to certain foods may provoke arthritis in certain patients'. A minority of patients with RA claim that their symptoms are alleviated by special diets or by elimination of certain constituents from their diet. Foods that most often are suspected to cause worsening of symptoms are red meat, spices, flour products, citrus fruits, chocolate, and alcohol[104].

Much of the data on food allergy and RA are anecdotal and originate in case reports[105–109]. In 1986, Panush et al.[108] reported on a patient, whose RA flared with peak of symptoms after 24–28 h, when challenged blindly with lyophilized milk products given in gelatin capsules. Immunological investigation showed a marked increase of IgG antimilk levels, increasing IgG milk circulating immune complexes, and *in vitro* cellular sensitivity to milk.

Also in 1986, Darlington et al.[110] reported that food allergy might contribute to the manifestations of polyarthritis more often than was usually believed. They had given 53 patients with RA an allergen-reduced diet for 1 week, followed by a reintroduction phase of 5 weeks, when foods were reintroduced one at a time. Foods that were identified to produce symptoms were excluded from the diet, and at the end of the 6-week diet period, every patient had adopted an individualized diet. This single-blind, controlled study, over 6 weeks of specific exclusion-diet therapy showed favorable effects on pain, on the number of painful joints, on the platelet counts, and on plasma levels of complement factor 3. Three of four patients felt improvement. The experiment is difficult to evaluate. The food challenges were not blinded. Obviously, in part, the positive results could represent a placebo response. The same authors have later reported that out of 70 rheumatoid patients who started an individualized elimination diet, 13 were still well, requiring no drug treatment after a mean follow-up period of 3 years[111].

According to several other investigations, food allergy is probably not a common factor in the pathogenesis of RA[13,108,112–115]. Panush et al.[108] reported that the prevalence of food sensitivity among rheumatoid patients was less than 5 per cent, and assumed that food intolerance of importance to the manifestations of RA was even less common.

Others reported a double-blind, randomized, 12-week study, completed by 78 patients[114]. After an initial observational period of 4 weeks they were randomized to one of two experimental diets for 4 weeks, allowing no other foods. The first diet was free from potential allergens including additives and preservatives. The second was also free from allergens except for milk and azo dyes. Both kind of diets contained all essential nutrients and were provided in tins, in different flavorings. During the remaining 4 weeks the patients were rechallenged to all foods and finally resumed their original diets. At the end of the artificial diet period, the patients had lost 2.7 kg of weight, on average. Nearly all patients showed some improvement while receiving one of the two diets. Both groups of patients were significantly improved in measurements of morning stiffness, tender and swollen joints, global assessment, Ritchie index, and fatigue. No laboratory parameters were affected. No difference was seen between the two diet groups. During the course of rechallenge back to an ordinary diet, essentially all beneficial effects were lost. Nine patients were identified for their markedly good responsiveness to the artificial exclusion diet (≥ 20 per cent improvement). Six of these were further studied using placebo-controlled rechallenges[115]. Intolerance for specific foodstuffs were finally diagnosed in four patients, and the authors concluded[115] that only a minority of patients showed evidence of food intolerance, that this was laborious to prove, and that therapeutic effects of clinical duration were unusual.

Profound diet intervention— adoption of a significantly 'new' diet

Ziff's[21] conclusion on diet and RA from 1983 is still valid: 'Whatever diet one chooses, its evaluation will be fraught with difficulties', and he recommended that: 'the choice of diet should be based on a concept that links intermediary metabolism with immunity and chronic inflammation, and there ought to be a clear idea of what the diet is designed to achieve metabolically'. Of course, the theory must be transformed into a concrete diet that is applicable to the participating patients.

There are few diet intervention studies motivated by scientific objectives with RA patients. The Danish study of Hansen *et al.*[26] is a rare example. They tested a diet containing 800 g weekly of fatty fish, and supplemented with vitamin and mineral additives, versus ordinary Danish food. The study design was controlled, randomized, and single-blinded, and lasted over 6 months. The drop-out rate was 25 per cent. Of the patients who fulfilled the trial, 36 had been randomly assigned to the diet and 45 to the control group. The participating patients tended to be highly selected on the basis of health consciousness and motivation. Yet, and very unexpectedly, prior to the study these Danish RA patients consumed little or no fish at all. In addition, their intakes of iodine, vitamin A, E, and D were also estimated to be very low.

At the end of the trial the patients of the fish diet group showed significant improvement in duration of morning stiffness, number of swollen joints, and in pain status as compared to the control group. No difference between groups of diet and control patients were seen in physicians assessment of global activity. HAQ-score, ESR, and radiograph. These results lend support to the hypotheses that a diet enriched with fish and antioxidative micronutrients is suppressive of rheumatoid inflammation.

The experimental diet was meant to contain a low fat content of < 30 energy per cent, with a ratio of saturated to unsaturated fat of 1. The intention was also to increase the protein intake to 1.5 g per kg body weight per day, mostly in the form of vegetables and fish. Food intakes were assessed and these results indicated some problems with compliance. Biological markers were not used. As expected, during the study the diet patients reported decreased intake of fats and meat, and increased intake of fish, cereals, and fruits. That they also consumed 50 per cent more of eggs and dairy products, and 30 per cent less of vegetables and roots was not commented on by the authors. Contrary to the intentions, the control patients reported almost 25 per cent increase of their fish consumption.

Motivated by utilitarian or philosophic objectives, various vegetarian diets have been tested on patients with RA4,[72,73,75,79,112,116,117]. Information on vegetarianism and RA is limited. The study designs have been open or single blinded. Most of them indicate that vegetarian diets may induce subjective improvement to patients with RA. However, the benefits from short terms of vegetarianism have mostly been small, and after the conclusion of formal studies a majority of patients have chosen to return to ordinary diets[72,79].

Considerable attention was devoted to the study of Kjeldsen-Kragh *et al.*[112]. They reported that a group of 27 Norwegian patients with RA, compared to a control group, gained extraordinary good benefit from a vegan diet followed by a lactovegetarian diet. Altogether the diet intervention lasted for 1 year. Both subjective and objective parameters of rheumatoid disease activity showed improvement. The study met with several methodological problems. The drop out rate was 36 per cent. The patients were a highly selected group of people with very strong beliefs in 'alternative' forms of treatment while their trust in ordinary medical therapies was low[118]. The question is whether placebo could have explained the very good results, or alternatively, if these Norwegian patients were more motivated than others to adhere to the prescribed diet? The diet per se was not significantly different from other vegan[79] or lactovegetarian diets[72], and the beneficial effect started early. Thus the length of the trial was not the critical factor. Nenonen *et al.*[4,117] in their study on extreme vegan diet ('living food') and RA, served food to the patients throughout the study period in order to achieve optimal compliance. Still, their results were very modest compared to the Norwegian study.

Large epidemiological studies on vegetarian diets and chronic disease have been done in Seventh-Day Adventist populations. Dwyer[119] summarized the results of these studies, prior to 1988, with respect to RA, with the words: 'at present there is little evidence that vegetarian diet play any significant role in treating rheumatoid arthritis'.

Conclusion

Rheumatoid artritis affects the nutritional status and body composition of patients[28-30]. More active disease is characterized by cachexia. In present day Western cohorts, only a minority of RA patients are underweight[32]. Many patients with RA have a poor dietary intake pattern[32,36], with a relative shift from carbohydrate to fat as source of the dietary energy content, and a concomitant deficient intake of several micronutrients.

Current methods to assess food intake tend to be rather inaccurate and, if possible, a complementary use of biological markers is recommended[31].

In patients with RA, the serum levels of antioxidative micronutrients reflect not only the nutritional intake, but also the intensity of inflammation. Plasma levels of vitamin A, C, and E, as well as plasma levels of iron, selenium, and zinc are regularly decreased in patients with active RA in direct relation to the degree of inflammatory activity[44-48].

It is evident that modulation of diet and caloric intake can have a marked effect on autoimmune disease in murine models[7,8]. Cross cultural epidemiological surveys[11-19] together with twin studies[9] indicate that environmental factors do effect the prevalence and severity of RA. More recent research has revealed that many nutrients and vitamins seem to bind to soluble intranuclear receptors and may, thereby, in a similar manner to hormones, affect regulatory mechanisms of gene transcription[6].

Certain PUFA of the n-6, and especially of the n-3, families have been recognized for their modulatory effects on RA inflammation[55,60-66], when given to the patients in capsules in the form of fish oil concentrates. A normal diet enriched in fish can induce similar changes in serum lipids[69]. The results of a recent population-based, case-control study showed, that a high consumption of broiled or baked fish was associated with a decreased risk of RA, and the relation was stronger for cases positive for rheumatoid factor[13]. Two other case-control studies indicate an association of low serum levels of antioxidants and later development of RA[49,50].

Fasting improves patients with RA[72-77], but the anti-inflammatory effect is lost within a week or two of return to regular eating habits. Food antigens can be detected in the human circulation and in blood immune complexes[91]. However, several studies indicate that food allergy is not a frequent factor in the pathogenesis of RA[13,112-115]. Such allergy is laborious to diagnose and the long-term clinical effects from specific antigen exclusion is uncertain[115].

Different vegetarian diets have been tested on patients with RA, in open studies[72,73,75,79,112,116,117]. The results indicate that vegetarianism may induce subjective improvement. The effect seems to be small, and a majority of patients tend to return to ordinary diets, after the conclusion of the formal studies[72,79]. Comparatively few diet interventional studies have been motivated by scientific objectives. Hansen *et al.*[26] tested a diet containing 800 g per week of fatty fish, and supplemented with vitamin and mineral additives, versus ordinary Danish food. Their results lend some support to the hypothes that a diet rich in n-3 PUFA and antioxidative micronutrients may be suppressive to rheumatoid inflammation.

References

1. Ames B.N., Gold L.S. Alternative therapies — medicine, magic, or quackery. Who is wining the battle? *J Rheumatol*, 1997;**24**:12, 2276–2279.
2. Wasner C.K. The art of unproven remedies *Rheum Dis Clin North America*, 1991;**17**:197–202.
3. Buchanan H.M., Preston S.J., Brooks P.M., Buchanan W.W. Is diet important in rheumatoid arthritis? *Br J Rheumatol*, 1991;**30**:125–134.
4. Nenonen M.T. *Vegan diet, rich in lactobacilli ('living food'): metabolic and subjective responses in healthy subjects and in patients with rheumatoid arthritis.* Doctoral dissertation, Kuopio 1995 Kuopio University Publications D. Medical Sciences 76.
5. Darlington LG. Dietary therapy for arthritis. *Rheum Dis Clin North America*, 1991;**17**:273–285.
6. Gustavsson J-Å. Fatty acids in control of gene expression. *Nutrition Reviews*, 1998;**56**:20–21.
7. Delafuwnte J.C. Nutrients and immune responses. *Rhem Dis Clin North America*, 1991;**17**:203–211.
8. Keen C.L., German B.J., Mareschi J-P, Gershwin M.E. Nutritional modulation of murine models of auto immunity. *Rheum Dis Clin North America*, 1991;**17**:223–234.
9. Järvinen P., Aho K. Twin studies in rheumatic diseases. *Semin Arthritis Rheum*, 1994;**24**:19–28.
10. Linos A., Kaklamanis P.H. The effect of olive oil and fish consumption on rheumatoid arthritis: a case control study. *Scand J Rheumatol*, 1991;**20**:419–426.
11. Drosos A.A., Alamonos I., Voulgari P.V., Psychos D.N. *et al.* Epidemiology of adult rheumatoid arthritis in northwest Greece 1987–1995. *J Rheumatol*, 1997;**24**:2129–2133.
12. Recht L., Helin P., Rasmussen J.O., Lithman T., Schersten B. Hand handicap and rheumatoid arthritis in a fish-eating society (the Faroe islands). *J Intern Med*, 1990;**227**:49–55.
13. Shapiro J.A., Koepsell T.D., Voigt L.F., Dugowson C.E., *et al.* Diet and rheumatoid arthritis in women: A possible protective effect of fish consumption. *Epidemilogy*, 1996;**7**:256–263.
14. Guillemin F., Briancon S., Klein J.-M., Sauleau E., *et al.* Low incidence of rheumatoid arthritis in France. *Scand J Rheumatol*, 1994;**23**:264–268.
15. Uhlig T., Kvien T., Glennås A., Smedstad L.M., *et al.* The incidence and severity of rheumatoid arthritis. Results from a county register in Oslo, Norway. *J Rheumatol*, 1998;**25**:1078–1084.
16. Beasley R.P., Retailliau H., Healey L.A. Prevalence of rheumatoid arthritis in Alaskan Eskimos. *Arthritis Rheum*, 1973;**16**:737–742.
17. Boyer GS, Benevolenskaya LI, Templin DW, Erdesz S, *et al.* Prevalence of rheumatoid arthritis in circumpolar native populations. *J Rheumatol*, 1998;**25**:23–29.
18. Mijiyawa M. Epidemilogy and semiology of rheumatoid arthritis in third world countries. *Rev Rhum* (Engl Edn), 1995;**62**: 121–126.
19. Mody G.M. Rheumatoid arthritis and connective tissue disorders: sub-Saharan Africa *Bailliéré s Clin Rheumatol*, 1995;**9**:31–44.
20. Johnsson K.. Efficacy assessment in trials of combination therapy for rheumatoid arthritis. *J Rheumatol*, 1996;**23**, suppl 44:107–109.
21. Ziff M.M. Diet in the treatment of rheumatoid arthritis. *Arthritis Rheum*, 1983;**26**:457–460.
22. Panush R.S., Carter R.L., Katz P., Kowsari B., Longley, S., Finnie S. Diet therapy for rheumatoid arthritis. *Arthritis Rheum*, 1986;**26**:462–471.
23. Dong C.H. and Banks J. *The arthritic's cookbook*. Bantam Nutrition Books, New York 1973.
24. Heinonen O.P., Albanes D., for the Alpha-Tocopherol, Beta-carotene, Cancer Prevention Study Group. The effect of vitamin E and beta-carotene on the incidence of lung cancer and other cancers in male smokers. *N Engl J Med*, 1994;**330**: 1029–1035.
25. Gey K.F. Cardiovascular disease and vitamins. In: *The scientific basis for vitamin intake in human nutrition*. Eds Walter B., Somogyi J.C., Bibl Nutr Dieta, Basel, Karger 1995, pp 75–91.
26. Hansen G.V.O., Nielsen L., Kluger E., Thysen M., *et al.* Nutritional status of Danish rheumatoid arthritis patients and effects of a diet adjusted in energy intake, fish-meal, and antioxidants. *Scand J Rheumatol*, 1996;**25**:325–330.
27. Shenkin A., Cederblad G., Elia M., Isaksson B. Laboratory assessment of protein-energy status International federation of clinical chemistry *Clinica Chimica Acta*, 1996;**253**:5–59.
28. Roubenoff R., Roubenoff R.A., Cannon J.G., Rosenberg I.H. Rheumatoid Cachexia: cytokine-driven hypermetabolism accompanying reduced body cell mass in chronic inflammation. *J Clin Invest*, 1994;**93**:2379–2386.
29. Streat S.J., Beddoe A.H., Hill G.L. Aggressive nutritional support does not prevent protein loss despite fat gain in septic intensive care patients. *J Trauma*, 1987;**27**:262–266.
30. Collins R., Dunn T.L., Walthaw J., Harrel P., *et al.* Malnutrition in rheumatoid arthritis. *Clin Rheumatol*, 1986;**6**:391–398.
31. Johansson G., Callmer E., Gustavsson J.-Å. Validity of repeated dietary measurements in a dietary intervention study. *Eur J Clin Nutrition*, 1992;**46**:717–728.
32. Morgan S.L., Andersson A.M., Hood S.M., Matthews P.A., *et al.* Nutrient intake patterns, body mass index, and vitamin levels in patients with rheumatoid arthritis. *Arthritis Care Res*, 1997;**10**:9–18.
33. Joint FAO/WHO Expert Consultation on Carbohydrates in Human Nutrition. FAO, Rome 1997; April 14–18, (Interim Report). http://www.fao.org/waicent/faoinfo/economic/esn/carbohyd/carbohyd.htm.
34. Astrup A., Flatt J.P. Carbohydrate and obesity. *J Obes*, 1995;**19** (suppl 5):27–37.
35. Nydahl M., Gustavsson I.B., Mohsen R., Vessby B. The food and nutrient intake of Swedish non-smokers *Scand J Nutrition*, 1996;**40**:64–69.

Table 31.1 Scores of health status in 1030 patients with RA from the RA county register in Oslo, Norway

Scales	Mean (SE) total, n = 1030	< 40 years (n = 110)	40–49 years (n = 93)	50–59 years (n = 157)	60–69 years (n = 265)	70–79 years (n = 317)	> 80 years (n = 88)
SF-36 (0–100, 0 worst health)							
Physical functioning	47.3 (0.83)	65.0 (2.44)	56.6 (2.41)	51.2 (1.95)	45.2 (1.52)	41.4 (1.49)	35.2 (2.76)
Role physical	27.0 (1.12)	46.8 (3.93)	35.7 (3.86)	32.4 (2.91)	23.4 (2.07)	20.3 (1.82)	16.4 (3.48)
Bodily pain	41.0 (0.69)	50.5 (2.29)	45.8 (2.04)	41.3 (1.57)	39.3 (1.32)	37.8 (1.28)	37.3 (2.43)
General health	42.0 (0.70)	47.7 (2.13)	45.7 (2.20)	44.7 (1.70)	39.2 (1.32)	39.5 (1.34)	42.8 (2.28)
Vitality	39.4 (0.71)	46.4 (1.84)	40.0 (2.24)	40.4 (1.75)	39.9 (1.32)	36.1 (1.41)	38.0 (2.41)
Social functioning	63.7 (0.92)	74.0 (2.32)	69.5 (2.60)	66.5 (2.15)	64.8 (1.83)	57.6 (1.73)	57.9 (3.56)
Role emotional	52.0 (1.32)	68.2 (3.62)	58.5 (4.32)	57.1 (3.39)	52.3 (2.54)	41.2 (2.31)	51.4 (5.11)
Mental health	68.1 (0.68)	74.9 (1.66)	69.0 (1.92)	68.6 (1.80)	68.1 (1.33)	65.4 (1.30)	66.5 (2.58)
Reported health transition	41.8 (0.80)	49.5 (2.58)	49.2 (2.82)	45.5 (2.06)	39.3 (1.45)	39.2 (1.44)	34.3 (2.68)
MHAQ (1–4, 4 worst health)	1.70 (0.02)	1.38 (0.04)	1.55 (0.05)	1.67 (0.04)	1.72 (0.04)	1.80 (0.04)	1.86 (0.08)
AIMS 2 (0–10, 10 worst health)							
Physical	2.88 (0.07)	1.70 (0.16)	2.03 (0.14)	2.40 (0.14)	2.95 (0.13)	3.40 (0.12)	4.05 (0.27)
Affect	3.45 (0.06)	2.92 (0.15)	3.40 (0.18)	3.45 (0.15)	3.43 (0.12)	3.60 (0.11)	3.66 (0.22)
Symptom (pain)	5.43 (0.08)	4.39 (0.24)	4.98 (0.26)	5.65 (0.20)	5.48 (0.17)	5.72 (0.15)	5.66 (0.28)
Social interaction	4.28 (0.05)	3.81 (0.12)	4.21 (0.15)	4.48 (0.14)	4.35 (0.10)	4.31 (0.10)	4.27 (0.19)
VAS (0–100, 100 worst health)							
Pain	46.0 (0.75)	38.2 (2.12)	39.6 (2.24)	47.4 (1.75)	48.3 (1.49)	48.0 (1.43)	47.2 (2.62)
Fatigue	49.9 (0.88)	43.1 (2.66)	52.0 (2.74)	51.6 (2.05)	49.8 (1.69)	50.7 (1.71)	51.2 (3.32)

29 per cent equaled or exceeded the cut-off point in at least 1 year. To put these findings in perspective Katz provided data on a comparison group of people without RA that were given the GDS between 1989 and 1991. The proportion of these people who exceeded the cut-off point of 7 between 1989 and 1991 ranged from 3 to 5 per cent[24].

A Norwegian group of 238 RA patients aged up to 70 years and with disease duration of maximum 4 years was examined for their levels of psychological distress and compared with 116 healthy controls matched with respect to sex, age, and geographical area[56]. Psychological distress was measured by a generic self-report instrument, namely the General Health Questionnaire. The patients reported significantly more severe mental distress than the controls. This was so for the GHQ sum score reflecting global mental distress as well as for each of the four subscales measuring symptoms of anxiety and depression, somatization, and social dysfunction, respectively. Twenty per cent of the patients had GHQ sum score values indicating possible psychiatric caseness compared to 6 per cent of the controls. The percentage of *possible* depressive cases among patients was 22 when the AIMS depressive subscale was used as an indicator of possible caseness, whereas 11 per cent were classified as *probable* psychiatric cases[56]. In another study, Gilboe et al.[57] found that 82 RA and SLE patients had consistently worse SF-36 health status scores compared with healthy individuals.

Psychological problems do not seem to be greater in rheumatoid arthritis than in other chronic medical conditions. Hawley and Wolfe used 19 122 AIMS depression scores to compare depressive symptoms and scores between various rheumatic diseases. Depressive symptoms and depression scores in RA did not differ from other clinical patients taken as a whole and were less pronounced than in patients with fibromyalgia[46]. Matched RA and SLE-patients had similar SF-36 scores within the dimension of mental health and role limitations due to emotional problems[57].

Social health status in RA

Some of the multidimensional generic and disease specific health status measures also capture the social functioning, which reflects the patients' social relationships rather than occupational aspects. SF-36 and AIMS-2 scores obtained by postal surveys to a community based RA sample in Oslo are shown in Table 31.1. In a comparative study, Gilboe et al.[57] have shown that the SF-36 social functioning score is similar between RA and SLE patients and lower (worse health) compared to matched, healthy controls.

Several studies have shown that the course of RA is associated with a considerable work disability and decreased earnings[51,58,59]. Wolfe[14] reviewed four studies of work disability in a total number of more than 2000 RA patients. These studies showed that approximately half of the patients were work disabled after about 10 years of disease. Pincus[60] has discussed the underestimated long-term medical and economic consequences of rheumatoid arthritis and documented that more than 50 per cent of patients with rheumatoid arthritis younger than 65 years and who were working at onset of disease received work disability payments.

Compared to studying full-time employees/workers, it is much more difficult to study work limitations in women working fully or partially in their homes. Reisine et al.[61] showed in a survey of 142 home makers that half of them reported limitations in their usual work roles.

Indirect costs account for activities that are foregone as a result of the disease. These activities may include paid or unpaid labor and tasks such as shopping, gardening, etc.[62]. Indirect costs in clinical samples of rheumatoid arthritis exceed direct costs and most of the indirect costs are related to wage losses[63]. Population studies have shown major earning gaps between individuals with symmetric polyarthritis and those in the general population[60].

However, the relation between direct and indirect cost may be related to age. Clarke *et al.*[64] found that direct costs were higher than indirect costs in a large sample of 1063 RA patients followed up to 12 and 4 years respectively in two center in Canada. The mean age was more than 60 years. Thus all the patients were closer to retirement and required more hospital stays, explaining that the direct costs could exceed the indirect costs.

Gabriel *et al.*[65] compared the indirect and non-medical costs among people with rheumatoid arthritis, osteoarthritis and non-arthritic controls. They found that both RA and OA incurred significantly more expenditures for home or childcare and other services compared to non-arthritics. Patients with rheumatoid arthritis were significantly more likely to have lost their jobs or to have retired early due to their illness. They were also the most likely to have reduced their work hours or stopped working entirely due to their illness, and they were three times more likely to have had a reduction in household family incomes than either individuals with OA or those without arthritis[65].

How are psychological variables related to disease factors?

Examinations of the relationships between psychological variables and disease factors have traditionally been examined as one-way directional effects; either by studying the disease impact in terms of psychological outcome, or by studying the impacts on clinical status by psychological variables. However, this idea of one-way directional effects between physical and psychological variables in RA may be overly simplistic. Thus, due to the complexity of the task, even prospective, longitudinal studies with multiple time points will have difficulties testing causal models which allow for reciprocal (two-way) causation and feedback loops. This is probably the main reason why studies exploring causal relationships between psychosocial and physical variables in RA are relatively scarce. Nevertheless, the question of directionality is a key issue as evidence of causality may have considerable impact on clinical practice. If, for example, depression is a factor that enhances the pain level and not vice versa, then drug management of depression would be a therapeutic option to improve pain. If, on the other hand, pain is a primary phenomenon and depression secondary, pain treatment would be the major challenge, and successful treatment of pain could be expected to lead to lower levels of depression. Studies exploring these relationships can be divided into cross-sectional and longitudinal studies. The cross-sectional design has limitations as only relations between variables can be explored, whereas causal relationships can only be examined in a longitudinal design.

Several cross-sectional studies have examined the relationships between pain and psychological distress and between disease activity variables and psychological measures. Most of these studies have, not surprisingly, found significant correlations between anxiety and depression on one side and pain and disability on the other side. Weaker, but also generally significant correlation has been found between the level of joint counts

acute phase reactants and depression/anxiety[66-70]. Multivariate analyses have also been used in these cross-sectional studies to identify primary versus secondary phenomena. Several studies have indicated that, for example, chronic pain adversely impact mood rather than the opposing hypotheses that negative mood is a predisposing factor in the development of chronic pain[67], but there are also exceptions. Hagglund *et al.*[69] examined how disease activity measures, radiographic ratings, and psychological variables could predict pain and functional impairment in 53 RA patients. Psychological variables explained the substantial proportion of the variance in outcome scores even after disease activity was taken into account.

Different designs have been used for the longitudinal studies. Krotty *et al.*[71] frequently examined 75 young women (median age 43 years) with early rheumatoid arthritis, with a wide range of disease activity and disability measures (HAQ) and psychosocial variables. The results showed that psychosocial variables were as important as disease and pain in determining function. They conclude that the result suggest interventions based on the importance of maintaining social relationships could have impact on function. However, this study also demonstrates the complicated statistical approach necessary to show directional relationships in longitudinal studies.

Hawley and Wolfe[72] studied psychological and clinical factors in 400 patients with rheumatoid arthritis examined at 6-month intervals over a mean of 3 years using the AIMS psychological scales. Development of depression was associated with socioeconomic but not clinical factors, and disease activity appeared to have a limited effect on psychological status. Initial psychological scores were associated with subsequent pain levels and number of physician visits. Some years later the same author group analyzed data from 713 patients with rheumatoid arthritis attending two subsequent clinic visits[73]. Six demographic and seven clinical variables were assessed including the AIMS depression score. They found that clinical changes explained about 20 per cent of depressive changes between visits, while 34 per cent of current depression scores were explained by demographic and clinical variables. Thus, changes in pain and disability score predicted changes in depression.

An Australian study of 30 RA patients examined on two occasions, 3 years a part, revealed few significant relationships between disease and psychological measures. The authors concluded that the psychological state of the patient needed to be assessed as a variable independent of physical impairment[74]. A more recent study showed that patients describing themselves as more depressed on a depression scale also reported more intense pain across the recording period, independent of the level of disease activity and disability[75].

Smedstad *et al.*[76] examined 216 RA patients annually for 2 years for symptoms of anxiety and depression measured by the Arthritis Impact Measurement Scales, tender joint counts, ESR, self-reported pain, measured by visual analogue scales, and disability measured by the Health Assessment Questionnaire. Strong cross-sectional relationships were found between symptoms of anxiety and depression respectively and the other clinical variables. Using a multivariate approach, pain and disability consistently were the two variables most strongly related therapy of the depressive symptoms without simultaneously considering adequate anti-inflammatory and or antirheumatic medication and relief of pain. Despite the lack of consistent causal relationships between psychological and traditional disease variables, there is more evidence suggesting that, for example, psychological distress appears as a phenomenon secondary to disease factors than as a factor aggravating arthritis activity[73,76]. However, it seems that all of these factors interact in complex reciprocal patterns that, so far, are poorly understood. As some of these variables represent opportunities for therapeutic interventions, it seems reasonable to have a wide therapeutic approach to hopefully counteract negative feed-back loops leading to excess dysfunction and suffering.

It has been documented that coping behavior may influence the psychological and social functioning[92]. Several studies have documented that cognitive behavioral patient education programs may improve health status[93–96]. In a controlled study of a cognitive-behavioral pain management program the patients received a comprehensive, 12-month pain management program that taught coping strategies such as problem-solving techniques, relaxation training, strategies for attention diversion, and training in family dynamics and communication. Outcome variables included pain, coping strategies, psychological status, functional status, and disease status. Data analysis revealed benefits for the intervention group in the area of enhanced coping strategies[97]. Lorig *et al.* found that improvement in health status subsequent to the arthritis self-management program was probably mediated through improved self-efficacy[94,98].

A possible consequence of the development of new, sophisticated drug management programs for rheumatoid arthritis patients is that less prestigious therapies such as rehabilitation medicine receive less attention and priorities in the clinics. Many studies have documented that various rehabilitation interventions are effective[99]. Furthermore, a biopsychosocial therapeutic approach also mean a multidisciplinary approach. The rheumatologists rarely have enough time to deal with all the disease-related psychosocial aspects. Therefore, other categories of health professionals have to be available to meet the patients' therapeutic needs within these dimensions.

Hill *et al.*[100] compared the effect on disease course of either a follow-up system with a rheumatology nurse practitioner or a consultant rheumatologist. In the patients managed by the nurse practitioner pain, morning stiffness, psychological status, patient knowledge, and satisfaction had all improved significantly, whereas similar improvement was not observed in the consultant rheumatologist group. It is probable that the patients under the care of the nurse practitioner were more widely informed about the disease and received educational material. More attention was probably also given to psychological factors as well as coping strategies. In line with this, Ahlmen *et al.*[101] documented, in a randomized controlled study, that the patient group under the supervision of a multidisciplinary team reached a better outcome than the control group.

In summary, these studies show that the organization of the health care system may be important and that the team work between nurse, rheumatologist, and other health professionals may lead to a more successful outcome when more time and attention are used to improve the psychosocial well being of the patient. As a minimum, it must be required that the therapeutic approach account for the present status of knowledge: RA is a chronic disease in which psychosocial variables represent important outcomes, but also act as predictors of an unfavorable outcome. As a consequence, the therapy has to target both biological and psychosocial aspects of the disease.

References

1. Pincus T., Callahan L.F. Reassessment of twelve traditional paradigms concerning the diagnosis, prevalence, morbidity and mortality of rheumatoid arthritis. *Scand J Rheumatol*, 1989;**18**(suppl. 79):67–96.
2. Liang M.H., Katz J.N. Measurement of outcome in rheumatoid arthritis. *Baillieres Clin Rheumatol*, 1992;**6**:23–37.
3. Engel G.L. The need for a new medical model: A challenge for biomedicine. *Science*, 1977;**196**:129–36.
4. Green S.A. Supportive psychologic care of the medically ill: a synthesis of the biosychosocial approach in medical care. In: (Stoudemire A, Ed) *Human behavior—an introduction for medical students*. J.B. Lippincott Company, Philadelphia, 1990;323–38.
5. Engel G.L. From biomedical to biopsychosocial. *Families, Systems and Health*, 1996;**14**:425–33.
6. Shipley M., Newman S.P. Psychological aspects of rheumatic diseases. *Baillieres Clin Rheumatol*, 1993;**7**:215–9.
7. Wegener S.T. Psychosocial aspects of rheumatic disease: the developing biopsychosocial framework. *Curr Opin Rheum*, 1991;**3**:300–4.
8. Pincus T. Formal education level-A marker for the importance of behavioral variables in the pathogenesis, morbidity and mortality of most diseases? *J Rheumatol*, 1988;**15**:1457–60.
9. Wells K.B., Golding J.M., Burnam M.A. Psychiatric disorder in a sample of the general population with and without chronic medical conditions. *Am J Psychiatry*, 1988;**145**:976–81.
10. Stewart A.L., Greenfield S., Hays R.D., Wells K., Rogers W.H., Berry S.D., McGlynn E.A., Ware J.E. Functional status and well-being of patients with chronic conditions. Results from the medical outcomes study. *JAMA*, 1989;**262**:903–13.
11. Magni G., Marchetti M., Moreschi C., Merskey H., Luchini S.R. Chronic musculoskeletal pain and depressive symptoms in the National Health and Nutrition Examination. I. Epidemiologic follow-up study. *Pain*, 1993;**53**:163–8.
12. Magni G., Caldieron C., Rigatti-Luchini S., Merskey H. Chronic musculoskeletal pain and depressive symptoms in the general population. An analysis of the 1st National Health and Nutrition Examination Survey data. *Pain*, 1990;**43**:299–307.
13. Fries J.F., Spitz P., Kraines R.G., Holman H.R. Measurement of patient outcome in arthritis. *Arthritis Rheum*, 1980;**23**:137–45.
14. Wolfe F. The natural history of rheumatoid arthritis. *J Rheumatol*, 1996;**23**(suppl. 44):13–22.
15. Wolfe F., Lasserre M., van der Heijde D., Stucki 6., Svarez-Almazon M., Pincus T., Erenhardt K., Kvien T.K., Symmoni D., Silman A., van Riel P., Tugwell P., Boers M. Preliminary core set of domains and reporting requirements for longitudinal observational studies in rheumatology. *J Rheumatol*, 1999;**26**:484–9..
16. World Health Organization. *International classification of impairments, disabilities and handicaps: a manual of classification related to the consequences of disease*. Geneva: World Health Organization. 1980; WHO.
17. Badley E.M. The genesis of handicap: definition, models of disablement, and role of external factors. *Disabil Rehabil*, 1995;**17**:53–62.
18. Fitzpatrick F., Badley E.M. An overview of disability. *Br J Rheumatol*, 1996;**35**:184–7.
19. Carr A.J., Thompson P.W. Towards a measure of patient-perceived handicap in rheumatoid arthritis. *Br J Rheumatol*, 1994;**33**:378–82.

20. Carr A.J., Thompson P.W., Kirwan J.R. Quality of life measures. *Br J Rheumatol*, 1996;**35**:275–81.

21. O'Boyle C.A., McGee H., Hickey A., O'Malley K., Joyce C.R. Individual quality of life in patients undergoing hip replacement. *Lancet*, 1992;**339**:1088–91.

22. Harwood R.H., Gompertz P., Ebrahim S. Handicap one year after a stroke: validity of a new scale. *J Neurol Neurosurg Psychiatry*, 1994;**57**:825–9.

23. Muldoon M.F., Barger S.D., Flory J.D., Manuck SB. What are quality of life measurements measuring? *Br Med J*, 1998;**316**:542–5.

24. DeVellis B.M. The psychological impact of arthritis: prevalence of depression. *Arthritis Care Res*, 1995;**8**:284–9.

25. Pincus T., Callahan L.F., Brooks R.H., Fuchs H.A., Olsen N.J., Kaye J.J. Self-report questionnaire scores in rheumatoid arthritis compared with traditional physical, radiographic, and laboratory measures. *Ann Intern Med*, 1989;**110**:259–66.

26. Wolfe F. Practical issues in psychosocial measures. *J Rheumatol*, 1997;**24**:990–3.

27. Blalock S.J., DeVellis R.F., Brown G.K., Wallston K.A. Validity of the Center for Epidemiological Studies Depression Scale in arthritis populations. *Arthritis Rheum*, 1989;**32**:991–7.

28. Peck J.R., Smith T.W., Ward J.R., Milano R. Disability and depression in rheumatoid arthritis. A multi-trait, multi-method investigation. *Arthritis Rheum*, 1989;**32**:1100–6.

29. Pincus T., Callahan L.F., Bradley L.A., Vaughn W.K., Wolfe F. Elevated MMPI scores for hypochondriasis, depression, and hysteria in patients with rheumatoid arthritis reflect disease rather than psychological status. *Arthritis Rheum*, 1986;**29**:1456–66.

30. DeVellis B.M. Depression in rheumatological diseases. *Baillieres Clin Rheumatol*, 1993;**7**:241–57.

31. Pincus T., Callahan L.F. Depression scales in rheumatoid arthritis: criterion contamination in interpretation of patient responses. *Patient Educ Couns*, 1993;**20**:133–43.

32. McDowell I., Newell C. *Measuring health* (2nd edn.) New York: Oxford University Press; 1996.

33. Bellamy N. *Musculoskeletal clinical metrology*. Dordrecht: Kluwer Academic Publishers; 1993.

34. Brooks P., McFarlane A.C., Newman S., Rasker J.J. Psychosocial measures. *J Rheumatol*, 1997;**24**:1008–11.

35. Goldberg D., Williams P. *A user's guide to the general health questionnaire*. Windsor: NFER-Nelson; 1998.

36. Ware J.E., Jr., Sherbourne C.D. The MOS 36-item short-form health survey (SF-36). I. Conceptual framework and item selection. *Med Care*, 1992;**30**:473–83.

37. McHorney C.A., Ware J.E., Jr., Lu J.F., Sherbourne C.D. The MOS 36-item Short-Form Health Survey (SF-36): III. Tests of data quality, scaling assumptions, and reliability across diverse patient groups. *Med Care*, 1994;**32**:40–66.

38. Kvien T.K., Kaasa S., Smedstad L.M. Performance of the Norwegian SF-36 health survey in patients with rheumatoid arthritis. II A comparison of the SF-36 with disease specific measures. *J Clin Epidemiol*, 1998; **51**:1077–86.

39. Bergner M., Bobbitt R.A., Kressel S., Pollard W.E., Gilson B.S., Morris J.R. The Sickness Impact Profile: Conceptual formulation and methodology for the development of a health status measure. *Int J Health Serv*, 1976;**6**:393–415.

40. Liang M.H., Larson M.G., Cullen K.E., Schwartz J.A. Comparative measurement efficiency and sensitivity of five health status instruments for arthritis research. *Arthritis Rheum*, 1985;**28**:542–7.

41. Sullivan M., Ahlmen M., Bjelle A. Health status assessment in rheumatoid arthritis. I. Further work on the validity of the sickness impact profile. *J Rheumatol*, 1990;**17**:439–47.

42. Sullivan M., Ahlmen M., Bjelle A., Karlsson J. Health status assessment in rheumatoid arthritis. II. Evaluation of a modified Shorter Sickness Impact Profile. *J Rheumatol*, 1993;**20**:1500–7.

43. Hunt S.M., McEwen J., McKenna S.P. Measuring health status: A new tool for clinicians and epidemiologists. *J R Coll Gen Pract*, 1985;**35**:185–8.

44. Meenan R.F., Gertman P.M., Mason J.H. Measuring health status in arthritis. The Arthritis Impact Measurement Scales. *Arthritis Rheum*, 1980;**23**:146–52.

45. Meenan R.F., Gertman P.M., Mason J.H., Dunaif R. The arthritis impact measurement scales. Further investigations of a health status measure. *Arthritis Rheum*, 1982;**25**:1048–53.

46. Hawley D.J., Wolfe F. Depression is not more common in rheumatoid arthritis: a 10-year longitudinal study of 6,153 patients with rheumatic disease. *J Rheumatol*, 1993;**20**:2025–31.

47. Meenan R.F., Mason J.H., Anderson J.J., Guccione AA, Kazis LE. AIMS2. The content and properties of a revised and expanded Arthritis Impact Measurement Scales Health Status Questionnaire. *Arthritis Rheum*, 1992;**35**:1–10.

48. Guillemin F., Coste J., Pouchot J., Ghezail M., Bregeon C., Sany J. The AIMS2-SF: a short form of the Arthritis Impact Measurement Scales 2. *Arthritis Rheum*, 1997;**40**:1267–74.

49. Frank R.G., Beck N.C., Parker J.C., Kashani J.H., Elliott T.R., Haut A.E., Smith E., Atwood C., Brownlee-Duffeck M., Kay D.R. Depression in rheumatoid arthritis. *J Rheumatol*, 1988;**15**:920–5.

50. Creed F. Psychological disorders in rheumatoid arthritis: A growing consensus? *Ann Rheum Dis*, 1990;**49**:808–12.

51. Eberhardt K., Larsson B.M., Nived K. Early rheumatoid arthritis–some social, economical, and psychological aspects. *Scand J Rheum*, 1993;**22**:119–23.

52. Darby P.L., Schmidt P.J. Psychiatric consultations in rheumatology: A review of 100 cases. *Can J Psychiatry*, 1988;**33**:290–3.

53. Kvien T.K., Glennås A., Knudsrød O.G., Smedstad L.M. The validity of self-reported diagnosis of rheumatoid arthritis: Results from a population survey followed by clinical examinations. *J Rheumatol*, 1996;**23**:1866–71.

54. Kvien T.K., Glennås A., Knudsrød O.G., Smedstad L.M., Førre Ø. The prevalence and severity of RA: Results from a county register and a population survey. *Scand J Rheumatol*, 1997;**26**:412–8.

55. Katz P.P., Yelin E.H. Prevalence and correlates of depressive symptoms among persons with rheumatoid arthritis. *J Rheumatol*, 1993;**20**:790–6.

56. Smedstad L.M., Moum T., Vaglum P., Kvien T.K. The impact of early rheumatoid arthritis on psychological distress: A comparison between 238 patients with RA and 116 matched controls. *Scand J Rheumatol*, 1996;**25**:377–82.

57. Gilboe I-M., Kvien T.K., Husby G. Health status in systemic lupus erythematosus compared to rheumatoid arthritis and healthy controls *J Rheumatol*, 1999;**26**:1694–700.

58. Kochevar R.J., Kaplan R.M., Weisman M. Financial and career losses due to rheumatoid arthritis: a pilot study. *J Rheumatol*, 1997;**24**:1527–30.

59. Van Jaarsveld C.H.M., Jacobs J.W.G., Schrijvers A.J.P., van Albada-Kuipers G.A., Hoffman D.M., Bijlsma J.W.J. Effects of rheumatoid arthritis on employment and social participation during the first years of disease in the Netherlands. *Br J Rheumatol*, 1998;**37**:848–53.

60. Pincus T. The underestimated long term medical and economic consequences of rheumatoid arthritis. *Drugs*, 1995;**50**(suppl. 1):1–14.

61. Reisine S.T., Grady K.E., Goodenow C., Fifield J. Work disability among women with rheumatoid arthritis. The relative importance of disease, social, work, and family factors. *Arthritis Rheum*, 1989;**32**:538–43.

62. Maetzel A. Costs of illness and the burden of disease. *J Rheumatol*, 1997;**24**:3–5.

63. Yelin E. The costs of rheumatoid arthritis: absolute, incremental, and marginal estimates. *J Rheumatol*, 1996;**23**(suppl. 44):47–51.

64. Clarke A.E., Zowall H., Levinton C., Assimakopoulos H., Sibley J.T., Haga M., Shiroky J., Neville C., Lubeck D.P., Grover S.A., *et al.* Direct and indirect medical costs incurred by Canadian patients with rheumatoid arthritis: a 12 year study. *J Rheumatol*, 1997;**24**:1051–60.

65. Gabriel S.E., Crowson C.S., Campion M.E., O'Fallon W.M. Indirect and nonmedical costs among people with rheumatoid

Needs assessment

Before planning a patient education program, it is essential to assess the needs and problems of those being served. These may vary among different age groups, cultures, customs, health-care systems, and geographical settings. Surveys have indicated disagreement as to the foremost complaints of arthritis patients. Some patients report dealing with pain as their main problem[21]. Others are concerned more with the origin of their disease and with diagnostic procedures. They find their greatest problems alleviated in learning to communicate with their physician, understanding medication, dealing with the impact of arthritis on work, and confronting their worries about the future[16]. In yet another study, when patients were asked to state spontaneously what troubled them the most, they cited functional disability, feeling dependent on others, and pain. Psychological, family, and marital problems were seldom mentioned. However, when the same patients were given a preformatted list, they did reveal psychological problems—the most prevalent one being uncertainty regarding the future course of their disease[22]. Disruption of leisure activities was often singled out as a distressing aspect of living with chronic arthritis[23-25]. Since the inability of patients to engage in activities which they formerly enjoyed and continue to value has been strongly linked to the development of depressive symptoms[26], this is an important issue to address in patient education programs.

There may be a discrepancy between what patients perceive as their needs and the physician's view of a patient's greatest problems[16,20,21]. Research has shown that individuals with more formal education know more about their disease before taking part in a patient education program[3,19,27,28] and are eager to learn even more[18]. Language barriers and cultural background may need to be addressed by other strategies. For example individuals who come as refugees from other countries or who live in remote areas may find it hard to sit down and discuss their problems in a group with other patients. In Java, leather puppets in 'Wayang Kulit,' a local cultural event, have been used as a basis for teaching villagers[29]. All the aforementioned factors should be borne in mind if one is to establish a successful patient education program.

Approaches to arthritis patient education (Table 32.1)

The best way to deliver patient education has yet to be determined. Local traditions and available resources play an important part in the choice of method. In some countries, group programs for the education of arthritis patients are administered by the overall health-care system. Shared care is a part of rheumatology units and involves a professional team with rheumatologists, nurses, physiotherapists, occupational therapists, social workers, and sometime dietitians and podiatrists as well[30,31]. This multidisciplinary team approach is increasingly prevalent in the out-patient management of arthritis. Patient

Table 32.1 Different methods of arthritis patient education

Type of education	First author	Publication year	Reference number
Groups led by health professionals	Althoff B	1977	32
	Cohen JL	1986	34
	Lindroth Y	1989	24
	Thaal E	1993	22
	Hammond A	1994	35
Groups led by lay-leaders	Lorig K	1985	36
	Goeppinger J	1989	28
	Cohen JL	1986	34
Home study	Goeppinger J	1989	28
Cognitive–behavioral groups	Keefe FJ	1996	45
	Calfas KJ	1992	38
Support groups	Potts M	1985	39
	Radojevic V	1992	44
Individual strategy	Lorish CD	1985	27
	Hammond A	1994	35
Telephone information service pamphlets, books	Weinberger M	1989	42
	Vignos PJ	1976	3
Computer-based programs	Wetstone SC	1985	43
'Wayang kulit', Leather puppets	Darmawan J	1992	29
Part of day care	Jacobsson L	1998	68

education is then one of the activities of the team[18,22,24,32-35]. Patient education can also be organized and led by lay leaders in the community as self-management courses[28,34,36].

Early patient education programs presented information in a didactic format to those with arthritis, and had three major goals: to enhance patients' understanding of their disease, to teach patients to make informed choices regarding the management of the disease, and to facilitate adherence to the recommendations of health-care providers.

On the other hand, cognitive–behavioral treatment focused on teaching patients how to correlate thought, feeling, and behavior to help them deal with pain and disability. Patients were also trained in a variety of cognitive and behavioral techniques such as relaxation, cognitive strategies, imagery, goal setting, and cognitive reconstructing in order to enhance coping skills in a wide variety of situations[37,38].

Today most programs use a combination of an informational and an educational–behavioral approach, since these two in combination have been found to be more effective than lecturing alone[4]. Small groups of six to ten participants allow enough time for individual patients to raise their own concerns. Discussions focused on problem-solving enhance self-management strategies. Experience from other participants and group leaders can help individuals handle their pain and functional impairment. Groups comprised of patients with the same diagnosis, similar age, and the same regional background may increase the individual's ability to identify with other members of the group. Some education programs, however, focus on arthritis irrespective of diagnosis, holding that problems such as pain, functional impairment, and psychosocial aspects are common to all cases of arthritis. The education program may follow a strict schedule, delivering exactly the same information to all groups[36]; it can consist of health professionals addressing the problems posed within each group[18]; or it may established a support group where health professionals facilitate discussion and handle topics that arise spontaneously[39].

Patients were found to prefer individual meetings with a health practitioner when they were asked to state their preferred method of learning about arthritis. The physician was their most valued source of information[16]. Individualized strategies, based on the patient's physical condition, emotional state, and arthritis knowledge level, resulted in greater learning, as compared with routine methods of teaching each group of patients the identical information using exactly the same format[27].

Inexpensive methods of education such as pamphlets and booklets have been shown to be effective in increasing patient knowledge about arthritis[3,40]. However, instruction from a health professional resulted in greater comprehension than distributing a booklet alone. Furthermore, increased knowledge alone had no effect on alleviating disability or improving quality of life[41]. Other low-cost methods of providing information to arthritis patients have been employed—such as telephone contacts, audio-visual tapes, and computer-based education[42,43].

Including the family in the education program increased the positive effect of such education on pain, psychological disability, and coping skills[39,44,45]. There is little information on the importance of reinforcement education, and what there is does not seem to indicate any enhancement of the long-term effect of patient education programs[46].

Outline of arthritis patient education

The patient's knowledge of arthritis

Understanding the nature of the disease, the theoretical background of different symptoms, and the rationale for treatment options is fundamental to all arthritis education programs (see Table 32.2). Nevertheless, knowledge by itself is not sufficient to change behavior and thereby affect the outcome of the disease[47]. Patients must be encouraged to relinquish the passive role they often assume when presenting themselves for medical treatment. In order to take an active part in rehabilitation programs and communicate better with health professionals, patients need and, in fact want, to know more about arthritis[16-18]. Because patients have developed their own ideas of their disease[20], certain clinical expressions used daily by health professionals may have different meanings to patients, and may even scare them. 'Seronegative' may imply that the person has a negative attitude; 'prosthesis' may symbolize a wooden leg, 'joint erosion' may suggest a picture of the whole joint being washed away. Fear and misunderstanding may be avoided if patients acquire

Table 32.2 Outline of arthritis patient education

Knowledge	Anatomy, medical aspects, inflammation
	Pharmacological and surgical treatment, effects, side-effects
	Disease monitoring, signs of progression of disease
	Mechanism of pain and possible way to relieve it
	Muscle function, contractures
	Joint protection
	Nutrition
	Community resources
Skills and behaviors	Exercise, TENS, acupuncture
	Pain management
	Practice of work simplification
	Taking extra medicine; adhering to lab check-ups
	Weight reduction, adequate nutrition intake
	Adjusting work situation
Psychological aspect and coping	Communicating with health professionals
	Problem solving
	Goal setting
	Self-efficacy
	Dealing with anxiety and depression
	Maintaining leisure activities
	Eliciting family support

knowledge of their disease, understand routine medical terminology, and realize the importance of asking about things they do not understand. It is also vital for patients to be acquainted with anatomical structure, inflammation, muscle function, and cartilage destruction in order to accept the role of anti-inflammatory therapy, regular muscle exercise, joint protection, and weight reduction. Knowing the rationale for laboratory check-ups, for example, may give patients better motivation to adhere to controls.

Behavior modification

Most arthritis education programs aim to develop patients skills and change their behavior. This has been proven to be more effective than cognitive change alone[4]. These modifications in a patient's life style involve exercise, rest, joint protection, and adherence to medication. Participatory sessions teach exercises to be performed daily, demonstrate technical aids, instruct in work simplification methods, and train the group in relaxation techniques.

Psychosocial aspects

For many patients, the mere fact of living with arthritis presents them with the difficult task of tolerating the uncertainties of a chronic disease. These individuals need to develop strategies to balance their fear of progressive worsening and the threat of dependency against their hopes for relief and remission[48]. To address these issues, many programs include sessions about self-awareness, communication skills, and stress management[22,24,36]. Modeling can be used effectively by allowing group members to help each other solve problems. The concept of self-efficacy has been found to be important in any attempt to change one's own behavior. Self-efficacy has been defined as people's judgments of their capabilities to organize and execute courses of action required to attain designated types of performance. It is concerned not with the skills one has, but with the judgment of what one can do with whatever skills one possesses[49]. Goal setting and feedback about performance have been shown to be effective in strengthening patients' self-efficacy and skill acquisition[22,50]. Inability to pursue hobbies and leisure activities is a main problem for many patients[24,25] and can be a strong risk factor for developing depression[26]. Addressing this should, therefore, be a high priority in patient education programs. Including family members in such sessions may result in increased emotional support and improve behavior modification[44].

Effects of arthritis patient education

The development of reliable and validated outcome instruments to measure pain, disability, depression, and quality of life has made it possible to study the effectiveness of different types of arthritis patient education programs. Multiple-choice questions are often used as tests of knowledge about the disease process and its treatment[51,52]. Pain can be measured using a visual analogue scale (VAS)[53]. There are scales which quantify disability and impairment, such as the Health Assessment Questionnaire (HAQ)[54]. Consequences of the disease can be ascertained by the Arthritis Impact Measurement Scales (AIMS)[55]. Psychological aspects can be evaluated by the degree of self-efficacy[49], helplessness[56], and depression[57]. Finally, quality of life measurements are ascertained by various instruments and are used in the study of a large number of diseases. These instruments include SF-36[58], Nottingham Health Profile[59], and Sickness Impact Profile[60]. Since the advent of such assessments, many patient education programs have been documented as having reduced pain, depression, and disability[10–14,61].

Change in patient knowledge

In a review of 76 patient education studies, 34 measured patient knowledge; of these, 94 per cent found an increase[10]. In a later review of 25 studies, eight of them studied change in knowledge and seven of the eight found an increase[61]. During the last few years, a trend away from studies measuring cognitive change has emerged, with the focus shifting toward studies that include three or more disease-outcome categories[12].

Change in behavior

The changes in behavior most frequently prescribed in arthritis patient education programs were the increased practice of exercise and compliance with medication[12]. Also recommended were relaxation techniques, joint protection, and work simplification. The above cited review examined 34 different behavior patterns in 25 studies; of which 29 showed some

positive changes. In long-term follow-up over 5 years[61], old habits of neglect with regard to exercise prevailed after 12 months, and remained unchanged after 5 years. In contrast, the practice of joint protection and work simplification remained in place, in both the short and long-term. It may be that individuals with a painful grip and significant limitations in physical performance are more motivated to practice joint protection in the hope of halting further disability, whereas engaging in physical exercise several times a week does not yield immediate pain relief, and may, in fact, cause real discomfort. A study on methods of work simplification and joint protection indicated that patients were still using 91 per cent of the assistive devices prescribed when surveyed from 6 months to 7 years after completing a joint protection education program[63]. Nevertheless, although patients with RA testified that they considered joint protection behavior important and stated that they believed they had altered their habits after receiving joint protection education, another study revealed that no change had actually taken place[35]. The failure of patients to continue an exercise program on their own suggests that more emphasis should be given to this component in the future. Since current views on exercise differ fundamentally from those held 10 years ago[64], programs offered today may have greater success than those in the past. Dynamic muscle training has yielded positive results in individuals with RA[65], and progressive relaxation training had an even greater impact on a patient's quality of life, as it reduced joint tenderness and improved muscle functioning in the lower extremities[66].

Change in health status

Does patient education have an impact on the outcome of rheumatic disease? There are as yet no studies regarding the effect of patient education programs on mortality, and only limited information is available on whether they can reduce the side-effects of drugs, or favorably alter the economic consequences of arthritis[46]. The impact of patient education with regard to pain is a matter of controversy. Some studies have reported a reduction in pain[28,35,45]; whereas others show either no effect[22,24]; or suggest increased pain[33]. On the whole, a majority of patients reported knowing how to deal with pain better after going through an education program[18]. In a review of 14 studies measuring pain, 50 per cent showed pain was reduced significantly after patient education[12]. A meta-analysis compared trials of patient education and NSAID treatments[13]. Patient education accounted for a diminution in pain approaching 20–30 per cent of that achieved by NSAID treatment. In most studies pain was measured using VAS, a visual analogue scale[53]. However, VAS gives a unidimensional measurement of a multidimensional symptom of arthritis. The values for pain which VAS had ascertained in patients with RA have been challenged by more sophisticated techniques of administering the same test[67]. 'Present Pain' was half of 'usual pain', and 'worst pain' was more than twice the intensity of 'usual pain'. It has been suggested that pain could be measured more accurately with VAS if readings were taken before and after the performance of a standardized task[63]. The somewhat vague inquiry as to a patient's 'pain experienced during the last week' which is routinely employed in clinical trials, elicits varying results and allows no precise interpretation. Teaching patients ways of dealing with pain may be more important than having them focus on the level of pain per se. A review of 19 trials found an average reduction of disability by 0.03, measured on a scale where NSAIDs were found to be reduced by 0.34 in NSAID trials[12]. It is believed that disability increases with age and the duration of the disease[54]. Thus, an intervention group remaining at the same level on the HAQ over a period of 5 years may indicate a relatively successful outcome[62].

Evaluating the success of patient education intervention on psychosocial status should be done with caution. Assessments have been difficult to quantify, and questions have therefore been raised about statistical reliability[10]. As psychosocial variables are often closely related to such things as disease activity, the progression of pain, and disability or depression from other causes, it may prove difficult to determine if alterations in these variables are the result of an intervention, or represent natural changes in the disease process. Reviews of studies in patient education have found positive change in about 50 per cent of the aforementioned variables[10], and meta-analysis of psychoeducational interventions show a modest effect size of 0.28 for depression[11]. Similar results are reported in a subsequent review[12].

The future of patient education

Patient education has undergone fundamental changes during the last 30 years, going from hand-out materials and lecture programs to cognitive, behavioral, and interactive educational–behavioral self-management courses. If a similar development continues, we can expect to see the emergence of better methods based on research from other fields such as education, sociology, and psychology. New approaches involving computer-based Internet technology may supplement personal interactive meetings. Problem-based programs have now appeared[18] and the further development of these strategies may better meet the needs of individual patients, as well as increase their motivation to learn. Further connections with hospital-based and perioperative treatment could be developed. Patient education has recently demonstrated its effectiveness as part of other day-care rehabilitation systems. Patients with recent onset of disease were found to benefit significantly from group education[68]. Economic analyses may look closer at the cost-effectiveness of patient education in the totality of the health-care system: does it reduce or add to the total cost? Comparisons between different types of programs will be necessary, that is telephone contact versus visiting a physician, community support groups as opposed to a multisession program of structured education, community-based self-management courses instead of multidisciplinary education. International and national standards using similar methods of evaluation will make it easier to compare the effectiveness of different programs. Until now, educational programs have mainly been offered to patients with rheumatoid arthritis and osteoarthritis. There are many other chronic conditions which fall into the area of rheumatology care and which may warrant consideration for arthritis patient education. Although there may be programs to address anchylosing spondylitis, psoriatic arthritis, and systemic connective tissue disorders, few appear in the literature. New methods also need to be developed for individuals with other ethnic backgrounds, as well as for those who cannot read, or who live in remote areas. It is to be hoped that patient education will be offered increasingly to a wider spectrum of patients suffering from rheumatic diseases and that such programs, designed to meet specific patient needs, will achieve acceptance as part of the total management of chronic illness.

References

1. Bartlett E.E. Forum: Patient education. Eight principles from patient education research. *Preventive Medicine*, 1985;14:667–9.
2. Bauman A., Lindroth Y., Daltroy L.H. Health promotion and patient education for people with arthritis. In *Rheumatology*, eds Klippel J.H. and Dieppe P.A. 1998. Mosby, London.
3. Vignos P.J., Parker W.T., Thompson H.M. Evaluation of a clinic education program for patients with rheumatoid arthritis. *J Rheumatol*, 1976;3:155–65.
4. Mazzuca S.A. Does patient education in chronic disease have a therapeutic value? *J Chron Dis*, 1982;35:521–9.
5. Funnel M.M., Arnold M.S., Fogler J., Merritt J.H., Anderson L.A. Participation in a diabetes education and care program: experiences from the diabetes care for older adults project. *Diabetes Educ*, 1998;24:163–7.
6. Braden C.J., Mishel M.H., Longman A.J. Self-help intervention project, Women receiving breast cancer treatment. *Cancer Pract*, 1998;6:87–98.
7. Mertens D.J., Shephard R.J., Kavanagh T. Long term exercise therapy for chronic obstructive lung disease. *Prespiration*, 1978;35:96–107.
8. Ordonez G.A., Phelan P.D., Olinski A., Robertson C.F. Preventable factors in hospital admissions for asthma. *Arch Dis Child*, 1998;78:143–7.
9. Nessman D.G., Carnahan J.E., Nugent C.A. Increasing compliance. Patient operated hypertension groups. *Arch Int Med*, 1980;140:1427–80.
10. Lorig K., Konkol L., Gonzales V. Arthritis patient education: a review of the literature. *Patient Educ Councel*, 1987;10:207–52.
11. Mullen P.D., Laville E.A., Biddle A.K., Lorig K. Efficacy of psycho-educational interventions on pain, depression, and disability in people with arthritis: A meta-analysis. *J Rheumatol*, 1987;(Suppl. 15)14:33–9.
12. Hirano P.C., Laurent D.D., Lorig K. Arthritis patient education studies, 1987–1991: a review of the literature. *Patient Educ Councel*, 1994;24:9–54.
13. Superio-Cabuslay E., Ward M.M., Lorig K.R. Patient education intervention in osteoarthritis and rheumatoid arthritis: A meta-analytic comparison with non steroid antiinflammatory drug treatment. *Patient Educ Councel*, 1996;9:292–301.
14. Taal E., Rasker J.J., Wiegman O. Group education for rheumatoid arthritis. *Sem Arthritis Rheum*, 1997;26:805–16.
15. Daltroy L.H., Liang M.H. Arthritis education: opportunities and state of the art. *Health Educ Q*, 1993;20:3–16.
16. Silvers I.J., Melbourne F.H., Weisman M.H., Mueller M.R. Assessing physician/patient perceptions in rheumatoid arthritis. A vital component in patient education. *Arthritis Rheum*, 1985;28:300–7.
17. Kay E.A., Punchak S.S. Patient understanding of the causes and medical treatment of rheumatoid arthritis. *Br J Rheumatol*, 1988;27:396–8.

18. Lindroth Y., Brattström M., Bellman I., Ekestaf G., *et al.* A problem-based education program for patients with rheumatoid arthritis: Evaluation after three and twelve months. *Arthritis Care Res*, 1997;10:325–32.

19. Hill J., Bird A., Hopkins R., Lawton C., Wright V. The development and use of a patient knowledge questionnaire in rheumatoid arthritis. *Br J Rheumatol*, 1991;30:45–9.

20. Donovan J.L., Blake D.R., Fleming W.G. The patient is not a blank sheet: lay beliefs and their relevance to patient education. *Br J Rheumatol*, 1989;28:58–61.

21. Lorig K., Cox T., Cuevas Y., Kraines R.G., Britton M.C: Converging and diverging beliefs about arthritis: caucasian patients, Spanish-speaking, and physicians. *J Rheumatol*, 1984;11:76–9.

22. Taal E., Remes R.P., Burs H.L., Seedy E.R., Rasker J.J., Wiegman O. Group education for patients with rheumatoid arthritis. *Patient Educ Counsel*, 1993;20:177–87.

23. Eberhardt K., Larsson, B.-M., Nived K. Early rheumatoid arthritis—some social, economic and psychological aspects. *Scand J Rheumatol*, 1993;22:119–

24. Lindroth Y., Bauman A., Barnes C., Mc Credie M., Brooks P.M. A controlled evaluation of arthritis education. *Br J Rheumatol*, 1989;28:7–12.

25. Fex E., Larsson B.M., Nived K., Eberhardt K. Effect of rheumatoid arthritis on work status and social and leisure time activities in patients followed 8 years from onset. *J Rheumatol*, 1998;25:44–50.

26. Kats P.P., Yelin E.H. The development of depressive symptoms among women with rheumatoid arthritis. *Arthritis Rheum*, 1995;38:49–56.

27. Lorish C.D., Parker J., Brown S. Effective patient education. A quasi-experiment comparing an individualized strategy with a routinized strategy. *Arthritis Rheum*, 1985;28:1289–97.

28. Goeppinger J., Arthur M.W., Baglioni A.J., Brunk S.E., Brunner C.M. A re-examination of the effectiveness of self-care education for persons with arthritis. *Arthritis Rheum*, 1989;32:706–16.

29. Darmawan J., Muriden K.D., Wigley R.D., Valkenburg H.A. Arthritis community education by leather puppet (wayang kulit) shadow play in rural Indonesia (Java). *Rheumatol Int*, 1992;12:97–101.

30. Brattström M. *Ledskydd och rehabilitering*. Studentlitteratur. Lund 1970.

31. Ahlmén M., Sullivan M., Bjelle A. Team versus non-team outpatient care in rheumatoid arthritis. *Arthritis Rheum*, 1988;31:471–479.

32. Althoff B., Nordenskiöld U., Hansen A.M. Ledskydd–ett skonsamt levnadssätt. *Riksförbundet Mot Reumatism*. Stockholm, 1977.

33. Parker J.C. *et al.* Educating patients with rheumatoid arthritis: A prospective analysis. *Arch Phys Med Rehab*, 1984;65:771–4.

34. Cohen J.L., Sauter S.H., De Vellis R.F., De Vellis B.M. Evaluation of arthritis self-management courses led by laypersons and by professionals. *Arthritis Rheum*, 1986;29:388–93.

35. Hammond A. Joint protection behavior in patients with rheumatoid arthritis following an education program. *Arthritis Care Res*, 1994;7:5–9.

36. Lorig K., Lubeck D., Kraines R.G., Seleznick M., Holman H.R. Outcomes of self-help education for patients with arthritis. *Arthritis Rheum*, 1985;28:680–5.

37. Keefe F.J., Van Horn Y. Cognitive-behavioral treatment of rheumatoid arthritis pain. Maintaining treatment gains. *Arthritis Care Res*, 1993;6:213–22.

38. Calfas K.J., Kaplan R.M., Ingram R.I. One-year evaluation of coginitive-behavioral intervention in osteoarthritis. *Arthritis Care Res*, 1992;5:202–9.

39. Potts M., Brandt K.D. Analysis of education-support groups for patients with rheumatoid arthritis. *Patient Councel Health Educ*, 1985;4:161–6.

40. Moll J.M.H., Wright V. Evaluation of the arthritis and rheumatism council handbook on gout. *J Chron Dis*, 1972;31:405–11.

41. Maggs F.M., Jubb R.W., Kemm J.R. Single-blind randomized controlled trial of an educational booklet for patients with chronic arthritis. *Br J Rheumatol*, 1996;35:775–7.

42. Weinberger M., Tierny W.M., Booher P., Katz B.P. Can the provision of information to patients with osteoarthritis improve functional status? *Arthritis Rheum*, 1989;32:1577–83.

43. Wetstone S.C., Sheehann T.J., Votaw R.G., Peterson M.G., Rothfield N. Evaluation of a Computer Based Education Lesson for Patients with Rheumatoid Arthritis. *J Rheumatol*, 1985;2:907–3.

44. Radojevic V., Nicassio P.M., Weisman M.H. Behavioral intervention with and without family support for rheumatoid arthritis. *Behavior Therapy*, 1992;23:13–30.

45. Keefe F.J., Caldwell D.S., Baucom D., Salley A., Robinson E., Timmons K., *et al.* Spouse-assisted coping skills training in the management of osteoarthritic knee pain. *Arthritis Care Res*, 1996;9:279–91.

46. Lorig K., Holman H.R.. Arthritis self-management studies. A twelve-year review. *Health Educ Q*, 1993;20:17–28.

47. Lorig K., Seleznick M., Lubeck D., Ung E., Chastain R.L., Holman H.R. The beneficial outcomes of the arthritis self-management course are not adequately explained by behavior change. *Arthritis Rheum*, 1989;32:91–5.

48. Wiener C.L. The burden of rheumatoid arthritis: Tolerating the uncertainty. *Soc Scien Med*, 1975;9:97–104.

49. Bandura A. Self-efficacy: Toward a unifying theory of Behavior change. *Psychol Rev*, 1977;84:191–215.

50. Lorig K., Chastain R.L., Ung E., Shoor S., Holman H.R. Development and evaluation of a scale to measure perceived self-efficacy in people with arthritis. *Arthritis Rheum*, 1989;32:37–44.

51. Hill J., Bird A., Hopkins R., Lawton C., Wright V. The development and use of a patient knowledge questionnaire in rheumatoid arthritis. *Br J Rheumatol*, 1991;30:45–49.

52. Edworthy A.M., Devins G.M., Watson M.M. The arthritis knowledge questionnaire. *Arthritis Rheum*, 1995;38:590–5.

53. Huskisson E.C. Measurement of pain. *J Rheumatol*, 1982;9:768–9.

54. Fries J., Spitz P., Kraines R., Holman H. Measurement of patient outcome in arthritis. *Arthritis Rheum*, 1980;23:137–45.

55. Meenan R.F., Gertman P.M., Mason J.H. Measuring health status in arthritis: Arthritis Impact Measurement Scales. *Arthritis Rheum*, 1980;23:146–52.

56. Nicassio P.M., Wallston K.A., Callahan L.F., Herbert M., Pincus T. The measurement of helplessness in rheumatoid arthritis. The development of the Arthritis Helplessness Index. *J Rheumatol*, 1980;12:462–7.

57. Zigmond A.S., Snaith R.P. The Hospital Anxiety and Depression Scale. *Acta Psyciatr Scand*, 1983;67:361–70.

58. Ware J.E., Sherbourne C.D. The MOS-item short-form health survey (SF-36):I. Conceptual framework and item selection. *Med Care*, 1992;30:473–83.

59. Hunt S.M., Mc Kenna S.P., Williams J. Reliability of a population survey tool for measuring perceived health problems: a study of patients with osteoarthrosis. *J Epidemiol Community Health*, 1981;35:297–300.

60. Bergner M., Bobbitt R.A., Pollard W.E., *et al.* The sickness impact profile: Validation of a health status measure. *Med Care*, 1976;14:57–67.

61. Hawley D.J. Psycho-educational interventions in the treatment of arthritis. *Bailliere's Clin Rheumatol*, 1995;9:803–23.

62. Lindroth Y., Bauman A., Brooks P.M., Priestley D. A 5-year follow-up of a controlled trial of an arthritis education program. *Br J Rheumatol*, 1995;34:647–52.

63. Nordenskiöld U. Evaluation of assistive devices after a course in joint protection. *Int J Tehchnol Asess Health Care*, 1994;10:293–304.

64. Minor Ma. Arthritis and exercise: The times they are a-changin'. *Arthritis Care Res*, 1996;9:79–81.

65. Ekdahl C., Eberhardt K., Andersson S.I., Svensson B. Assessing disability in patients with rheumatoid arthritis. *Scand J Rheumatol*, 1988;17:263–71.

66. Stenström C.H., Arge, Sundbom A. Dynamic training versus relaxation training as home exercise for patients with inflammatory rheumatic diseases. *Scand Rheumatol*, 1996;25:28–33.

67. Gaston-Johansson F., Gustavsson M. Rheumatoid Arthritis: determination of pain characteristics and comparison or RAI and VAS in its measurement. *Pain*, 1990;41:35–40.

68. Jacobsson L., Fritiof M., Olofsson Y., Runesson I., Strömbeck B., Wikström I. Evaluation of a structured multidisciplinary day care program in rheumatoid arthritis. *Scand J Rheumatol*, 1998;27:117–24.

33 | Non-drug management of chronic pain

W. Hamann

Introduction

Pain is an unpleasant sensation following tissue damage or a sensory experience expressed in terms of tissue damage (International Association for the Study of Pain, IASP). In neurophysiological terms, pain is experienced when selected areas in the limbic system, particularly neurones in the cingulate gyrus and related areas of the somatosensory cortex are excited at the same time[1]. Physiologically, this condition arises when nociceptors in peripheral tissues are stimulated as is the case following trauma in acute pain or in inflammatory pain (**nociceptive pain**). However, it is not uncommon that excitation of limbic and related somatosensory cortical neurones originate from abnormal, usually damaged, peripheral or central nervous tissue (**neuropathic pain**) or as the consequence of psychological mechanisms (**psychogenic pain**). For the individual it does not matter how the typical state of limbic and somatosensory cortex excitation comes about, because the end result is just as unpleasant. In order to control chronic pain successfully, it is important to establish first which combination of the above mechanisms one is dealing with in the individual patient. The final treatment plan needs to be multidisciplinary taking account of all aspects of a particular pain condition[2].

It is a feature of the pain pathway that at each synaptic relay there are mechanisms for amplification as well as inhibition. Pain control in clinical practice is targeted at the extensive variety of the inhibitory mechanisms which may be segmental, descending from higher centers or within the brain itself. Before concentrating on specific techniques or methods of pain control, it is helpful to follow the pain pathway from the periphery to the brain, looking out for the target points of known methods of pain relief.

Pain pathway

A schematic outline of the pain pathway is given in Fig. 33.1. The major functional compartments are: a) the somatosensory receptors; b) the primary afferent fibers including c) dorsal root ganglia, d) the dorsal horn/trigeminal nuclei and the ascending tracts, e.g. spinothalamic tract, the descending inhibitory or facilitatory tracts; e) the brain stem, the thalamus; f) the limbic system, in particular the cingulate gyrus; and h) the somatosensory cortex. Pain relieving techniques have targeted almost all of these structures.

Peripheral sensory receptors

Nociceptors (pain receptors) are the source of nociceptive pain. Their sensitivity is increased by the action of inflammatory substances. They are the main target of anti-inflammatory analgesia in rheumatoid arthritis (see Chapter 22). It is worth noting that some of these sensory receptors cannot be excited in the absence of inflammation (silent nociceptors).

Tactile and temperature receptors are the targets for some physical therapies in pain control. In the dorsal horn, inhibition is exerted by primary afferents from these receptors at post- and presynaptic terminals of nociceptor afferents. These inhibitory mechanisms may be activated by treatment with warmth, cold, or massage.

Primary afferent fibers

They may be the source of pain following nerve damage or following transection of peripheral nerves. In their search for peripheral sections of a severed peripheral nerve, sprouting nerve fibers may form neuromata. The increased number of Na^+ channels in the tips of sprouts are probably the reason for the increased nervous discharge that may originate form neuromata. More than 50 per cent of the individuals with large peripheral nerves severed in limb amputations will develop neuropathic pain in the form of phantom limb pain. Sodium channel antagonists such as carbamazepine or mexilitine may be helpful in this condition. For temporary analgesia, peripheral nerves can be blocked by infiltration with local anesthetics.

Terminal parts of primary afferent nerve fibers are also the target of two types of often very effective types of physical treatments, transcutaneous nerve stimulation (TENS) and acupuncture. In TENS low threshold afferent nerve fibers are stimulated electrically. Nervous activity in these fibers will activate segmental inhibition as well as long inhibitory loops reaching up to the brainstem, both targeting nervous transmission through the pain pathway.

Dorsal root ganglia

Dorsal root ganglia have gained much more prominence recently, because they are not only the nutritive cell bodies for primary afferent fibers but they are also the place of manufacture of many chemical mediators released either centrally or peripherally. Substance P is of particular interest. The majority of this substance is released peripherally. Centrally, it serves as

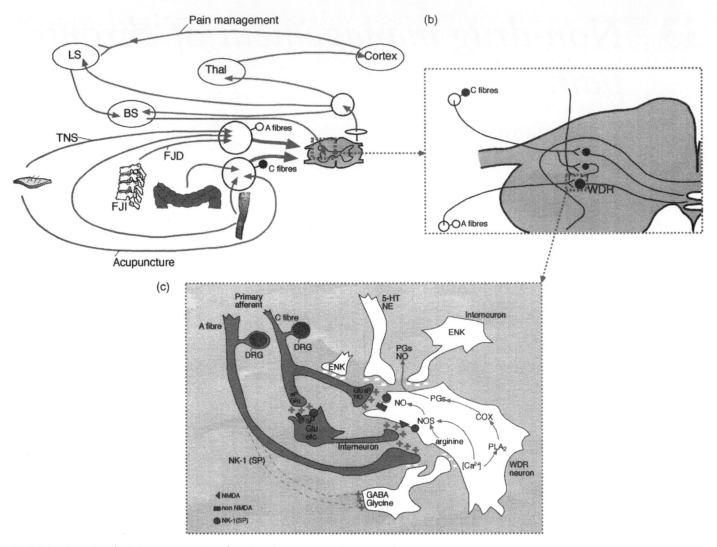

Fig. 33.1   Overview depicting access points of modes of treatment to the pain pathway.
(a)   Primary afferent fibers from skin, muscle, bone and other soft tissues and viscera. The term C-fiber includes small myelinated fibers. A-fibers are large myelinated fibers. Ascending pathways connect to the brainstem (BS), thalamus (Thal, cortex, and limbic system (LS). Transcutaneous electrical nerve stimulation (TNS), facetjoint injection (FJI), facetjoint denervation (FJD).
(b)   Postsynaptic projections of primary afferent fibers in the dorsal horn. WDR wide dynamic range neurons.
(c)   Excitatory and inhibitory synaptic connections to WDR-cell (white), excitatory neurones (blue), inhibitory neurons (yellow). Abbreviations DRG = dorsal root ganglion; ENK = enkephalin; NO = nitric oxide; NOS nitric oxide synthetase; PG = prostaglandin; COX = cyclo-oxygenase; NK-1 = neurokine 1; SP = substance P. (Modified from Yak S. (4).) See also Plate 34.

an excitatory modulator substance in the dorsal horn. Topical application of capsaicin to the skin can deplete primary afferents of substance P. This phenomenon is used in the topical application of capsaicin in a variety of neuropathic pain conditions and in osteoarthritis.

Dorsal horn

The principal synaptic connections of nociceptor afferents in the dorsal horn can be summarized into reflex and ascending (pain pathway). Pre and postsynaptically, they are under the control of powerful segmental and descending inhibitory systems as described in the gate theory[3]. Nervous activity in large diameter afferent nerve fibers (touch and proprioception) has a strongly

inhibitory effect on input from the population of small afferent fibers which contains the nociceptor (pain) fibers. The main excitatory transmitter substance is glutamate together with other substances such as substance P, which are continuing to be discovered. Two types of excitatory terminals are known:

(1)   the nociception-specific small neurons in lamina I; and

(2)   the so-called wide dynamic range neurons (WDR) in lamina V of the dorsal horn which can be excited by tactile thermal proprioceptive and noxious stimuli. The WDR neurons have been widely investigated and much of the present knowledge about processing of nociceptive information comes from studies on these cells[3].

It is a significant feature of WDR cells that nervous impulses from non-myelinated nociceptor fibers result in depolarization and increased excitability outlasting the afferent activity by many seconds. This so called wind-up phenomenon is mediated through glutamate released on to NMDA (N-methyl-D-aspartate) receptors on the WDR cells. Wind-up is an important functional mechanism of the gate theory[3] which states that increased activity in small afferent nerve fibers opens the gate to the pain pathway and, conversely, increased nervous activity in large diameter (tactile) nerve fibers has the opposite effect. Large afferent nerve fibers are the target of TENS (see below).

The number of chemical mediators affecting transmission through the pain pathway is considerable. Here we can only mention the substances that are directly implicated in current methods of pain control. Seventy-five per cent of opioidergic inhibition at the level of the dorsal horn is presynaptic. Mu receptor agonists are clinically the most significant analgesic drugs. Morphine and morphine-like drugs are, however, often not effective in neuropathic pain conditions because cholecystokinine is up-regulated and counteracts the effect of mu-receptor agonists. Opioidergeic inhibitory mechanisms are utilized in acupuncture. The insertion and manipulation of acupuncture needles is a mildly nociceptive stimulus activating small nociceptor afferents. Either directly or through the Descending Nonspecific Inhibitory Complex (DNIC)[4] endorphinergic inhibition is produced. The role of endorphines in acupuncture is underlined by the fact that pain relief through acupuncture is frequently accompanied by nausea. GABA (gamana-amino-butyric acid)-ergic inhibition is activated by benzodiazepines. Adrenergic and 5-hydroxy-tryptaminergic mechanisms are amplified by tricyclic antidepressants. NMDA-effects of glutamate may be antagonized by, for example, ketamine. Descending inhibitory mechanisms are often effectively activated by spinal cord stimulation. This technique is most effective in neuropathic pain conditions. It has therefore no role in the control of RA pain.

Brainstem and brain

The brainstem is the origin of powerful descending inhibition originating, in particular, from the periaquaeductal grey. Strong binding sites for mu-receptor agonists can be found in the brainstem and in the thalamus. Anxiolytics may be useful in curtailing the limbic aspects of pain perception. Finally, pain management, a combination of behavioral techniques with physical therapy addresses, at the same time, limbic as well as cortical mechanisms in combination with improvement of physical parameters and peripheral sensory perception.

Stimulation analgesia

Stimulation analgesia targets either segmental inhibitory mechanisms activated by a-β afferent fibers (TENS, peripheral nerve stimulation, and vibration), or small afferent fibers to causing release of endorphins (acupuncture, acupuncture-like TENS), or descending inhibitory systems (spinal cord stimulation). Spinal cord stimulation will not be discussed any further, because its main indication are neuropathic and ischemic pain conditions.

Transcutaneous electrical nerve stimulation (TENS)

TENS is a commonly used form of stimulation analgesia. It has also proved itself as a pain control method in rheumatoid arthritis (RA). For a more detailed review of this method of pain control the reader is referred to the excellent chapter by Wolf and Thompson in the *Textbook of Pain*[5].

The technique

Transcutaneous nerve stimulation is a form of pain control that mobilizes the bodies own analgesic mechanisms. When it is used successfully there are few side-effects and almost no complications. It therefore deserves an optimal chance of success. This can only be guaranteed if time is spent by qualified staff first to explain in layman's terms what this technique is concerned with and secondly to explain in detail how to test for efficacy and how to manage TNS on a daily basis. Wynn Perry[6] feels it often necessary to admit a patient for assessment purposes, although this is a minority view. There are no reliable criteria predicting that TENS will control a particular pain condition[7]. A detailed guide has been published by Filshie and Thompson[8] on how to establish whether TENS is effective and how to start treatment.

Equipment

The equipment consists of a set of electrodes connected through a set of highly flexible leads to a battery-driven electrical stimulator. Modern transistorized stimulators can be quite small, even to the point that patients with hand deformities may not be able to operate them. It is important to select a model of appropriate dimensions for the individual. The price of transcutaneous nerve stimulators has come down dramatically over the years, so that all the equipment needed costs less than one consultant outpatient appointment.

TENS machines are designed as one or two channel devices with independent controls. The device used must at least offer the stimulation options: (1) regular repetitive; (2) burst mode; and (3) random stimulation. Stimulation frequencies available should cover the range between 3 and 120 Hz as well as stimulus durations between 0.1 and 1 ms. The device should also be equipped with rechargeable batteries.

The choice of electrodes is essentially between carbonized silicone rubber or adhesive electrodes. Silicone rubber electrodes have the advantage that they can be reused many times. They have to be kept in position with micropore tape and some times do not stay as securely fixed as necessary. Particularly during physical activity, they may be dislodged. It is important that proper saline gel is used. Without a proper contact gel there may be unreliable electrical contact and current sinks and sources may develop resulting in irritation of the skin.

An occasionally encountered complication is skin reactions. This occurrence can be minimized by the use of purpose-designed TENS gel, which are based on normal saline. Do not use hypertonic gels such as ECG gel. Occasionally, it may also be necessary to use a low allergy gel to overcome sensitivity problems.

Parameters of stimulation

There is no way of predicting which particular pattern of stimulation a patient will find most effective[5]. Several studies concentrating on this point, have been unsuccessful in predicting whether continuous, burst, or random stimulation are most effective in certain situations. Physiologically, it is known that different patterns of afferent nervous discharge may result in the release of different transmitter substances. Empirically, it is important that any pattern tried needs to be used for at least 1 hour three times a day[8]. In terms of frequencies preferred, this is best left to the patient himself. Usually, frequencies between 30 and 70 Hz are chosen. The strength of stimulation should be as high as tolerated comfortably. Ordinary TENS should not be painful, and there should be no muscle twitching.

Other parameters offered on some devices are ramped or high frequency stimulation. Ramped stimuli my be experienced as more pleasant. They are functionally not different from the above types. High frequency stimulation aims to make use of the phenomenon that this type of stimulation is known to block nervous conduction in the fibers stimulated. Practically, this can be seen to apply only to large afferent nerve fibers, because the strength of stimulation needed to excite C-fibers would have to be quite high and quite unpleasant. In the absence of nerve damage it is not helpful to block conduction in large sensory nerve fibers, because it is these fibers that mediate segmental inhibition of the pain pathway. Theoretically, high frequency fiber block may be useful in situations where pain is mediated through large fibers, as is the case in some forms of allodynia. More research is needed on this topic.

Positioning of electrodes

The aim is to position the electrodes in the inhibitory cutaneous receptive field. The most powerful inhibitory mechanisms are segmental. The electrodes must therefore be placed in the same nervous segment[8]. This may be quite distant from the site of pain. Electrodes must never be placed on skin that is not intact.

Effectiveness of TENS

A meta-analysis[9] found that the use of TENS to control chronic pain 'may well be justified but it cannot be proved' with clinical trials available. Experimentally, it is very difficult to design placebo TENS which would be required for a double-blind, controlled study. There are two components in pain control with TENS, the segmental inhibition and the placebo effect. The placebo effect is significant during the first month of use. Research using placebo TENS has shown that afterwards pain relief relies solely on segmental inhibition[5]. There is also a significant decline over time in the number of individuals who respond to TENS. Whilst at the beginning, 60–80 per cent of all individuals tested respond positively to TENS, this figure declines to 20–30 per cent after 1 year[5].

It is important to appreciate that TENS is pain control and not cure. Pain relief is most commonly experienced when the stimulator is used. In some patients, pain relief outlasts use of the stimulator by 10–30 min or even longer. In others two or more sessions are needed before significant pain relief is experienced. Except for patients with purely psychogenic pain who tend not to respond to TENS, there are no distinct groups of chronic pain sufferers who do or do not respond[7]. Responsiveness to TENS needs to be established through a trial. It may, of course, still be necessary to supplement with other forms of pain control.

Acupuncture-like TENS

This form of TENS is different from the above techniques, because stronger stimuli are employed with the aim of exciting small nociceptor afferent nerve fibers to effect spinal release of endogenous opioids, similar to the use of acupuncture. The electrodes are placed over known acupuncture points. This form of acupuncture may be mildly painful and there may also be some local contraction of muscle[5].

Acupuncture

Acupuncture is a form of stimulation analgesia targeting the small primary afferent fibers from nociceptors. Stimulation of this fiber group causes release of endogenous opioids through activation of the DNIC in the central nervous system[4], and increased levels of the inhibitory transmitter substances enkaphaline, as well as 5-hydroxytryptamine and catecholamines have been found in the CSF following acupuncture. The significance of this finding is, however, reduced by the observation that the placebo response is also mediated through an opioidergic link[10].

Although there is a sizable literature on the use of acupuncture in musculosceletal pain, reports of its use in rheumatoid arthritis are not common. The various forms of acupuncture used are the traditional acupuncture where specific points have been identified for specific effects. Probably for mnemonic convenience, a system of meridians has been introduced for the description of the location of individual points[11]. In Western acupuncture, needles are positioned in the dermatome where the pain is localized. The needles are either manipulated in the traditional fashion between thumb and index finger or they are connected to a low current source of repetitive electricity. Acupuncture is now widely used for pain control. Initially, 49 per cent of patients with nociceptive pain experienced pain relief in the study by Carlsson and Sjolund[12], decreasing to under 17 per cent after 6 months. Two meta-analyses[13,14] and a clinical update[15] produced equivocal results. The absence of support by meta-analysis can be explained partly by the difficulty of designing a placebo acupuncture technique. Needling in apparently non-effective points will still set a small tissue injury and activate the DNIC system.

Pain management

The experience of pain is based on simultaneous excitation of neurons in the somatosensory cortex and the limbic system. So far we have discussed pain control mechanisms targeting primary afferent fibers, the dorsal horn, and descending inhibitory systems. Pain management targets the cortex and the limbic system. The techniques employed are psychological, and the cognitive–behavioral approach appears to be the most successful method[16].

The adaptation to chronic pain may be studied using the model of stress and coping. Chronic pain represents the stressor to which individuals respond with widely divers adaptations ranging from almost normal function to catastrophizing and complete disability. Rheumatoid arthritis is a good test condition for this model, because the disease level can be quantified relatively well. In RA it has been found that adjustment to pain and functional impairment correlates more strongly with psychosocial factors such as depression and anxiety than with disease activity[17], which can be altered using techniques of cognitive evaluation and coping strategies. It has also been shown that pain-coping strategies predict perceived control of pain[18]. Severity of pain is unfortunately not easily controlled with cognitive evaluation and coping strategies. Keefe *et al.*[19] showed that higher levels of pain are related to lower levels of self-efficacy. However, after eliminating pain intensity as a component, pain-coping strategies were found to explain 8–15 per cent of self efficacy.

A great variety of topics are taught including an educational overview of RA, a simplified version of the gate theory, information about acute versus chronic pain, information about medical management of pain, specific coping strategies such as problem solving, relaxation, awareness of pain behavior, strategies for attention diversion, and training in family dynamics and communication. Programs are either residential or out-patient based. For patients with musculoskeletal impairment they are frequently run in combination with physiotherapists, who are assisting in realistically increasing goal setting and regaining of mobility. The establishment of a pain management program is a specialist task, however, and is possible in the setting of a district general hospital[20].

For how long do the benefits last following a course? Lorig and Halsted[21] looked at the long-term outcomes of an arthritis self-management study. They found the beneficial effects of the program sustained after 20 months. There were no differences between test groups with or without exposure to reinforcement. Patient education is discussed further in Chapter 32.

Nerve blocks and radiofrequency procedures

Nerve blocks may be indicated in situations of entrapment, for example carpal tunnel syndrome or radiculopathy. In entrapment it is often useful to add steroid to the local anesthetic, to reduce inflammatory swelling. Detailed descriptions of techniques can be found in Cousins and Bridenbaugh[22] and Wedley and Gauci[23]. Surgical transection of large nerves or nerve roots for pain relief should be performed only after very careful considerations, because it may result in neuropathic pain. More than 50 per cent of limb amputees experience phantom limb pain[24]. Using radiofrequency or cryolesioning, nerves retain their physical continuity. Nerve fibers can regenerate and nerve pains in the form of anesthesia dolorosa are less likely to occur. Radiofrequency lesioning is the technique that permits the greatest amount of precision in targeting. It is also the least invasive technique. It is used for a variety of indications of which facet joint denervation is the most relevant to RA.

Pain originating from the zygo apophyseal (facet) joints

Rheumatoid arthritis can affect any joint in the body. However, joints rarely involved are the distal interphalangeal, sacroiliac, and lumbar facet joints. Among the facet joints, the atlanto-occipital joints are a well recognized site giving rise to sometimes severe problems in the form of atlanto-occipital instability. The bulk of the literature about facet joints in rheumatoid arthritis is concerned with this problem, for which the reader is referred to the Chapter 37.

Like any other joint, facet joints may give rise to pain. Kaplan and coworkers[25] where able to show that distension of the capsule of facet joints causes pain and that this pain can be abolished reversibly by conduction block of the nerve supplying the facet joint with local anesthetic. Dolan and coworkers[26] showed a good correlation between pain relief caused by injection of facet joints with local anesthetic, which exhibited an increased uptake of technetium in single photon emission computerized tomography (SPECT). Pain relief was less likely to occur in apparently painful joints which did not show up on SPECT scanning. The physiological parameter measured with SPECT is an increase in localized blood flow as is present in inflammation. Facet joint injections, nerve blocks and denervations have been performed for many years. The effectiveness of facet joint denervation for pain control has been established by double-blind, controlled trial[27].

Diagnosis of facet joint arthropathy

Facet joint pain may be episodic or continuous. It usually has a local component that may be sharp or aching and often a referred component that must not be of a radicular distribution. Movements that increase the pressure on the joint tend to aggravate the pain. At the same time, not to have any movement in an affected joint is often very unpleasant, resulting in the typical phenomenon that individuals with facet joint pain find it uncomfortable to be in positions that puts even slight loading on an affected joint. Patients with cervical facet joint pain present with a stiff and painful neck, possibly even torticollis. The pain may radiate into the head, shoulder, and even the arm in a non-radicular fashion. The pain is exacerbated particularly by extension rotation and lateral flexion. There should be no neurological abnormalities.

Radiographs, CT scans, or MRI scans often show degeneration or appositional bone growth producing lipping of joints and various forms of misalignment of the joint surfaces. However, none of the structural radiological signs are sufficiently pathognomonic, because all these observations may be present without pain. As shown above, a positive SPECT scan strengthens the diagnosis[26].

It is not always easy to differentiate facet joint pain from surrounding soft tissue pain such as bursitis. It is the absence of more clearly-defined diagnostic criteria in some published work that may be responsible for the present unequivocal data for the effectiveness of facet joint injection as a mode of treatment.

Aims and outcome of injections

Facet joint injections are performed either with the aim of curbing an episode of facet joint pain or as a diagnostic procedure to decide on a denervation of the joint in question. Several open studies give a wide range of outcome of this treatment. In most studies, the diagnosis of facet joint pain is based on clinical criteria or on the exclusion of other more clearly-defined conditions. Lilius and coworkers[28] performed a randomized controlled study on 109 subjects with three types of injections: (1) cortisone and local anesthetic into facet joints; (2) the same mixture as a periarticular injection; and (3) physiological saline injected into two joints. A significant but treatment-independent improvement was noted in pain and disability scores but not in movements of the lumbar spine. Carette and coworkers[29] performed a double-blind, controlled study comparing injection with methyl prednisolone with saline in patients diagnosed as suffering from facet joint arthropathy by successful facet joint injection with lidocaine. No difference was found between the two groups that could be related to the use of methyl prednisolone. In this study the correct needle position in the joint to be injected was checked by injecting 0.5 ml of omnipaque contrast before injection of the test substance, so that the joint was largely filled with contrast medium before the test substance could be injected (see below). Roy and coworkers[30] did observe good but temporary pain relief following intra or periarticular facet joint injection. Using a small volume of 1.5 ml local anesthetic Moran and coworkers[31] observed pain relief in only 16.7 per cent of their total sample of 143 facet joints in 54 patients.

Techniques employed

Two techniques with slightly different aims are used:

1. Medial branch block[32]: the aim of this block is to identify facet joints suitable for denervation. The medial branches of the dorsal rami of spinal roots innervate the segmental facet joints with no fibers supplying skin. Under fluoroscopic control and with the determination of sensory electrical thresholds it is easily possible to identify the medial branch functionally. A small amount of local anesthetic is injected in order to block this nerve, and the subject is asked to observe whether or not there is short-lasting pain relief for the duration of the effectiveness of the local anesthetic. There is no treatment value in itself in this procedure.

2. Facet joint injection[23,31]: the aim of this procedure is to identify facet joints suitable for denervation as well as to provide pain relief for more than a few hours, under fluoroscopic control.

Two procedural questions have attracted attention in the literature, namely the volume of substrate to be injected and whether contrast should be used or not. The volume of the extended joint capsule of a facet joint is probably less than 1 ml. Any volume injected in excess of the capsular capacity will either result in the rupture of the joint capsule with part of the injected substrate ending up periarticular or part of the injection will have to be deposited periarticularly after slight withdrawal of the needle to overcome increasing resistance to injection. The differentiation between intra and periarticular injection with volumes in excess of the capsular capacity is therefore a spurious one. Secondly, contrast used to verify intra-articular positioning of the needle will itself fill up capsular space and needs to be added to the total volume injected.

Denervation of cervical facet joints

The technique of radiofrequency (RF) denervation of facet joints was first described by Shealey[33]. RF-denervation does frequently provide long lasting pain relief[27,34], although it is followed by nerve regeneration which can be quite rapid[35].

For cervical facet joint denervation, the patient is positioned in a supine position on a radiotranslucent table. The procedure is carried out under local anesthesia and sedation as required. Under fluoroscopic control the facet joint in question is displayed with the fluoroscope in an oblique position. Under local anesthesia with or without sedation the tip of a needle, insulated except for the last 5 mm of the tip (Sluiter Mehta needle), is positioned on the facet joint 1–2 mm dorsal of the foramen. The target is the medial branch of the dorsal ramus of the spinal root where it runs around the superior margin of the transverse process. Following anatomical positioning of the needle tip, the proper positioning is the ascertained functionally by electrical stimulation through the tip of the needle. A local change in sensation, for example a feeling of heaviness or tingling should be felt during stimulation with not more than 0.5 V at a rate of 50 /s. The rate of stimulation is then reduced to 2/s. The sensory threshold at this rate of stimulation should exceed the 50/s value by 50 per cent or more and no stimulation synchronous distant muscle twitching should occur. The purpose of the low frequency stimulation is to make sure that no motor nerve is within reach of the tip of the needle. Following the identification process, 1 ml of 2 per cent lidocaine is injected and after 2 min a radiofrequency current is passed through the needle raising the temperature to 80°C.

References

1. Derbyshire S.W., Jones A.K. Cerebral responses to a continual tonic pain stimulus measured using positron emission tomography. *Pain*, 1998;76:127–135.
2. Flor H., Fydrich T., Turk D.C. Efficacy of multidisciplinary pain treatment centers: a meta-analytic view. *Pain*, 1992;49:221–230.
3. Melzack R., Wall P.D. Pain transmission: A new theory. *Science*, 1965;150:971–979.
4. Le Bars D., Dickenson A.H., Besson J.M., Villanueva L. Aspects of sensory processing through convergent neurons. In: *Spinal afferent*

processing, ed. T.L. Yaksh, Plenum, New York, 1986; pp. 467–504.

5. Woolf C.J., Thompson J.W. Stimulation-induced analgesia transcutaneous electrical nerve stimulation (TENS) and vibration. In: *Textbook of pain*, ed. Wall P.D. and Melzack R. 1994. Churchill Livingstone, Edinburgh, pp. 1191–1208.

6. Wynn P. Pain in avulsion lesions of the brachial plexus. *Pain*, 1980;9:41–53.

7. Bates J.A.V., Nathan P.W. Transcutaneous electrical nerve stimulation for chronic pain. *Anaesthesia*, 1980;35:817–822.

8. Thompson J.W., Filshie J. Transcutaneous electrical nerve stimulation (TENS) and acupuncture. In: *Oxford texbook of palliative medicine*, eds Doyle D., Hanks G., MacDonald N. Oxford University Press, 1993:229–244.

9. McQuay H.J., Moore R.A. Transcutaneous electrical nerve stimulation. In: *An evidence-based resource for pain relief*. Oxford University Press, 1998, pp. 207–211.

10. ter Riet G., de Craen A.J.M., de Boer A., Kessels A.G.H. Is placebo analgesia mediated by endogenous opioids? A systematic review. *Pain*, 1998;76:273–275.

11. Lim J. *Understanding acupuncture*. PhD Thesis, Cambridge, 1989.

12. Carlsson C.P., Sjolund B.H. Acupuncture and subtypes of chronic pain: assessment of long-term results. *Clin J Pain*, 1994;10:290–295.

13. Ernst E., White A.R. Acupuncture for back pain. A meta-analysis of randomized controlled trials. *Arch Intern Med*, 1998;158:2235–2241.

14. ter Riet G., Kleijnen J., Knipschild P. Acupuncture and chronic pain: a criteria based meta-analysis. *J Clin Epidemiol*, 1990;43:1191–1199.

15. Thomas M., Lundeberg T. Does acupuncture work? *Pain Clinical Updates*, 1996;4 Issue 3, pp. 1–4.

16. Parker J.C., Frank R.G., Beck N.C., Smarr K.L., Buescher K.L., Phillips L.R., Smith E.I., Anderson S.K., Walker S.E. Pain management in rheumatoid arthritis patients, A cognitive-behavioral approach. *Arthritis Rheum*, 1988;31:593–601.

17. Hagglund K.J., Roth D.L., Haley W.E., Alarcon G.S. Discriminant and convergent validity of self-report measures of affective distress in patients with rheumatoid arthritis. *J Rheumatol*, 1989;16:1428–1432.

18. Haythornthwaite J.A., Menefee L.A., Heinberg L.J., Clark M.R. Pain coping strategies predict perceived control over pain. *Pain*, 1998;77:33–39.

19. Keefe F.J., Affleck G., Lefebvre J.C., Starr K., Caldwell D.S., Tennen H. Pain coping strategies and coping efficacy in rheumatoid arthritis: a daily process analysis. *Pain*, 1997;69:35–42.

20. Luscombe F.E., Wallace L., Williams J., Griffiths D.P.G. A district general hospital pain management programme. First year experiences and outcomes. *Anaesthesia*, 1995;50:114–117.

21. Lorig K., Halsted H.R. Long-term outcomes of an arthritis self-management study: Effects of reinforcement efforts. *Soc Sci Med*, 1989;29:221–224.

22. Cousins M.J., Bridenbaugh P.O. *Neural blockade in clinical anaesthesia and pain management*, 1980. J.B. Lippincott, Philadelpia, 1002–1007.

23. Wedley J.R., Gauci C.A. *Handbook of clinical techniques in the management of chronic pain*. Harwood Academic Publ., Chur, 1994.

24. Wartan S.W., Hamann W., Wedley J.R., McColl I. Phantom pain and sensation among british veteran amputees. *British J Anaesth*, 1997;78:652–659.

25. Kaplan M., Dreyfuss P., Halbrook B., Bogduk N. The ability of lumbar medial branch block to anesthetize the zygapophyseal joint. *Pain*, 1998;23:1847–1852.

26. Dolan A.L., Ryan P.J., Arden N.K., Stratton R., Wedley J.R., Hamann W., Foglman I., Gibson T. The value of SPECT scans in identifying back pain likely to benefit from facet joint injection. *Br J Rheumatol*, 1996;35:1269–1273.

27. Gallagher J., Pettricioni di Vadi P.L., Wedley J.R., Hamann W., Ryan P., Chikanza B., Kirkham B., Price R., Watson M.S., Graham R., Wood S. Radiofrequency facet joint denervation in the treatment of low back pain: a prospective controlled double-blind study to assess its efficacy. *Pain Clinic*, 1994;7:193–198.

28. Lilius G., Laasonen E.M., Myllynen P. Chronic unilateral low-back pain. Predictors of outcome of facet joint injections. *Spine*, 1990;15:780–782.

29. Carette S., Marcoux S., Truchon R., Grondin C., Gagnon J., Allard Y., Latulippe M. A controlled trial of corticosteroids into facet joints for chronic low back pain. *New Eng J Med*, 1991;325:1002–1007.

30. Roy D.F., Fleury J., Fontaine S.B., Dussault R.G. Clinical investigation of cervical facet joint infiltration. *Can Assoc Radio J*, 1988;39:118–120.

31. Moran R., O'Connel D., Walsh M.G. The diagnostic value of facet joint injections. *Spine*, 1988;13:1407–1410.

32. Dreyfuss P., Schwarzer A.C., Lau P., Bogduk N. Specificity of lumbar medial branch and L5 dorsal ramus blocks. A computed tomography study. *Spine*, 1997;22:895–902.

33. Shealy C.N. Percutaneous radiofrequency denervation of spinal facets: Treatment of chronic back pain and sciatica. *J Neurosurg*, 1975;43:448–451.

34. Lord S.M., Barnsley L., Wallis B.J., McDonald G.J., Bogduk N. Percutaneous radiofrequency neurotomy for chronic cervical zygapophyseal-joint pain. *New Eng J Med*, 1996;335:1721–1726.

35. Hamann W., Hall S. Acute effect and recovery of primary afferent nerve fibres after graded radiofrequency lesions in anaesthetised rats. *Br J Anaesth*, 1992;68:443.

34 | *Health economics*

Leigh F. Callahan

Introduction

Arthritis and musculoskeletal disorders are among the most prevalent chronic conditions and a leading cause of disability [1-11]. In addition, the economic consequences of arthritis are enormous[11-13]. In the most recent comprehensive economic study in the United States (US), the estimated costs of arthritis and musculoskeletal conditions were $149 billion in 1992 US dollars or 2.5 per cent of the gross domestic product (GDP)[12]. In Canada, the most recent estimate of the total costs of musculoskeletal disorders was $25.6 billion 1994 Canadian dollars or 3.4 per cent of the GDP[11]. Of the total costs of these diseases, about half were due to expenditures for medical care and about half were due to expenditures for medical care and about half were due to lost wages and disability[11,12].

Rheumatoid arthritis (RA), the second most prevalent form of arthritis, is a progressive, systemic, chronic disease affecting 0.5–1 per cent of the population[1,14-16]. The impacts of RA on the individual and society are substantial (Table 34.1). RA results in significant disability, functional loss, pain and fatigue[17-39], substantial psychological and social effects[12,40-55], and may lead to increased mortality[21,56-72]. There are also significant economic consequences for both individual patients, their families, and society[12,44,51,73-84] associated with RA. The costs of RA have been estimated at up to $14 billion dollars per year[85]. Yet despite the documentation of the enormous impact of RA, the consequences and 'side-effects' of the disease have often been underestimated[86,87].

The changes in the health care environment demand the concomitant evaluation and measurement of the costs and benefits of interventions for RA[81,88-91]. Assessment of health outcomes and economic evaluation essentially address the problem. It has become necessary for health care providers, hospitals, and systems of delivery to demonstrate that they achieve appropriate patient outcomes in a cost-effective manner[90]. Cost of illness studies are generally used to estimate the different types of costs associated with a specific disease (Table 34.2) and economic evaluations are used to study the relationship between the effec-

Table 34.1 Impact of rheumatoid arthritis on the individual and society

Increased mortality
Reduced quality of life
Disability
Psychological and social effects
Economic consequences

Table 34.2 Categories of cost-of-illness studies

Direct costs—expenditures for medical care and related items
Indirect costs—costs due to lost wages
Intangible costs—costs of an individual foregoing the activities they and society value

Table 34.3 Types of economic analyses

Cost-benefit—values the consequences or benefits in monetary terms
Cost-effectiveness—all costs are related to a single, common effect
Cost-utility—type of cost-effectiveness analysis in which benefits are expressed as quality-adjusted life years

tiveness of interventions and their costs (Table 34.3)[81,91-94]. These studies and evaluations are receiving increasing attention as health care budgets are limited and decision makers in reimbursement agencies are forced to regulate the allocation of health care resources[95].

Cost of illness studies are generally divided into three categories (Table 34.2). The three categories include direct costs, indirect costs, and intangible costs[96,97]. Direct costs are the costs that accrue when people receive medical care, such as physician visits, hospitalizations, medications, and diagnostic tests. Direct costs also include expenditures for other items such as adaptations to the home environment and transportation costs to visit health care providers, but it is often difficult to estimate accurately these other expenditures. Indirect costs are usually calculated as the costs due to lost wages from a reduction or cessation in work. Intangible costs are the costs of individuals foregoing the activities they and society value. Intangible costs include the costs associated with a decline in functional capacity, increased pain, and reduced quality of life.

The purpose of an economic analysis is to identify, measure, value, and compare the costs and consequences of interventions. Three methods are commonly used for economic analyses: cost-benefit, cost-effectiveness, or cost-utility studies (Table 34.3)[81,92-94]. Cost-benefit analyses value the consequences of benefits in monetary terms. With cost-benefit analysis, outcomes or benefit are assigned a monetary value. Due to the reluctance of many clinicians to value human life in dollars, cost-benefit analyses are rarely done in rheumatology[92]. Cost-effectiveness analyses relate all costs to a single, common effect. These analyses highlight the aggregate benefits conferred in non-economic terms[92,93]. These are the type of economic analyses most commonly performed in the health arena. Cost-utility analyses are a type of cost-effectiveness analysis in which benefits are expressed as quality-adjusted life years[92,93].

This chapter will focus on the economic consequences of RA, reviewing the components and estimates of the costs of disease and discussing some of the limitations in the methods for estimating cost. In addition, some of the studies where the costs of RA have been evaluated in economic analyses will be discussed.

Direct costs

The economic costs of RA are high, approximately those of coronary heart disease[73–80,82,98]. The direct costs of RA are, on average, three times the costs of medical care for persons of the same age and gender who do not have RA in the United States[78] and 2.5 times the costs of age and gender matched individuals in Sweden[99]. And, it has been estimated that the costs associated with caring for individuals with RA are increasing at twice the rate of the Medical Care Price Index in the United States[78,100].

The majority of studies examining costs of RA have been conducted in clinical populations. The studies can not be compared directly due to different costing methods, but some trends and similarities can be seen among the studies. A summary of four studies conducted in the late 1970s and early to mid 1980s is presented in Table 34.4[98]. The cost estimates from the original studies were updated to 1990 dollars by using the Consumer Price Index[98]. The annual directs costs of an RA patient averaged $6000 in 1990 dollars[73,76,85,98].

Hospitalization rates accounted for 40 per cent to more than 60 per cent of direct costs[73,76,77,85,98,101]. Fifty-four per cent of the admissions were accounted for by surgery, which was responsible for 70 per cent of the cost[101]. Medical admissions were distributed according to evaluation and treatment (47 per cent), management of adverse effects of therapy (43 per cent), and complications of RA (11 per cent)[101]. Direct costs for laboratory tests and medications were in the range of physician fees[78,80]. Both out-patient and in-patient direct costs were corre-

lated significantly with self-reported scores for global health status and functional status on the Health Assessment Questionnaire (HAQ)[76,101].

The medical charges for all health services used in a 1-year period were computed for a community-based cohort of individuals with RA in Olmstead Country, Minnesota[82]. The average direct medical charges were $3802 in 1987[82]. Of the total charges, $2554 were for in-patient charges and $1248 were for outpatient charges. These charges were significantly greater than the direct medical charges for individuals with osteoarthritis (OA) or no arthritis[82]. When the costs of medical services over a 1-year period for patients with RA were evaluated in a managed care setting in the US, the average individual cost rate of arthritis-related care was $2162 (1993 US dollars) per year[102]. Hospital visits accounted for 16 per cent of the total costs of RA care, while ambulatory care accounted for 21 per cent, and prescription medications for 62 per cent[102].

When the costs of RA were estimated in two Canadian provinces, the annual direct costs were $3788 (1994 Canadian dollars) in the late 1980s and $4656 (1994 Canadian dollars) in the early 1990s[103]. Institutional stays and medications made up at least 80 per cent of the total direct costs. The total economic impact of RA in England was estimated to be £1.256 billion in 1992, of which 48 per cent was due to direct costs[104]. The largest portion of direct costs were accounted for by hospital days, 28.3 per cent, followed by living in nursing home or residential establishments, 21.8 per cent[104]. Drugs accounted for 15.5 per cent of direct costs, nurse visits 13.7 per cent, home help visits 10 per cent, out-patient visits 6.4 per cent, general practitioner surgery visits 2.5 per cent, and daily living aids 1.8 per cent[104].

The mean annual direct cost due to RA in the Netherlands in 1996 was estimated to be Dfl. 11 550 per patient (i.e. £3680)[105]. There was no direct association with disease duration, but patients with higher levels of disease activity exhibited significantly higher costs compared to patients with lower disease activity[105].

Table 34.4 Economic costs of rheumatoid arthritis, by study (in 1990 dollars)

Author, year	Direct costs	Indirect costs	Total costs
Meenan *et al.*, 1978	5767 (25 %)	16 936 (75 %)	22 703 (100 per cent)
Liang *et al.*, 1984	1776 (15 %)	10 230 (85 %)	12 006 (100 per cent)
Stone, 1984	10 938 (18 %)	50 764 (82 %)	61 702 (100 per cent)
Lubeck *et al.*, 1986	5064	NR	NR

Source: Lubeck D.P., *Arth Care Res* 1995;8:304–310.

Table 34.5 Average medical care costs among patients with RA (1994 dollars)

Category	RA related cost	Non-RA related cost	Total costs
Physician visits	$911	$275	$1186
Other health providers	$261		$261
Out-patient surgery	$280	$900	$1180
Hospital admissions	$2188	$2086	$4274
DMARD	$323		$323
NSAID	$365		$365
Total	$4328	$3261	$7589

Source: Yelin E.H. *J Rheumatol* 1996;23:47–51.

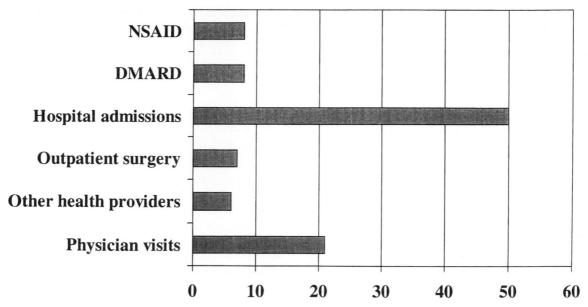

Fig. 34.1   RA related direct costs in per cent among 1025 patients in California, USA. Data from Ref. 20.

In a study of the average medical care costs among individuals with RA employing utilization data from a panel of 1025 patients followed by the University of California, San Francisco, both RA and non-RA related medical care are documented (Table 34.5) (Fig. 34.1)[79]. In this study, the costs are summarized in 1994 dollars. The total direct costs of medical care for RA and non-RA related care were $7589 (Table 34.5). RA medical care costs were $4328 and non-RA related care costs were $3261. Of the RA related costs, 50 per cent of the costs, $2188, were due to hospital admissions (Fig. 34.1). Of this amount, approximately 80 per cent was for surgical admissions. It is important to note though, that although hospitalizations accounted for slightly more than half of all costs, only slightly more than 12 per cent of the patients with RA were hospitalized in any one year. Disease modifying antirheumatic drugs (DMARD) and non-steroidal anti-inflammatory drugs (NSAIDs) each accounted for 8 per cent of the total RA related costs (Figs. 34.1). Physician visits accounted for 21 per cent of the costs.

To account for the potential upward bias in the cost estimates derived from clinical samples which might have individuals with greater disease severity, the absolute and incremental national costs of RA were analyzed using the 1989–91 National Health Interview Surveys[79]. The Health Interview Survey (HIS) is a population-based national probability sample of the non-institutionalized population in the United States. The medical coding in the HIS is purposefully conservative, so the HIS probably underestimates the true prevalence of RA. It does however provide a representative sample of those who meet the criteria for RA.

The absolute total direct costs for RA, in 1994, in the national community-based sample were $4.76 billion (Table 34.6). Physician visits accounted for $1.47 billion and hospital admissions accounted for $3.29 billion. Estimates of the absolute costs assume that individuals would incur no costs of illness in the absence of RA. Since this is not a reasonable assumption given the demographics of the population, the incremental costs expe-

rienced by those with RA were computed (Table 34.6). The incremental direct costs of RA were estimated to be $0.62 billion dollars (13 per cent of the total medical care), with $0.48 billion dollars attributed to hospital admissions and $0.14 billion dollars attributed to physician visits.

A recent study in the United States used individual utilization data from a managed health care plan to assess the total direct cost of diagnosing and treating RA[102]. The average individual cost rate of arthritis-related care was $2162 per year. In contrast to other studies, in this setting prescription medications accounted for 62 per cent of the total cost of RA care, and hospital visits for 16 per cent[102].

In summary, with the exception of one study[102], data from both the clinical studies and the population based estimates indicate that the majority of the direct costs of RA are due to hospitalizations[73,76,78–80,82,85,98,101–105]. It is clear that although only a small percentage of patients are hospitalized and most patients receive out-patient treatment and medications, the costs of medications, diagnostic tests, and physician visits reflect less than 50 per cent of the total direct costs of care for patients with RA.

Table 34.6   Estimates of the absolute and incremental costs of RA among 1.74 million patients with RA and 1.05 million patients with RA of working age (18–64), in 1994 dollars, US, 1989–1991

	Absolute costs[a]	Incremental costs[a]
Direct (n = 1.74 million)		
MD visits	$1.47	$0.14
Hospital admissions	$3.29	$0.48
Total	$4.76	$0.62
Indirect (n = 1.05 million)	$3.98	$2.45
Total	$8.74	$3.07

[a] in billions of US dollars.
Source: Yelin E.H. *J Rheumatol* 1996;**23**:47–51.

Indirect costs

Estimates of the indirect costs of RA, primarily lost income from work measured by the human capital approach, are three to four times higher than the direct costs of RA (Table 34.4)[73,76,78,85,98]. Indirect costs in clinical studies ranged from $10 000 to $50 000 in 1990 dollars (Table 34.4). Work disability has been reported after 5 years in 60 to 70 per cent of patients with RA younger than 65 years who had been working at disease onset[17]. Of the individuals who stopped working, 10 per cent indicated they had tried changes such as reducing their hours before stopping work[17].

In a recent clinical study in Minnesota of the indirect and non-medical costs among people with RA and OA compared to non-arthritic controls, patients with RA were significantly more likely to have lost their job or to have retired early due to their illness[83]. They were also more likely to have reduced their work hours or stopped working entirely due to their illness, and they were three times more likely to have had a reduction in household family income than either individuals with OA or those without arthritis[83]. Fifteen per cent of the individuals with RA were unable to get a job because of their illness. In addition to the costs associated with labor force participation, the individuals with RA incurred significantly more expenditures for home or child care compared to individuals without arthritis[83].

When the absolute and incremental indirect costs of RA were estimated in a national community-based sample in the United States, the absolute indirect costs were estimated to be $3.98 billion (Table 34.6). The incremental indirect costs that were due to RA were estimated to be $2.45 billion, more than 60 per cent of the total lost wage costs of this condition (Table 34.6). Eighty per cent of the increment of the costs of RA is due to wage losses.

In England in 1992, the indirect costs resulting from production loss were estimated to be £651.5 million, 52 per cent of the total costs[104]. Lost production among males and females was £177.2 million and £474.3 million, respectively[104]. The higher loss among the female population is a result to the higher prevalence of RA among females.

In a study of the effect of RA on working capabilities and social participation during the first 6 years of disease in the Netherlands, the employment rate was low in the RA population compared to the Dutch population[106]. In the male 45- to 64-year old group, 63 per cent of RA patients were not employed compared to 32 per cent of the Dutch population. Of the employed patients, 59 per cent reported that RA affected their working capabilities. And, of the patients without a paying job, 41 per cent believed that this was partly due to RA[106]. In addition, fewer RA patients had non-paying jobs and they performed fewer household activities compared to the Dutch population.

Although the indirect cost estimates of RA are substantial, they are an underestimate of the true indirect costs of the condition. The human capital approach to estimating indirect costs tends to underestimate the work loss or disability days of older individuals and females. Homemaker costs are estimated using the wages of house cleaners and day care workers, not teachers or counselors. Also, older women have lower labor force participation rates, resulting in lower estimates of the economic impact.

Intangible costs

The costs of RA extend far beyond the medical care costs, work loss, and changes in economic status. The intangible costs of RA include pain, depression, anxiety, changes in family structure, limitations in instrumental and nurturant activities, and changes in appearance resulting from deformity[12,40–42,44–52,54,55,78,107–110]. The amount of time individuals spend engaging in activities such as shopping, visiting the bank and supermarket, as well as the amount of time spent actively participating in hobbies, is significantly reduced in individuals with RA. Studies by Reisine[111] and by Allaire[112] showed that women with RA report limitations in numerous aspects of homemaking (Table 34.7). Reported limitations in instrumental activities, such as cleaning, laundry, shopping, cooking, and organizing finances range from 16 to 73 per cent (Table 34.7). The range of reported limitations in nurturant activities including listening, making arrangements, maintaining ties, care for the sick, and teaching is from 16 to 42 per cent. It is very difficult to put a price on these limitations.

The impact of RA on psychological status has been measured in terms of depression, coping strategies, anxiety, cognitive changes, self-efficacy, and learned helplessness[52,54,113–119]. Most studies indicate higher levels of psychological distress in individuals with RA than in the general population. This higher level of distress is comparable with levels found among clinical samples of individuals with other chronic conditions[49].

Studies evaluating the rates of divorce in individuals with RA have yielded equivocal findings[120,121]: some studies have found that divorce rates are higher in individuals with RA compared with the general population, whereas others show no significant difference[120]. Hawley and colleagues did note a significant reduction in the rate of remarriage after divorce in individuals with RA[121]. Moreover, the studies in the literature have consistently shown that RA creates stress on marriage and on the healthy spouses[120].

There are no national data summarizing the psychological and social impacts of RA. Perhaps this is because it is difficult to quantify these consequences in a traditional population-based

Table 34.7 Intangible impacts of rheumatoid arthritis

Limitations in instrumental activities		Limitations in nurturant activities	
Cleaning	73%	Making arrangements	42%
Laundry	65%	Maintaining ties	42%
Shopping	61%	Caring for the sick	39%
Cooking	42%	Teaching, guiding	23%
Finances	16%	Listening	16%

Source: Reisine *et al. Soc Sci Med.* 1987;25:89–95.

survey format, let alone price them in economic terms. The difficulty of data collection notwithstanding, information is needed to increase awareness of the many intangible costs of RA.

Conclusion

The direct, indirect, and intangible costs associated with RA are enormous. The long-term economic consequences include medical costs, lost wages due to frequent work disability and reductions in work capacity, psychological distress, and social dislocation. The indirect costs of RA are probably underestimated substantially with current costing methods, but even with underestimations they are significantly higher than the direct costs of RA. The majority of direct medical costs are due to hospitalizations and long-term care, with surgery comprising the largest part of the hospitalization costs. The intangible costs of RA are considerable, but difficult to quantify and price. Therapies and treatment of RA should be evaluated in terms of the many consequences of the disease.

References

1. Lawrence R., Helmick C., Arnett F., Deyo R., Felson D., Giannini E., Heyse S., Hirsh R., Hochberg M., Hunder G., Liang M., Pillemer S., Steen V., Wolfe F.: Estimates of the prevalence of arthritis and selected musculoskeletal disorders in the united states. *Arthritis Rheum*, 1998;**41**:778–799.
2. Helmick C.G., Lawrence R.C., Pollard R.A., Lloyd J.C., Heyse S.P.: Arthritis and other rheumatic conditions: who is affected now, who will be affected later? *Arthritis Care Res*, 1995;**8**:203–211.
3. Badley E.M., Rasooly I., Webster G.K.: Relative importance of musculoskeletal disorders as a cause of chronic health problems, disability, and health care ultilization: findings from the 1990 Ontario health survey. *J Rheumatol*, 1994;**21**:505–514.
4. Badley E.M., Tennant A.: Impact of disablement due to rheumatic disorders in a British population: estimates of severity and prevalence from the Calderdale Rheumatic Disablement Survey. *Ann Rheum Dis*, 1993;**52**:6–13.
5. Reynolds D., Chambers L., Badley E., Bennett K., Goldsmith C., Jamieson E., Torrance G., Tugwell P.: Physical disability among Canadians reporting musculoskeletal diseases. *J Rheumatol*, 1992;**19**:1020–1030.
6. Reynolds D., Torrance G., Badley E., Bennett K., Chambers L., Goldsmith C., Jamieson E., Tugwell P., Wolfson M.: Modelling the population health impact of musculoskeletal diseases: arthritis. *J Rheumatol*, 1993;**20**:1037–1047.
7. Badley E.M.: The impact of disabling arthritis. *Arthritis Care Res*, 1995;**8**:221–228.
8. Verbrugge L.M., Gates D.M., Ike R.W.: Risk factors for disability among U.S. adults with arthritis. *J Clin Epidemiol*, 1991;**44**:167–182.
9. Verbrugge L.M., Lepkowski J.M., Konkol L.L.: Levels of disability among U.S. adults with arthritis. *J Gerontol*, 1991;**46**:S71–S83.
10. Verbrugge L., Patrick D.: Seven chronic conditions: their impact on U.S. adults' activity levels and use of medical services. *Am J Public Health*, 1994;**85**:173–182.
11. Coyte P.C., Asche C.V., Croxford R., Chan B.: The economic cost of musculoskeletal disorders in Canada. *Arthritis Care Res*, 1998;**11**:315–325.
12. Yelin E., Callahan L.F.: The economic cost and social and psychological impact of musculoskeletal conditions. *Arthritis Rheum*, 1995;**38**:1351–1362.
13. Badley E.M.: The economic burden of musculoskeletal disorders in Canada is similar to that for cancer, and may be higher (editorial). *J Rheumatol*, 1995;**22**:204–206.
14. Silman A., Hochberg M.: *Epidemiology of rheumatic diseases.* Oxford, Oxford University Press, 1993.
15. Abdel-Nasser A.M., Rasker J.J., Valkenburg H.A.: Epidemiological and clinical aspects relating to the variability of rheumatoid arthritis. *Semin Arthritis Rheum*, 1997;**27**:123–140.
16. Kvien T.K., Glennas A., Knudsred O.G., Smedstad L.M., Mowinckel P., Forre O.: The prevalence and severity of rheumatoid arthritis in Oslo. *Scand J Rheumatol*, 1997;**26**:412–418.
17. Yelín E., Meenan R., Nevitt M., Epstein W.: Work disability in rheumatoid arthritis: effects of disease, social, and work factors. *Ann Intern Med*, 1980;**93**:551–556.
18. Pincus T., Mitchell J.M., Burkhauser R.V.: Substantial work disability and earnings losses in individuals less than age 65 with osteoarthritis: comparisons with rheumatoid arthritis. *J Clin Epidemiol*, **42**:449–457, 1989.
19. Sherrer Y.S., Bloch D.A., Mitchell D.M., Roth S.H., Wolfe F., Fries J.F.: Disability in rheumatoid arthritis: comparison of prognostic factors across three populations. *J Rheumatol*, 1987;**14**:705–709.
20. Yelin E.H., Henke C.J., Epstein WV: Work disability among persons with musculoskeletal conditions. *Arthritis Rheum*, 1986;**29**:1322–1333.
21. Pincus T., Callahan L.F., Sale W.G., Brooks A.L., Payne L.E., Vaughn W.K.: Severe functional declines, work disability, and increased mortality in seventy-five rheumatoid arthritis patients studied over nine years. *Arthritis Rheum*, 1984;**27**:864–872.
22. Siegert C.E.H., Vleming L.J., Vandenbroucke J.P., Cats A.: Measurement of disability in Dutch rheumatoid arthritis patients. *Clin Rheumatol*, 1984;**3**:305–309.
23. Tugwell P., Bombardier C., Buchanan W.W., Goldsmith C.H., Grace E., Hanna B.: The MACTAR Patient Preference Disability Questionnaire—an individualized functional priority approach for assessing improvement in physical disability in clinical trials in rheumatoid arthritis. *J Rheumatol*, 1987;**14**:446–451.
24. Reeback J., Silman A.: Predictors of outcome at two years in patients with rheumatoid arthritis *J R Soc Med*, 1984;**77**:1002–1005.
25. Isomäki H., Martio J., Sarna S., Kiviniemi P., Akimova T., Ievleva L., Mylov N., Trofimova T.: Predicting the outcome of rheumatoid arthritis: a Soviet-Finish co-operative study. *Scand J Rheumatol*, 1984;**13**:33–38.
26. Yelin E., Nevitt M., Epstein W.: Toward an epidemiology of work disability. *Milbank Mem Fund Q Health Soc*, 1980;**58**:386–415.
27. Anderson K.O., Keefe F.J., Bradley L.A., McDaniel L.K., Young L.D, Turner R.A., Agudelo C.A., Semble E.L., Pisko E.J.: Prediction of pain behavior and functional status of rheumatoid arthritis patients using medical status and psychological variables. *Pain*, 1988;**33**:25–32.
28. Fries J.F., Spitz P.W., Young D.Y.: The dimensions of health outcomes: the health assessment questionnaire, disability and pain scales. *J Rheumatol*, 1982;**9**:789–793.
29. Ekdahl C., Eberhardt K.B., Andersson S.I., Svensson B.: Assessing disability in patients with rheumatoid arthritis. *Scand J Rheumatol*, 1988;**17**:263–271.
30. Wolfe F., Hawley D.J., Cathey M.A.: The risk of functional disability and the rate of its development in patients with rheumatoid arthritis. *Arthritis Rheum*, 1989;**32**:S88(Abstract).
31. Reisine S.T., Grady K.E., Goodenow C., Fifield J.: Work disability among women with rheumatoid arthritis: the relative importance of disease, social, work, and family factors. *Arthritis Rheum*, 1989;**32**:538–543.
32. Callahan L.F., Bloch D.A., Pincus T.: Identification of work disability in rheumatoid arthritis: physical, radiographic and laboratory variables do not add explanatory power to demographic and functional variables. *J Clin Epidemiol*, 1992;**45**:127–138.

33. McFarlane A.C., Brooks P.M.: Determinants of disability in rheumatoid arthritis. *Br J Rheumatol*, 1988;27:7–14.

34. Leigh J.P., Fries J.F., Parikh N.: Severity of disability and duration of disease in rheumatoid arthritis. *J Rheumatol*, 1992;19:1906–1911.

35. Yelin E.H.: Work disability and rheumatoid arthritis. In: *Rheumatoid arthritis: pathogenesis, assessment, outcome, and treatment*. Eds F. Wolfe, T. Pincus. New York, Marcel Dekker, 1994, p. 261.

36. van der Heide A., Jacobs J.W.G., van Albada-Kuipers G.A., Kraaimaat F.W., Geenen R., Bijlsma J.: Self report functional disability scores and the use of devices: two distinct aspects of physical function in rheumatoid arthritis. *Ann Rheum Dis*, 1993;32:497–502.

37. Ward M.M., Leigh J.P., Fries J.F.: Progression of functional disability in patients with rheumatoid arthritis: associations with rheumatology subspeciality care. *Arch Intern Med*, 1993;153:2229–2237.

38. Reisine S., Mcquillan J., Fifield J.: Predictors of work disability in rheumatoid arthritis patients. *Arthritis Rheum*, 1995;38:1630–1637.

39. Smedstad L.M., Kvien T.K., Moum T., Vaglum P.: Life events, psychosocial factors, and demographic variables in early rheumatoid arthritis: relations to one-year changes in functional disability. *J Rheumatol*, 1995;22:2218–2225.

40. Bradley L.A.: Psychological aspects of arthritis. *Bull Rheum Dis*, 1985;35:1–12.

41. Smith T.W., Peck J.R., Milano R.A., Ward J.R.: Cognitive distortion in rheumatoid arthritis: relation to depression and disability. *J Consult Clin Psychol*, 1988;56:412–416.

42. Ehrlich G.E.: Social, economic, psychologic, and sexual outcomes in rheumatoid arthritis. *Am J Med*, 1983;75(suppl. 6A):27–34.

43. Mewa A.A., Rosenbloom D., Grace E.M., Brooks P., Bellamy N., Denko C., Norman G., Buchanan W.W.: Effects of aspirin, naloxone and placebo. *Clin Rheumatol*, 1987;6:526–531.

44. Meenan R.F., Yelin E.H., Nevitt M., Epstein W.V.: The impact of chronic disease: a sociomedical profile of rheumatoid arthritis. *Arthritis Rheum*, 1981;24:544–549.

45. Skevington S.M.: Psychological aspects of pain in rheumatoid arthritis: a review. *Soc Sci Med*, 1986;23:567–575.

46. Revenson T.A., Felton B.J.: Disability and coping as predictors of psychological adjustment to rheumatoid arthritis. *J Consult Clin Psychol*, 1989;57:344–348.

47. Fitzpatrick R., Newman S., Archer R., Shipley M.: Social support, disability and depression: A longitudinal study of rheumatoid arthritis. *Soc Sci Med*, 1991;33:605–611.

48. Parker J.C., Wright G.E.: The implications of depression for pain and disability in rheumatoid arthritis. *Arthritis Care Res*, 1995;8:279–283.

49. De Vellis B.: Depression in rheumatological diseases. *Bailliere's Clin Rheum*, 1993;7:241–257.

50. Katz P.P., Yelin E.H.: Prevalence and correlates of depressive symptoms among persons with rheumatoid arthritis. *J Rheumatol*, 1993;20:790–796.

51. Eberhardt K., Larson B., Nived K.: Early rheumatoid arthritis—some social, economical, and psychological aspects. *Scand J Rheumatol*, 1993;22:119–123.

52. Zautra A., Manne S.: Coping with rheumatoid arthritis: Review of a decade of research. *Ann Behav Med*, 1992;14:31–39.

53. Zautra A.J., Burleson M.H., Matt K.S., Roth S., Burrows L.: Impersonal stress, depression, and disease activity in rheumatoid arthritis and osteoarthritis patients. *Health Psychol*, 1994;13:139–148.

54. Blalock S.J., De Vellis B.M., De Vellis R.F., Giorgino K.B., van H. Sauter S., Jordan J.M., Keefe F.J., Mutran E.J.: Psychological well-being among people with recently diagnosed rheumatoid arthritis. Do self-perceptions of abilities make a difference? *Arthritis Rheum*, 1992;35:1267–1272.

55. Blalock S.J., De Vellis B.M., De Vellis R.F.: Social comparison among individuals with rheumatoid arthritis. *J Appl Soc Psychol*, 1989;19:665–680.

56. Cobb S., Anderson F., Bauer W.: Length of life and cause of death in rheumatoid arthritis. *N Engl J Med*, 1953;249:553–556.

57. Koota K., Isomäki H., Mutru O: Death rate and causes of death in RA patients during a period of five years. *Scand J Rheumatol*, 1977;6:241–244.

58. Rasker J.J., Cosh J.A.: Cause and age at death in a prospective study of 100 patients with rheumatoid arthritis. *Ann Rheum Dis*, 1981;40:115–120.

59. Mitchell D.M., Spitz P.W., Young D.Y., Bloch D.A., McShane D.J., Fries J.F.: Survival, prognosis, and causes of death in rheumatoid arthritis. *Arthritis Rheum*, 1986;29:706–714.

60. Allebeck P., Ahlbom A., Allander E.: Increased mortality among persons with rheumatoid arthritis, but where RA does not appear on death certificate: eleven year follow-up of an epidemiological study. *Scand J Rheumatol*, 1981;10:301–306.

61. Monson R.R., Hall A.P.: Mortality among arthritics. *J Chronic Dis*, 1976;29:459–467.

62. Pincus T., Callahan L.F., Vaughn W.K.: Questionnaire, walking time and button test measures of functional capacity as predictive markers for mortality in rheumatoid arthritis. *J Rheumatol*, 1987;14:240–251.

63. Pincus T., Callahan L.F.: Taking mortality in rheumatoid arthritis seriously—predictive markers, socio-economic status and comorbidity. *J Rheumatol*, 1986;13:841–845.

64. Pincus T., Callahan L.F.: Early mortality in RA predicted by poor clinical status. *Bull Rheum Dis*, 1992;41,4:1–4.

65. Pincus T., Brooks R.H., Callahan L.F.: Prediction of long-term mortality in patients with rheumatoid arthritis according to simple questionnaire and joint count measures. *Ann Intern Med*, 1994;120:26–34.

66. Callahan L.F., Pincus T.: Mortality in rheumatic diseases. *Arthritis Care Res*, 1995;8:229–241.

67. Callahan L.F., Cordray D.S., Wells G., Pincus T.: Formal education and five-year mortality in rheumatoid arthritis: Mediation by helplessness scale scores. *Arthritis Care Res*, 1996;9:463–472.

68. Symmons D.P.: Mortality in rheumatoid arthritis *Br J Rheumatol*, 1988;27:44–54.

69. Rasker J.J., Cosh J.A.: The natural history of rheumatoid arthritis over 20 years. Clinical symptoms, radiological signs, treatment, mortality and prognostic significance of early features. *Clin Rheumatol*, 1987;6(suppl. 2):5–11.

70. Scott D.L., Symmons D.P., Coulton B.L., Popert A.J.: Long-term outcome of treating rheumatoid arthritis: Results after 20 years. *Lancet*, 1987;16:1108–1111.

71. Abruzzo J.L.: Rheumatoid arthritis and mortality. *Arthritis Rheum*, 1982;25:1020–1023.

72. Isomaki H.A., Mutru O., Koota K.: Death rate and causes of death in patients with rheumatoid arthritis. *Scand J Rheumatol*, 1975;4:205–208.

73. Meenan R.F., Yelin E.H., Henke C.J., Curtis D.L., Epstein W.V.: The costs of rheumatoid arthritis: a patient-oriented study of chronic disease costs. *Arthritis Rheum*, 1978;21:827–833.

74. Liang M.H., Larson M., Thompson M., Eaton H., McNamara E., Katz R., Taylor J.: Costs and outcomes in rheumatoid arthritis and osteoarthritis. *Arthritis Rheum*, 1984;27:522–529, 1984.

75. Stone C.E.: The lifetime economic costs of rheumatoid arthritis. *J Rheumatol*, 1984;11:819–827.

76. Lubeck D.P., Spitz P.W., Fries J.F., Wolfe F., Mitchell D.M., Roth S.H.: A multicenter study of annual health service utilization and costs in rheumatoid arthritis. *Arthritis Rheum*, 1986;29:488–493.

77. Jacobs J., Keyserling J.A., Britton M., Morgan G.J., Jr, Wilkenfeld J., Hutchings H.C.: The total cost of care and the use of pharmaceuticals in the management of rheumatoid arthritis: the Medi-Cal program. *J Clin Epidemiol*, 1988;41:215–223.

78. Allaire S.H., Prashker M.J., Meenan R.F.: The costs of rheumatoid arthritis. *PharmacoEconomics*, 1994;6:513–522.

79. Yelin E.: The costs of rheumatoid arthritis: absolute, incremental, and marginal estimates. *J Rheumatol*, 1996;23(Suppl. 44):47–51.

80. Pincus T.: The underestimated long term medical and economic consequences of rheumatoid arthritis. *Drugs*, 1995;50:1–14.

81. Lambert C.M., Hurst N.P.: Health economics as an aspect of health outcome: basic principles and application in rheumatoid arthritis. *Br J Rheumatol*, 1995;34:774–780

82. Gabriel S.E., Crowson C.S., Campion M.E., O'Fallon W.M.: Direct medical costs unique to people with arthritis. *J Rheumatol*, 1997;24:719–725.

83. Gabriel S.E., Crowson C.S., Campion M.E., O'Fallon W.M.: Indirect and nonmedical costs among people with rheumatoid arthritis and osteoarthritis compared with nonarthritic controls. *J Rheumatol*, 1997;24:43–48.

84. Mitchell J.M., Burkhauser R.V., Pincus T.: The importance of age, education, and comorbidity in the substantial earnings losses of individuals with symmetric polyarthritis. *Arthritis Rheum*, 1988;31:348–357.

85. Lubeck D.P.: The economic impact of rheumatoid arthritis. In: *Rheumatoid arthritis: pathogenesis, assessment, outcome, and treatment*. Eds F. Wolfe, T. Pincus. New York, Marcel Dekker, 1994, p. 247.

86. Strober S., Okada S., Oseroff A.: Role of natural suppressor cells in allograft tolerance. *Fed Proc*, 1984;43:263–265.

87. Pincus T., Callahan L.F.: The 'side effects' of rheumatoid arthritis: joint destruction, disability and early mortality. *Br J Rheumatol*, 1993;32(suppl. 1):28–37, 1993.

88. Katz J.N., Sangha O.: Assessment of the quality of care. *Arthritis Care Res*, 1997;10:359–369.

89. Katz P.P., Showstack J.A.: Choosing quality and outcomes measures for rheumatic diseases. *Arthritis Care Res*, 1997;10: 370–380.

90. Mason J.H.: Outcomes measurement in today's health care environment. *Arthritis Care Res*, 1997;10:355–358.

91. Ferraz M.B., Maetzel A., Bombardier C.: A summary of economic evaluations published in the field of rheumatology and related disciplines. *Arthritis Rheum*, 1997;40:1587–1593.

92. Ruchlin H.S., Elkin E.B., Paget S.A.: Assessing cost-effectiveness analyses in rheumatoid arthritis and osteoarthritis. *Arthritis Care Res*, 1997;10:413–421.

93. Haddix A.C., Teutsch S.M., Shaffer P.A., Dunet D.O., eds. *Prevention effectiveness: a guide to decision analysis and economic evaluation*. New York, Oxford University Press, 1996.

94. Gold M.R., Siegel J.E., Russell L.B., Weinstein M.C., eds. *Cost-effectiveness in health and medicine*. New York, Oxford University Press, 1996.

95. Maztzel A.: Costs of illness and the burden of disease. *J Rheumatol*, 1997;24:3–5.

96. Hall J., Mooney G.: What every doctor should know about economics. Part I. The benefits of costing. *Med J Aust*, 1990;152:29–31.

97. Savage R.L., Moller P.W., Ballantyne C.L., Wells J.E.: Variation in the risk of peptic ulcer complications with nonsteroidal antiinflammatory drug therapy. *Arthritis Rheum*, 1993;36:84–90.

98. Lubeck D.P.: The economic impact of arthritis. *Arthritis Care Res*, 1995;8:304–310.

99. Jonsson B., Rehnberg C., Borgquist L., Larsson S.-E: Locomotion status and costs in destructive rheumatoid arthritis: A comprehensive study of 82 patients from a population of 13 000. *Acta Orthop Scand*, 1992;63:207–212.

100. Polley H.F., Hunder G.G.: *Rheumatologic interviewing and physical examination of the joints*, 2nd edn. Philadelphia, W.B. Saunders, 1978.

101. Wolfe F., Kleinheksel S.M., Spitz P.W., Lubeck D.P., Fries J.F., Young D.Y., Mitchell D.M., Roth S.H.: A multicenter study of hospitalization in rheumatoid arthritis: effect of health care system, severity, and regional difference. *J Rheumatol*, 1986;13:277–284.

102. Lanes S.F., Lanza L.L., Radensky P.W., Yood R.A., Meenan R.F., Walker A.M., Dreyer N.A.: Resource utilization and cost of care for rheumatoid arthritis and osteoarthritis in a managed care setting. *Arthritis Rheum*, 1997;40:1475–1481.

103. Clarke A.E., Zowall H., Levinton C., Assimakopoulos H., Sibley J.T., Haga M., Shiroky J., Neville C., Lubeck D.P., Grover S.A., Esdaile J.M.: Direct and indirect medical costs incurred by Canadian patients with rheumatoid arthritis: a 12 year study. *J Rheumatol*, 1997;24:1051–1060.

104. McIntosh E.: The cost of rheumatoid arthritis. *Br J Rheumatol*, 1996;35:781–790.

105. van Jaarsveld C.H.M., Jacobs J.W.G., Schrijvers H.J.P., Heurkens A.H.M., Haanen H.C.M., Bijlsma J.W.J.: Direct cost of rheumatoid arthritis during the first six years: A cost-of-illness study. *Br J Rheumatol*, 1998;37:837–847.

106. van Jaarsveld C.H.M., Jacobs J.W.G., Schrijvers A.J.P., van Albada-Kuipers G.A., Hofman D.M., Bijlsma J.W.J.: Effects of rheumatoid arthritis on employment and social participation during the first years of disease in the Netherlands. *Br J Rheumatol*, 1998;37:848–853.

107. Katz P.P., Yelin E.H.: Life activities of persons with rheumatoid arthritis with and without depressive symptoms. *Arthritis Care Res*, 1994;7:69–77.

108. Spitz P.W.: The medical, personal, and social costs of rheumatoid arthritis. *Nurs Clin North Am*, 1984;19:575–582.

109. Erslev A.J., Wilson J., Caro J.: Erythropoietin titers in anemic, non-uremic patients. *J Lab Clin Med*, 1987;109:429–433.

110. Mossey J.M., Knott K., Craik R.: The effects of persistent depressive symptoms on hip fracture recovery. *J Gerontol*, 1990;45:M163–M168.

111. Reisine S.T., Goodenow C., Grady K.E.: The impact of rheumatoid arthritis on the homemaker. *Soc Sci Med*, 1987;25:89–95.

112. Allaire S.H., Meenan R.F., Anderson J.J.: The impact of rheumatoid arthritis on the household work performance of women. *Arthritis Rheum*, 1991;34:669–678.

113. Manne S., Zautra A.: Coping with arthritis: Current status and critique. *Arthritis Rheum*, 1992;35:1273–1279.

114. Blalock S.J., De Vellis B.M., Holt K., Hahn P.M.: Coping with rheumatoid arthritis: Is one problem the same as another? *Health Educ Q*, 1993;20:119–132.

115. Blalock S.J., Afifi R.A., De Vellis B.M., Holt K., De Vellis R.F.: Adjustment to rheumatoid arthritis: the role of social comparison processes. *Health Educ Res*, 1990;5:361–370.

116. Lorig K.R., Chastain R.L., Ung E., Shoor S., Holman H.R.: Development and evaluation of a scale to measure perceived self-efficacy in people with arthritis. *Arthritis Rheum*, 1989;32:37–44.

117. Nicassio P.M., Wallston K.A., Callahan L.F., Herbert M., Pincus T.: The measurement of helplessness in rheumatoid arthritis. The development of the Arthritis Helplessness Index. *J Rheumatol*, 1985;12:462–467.

118. Callahan L.F., Brooks R.H., Pincus T.: Further analysis of learned helplessness in rheumatoid arthritis using a 'Rheumatology Attitudes Index'. *J Rheumatol*, 1988;15:418–426.

119. Callahan L.F., Kaplan M.R., Pincus T.: The Beck Depression Inventory, Center for Epidemiological Studies Depression Scale (CES-D), and General Well-being Schedule Depression Subscale in rheumatoid arthritis: criterion contamination of responses. *Arthritis Care Res*, 1991;4:3–11.

120. Revenson T.A.: The role of social support with rheumatic disease. *Bailliere's Clin Rheum*, 1993;7:377–396.

121. Hawley D.J., Wolfe F., Cathey M.A., Roberts F.K.: Marital status in rheumatoid arthritis and other rheumatic disorders: a study of 7293 patients. *J Rheumatol*, 1991;18:654–660.

SECTION
6

Surgical therapy

35 | *Large joints and feet*

Urban Rydholm

Joint surgery in RA was pioneered in Heinola in Finland in the early 1960 and has been in common use in the last 30 years. It is now considered an essential component of rheumatological rehabilitation, in particular large joint replacement procedures. Surgical synovectomy, however, has largely been replaced by intra-articular glucocorticoids and by systemic pharmacotherapy (see Section 4). An increasing number of joint prostheses are now in use. Immediate results are often dramatic, but, as will become apparent, long-term, controlled trials are scarce.

The outcome of surgical procedures in the large joints and feet differ between patients with RA and OA, due to the systemic and progressive character of RA. On the other hand, the average RA patient puts less weight on the operated joint(s) which will reduce wear of prosthetic components.

Indications and contraindications

Indications

Indications for surgery are mainly as follows:

- *pain relief* when conservative measures have failed;
- *prevention* of nerve compression, tendon rupture, or further functional joint deterioration;
- *reconstruction* of damaged joints with the aim of improving function.

Relieving pain is the most important and most frequent indication.

The decision to perform surgery must always be based on a careful analysis of the origin of the pain. It may be caused by synovial inflammation in an intact joint, by destructive changes, or by a combination of inflammation and destruction. The radiographic appearance of the painful joint is of interest, since it is less likely that advanced radiographic changes will be reversible with non-surgical treatments. Surgical procedures involving removal of synovial tissue from tendon sheaths may prevent tendon rupture. Correction of deformity and fusion of the ankle and small joints in the foot may also prevent unfavorable loading conditions in proximal joints. Isolated correction of deformities is, however, often superfluous, since neighboring joints have commonly adapted to surrounding deformities. Reconstructive surgery can consist of replacement of destroyed joint surfaces with artificial materials, endoprostheses, or autologous tissue. Arthrodesis is also still useful, for example in the hindfoot where it may improve loading conditions for the knee and foot. Often a combination of indications is present.

Table 35.1 Risk factors related to rheumatoid arthritis

Increased disease or therapy related risk of infection
Nutritional difficulties (temporomandibular arthritis, dysphagia
Secondary to cervical spine involvement)
Cardiovascular problems (vasculitis, valvular heart disease)
Renal insufficiency (*e.g.* amyloidosis)
Impaired bone quality (osteopenia)
Anesthesiological risks related to the cervical spine and
Temporomandibular joints

Contraindications and risk factors

There are some risk factors related to rheumatoid disease that always should be taken into consideration in the planning of surgery (Table 35.1). Certain drugs may increase the risks associated with surgery. Conventional COX inhibitors inhibit platelet function and increase the risk of bleeding which, however, can be partly counteracted by meticulous surgical technique. Bleeding may also be reduced by the preoperative use of tranexamic acid[1]. Maintaining NSAIDs avoids exacerbation of pain and stiffness and prevents heterotopic bone formation[2], and decreases the risk of postoperative thromboembolism. Immune suppressive therapy is increasingly used in the treatment of RA and may or may not affect wound healing[3,4]. Old age, wide spread and active disease, lack of motivation, and unrealistic patient expectations are relative contraindications.

Strategic considerations

In order to optimize surgery in patients with several potential options for joint surgery during decades of disease, it is essential to asses the indications and priorities in combined clinics involving rheumatologists, orthopedic surgeons, hand surgeons, and health professionals. The experienced team will be aware of the many paradoxical effects that may result from individual joint procedures in patients with RA. Total knee replacement in a patient with valgus deformities of the knee may result in pain relief not only in the knee but also in the ankle and foot, due to improved loading position. On the other hand, replacement of the knee joints in a previously wheel-chair restricted patient may give rise to increased hip and foot pain caused by resumed walking ability, and thus require further surgery. Another example is ameliorating elbow pain in patients dependent on assistive walking devices, by improving lower extremity function and eliminating the need for such devices.

The first in a series of planned operations should, if possible, be a small procedure, that is forefoot surgery or arthrodesis of a thumb. This will facilitate knowledge of the patients' capacity to participate in postoperative rehabilitation after more complex procedures.

General anesthesia in patients with instability of the cervical spine and/or limited mouth opening due to temporomandibular arthritis need special equipment and competence. In these patients the possibility of multiple joint surgery during the same sitting should always be considered in order to minimize the need for anesthesia. Bilateral total hip or knee replacement and ipsilateral shoulder and elbow replacement may be performed without increased per- or postoperative morbidity[5].

Non-cemented joint implants and conventional osteosynthetic devices may be impossible to use in RA patients with severe osteopenia. The risk for permanent deformities and osteopenia also contraindicates prolonged postoperative bed rest or joint immobilization in these patients. Postoperative exercises are possibly an important component for a good outcome.

Surgery of the shoulder

Between 80 and 90 per cent of hospitalized rheumatic patients or patients with more than 15 years of illness have radiographic changes and more or less severe symptoms from the shoulder[6]. Arthritis in the glenohumeral (GH) joint and the acromioclavicular (AC) joint are both common. Radiographic deterioration of the GH joint progresses as mobility is lost. Disease in the AC joint is an often-overlooked cause of shoulder pain. Clinical signs of AC joint arthritis have been reported in 34 per cent and radiographic changes in 85 per cent in one report[6].

Indications and surgical methods

Swelling of the subacromial bursa resistant to conservative therapy may indicate a bursectomy. Often there is concurrent AC joint arthritis and the procedure can then be combined with a lateral clavicle resection. Isolated painful AC joint arthritis can be treated by clavicle resection, possibly in combination with anterior acromioplasty, a procedure which can provide good pain relief in patients with massive rotator cuff rupture. Lateral clavicle resection should probably be considered more often than is currently the case. The procedure is relatively minor and may possibly replace prosthetic surgery in some patients where the shape of the head of the humerus is retained and the articular cartilage of the glenohumeral joint is somewhat preserved[7].

Synovectomy

Synovectomy in the GH joint is seldom warranted, because when non-remitting shoulder problems develop, pronounced joint destruction is usually present. A patient with pain at rest, somewhat well preserved joint surfaces, and a proliferative synovitis could be a candidate for synovectomy, but there is no good published evidence for this. Arthroscopic synovectomy is also unexplored.

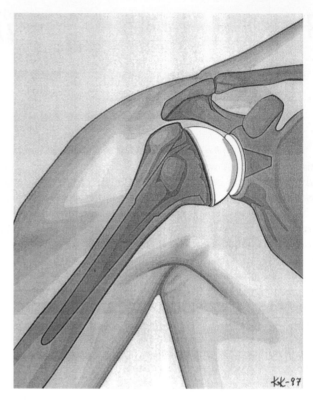

Fig. 35.1 The typical shoulder prosthesis is a design with a cemented or non-cemented stem, a modular head, and an optional glenoid component. As in the normal shoulder the joint is stable through the tension of the joint capsule and muscles. Reprinted with permission from Knutson K. (1998). Arthroplasty and its complications. In: Osteoarthritis (eds K.D. Brandt, M. Doherty, L.S. Lohmander). Oxford University Press, pp. 388–402.

Resection interposition arthroplasty

Resection interposition arthroplasty involves trimming the joint surfaces and interposing a membrane, usually Lyodura®, between the head of the humerus and the glenoid. The postoperative course is often long and troublesome and there is a risk of instability[8]. A prosthesis is most likely the superior material for interposition.

Shoulder replacement

Arthroplasty by endoprosthesis, either in form of a hemiprosthesis, or as a total joint prosthesis with a glenoid component (Fig. 35.1), has become an increasingly common procedure on the indication of painful motion of the shoulder with deterioration in the glenohumeral joint. The functional outcome of prosthetic surgery is determined by the quality of the soft tissue parts, not least the rotator cuff, in addition to the correct positioning of the prosthesis. Recent trends have favored modular humeral prostheses of various styles, with a conical connection between the humerus component's shaft and the articular head, making it possible to vary the humeral head size while keeping the same prosthetic humeral shaft. It is too early to determine the durability of these prostheses. Hemiprostheses, rather than total joint replacement, are still widely used, due to the lack of good methods for the fixation of a glenoid component.

Table 35.2 Average clinical results and radiographic findings in 558 replaced shoulders

Pain relief	89 (78–100) %
Pre- or postoperative complications	10 (0–24) %
Loosening of humeral component	6 (0–25) %
Loosening of glenoid component	8 (0–25) %

There is agreement that arthroplasty with a prosthesis usually provides reliable pain relief and functional gain. The need to replace the glenoid is, however, controversial[9,10,11]. A disadvantage with hemiarthroplasty is that pain relief may be less reliable than after total shoulder replacement and that bone loss in the glenoid accelerates, which may make revision difficult. However, the bone quality of patients with extensive preoperative bone loss is such that safe fixation of a glenoid component may be nearly impossible. This is reflected by the rather high frequency of development of radiolucent zones, probably a prostage to loosening, in many studies. Preservation of the original glenoid also excludes that plastic wear products would cause or accelerate prosthetic loosening.

Shoulder prostheses of various styles have now been used to treat rheumatic patients for several decades. Nevertheless, long-term follow-up is lacking. It is difficult to extract reliable data from the literature since different authors mix both diagnoses and prosthetic types in their studies. The majority of such mixed studies have average follow-up periods of 3–4 years. Since it is difficult to measure isolated mobility of the GH joint, usually total shoulder mobility is reported. Pain relief is good, and approximately 90 per cent outcome of 'good–excellent' is standard. Table 35.2 shows achieved average pain relief and radiographic findings in 558 procedures from 14 studies with a follow-up period exceeding 3 years[12]. None of the studies used randomized controlled protocols.

Radiographic loosening of the components is common, but causes insignificant symptoms. An association between loosening of the glenoid component and concurrent occurrence of rotator cuff injury has been proven[13]. Proximal migration of the humerus is common, and may change the kinetics of the shoulder and increase the risk of prosthetic loosening. There is, however, no relationship between the clinical outcome and the degree of progressive proximal migration of humerus[14].

The only severe complications to shoulder arthroplasty are fracture, the incidence of which is less than 2 per cent, nerve damage with an incidence of less than 1 per cent, and infection with a risk of approximately 0.5 per cent[15]. Use of a glenoid component may increase the risk of complications.

Modular and non-cemented prostheses have recently been introduced. The former provide better possibilities for achieving an optimal tension in soft tissues and restoring the center of mobility, but they also involve a risk for dislocations between the components and corrosion of the taper. There are no long-term results yet. Non-cemented glenoid components have shown promising short-term results, but have the disadvantage of potentially causing plastic wear[16]. Bipolar prostheses with a small head articulating with polythene inside a larger metallic shell articulating against the glenoid, have also been introduced[17].

The results of prosthetic surgery in the shoulder can be evaluated in terms of pain relief, improved mobility, functional improvement of the upper extremity, radiographic results, and complication frequency. There are several scoring systems for evaluating shoulder function, but there is no consensus on which is best suited for RA. It appears most reasonable to evaluate the outcome based on function. (Table 35.3)[14,18,19,20].

Arthrodesis

Arthrodesis is an option in young patients with severe bone destruction, which precludes secure prosthetic fixation, or, rarely, when severe pain is present despite very limited range of motion. Long-term postoperative immobilization is required, with the risks involved of stiffening of the other joints in the upper extremity.

The elbow

Elbow synovitis particularly limits joint extension. Instability of the elbow is unusual and generally a sign of severe bone loss. The ulnar nerve passes close to the articular capsule, and nerve compression is not uncommon. Approximately half of all hospitalized rheumatics experience elbow problems, often at an early stage[21]. Radiographically, rheumatic destruction of the elbow progresses

Table 35.3 Upper limb function following shoulder arthroplasty in patients with RA

	Can manage personal hygiene		Can use a comb	
	Preop (%)	Follow-up (%)	Preop (%)	Follow-up (%)
Kelly (1987) n = 41	41	83	12	54
Barrett *et al.* (1989) n = 134	46	84	28	66
Rydholm and Sjögren (1993) n = 71	30	78	6	56
vanCappelle and Visser (1994) n = 41	39	71	29	61

n = number of shoulders.

slowly[22]. Although pain and limitation of movement of the rheumatic elbow is a common clinical problem, surgery seldom comes into question until there is significant loss of cartilage.

Indications and surgical methods

Patients with instability may be helped by a stabilizing orthoses that allow full motion. A sound method to alleviate symptoms from the elbow in patients who are using walking devices is to take measures in the lower extremities to make the patient independent of these devices and thereby avoid pressure on the elbow.

Synovectomy

The stable, somewhat movable, but painful elbow is well suited for synovectomy with concurrent removal of the radial head. Synovectomy may be performed both early and late in the course, and provides good pain relief with only minor effects on mobility. Removal of the radial head has been considered a condition for radical synovectomy, and is likely to contribute to the pain relief by disconnecting the radiohumeral and radioulnar joints. Since the stability of the elbow is largely dependent on the congruence of the humeroulnar joint, instability problems after extirpation of the radial head are uncommon. However, synovectomy can also be performed radically with preservation of the radial head. Thus, the risk for a potential sense of weakness in the forearm, which occurs in some cases and is troublesome to the patient, may be avoided. Compression of the ulnar nerve at the elbow may, at times, also be an indication for synovectomy of the elbow, with or without concurrent neurolysis and nerve transposition. There are few long-term follow-ups of elbow synovectomy in patients with RA[23]. Synovectomy seems to provide long-term pain relief and minor improvement in flexion in approximately two-thirds of the patients. Synovectomy is not followed by progressive bone loss, and hence any subsequent prosthetic surgery is not rendered more difficult. It also appears that the results are not appreciably affected by the degree of preoperative destruction.

Some hold the opinion that synovectomy is an alternative superior to prosthesis, since it is easier and less expensive to perform and has fewer complications, but still with long-term results comparable to those of prostheses[23,24]. The results concerning pain relief are, however, inferior to those achieved by prosthetic surgery.

Resection interposition arthroplasty

Resection interposition arthroplasty has been used to treat patients with an elbow which is painful and limited in mobility, but reasonably stable and radiographically intact. The affected joint surfaces are trimmed and covered with a material to prevent adhesion. A number of interposition materials have been used over the years. Usually, Lyodura®, abdominal skin, or muscle fascia from the thigh is used. The disadvantages of the method is the risk of progressive loss of bone with subsequent instability. Pain relief has generally been reported as good. Mobility and stability are, however, not helped[25,26] and ulnar

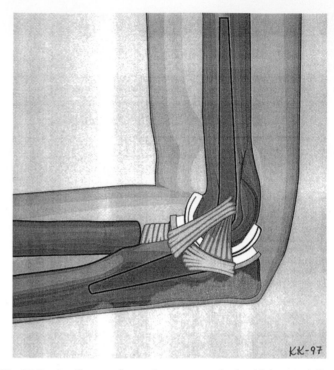

Fig. 35.2   An elbow surface replacement prosthesis with intramedullary humeral and ulnar stems. Some constraint is achieved by the anatomy of the prosthetic joint surfaces. The ulnar component has an articulating surface from polyethylene. Joint stability is achieved by tension in ligaments and muscles. Reprinted with permission from Knutson K. (1998). *Arthroplasty and its complications*. In: *Osteoarthritis* (eds K.D. Brandt, M. Doherty, L.S. Lohmander). Oxford University Press, pp. 388–402.

nerve damage and fractures are relatively common. Loss of bone may, in the long run, be such that reoperation by prosthesis is rendered impossible. In view of the improved results with prosthetic surgery the method has slowly lost ground.

Elbow replacement

For elbows with severe pain at motion, limited range of motion, and pronounced loss of cartilage and bone, joint replacement is a well established alternative. Development has been from hinged prostheses to prostheses with a sloppy hinge permitting some rotation and valgus–varus laxity, in order to decrease the forces on the bone–cement and cement–prosthesis interface. The most commonly used implants today are stemmed surface replacement prostheses of the same basic type as knee prostheses (Fig. 35.2). More than 90 per cent of the patients are completely free from pain after surgery[27]. Flexion and rotation is usually improved postoperatively. Correct positioning of the prosthesis and careful handling of the soft tissues is critical for the outcome. The surgical technique is difficult, and the procedure is associated with a relatively high frequency of complications. Transient impairment of ulnar nerve function is common, but permanent ulnar nerve injury is uncommon[28].

Results of 1495 procedures reported in 18 studies are shown in Table 35.4[12].

Although the average gain in flexion was only 15° (8°–25°), this may represent a substantial functional gain, allowing the

Table 35.4 Average clinical results of prosthetic surgery in the elbow

Pain relief	89 (70–100) %
Gain of flexion	15 (8–25) °
Gain of extension	8 (–2–21) °
Gain of supination	16 (4–28) °
Gain of pronation	14 (8–25) °

patient to reach the mouth with the hand. The gain in extension of 8° (–2°–21°) usually has little impact on function, in contrast to improved rotation of the forearm. For an elbow to be useful during daily activities, freedom from pain, mobility, and stability are required. It has been reported[29] that 43/50 surface replaced elbows after 3 years showed negligible pain, a range of motion exceeding 100°, and instability less than 10°.

The predominant complication is ulnar nerve damage, which, as a rule, is reversible and which may possibly be minimized by modification of the surgical technique. It is characteristic of surface replacement prostheses that early complication risks are frequent (ulnar nerve injury, dislocation, and infection) while long-term risks are low. For the linked prostheses, on the contrary, the long-term results are jeopardized by both wear of the coupling mechanism and mechanical prosthetic loosening. Due to the superficial location of the elbow, impaired wound healing involves a significant risk of deep infection. The average risk of deep infection is 3 per cent[28], which is in the same range as the risk after a knee prosthesis, but significantly higher than the risk for infection after hip or shoulder prostheses. The probability for survival of the prosthesis after synovectomy and vigorous antibiotic treatment is low. It is generally considered too risky to attempt a reimplantation after deep infection. These patients are submitted to a resection arthroplasty, which generally involves significant loss of function. The results after revision performed due to aseptic prosthetic loosening, instability, material defects, or fracture are significantly better.

Surgery of the hip

The rate of involvement of the hip in patients with RA is difficult to assess, since ultrasound screening shows that asymptomatic synovitis is as common as symptomatic[30]. Nevertheless, manifest hip problems occur in 20–40 per cent of all patients with RA[31]. Pain, synovitis, and effusion will often result in flexion contracture, outward rotation, and adduction, and may cause functional shortening of the limb, valgus stress in the knee joint, and malpositioning of the foot. Early in the course, radiographs may appear normal. Radiographic changes occur with time, but do not correlate closely with symptoms. RA of the hip may progress in an explosive way, when combined with infarction of the femoral head. Bone loss in the acetabulum results in protrusion of the head of the femur into the pelvis. This may not cause symptoms but, with progress, follows loss of mobility. Protrusion is observed in up to 40 per cent of patients with RA[32]. Progression is usually slow, but may be explosive in some cases. Shortening of a limb can be accentuated by protrusion. Patients with protrusion should undergo regular radiographic

check ups so that bone loss does not reach a stage where prosthetic implantation becomes difficult or impossible.

Indications for surgery include severe pain on weight-bearing or at rest. Limited range of motion and/or advanced protrusion occasionally indicate need for surgery.

Hip replacement

Total hip replacement (THR) was made practical by Sir John Charnley, and its astounding success has made other surgical alternatives most uncommon. In the absence of long-term follow-up studies of uncemented prostheses, prosthetic anchorage using bone cement (Fig. 35.3) is considered to be the gold standard. Osteopenia and subchondral cyst formation reduce the chances for successful prosthetic anchorage, especially on the acetabular side. Even if the long-term loosening rate of cemented cups has been reduced with the most modern cementation technique[33], a trend has developed toward using non-cemented cups aiming at osseointegration through press–fit fixation to bone. No evidence, however, supports the use of uncemented femoral components.

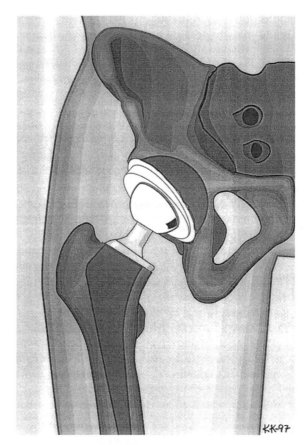

Fig. 35.3 Conventional hip prostheses have a cobalt–chromium stem fixed with bone cement to the femoral shaft. The head may be modular and made from cobolt–chromium alloy or ceramics. It is fixed to the neck with a taper lock. The polyethylene acetabular cup is fixed with bone cement. Reprinted with permission from Knutson K. (1998). Arthroplasty and its complications. In: *Osteoarthritis* (eds K.D. Brandt, M. Doherty, L.S. Lohmander). Oxford University Press, pp. 388–402.

pseudarthrosis. The treatment principles involve observing the risk for prosthetic complications from persistent malalignment.

Deep infection presents a serious complication since there is a risk of jeopardizing the knee joint. The infection risk has been estimated at two to three times higher than in OA. The risk of infection is greater when using large prostheses with intramedullary stems[50]. Furthermore, RA patients may acquire deep infections later than 3 years after the surgery, probably via blood-borne infection, in particular when leg ulcers are present[32,48,51]

Loosening is less frequent when tricompartmental prostheses are used[50]. Component designs and cementing techniques have also improved results[51]. The claimed advantages of biological anchoring have not been confirmed concerning the attachment of the tibial component, which is most often affected by loosening[51].

Patellar problems have become more dominant as other complications decrease[50]. If a patellar component is not used, the risks for continued patellofemoral joint pain, attrition of the patella, and subsequent patellar instability or subluxation remain. If a patellar component is used, yet another particle-generating, thin plastic part is introduced, which may wear and loosen. Furthermore, the osteopenic patella may be weakened by surgical preparation, hence increasing the risk for fracture[52]. Opinions on the use of the patellar component are divergent and attempts to predict postoperative patellar pain for selective use of patellar components have been made[53].

In conclusion good results regarding pain relief, stability and mobility can be expected after TKR with currently used tricompartmental prostheses, and the risk for revision within 10 years should be less than 10 per cent (Table 35.6). The problem of persistent patellar pain, however, remains to be solved.

Surgery of the ankle

Arthritis of the ankle seldom occurs in isolation, but follows arthritis of the hindfoot and middle foot. It may be severely debilitating and is perhaps the most common cause of more significant gait difficulties among rheumatics[62,63]. After 10 years of disease, nearly all patients show clinical signs of arthritis in one or more joints of the feet.

The ankle is affected by malalignment of the hind and forefoot to a high degree, and it is usually appropriate to manage these (see below) before considering surgery of the ankle. It should also be remembered that pain from the hind and middlefoot joints may cause symptoms which are perceived as originating from the ankle joint. A non-corrected malposition of the ankle or hindfoot may jeopardize gait improvement after a hip and knee arthroplasty.

Indications and surgical methods

Synovectomy

Synovectomy of the ankle is rarely performed. The opportunity for radical treatment is small, and joint destruction has usually progressed too far when the patient's symptoms begin. Tenosynovectomy around the medial tendons is likely to be valuable in preventing rupture of the tibialis posterior tendon[64]. Such rupture is, however, uncommon and not the genesis of rheumatic valgus foot, but may cause an acute and further accentuated valgus malalignment of the foot.

Arthrodesis

Arthrodesis is the most established treatment for rheumatic destruction of ankle joints. The choice of surgical method is

Table 35.6 Survival analysis showing the cumulative risk of revision for a knee prosthesis in patients with RA

Author	No	Revised (%)		
		5 years	7 years	10 years
Knutson *et al.* (1986)	270	15	–	–
	1962	9	–	–
	296	10	–	–
	170	16	–	–
Ranawat *et al.* (1989)	73	–	–	0
Scuderi *et al.* (1989)	193	0	5	11
	193	3	3	3
	193	0	0	–
Laskin (1990)	80	6	10	19
Moran *et al.* (1991)	73	17	–	–
Rand and Ilstrup (1991)	2876	7	–	18
	779	2	–	–
Aglietti *et al.* (1995)	65	1	–	4
Elke *et al.* (1995)	61	9	–	19
Kolstad *et al.* (1996)	55	8	27	–
Robertsson *et al.* (1996)	1776	4	–	5
	1976	2	–	–
	189	16	–	–

Table 35.7 Clinical and radiographic results of ankle arthrodesis in patients with RA

Author	No	Mobility of foot (°)	Pain free (%)	Radiographically fused (%)
Sowa and Krackow (1989)	6	18 (0–30)		100
Smith and Wood (1990)	11	4 (0–20)	91	82
Moran *et al.* (1991)	30	12	96	60
Cracchiolo *et al.* (1992)	32		71	78
Turan *et al.* (1995)	10		100	100

probably of lesser significance for healing, but may influence the degree and type of complications. Special consideration should be given to inferior bone quality and possible malalignment in adjacent joints in rheumatic patients. A malaligned heel can be corrected and fixed in the same session as the ankle arthrodesis by driving the fixation screws down through the talus and into the calcaneus. Mechanical studies have shown that good fixation is achieved by two or three crossed screws, and is fully comparable to that achieved with external fixation[65]. A recent method involves arthroscopic cleansing of the joint followed by percutaneous screwing, aiming to minimize the risk of disrupting healing in the skin and bone[66]. Arthroscopic methods aim at decreasing surgical trauma and hence postoperative complications in cases where there is minor malalignment, and percutaneous screw fixation, *per se*, may offer the same advantages[67].

Arthrodesis of the ankle usually relives pain (Table 35.7) and is a good alternative in patients with somewhat well maintained hind and middle foot, with possibility for these joints to overtake some of the lost flexion and extension capacity of the ankle. Through these movements of the middle foot, the patient retains a good walking ability on flat ground. However, a long-term risk with ankle arthrodesis is progression of pathological changes in the middle foot due to such compensatory mobility. If middle foot movement is lacking due to earlier arthrodesis or spontaneous ankylosis, walking following ankle arthrodesis may still function with the help of adapted shoes. Arthrodesis remains a safer surgical option than arthroplasty, since late complications are seldom observed in a primarily successful arthrodesis.

Ankle replacement

Arthroplasty using endoprosthesis of the ankle is an appealing alternative since postoperative rehabilitation is short and retaining mobility of the ankle is functionally beneficial. A stiff ankle involves a risk for compensatory hypermobility of the joints in the middle foot with the risk for secondary osteoarthritis, a risk which may be avoided by using a prosthesis. However, implantation of a prosthesis involves a risk for deep infection after disturbed wound healing, prosthetic loosening, migration, and wear. Ankle prostheses have yielded poor outcome results,[12] and their use is still in an experimental stage. Prosthetic survival after 10 years has been estimated at 60 per cent in a mixed ankle study, where patients below the age of 57 years had only 42 per cent prosthetic survival[72]. 78 per cent prosthetic survival at 5 years has been reported for RA patients[73].

The ankle is more prone to disturbances in wound healing than other joints, and frequency of infection is high regardless of the type of implant. Late infection via blood-borne contamination occurs also in the ankle. Cases where loosening occurs can be made to heal only by arthrodesis involving massive bone transplantation and extended fixation[74]. Revision surgery after loose or infected ankle prostheses is technically difficult and often demanding for the patient. Non-healed arthrodesis on the other hand can, in some cases, be fairly pain-free and may be compensated by an orthosis or sturdy shoes.

Surgery of the foot

The prevalence of the onset of RA symptoms are the same for the hand and foot[75]. In a cross-sectional study of 99 non-hospitalized patients, 94 per cent reported foot pain[63]. The percentage with foot pain increased with duration of the disease.

Many rheumatic foot problems can be solved with adapted shoes with or without different kinds of insoles. Some patients with ankle and hindfoot pain manage well with a stiff ankle joint cap.

Indications and surgical methods

The most important indication for surgery is pain on weight-bearing, which threatens walking ability. However, there is also a preventive indication, partly to avoid progressive malalignment and partly to avoid wound formation. Pressure from shoes can cause troublesome wounds and infections in such pressure sores may be a cause of late, hematogenously spread prosthetic infections, mainly to the knee joint. Hence, it is always wise to try to provide rheumatic patients with a foot free from infection and weight-bearing pain, prior to proceeding to prosthetic surgery in the knee or hip. It is also recommended that forefoot problems are managed prior to or concurrently with the ankle joint.

Surgery of the hindfoot

Since arthritis in the talonavicular joint is a common and early finding in RA, arthrodesis in this joint can be used to prevent development of pes planovalgus. An isolated talonvicular arthrodesis has been shown to limit mobility even in the remaining two hindfoot joints[76]. Joint destruction, with a reduction in joint space, is easy to detect radiographically in the talonavicular and calcaneocuboid joints, but much more difficult in the talocalcanear joint.

Table 35.8 Outcome of hind and middle foot arthrodeses

Author	No of feet	Results (%)	Fusion (%)	Complications (%)
Talonavicular arthrodesis				
Elboar et al. (1976)	26	85 better	?	19 (Preop.)
Ruff and Turner (1984)	10	70 good	70	0
Ljung et al. (1992)	19	89 good	63	0
Talocalcanear arthrodesis				
Russoti et al. (1988)	45	90 satisfied	98	2 (infection)
Triple arthrodesis				
Ruff and Turner (1984)	8	88 good	88	0
Figgie et al. (1989)	49	86 good	96	12 (wound problems)
Cracchiolo et al. (1990)	24	88 satisfied	100	21 (wound problems)

If the heel is already in a valgus position or if pain originates mainly in the talocalcanear joint, a complete triple arthrodesis should be considered, involving the joints between talus and the heel bone, between the talus and the navicular bone, and between the heel bone and the cuboid bone. In patients having major malalignment, corrective talocalcanear arthrodesis must be performed by removing a wedge of bone during the procedure. Arthrodeses of the hindfoot are often performed with transplantation of iliac crest bone.

The effect of arthrodesis on hindfoot pain is good (Table 35.8), regardless whether or not radiographs show the arthrodesis to be healed, that is fibrous healing appears to be sufficient for relieving pain. Painful, unhealed arthrodesis requiring reoperation is unusual. Bone transplantation can be performed by simply using the dowel technique, which works well if autologous bone is used. The fixation method *per se* (staple, screw, or pin) is of less importance. Progression of ankle pain does occur, and seems to be correlated with persistent valgus malalignment of the hindfoot[81].

Surgery of the forefoot

Surgical treatment of forefoot problems includes everything from bursectomy, chiseling of exostoses, hallux valgus procedures, arthrodeses, joint resections, and osteotomies, to forefoot amputation. The two main types of surgical methods are joint preserving metatarsal osteotomies, and joint resections possibly in combination with arthrodesis of the great toe.

Joint resections can be performed completely or partially involving one of the metatarsal articular heads or the toe base, and the joints can be reached via dorsal or plantar incisions. These procedures can be completed with volar plate arthroplasty, flexor tendon centralization, and medial capsuloraphy. Several corrective hallux valgus procedures have been described, but the methods mainly used in RA include resection of the proximal first phalanx with or without capsuloplasty, metatarsal head resection, arthrodesis, metatarsal osteotomy, or implantation of silicone prostheses.

Forefoot surgery belongs to the most common rheumatic surgical procedures and the results are reported to be rather satisfactory[82-87]. The foot may, however become shorter, and the toes functionally detached, which in turn affects walking ability. There is also a risk of relapse of hallux valgus due to poor lateral support from the other toes, which may be an argument for arthrodesis in the metatarsophalangeal joint of the great toe.

When the MTP joints of the toes are relatively well preserved, osteotomy of the metatarsal bones may be a good alternative. Most surgical methods, however, involve resection of the MTP joints. These procedures yield clinical improvement in approximately 80 to 90 per cent of the cases. Walking distance improves and it is easier to fit shoes[85,88]. The early gains in function and pain relief decline with time[89]. Isolated resection of the MTP joints of the small toes creates a risk for later problems in the first MTP joint, due to poor lateral support, even if the great toe appears to be unaffected at the time of surgery.

A comparative study[90] shows a high frequency of relapse of metatarsalgia after forefoot arthroplasty, and results comparable to those obtained by conservative treatment with orthopedic technical devices, for example shoe insoles. What is needed in the future is both randomized prospective studies to compare different surgical methods and longer follow-up studies after forefoot surgery.

The literature offers no clear answers regarding the optimum method for treating rheumatic hallux valgus. A retrospective study[86] shows similar results with and without arthrodesis of the great toe. Resection of the first MTP joint offers pain relief, but poor function of the great toe, decreased ability to bear weight on the medial forefoot, poorer balance, and a significant risk of hallux valgus relapse with the risk for lateralization of the small toes. In this respect, arthrodesis seems preferable. A disadvantage of arthrodesis is the increased risk for interphalangeal joint degeneration, either by peroperative trauma of axial pins or later by increased load as the foot concludes the stepping motion. Results after great toe arthrodesis are poorest in fibrous healing of the arthrodesis.

Good results have been reported with silicone prostheses[91]. However, some silicone implants fracture, and prosthetic surgery of the great toe do not work well in conjunction with concurrent small toe resection, due to a loss of lateral support for the great toe.

Problems with overall outcome assessment of surgery in RA

It is unfortunate that it is still common that reports on the results of joint surgery are based on a mixture of patients with different types of joint diseases. Results of joint surgery are probably less dramatic in patients with RA than OA due to the systemic and more progressive type of disease.

There exist many systems for assessment of joint function in patients with monarticular disease, notably OA. When reporting the outcome of surgery in patients with polyarticular disease it is, however, necessary to use some measurement of total loco-motor function. The effects of surgery in patients with RA should be assessed by means of one of the established functional scales for RA. Ideally the patient groups should also be stratified for medical therapy. This may only be possible using prospective randomized protocols.

The outcome is often reported as improvements in some kind of score, which combines the patients subjective opinion with radiographic findings and objective parameters such as stability and mobility of the actual joint. Most reports are retrospective and short-term. Long-term follow-up studies in RA are further complicated by heterogeneity in disease course between individual patients. There is a general lack of reports which include measurements of the level of overall function and quality of life as well as cost-benefit analyses.

The future of total joint replacement

Alternatives to bone cement fixation of prosthetic components are continuously introduced to solve the problem of long-term implant fixation. Different surface finishes give the option of bone ingrowth, but retrieval studies have so far been able to show only partial success. Such microstructured or porous ingrowth prostheses require good bone quality and proper prosthetic fit, which may not be realistic to achieve in every patient with RA. In the 1980s titanium alloys were introduced because of good biocompatibility, and the possibility of so called osseointegration. The bearing surface of a titanium implant must, however, be prepared to allow for articulation with poly-ethylene or it must a modular implant with a Co–Cr or ceramic bearing. A cemented titanium implant also means a risk of release of high concentrations of local and systemic metallic particles upon micromotion of the prosthesis inside the cement mantle[92]. The use of titanium alloys for joint implants has steadily decreased during later years.

Hydroxyapatite (HA) and tricalcium phosphate can be coated to an implant to enhance fixation to bone[93]. HA is bioactive, allowing bone ingrowth and it has even been shown that gaps less than 2 mm can be bridged. HA coating also reduces the metallic contact surface to bone. HA will undergo dissolution, but the effects of the amount or rate of dissolution on prosthetic fixation is not known. There is also a risk of loose HA particles creating third body wear in the articulation.

Bone morphogenic proteins and transforming growth factor-β to enhance the attachment of prostheses to bone represents a recent development[94].

Metal-on-metal articulations for the hip were already available in the 1950s. However, their use was abandoned due to the unsolved problem of fixation, and manufacturing problems with regard to the congruity between the ball and socket. The idea has been taken up again in later years with implants of very high quality. The substantial metal release is, however, a concern, and the CoCr–CoCr articulation is hardly the final solution to the wear problem in total hip arthroplasty[95].

Ceramic materials (alumina, zirconium oxide) have been used for several decades as a material for bearing surfaces in THR. Their use has been limited chiefly due to the risk for fracture of the material. Alumina–polyethylene articulation however results in low wear rates and ceramic–ceramic couplings shown almost no wear, that is particle production. With the introduction of zirconium oxide it has been possible to manufacture even small 22 mm femoral heads, and the risk for fracture of the material is negligible. Metal-backed ceramic acetabular cups as well as polyethylene cups with a ceramic bearing surface have recently been introduced to give the possibility of ceramic–ceramic artic-ulation. Improved quality control will perhaps result in an increased use of ceramics as prosthetic material in the future[96].

High density polyethylene has been used for decades as the plastic material in all kinds of total joint prostheses, but modifications to improve its performance are in progress. Wear characteristics may be improved by irradiation or by using cross-linking agents. Heat and high pressure during the manufacturing may help to form a more resistant structure of the material[97].

References

1. Benoni, G., and Fredin, H. Fibrinolytic inhibition with tranexamic acid reduces blood loss and blood transfusion after knee arthro-plasty. A prospective, randomized double-blind study of 86 patients. *Journal of Bone and Joint Surgery (British)*, 1996; 78-B:434–40.

2. Dorn, U., Grethen, C., Effenberger, H., Berka, H., Ramsauer, T., and Drekonja, T. Indomethacin for prevention of heterotopic ossification after hip arthroplasty. A randomized comparison between 4 and 8 days of treatment. *Acta Orthopaedica Scandinavica*, 1998;69:107–10.

3. Kasdan, M.L., June, L. Postoperative results of rheumatoid arthri-tis patients on methotrexate at the time of reconstructive surgery of the hand. *Orthopaedics*, 1993;16:1233–35.

4. Perhala, R.S., Wilke, W.S., Clough, J.D., and Segal, A.M. Local infectious complications following large joint replacement in rheumatoid arthritis patients treated with methotrexate versus those not treated with methotrexate. *Arthritis & Rheumatism*, 1991;34:146–52.

5. Worland, R.L, Jessup, D.E., and Clelland, C. Simultaneous bilat-eral total knee replacement versus unilateral replacement. *American Journal of Orthopaedics*, 1996;25:292–5.

6. Petersson, C.J. Painful shoulders in patients with rheumatoid arthritis. *Scandinavian Journal of Rheumatology*, 1986;15:275–9.

7. Kelly, I.G. The source of shoulder pain in rheumatoid arthritis-usefulness of local anaesthetic injections. *Journal of Shoulder and Elbow Surgery*, 1994;3:62–5.

8. Milbrink, J., and Wigren, A. Resection arthroplasty of the shoulder in rheumatoid arthritis. A follow-up study. *Journal of Orthopaedic Rheumatology*, 1990;19:432–6.

9. Kechele, P., Bamania, C., Wirth, M.A., Seltzer, D.G., and Rockwood C.A. Rheumatoid shoulder: hemiarthroplasty *vs* total shoulder arthroplasty. *Journal of Shoulder and Elbow Surgery*, 1995;4:13.

10. Pollock, R.G. ,Deliz, E.D., McIlveen, S.J. Flatow, E.L. and Bigliani, L.U. Prosthetic replacement in rotator cuff-deficient shoulders. *Journal of Shoulder and Elbow Surgery*, 1992;1:173–86.

11. Rodosky, M.W. and Bigliani, U. Indications for glenoid resurfacing in shoulder arthroplasty. *Journal of Shoulder and Elbow Surgery*, 1996;5:231–248.

12. Arthritis surgery. *Acta Orthopaedica Scandinavica,* Suppl 30 (in press).

13. Franklin, J.L., Barret, W.P., Jackins, S.E., and Matsen, F.A. III (1988). Glenoid loosening in total shoulder arthroplasty. *Journal of Arthroplasty*, 1:39–46.

14. Rydholm, U., and Sjögren, J. Resurfacing of the humeral head in rheumatoid arthritis. *Journal of Shoulder and Elbow Surgery*, 1993;2:286–95.

15. Wirth, M.A., and Rockwood, C.A. Complications of total shoulder-replacement arthroplasty. *Journal of Bone and Joint Surgery (American)*, 1966;78-A:603–616.

16. Cofield, R.H. Uncemented total shoulder arthroplasty. A review. *Clinical Orthopaedics and Related Research*, 1994;307:86–93.

17. Lee, D.H., and Niemann, K.M.W. Bipolar shoulder arthroplasty. *Clinical Orthopaedics and Related Research*, 1994;304:97–107.

18. Barret, W.P., Thornhill, T.S., Thomas, W.H., Gebhart, E.M., and Sledge, C.B. Nonconstrained total shoulder arthroplasty in patients with polyarticular rheumatoid arthritis. *Journal of Arthroplasty*, 1989;4:91–6.

19. Kelly, I.G. Unconstrained shoulder arthroplasty in rheumatoid arthritis. *Clinical Orthopaedics and Related Research*, 1994;307:94–102.

20. van Cappelle, H.G.J., and Visser J.D. Hemiarthroplasty of the shoulder in rheumatoid arthritis. *Journal of Orthopaedic Rheumatology*, 1994;7:43–7.

21. Amis, A.A., Hughes, S.J., Miller, J.H., and Wright W. A functional study of the rheumatoid elbow. *Rheumatology and Rehabilitation*, 1982;21:151–7.

22. Ljung, P., Jonsson, K., Rydgren, L., and Rydholm, U. The natural course of rheumatoid elbow arthritis: a radiographic and clinical 5-year follow-up. *Journal of Orthopaedic Rheumatology*, 1995; 8:32–6.

23. Herold, N., and Schröder, H.A. Synovectomy and radial head excision in rheumatoid arthritis. *Acta Orthopaedica Scandinavica*, 1995;66:252–4.

24. Wanivenhaus, A., and Bretschneider, W. (1995). Late synovectomy of the elbow joint. In *The elbow. Endoprosthetic replacement and non-endoprosthetic procedures* (ed. W. Rüther) pp. 48–56. Springer Verlag, Berlin.

25. Ljung, P., Jonsson, K., Larsson, K., and Rydholm, U. Interposition arthroplasty of the rheumatoid elbow. *Journal of Shoulder and Elbow Surgery*, 1996;5:81–5.

26. Milbrink, J., and Wigren, A. Resection interposition arthroplasty of the elbow in rheumatoid arthritis. *Journal of Orthopaedic Rheumatology*, 1990;3:95–106.

27. Ewald, F.C., Simmons, E.D., Sullivan, J.A., Thomas, W.H., Scott, R.D., Poss, R. *et al.* Capitellocondylar total elbow replacement in rheumatoid arthritis. Long-term results. *Journal of Bone and Joint Surgery(American)*, 1993;75-A:498–507.

28. Ljung, P. (1995). *Arthroplasty of the rheumatoid elbow. With special reference to non-constrained replacement and its complications*. Thesis, University of Lund, Sweden.

29. Ljung, P., Jonsson, K., and Rydholm, U. Short-term complications of the lateral approach for non-constrained elbow replacement. *Journal of Bone and Joint Surgery (British)*, 1995;77-B:937–42.

30. Eberhardt, K., Fex, E., Johnsson, K., and Geborek, P. Hip involvement in early rheumatoid arthritis. *Annales of the Rheumatic Diseases*, 1995;54:45–8.

31. Lehtimäki, M.Y., Kaarela, K., and Hämäläinen M.M.J. Incidence of hip involvement and need for total hip replacement in rheumatoid arthritis. An eight-year follow-up study. *Scandinavian Journal of Rheumatology*, 1986;15:387–91.

32. Poss, R., Maloney, J.P., Ewald, F.C., Thomas, W.H., Batte, N.J., Hartness, C., and Sledge C. 6 to 11 years results of total hip arthroplasty in rheumatoid arthritis. *Clinical Orthopaedics and Related Research*, 1984;182:109–16.

33. Önsten, I., Besjakov, J., and Carlsson. Å.S. Improved radiographic survival of the Charnley prosthesis in rheumatoid arthritis and osteoarthritis-results of new versus old operative techniques in 402 hips. *Journal of Arthroplasty*, 1994;9:3–8.

34. Kinzinger, P.J.M., Karthaus, R.P., and Sloof, T.J.H. Bone grafting for acetabular protrusion in hip arthroplasty: 27 cases of rheumatoid arthritis followed for 2–8 years. *Acta Orthopaedica Scandinavica*, 1991;62:110–2.

35. Severt, R., Wood, R., Cracchiolo, A., and Amstutz. H.C. Long-term follow-up of cemented total hip arthroplasty in rheumatoid arthritis. *Clinical Orthopaedics and Related Research*, 1991;265:137–45.

36. Malchau, H., Herberts. P., and Ahnfelt, L. Prognosis of total hip replacement in Sweden: follow-up of 92 675 operations performed in 1978–1990. *Acta Orthopaedics Scandinavica*, 1993;64:497–506.

37. Whittle, J., Steinberg, E.P., Anderson, G.F., Herbert, R., and Hochberg, M.C. Mortality after elective total hip arthroplasty in elderly Americans-age, gender, and indication for surgery predict survival. *Clinical Orthopaedics and Related Research*, 1993;295:119–26.

38. Joshi A.B., Porter M.L., Trail, I.A., Hunt, L.P., Murphy, J.C.M., and Hardinge, K. Long-term results of Charnley low-friction arthroplasty in young patients. *Journal of Bone and Joint Surgery (British)*, 1993;75-B:616–23.

39. Partio, E., Von Bonsdorff, H., Wirta, J., and Avikainen, V. Survival of the Lubinus prosthesis. *Clinical Orthopaedics and Related Research*, 1994;303:140–6.

40. Gie, G.A., Linder, L., and Ling, R.S.M. Impacted cancellous allografts and cement revision total hip arthroplasty. *Journal of Bone and Joint Surgery (British)*, 1993;75-B:14.

41. Önsten, I., Bengnér, U., and Besjakov, J. Socket migration after Charnley arthroplasty in rheumatoid arthritis and osteoarthritis. A roentgen stereophotogrammetric study. *Journal of Bone and Joint Surgery (British)*, 1993;75-B:677–80.

42. Önsten, I., Åkesson, K., Besjakov, J., and Obrant K.J. Migration of the Charnley stem in rheumatoid arthritis and osteoarthritis. A roentgen stereophotogrammetric study. *Journal of Bone and Joint Surgery (British)*, 1995;77-B:18–22.

43. Schmalzried, T.P., Jasty, M., and Harris, W.H. Periprosthetic bone loss in total hip arthroplasty. Polyethylene wear debris and the concept of the effective joint space. *Journal of Bone and Joint Surgery (American)*, 1992;74-A:849–63.

44. Ogilvie-Harris, D.J., and Basinski, A. Arthroscopic synovectomy of the knee for rheumatoid arthritis. *Arthroscopy*, 1991;7:91–7.

45. Doets, H.C. Bierman, B.T. and Von Soesbergen R.M. Synovectomy of the rheumatoid knee does not prevent deterioration. 7-year follow-up of 83 cases. *Acta Orthopaedica Scandinavica*, 1989;60:523–5.

46. Johnson, D.P. The effect of continous passive motion on wound healing and joint mobility after knee arthroplasty. *Journal of Bone and Joint Surgery (American)*, 1990;72-A:421–6.

47. Harvey I.A. Barry, K. Kirby, S.P. Johnson, R. and Elloy, M.A. Factors affecting the range of movement of total knee arthroplasty. *Journal of Bone and Joint Surgery (British)*, 1993;75-B:950–5.

48. Wilson, M.G., Kelley, K., and Thornhill, T.S. Infection as a complication of total knee-replacement arthroplasty:risk factors and treatment in sixty-seven cases. *Journal of Bone and Joint Surgery (American)*, 1990;72-A:878–83.

49. Vlasak, R., Gearen, P.F., and Petty, W. Knee arthrodesis in the treatment of failed total knee replacement. *Clinical Orthopaedics and Related Research*, 1998;321:138–44.

50. Knutson, K., Lindstrand, A., and Lidgren, L. Survival of knee arthroplasties: a nation-wide multicentre investigation of 8000 cases. *Journal of Bone and Joint Surgery (British)*, 1986; 68-B:795–803.

51. Robertsson, O., Knutson, K., Lewold, S., Goodman, S., and Lidgren, L. (1996). Knee arthroplasty in rheumatoid arthritis. A report from the Swedish Knee Arthroplasty Register on 4 381 primary operations 1985–1995. *Acta Orthopaedics Scandinavica*, 1997, 68:545–53.

52. Grace, J.N. and Sim, F.H. Fracture of the patella after total knee arthroplasty. *Clinical Orthopaedics and Related Research*, 1988;230:168–75.

53. Fern, E.D., Winson, I.G., and Getty, C.J. Anterior knee pain in rheumatoid patients after total knee replacement. Possible selection criteria for patellar resurfacing. *Journal of Bone and Joint Surgery (British)*, 1992;74-B:745–8.

54. Ranawat, C.S., Padgett, D.E., and Ohashi, Y. Total knee arthroplasty for patients younger than 55 years. *Clinical Orthopaedics and Related Research*, 1989;248:28–33.

55. Scuderi, G.R., Insall, J.N., Windsor, R.E., and Moran, M.C. Survivorship of cemented knee replacements. *Journal of Bone and Joint Surgery (British)*, 1989;71-B:798–803.

56. Laskin, R.S. Total condylar knee replacement in patients who have rheumatoid arthritis. A ten-year follow-up study. *Journal of Bone and Joint Surgery (American)*, 1990;72-A:529–35.

57. Moran, C.G., Pinder, I.M., Lees, T.A., Midwinter, M.J. Survivorship analysis of the uncemented porous-coated anatomic knee replacement. *Journal of Bone and Joint Surgery (American)*, 1991;73-A:848–57.

58. Rand, J.A., and Ilstrup D.M. Survivorship analysis of total knee arthroplasty. *Journal of Bone and Joint Surgery (American)*, 1991;73-A:397–409.

59. Aglietti, P., Buzzi, R., Segoni, F., and Zaccherotti, G. Insall-Brustein posterior-stabilized knee prosthesis in rheumatoid arthritis. *Journal of Arthroplasty*, 1995;10:217–212.

60. Elke, R., Meier, G., Warnke, K., and Morscher, E. Outcome analysis of total knee-replacements in patients with rheumatoid arthritis versus osteoarthrosis. *Archives of Orthopaedic and Traumatic Surgery*, 1995;114:330–4.

61. Kolstad, K., Sahlstedt, B., and Bergström, B. Marmor modular knee plateau positioning and prosthesis survival in 55 knees with rheumatoid arthritis. *Archives of Orthopaedic and Traumatic Surgery*, 1996;115:17–21.

62. Kerry, R.M., Holt, G.M., and Stockley, I. The foot in chronic rheumatoid arthritis: a continuing problem. *Foot*, 1994;4:201–3.

63. Michelson, J., Easley, M., Wigley, F.M., and Hellmann, D. Foot and ankle problems in rheumatoid arthritis. *Foot and Ankle International*, 1994;15:608–13.

64. Johnson, K.A., Strom, D.E. Tibialis posterior tendon dysfunction. *Clinical Orthopaedics and Related Research*, 1989;239:196–206.

65. Thordarson, B.D., Markolf, K.L., and Cracchiole IIIA. Arthrodesis of the ankle with cancellous-bone screws and fibular strut graft: biomechanical analysis. *Journal of Bone and Joint Surgery (American)*, 1990;72-A:1359–63.

66. Turan, I., Wredmark, T., and Felländer-Tsai, L. Arthroscopic ankle arthrodesis in rheumatoid arthritis. *Clinical Orthopaedics and Related Research*, 1995;320:110–4.

67. Lauge-Pedersen, H., Knutson, K., and Rydholm, U. (1998). Percutaneous ankle arthrodesis in the rheumatoid patient without debridemenet of the joint. *Foot*, (in press).

68. Sowa, D.T., and Krackow, K.A. Ankle fusion: a new techniqui of internal fixation using a compression blade plate. *Foot and Ankle*, 1989;9:222–40.

69. Smith, E.J., and Wood, P.l. Ankle arthrodesis in the rheumatoid patient. *Foot and Ankle*, 1990;10:252–6.

70. Moran, C.G., Pindler, I.M., and Smith, SR. Ankle arthrodesis in rheumatic arthritis: 30 cases followed for 5 years. *Acta Orthopaedica Scandinavica*, 1991;62:538–43.

71. Cracchiolo III, A., Cimino, W.R., and Lian, G. Arthrodesis of the ankle in patients who have rheumatoid arthritis. *Journal of Bone and Joint Surgery (American)*, 1992;74-A:903–9.

72. Kitaoka, H.B., Patzer, G.L., Ilstrup, D.M., and Wallrichs, S.L. Survivorship analysis of the Mayo total ankle arthroplasty. *Journal of Bone and Joint Surgery (American)*, 1994;76-A: 974–9.

73. Carlsson, Å.S., Henricson, A., Linder, L., Nilsson, J.Å., and Redlund-Johnell, I. A survival analysis of 52 Bath&Wessex ankle replacements. A clinical and radiographic study in patients with rheumatoid arthritis and a critical review of the literature. *Foot*, 1994;4:34–40.

74. Carlsson, A.S., Montgomery, F., and Besjakov, J. Arthrodesis of the ankle secondary to replacement. *Foot and Ankle International*, 1998;19:240–5.

75. Heijde, Van Der D.M.F.M., Van Leeuwen, M.A., Van Riel, P.L.C.M., Koster, A.M., Van't Hof, M. Van Rijswijk MH, *et al.* Biannual radiographic assessment of hands and feet in a three-year prospective follow-up of patients with early rheumatoid arthritis. *Arthritis & Rheumatism*, 1992;35:26–34.

76. Carlsson. Å.S., Önsten, I., Besjakov, J., and Sturesson, B. Isolated talonavicular arthrodesis performed for non-inflammatory conditions block motion in healthy adjacent joints-a radiostereometric analysis of 3 cses. *Foot*, 1995;5:80–3.

77. Elboar, J.E., Thomas, W.H., Weinfeld, M.S. *et al.* Talonavicular arthrodesis for rheumatoid arthritis of the hindfoot. *Orthopaedic Clinics of North America*, 1976;7:821–6.

78. Ruff, M.E., and Turner, R.H. Selective hindfoot arthrodesis in rheumatoid rthritis. *Orthopaedics*, 1984;7:49–54.

79. Ljung, P., Kaij, J., Knutson, K., Pettersson, H., and Rydholm, U. Talonavicular arthrodesis in the rheumatoid foot. *Foot and Ankle*, 1992;13:313–6.

80. Russotti, G.M., Cass, J.R., and Johnson, K.A. Isolated talocalcaneal arthrodesis: A technique using moldable bone graft. *Journal of Bone and Joint Surgery (American)*, 1988;70-A:1472–8.

81. Figgie, M.P., O'Malley, M.J., Ranawat, C., Inglis, A.E. and Sculco, T.P. Triple arthrodesis in rheumatoid arthritis. *Clinical Orthopaedics and Related Research*, 1993;292:250–4.

82. Cracchioleo, III. A. Pearson, S. Kitaoka, and H. Grace, D. Hindfoot arthrodesis in adults utilizing a dowel graft technique. *Clinical Orthopaedics and Related Research*, 1990;257:193–203.

83. Helal, B., and Greiss, B. Telescoping osteotomy for pressure metatarsalgia. *Journal of Bone and Joint Surgery (British)*, 1984;66-B:213–7.

84. Åström, M., and Cedell, C-A. Metatarsal osteotomy in rheumatoid arthritis. *Acta Orthopaedica Scandinavica*, 1987;58:398–400.

85. Stockley, I., Betts, R.P., Getty, C.J.M., Rowley, D.I., and Duckworth, T. A prospective study of forefoot arthroplasty. *Clinical Orthopaedics and Related Research*, 1989;248:213–8.

86. Hughes, J., Grace, D., Clark, P., and Klenerman, L. Metatarsal head excision for rheumatoid arthritis. *Acta Orthopaedica Scandinavica*, 1991;62:63–6.

87. Heijden, Van Der K.W.A.P., Rasker, J.J., Jakobs, J.W.G., and Dey, K. Kates forefoot arthroplasty in rheumatoid arthritis. *Journal of Rheumatology*, 1992;19:1545–50.

88. Mann, R.A., and Schakel, M.E. Surgical correction of rheumatoid forefoot deformits. *Foot and Ankle*, 1995;16:1–6.

89. Patsalis, T., Georgousis, H., and Göpfert, S. Long-term results of forefoot arthroplasty in patients with rheumatoid arthritis. *Orthopaedics*, 1996;19:439–47.

90. Craxford, A.D., Stevens, J., and Park, C. Management of the deformed rheumatoid forefoot: a comparison of conservative and surgical methods. *Clinical Orthopaedics and Related Research*, 1981;166:121–6.

91. Cracchioleo, III A., Weltmer Jr, J.B., Lian, G., Dalseth, T., and Dorey, F. Arhtroplasty of the first metatarsophalangeal joint with a double-stem silicone implant-results in patients who have degenerative joint disease, failure of previous operations or rheumatoid arthritis. *Journal of Bone and Joint Surgery (American)*, 1992;74-A:552-63.

92. Kärrholm, J., Frech, W., Nivbrant, B., Malchau, H., Snorrason, F., and Herberts, P. Fixation and metal release from the Tifit femoral stem prosthesis. 5-year follow-up of 64 cases. *Acta Orthopaedica Scandinavica*, 1998;69:369–378.

93. Önsten, I., Nordqvist, A., Carlsson, Å.S., Besjakov, J., and Shott, S. Hydroxiapatite augmentation of the porous coating improves fixation of tibial components. A randomized RSA study in 116

patients. *Journal of Bone and Joint Surgery (British)*, 1998; **80-B**:417–25.

94. Sumner, D.R., Turner, T.M., Purchio, A.F., Gombotz, W.R., Urban, R.M., and Galante, J.O. Enhancement of bone ingrowth by transforming growth factor-β. *Journal of Bone and Joint Surgery (American)*, 1995;77-A:1135–47.

95. Saikko, V., Nevalainen, J., Revitzer, H., and Ylinen, P. Metal release from total hip articulations in vitro. *Acta Orthopaedica Scandinavica, 1998;69*:449–54.

96. Saikko, V., and Pfaff, HG., Low wear and friction in alumina/alumina total hip joints. *Acta Orthopaedica Scandinavica*, 1988;69:443–48.

97. Jazrawi, L.M., Kummer, F.J., and DiCesare, PE. Alternative bearing surfaces for total joint arthroplasty. *Journal of the American Academy of Orthopaedic Surgeons*, 1998;6:198–203.

36 | *The hand*

Christer Sollerman

Introduction

The human hand is mainly a prehensile organ of prime importance for both occupational capacity and for performing activities of daily living. The hand and its function, however, is also part of the body language affecting social life and interpersonal relations to a very significant degree. A painful, swollen hand with deformities is therefore not only a prehensile disaster but might also lead to a most disabling psychosocial handicap.

Hand function is based upon certain properties of the hand which can be characterized as:

- freedom from pain;
- perceptual skin sensibility;
- optimal joint stability;
- functional range of motion;
- muscle strength.

These properties are listed in order of significance, freedom from pain and tactile sensibility being more important than range of motion and strength. This fact forms the basis for many of the surgical procedures used in rheumatoid arthritis, for example when arthrodesis of a joint improves hand function through transforming a painful and unstable joint into a pain-free and stable fusion. The loss of joint motion after such a procedure is for certain joints, for example the wrist joint and the metacarpophalangeal joint of the thumb, of minor importance compared to the improvement due to stability and pain relief.

Being unable to perform activities of daily living because of impaired hand function is often the main reason why institutional care is needed for a rheumatoid patient. Hand surgery might, in such cases, be of importance—even simple surgical procedures might significantly improve hand function and contribute to the patients' independency. The most common indication for surgery in rheumatoid arthritis is uncontrolled pain, which patients consider the main reason for treatment. The timing, order, and type of surgical procedures must be discussed with the patient in detail. The patients are often well aware of the expected postoperative result, but often they are mainly informed by their fellow patients. Rheumatoid patients often have strong feelings about the advantages and disadvantages with various procedures, and they must be allowed to have a main influence on the decision. Such a discussion is preferably performed in a team consisting of hand surgeon, rheumatologist, physical therapist, and occupational therapist.

Surgical procedures

The surgical options in RA include tenosynovectomy (i.e. excision of synovitis from a tendon sheath), tendon transfer or tendon repair, soft tissue stabilizing procedures, excision of painful nodules, peripheral nerve release, arthrosynovectomy (implying removal of synovitis from a joint), arthrodesis, and arthroplasty (consisting of excision of a joint with or without endoprosthetic replacement). The main goals of hand surgery for RA patients are to obtain:

- pain relief
- improved hand function
- correction of deformities
- prophylactic effects.

A combination of these goals is often achieved; endoprosthetic replacement of destroyed metacarpophalangeal (MCP) joints results, for example, in both pain relief, improved function, and correction of deformity.

The indication for surgery is based mainly on symptoms and clinical findings rather than the radiographic appearance. The radiographs, however, are essential for the choice between different surgical alternatives. All patients in whom hand surgery is considered therefore have to be radiographically examined. Rheumatoid joint destruction is commonly classified according to Larsen–Dale–Eek[1] in stages 1–6; stage 1 corresponding to a normal radiographic appearance, stage 6 to a totally destroyed joint. Surgical treatment in RA has a long tradition, but many of commonly used procedures are based on empiric data and not controlled data. In a recent meta-analysis by the Swedish Council on Technology Assessment in Health Care[2] the main conclusion was that better documentation of both new and established surgical procedures is needed.

Tenosynovectomy and tendon repair

Tenosynovitis is common around the extensor tendons at the wrist, the flexor tendons in the carpal canal, and in the flexor tendon sheaths of the fingers. Tenosynovitis impairs the range of motion, but gives rise to pain mainly when peripheral nerves are involved as in the carpal canal. Tenosynovitis may take the form of inflammatory tissue on the tendon surface and of intratendinous rheumatoid nodules. Such nodules may impair the strength of the tendon; ruptures seem to increase in RA[3]. Tendon ruptures may also be a consequence of wear against sharp bony edges, so called attrition ruptures. These are seen around the ulnar head (caput ulna syndrome), in the carpal canal against the carpal bones, and volar to the MCP joints when the proximal phalanx is subluxated.

Surgical excision of the synovial sheath and intratendineous nodules (i.e., tenosynovectomy) improves the range of motion and probably minimizes the risk of rupture[4]. The technique should take great care of important structures, not severing tendons or the fibrous parts of the tendon sheath, the pulleys. Immediately postoperative, exercises are performed under supervision of a physical or occupational therapist.

Tenosynovectomy results in improved range of motion, improved strength, and possibly less risk of rupture, though this has not been proven[4–6]. Tendon ruptures result in sudden loss of active motion. Ruptures of the finger extensors in the wrist region cause impaired active extension of the MCP joints, ruptures of flexor tendons in the carpal canal cause impaired active flexion of one or more finger joints depending on how many tendons that are involved. In cases of isolated rupture of the deep flexor tendons or the long thumb flexor, active flexion of the distal interphalangeal (DIP) and/or interphalangeal (IP) joints is lost. Fusion of the involved joints is a simple method to restore stability and strength, since active motion in a single DIP joint is not important for a functional hand grip. However, if multiple tendons are ruptured, a tendon repair is required. Reconstruction of ruptured tendons with the help of tendon grafts implies an intact proximal muscle and a time-consuming and sometimes complicated postoperative rehabilitation. Most rheumatoid patients are better served with a transfer of one or more intact tendons to compensate for the loss of motion. The results of such tendon transfers are improved range of motion, although it is not normalized[7].

Soft tissue procedures

A variety of surgical procedures, including reefing of ligaments, shortening or changing direction of tendons, and releasing contracted joint capsules may be used to correct deformities, and achieve improved hand function. In early stages of the disease, soft tissue stabilization may help to achieve joint stability when combined with synovectomies or other procedures. Excision of painful subcutaneous nodules are popular among patients because of the beneficial effects on tenderness and pain, but the recurrence rate is high. Most subcutaneous nodules are, however, not tender.

Peripheral nerve surgery

Synovitis in joints and tendon sheaths may affect neighboring peripheral nerves. Raised tissue pressure may impair nerve function—compression neuropathy. The symptoms are paresthesis and pain, and later loss of sensibility and/or motor function. Compression neuropathies are common in RA, the symptoms of pain and tingling are, however, often masked by other kinds of chronic pain and one has to ask specifically for paresthesis during the night, which are the main signals distinguishing nerve compression symptoms from joint pain. Compression of periph-

eral nerves may be caused by synovitis in nearby joints or tendon sheaths. The most common location is in the carpal tunnel where the median nerve is prone to be compressed by tenosynovitis of the flexor tendons resulting in paresthesies in the radial two-thirds of the hand. The prevalence of this condition is reported to be as high as 10–69 per cent[8]. A carpal tunnel release with a careful tenosynovectomy is a reliable procedure which will restore nerve function and finger flexor capacity.

Synovitis of the elbow joint may involve the ulnar nerve, causing paresthesis in the ulnar part of the lower arm and hand[9]. Release of the nerve from the sulcus cubiti may relieve symptoms, but preferably a nerve transposition should be performed. This will prevent recurrence of the nerve compression. Elbow synovitis may also influence the function of the median nerve in the elbow region (anterior interosseous syndrome)[10] or the posterior branch from the radial nerve[11].

Joint synovectomy

Surgical synovectomy may be performed to achieve pain relief and to reduce swelling and tenderness. The feasibility of complete surgical removal of synovial tissue between joints varies. In multichamber joints such as the hand, complete synovectomy is difficult or impossible.

Synovectomy should be performed in early stages when radiographic changes are minimal (Larsen stage 1–3) and the result is influenced by the radicality of the removal, the degree of radiographic destruction, and also with the general disease development. Postoperatively, the joint is immobilized for a few days followed by a period of active physiotherapy. Satisfactory pain relief has been reported[12] but relapses do occur and long-term studies have not shown any retarding effect on radiographic progression[13,14]. Consequently, synovectomy is rarely performed as an isolated surgical procedure.

Arthrodesis (fusion)

Arthrodesis implies removal of all cartilage and subchondral bone from a joint, necessary to achieve bony healing between joint surfaces. The joint has to be immobilized internally with wires, pins, screws, or plates during the healing period. The osteosynthesis material can be removed after healing if local tenderness occur. The surgical procedure should aim at achieving maximum stability with internal fixation in order to minimize the need of plaster or external splints. In some joints [i.e. the MCP and proximal interphalangeal (PIP) joints of the fingers] fusion impairs function to a significant degree, even if pain relief is achieved, and is thus rarely performed. In other joints, however, [i.e. the wrist, the metaparpophalangeal (MCP) joint of the thumb, the DIP joints of the fingers] fusion is an effective way of improving hand function because stability in these joints is more important for function than range of motion.

Arthroplasty

Destroyed joints with deformity, impaired range of motion, and with pain can be resected and replaced by soft tissues (interposition arthroplasty) or with implants (endoprostheses). Interposition arthroplasty may be performed in joints without too much loading. Tendons, fascia, or fibrocartilage material can be interposed between the resected joint surfaces in order to obtain a joint-like function. The advantages with these procedures are low cost and low incidence of foreign body reactions. Arthroplasty with endoprostheses is, however, a more common procedure, although development of implants for hand surgery has been slow, compared with devices for larger joints. The problems in arthroplastic surgery are to achieve implant fixation to surrounding bone and to find a joint mechanism which combines optimal range of motion with stability. All joint prostheses are prone to tear and wear, particularly in joints exposed to load.

A detailed description of the various procedures and their reported results in the different joints is given below.

The wrist joint

The wrist joint is very important for hand function, especially in RA. The wrist joint is the fundament of the hand and any wrist disability will significantly affect the function of the hand.

The wrist joint has a complex anatomy involving many joints allowing motion between radius, ulna, and the eight carpal bones. The wrist consists of three different parts:

(1) The **radiocarpal joint** is the main wrist joint between the distal surface of the radius and the proximal surfaces of the proximal row of carpal bones. About half of the flexion–extension capacity depends on this joint.

(2) The **intercarpal joints** link the eight carpal bones together. About half of the range of motion in flexion–extension depends on motion between the carpal bones, as does the ability of radial and ulnar deviation.

(3) The **distal radioulnar (DRU) joint** is part of the rotating joints of the lower arm enabling pronation and supination of the hand.

In RA of the wrist the stabilizing structures (ligaments, tendons, and joint capsule) often become weakened by the synovitis. Instability and subsequent deformity follow. Volar subluxation (Fig. 36.1) and reduced range of motion are typical for RA[15,16]. The intercarpal joints may develop either ankylosis or instability. In the DRU joint, synovitis causes destruction of stabilizing structures, leading to displacement between the ulnar head and radius. Such a displacement impairs pronation–supination and may interfere with the surrounding tendons, especially the ulnarly located finger extensors tendons which may rupture. The caput ulna syndrome[17] is characterized by weakness in the hand and wrist joint, pain and limited prosupination and a dorsal protrusion of the ulnar head with crepitations and clicking. About 30 per cent of patients with rheumatoid arthritis may become affected by a caput ulna syndrome[18].

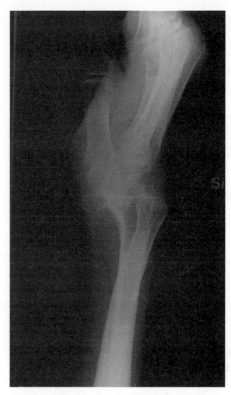

Fig. 36.1 Radiographic lateral view of a wrist joint with volar subluxation.

The radiocarpal and intercarpal joints

Simmen[19] has defined three types of natural courses for the wrist joint in rheumatoid arthritis, which affect the indication for surgery and choice of surgical alternatives:

Type I: progressive destruction with moderate pain at loading leading to subsequent ankylosis without pain. This is a favorable development since stability is more important than range of motion in the wrist. Surgery is rarely indicated. In type I disease, fusion of the intercarpal joints occurs spontaneously. Treatment is aimed at achieving a functional position for the ankylosis and splints are useful to prevent flexion or ulnar deformity. After spontaneous ankylosis the wrist becomes stable and pain-free.

Type II: progressive erosive destruction; severe pain, ankylosis will not occur spontaneously. A progressive destruction with severe pain at loading may necessitate surgical arthrodesis which is the method of choice in this type of disease. Range of motion after arthroplasty or partial wrist fusion is often limited.

Type III: progressive destruction with severe instability and/or deformity. The patient often experiences inflammatory symptoms and without treatment the end result is a grossly deformed wrist joint with major impairment of hand function. Surgery is strongly indicated to prevent disabling deformity with impaired range of motion. The aims of surgical intervention are to achieve pain relief and stability, and to prevent secondary tendon ruptures. Synovectomy, often combined with ulnar head resection or a ligament stabilizing procedure, total or partial fusion, and arthroplasty are the surgical alternatives of choice.

The distal radioulnar joint

Synovitis in the DRU joint often causes destruction of ligaments and joint surfaces of both ulna and radius resulting in displacement and destruction of the joint. If the joint surfaces are intact, a synovectomy combined with ligament reconstruction around the ulnar head may restore function, but in most cases a resection of the ulnar head, (Darrach procedure) is needed. The Darrach procedure is effective in relieving pain, improving prosupination and preventing tendon ruptures, but should not be performed in wrists with ulnar translocation, in which severe ulnar deviation may develop. Ulnar head resection is often combined with soft tissue stabilization in order to avoid instability of the distal end of the ulna, fascia, capsular structures or tendons (extensor carpi ulnaris or flexor carpi ulnaris) can be utilized for this purpose[20].

Although ulnar head resection helps to improve wrist function, complications do occur. Instability of the ulnar end is, in spite of stabilizing procedures, frequent, but rarely disabling. In wrist joints with ulnar translocation of the carpus, the ulnar head plays an important role as a support for the carpal bones; ulnar head resection in such individuals may result in severe ulnar deviation of the wrist. An alternative to ulnar head resection is the Sauvée–Kapandji procedure, which comprises of a fusion between the ulnar head and the radius in order to preserve the ulnar support for the carpus, prosupination is achieved through an osteotomy of the ulna proximal to the fusion. The Sauvée–Kapandji procedure was originally designed for post-traumatic problems of the DRU joint, but good results in RA have also been reported[21].

Synovectomy of the wrist

In early stages of rheumatic arthritis (Larsen stage 1–3) synovectomy can be an effective treatment to achieve pain relief in the wrist joint. Synovectomy is performed through a dorsal approach and should always include tenosynovectomy of the extensor tendons and arthrosynovectomy of the radiocarpal, intercarpal, and distal radioulnar joints. This implies a broad surgical exposure of the wrist joint with expanded healing time and postsurgical loss of motion as a consequence. Arthroscopic synovectomy has been introduced to minimize the surgical trauma[22], but this technique is still not accepted as a routine procedure because it is time- and resource-consuming.

The initial result of wrist synovectomy is pain relief, but the range of motion in terms of flexion–extension capacity is always impaired; the prosupination is, however, often improved, especially if ulnar head resection is performed. Long-term studies have shown pain relief, but no preventive effect on progressive destruction[12]. Since the preventive effect of wrist synovectomy is doubtful, this procedure is rarely performed. Wrist tenosynovectomy has, however, proven effective in preventing tendon ruptures[23] and should therefore be considered in cases of wrist tenosynovitis.

Proximal carpectomy

In later stages of RA (Larsen 3–6) resection of the proximal carpal row might be an alternative to fusion in order to preserve some range of motion in the wrist joint. After bone resection, soft tissue interposition is sometimes performed to achieve stability and mobility[24].

Arthrodesis of the wrist

Fusion is a reliable procedure to achieve pain relief and stability together with correction of any deformity of the wrist joint[25–27]. Restored stability and pain relief always improve hand function, even when bilateral wrist fusions are performed. Various fusion techniques are described, using Steinmann pins, screws and plates, or bone grafts to achieve internal stability. It avoids prolonged external fixation, a method that should be avoided in patients with RA. The clinical results of wrist fusions are very satisfying, since the pain-free and stable wrist improves hand function[28]. Complications comprise failed healing, persisting pain, or median nerve compression, a complication seen especially when severe volar subluxation of the wrist joint is reduced by the fusion.

Limited wrist fusion

When only limited parts of the wrist is destroyed, a partial fusion of the wrist may be considered as an alternative to total wrist fusion in order to preserve some range of motion. Partial wrist fusion can be performed both in the radiocarpal joint with preservation of the intercarpal joints, or in the intercarpal joints with preservation of the radiocarpal joint[29]. Fusion between os lunatum and radius is advocated in ulnar head resection to prevent deviation of the wrist joint in cases of ulnar translocation of the carpus[30,31].

Arthroplasty of the wrist

Replacement of the wrist joint with endoprosthesis is still a controversial procedure, mainly because fusion is the gold standard for reconstruction of an unstable and painful wrist joint. However, when surgical intervention of both the right and left wrist joint is indicated, arthroplasty might be an alternative for one of the joints, taking into account that some range of wrist motion is useful when performing activities of daily living[32]. There are three problems with endoprosthetic replacement of the wrist: to define the center of rotation in the wrist; to achieve implant fixation to bone; and to balance the forces acting on the wrist joint[33]. Both constrained hinge joints and non-constrained ball-in-socket joints have been advocated.

Constrained wrist implants

Silicone implants of Swanson's design have been in use for 20 years. Early results were encouraging with immediate pain relief and a functional range of motion[34–39]. The implant is merely a spacer with silicone stems introduced into the marrow channels of the third metacarpal bone and the radius. Increasing reports of bone resorption and subsidence (70–100 per cent in some studies), frequent fractures of the silicone implant and development of foreign body reactions, 'silicone synovitis', have tempered the initial enthusiasm with this implant[40,41]. Titanium shields (grommets) have been introduced in order to improve the results, but their effect is unproven. Silicone implants for replacement of the wrist joint is now considered an almost abandoned method, though some authors still advocate them.

Non-constrained wrist implants

Various designs of ball-in-socket implants in the wrist joint have been suggested, the Volz and Meuli prostheses being the most used non-constrained implants. Both implants have spherical metal balls, articulating against sockets of polyethylene with titanium stems enabling bone fixation with or without cement. Pain relief and 60–70 degrees of flexion–extension is often achieved[42,43]. Loosening of the components, especially the distal stem, is however a problem. Frequently the implant's center of rotation is malplaced in the wrist joint leading to ulnar deviation and/or flexion deformity of the wrist. Complications occurred in 44 per cent of the procedures with a total revision rate of 33 per cent due to loosening, dislocation, or imbalance[44]. Beckenbaugh and Menon have presented an alternative non-constrained implant with ellipsoid balls (Fig. 36.2), aimed at improving the balance of the arthroplasty[45]. These implants can be used with or without cement fixation. Preliminary experiences are encouraging but no long-term results are available. Thus no implants for the wrist joint are at present documented as alternatives to fusion.

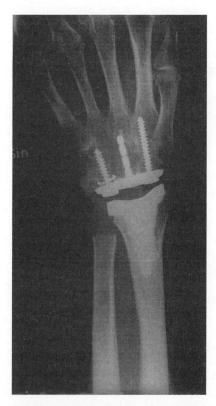

Fig. 36.2 Radiographic anterioposterior view of the Universal Total Wrist Implant (KMR[R]).

The MCP joint and ulnar drift

The MCP joints of the fingers are ball-in-socket joints allowing some 90 degrees of extension–flexion and 25 degrees of ulnar–radial deviation. The range of motion of the MCP joints is important, both for opening the hand and for the grasping of objects. Lateral stability is needed, especially in the index finger when used in the lateral pinch.

Isolated synovectomy of the MCP joints was a frequent procedure in the past, but is now usually performed only as adjunct to soft tissue stabilizing procedures. Ulnar drift and volar subluxation is often both functionally and psychologically a dominating problem for the RA patient. The hands are, together with the face, the only parts of the body that are not covered by clothes making deformities of the hand most obvious. In most cases, ulnar drift causes impaired prehensile function, the destroyed MCP joints loosing their extension capacity with inability to open the hand in order to grasp a glass or to shake hands as a result. In some cases, the pinch grip between the thumb and the finger tips is lost, leaving the lateral pinch between the thumb and the radial side of the index finger as the only remaining grip for manipulation[46]. Even if the prehensile function of the hand is not impaired, patients often experience ulnar drift as cosmetically disturbing and strongly urge a surgical correction.

The development of ulnar drift has many reasons including:

- radial deviation of the wrist joint leading to hand scoliosis with secondary ulnar deviation of the fingers;
- tenosynovitis of the flexor tendon sheath leading to weakening of annular ligaments with subsequent ulnarly directed forces of the flexor tendons onto the index and middle fingers;
- synovitis of MCP joints leading to weakening of the transverse ligaments of the extensor tendon 'hood' with subsequent ulnar luxation of the extensor tendons;
- common use of lateral pinch in which the thumb creates ulnarly-directed forces to the radial side of the index finger.

These different forces produce not only ulnar deviation of the fingers but also volar subluxation of the proximal phalanx from the metacarpal heads, which is a mandatory part of the deformity and the main cause of extension loss of the MCP joints.

Ulnar drift is classified into three stages[47]. The early stage (Fearnley 1: active reduction is possible = minor deformity which might be corrected by the muscle activity of the hand itself) is often treated with dynamic splinting with rubber bands counteracting both the ulnar deviation and the volar subluxation of the fingers. In the next stage (Fearnley 2: passive reduction is possible = more severe deformity which can be corrected with splints or with the help of the contralateral hand), the MCP joints are still radiographically normal and soft tissue surgical procedures might be used to correct the ulnar deviation. In the last stage (Fearnley 3: fixed deformity combined with subluxation and/or radiographic destruction of the MCP joints), soft tissue procedures are no longer successful; arthroplasty of the MCP joints is the recommended surgical correction.

Soft tissue procedures in ulnar drift

The ulnar drift deformity often includes luxation of the extensor tendons ulnarly to the metacarpal heads due to synovitis of the MCP joint which causes destruction of the tendon's stabilizing structures. Extension movements of the MCP joints will then cause ulnar deviation of the fingers due to the ulnarly luxated tendons. Early surgical correction of the tendon displacement may prevent ulnar drift in these cases[48]. Such a procedure, called centralization of the extensor tendons, can be done in Fearnley stage 1 or 2 and is performed with a release of the ulnar transverse ligament and a duplication of the radial transverse ligament of each of the MCP joints.

Correction of ulnar drift in Fearnley stage 2 can also be performed through transfer of the interosseous tendons from one proximal finger phalanx to its ulnarly situated neighbor, so called crossed intrinsic transfer or Straub[49]. The interosseous muscles, which act on the lateral bands, produces ab- and adduction movements of the fingers and transfer of the ulnar lateral band (i.e. the intrinsic tendon) from each of the index, middle, and fourth finger to the radial side of the middle, fourth, and fifth finger respectively, radial correction of ulnarly deviating fingers can be achieved.

After both procedures, post operative early controlled motion is performed with the help of a dynamic splint which prevents the ulnar deviation of the fingers. Dynamic splinting is used for 6 weeks and a static splint worn at night is then used for 3 months or longer. About 80 per cent good or excellent early results are reported with centralization when used in Fearnley stage 1 or 2[48].

Arthrodesis of the MCP joints

A functional hand grip depends on proper range of motion in the MCP joints of the fingers, both for opening of the hand and for grasping. The adaptation of the fingers to different shapes of objects also depend on the ulnar–radial deviation of the fingers. Fusion of the MCP joints II–V is therefore not recommended, at least not for the three ulnar fingers. In the thumb, however, fusion of the MCP joint is useful. Fusion of the MCP joint of the index finger is sometimes performed in conjunction with arthroplasty of the remaining fingers, in order to achieve radial stability in the lateral pinch.

Arthroplasty of the MCP joints

In Fearnley stage 3 surgical procedures of the MCP joint itself are needed to improve joint function and to correct the ulnar drift. Since fusion is not a useful procedure for the MCP joints, except the thumb and perhaps the index finger, surgical alternatives are arthroplasties with or without endoprostheses.

Interposition arthroplasty

Various concepts of arthroplasties using different kinds of soft tissues for interposition and stabilization of the MCP joints have been described, commonly using the extensor tendon[50] or the volar plate[51] as the interposed structure. A disadvantage is that

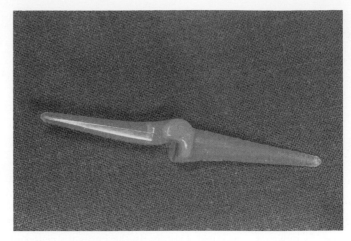

Fig. 36.3   Silicone MCP implant of Swanson type.

the range of motion is often limited and tends to deteriorate with time. Published data with these procedures are sparse.

Arthroplasty with endoprostheses

The first reported surgical procedure using an endoprosthesis for replacement of the MCP joints was performed in the beginning of 1950 and since then a variety of endoprosthesis have been presented[52]. The joint mechanism might be constrained using a polymer (silicone) as the flexible hinge, or non-constrained using a ball-in-socket concept. The stem of the endoprosthesis might be fixed into the bone marrow channels, with or without cement, or might be encapsulated by soft tissues as the main fixation. A new principle of non-cemented fixation is the osseointegration concept, in which titanium fixtures anchored to the surrounding bone tissue are used for implant fixation.

Silicone implants

Swanson's arthroplasty using silicone implants has, for more than 20 years, been the gold standard for endoprosthetic replacement of the MCP joints[53–56]. The concept is based on the flexible silicone spacer with proximally and distally directed stems (Fig. 36.3), which after resection of the metacarpal head are introduced into the marrow channels of the metacarpal bone and the proximal phalanx respectively. The spacer is subsequently 'encapsulated' into surrounding soft tissues for implant fixation. The radial collateral ligaments, at least for the index finger, are reinserted to bone before implantation of the spacers. With the Swanson arthroplasty immediate pain relief, proper correction of deformity, and adequate range of motion is often obtained. With time, however, bone reactions tend to occur around the implants, both as new bone formation and as bone resorption due to movements between implant and bone, described as early as 1975[57]. The range of motion deteriorates due to subsidence of the implants into the surrounding bone. Silicone particle induced synovitis has mainly been described around silicone implants in larger joints, but it can occasionally occur in MCP joints as well[41]. A range of motion varying between 25 and 66 degrees can be achieved, the fracture rate of the silicone can be up to 39 per cent[58,38].

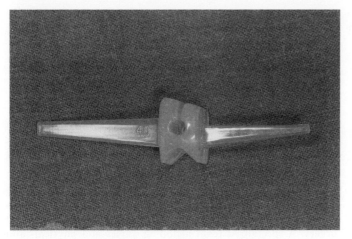

Fig. 36.4 Silicone MCP implant of Sutter (Avanta) type.

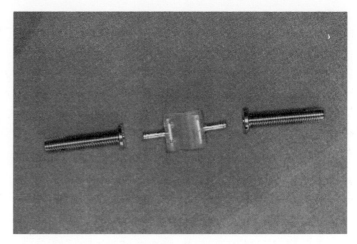

Fig. 36.5 Silicone MCP implant with titanium fixtures a.m. Brånemark.

A new design of silicone implants has been introduced in which the implant surface against the resected bone ends is larger in order to prevent subsidence of the implant, and the axis of motion being placed more volarly to improve the range of motion (Fig. 36.4). High fracture rates have, however, been reported with this implant[59]. No long–term studies are available. Other polymeric materials such as polyurethane have been used in limited series as an alternative to silicone, but experience is limited[60].

Many authors are, in spite of obvious disadvantages with silicone implants, still recommend this technique as the standard procedure for MCP joint replacement because of it reliable and well-known initial functional results.

Non-constrained implants

A non-constrained implant with a metal ball articulating in a plastic socket with implant stems fixed to surrounding bone with the help of bone cement has been described[61]. Extensive periarticular ectopic bone formation in 32 per cent, and loosening of the distal stem in 17–18 per cent have contributed to a very limited use of this implant design. There are also a few reports published on various kinds of non-cemented non-constrained implants, for example with alumina–ceramic material[62] or polyester[63]. None of these implant designs can be recommended at present.

Osseointegrated implants

A new concept of implant fixation is based on the osseointegration principle using titanium fixtures. The osseointegration concept has been introduced by Brånemark and has been used extensively for fixation of artificial teeth[64]. Preliminary experience from silicone implants with titanium stems anchored to titanium screw-shaped fixtures in the marrow channels of the surrounding bone (Fig. 36.5) indicate that this concept may be an encouraging way of obtaining implant fixation with cement. Osseointegrated MCP implants were used 1980 by Hagert, but the joint mechanism in this series was complicated and the clinical result was bad[65]. In a new series, a constrained hinge joint made of silicone was used and preliminary results showed 100 per cent osseointegration (measured from radiographic

examinations) and excellent clinical results. The fracture rate of the silicone is still a problem with this implant design, 6 per cent of the silicone fracture after 2.5 years, but this increases with time. However, it is easy to exchange the silicone hinge in the osseointegrated titanium fixtures[66].

The PIP joint

The PIP joint is a hinge joint with about 100 degrees of flexion–extension and with no lateral motion. Synovectomy is sometimes performed, sometimes in addition to reefing the central tendon in order to treat button hole deformity. Impaired range of motion after synovectomy is however common, as are relapses of synovitis, making synovectomy subsequently more and more rarely performed.

Arthrodesis of the PIP joint

Since range of motion in the PIP joints is important for a functional hand grip, fusion is not an attractive alternative in these joints. Fusion is, however, widely used in spite of its obvious drawbacks, since results of arthroplasties are not consistent[67]. The surgical technique should imply rigid internal fixation in order to avoid prolonged splinting of the fingers with subsequent loss of motion in neighboring joints.

Arthroplasty of the PIP joint

Replacement of the PIP joint is commonly performed with silicone implants, for example Swanson-, Niebauer- or Sutter-type[68,69]. The pain relieving effect is reasonably good, but range of motion and correction of deformities is unsatisfactory[70]. Non-constrained implants with cement fixation have been used without success[71,72]. A bicondylar non-constrained implant which can be used both with or without cement shows encouraging initial results[73]. Such an implant may be an attractive alternative to fusion in the future (Figs. 36.6 and 36.7).

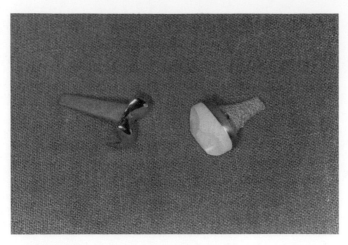

Fig. 36.6 Avanta Anatomic Poly PIP implant[R].

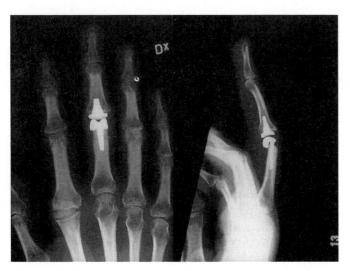

Fig. 36.7 Radiographic view of the Avanta Anatomic Poly PIP implant[R].

The DIP joint

Engagement of the DIP joints is not common in RA, but is frequent in psoriatic arthritis. As range of motion in these joints is not important for hand function, fusion is the method of choice to achieve pain relief and to correct deformities. Bone resorption is often severe, necessitating the use of bone grafts when performing a DIP joint fusion.

The thumb

The main property of the thumb is to provide a stable pose against the fingers in grasping and pinching. Fusion is therefore commonly used in the MCP and IP joints, even when both joints are operated simultaneously. The CMC joint is rarely fused in RA, but arthroplasty with or without endoprostheses is, in most cases, a reliable method to achieve pain relief and stability with

preserved range of motion[74]. Soft-tissue stabilization of the MCP joint may be considered when the joint surfaces still allow motion[18].

Postoperative rehabilitation

Rigorous rules have to be followed in the postoperative phase in order to avoid complications. The rheumatoid patient is sensitive to prolonged bed rest, the use of wheel–chair, and prolonged splinting, therefore these should be avoided. The surgical technique must include rigid internal fixation of fusions, fractures, and soft tissue stabilization procedures. Early mobilization, often controlled with splints, is commonly used after hand surgery. A specialized team including nurses and physical- and occupational therapists is essential in the postoperative period.

Splints

Immobilization of the hand and wrist is often performed with the help of splints, that are lighter and more easy to use than plaster. Splints are custom-made from various plastic materials by occupational therapists. Static splints are used for immobilization. Dynamic splints use rubber bands acting on fingers or finger joints in order to counteract muscle forces or to facilitate range of motion. After correction of ulnar drift, for example, a dynamic splint with rubber bands providing radial traction of the fingers is used for 6–8 weeks postoperatively. The use of dynamic splints has to be supervised by an occupational therapist.

Functional assessment

The indication for many hand surgical procedures is to improve hand function which might be essential for a patient's occupation, independence, and ability to perform activities of daily living. Exercises to improve hand function are an important part of a treatment program in rheumatoid arthritis. Certain methods are available for measuring hand function and to register function before a surgical procedure and during the postoperative training period[75].

References

1. Larsen A., Dale K., Eek M. Radiographic evaluation of rheumatoid arthritis and related conditions by standard reference films. *Act Radiol (Diagn)* 1977;**18**:481–491.
2. SBU TSCoTAiHC (The Swedish Council Technology Assessment in Health Care). *Rheumatoid arthritis–Surgical treatment* (in Swedish). SBU-rapport 1998;136(1+2).
3. Ferlic D. Rheumatoid flexor tenosynovitis and rupture. *Hand Clinic* 1996;**12**:561–572.
4. Connor J., Nalebuff E.A. Current recommendations for surgery of the rheumatoid hand and wrist. *Current Opin Rheumatol* 1995;7:120–124.
5. Leslie B.M. Rheumatoid extensor tendon ruptures. *Hand Clinics*, 1989;5:191–202.
6. Ertel A.N. Flexor tendon ruptures in rheumatoid arthritis. *Hand Clinics*, 1989;5:177–190.

7. Moore J.R., Weiland A.J., Valdata L. Tendon ruptures in the rheumatoid hand: analysis of treatment and functional results in 60 patients. *J Hand Surg* (Am), 1987;**12**:9–14.

8. Chang D.J., Paget S.A. Neurologic complications of rheumatoid arthritis. *Rheum Dis Clinics*, 1993;**19**:955–973.

9. Schmidt V.A. Nervenkompressionssyndrome in Bereich des Ellenbogengelenkes bei Patienten mit chronischer Polyarthritis. Eine Literaturübrsicht. *Handchir Mikrochir Plast Chir*, 1993;**25**:70–75.

10. Rask M.R. Anterior interosseous nerve entrapment: (Kiloh-Neven-syndromet). Report of seven cases. *Clin Orthop*, 1979;**142**: 176–181.

11. Ishikawa H., Hirohata K. Posterior interosseous nerve syndrome associated with rheumatoid synovial cysts of the elbow joint. *Clin Orthop*, 1990;**254**:134–139.

12. Vahvanen V, Patiala H. Synovectomy of the wrist in rheumatoid arthritis and related disease. A follow-up study of 97 consecutive cases. *Arch Orthopaedic Traumatic Surgery*, 1984;**102**:230–237.

13. Allieu Y., Lussiez B., Asencio G. Long-term results of surgical synovectomies of the rheumatoid wrist. Apropos 60 cases. *Revue de Chirugie Orthopedique et Reparatrice de 1 Appareil Moteur*, 1989;**75**:172–178.

14. Bohler N., Lack N., Schwagerl W., Sollerman C.T., J., Thabe H., Tillmann K. Late results of synovectomy of wrist, MP, and PIP joints. Multicenter study. *Clin Rheumat*, 1985;**4**:23–25.

15. Evan J.S., Blair W.F., Andrews J.G., Crowninshield R.D. The in vivo kinematics of the rheumatoid wrist. *J Orthop Research*, 1986;**4**:142–151.

16. Stanley D., Norris S.H. The pathogenesis and treatment of rheumatoid wrist and hand deformities. *Br J Hosp Med*, 1988;**39**:156–160.

17. Backdahl M. The caput ulnae syndrom in rheumatoid arthritis: A study of the morphology, abnormal anatomy and clinical picture. *Acta Rheumatol Scand*, 1963;**5**:1–75.

18. Nalebuff E.A., Feldon P.G., Millender L.H. Rheumatoid arthritis in hand and wrist. In: Green D.P., ed. *Operative Hand Surgery*. 2nd edn: New York: Churchill Livingstone, 1988:1655–1766. vol 3).

19. Simmen B.R., Huber H. The Rheumatoid Wrist: A new classification related to the type of natural course and its consequences for surgical therapy. *Rheumatology*, 1992;**17**:13–25.

20. Melone C.P., Jr. Taras J.S. Distal ulna resection, extensor carpi ulnaris tenodesis, and dorsal synovectomy for the rheumatoid wrist. *Hand Clinics*, 1991;**7**:335–343.

21. Taleisnik J. The Sauvée-Kapandji procedure. *Clinical Orthopaedics Related Research*, 1992;**275**:110–123.

22. Adolfsson L, Nylander G. Arthroscopic synovectomy of the rheumatoid wrist. *J Hand Surg* Br, 1993;**18**:92–96.

23. Brown F.E., Brown M.L. Long-term results after tenosynovectomy to treat the rheumatoid hand. *J Hand Surg*, 1988;**13**:704–708.

24. Culp R.W., McGuigan F.X., Turner M.A., Lichtman D.M., Osterman A.L., McCarrol H. Proximal row carpectomy. *J Hand Surg* (Am), 1993;**18**:19–25.

25. Mannerfelt L, Malmsten M. Arthrodesis of the wrist in rheumatoid arthritis. A technique without external fixation. *Scand J Plast Reconstr Surg*, 1971;**5**:124–130.

26. Millender L.H., Nalebuff E.A. Arthrodesis of the rheumatoid wrist. An evaluation of sixty patients and a description of a different surgical technique. *J Bone Joint Surg*, 1973;**55A**:1026–1034.

27. Rayan G.M., Brentlinger A., Purnell D., Garcia-Moral C.A. Functional assessment of bilateral wrist arthrodesis. *J Hand Surg* (Am), 1987;**12**:1020–104.

28. Vicar A.J., Burton R.I. Surgical management of the rheumatoid wrist-fusion or arthroplasty. *J Hand Surg*, 1986;**11A**:790–797.

29. Ishikawa H, Hanyu T., Saito H., Takahashi H. Limited arthrodesis for the rheumatoid wrist. *J Hand Surg*, 1992;**17A**:1103–1109.

30. Della Santa D., Chamay A. Radiological evolution of the rheumatoid wrist after radio-lunate arthrodesis. *J Hand Surg*, 1995;**20B**:146–54.

31. Stanley J.K., Boot D.A. Radio-lunate arthrodesis. *J Hand Surg* (Br), 1989;**14**:283–7.

32. Palmer A.K., Werner F.W., Eng M.M. Functional wrist motion; a biomechanical study. *J Hand Surg*, 1985;**19A**:39.

33. Cooney W.P.I., Beckenbaugh R.D., Linscheid R.L. Total wrist arthroplasty: problems with implant failures. *Clin Orthop*, 1984;**187**:121.

34. Jolly S.L., Ferlic D.E., Clayton M.L., Dennis D.A., Stringer E.A. Swanson silicone arthroplasty of the wrist in rheumatoid arthritis: A long-term follow-up. *J Hand Surg*, 1992;**17A**:142–149.

35. Lundkvist L., Barfred T. Total wrist arthroplasty. Experience with Swanson flexible silicone implants 1982–1988. *Scand J Plast Reconstr Hand Surg*, 1992;**26**:97–100.

36. Nylén S., Sollerman C., Haffajee D., Ekelund L. Swanson implant arthroplasty of the wrist in rheumatoid arthritis. *J Hand Surg*, 1984;**9B**:295–299.

37. Simmen B.R., Gschwend N. Swanson silicone rubber interpositional arthroplasty of the wrist and of the metacarpophalangeal joints in rheumatoid arthritis. I. Wrist arthroplasty. *Acta Orthopaedica Belgica*, 1988;**54**:196–209.

38. Stanley J.K., Tolat A.R. Long-term results of Swanson silastic arthroplasty in the rheumatoid wrist. *J Hand Surg*, 1993;**18B**: 381–388.

39. Swanson A.B., De Groot Swanson G., Maupin B.K. Flexible implant arthroplasty of the radiocarpal joint. Surgical technique and long-term study. *Clin Orthop Rel Res*, 1984;**187**:94–106.

40. Smith R.J., Atkinson R.E., Jupiter J.B. Silicone synovitis of the wrist. *J Hand Surg*, 1985;**10A**:47–60.

41. Peimer C., Medige J., Eckert B., Wright J., Howard C. Reactive synovitis after silicone arthroplasty. *J Hand Surg* Am, 1986;**11A**:624–638.

42. Volz R.G. Total wrist arthroplasty. A clinical review. *Clin Orthop*, 1984;**187**:112–120.

43. Meuli H.C., Fernandex D.L. Uncemented total wrist arthroplasty. *J Hand Surg*, 1995;**20A**:115–122.

44. Menon J. Total wrist replacement using the modified Volz prosthesis. *J Bone Joint Surg*, 1987;**69A**:998–1006.

45. Beckenbaugh R. Preliminary experience with a noncemented nonconstrained total joint arthroplasty for the metacarpophalangeal joints. *Orthopedics*, 1983;**6**:962–965.

46. Wilson R.L., Carlblom E.R. The rheumatoid metacarpophalangeal joint. *Hand Clinics*, 1989;**5**:223–237.

47. Fearnley G.R. Ulnar deviation of fingers. *Ann Rheum Dis*, 1951;**10**:126–136.

48. Wood V.E., Ichtertz D.R., Yahiku H. Soft tissue metacarpophalangeal reconstruction for treatment of rheumatoid hand deformity. *J Hand Surg* (Am), 1989;**14**:163–174.

49. Straub L.R. Surgical rehabilitation of the hand and upper extremity in rheumatoid arthritis. *Bull Rheumat Dis*, 1962;**12**: 265–8.

50. Vainio K. Vainio arthroplasty of the metacarpophalangeal joints in rheumatoid arthritis. *J Hand Surg*, 1989;**14A**:367–368.

51. Tupper J.W. The metacarpophalangeal volar plate arthroplasty. *J Hand Surg*, 1989;**54A**:371–375.

52. Beevers D.J., Seedhom B.B. Metacarpophalangeal joint prosthesis. *J Hand Surg*, 1995;**20B**:125–36.

53. Gschwend N., Zimerman. Analyse von 200 MCP-Artroplastiken. *J Handchirurgie*, 1974;**6**:7–14.

54. Kirschenbaum D., Schneider L.H., Adams D.C., Cody R.A. Arthroplasty of the metacarpophalangeal joints with use of silicone rubber implants in patients who have rheumatoid arthritis. *J Bone Joint Surg*, 1993;**75A**:3–12.

55. Maurer R., Ranawat C., McCormack R., Inglis A. Long-term follow-up of the Swanson MP arthroplasty for rheumatoid arthritis. *J Hand Surg*, 1990;**15A**:810–811.

56. Swanson A.B. Flexible implant arthroplasty for arthritic finger joints: Rationale, technique and results of treatment. *J Bone Joint Surg*, 1972;**54A**:435–455.

57. Hagert C., Eiken O., Ohlsson N., Aschan W., Movin A. Metacarpophalangeal joint implants. I. Roentgenographic study of the silastic finger joint implant, Swanson design. *Scan J Plast Reconstr Surg*, 1975;**9**:147–157.

58. Wilson Y.G., Sykes P.J., Niranjan N.S. Long-term follow-up of Swanson's silastic arthroplasty of the metacarpophalangeal joints in rheumatoid arthritis. *J Hand Surg*, 1993;**18B**:81–91.

59. Bass R.L., Stern P.J., Nairus J.G. High implant fracture incidence with Sutter silicone metacarpophalangeal joint arthroplasty. *J Hand Surg*, 1996;21A:813–818.

60. Sollerman C.J., Geijer M. Polyurethane versus silicone for endoprosthetic replacement of the metacarpophalangeal joints in rheumatoid arthritis. *Scand J Plast Reconstr Hand Surg* 1996;**30**,:145–150.

61. Steffee A., Beckenbaugh R., Lindsheid R. The development, technique and early results of total joint replacement for the metacarpophalangeal joint of the fingers. *Orthopedics* 1981;4,: 175–80.

62. Minami M., Yamasaki J., Kato S., Ishii S. Alumina ceramic prosthesis arthroplasty of the metacarpophalangeal joint in the rheumatoid hand. A 2–4 year follow-up study. *J Arthroplasty* 1988;3,:157–166.

63. Vermeiren J.A.M., Dapper M.M., Schoonhoven L.A., Merx P.W.J. Isoelastic arthroplasty of the metacarpophalangeal joints in rheumatoid arthritis: A preliminary report. *J Hand Surg*, 1994;**19A**:319–324.

64. Brånemark P.I., Breine U., Lindström J., Adell R., Hansson B.O., Ohlsson Å. Intraosseus anchorage of dental prosthesis. I. Experimental studies. *Scand J Plastic Reconstr Surg*, 1969;3: 81–100.

65. Hagert C-G., Brånemark P-I., Albrektsson T., Strid K-G., Irstam L. Metacarpophalangeal joint replacement with osseointegrated endoprosthesis. *Scand J Plast Reconstr Hand Surg*, 1986;20: 207–218.

66. Lundborg G., Brånemark P-I., Carlsson I., Metacarpophalangeal joint arthroplasty based on the osseointegration concept. *J Hand Surg*, 1993;**18B**:693–703.

67. Osterman A.H. Synovectomy, arthroplasty, and arthrodesis in the reconstruction of the rheumatoid wrist and hand. *Current Opin Rheumatol*, 1991;3:102–108.

68. Pellegrini V.D., Burton R.I. Osteoarthritis of the proximal interphalangeal joint of the hand: Arthroplasty or fusion? *J Hand Surg*, 1990;**15A**:194–209.

69. Swanson A.B., de Groot Swanson G. Flexible implant arthroplasty of the proximal interphalangeal joint. *Hand Clinics*, 1994;**10**: 261–266.

70. Adamson G.J., Gellman H., Brumfield R.H., Kuschner S.H., Lawler J.W. Flexible implant resection arthroplasty of the proximal interphalangeal joint in patients with systemic inflammatory arthritis. *J Hand Surg*, 1994;**19A**:378–384.

71. Beckenbaugh R.D. New concepts in arthroplasty of the hand and wrist. *Arch Surg*, 1977;**112**:1094–1098.

72. Linscheid R.I., Dobyns J.H., Beckenbaugh R.D., Cooney W.P. Proximal interphalangeal joint arthroplasty with a total joint design. *Mayo Clin Proc*, 1979;**54**:227–240.

73. Linscheid R.L. M.P., Vidal M.A., Beckenbaugh R.D. Development of a Surface Replacement Arthoplasty for Proximal Interphalangeal Joints. *J Hand Surg* (Am), 1997;**22A**:286–298.

74. Amadio P., Millender L., Smith R. Silicone spacer or tendon spacer for trapezium resection arthroplasty-Comparison of results. *J Hand Surg*, 1982;7:273–244.

75. Sollerman C., Ejeskär, A. Sollerman hand function test—a standardised method and its use in tetraplegic patients. *Scand J Plast Reconstr Hand Surg*, 1995;**29**:167–176.

37 | *The cervical spine*

A.T.H. Casey and H.A. Crockard

Introduction

Rheumatoid arthritis is a chronic, systemic, inflammatory disorder of unknown etiology characterized by an erosive synovitis. It affects 0.8 per cent of the population. Articular inflammation may be remitting, but if continued usually results in progressive joint destruction, deformity, and ultimately variable degrees of incapacitation. Cervical spine involvement characteristically involves the atlantoaxial complex, the most mobile part of the spine, with the radiological abnormalities being classified into those of atlantoaxial subluxation (AAS) which may be horizontal or vertical in direction. Significant subaxial disease is less common and usually coexists with the above deformities (Fig. 37.1).

In many cases these radiological abnormalities remain asymptomatic for years, but these patients nonetheless are at continued risk from a range of neurological complications and even sudden death from medullary compression. Despite the predilection that rheumatoid arthritis has for the cervical spine and the severe consequences that may ensue, there has been surprisingly little work in determining the factors that influence which patients will become myelopathic and, if and when they do, what role has surgery to play.

The purpose of this chapter is to review the available surgical knowledge from the medical literature examining the clinical features, the size of the problem, and also the current surgical approaches and possible instrumentation solutions. Finally we will audit the results of surgery comparing the surgical results with the natural history of the condition.

Radiographic patterns of disease

Common radiographic patterns of disease are illustrated below. Although some authors have tried to implicate cranial nerve findings with vertical translocation (also known as cranial settling or basilar invagination or impression) the symptoms of dysphagia and dysarthria are no more common in uncomplicated

Table 37.1 The incidence and prevalence of cervical rheumatoid arthritis and calculated estimates of the potential surgical workloads in the United Kingdom and United States of America (data extrapolated from Refs 9, 40, and 41)

Demographics	UK	USA	Comment
1. Population	57 M	248 M	Census data
2. Prevalence of RA	1.1%	0.9%	Based on Lawrence and Cathcart population studies
3. Number with RA	627 000	2.2 M	Calculated from the above
4. Incidence of RA	25 per 100 000	29 per 100 000	Based on large population studies in Norfolk, UK and Rochester, USA
5. Per cent with AAS at 3 years	15 %	N/A	Personal communication A. Young on behalf of the ERAS group (prospective study of 650 patients)
6. Annual incidence at 3 years	2325(*)	10 788(*)	* calculated from 1. and 5.
7. Prevalence	206 910	726 000	Based on point prevalence population study in Finland % shown in brackets.
a) AAS (33 %)	169 000	594 000	
b) VS (27 %)	62 700	220 000	AAS of > 9 mm was found
8. Potential surgical candidates fulfilling radiological criteria for surgery—10 %.			in 4% and a combination of ASS of 6–9 mm and vertical translocation in 6%. Subaxial subluxation > 4 mm was present in 1%.

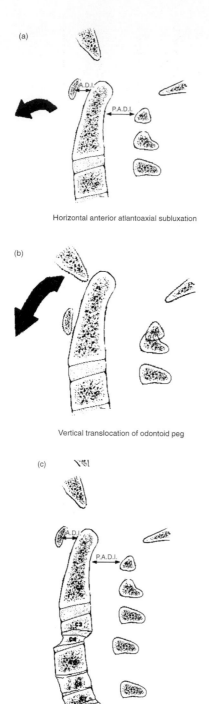

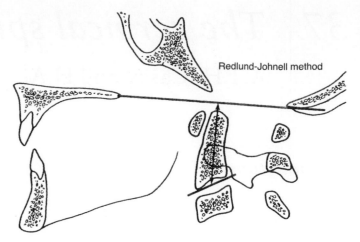

Fig. 37.2 Method of measuring vertical translocation by Redlund–Johnell. The disease from the base of C2 (axis) to McGregor's palato-occipital line is measured. As vertical translocation (also known as cranial setting) progresses this distance gets smaller.

of C2 to the McGregor's palato-occipital line. If this measurement is less than a certain length, which is different for men and women (males < 34 mm: females < 29 mm) it implies that there has been collapse of the lateral masses of C1 and C2 and vertical translocation is present [3].

Epidemiology

There are few epidemiological studies concentrating purely on rheumatoid manifestations in the cervical spine and many have serious methodological problems with bias introduced by selecting only hospital-based patients or those who have a cervical spine radiograph for various reasons. There is one good quality study from Finland with a captive, geographically isolated population[9]. Their results are summarized in Table 37.1, with extrapolated figures for the United Kingdom and United States. One problem with this study and most of the others is that it only provides a snap-shot in time of the incidence (point incidence) and this depends very much on the disease duration and age distribution of the selected patient population. What is lacking from the literature is a prospective, community-based study that gives information about the prevalence of AAS, VT, or other important manifestations of rheumatoid involvement of the cervical spine at predefined time intervals, that is 2 years, 5 years, 10 years, 15 years, etc. Also, more importantly, what percentage of patients with these radiographic abnormalities develop neurological symptoms or signs?

A literature meta-analysis is provided in Tables 37.2 and 37.3, but problems with retrospective data, biased population groups, and the lack of any agreement on what constitutes a neurological problem allow only broad conclusions to be drawn. Atlantoaxial subluxation (AAS) has been recorded in a range of 5.5 per cent to 73 per cent (mean 32 per cent)! The average incidence of neurological problems is 17 per cent. These epidemiology studies do not bring out the fact that is so obvious, from the

Fig. 37.1 (a) Horizontal atlantoxial subluxation as the ADI (atlantodens interval) increases the space available for the cord (posterior atlantodens interval—PADI) decreases. (b) Vertical translocation—the odontoid peg has transgressed the foramen magnum. (c) Subaxial diseases—staircase deformity.

horizontal atlantoaxial subluxation than vertical translocation[1]. There are different definitions of vertical translocation (VT)[2–8]. Many of these are historical (McRae, McGregor's method). We prefer the Redlund Johnell method which measures from the base

Table 37.2 Incidence of atlantoaxial subluxation in rheumatoid arthritis reported in non-surgical series

Author	Total no. of patients	Number with AAS	% with AAS	Vertical translocation (VT)	% with VT	Neurologically affected	% with neurological symptoms or signs	Source of patients
Serre 1964[42]	60	23	38	n/a	n/a	n/a	n/a	n/a admissions
Cabot 1978[43]	53	19	36	4/53	7.5	6/19	32	Hospital admissions
Conlon 1966[45]	333	84	25	n/a	n/a	11/84	13	Hospital admissions
Martel 1961[44]	34	24	73	n/a	n/a	n/a	n/a	n/a
Halla 1990[46]	650	36	5.5	8/650	1.2	3/61	4.9	Out-patient study admissions
Mathews 1969[47]	76	19	25	6/76	18	5/76	6.6	Hospital admissions
Meikle 1971[48]	118	44	37.3	n/a	n/a	n/a	n/a	Out-patients with neck pain
Ornilla 1972[49]	100	14	14	n/a	n/a	n/a	n/a	Arthroplasty patients
Pellici 1981[12]	163	40	25	4/163	2.5	11/74	15	Out-patients with radiographs
Rasker 1978[50]	62	26	42	20/62	32	n/a	n/a	In-patients (age 55–64)
Stevens 1971[10]	100	36	36	n/a	n/a	24/36	67	Out-patient clinic
Meta-analysis	1749	365	32	42/1004	4.2	60/350	17	Mixture

Table 37.3 Natural history studies on atlantoaxial subluxation in the rheumatoid cervical spine

Author	Length of follow-up (years)	Total number in series	% follow-up achieved	Source of patients	Neurological problems	% with neurological problems	Number with AAS	% with AAS	Radiological progression	
									Horizontal	*Vertical*
Isdale 1971[51]	6	171	62	Hospital admissions	'no change in 49 pts. by 3 years'	n/a	79	46	14/171 (8%)	n/a
Mathews 1974[11]	5	54	71	Out-patient clinic	12/54	22	6	11	9/54 (17%)	18/54 (33%)
Pellici 1981[12]	5	106	65	Out-patient clinic	33/106	31	41	39	28/106 (27%)	10/106 (9.4%)
Rana 1989[13]	10	41	100	Clinic and hospital patients with AAS	6/41	15	41	n/a	11/41 (27%)	4/41 (9.8%)
Smith 1972[14]	7.8	84	65	Cervical luxation cohort	10/130	7.7	55	65	19/55 (35%)	n/a
Winfield 1981[15]	7.2	100	100	Prospective study Patients within 1 year of diagnosis	0	0	12	12	12/100	3/100 (3%) (12%)
Meta-analysis	6.8 (mean)	556 (total)	77 (mean)	Mixed	61/431	15	234	35 (mean)	21% (mean)	14% (mean)

Several discrepancies appear to exist in the baseline number of patients (denominator). This is due to the fact that not all patients were followed up for both radiological and clinical examination. The abbreviation n/a is used when the authors of the original paper did not analyze their data for the relevant reading or value.

surgical papers, that neurological complications are a late manifestation of the disease process, *vide infra*.

Natural history

The findings of the major non-surgical series have been summarized in Table 37.3[10-14]. There is an overall fall-out rate of 33 per cent, with many patients lost to follow-up.

One prospective study, which originated from the Middlesex Hospital, found subluxation to be an early complication of the rheumatoid process[15]. In this series, 12 per cent of patients developed AAS, a further 20 per cent developed subaxial subluxation whilst 3 per cent developed vertical translocation. Over 80 per cent of these patients showed the first evidence of subluxation within 2 years of the disease presentation, and all these cases it was apparent within 5 years[15]. Their message that atlantoaxial subluxation was not a late development of the disease contradicted the perceived wisdom of that time, and in many ways was an unexpected finding. A dilemma is therefore created—why are these individuals neurologically normal, despite the fact that they have an obvious radiographic abnormality, and why do patients present with myelopathy, at average of 19 years after the disease onset, when subluxation has been present since 'year 2' in many individual cases? We hypothesize that the damage is due to multiple repetitive microtrauma over many years. Our neuropathological analysis bears this out[1,16].

The Swedish post-mortem study by Mikulowski of 104 patients with RA is an important contribution. This revealed 11 patients with unexpected AAS and cord compression. Seven of the 11 experienced sudden death; medullary compression by a translocated peg was clearly demonstrable in all these individuals [17]. The findings of this study raises serious doubts about the benign nature of the disease as suggested by the natural history studies detailed in Table 37.3.

Once cervical myelopathy is established mortality appears to be common. A report on 31 patients with RA and cervical myelopathy revealed that 19 died, with 15 deaths, nearly half, occurring within 6 months of presentation. All of those who were untreated died, and half of those treated by collar alone died[18]. In another study, nine patients with myelopathy treated non-operatively all died within 12 months, with four deaths directly attributable to cord compression, according to their death certificate[19]. However, the latter are unreliable in a multisystems disease and may seriously underestimate the incidence of cervical myelopathy as a cause of death[20,17]. Evidence from our own series of patients selected for surgery who refused decompression and fixation also suggests a very poor outcome once myelopathy is established with all seven patients dead within 5 years[21]. These findings are echoed by 21 rheumatoid arthritis patients with myelopathy resulting from atlantoaxial dislocation who were studied by Sunahara N., *et al*. from Kagoshima University, Japan[22]. All of these patients were recommended for surgery, but they refused. Patients were reviewed by direct examination yearly. Radiographic changes and clinical course, including the survival rate, were observed. All patients became bedridden within 3 years of the onset of myelopathy. Seven of the 21 patients died suddenly for unknown reasons, three died of pneumonia, and one died of multiple organ failure. The three sudden-death cases showed progressive upward migration of the odontoid process.

The overall impact of cervical spine involvement is highlighted in Corbett's prospective study of 102 patients[23], this is a follow-up to her original paper in 1981[15]. In this she has demonstrated, for the first time, that cervical subluxation appearing within the first 2 years of disease onset is a predictor of eventual poor functional outcome.

All these studies, therefore, seem to provide conflicting evidence. On the one hand there are reports of only modest radiographic progression over time with only 15 per cent of patients developing neurological problems. On the other hand we are presented with fairly compelling evidence that the incidence of myelopathy is probably underestimated and that once it develops the outlook is grim.

These apparent contradictions arise from the difficulty in diagnosing cervical myelopathy in the presence of a painful deforming arthritis with an often associated peripheral neuropathy and myopathy. Also, it is important to bear in mind that the radiographic abnormalities described in many of these studies are plain radiographs. Many deal solely with horizontal atlantoaxial subluxation and fail to take into account the less common manifestations of rheumatoid involvement of the cervical spine, that is vertical translocation, lateral and rotatory atlantoaxial subluxation, and subaxial disease. Plain radiographs cannot visualize compression by soft tissue, notably pannus. These facts, in part, explain the poor correlation of radiographic abnormalities and the development of cervical myelopathy described in the literature.

One of the issues that we have tried to address in this work is the more accurate characterization of the radiographic abnormalities associated with cervical myelopathy, taking into account findings from CT myelography which can visualize the neuraxis and soft tissue compression. Many of these radiographic parameters can be measured directly or via computerized morphometric analysis. Efforts had been made to quantify the level of disability secondary to rheumatoid cervical myelopathy[24].

Surgical indications

There is a consensus view that surgery should be offered to those individuals with neurological symptoms or signs. Patients with atlantoaxial instability and severe unremitting pain, unresponsive to conservative measures, are also usually offered surgery.

There is a significant grey area. This is whether prophylactic surgery should be offered to patients with severe radiographic abnormalities, for example a large atlantodens interval (> 6–10 mm), who are at risk of imminent neurological catastrophe[25,26]. There is no compelling evidence to support prophylactic surgery. Circumstantial evidence in its favor comes from several sources. Agarwal's group have demonstrated that patients who undergo surgery at an early stage of disease (atlantoaxial fixation) fare better in the long run than patients who have surgery at a later stage of their disease (occipitocervical fixation). Our group has highlighted the very poor prognosis for the end-stage patient (Ranawat class IIIB)[2]. The incidence of surgical complications is double that of Ranawat class IIIA patients. Finally the post-mortem studies of Mikulowski, Wollheim et al. reveal that sudden death is a not infrequent complication[17].

Boden has suggested the posterior atlantodens interval (PADI or ADI) (space available for the cord) as an alternate radiographic indicator based on an analysis of 73 patients over a 20-year period [27]. The problem with relying on the atlantodens interval is that it takes no account of soft tissue inflammation (pannus) or that the ADI actually decreases with advanced disease as vertical translocation occurs[1,28]. The presence of vertical translocation is an ominous sign and in our analysis of 116 patients with this condition they were more severely disabled than those patients with simple horizontal atlantoaxial subluxation, and ultimately had a poorer long-term. survival as assessed by Kaplan–Meier survival curves[1,29,30]. Dvorak has suggested that a spinal cord diameter of less than 6 mm in flexion[31] as assessed by MRI should be an indication for surgery. Our own analysis of spinal cord morphometry has shown that once the spinal cord area is below 45 mm[2] the chances of a neurological recovery are very poor indeed[28].

Surgical techniques

A full description of all the surgical approaches and methods of fixation is beyond the scope or remit of this chapter. A transoral decompression of the dens is illustrated, along with a posterior occipitocervical fixation Figs 37.3 and 37.4.

From careful inspection of the preoperative radiological studies the surgeon has to decide where the major area of compression *anterior or posterior* is, and at what level(s) is it occurring, that is *cervicomedullary, atlantoaxial, subaxial, or a combination of these.* The next problem is to decide whether there is instability present preoperatively, or will it be created following surgical decompression? The influence of resection of the dens has been formally studied by Dickman *et al.* but the answer to these questions almost by definition is yes as the rheumatoid inflammatory process will destroy both ligaments and bone alike. For the atlantoaxial region this will involve the transverse ligament with atlantoaxial subluxation occurring, and this would have been the indication for surgery originally.

Anterior approaches include the transoral approach for resection of the dens or associated pannus; and the standard Cloward anterolateral approach to the anterior subaxial spine [32,33].

The **posterior approach** to either the posterior craniocervical junction or cervical spine is through the standard midline approach with subperiosteal dissection of the muscles from the spinous processes, lamina, and occipital bone.

Healing in the rheumatoid patient is poor due to a combination of steroids, cytotoxic agents, osteopenia, and general debility. Therefore careful attention has to be paid to stabilization. In the opinion of the authors, too much attention has been given to achieving bony fusion. This is important but an instrumented fixation will rarely fail in the elderly rheumatoid patient

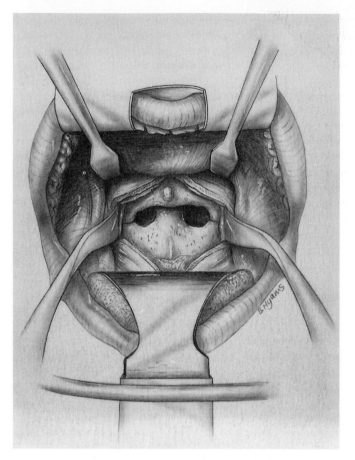

Fig. 37.3   Schematic drawing of transoral exposure. A midline vertical incision in the pharynx exposes the arch of C1 and anterior bony of C2.

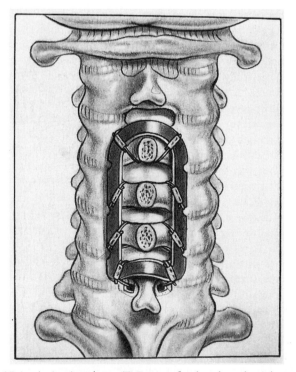

Fig. 37.4   A titanium loop (Ti-Frame) fixed to be subaxial cervical spine with titanium multistranded cables (Sof'wire). This can be attached to occiput to effect an occipitocervical fixation.

who will place little demands on the spinal instrumentation. Harvesting a bone graft is not without complications and will cause significant pain. For occipitocervical fixations we rely purely on instrumentation and do not supplement this with a bone graft in order to decrease operative morbidity. In our prospective follow-up of 256 patients there have been very few instances of instrumentation failure (only 3 per cent of patients had broken wires, there were no instances of failure of Ransford loop—unpublished data). We currently use posterior transarticular screw fixation method to stabilize the atlantoaxial joint. This technique is inappropriate in 20 per cent of patients due to variations of the vertebral artery groove [34] and also in patients with significant vertical translocation [35]. Nonetheless, this provides true three-point fixation and is superior to the previously used methods of Brooks and Gallie [36].

Surgical results

There are many ways of assessing outcome following spinal fixation. These would include the fusion rates, and standard operative morbidity and mortality figures which are summarized in Tables 37.4 and 37.5. But surely patients are interested in more than this? They would be interested to know whether their pain will improve, will their neurological deficit get better, and if so, by how much? A summary of the findings in the literature is presented in Table 37.6. The use of neurological outcome scales, such as the Ranawat class or Steinbrocker's grades used by previous investigators, has the advantage of standardization but really only provides a thumb-nail sketch of outcome (Table 37.7).

A useful way of describing outcome is by the use of functional questionnaires. A popular questionnaire which has been well validated is the Stanford Health Assessment Questionnaire HAQ devised by Fries *et al.*[37]. Wollheim's group used this to characterize functional recovery following occipitocervical fixation in 20 patients[38] and found there was little functional improvement. We have also used the Stanford HAQ and reported the change in function following surgery for 134 Ranawat class IIIA-B

Table 37.5 Documented mortality rates for cervical spine surgery on patients with rheumatoid arthritis

Authors	Series	Percentage mortality (%)
Boden[27]	7/42	18
Clark[52]	0/41	0
Conaty and Mongan[53]	3/38	8
Crellin[61]	2/11	18
Fehring[54]	1/17	6
Ferlic[55]	2/15	13
Heywood[25]	2/26	8
Papadopoulos[26]	1/17	6
Peppelman[57]	4/110	4
Ranawat[2]	3/33	9
Santavirta[62]	0/34	0
Stanley[63]	2/25	8
Stirrat[64]	0/28	0
Thompson[59]	1/12	8
Zoma[60]	3/32	10
Overall	31/481	6.4 %

patients[21]. We then attempted to reduce the extraneous noise or redundant questions from the original instrument by statistical maneuvres including Principal Components Analysis. The resulting questionnaire, which we have called the Myelopathy Disability Index (Table 37.8), has good psychometric properties including reliability, validity, and responsiveness. Eigen analysis shows that it is measuring mainly one dimension of disability. There are statistical associations with the Myelopathy Disability Index and spinal cord area, response to surgery, and indeed long-term survival (Kaplan-Meier Analysis)[24]. Occipitocervical pain is best assessed by means of a visual analogue scale and the results of surgery are very good indeed in this respect. Unfortunately there is no literature on the success of C2 nerve blocks with local anesthetic and steroid which these two authors have found to be successful for both surgical and non-surgical patient alike.

New frontiers

The management of the rheumatoid spine is an exciting area with many still unresolved issues. Surgical technique is fairly well established, indications and complication management is not. Future developments are likely in the field of surgical instrumentation but will essentially be refinements rather than any radical change of direction. It should be emphasized that surgery to the rheumatoid spine is not commonly performed and should stay concentrated in centers of excellence as there is little margin for error in these frail, debilitated patients. The concentration of surgical experience will hopefully continue to produce dividends. Other areas of interest are in the commercial availability of human bone morphogenic protein. In animal experiments, this evokes very prompt bony fusion[39]. Phase 1 clinical trials are currently underway. Neuroprotective agents are been developed for use following spinal cord injury with much of the research background to the development of these new agents being common to traumatic brain injury.

Table 37.4 Fusion rates reported in the literature from 'pure rheumatoid' series

Author	Successful osseous fusion	Fusion rate %
Boden[27]	32/35	91
Clark[52]	36/41	88
Conaty and Mongan[53]	25/31	81
Fehring[54]	12/16	75
Ferlic[55]	6/12	50
Heywood[25]	21/30	70
Milbrink[56]	11/12	92
Papadopoulos[26]	13/17	76
Peppelman[57]	67/77	87
Ranawat[2]	20/25	80
Santavirta[58]	16/18	89
Thompson[59]	10/11	91
Zoma[60]	18/30	60
Overall	287/355	83%

Table 37.6 Outcome in several recent surgical series

Author	No. with neurological improvement	% with neurological improvement	No. with significantly reduced pain	% with pain reduction	No. with overall non-specified improvement
Boden[27]	25/42	60	–	–	–
Clark[52]	11/41	27	21/23	91	27/41 'clinical'
Conaty[53]	12/22	55	31/35	89	22/35 'satisfactory'
Fehring[54]	8/11	73	7/11	63	10/14
Ferlic[55]			8/15	53	8/15
Heywood[65]	7/8	88	12/12	100	–
Milbrink[56]	8/9	75			5/12 by 1 ARA grade
Milbrink[56]	10/12	83	16/19	84	–
Peppelman[57]	78/90	87		–	–
Ranawat[2]	8/17	47		–	18/33
Santavirta[62]	8/14	57	12/15	80	–
Santavirta[66]	6/8	75	30/36	83	–
Thompson[59]	3/6	50			84 per cent 'satisfactory'
Zoma[60]	19/29	66	23/32	72	23/40 'overall success'
Total	203/309	66%	160/199	80%	N/A

Table 37.7 Ranawat neurological disability classification and the American Rheumatism Association grading system (ARA) for functional disability[2, 67]

STEINBROCKER or ARA grading system for functional disability
I—Complete ability to carry out all the usual duties without handicaps.
II—Adequate for normal activities despite handicap of discomfort or limited motion of one of the joints.
III—Limited to little or none of the duties of usual occupation or self-care.
IV—Incapacitated largely or wholly bed-ridden or confined to a wheelchair with little or no self-care.

RANAWAT'S neurological classification
I—No neurological deficit (normal neurological condition)
II—Subjective weakness with hyperreflexia and dyesthesias
III A—Objective weakness and long-tract signs but able to walk
III B—Quadraparetic and non-ambulatory

References

1. Casey A.T., Crockard H.A., Geddes J.F., Stevens J. Vertical translocation: the enigma of the disappearing atlantodens interval in patients with myelopathy and rheumatoid arthritis. Part I. Clinical, radiological, and neuropathological features. *J Neurosurg*, 1997;87:856–62.
2. Ranawat C.S., O'Leary P., Pellicci P., Tsairis P., Marchisello P., Dorr L. Cervical spine fusion in rheumatoid arthritis. *J Bone Joint Surg Am*, 1979;61:1003–10.
3. Redlund J.I., Pettersson H. Radiographic measurements of the cranio-vertebral region. Designed for evaluation of abnormalities in rheumatoid arthritis. *Acta Radiol Diagn Stockh*, 1984;25:23–8.
4. Teigland J., Ostensen H., Gudmundsen T.E. Radiographic measurements of occipito-atlanto-axial dislocation in rheumatoid arthritis. *Scand J Rheumatol*, 1990;19:105–14.
5. McRae D.L. The significance of abnormalities of the cervical spine. *Am J Roentgenol*, 1960;84:3–25.

Table 37.8 Example of a myelopathy disability index[24] derived from the Stanford HAQ[37]

Please tick the response which best describes your usual abilities over the past week	Without ANY difficulty	With SOME difficulty	With MUCH difficulty	Unable to do
Score (office use only)	0	1	2	3
STANDING Are you able to:				
• Get in and out of bed?		√		
• Stand up from an armless chair?	√			
EATING Are you able to:				
• Cut your meat?		√		
• Lift a full cup or glass to your mouth?	√			
WALKING Are you able to:				
• Walk outdoors on flat ground?	√			
• Climb up five steps?	√			
HYGIENE Are you able to:				
• Wash and dry your entire body?	√			
• Get on and off the toilet		√		
GRIP Are you able to:				
• Open jars which have previously opened?		√		
ACTIVITIES Are you able to:				
• Get in and out of car?	√			
DRESSING Are you able to:				
• Dress yourself, –including tying shoelaces, and doing buttons on a shirt or blouse?			√	
• **TOTAL** (office use only)	0	4	2	0

6. McRae D.L., Barnum A.S. Occipitalization of the atlas. *Am J Roentgenol*, 1953;70:23–46.

7. McGregor M. The significance of certain measurements of the skull in the diagnosis of basilar impression. *Br J Radiol*, 1948;21:171–181.

8. Clark C.R. Cervical spine involvement in rheumatoid arthritis. *Iowa Med*, 1984;74:57–62.

9. Kauppi M., Hakala M. Prevalence of cervical spine subluxations and dislocations in a community-based rheumatoid arthritis population. *Scand J Rheumatol*, 1994;23:133–6.

10. Stevens J.C., Cartlidge N.E., Saunders M., Appleby A., Hall M., Shaw D.A. Atlantoaxial subluxation and cervical myelopathy in rheumatoid arthritis. *Q J Med*, 1971;40:391–408.

11. Mathews J.A. Atlanto-axial subluxation in rheumatoid arthritis. A 5-year follow-up study. *Ann Rheum Dis*, 1974;33:526–31.

12. Pellicci P.M., Ranawat C.S., Tsairis P., Bryan W.J. A prospective study of the progression of rheumatoid arthritis of the cervical spine. *J Bone Joint Surg Am*, 1981;63:342–50.

13. Rana N.A. Natural history of atlanto-axial subluxation in rheumatoid arthritis. *Spine*, 1989;14:1054–6.

14. Smith P.H., Sharp J., Kellgren J.H. Natural history of rheumatoid cervical subluxations. *Ann Rheum Dis*, 1972;31:222–3.

15. Winfield J., Cooke D., Brook A.S., Corbett M. A prospective study of the radiological changes in the cervical spine in early rheumatoid disease. *Ann Rheum Dis*, 1981;40:109–14.

16. Henderson F.C., Geddes J.F., Crockard H.A. Neuropathology of the brainstem and spinal cord in end-stage rheumatoid arthritis: implications for treatment. *Annals Rheum Dis*, 1993;52:629–37.

17. Mikulowski P., Wollheim F.A., Rotmil P., Olsen I. Sudden death in rheumatoid arthritis with atlanto-axial dislocation. *Acta Med Scand*, 1975;198:445–51.

18. Marks J.S., Sharp J. Rheumatoid cervical myelopathy. *Q J Med*, 1981;50:307–19.

19. Meijers K.A., van B.G., Luyendijk W., Duijfjes F. Dislocation of the cervical spine with cord compression in rheumatoid arthritis. *J Bone Joint Surg Br.* 1974;56-B:668–80.

20. Allebeck P., Ahlbom A., Allander E. Increased mortality among persons with rheumatoid arthritis, but where RA does not appear on the death certificate. *Scand J Rheumatol*, 1981;10:301–306.

21. Casey A.T., Crockard H.A., Bland J.M., Stevens J., Moskovich R., Ransford A.O. Surgery on the rheumatoid cervical spine for the non-ambulant myelopathic patient-too much, too late? *Lancet*, 1996;347(9007):1004–7.

22. Sunahara N., Matsunaga S., Mori T., Ijiri K., Sakou T. Clinical course of conservatively managed rheumatoid arthritis patients with myelopathy. *Spine*, 1997;22:2603–7.

23. Corbett M., Dalton S., Young A., Silman A., Shipley M. Factors predicting death, survival and functional outcome in a prospective study of early rheumatoid disease over fifteen years. *Br J Rheumatol*, 1993;32:717–23.

24. Casey A.T., Bland J.M., Crockard H.A. Development of a functional scoring system for rheumatoid arthritis patients with cervical myelopathy. *Ann Rheum Dis*, 1996;55:901–6.

25. Heywood A.W., Learmonth I.D., Thomas M. Cervical spine instability in rheumatoid arthritis. *J Bone Joint Surg Br*, 1988;70:702–7.

26. Papadopoulos S.M., Dickman C.A., Sonntag V.K. Atlantoaxial stabilization in rheumatoid arthritis. *J Neurosurg*, 1991;74:1–7.

27. Boden S.D., Dodge L.D., Bohlman H.H., Rechtine G.R. Rheumatoid arthritis of the cervical spine. A long-term analysis with predictors of paralysis and recovery. *J Bone Joint Surg (Am)*, 1993;75:1282–97.

28. Casey A.T., Crockard H.A., Bland J.M., Stevens J., Moskovich R., Ransford A. Predictors of outcome in the quadriparetic nonambulatory myelopathic patient with rheumatoid arthritis: a prospective study of 55 surgically treated Ranawat class IIIb patients. *J Neurosurg*, 1996;85:574–81.

29. Casey A.T., Crockard A. In the rheumatoid patient: surgery to the cervical spine. *Br J Rheumatol*, 1995;34:1079–86.

30. Casey A.T., Crockard H.A., Stevens J. Vertical translocation. Part II. Outcomes after surgical treatment of rheumatoid cervical myelopathy. *J Neurosurg*, 1997;87:863–9.

31. Dvorak J., Grob D., Baumgartner H., Gschwend N., Grauer W., Larsson S. Functional evaluation of the spinal cord by magnetic resonance imaging in patients with rheumatoid arthritis and instability of upper cervical spine. *Spine*, 1989;14:1057–64.

32. Crockard H.A., Essigman W.K., Stevens J.M., Pozo J.L., Ransford A.O., Kendall B.E. Surgical treatment of cervical cord compression in rheumatoid arthritis. *Ann Rheum Dis*, 1985; 44:809–16.

33. Crockard H.A., Pozo J.L., Ransford A.O., Stevens J.M., Kendall B.E., Essigman W.K. Transoral decompression and posterior fusion for rheumatoid atlanto-axial subluxation. *J Bone Joint Surg Br*, 1986;68:350–6.

34. Madawi A.A., Casey A.T., Solanki G.A., Tuite G., Veres R., Crockard H.A. Radiological and anatomical evaluation of the atlantoaxial transarticular screw fixation technique. *J Neurosurg*, 1997;86:961–8.

35. Casey A.T.H., Madawi A.A., Veres R., Crockard H.A. Is the technique of posterior transarticular screw fixation suitable for rheumatoid atlantoaxial subluxation. *Br J Neurosurg*, 1997;11508–519.

36. Montesano P.X. Biomechanics of Cervical Spine Internal Fixation. *Spine*, 1991;16(3 suppl.):S10–S16.

37. Fries J.F., Spitz P.W., Young D.Y. The dimensions of health outcomes: the health assessment questionnaire, disability and pain scales. *J Rheumatol*, 1982;9:789–93.

38. Hultquist R., Zygmunt S., Saveland H., Birch I.M., Wollheim F.A. Characterization and functional assessment of patients subjected to occipito-cervical fusion for rheumatoid atlanto-axial dislocation. *Scand J Rheumatol*, 1993;22:20–4.

39. Urist M., Hudak R. Radioimmunoassay of bone morphogenetic protein in serum: a tissue-specific parameter of bone metabolism. *Proc Soc Exp Biol Med*, 1984;4:472–475.

40. Lawrence J.S. Radiological cervical arthritis in populations. *Ann Rheum Dis*, 1976;35:365–71.

41. Symmons D.P.M., Barrett E.M., Bankhead C.R., Scott D.G.I., Silman A.J. The incidence of Rheumatoid Arthritis in the United Kingdom: Results from the Norfolk Arthritis Register. *Br J Rheumatol*, 1994;33:735–739.

42. Serre H., Simon L. Atlanto-axial dislocation in rheumatoid arthritis. *Rheumatism*, 1966;22:53–8.

43. Cabot A., Becker A. The cervical spine in rheumatoid arthritis. *Clin Orthop*, 1978.

44. Martel W. The occipito-atlanto-axial joints in rheumatoid arthritis and ankylosing spondylitis. *Am J Roentgenol*, 1961;86:230–240.

45. Conlon P.W., Isdale I.C., Rose B.S. Rheumatoid arthritis of the cervical spine. An analysis of 333 cases. *Ann Rheum Dis*, 1966;25:120–6.

46. Halla J.T., Hardin J.J. The spectrum of atlantoaxial facet joint involvement in rheumatoid arthritis [see comments]. *Arthritis Rheum*, 1990;33:325–9.

47. Mathews J.A. Atlanta-axial subluxation in rheumatoid arthritis. *Ann Rheum Dis*, 1969;28:260–6.

48. Meikle J.A., Wilkinson M. Rheumatoid involvement of the cervical spine. Radiological assessment. *Ann Rheum Dis*, 1971;30:154–61.

49. Ornilla E., Ansell B.M., Swannell A.J. Cervical spine involvement in patients with chronic arthritis undergoing orthopaedic surgery. *Ann Rheum Dis*, 1972;31:364–8.

50. Rasker J.J., Cosh J.A. Radiological study of cervical spine and hand in patients with rheumatoid arthritis of 15 years' duration: an assessment of the effects of corticosteroid treatment. *Ann Rheum Dis*, 1978;37:529–35.

51. Isdale I.C., Conlon P.W. Atlanta–axial subluxation. A six-year follow-up report. *Ann Rheum Dis*, 1971;30:387–9.

52. Clark C.R., Goetz D.D., Menezes A.H. Arthrodesis of the cervical spine in rheumatoid arthritis. *J Bone Joint Surg Am*, 1989; 71:381–92.

53. Conaty J.P., Mongan E.S. Cervical fusion in rheumatoid arthritis. *J Bone Joint Surg Am*, 1981;**63**:1218–27.

54. Fehring T.K., Brooks A.L. Upper cervical instability in rheumatoid arthritis. *Clin Orthop*, 1987;**2**:137–148.

55. Ferlic D.C., Clayton M.L., Leidholt J.D., Gamble W.E. Surgical treatment of the symptomatic unstable cervical spine in rheumatoid arthritis. *J Bone Joint Surg Am*, 1975;**57**:349–54.

56. Milbrink J., Nyman R. Posterior stabilization of the cervical spine in rheumatoid arthritis: clinical results and magnetic resonance imaging correlation. *J Spinal Disord*, 1990;**3**:308–15.

57. Peppelman W.C., Kraus D.R., Donaldson W., Agarwal A. Cervical spine surgery in rheumatoid arthritis: improvement of neurologic deficit after cervical spine fusion. *Spine*, 1993;**18**:2375–9.

58. Santavirta S., Slatis P., Kankaanpaa U., Sandelin J., Laasonen E. Treatment of the cervical spine in rheumatoid arthritis. *J Bone Joint Surg Am*, 1988;**70**:658–67.

59. Thompson R.J., Meyer T.J. Posterior surgical stabilization for atlantoaxial subluxation in rheumatoid arthritis. *Spine*, 1985;**10**:597–601.

60. Zoma A., Sturrock R.D., Fisher W.D., Freeman P.A., Hamblen D.L. Surgical stabilisation of the rheumatoid cervical spine. A review of indications and results. *J Bone Joint Surg Br*, 1987;**69**:8–12.

61. Crellin R.Q., MacCabe J.J., Hamilton E.B. Surgical management of severe subluxations of the rheumatoid cervical spine. *Ann Rheum Dis*, 1970;**29**:565.

62. Santavirta S., Konttinen Y.T., Laasonen E., Honkanen V., Antti P.I., Kauppi M.. Ten year results of operations for rheumatoid cervical spine disorders. J Bone Joint Surg Br, 1991;73(1):116–20.

63. Stanley D., Laing R.J., Forster D.M., Getty C.J. Posterior decompression and fusion in rheumatoid disease of the cervical spine: redressing the balance. *J Spinal Disord*, 1994;**7**(5):439–43.

64. Stirrat A.N., Fyfe I.S. Surgery of the rheumatoid cervical spine. Correlation of the pathology and prognosis. *Clin Orthop*, 1993;**293**:135–143.

65. Heywood A.W., Meyers O.L. Rheumatoid arthritis of the thoracic and lumbar spine. *J Bone Joint Surg Br*, 1986;**68**(3):362–8.

66. Santavirta S., Konttinen Y.T., Sandelin J., Slatis P. Operations for the unstable cervical spine in rheumatoid arthritis. Sixteen cases of subaxial subluxation. *Acta Orthop Scand*, 1990;**61**(2):106–10.

67. Steinbrocker O., Traeger C.H., Batterman R.C. Therapeutic criteria in rheumatoid arthritis. *J Am Med Assoc*, 1949;**140**:659–662.

38 | Medical synovectomy (synoviorthesis)

C.J. Menkes and S. Diallo

Rheumatoid arthritis is not only a systemic disease but also a conjunction of local disorders. In many patients, the systemic therapy is unable to induce a complete remission and in cases of persistent synovitis the local treatment is an important part of a good management of the disease. The first step of local measures is the injection of short-acting or long-acting corticosteroids such as triamcinolone hexacetonide. Local measures are especially well suited to the treatment of patients with rheumatoid monoarthritis or oligoarthritis occurring as the only manifestation of the disease or persisting under systemic therapy.

Synovectomy

Earlier attempts of precocious and multiple synovectomy with the hope of preventing the extension and evolution of the disease failed[1,2]. Synovectomy is currently accepted as a symptomatic treatment of joint or tendon sheath involvement before the occurrence of local destruction, at an early stage of the disease. The surgical removal of an inflamed tendon sheath can often prevent the tendon from rupturing. It is especially indicated at the hand level for extensor and flexor tendon involvement. This may be combined with an articular synovectomy and joint stabilization, and results in substantial improvement in hand function[3]. Synovectomy gives significant pain relief and usually a functional improvement of the affected joint[4–7]. The long-term benefit of the procedure is, however, not established[7,8]. A multicenter, controlled evaluation of synovectomy of the knees, metacarpophalangeal joints , and proximal interphalangeal joints of the fingers showed, 3 years later, no statistically significant differences in the progression of either marginal or subchondral erosions. Nevertheless, the synovectomized joints fared better than the controls in a number of features at the end of 1 year. During the 3-year observation period, exacerbations of active rheumatoid arthritis occurred with essentially equal frequency in synovectomized and control finger joints, but were somewhat less frequent in synovectomized knees[9,10]. Synovectomy has little place in the general treatment of rheumatoid arthritis or as a measure to prevent recurrent articular damage. It is still of value in selected joints, especially of the hand, and as help to prevent rupture of extensor tendons[3,9].

The main disadvantages of conventional surgical synovectomy are the relatively major surgical trauma with consequent discomfort to the patient, the presence of a scar, the necessity of rehabilitation, the risk of postoperative stiffness of the joint[11], and the cost.

Arthroscopic synovectomy

With the exception of hand surgery and especially of tendon sheath involvement, conventional synovectomy has been progressively replaced in the last years by percutaneous arthroscopy-assisted synovectomy with the hope of reducing the disadvantages of open surgery. It is mostly used in the knee, shoulder, and elbow joint. Smaller joints such as the wrist can also be treated, but this requires specially trained and skillful surgeons[3,11–16]. Arthroscopic synovectomies are most often performed under general or spinal anesthesia but sometimes under local anesthesia. After introduction of a motor-driven resector, a subtotal synovectomy of the anterior part of the knee (that is the suprapatellar bursa, femoral gutters, fat pad, intercondylar notch, and perimeniscal areas) is performed as completely as possible, considering that the maximum time of a pneumatic tourniquet is 90 minutes[12]. The approach of the posterior part of the knee is more difficult, with possible complications due to the presence of neurovascular structures[17]. We try to avoid it. At the end of the procedure a draining tube is sometimes left in the joint for a few hours. The patient is discharged the same day or preferably after 3 or 4 days of bedrest in the hospital. Comparing long-term results of randomized open or arthroscopic synovectomy, Ryu et al.[18] found a recurrence rate of 73 per cent after arthroscopy with an effect of the procedure for only 18 months on average compared to a recurrence rate of only 37 per cent with open surgery, persisting for an average of 75 months. Arthroscopic synovectomy resulted in less postoperative pain, no loss of range of motion, no need for prolonged rehabilitation, shorter hospital stay, lower incidence of osteoarthritic changes, perhaps as a consequence of the partial synovectomy, and earlier return to the daily life, compared to open synovectomy. After a mean follow-up of 32 months, Ayral et al.[12] found good and very good overall results in 61 per cent of 23 patients. Efficacy of arthroscopic synovectomy in relation to Larsen's radiological stage at baseline failed to disclose any correlation with outcome, but there was a bias of selection, since only four patients were in Larsen's stage 4 or 5. The mean time needed to recover adequate function was 4.6 weeks and the procedure was rated very acceptable by 32 per cent of patients, acceptable by 61 per cent unpleasant by 3.5 per cent, and very unpleasant by 3.5 per cent One case each of hemarthrosis and stiffness of the knee were recorded, with a full recovery in both cases[12]. Ogilvie-Harris et al.[17] treated 112 patients with a mean follow-up of 3 years. There was no significant difference in the range of movement pre- and postoperatively and long-term results were stable, as 80 per cent of patients still had either no or very mild recurrence of synovitis. Persistent good results were also reported by Fiocco et al.[19] at 36 months with a clinical remission in 45.7 per cent of the 17 knees treated.

Arthroscopic synovectomy currently used for the knee was also indicated for smaller joints but experience is still limited and there is a doubt about the innocuity of the method. There was a short-term improvement for the 18 wrists treated by Adolfsson and Nylander[11] but only early involvement without tenosynovitis was included and the effect of a previous intra-articular corticosteroid injection is not considered. For the elbow, Lee and Morrey[20] reported, in 11 patients and 14 arthroscopic synovectomies, 93 per cent short-term rating of excellent or good on the Mayo Elbow Performance Score. Unfortunately, after an average of 42 months, only 57 per cent maintained excellent or good results. The results deteriorate more rapidly than after open synovectomy. Recognition of the short-term gain and the potential for serious nerve injury should be considered when discussing arthroscopic synovectomy of the elbow with patients[20]. Arthroscopic synovectomy of the shoulder is generally performed by following the standard techniques for shoulder arthroscopy. Drains are not placed routinely and complications include transient synovial fistulas and bleeding[21].

Recently, conventional arthroscopic synovectomy was compared to a laser assisted technique using the holmium YAG laser. The arthroscopist may use a cutting, coagulation, or tissue ablation mode. The laser allows a shorter time for procedures, a reduction in postoperative pain, and a decreased incidence of hemarthrosis. There is a concern of the possible linkage of laser use with the subsequent development of avascular necrosis The cost is also a major barrier[22].

Joint lavage

The rationale of articular irrigation is removal of cartilage debris, rice bodies, fibrin deposits, and cellular elements, and also reduction of the concentrations of proinflammatory cytokines, proteolytic enzymes, and other inflammatory agents[23,24]. It may be tried after failure of joint aspiration and simple corticosteroid injection. Lindsay et al.[25] performed a double-blind, controlled trial to compare joint lavage of rheumatoid knee with simple aspiration. A cannula with an internal diameter of 1.45 mm was introduced into the joint from the lateral side under local anesthesia. A total volume of 500 ml of a solution of dextrose and sodium chloride was injected into the joint. The fluid was reaspirated and discarded. In the control group the lavage solution by-passed the joint before being discarded. Both groups of patients had improved at 42 days, and joint irrigation did not provide extra benefit. When combining joint lavage and intra-articular triamcinolone acetonide injec-

tion, Fitzgerald et al.[26] found that the lavage group responded better compared with aspiration of the synovial fluid and intra-articular triamcinolone alone. Aspiration was performed using a 14 gauge needle and the lavage was performed through the same needle with 60–120 ml of 0.9 per cent saline. Both groups of 10 patients were assessed at 12 weeks. Srinivasan et al.[27] randomly allocated 60 rheumatoid knee joints to receive one of three treatments: a steroid injection without washout, a joint washout only, or a joint washout with steroid injection. Due to time limitation in the outpatient department only 40 ml of normal saline was used in these patients. Patients who had a joint washout alone showed significantly less improvement compared to the other two groups, but there was no significant additional benefit from performing a joint washout prior to a corticosteroid injection. These results are not in agreement with the findings of Sharma et al.[23]. They found that office arthroscopic lavage with 750–1500 ml of sterile isotonic saline with the injection at the end of the procedure of 40 mg triamcinolone hexacetonide, was beneficial for at least 12 weeks in eight of the nine patients so treated, but there were no controls.

There is no clearcut and established indication for joint lavage. Different techniques have been used and comparison of the results is difficult. For instance, closed needle lavage probably does not allow a complete irrigation of the joint[23]. Washout should be considered in patients who have not responded to repeated steroid injections[27] and before prescribing a chemical or radioactive synoviorthesis. It has the advantage of allowing a synovial biopsy at the same time, to confirm the rheumatoid involvement of the joint and exclude the rare possibility of an associated non-RA lesion such as tuberculosis or sarcoidosis.

Medical synovectomy (synoviorthesis)

The term synoviorthesis was proposed by F. Delbarre[28] to designate chemical or radioactive intra-articular injections, which could induce a beneficial effect on the diseased synovium. Synoviorthesis should be considered when intra-articular injection of a long-acting corticosteroid has failed, and before attempting invasive procedures such as open or arthroscopic synovectomy. It consists of a symptom-reducing local treatment, applied to joints with active synovitis, persisting in spite of the systemic treatment. Synoviorthesis alone, should only be considered in patients with monoarticular or perhaps oligoarticular and histologically confirmed rheumatoid involvement.

Chemical synoviorthesis

Intra-articular injection of osmic acid was originally proposed by von Reiss and Swensson in 1951[29]. They were looking for a substance with a potential to suppress joint pain by the destruction of nerve endings in the synovium. The first attempts of local treatment were rapidly abandoned due to severe, painful, inflammatory reactions immediately following the injection. A

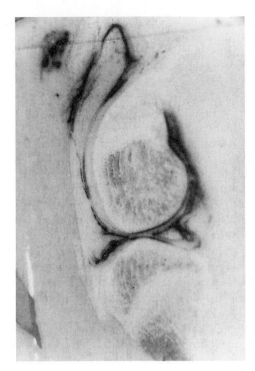

Fig. 38.1 Intra-articular injection of osmic acid in a rabbit joint showing the black coloration of synovium and cartilage. See also Plate 33.

few years later, the idea came of combining osmic acid with a local anesthetic and, in particular, with a local corticosteroid, to suppress or at least reduce the local reaction[30]. Osmic acid was for several years much used in the Scandinavian countries. Kajander and Ruotsi[31] treated 447 knee joints with 46 per cent having a very good improvement after 1 year; similar results were reported by Martio *et al.*[32] and Virkkunen *et al.*[33].

Osmium is transformed by oxidation into osmium tetroxide (O_sO_4) which gives rise to osmic acid in aqueous solution. The product reacts with proteins in the synovium, and with cell membrane lipids, resulting in the formation of black-colored, very stable oxides (Fig. 38.1). The intra-articular injection produces necrosis of inflamed synovial tissue. Synovial repair is accomplished initiated by histiocytic phagocytosis, with a storage of reduced osmium, and fibroblast stimulation. In some instances osmium is also permanently fixed in the adipose tissue. The presence of this heavy metal with the atomic number 76 may cause radiological opacities without clinical significance[34,35]. Some of the injected osmium is rapidly cleared into the circulation and subsequently excreted in the urine, which attains a blackish color. Transient proteinuria, microscopic hematuria, or glycosuria was often noted. This reverted rapidly and had disappeared 3 days after the injection, leaving no permanent renal damage[36,37].

The aqueous solution of osmic acid is injected in a concentration of 1 per cent. The volume of the solution depends on the joint to be treated: 10 ml are injected in an adult knee, 10 ml in a hip, 5 ml in an elbow or ankle, and 3 ml in a wrist. The injection must be strictly intra-articular, and radiological control of the position of the needle for joints other than the knee is mandatory. Osmic acid is not used for finger joints due to the

risk of skin necrosis by leakage of the product in the soft tissues after the injection. For the same reason one should avoid injecting joints other than the knee and the hip[38]. Injected joints are immobilized for a couple of hours, and weight bearing is allowed after 2 days[39].

Satisfactory results were reported in approximately 55 to 70 per cent of the patients 6 months after treatment and in 45 to 70 per cent of the patients after 1 year[31,32,38,40–43], mainly at an early stage of the disease.

Chemical synoviorthesis is cheap and relatively easy to apply. The limited experience in some countries may relate to availability of local expertise and safety concerns, and to perceived lack of efficacy[43]. There is a need for more controlled studies. Comparing intra-articular triamcinolone hexacetonide alone and osmic acid combined with triamcinolone hexacetonide in two groups of patients with persistent synovitis of the knee, Anttinen and Oka[44] found that both treatments produced long-lasting improvement in the treated knee but osmic acid seemed to potentiate the effect of the steroid.

Nissilä *et al.*[39] randomized 99 rheumatoid knee joints to receive either 10 ml of 1 per cent osmic acid solution or 10 ml of physiological sodium chloride solution and 50 mg of hydrocortisone acetate. After 6 months, effusion was found in 17 out of 52 joints treated with osmic acid (33 per cent) and in 27 out of 47 joints treated with placebo (57 per cent), the difference in the percentages being statistically significant.

The concern about safety is mainly based on animal experiments demonstrating cartilage damage after intra-articular injection of osmic acid[45–47]. In young animals, a dose-ranging effect on the cartilage was clearly demonstrated with, perhaps, a protective effect of the carragenan induced experimental arthritis[45]. In clinical practice, osmic acid causes limited superficial damage to the cartilage. Nissilä *et al.*[48] compared punch biopsy specimens from the cartilage of the lateral condyle of the femur taken from patients during open knee synovectomy. Eleven patients had never received osmic acid injections, whereas 18 had had such injections 1–24 months prior to surgery. By light microscopy only minor differences could be seen. On electron microscopy, changes in the cartilage were visible only in samples treated with osmic acid with increased amounts of dark-staining cell debris. The perilacunar matrix appeared normal and there was no irregularity of collagen fibers at the surface of the cartilage. The superficial lesion of the cartilage does not necessarily imply any clinical consequences in the form of subsequent degenerative joint disease[48]. An extensive radiological follow-up was performed by Nissilä[49], in 52 adults and 31 children treated with osmic acid in one knee joint 8–18 years previously. On the bases of the study it was concluded that no clinically significant cartilage damage was caused by osmic acid.

We currently use osmic acid for chemical synoviorthesis after the failure of intra-articular injection of triamcinolone hexacetonide alone, combining the two products, as suggested by Anttinen and Oka[44], particularly in young patients with hip or knee involvement, thereby avoiding the injection of radioactive compounds. In view of the experimental findings, osmic acid must be carefully handled. The given dose must be related to the age of the patient and the volume of the joint. It is not necessary to inject more than 100 mg (10 ml of 1 per cent solution) in the knee of an adult. The injection can be repeated once, in case of failure, after a delay of a minimum of 6 months.

Radiation synoviorthesis

It had been known for a long time that injection of a radioactive suspension, mainly radioactive gold, was useful in the treatment of malignant effusions in serous membranes. The first reported intra-articular injection of radioactive material was in 1952[50]. Ansell *et al.* in 1963[51] and Makin *et al.* in 1964[52] reported on extensive use of radioactive gold to treat chronic effusion of the knee. Ansell *et al.*[51] noted that the patients with marked effusion and relatively little soft tissue swelling showed the best results. After 1 year, a comparison of bilateral knee injection, where one knee had received the active preparation and the other had received a placebo, demonstrated a better clinical effect on the treated side. It was suggested that due to deeper penetration of radiation, yttrium should be more suitable to treat the thick rheumatoid synovium of the knee.

Radiation synovectomy requires only the injection into the synovial cavity of an isotope with the appropriate nuclear, chemical, and biochemical characteristics. It is regularly practiced in Europe, Australia, and Canada. Due to the fear of potential local or general adverse effects, the technique is virtually unused in the United States[53]. In spite of a very large clinical experience, extending over the last 30 years, with a quantity of clinical reports, there is still an urgent need for well-constructed, prospective controlled studies, evaluating results and hazards.

The isotope used for radiation synoviorthesis should be easy to obtain, non-toxic, and chemically pure. Tissue destruction should be effected by a beta emission of sufficient energy to penetrate the synovium. To minimize unwanted whole-body irradiation, there should be little or no associated gamma emission as its energy is released not only in the joint but also far away from it. Whole-body radiation, one of the main concerns in connection with this treatment, can be reduced considerably by using an isotope with a short half-life[54,55].

The isotope must be linked to a colloid to impede its escape from the joint. A metal transformed to a colloidal form loses the biochemical and physiological properties of its soluble form, and is transformed into a radioactive carrier, only active locally[55]. The ideal colloidal particles should be biodegradable, have strong affinity for synovium, and undergo little or no leakage from the joint. The ideal preparation should be fast and easy to formulate, reproducible, non-toxic, non-allergenic, and stable *in vitro*[54,55]. After injection, radioactive colloids are distributed in the joint in conformity with the synovium. In rabbit knees, the cartilage surface is usually devoid of radioactivity[56].

The effect on synovitis depends essentially on the energy absorbed at the surface of, and within, the synovium. The homogeneity of the irradiation depends on the size of the colloidal particles. With small particles one obtains a more uniform irradiation, but also a high incidence of extra-articular spread. The ideal particle size is around 100 nm[55].

Currently, therapeutic applications of pure beta emitters are confined to three radionuclides with a short half-life: yttrium 90, rhenium 186, and erbium 169[57] (Table 38.1). Yttrium is very penetrating (3.6 mm) and should be used for severe proliferative forms of synovitis, specially of the knee. Rhenium ([186]Re) has the same physical characteristics as [198]Au but without unwanted gamma emission and is suitable for the treatment of medium sized joints, such as the shoulder, the elbow, the wrist, the hip, and the ankle. Erbium ([169]Er) has a low radiation energy and is mainly used for digital joints[55,57,59,60].

Radiocolloids are injected in combination with a corticosteroid derivative. Except for the knee, X-ray contrast medium is used to check correct position of the needle and to visualize any communication with serous bursas or synovial tendon sheaths. A three-way tap is used and the needle is flushed before removal to avoid back flow and skin necrosis due to radiation. Use of local steroids and immobilization of the treated joint for 3 days, reduce the escape of radioactivity and prevent painful local post-injection flare-up. The upper limbs are splinted but on lower limb joints we usebed rest only, since knee splinting can cause pulmonary embolism[61,62].

Since in-patient care is costly, inconvenient, and increasingly difficult to arrange in some centers, a comparison was made between early discharge with 3 days bed rest at home and in-patient immobilization for 3 days; leakage rate of ^{90}Y from the joint was measured and its uptake in extra-articular sites, that is lymph nodes, liver, blood, and urine. Home patients were discharged after 6 hours with the knee in a firm crepe bandage. The retained knee activity was calculated using a gamma camera with a high energy collimator able to detect the Brems-strahlung induced by the beta-emitter radioisotope. Retention rates ranged from 72–100 per cent and retained knee activity of ^{90}Y was significantly reduced in patients discharged to rest at home. The retention of the radioisotope was not modified by intra-articular steroid but it correlated with the degree of joint inflammation as

Table 38.1 Radioisotopes for intra-articular therapy

Radioisotope	Half-life (days)	Emission	Max. radiation energy (MeV)	Soft tissue penetration (mm)	
				Average	Maximum
Yttrium 90	2.7	beta	2.20	3.6	11
Rhenium 186	3.7	beta + Erbium 169	0.98	1.2	3.7
Erbium 169	9.5	beta	0.34	0.3	1
Dysprosium 165	140 min	beta + gamma rare	1.30		5.7
Samarium 153	1.95	beta + gamma rare	0.70		2.5

assessed by radionuclide blood pool scan of Technetium 99 in methylene bisphosphonate.

Dosimetry

The appropriate radiation dose for each clinical situation is difficult to define and the therapeutic doses actually administered are for a large part empirical, even though a mathematical model of the rheumatoid joint was recently proposed to estimate absorbed dose and dose rate distribution in treated joints[64]. It is not easy to define an adequate radiation dose. The adsorbed dose, calculated in Grays, depends not only on the radioisotope (energy of beta-emission and half-life) and the injected amount (activity in MBq), but also on the final distribution of the radioactivity. The thickness of the pannus and the folds of the synovium influence the volume of tissue irradiated[55].

The first attempt of intra-articular knee injection with 37 MBq (1 mCi) of ^{198}Au was not effective[50] but Ansell *et al.*[51] estimated, based on the volume of the joint cavity, that a dose of 370 MBq (10 mCi) would be required . Compared to gold 198, Yttrium 90 was more effective with no statistical difference between a low dose of 111–148 MBq (3–4 mCi) and a higher dose of 222 MBq (6 mCi) but with less local side-effects[65,66]. We also compared the effect of 37 or 74 MBq of ^{198}Au for the treatment of rheumatoid wrist and found a significant increase of efficacy by doubling the dose[67].

The dosimetry that we currently use is mostly based on clinical experience, demonstrating a clinical result with the lowest possible dose of radiation (Table 38.2). In general, we use 148 MBq (4 mCi) of ^{90}Y in synovitis of the knee; ^{186}Re is given in doses of 74 MBq (2 mCi) in the wrist, elbow, shoulder, and ankle, and 111 MBq (3 mCi) in the hip; ^{169}Er is given in doses of 37 MBq (1 mCi) in the metacarpophalangeal (MCP) joint and 18 MBq (0.5 mCi) in the proximal interphalangeal (PIP) joint[57].

Clinical experience

The efficacy of radiosynoviorthesis is generally accepted, although there still is some doubts regarding long-term safety with regard to possible leakage of the beta-emitter from the joint. The efficacy of ^{90}Y was first demonstrated by the statistical comparison of 146 knee rheumatoid arthritis randomized

between saline, non-radioactive yttrium (^{89}Y), and radio-active ^{90}Y. The difference was also significant in patients who received ^{90}Y in one knee and saline or ^{89}Y in the other[70]. A double-blind study of ^{169}Er injection into rheumatoid digital joints was carried out with saline as control; 201 joints in 36 patients were studied and prednisolone acetate was added to ^{169}Er in both groups. A definite improvement was observed in 55–58 per cent of cases with ^{169}Er and in 26–28 per cent of cases with saline, the difference being highly significant[71]. In another double blind study, Boussina *et al.*[72] used 35 paired joints injecting one joint of each pair with ^{169}Er and the other one with saline. Six months after synoviorthesis, good and excellent results were observed in 71 per cent of the joints treated with ^{169}Er compared with 40 per cent of controls (p < 0.01). The efficacy was present after 1 year. These patients had not responded to corticosteroid injections. The histological examination of the synovium of two joints 10 months after treatment showed large areas of fibrosis and no signs of inflammation in contrast to the control synovium, which still showed all the histological characteristics of rheumatoid synovitis. Ruotsi *et al.*[73] compared 83 digital joints injected with ^{169}Er and 54 digital joints injected with triamcinolone hexacetonide and found that both treatments produced alleviation of joint pain and swelling and improvement of grip strength. The remission rate was significantly higher at 1, 3, and 6 months after the long corticosteroid but the radiation dose was only half of the dose currently used[71,72]. No difference was found between ^{169}Er and methylprednisolone acetate at the usual doses, when digital joints were combined with wrists, with no previous steroid injections[74].

A randomized, prospective, controlled trial was recently published using ^{186}Re[75]. Three different treatment regimens for shoulder, elbow, wrist, hip, and ankle joints were compared, each including 50 joints. One group received ^{186}Re only, one a combination of ^{186}Re and triamcinolone hexacetonide, and one triamcinolone hexacetonide only. The combined injection of ^{186}Re and triamcinolone hexacetonide resulted in better clinical results and slower radiological progression after 3 years.

A number of uncontrolled studies indicate efficacy in the shoulder, elbow and hip, provided the joints were not destroyed. Thus in uncontrolled open studies ^{186}Re seemed to reduce pain in non-destroyed shoulder joints[76], elbows[77], and hips[78].

Two studies attempted repeat injections after poor initial response or relapse[79,68]. Although some effects were observed,

Table 38.2 Current dosimetry (MBq)

Joint	Source of beta-emitter		
	^{90}Y (citrate or silicate)	^{186}Re (sulfide)	^{169}Er (citrate)
knee	148–185 (4–5 mCi)		
hip		111 (3 mCi)	
shoulder		74 (2 mCi)	
elbow		74	
ankle		74	
wrist		74	
MCP			37 (1 mCi)
PIP			18 (0.5 mCi)

these were not impressive, in particular in non-responders to the first injection. Stucki *et al.*[68] observed beneficial effects of repeated injections only in those patients who had responded to the initial injection. Before repeating intra-articular injection of beta-emitters it is essential to consider the total dose of radiation already received by the patient, the potential risks of radiosynoviorthesis and the chance of success in comparison with open or arthroscopic synovectomy.

The long-term effect of ^{90}Y in knee-joint arthritis was evaluated by Szanto[80]; 33 patients with long-standing synovitis and effusion of the knee were treated by 3–4 mCi (111–148 MBq) of ^{90}Y with strict bed rest during the first 3 days after the injection. Excellent (resolution of all symptoms) or good results were recorded in 74 per cent at 3 months, in 77 per cent at 6 months, in 59 per cent at 1 year, in 44 per cent at 2 years, and in 40 per cent at 3.5 years. Of the 33 treated patients, three died and three others were excluded from the study. There was no radiological deterioration due to the treatment but the results were unsatisfactory in patients with severe articular destruction and instability prior to therapy.

Precautions and side-effects

Radiation synovectomy should be performed before the onset of joint destruction and is not indicated for patients with severe articular damage, dislocation, or instability. The radioisotope must be selected according to the joint to be treated. Accordingly, ^{90}Y is only suitable for the knee joint. Radiation necrosis was reported after injection of ^{9}Y in the ankle joint[81]. We are also aware of a case of radionecrosis of finger joints and of a wrist joint with median nerve radioneuritis after ^{90}Y injection.

The potential for leakage of radioactive particles from the joint is an important consideration when administering an intra-articular beta-emitter. Isomäki *et al.*[82] detected radioactive particles in vacuolar cavities in the knee joint synovium up to 6 days following intra-articular injection of ^{90}Y, probably indicating leakage to the lymphatics.

After intra-articular injection of ^{198}Au, Stevenson *et al.*[83] reported an 8.5 per cent incidence of chromosomal abnormalities with a 7.1 per cent incidence of dicentric forms in circulating blood lymphocytes. The incidence of chromosomal abnormalities was reduced by splinting the treated joint[84]. Colloid ^{90}Y may cause more lymphocyte abnormalities than silicate according to a small pilot study[85]. Chromosomal abnormalities and changes in peripheral lymphocytes are not uncommon after radiosynoviorthesis but the significance of these findings is unknown. It is reassuring that there has been no reported increase of cancer in association with this procedure after more than 30 years of use[86,87]. A case of chronic myeloid leukemia in a woman with Still's disease treated with ^{198}Au synoviorthesis[88] and a case of sarcoma of the groin lymph nodes[57] 2 years after ^{90}Y injection in the knee were reported but they could not be linked explicitly to the treatment.

Whole-body irradiation is due to a possible leakage (5–25 per cent) of radiocolloids. It can be reduced by strictly controlling the total dose of radioactivity administered to a patient and the technique of injection, especially in young patients, under 45 years. Dysprosium 165, a beta-emitter with a very short half-life of 140 min and a range in tissue of 5.7 mm, has been proposed to limit tissue irradiation[89]. The isotope was fixed on macroaggregates of ferric hydroxide. These are known to be taken up and enzymatically degraded by synovial tissue[90]. The comparison of ^{90}Y and ^{165}Dy showed that both were effective and equally safe[91]. The induction of micronuclei in peripheral lymphocytes of patients treated with ^{165}Dy ferric hydroxide macro aggregates (FHMA) or ^{90}Y silicate was not significantly increased, in either groups. The maximum increase in micronucleus frequency observed corresponded to a radiation dose to circulating cells of approximately 0.3 Gray[92].

FHMA may not be the ideal carrier system for long-lived radionuclides with low specific activities, and[165]Dy is not easily available due to its very short half-life[90]. A new class of agents for radiosynoviorthesis was developed using particles made from hydroxyapatite from bone with good biocompatibility features. Low levels of activity leaked from rabbit joints injected with samarium-153 (^{153}Sm) labeled particulate hydroxyapatite. Samarium-153 has a half-life of 46.3 h, maximum beta energy of 0.81 MeV, and an average soft-tissue penetration of 0.8 mm. There is also a spectrum of gamma decay including a 20 per cent abundant 130-keV photon. Eighteen patients with persistent rheumatoid knee synovitis were injected with 555 MBq (15 mCi) of ^{153}Sm particulate hydroxyapatite combined with triamcinolone hexacetonide. Symptom relief was maintained in 56 per cent of patients at 6 months and in 46 per cent of patients at 12 months following treatment. Mean extra-articular activity calculated from serial whole-body scans in 13 patients was 0.74 per cent of injected activity (range 0–3 per cent). Some difficulty was recognized in injecting a constant amount of activity due to the large size of the particles (5–45 micrometer). There is uncertainty as to whether the synovium irradiation will be as homogeneous as the irradiation obtained with the usual radiocolloids[90,93,94].

Conclusion

Medical synovectomy (synoviorthesis) is a symptomatic treatment, mainly effective on pain, swelling, and joint effusion. No ability to retard joint damage has been documented[69]. Concerns regarding local or general adverse effects have not been confirmed despite more than 30 years of clinical use. Practicing medical synovectomy requires careful selection of patients and a perfect technique to ensure strictly intra-articular injection. It is mandatory to consider the total dose of radioactive beta-emitter that a patients has received with a prudent limitation, empirically determined, to 555 MBq (15 mCi). In patients less than 45-years-old, radiosynoviorthesis is not recommended for knee joints or hip joints but can be applied to one or two small upper limb joints. The limitation of the radiation risk is facilitated by a step-up procedure, beginning with a long-acting corticosteroid, using chemical synovectomy in young patients for inferior limb joints, and open or arthroscopic synovectomy in case of joint relapse[95]. Medical synoviorthesis should not be repeated more than once before considering surgical synovectomy.

Only new trials using a uniform methodology and new radiological possibilities will confirm the efficacy and innocuity of chemical and radioactive synoviorthesis with an accurate comparison between the numerous preparations that have been suggested[96,97].

References

1. McEwen C. Early synovectomy in the treatment of rheumatoid arthritis. *N Engl J Med*, 1968;279:420–1.

2. Göbel D., Schultz W. Systemic effects of open and arthroscopic articulosynovectomy compared to radiosynoviorthesis in patients with rheumatoid arthritis. *Br J Rheumatol*, 1997;36: 402–3.

3. Tubiana R. Indications du traitement chirurgical de la polyarthrite rhumatoïde au niveau de la main et du membre supérieur. In: Tubiana R ed. *Traité de chirurgie de la main*, vol 5. Paris: Masson, 1995;490–515.

4. Ranawat C.S,. Ecker M.L., Straub L.R. Synovectomy and debridement of the knee in rheumatoid arthritis (a study of 60 knees). *Arthritis Rheum*, 1972; 15:571–81.

5. Graham J., Checketts R.G. Synovectomy of the knee-joint in rheumatoid arthritis. A long term follow-up. *J Bone Joint Surg*, 1973;55 B:786–95.

6. Ishikawa H., Ohno 0., Hirohata K. Long term results of synovectomy in rheumatoid patients. *J Bone Joint Surg*, 1986;68 A:198–205.

7. Böhler N., Lack N., Schwägerl W., Sollerman C., Teigland J., Thabe H., Tillmann K. Late results of synovectomy of wrist, MP, PIP joints: multicenter study. *Clin Rheumatol*, 1985;4:23–5.

8. Aschan W., Moberg E. A long term study of the effect of early synovectomy in rheumatoid arthritis. *Bull Hosp Joint Dis Orthop Inst*, 1984;44:106–21.

9. Arthritis Foundation Committee on Evaluation of Synovectomy. Multicenter evaluation of synovectomy in the treatment of rheumatoid arthritis. Report of results at the end of three years. *Arthritis Rheum*, 1977;20:765–71.

10. Arthritis and Rheumatism Council and British Orthopaedic Association. A controlled trial of synovectomy of the knee and metacarpophalangeal joints in rheumatoid arthritis. *Ann Rheum Dis*, 1976;35:437–42.

11. Adolfsson L., Nylander G. Arthroscopic synovectomy of the rheumatoid wrist. *J Hand Surg*, 1993;18 B:92–6.

12. Ayral X., Bonvarlet J.P., Simonnet J., Amor B., Dougados M. Arthroscopy assisted synovectomy in the treatment of chronic synovitis of the knee. *Rev Rhum* (Engl ed), 1997;64:215–26.

13. Smiley P. Wasilewski S.A. Arthroscopic synovectomy. *Arthroscopy*, 1990; 6:18–23.

14. Matsui N., Taneda Y., Ohta H., Itoh H., Tsubogushi S. Arthroscopic versus open synovectomy in the rheumatoid knee. *Int Orthop*, 1989;13:17–20.

15. Klein W., Jensen K.U. Arthroscopic synovectomy of the knee joint: indication, technique and follow-up results. *Arthroscopy*, 1988;4: 63–71.

16. Schmidt von K., Miehlke R.K. Die Arthroskopische Sunovektomie von Schulter und Ellenbogengelenk. *Beit Orth Traumatol*, 1990;37:11–12, 637–41.

17. Ogilvie-Harris D.J., Weisleder L. Arthroscopic synovectomy of the knee: is it helpful? *Arthroscopy*, 1995;11:91–5.

18. Ryu J., Saito S., Honda T., Shimakura Y., Sano S. Comparison between the arthroscopic and open synovectomies for rheumatoid knee. A retrospective and random study on the results of the two methods. *Ryumachi*, 1995;35:880–8.

19. Fiocco U., Cozzi L., Rigou C. Arthroscopic synovectomy in rheumatoid and psoriatic knee joint synovitis: long term outcome. *Br J Rheumatol*, 1996;35:463–470.

20. Lee B.P.H., Morrey B.F. Arthroscopic synovectomy of the elbow for rheumatoid arthritis: a prospective study. *J Bone Joint Surg*, 1997;79 B:770–2.

21. Matthews L.S., Labudde J.K. Arthroscopic treatment of synovial diseases of the shoulder. *Orthop Clin North Am*, 1993;24:101–9.

22. Wei N., Delauter S.K., Erlichman M.S. The holmium YAG laser in office based arthroscopy of the knee: comparison with standard interventional instruments in patients with arthritis. *J Rheumatol*, 1997;24:1806–8.

23. Sharma A., Baethge B.A., Acebes J.C., Lisse J.R. Arthroscopic lavage treatment in rheumatoid arthritis of the knee. *J Rheumatol*, 1996;23:1872–4.

24. Popert A.J., Scott D.L., Wainwright A.C., Walton K.W., Williamson N., Chapman J.H. Frequency of occurence, mode of development and significance of rice bodies in rheumatoid joints. *Ann Rheum Dis*, 1982;41:109–17.

25. Lindsay D.J., Ring E.F.J., Coorey P.F.J., Jayson M.I.V. Synovial irrigation in rheumatoid arthritis. *Acta Rheum Scand*, 1971;17:169–74.

26. Fitzgerald 0., Hanley J., Callan A., McDonald K., Molony J., Bresnihan B. Effects of joint lavage on knee synovitis in rheumatoid arthritis. *Br Rheumatol*, 1985;24:6–10.

27. Srinivasan A., Amos M., Webley M. The effects of joint washout and steroid injection compared with either joint washout or steroid alone in rheumatoid knee effusion. *Br J Rheumatol*, 1995;34:771–3.

28. Delbarre F., Cayla J., Menkes C.J., Aignan M., Roucayrol J.C., Ingrand J. Le traitement des rhumatismes par les synoviorthéses. *Rev Prat*, 1969;19:2737–58.

29. Von Reiss G., Swensson A. Intraarticular injection of osmic acid in painful joint affections. Acta Med Scand (suppl), 1951;259:27–32.

30. Berglof F.E. Osmic acid in arthritis therapy. *Acta Rheum Scand*, 1959;5:70–4.

31. Kajander A., Ruotsi A. The effects of intra-articular osmic acid on rheumatoid joint affections. *Ann Med Intern Fenn*, 1967;57:87–91.

32. Martio J., Isomäki H., Heikkola T., Laime V. The effect of intra-articular osmic acid in juvenile rheumatoid arthritis. *Scand J Rheumatol*, 1972;1:5–8.

33. Virkkunen M., Krusius F.E., Muroma A., Voutilainen A.V. Erfahrungen mit unblutiger synovectomie. *Med Hyg* (Genéve), 1965;23:423–4.

34. Lagier R., MacGee W., Boussina I. Synovial deposit of osmic acid after intra-articular injection. *Virchows Arch Path Anat Histol*, 1976;372:237–44.

35. Boussina I., Lagier R., Ott H., Fallet G.H. Osmium deposits detected by x-ray after synoviorthesis of the knee. Radiological, clinical and anatomical study. Scand J Rheumatol, 1976;5:53–9.

36. Nissilä M., Isomäki H., Jalava S. Reversible renal side effects of intra-articular osmic acid injection. *Scand J Rheumatol*, 1978;7:79–80.

37. Oka M., Rekonen A., Ruotsi A. The fate and distribution of intra-articularly injected osmium tetroxide ([191]OS). Acta Rheum Scand, 1969;15:35–42.

38. Menkes C.J., Verrier P., Aignan M., Delbarre F. La synoviorthèse à l'acide osmique. *Rhumatologie*, 1974;26:187–91.

39. Nissilä M., Isomäki H., Koota K., Larsen A., Raunio K. Osmic acid in rheumatoid synovitis. A controlled study. *Scand J Rheumatol*, 1977;6:158–60.

40. Delcambre B., Duquesnoy B., Deremau J.J., Siame J.L., Cocheteux P. Résultats à plus de cinq ans des synoviorthèses à l'acide osmique du genou rhumatoïde. *Rev Rhum*, 1982;49:537–43.

41. Bontoux D., Alcalay M., Reboux J.F., Puthon A. Synoviorthèses du genou par l'acide osmique. *Rev Rhum*, 1978;45:101–5.

42. Ott H., Boussina I., Fallet G.H. La synoviorthèse du genou à l'acide osmique (OsO4). Résultats à moyen terme. *Schweiz Med Wschr*, 1977;107:1165–70.

43. Steuer A., Bessant R., Rigby S.P., Gumpel J.M. Intra-articular osmic acid for persistent synovitis of the knee. A retrospective analysis of 99 treatments. *Br J Rheumatol*, 1998;abst 37:116.

44. Anttinen J., Oka M. Intra-articular triamcinolone hexacetonide and osmic acid in persistent synovitis of the knee. *Scand J Rheumatol*, 1975;4:125–8.

45. Menkes C.J., Piatier-Piketty D., Zucman J., Delbarre F. Effet des injections articulaires d'acide osmique chez le lapin. Répercussion sur la croissance osseuse *Rev Rhum*, 1972;39:513–21.

46. Goldberg V.M., Rashbaum R., Zika J. The role of osmic acid in the treatment of immune synovitis. *Arthitis Rheum*, 1976;19:737–42.

47. Wollheim F.A., Ahlberg A., Techag H. Osmium tetroxyde and radiogold in antigen induced arthritis: effect on cartilage. *Scand J Rheumatol* (suppl), 1975;abst 8:23.

48. Nissilä M., Ahlqvist J., Collan Y., Raunio P. Isomäki H. Morphological findings in joint cartilage after osmic acid treatment. *Scand J Rheumatol*, 1977;5:231–6.

49. Nissilä M. Absence of increased frequency of degenerative joint changes after osmic acid injections. *Scand J Rheumatol*, 1978;7:81–4.

50. Fellinger K., Schmid J. Die lokale Behandlung der rheumatischen Erkrankungen. *Wien Z Inn Med*, 1952;33:351.

51. Ansell B.M., Crook A., Mallard J.R., Bywaters G.L. Evaluation of intra-articular colloidal gold, [198]Au, in the treatment of persistent knee effusion. *Ann Rheum Dis*, 1963;22:435–9.

52. Makin M., Robin G.C. Chronic synovial effusion treated with intra-articular radioactive gold. *JAMA*, 1964;188:725–8.

53. Deutsch E., Brodack J.W., Deutsch K.F. Radiation synovectomy revisited. *Eur J Nucl Med*, 1993;20:1113–27.

54. Sledge C.B., Noble J., Hnatowich D.J., Kramer R., Shortkroff S. Experimental radiation synovectomy by [165]Dy ferric hydroxyde macroaggregate. *Arthritis Rheum*, 1977;20:1334–42.

55. Ingrand J. Characteristics of radioisotopes for intraarticular therapy. *Ann Rheum Dis* (suppl), 1973;32:3–9.

56. Bonneton C. Injection intraarticulaire de colloïdes radioactifs. Etude chez l'animal. 'R' *Intern Rev Rhum*, 1972;suppl 1,2:39–44.

57. Menkes C.J. Is there a place for chemical or radiation synovectomy in rheumatic diseases? *Rheumatol Rehabil*, 1979;18:65–77.

58. Bergmann H., Höfer R. Physical and technical basis of radiosynoviorthesis. In: Kolarz G., Thumb N eds. *Methods of nuclear medicine in rheumatology*. Stuttgart: Schattauer Verlag, 1982:123–7.

59. Roucayrol J.C. Introduction à la biophysique de la synoviorthése par les isotopes bêta émetteurs. 'R' *Intern Rev Rhum*, 1972;suppl 1,2:19–24.

60. Delbarre F., Roucayrol J.C., Menkes C.J., Ingrand J., Aignan M., Sanchez A. Une nouvelle preparation radio-active pour la synoviorthése: le Rhénium[186] colloïdal. *Nouv Presse Méd*, 1973;2:1372.

61. Menkes C.J., Ingrand J., Paris M.N. Clinical results with radiosynoviorthesis. In: Kolarz G., Thumb N. eds. *Methods of nuclear medicine in rheumatology*. Stuttgart: Schattauer Verlag, 1982:131–143.

62. Rekonen A., Kuikka J., Oka M. Retention and extra-articular spread of intraarticularly injected [90]Yttrium silicate. *Scand J Rheumatol*, 1976;5:47–8.

63. Jaworsi R., McLean R., Choong K., Smart K., Edmonds J. Re-evaluating the need for hospitalization following synovectomy using yttrium-90 silicate. *Br J Rheumatol*, 1993;32:1012–17.

64. Johnson L.S., Yanch J.C., Shortkroff S., Barnes C.L., Spitzer A.I., Sledge C.B. Beta particle dosimetry in radiation synovectomy. *Eur J Nucl Med*, 1995;22:977–989.

65. Menkes C.J., Aignan M., Galmiche B., Le Gô A. Le traitement des rhumatismes par les synoviorthéses: choix des malades, choix des articulations, modalités pratiques, résultats, indications, contre-indications. 'R' *Intern Rev Rhum*, 1972;suppl 1,2:61–80.

66. David-Chaussé J., Reboul J., Dehais J., Gillet M. Résultats personnels de l'introduction intra-articulaire de corps radioactifs pour le traitement des affections rhumatismales. 'R' *Intern Rev Rhum*, 1972;suppl 1,2:99–106.

67. Menkes C.J., Verrier P., Paris M.N. La synoviorthése des poignets. *Méd Hyg*, 1982;40:1190–2.

68. Stucki G., Bozzone P., Treuer E., Wassmer P., Felder M. Efficacy and safety of radiation synovectomy with yttrium 90: a retrospective long term analysis of 164 applications in 82 patients. *Br J Rheumatol*, 1993;32:383–6.

69. Delbarre F., Menkes C.J., Roucayrol J.C., Ingrand J. *Les synoviorthéses dans le traitement des maladies rhumatismales*. Paris: FDP éditeur, 1972.

70. Delbarre F., Le Gô A., Menkes C.J., Aignan M. Preuve par étude statistique 'en double aveugle' de l'effet thérapeutique d'un colloïde chargé d'yttrium radioactif (^{90}Y) dans l'arthrite rhumatoïde du genou. *C R Acad Sc Paris*, 1974;279:1051–4.

71. Menkes C.J., Le Gô A., Verrier P., Aignan M., Delbarre F. Double blind study of Erbium-169 injection (synoviorthesis) in rheumatoid digital joints. *Ann Rheum Dis*, 1977;36:254–6.

72. Boussina I., Toussaint M., Ott H., Hermans P., Fallet G.H. A double blind study of Erbium-169 synoviorthesis in rheumatoid digital joints. Results after one year. *Scand J Rheumatol*, 1979;8:71–4.

73. Ruotsi A., Hypen M., Rekonen A., Oka M. Erbium-169 versus triamcinolone hexacetonide in the treatment of rheumatoid finger joints. *Ann Rheum Dis*, 1979;38:45–7.

74. Gumpel J.M., Matthews S.A., Fisher M. Synoviorthesis with Erbium-169: a double blind comparison of Erbium-169 with corticosteroid. *Ann Rheum Dis*, 1979;38:341–3.

75. Göbel D., Gratz S., Rothkirch von T., Becker W., Willert H.G. Radiosynoviorthesis with Rhenium-186 in rheumatoid arthritis: a prospective study of three treatment regimens. *Rheumatol Int*, 1997;17:105–8.

76. Menkes C.J., Millet B. Synoviorthesis of the shoulder joint in rheumatoid arthritis. In: Lettin A.W.F, Petersson C. eds. *Rheumatoid arthritis surgery of the shoulder. Rheumatology*. Basel: Karger, 1989:46–51.

77. Gregoir C., Menkes C.J. The rheumatoid elbow: patterns of joint involvement and the outcome of synoviorthesis. *Ann Hand Surg*, 1991;10:243–6.

78. Menkes C.J., Paris M.N., Verrier P., Aignan M., Delbarre F. Le traitement des coxites rhumatismales par la synoviorthése médicale. 'R' *Intern Rev Rheumatol*, 1981;11:471–7.

79. Winfield J., Gumpel J.M. An evaluation of repeat intra-articular injections of Yttrium-90 colloids in persistent synovitis of the knee. *Ann Rheum Dis*, 1979;38:145–7.

80. Szanto E. Long-term follow-up of [90]Yttrium treated knee joint arthritis. *Scand J Rheumatol*, 1977;6:209–12.

81. Peters W., Lee P. Radiation necrosis overlying the ankle joint after injection with Yttrium-90. *Ann Plast Surg*, 1994;32:542–3.

82. Isomäki A.M., Inoue H., Oka M. Uptake of ^{90}Y resin colloid by synovial fluid cells and synovial membrane in rheumatoid arthritis. *Scand J Rheumatol*, 1972;1:53–60.

83. Stevenson A.C., Bedford J., Hill A.G.S, Hill H. Chromosome damage in patients who have had intra-articular injections of radioactive gold. *Lancet*, 1971;1:837–9.

84. De la Chapelle A., Oka M., Rekonen A., Ruotsi A. Chromosome damage after intra-articular injections of radioactive Yttrium. *Ann Rheum Dis*, 1972;31:508–12.

85. Gumpel J.M., Stevenson A.C. Chromosomal damage after intraarticular injection of different colloids of Yttrium-90. *Rheumatol Rehabil*, 1975;14:7–12.

86. Houvenagel E., Debouvry L., Leloire O., Croquette M.F, Vincent G., Carpentier P. et al. Anomalies cytogénétiques après synoviorthése isotopique au cours de la polyarthrite rhumatoïde. *Rev Rhum*, 1991;58:31–4.

87. Sholter D., Davis P. Radiochemical synovectomy. *Scand Rheumatol*, 1997;26:337–41.

88. Lipton J.H., Messner H.A. Chronic myeloid leukemia in a woman with Still's disease treated with [198]Au synoviorthesis. *J Rheumatol*, 1991;18:734–5.

89. Sledge C.B., Noble J., Hnatowich D.S., Kramer R., Shortkroff S. Experimental radiation synovectomy by [165]Dy ferric hydroxide macroaggregate. *Arthritis Rheum*, 1977;20:1334–42.

90. Chinol M., Vallabhajosula S., Goldsmith S.J., Klein M.J., Deutsch K.F., Chinen L.K., *et al.* Chemistry and biological behavior of Samarium-153 and Rhenium-186 labeled hydroxyapatite particles: potential radiopharmaceuticals for radiation synovectomy. *J Nucl Med*, 1993;34:1536–42.

91. Edmonds J., Smart R., Laurent R., Butler P., Brooks P. Hoschl R., et al. A comparative study of the safety and efficacy of dysprosium-165 hydroxide macro-aggregate and yttrium-90 silicate colloid in radiation synovectomy. A multicentre double-blind trial. *Br J Rheumatol*, 1994;39:947–53.

92. Prosser J.S., Izard B.E., Brown J.K., Hetherington E.L., Lambrecht R.M., Cato L., *et al.* Induction of micronuclei in peripheral blood lymphocytes of patients treated for rheumatoid or osteoarthritis of the knee with dysprosium-165 hydroxide macroaggregate or yttrium-90 silicate. *Cytobios*, 1993;73:7–15.

93. Clunie G., Lui D., Cullum I., Edwards J.C.W, Ell P.J. Samarium-153- particulate-hydroxyapatite radiation synovectomy: biodistribution data for chronic knee synovitis. *J Nucl Med*, 1995;36: 51–7.

94. Clunie G., Lui D., Cullum I., Ell P.J., Edwards J.C.W. Clinical outcome after one year following Samarium-153 particulate hydroxyapatite radiation synovectomy. *Scand J Rheumatol*, 1996;25:360–6.

95. Combe B., Krause E., Sany J. Treatment of chronic knee synovitis with arthroscopic synovectomy after failure of intraarticular injection of radionuclide. *Arthritis Rheum*, 1989;32:10–4.

96. Ostergaard M., Stoltenberg M., Gideon P. Wieslander S., Sonne-Holm S., Kryger P., et al. Effect of intraarticular osmic acid on synovial membrane volume and inflammation, determined by magnetic resonance imaging. *Scand J Rheumatol*, 1995;24:5–12.

97. Creamer P., Keen M., Zananiri F., Watertow J.C., Maciewicz R.A., Oliver C., et al. Quantitative magnetic resonance imaging of the knee: a method of measuring response to intra-articular treatments. *Ann Rheum Dis*, 1997;56:378–81.

39 | *Anticytokine therapy: TNF inhibitors and other novel approaches*

Tom W.J. Huizinga and Ferdinand C. Breedveld

Introduction

Cells in the immune system communicate via cell–cell contact, proteins and small non-protein molecules. Proteins produced by the immune system that were designed to perform the communication were originally described as biological response modifiers and later as cytokines. A detailed review of the cytokines relevant for the pathogenesis of rheumatoid arthritis (RA) is given in Chapter 11. Cytokines can be divided into cytokines that enhance inflammation (proinflammatory cytokines, e.g. TNF-α or IL-1) and cytokines that decrease inflammation (anti-inflammatory cytokines, e.g. IL-4 or IL-10). In RA a dysbalance is observed at the site of inflammation between pro- and anti-inflammatory cytokines in the rheumatoid synovial tissue in favor of the proinflammatory cytokines[1]. This dysbalance is considered to play an important role in the perpetuation of RA and in the induction of destruction[2]. This has resulted in the investigation of therapies with compounds that either block the effects of proinflammatory cytokine action or that induce the effect of anti-inflammatory cytokines.

Strategies to block proinflammatory cytokines

In order to achieve therapeutic goals with cytokine-targeted therapies, it might be envisioned that a strict hierarchy of cytokines is easier to disrupt than a redundant system in which many different proinflammatory cytokines mediate similar functions. Several data support the concept that such a hierarchy exists in the organization of the proinflammatory cytokine network. First, experiments in which synovial tissue was cultured *in vitro* showed that the addition of monoclonal antibodies against TNF-α (TNF-α mAb) inhibited the production of IL-1, IL-6 and IL-8 but IL-1 mAb did not inhibit the production of TNF-α[3]. The possible caveat to this set of data is that complete IgG TNF-α mAb were used allowing antibody-dependent cytotoxicity to occur. Second, experiments in TNF-α-transgenic mice showed that blockade of IL-1 prevented destructive arthritis[4]. This shows that in a TNF-α transgene-driven arthritis model, TNF-α acts in series with IL-1. However, these observations do not exclude independent effects of IL-1 in RA. The view that a strict hierarchy in proinflammatory cytokines is present has been challenged by studies on collagen arthritis in DBA/1 mice. In this model, TNF-α and IL-1 both had a central role in different stages of the disease[5]. Despite the fact that the issue of cytokine hierarchy is not yet completely resolved, the clear preponderance of the proinflammatory cytokines has led to studies on new therapies targeting these cytokines.

Cytokines have strong biological effects at a low concentration. Therefore cytokine production, cytokine degradation in the extracellular environment, biological availability, and cytokine receptor function are tightly regulated. Each of these steps has been exploited in order to disrupt proinflammatory cytokine action. The most straightforward way to target proinflammatory cytokines is to administer proteins that bind to the proinflammatory cytokines. This approach can be achieved by administration of monoclonal antibodies (mAb), soluble receptors binding the cytokine, or by administration of naturally-occurring decoy proteins that regulate biological availability *in vivo*.

The biological availability of TNF-α is regulated by soluble TNF-α receptors[6]. Since the molar ratio of TNF-α receptors/TNF-α is in general high, a large proportion of the TNF-α produced *in vivo* will be receptor bound[7]. Similarly, the biological availability of IL-1 is regulated by soluble IL-1 receptors. In addition, the IL-1-induced cellular responses are regulated by a unique protein (IL-1-receptor antagonist = IL-1Ra) that binds to the IL-1 receptor but does not lead to IL-1-receptor signaling[8,9]. A potential advantage of exploiting receptors or natural antagonists in order to correct the cytokine balance is RA is the fact that these molecules are of human origin, thus obviating the fear of patient immunization. However there are drawbacks. Soluble receptors bind to their ligands with a defined affinity, which is lower than the affinity of antigen–antibody interactions. Furthermore, receptors or receptor antagonists have a short half-life *in vivo*; thus IL-1-RA, in particular, has to be administered in a quantity that greatly exceeds the level of IL-1 produced in order to inhibit efficacy. Another possible problem, which also applies to anticytokine antibodies, is that cytokine-binding proteins may stabilize the cytokines and increase their half-life. Thus, the half-life of IL-6 in rats is 20 min in contrast to IL-6-anti-IL-6 complexes which have a half-life of 3.5 days[10]. At present, no data have been published on the biological implication of this longer half-life.

Despite the incomplete insight into the nature of the cytokine hierarchy and the pharmacodynamics of cytokine-targeted biologicals, interventions with TNF-α, or IL-6-mAb, soluble TNF or IL-1 receptors, or IL-1 receptor antagonist have reached various stages of clinical development.

Strategies to enhance anti-inflammatory cytokines

The disbalance between pro- and anti-inflammatory cytokines can also be corrected by administration of antiinflammatory cytokines such as IL-4, IL-10, and IL-13. This has the theoretical advantage of the administration of a 'naturally occurring protein'. Administration of anti-inflammatory cytokines may correct the disbalance between pro- and anti-inflammatory cytokines and may have an additional advantage in disrupting the mechanisms that drive the preponderance of proinflammatory cytokines. *In vitro* cell culture studies showed that physical cell–cell contact between T cells and macrophages contribute to the continuous excessive production of proinflammatory cytokines in RA[11]. The acquisition of this monocyte-activating capacity by T cells was dependent on T-cell activation[11]. Although it is not yet known which surface markers on activated T cells are responsible for monocyte activating capacity, a large body of knowledge is available on subsets of T cells that orchestrate inflammation.

During the 1980s detailed analysis of the cytokines produced by mouse T-cell clones revealed a dichotomy between T helper (Th)1 and Th2 clones. The Th1 clones produced IFN-γ, IL-2, and lymphotoxin whereas Th2 clones produced IL-4 and IL-5. The immune response mediated by Th 1 and Th 2 cells is completely different. Central to the function of Th 1 cells is the activation of macrophages by IFN-γ, leading to an increased ability of macrophages to kill a wide variety of extracellular and intracellular pathogens. Th2 cells stimulate production of mast cells, eosinophils, and IgE antibodies. Furthermore, Th1 and Th2 cells downregulate each other.

This dichotomy in Th-cell function seems relevant for autoimmune disease because of data from animal models showing that Th2 cytokines can delay disease onset and diminish disease activity[12]. Moreover, dominance of Th1 over Th2 cells has been demonstrated in T cells isolated from joints of patients with RA[13]. Furthermore, preliminary data exist showing that a low Th1/Th2 ratio is of prognostic value in patients with early RA[14].

IL-4, IL-10, and IL-13 stimulate Th2 cells and downregulate synthesis of proinflammatory cytokines. Therefore, administration of these cytokines may restore the disbalance between pro- and anti-inflammatory cytokines in RA. Both IL-4 and IL-10 have reached various stages of clinical development; and details for IL-10 are given below.

Blockade of proinflammatory cytokines

TNF-α

TNF-α is a proinflammatory cytokine that was originally described as a monocyte product that induced tumor lysis[15].

Several properties of TNF-α overlap with those of other cytokines, particularly IL-1[16]. Both stimulate metalloproteinase and PGE$_2$ production by synovial fibroblasts. This, together with the suppression of synthesis of matrix components by mesenchymal cells and the activation of osteoclasts, explains their capacity to promote cartilage and bone destruction. IL-1 and TNF-α are also potent activators of endothelial cells with the promotion of adhesion molecule expression and subsequent leukocyte transmigration into the tissue. They also stimulate the production of other cytokines and chemokines[17,18], increase the phagocytic function of leukocytes, and stimulate proliferation of fibroblasts and endothelial cells.

An important role of TNF-α in arthritis was further supported by the observations that mice transgenic for TNF-α developed destructive arthritis spontaneously[19]. The administration of TNF-α monoclonal antibodies prevented this form of arthritis. Other animal work further strengthened the view that TNF-α plays a key role in the pathogenesis of RA. TNF-α administered intra-articularly induces synovitis. Similarly in collagen-induced arthritis, TNF-α administered during the development of arthritis leads to a more severe form of joint inflammation whereas mice receiving anti-TNF-α monoclonal antibodies in the same time period show significant amelioration of the disease process[20]. TNF-α may also contribute to systemic features of RA by stimulating acute phase protein synthesis and inhibiting erythropoiesis[21].

Therapy with anti-TNF-α antibodies

In the first half of this decade, clinical trials using chimeric human/mouse or humanized anti-TNF-α mAb in RA patients provided the first direct evidence that inhibitors of TNF might be useful therapeutic agents. An open label trial of TNF-α mAb, cA2 (now called infliximab)[22], showed that cA2 induced significant improvements in swollen joint counts and falls in serum C-reactive protein levels in all RA patients. In a subsequent double-blind, multicenter European trial, 73 patients were randomly assigned to single infusions of either placebo, low-dose cA2 (1 mg/kg), or high dose cA2 (10 mg/kg). Seventy nine per cent of patients treated with high dose cA2 showed a 20 per cent Paulus response at 4 weeks after treatment and 44 per cent of the patients treated with the low dose, which both clearly contrasted with the 8 per cent placebo responders[23]. This response was substantial as over 50 per cent of the high dose cA2 group achieved the more stringent 50 per cent Paulus response.

Duration of response was related to the persistence of serum levels of cA2 and the original antibody dose, with those who received a single infusion of 10 mg/kg having a median response duration of 8 weeks. The antibody was well tolerated with minor infections and rashes being the most common side-effects.

In addition to these short-term studies, a repeated therapy study, involving eight patients included in the open-label trial, also indicated that cA2 may be useful for controlling disease flares during the long-term management of RA[24]. During this study, human antichimeric antibody responses to cA2, which may limit the efficacy of repeated cycles of cA2 therapy, were noted in several patients[24].

The development of a humanized monoclonal anti-TNF-α antibody (CDP571) has been part of a strategy directed towards minimizing the development of anti-idiotypic responses (which may cause accelerated clearance of the antibody, interference with the antibody–target interaction, or induce allergy)[25]. A double-blind study performed with CDP571 in 36 patients with RA demonstrated clinical benefit over 8 weeks at the 10 mg/kg dose level[26]. These trials provide the first convincing evidence that blockade of a specific cytokine could be an effective treatment in human autoimmune inflammatory disease.

To determine whether anti-TNF-α therapy is efficacious long term and may reduce disease activity not responding to methotrexate (MTX) therapy, 101 patients with active RA during MTX therapy were randomized to receive intravenous infliximab at 1, 3, or 10 mg/kg, with or without MTX 7.5 mg weekly at week 0, 2, 6, 10, and 14; patients were followed through to week 26[27]. Sixty to seventy per cent of patients receiving 1, 3, or 10 mg/kg infliximab with MTX therapy and 3 or 10 mg/kg cA2 without MTX achieved the 20 per cent Paulus criteria which was sustained during the 14 week period and in most cases also during the 12 weeks of follow-up. It was found that low-dose weekly MTX potentiates the magnitude and duration of the action of infliximab given repeatedly and decreases the immunogenicity of infliximab. The data suggest that the continuation of TNF-α blocking agents and MTX provides a novel strategy for long-term treatment of RA. Furthermore, recent data suggest that the antibody can arrest progression of bone erosions. Infliximab has been approved for use in combination with MTX in the United States.

Overall, the safety profile for infliximab administration at this point suggests that it is well tolerated and that suppression of this cytokine does not, as previously predicted, lead to an increase of serious infections. Nevertheless, the safety aspects of anti-TNF-α therapy need further evaluation in long-term regimens, particularly because of the following observations. Human antichimeric antibody responses occur in a considerable number of patients which may lead to shortening of clinical responses and side-effects. In addition, up to 10 per cent of the infliximab treated-patients developed anti-double-stranded DNA antibodies and one of these patients showed symptoms of a drug-induced lupus syndrome. Follow-up studies show that these autoantibodies disappear spontaneously during or after therapy. Finally, some of the more than 500 patients now treated with infliximab developed a malignancy. Seeking causal relationships between therapy and malignancy is complicated by the higher risk of malignancy in RA patients compared with the general population. To assess the risk of major infections or malignancy following anti-TNF-α therapy, a long-term registry has been established.

Therapy with soluble TNF-α receptors

Recently, investigators have studied the effects of a soluble TNF-α receptor (p75) Fc fusion protein (sTNFR-Fc: etanercept). This molecule is a dimer composed of two molecules of the recombinant form of the human p75 sTNFR fused to an Fc fragment of human immunoglobulin G1[28]. According to Murray and Dahl[29], sTNFR-Fc is a potent antagonist of TNF-α biological activity *in vitro* and *in vivo*, and it has been effective in many models of inflammation, including animal models of RA, and in clinical trials in RA patients.

The safety, pharmacokinetics, and potential clinical efficacy of lenercept were first evaluated in a double-blind, placebo-controlled, dose-escalation study in patients with active refractory RA[30]. In this study, sTNFR-Fc was administered in doses of 2, 4, or 16 mg/m² twice-weekly by subcutaneous injection for 4 weeks, following a single intravenous loading dose. In the double-blind phase of the study, four patients were evaluated in each dose group (three received active drug and one received placebo injection). After 4 weeks' treatment, the placebo patients in each group also received the active treatment for a further 4 weeks. An over 50 per cent reduction in individual response variables such as swollen joint count, tender joint count, and CRP was observed in patients receiving the sTNFR-Fc.

Pharmacokinetic data showed that the twice-weekly dosage schedule, in all four dose groups, resulted in an elevation of receptor concentration compared with baseline in all patients through day 35 (i.e. up to 6 days after the last injection). No serious adverse events were reported, with the most common side-effect being mild injection site reactions which did not necessitate discontinuation of the drug, and, importantly, no antibodies to lenercept were detected.

These initial encouraging clinical results were confirmed in a multicenter, randomized, double-blind, placebo-controlled study in 180 patients with RA[31]. In this study, patients receive 0.25, 2, or 16 mg/m² of sTNFR-Fc or placebo twice-weekly, subcutaneously for 3 months. Patients who received the highest dose had the greatest decrease in the number of swollen and tender joints. A 20 per cent clinical response according to the ACR response criteria was observed in 75 per cent of patients receiving the highest dose of lenercept versus only 14 per cent with placebo (p<0.001). Similarly, 57 per cent of the lenercept 16 mg/m² group had at least 50 per cent improvement, according to ACR criteria, versus only 7 per cent with placebo (p<0.001). Mean erythrocyte sedimentation rate and C-reactive protein were improved with lenercept at doses of 2 and 16 mg/m². sTNFR-Fc was also well tolerated in this study, and no dose-limiting toxic effects were observed. Only one patient withdrew, because of a mild injection site reaction. In both of the clinical studies, no human antibodies to sTNFR-Fc were detected.

Recently, the results of another multicenter trial were presented where patients were treated during 6 months with placebo (n = 80), 10 mg (n = 76), and 25 mg (n = 78) of lenercept subcutaneously, twice weekly[32]. At the end of the treatment 51 and 59 per cent of the 10 and 25 mg treated group fulfilled the ACR 20 per cent response criteria which was significantly more frequent than the 11 per cent of the placebo-treated patients. The data on extended treatment for more than 18 months so far indicate that lenercept is non-immunogenic and that the treatment is well tolerated.

Thus, clinical studies based on the use of anti-TNF-α antibodies or soluble receptors have suggested a potential beneficial effect of anti-TNF-α therapy in inducing amelioration of inflammatory parameters in patients with long-standing active RA. In these patients, anti-TNF-α therapy induces a rapid improvement in multiple, clinical assessments of disease activity and associated improvements in serological parameters.

The precise mechanisms of action remain to be defined. These include:

(1) binding and inactivation of TNF-α in the fluid phase;

(2) binding to transmembrane TNF-α;

(3) down-regulation of the expression of proinflammatory cytokines (suggested by the rapid reduction of C-reactive protein production);

(4) blockage of cell trafficking (suggested by the significant suppression of circulating levels of adhesion molecules and the reduced expression of adhesion molecules in synovial tissue following treatment)[33,34].

It is not yet certain whether there are significant differences among the most important biological agents being developed. The mAb might have the added advantage of cytotoxicity to cells that express membrane-bound TNF-α. Whether the high affinity of the TNFα-Fc fusion proteins and the possibility to bind TNF-β in addition to TNF-α are relevant to the efficacy remains to be seen. Because of the differences in protocols and presentation of results it is not easy to perform direct clinical comparison of cA2 with TNF-R (p75) Fc fusion protein.

Another important issue is whether blockade of TNF-α is merely anti-inflammatory or whether it is able to prevent destruction of the joints. Further clinical research parallel to TNF-α blockade is necessary to provide the answer. An inhibitory effect on joint destruction is suggested by reduced serum levels of metalloproteinases and reduced excretion of surrogate markers of cartilage and bone turnover following treatment[35].

How anti-TNF-α therapy will be used in RA remains to be defined. Long-term monotherapy is less likely than treatments in which new agents are used in conjunction with existing drugs. Alternatively, short-term treatments may be used to control aggressive disease thus allowing conventional drugs to exert their beneficial effects.

IL-1 blockade

Two approaches to IL-1 blockade have been used on a trial basis in the treatment of RA. The first therapeutic approach has been the intra-articular and subcutaneous administration of recombinant human IL-1 receptor. This treatment achieved a limited therapeutic efficacy. More recently, IL-1 blockade was pursued by the subcutaneous administration of recombinant IL-1 receptor antagonist (IL-1Ra), for review see Ref. 9. Treatment effects of IL-1Ra proved to be successful in the collagen-induced model of arthritis and with various results in antigen-induced arthritis[36]. In a preliminary trial, 15 RA patients received daily injections of IL-1Ra for a total of 28 days. After 7 days of treatment there were reductions in the mean joint counts and acute phase reactants with 12 of 15 patients showing a greater than 50 per cent reduction in serum CRP levels[37]. In a subsequent double-blind, placebo-controlled, multicenter trial, 175 RA patients were randomized to receive 20, 70, or 200 mg of rIL-1Ra with dose intervals varying from daily to once a week for 3 weeks[38] followed by weekly maintenance for 4 weeks. At the end of the 3 weeks treatment, daily dosing appeared more effective with patients showing a 50 per cent or more improvement in clinical outcome such as painful and swollen joint counts and general assessments of

disease activity by patient or doctor. This improvement was maintained when patients continued with rIL-1Ra treatment once daily for 4 weeks. The most frequent side-effects were reactions at the site of injection. In a follow-up study, 472 patients with early active RA received daily injections of 30, 75, and 150 mg rIL-1Ra or placebo for 24 weeks. In the 150 mg group, a significant improvement of clinical parameters ranging from 20 to 35 per cent was reported[39]. In addition, preliminary data on the evaluation of joint radiographs of treated patients were suggestive that a significant slowing of the progression of the disease with regard to cartilage and bone destruction occurred in the rIL-1Ra treated groups[40,41]. Studies on synovial biopsies demonstrated a strong decrease in lymphocyte infiltration during treatment[42].

IL-6 blockade

IL-6, like TNF-α and IL-1 is produced in high concentrations in the synovial fluid and synovial tissue. Serum levels of IL-6 strongly correlate with disease activity. IL-6 has diverse activating effects on a variety of cells, particularly on hepatocytes where it induces biosynthesis of acute phase proteins. Evidence for the role of IL-6 in cartilage degradation is conflicting. IL-6 together with IL-1 was shown to inhibit proteoglycan synthesis *in vitro* and may increase the catabolism of connective tissue[43,44]. However, in arthritis models administration of IL-6 ameliorated the disease[45]. In an open-label study five RA patients were treated with daily infusions of 10 mg of a murine IL-6 mAb over a 10-day period. On average the patients showed strong improvements of clinical variables such as morning stiffness, joint counts for pain and stiffness, as well as reduced production of acute phase proteins[46]. No side-effects were observed. Further clinical experience has not been presented. A humanized anti-human IL-6 receptor monoclonal antibody that was shown to inhibit collagen arthritis on monkeys has been developed in Japan and at present is being studied in RA.

Modulation of anti-inflammatory cytokines

Influencing the Th1–Th2 balance

Therapeutic strategies aimed at blockade of proinflammatory cytokines are relatively non-selective with regard to the rheumatoid disease process. Therefore, strategies that exploit the possibility that cytokine production by T cells can be redirected to a Th2-like production profile have been studied[47]. It has been demonstrated that particular antigens may, in the context of a particular MHC molecule, induce either a Th 1 response of a Th2 response. This implies that knowledge of the autoantigens involved may permit selective vaccination with 'protective' fragments. In a number of animal models this strategy has been shown to be successful. Apart from administration of particular parts of antigen, the cytokine environment in which the antigen is presented to naïve or quiescent T cells has been analyzed. Immature dendritic cells cultured in IL-10 for 2 days induced T cells that are non-responsive to the antigen[48]. This indicates that the biological environment of antigen presentation could induce tolerance-inducing T cells. The route of administration of the antigen is essential as well. In mice treated with auto-antigens that were delivered orally autoantigen-specific T cells that produced IL-10, IL-4, and TGF-β were identified[49], indicating that tolerance-inducing T cells exist. Immunohistochemical analysis showed that the cytokines produced in the gut-associated lymphoid tissue in autoantigen treated mice were primarily IL-10, IL-4, and TGF [50], supporting the concept that the gut is the right environment to present autoantigens in order to induce tolerance. In summary, oral administration of the right antigen in the right immunological environment may induce tolerance-inducing T cells that enhance production of anti-inflammatory cytokines. The T cells may also down-regulate the production of proinflammatory cytokines.

The relevance of this approach has been demonstrated in animal models of arthritis such as collagen-induced arthritis. In these models, the antigen that causes arthritis is known as well as the immunodominant peptide (in collagen-induced arthritis the peptide 250–270 of the collagen molecule). Oral administration of this peptide diminishes T cell proliferation against this peptide and abolishes anticollagen antibodies[15]. Moreover arthritis severity was reduced markedly.

Three different trials with human collagen have been performed in order to redirect the immune system to abort sustaining inflammation in RA[52–54]. One European trial included 90 patient with RA with a disease duration of less than 3 years[52] who were treated for 12 weeks; 30 were treated with oral type II collagen at 1 mg/day, 30 with 10mg/day, and 30 with placebo. The differences were not significant but a trend was seen: seven responders in the 10 mg group, six in the 1 mg group, and four in the placebo group. No data were generated to support the hypothesis that the treatment could indeed induce a shift to anti-inflammatory cytokine production by T cells. The results of two trials performed in the United States have been published[54,53]. In the first trial, 28 patients were treated with collagen (1 month 100 mg/day followed by 2 months 500 mg/day), and 30 with placebo[54]. The group on collagen did slightly, but significantly, better that the group on placebo. The second American trial was a large trial in which 274 patients with active RA were enrolled[53] at different sites and randomized to receive placebo or one of four dosages (20, 100, 500, or 2500 mg/ day) of oral collagen type II for 24 weeks. Eighty-three per cent of the patients completed 24 weeks of treatment. In the 20 mg/day treatment group 39 per cent of the patients showed a response in contrast to 19 per cent in the placebo group. A decrease in the proportion of patients that responded was seen with the larger dosages of oral collagen. In fact the patients on the 100 or 500 mg/day dose (initially reported to be an effective dose) did no better that the group on placebo. Interestingly, the presence of antibodies to collagen II was associated with an increased likelihood of achieving a response to collagen II, suggesting immunological differences between the patients who respond and those do not.

IL-4, IL-10, and IL-13

The dysbalance between pro- and anti-inflammatory cytokines in RA can also be corrected by anti-inflammatory cytokines.

Three different anti-inflammatory cytokines have been identified as inhibiting production of proinflammatory cytokines: IL-4, IL-10, and IL-13. These cytokines exhibit numerous effects other than down-regulation of synthesis of IL-1 and TNF-α. In this section the focus will be on the effects of IL-4, IL-10, and IL-13 on cells or tissue from rheumatoid joints. Next, the effects on animal models of arthritis will be reviewed. Finally, the first clinical observations with IL-10 in patients with RA will be presented.

IL-4 downregulates PGE production by synoviocytes[55]. Both IL-4 and IL-10 inhibit expression of proinflammatory (IL-1, IL-6, IL-8, TNF-α) genes by rheumatoid synovial cells[56]. IL-4 is more potent than IL-10 but the combination has the most profound effects. The inhibitory effect of IL-10 on the production of TNF-α by synovial fluid mononuclear cells was further substantiated by the fact that addition of anti-IL-10 to synovial fluid cells increased TNF production dramatically[57]. The effect of recombinant IL-13 on the production of IL-1/ TNF-α by these cells was similar to the effects of IL-4[58,59]. IL-4 and IL-10 when incubated with pieces of synovium, reduced IL-1 production[60]. However, IL-4 in contrast to IL-10 increased production of IL-1-RA about three-fold, suggesting that IL-4 may be able to shift the IL-1/IL-1Ra production ratio towards an anti-inflammatory profile. Both IL-4 and IL-10 added to cultures of synovial fluid mononuclear cells inhibit the ability of these supernatants to induce cartilage damage[61,62]. IL-10 seems to be of special importance for joint protection since IL-10 also directly stimulates cartilage proteoglycan synthesis[62]. Moreover, in cultures of human rheumatoid synovial cells that are cultured on human cartilage under the renal capsule of SCID mice, IL-10 inhibited both the influx of mononuclear cells and had a chondroprotective effect[63]. Apart from the cartilage protecting effects, IL-10, in contrast to IL-4 strongly inhibits the antigen-presenting function of synoviocytes[64].

In experimental animal models of arthritis, IL-10 has more potent anti-inflammatory effects than IL-4. IL-10 suppresses development of collagen-induced arthritis and ameliorates chronic arthritis in rats[65] and inhibits several different murine models of arthritis[12,66,67]. Interestingly, IL-4 had little effect in these models but the combined effects of IL-4 and IL-10 were larger than the effects of IL-10 administered alone. In collagen-induced arthritis in DBA/1 mice, the effects on cartilage destruction were studied in detail. IL-10 and/or IL-4 was administered from onset of arthritis to 10 days after onset. Administration of the combination of IL-4 and IL-10 had the best effects on protection against cartilage destruction. In this model, administration of anti-IL-10 accelerate the onset of disease, indicating a pivotal role for endogenous IL-10 in regulating arthritis activity[12]. A different approach to inhibit arthritis in animals was to administer CHO-cells that are genetically modified to produce IL-4, IL-10 or IL-13[68,69]. These treatments slightly attenuated development of arthritis and decreased the production of proinflammatory cytokines.

Based upon the above-mentioned animal data, IL-10 seems to be an attractive anti-inflammatory cytokine in the treatment of RA. Administration of IL-10 was safe in human volunteers and attenuated the proinflammatory cytokine response in healthy volunteers challenged with endotoxin[70]. The phase 1 study of recombinant human IL-10 in 72 subjects with active RA was a placebo-controlled, multicenter, randomized, double-blind, multidose study[71]. RA patients received, after a 4 week washout period of disease modifying antirheumatic drugs, IL-10 at doses of 0.5, 1, 5, 10, 20, mg/kg or placebo, by daily subcutaneous injections for 4 weeks. IL-10 was well tolerated and no anti-IL-10 antibodies were detected. A small drop in platelet counts was detected which returned to normal immediately after cessation of therapy. The biological effect was confirmed by a decrease in plasma concentration of soluble TNF-α-receptor and increase in IL-1-Ra concentration. In addition, trends towards decreased *ex vivo* production of IL-1 and TNF-α following PHA or LPS stimulation were observed. The clinical effects were not clear. The following proportion of patients reached the 20 per cent ACR response criteria: placebo 3/19, 0.5 mg/kg 0/8, 1 mg/kg, 0/9, 5 mg/kg 3/8, 10 mg/kg 2/14, and 20 mg/kg 2/14. A phase II study is currently under way.

Future prospects

Pharmacological strategies to inhibit TNF-α

The pharmacological agents that inhibit TNF-α production can be classified into drugs which inhibit signal transduction (see Chapter 44) TNF-α gene transcription, TNF-α mRNA stabilization and TNF-α processing.

Inhibition of transcription of the TNF-α gene can be mediated via the adenosine pathway that increases intracellular cyclic adenosine monophosfate (cyclic AMP). Several new compounds that increase adenosine concentration and subsequently reduce TNF-α production have been described[72–77]. As expected, the effects of compounds that affect intracellular adenosine concentration are broader than inhibition of TNF-α production. An interesting effect of an increase in adenosine concentration is enhancement of IL-10 secretion[78,79] and inhibition of collagenase gene expression[77]. An example of the beneficial effects of these agents in an animal model of arthritis are the effects of a particular adenosine A3R antagonist that blocks nuclear translocation of active p50/p65 subunits of nuclear factor kappa B (MDL 201,449A)[80]. This agent reduced TNF-α levels in serum of MRL-lpr/lpr mice and simultaneously inhibited inflammatory arthritis. In patients with RA, two open trials have been performed with another drug which is supposed to raise adenosine concentration—pentoxifylline. In these studies no relation between the decrease in an *ex vivo* TNF-α production and changes in arthritis activity was seen[81,82].

The half-life of TNF-α messenger RNA can be regulated by drugs such as thalidomide[83]. Structural analogues of thalidomide have been selected[84,85]. A detailed analysis of these analogues has revealed that inhibition of TNF-α production by these analogues is both inducer-specific and cell-type specific[86]. This hampers clinical use of these compounds since the stimuli leading to enhanced TNF-α production in RA are unknown. This is in agreement with the different data reported from clinical trials with thalidomide. In general, thalidomide is effective in a number of conditions with dysregulated TNF-α production such as aphthous ulcerations of the mouth of HIV patients[87]. However, the open-trials with thalidomide in RA suggested limited efficacy[82] although the *ex vivo* LPS-induced TNF-α production was inhibited at the dosage used in RA patients. The new analogues of thalidomide have not yet been tested in RA.

TNF-α is transported to the cell membrane and subsequently cleaved into the supernatant. Inhibitors, designated TNF-α converting enzyme (TACE) inhibitor, have been described that interfere with the protease that cleaves TNF-α from the cell membrane. TACE inhibitors reduced mortality in mice challenged with a lethal dose of LPS. Furthermore TACE inhibitor was effective in animal models of arthritis such as adjuvant arthritis[88]. These compounds are currently under clinical development.

TNF-α blockade—currently most promising therapeutic avenue

TNF-α blockade by biologicals is, at present, the most promising cytokine-targeted therapy in the treatment of RA. Definitive proof for clinical efficacy of the other treatment modalities remains to be provided. The successful, but temporary, therapeutic effect of TNF-α blockade by biologicals raises many questions that need to be addressed, such as the optimal dosage regimen, the management of human antibody responses, long-term side-effects, possibilities for combination therapy, and its place in the therapeutic strategy in RA. The most important lesson obtained so far is that manipulation of cytokines is beneficial in the treatment of organ-specific autoimmune diseases such as RA.

Gene therapy

The biologicals that are currently in phase II/III trials are proteins that disrupt TNF-α or IL-1 activity. Instead of administration of these proteins, administration of the gene encoding these proteins has several theoretical advantages, such as continuous production of the protein, localized production with high local concentration, and less systemic side-effects. Moreover, continuous long-term treatment may establish disease modification. Several different methods of delivering the genes encoding anti-inflammatory cytokines or decoy proteins for TNF-α or IL-1, are available. The methods of gene delivery are rapidly improving. At this moment it is not yet clear which gene delivery system is most appropriate for arthritis.

Advantage and disadvantages of gene delivery systems

The methods of gene delivery include the administration of naked DNA, DNA wrapped in chemical compounds such as liposomes, DNA inserted in replication-defective viral vectors, or DNA engineered into autologous cells[89–91]. Naked DNA has the advantage that any potentially immunogenic material is not introduced. However, it may be inefficient since DNA is degraded rapidly in the extracellular environment, uptake is low, and once the DNA has entered the cells a low nuclear expression is achieved. Nevertheless, in rabbits injection with naked DNA in the joint resulted in transient (2–5 days) expression of the injected DNA in the synovium[89].

Chemical compounds such as liposomes diminish loss of DNA in the extracellular space and are non-toxic, non-antigenic, and have no limit to the size of the DNA transferred. Liposomes will be taken up by phagocytic lining cells in the joints[92], conferring some cell specificity for this method of gene transfer.

Numerous viral vectors have been evaluated for gene transfer[89,93,91,94]. The most commonly used are retroviral and adenoviral vectors. Retroviral vectors are able to insert their genetic material stably into the host's chromosomal DNA. The limitations are the inability to infect non-dividing cells and the possibility of insertional mutagenesis. Thus most gene therapy protocols using retroviral vectors isolate cells, culture them *ex vivo*, transduce the cells with the retroviral vector, perform all safety evaluations, and subsequently transplant the engineered autologous cells back into the body. Adenoviral vectors infect a wide range of non-dividing and dividing cells and are extremely efficient in delivering DNA to the nucleus. The obvious limitations of viral gene delivery are expression of viral proteins by the cells the subsequently causes an immune response against the infected cells. This situation can be circumvented by genetic manipulation of the adenoviral vectors (e.g. deleting the genes that encode proteins that are presented by HLA-class I and induce and immune response), the so-called adenoassociated viral vectors[94–96]. Another approach is administration of immunosuppressive agents to dampen the immune response[97–99] or by inducing tolerance to adenoviral proteins[100].

Gene therapy of arthritis: animal models

In animal models (rabbits or several strains of mice), it has been demonstrated that synoviocytes could be infected after intra-articular injection of adenoviral vectors[101,102]. Interestingly the duration of the expression of the transgene (a reporter gene such as lac-Z or an immunologically active gene such as IL-1Ra) was more than 28 days[89,103] suggesting that relatively long-term gene expression is achievable with adenoviral vectors. The effectiveness of the approach was demonstrated using adenoviral vectors that harbor the gene for TNF-α-binding protein[104]. Treatment with the adenoviral vectors harboring these gene constructs yielded some positive effect on arthritis activity in rats. Another approach was selective killing of disease-causing lymphocytes by induction of expression of fas-ligand on synoviocytes induced by intra-articular administration of adenoviral vector encoding fas-ligand[105]. This treatment prevented collagen-induced arthritis in the treated joints.

The *in vivo* use of retroviral vectors is hindered by the low percentage of dividing cells that are able to be infected by these vectors. Nevertheless, in bacterial cell wall-induced arthritis in rats, the arthritic joints were shown to contain a population of cells that could be infected with retroviral vectors *in vivo*[106]. Retroviral vectors have been used in *ex vivo* approaches in which synoviocytes, fibroblasts, or hematopoietic cells have be transduced with a retrovirus carrying an immunomodulating protein such as IL-1-Ra, IL-4, IL-10 or IL-13 which leads to systemic production of these proteins[68,107,108]. Effectiveness was demonstrated in rabbits with synovial tissue *ex vivo* transduced by the retrovirus containing the IL-1Ra gene that were subsequently injected intra-articularly in rabbits that developed arthritis[108]. In these rabbits high IL-1Ra levels were found in the arthritic joints. In these joints a clear inhibition of cartilage matrix catabolism and increase of matrix synthesis were observed that was presumably caused by the IL-1Ra produced by the synoviocytes. In mice, local production of human IL-1Ra by synoviocytes *ex vivo* transduced with the IL-1Ra gene prevented arthritis in the joint in which the synoviocytes were injected[109]. A systemic effect was also observed because the joints of the ipsilateral paw also exhibited a reduced arthritis activity[109]. In dogs, IL-1Ra produced by *ex vivo* transduced cells reduced osteoarthritic lesions[110]. Therapeutic efficacy of engineered fibroblasts that express IL-10, IL-4, or IL-13 was demonstrated in two arthritis models in mice[68,69]. An interesting model to evaluate viral vectors that are designed to infect human tissue is the coimplantation of normal human cartilage with RA synovial fibroblast in a SCID mice[111]. In this model, transduction of the synovial fibroblasts with the IL-1Ra gene prevented chondrocyte-mediated cartilage degradation.

Gene therapy of arthritis: experience in humans

The first clinical protocol to assess safety, feasibility, and efficacy of gene therapy in RA has been approved[112] and the trial has started[113]. The trial includes post menopausal females with RA requiring total joint replacement of metacarpophalangeal joints 2–5, and prior surgery on at least one other joint. The latter provide synovial fibroblasts that are transduced *in vitro* with retrovirus containing the IL-1Ra gene. After confirming that the cells secrete IL-1Ra, either non-transduced or transduced synovial fibroblasts are injected into the MCP joints in a double-blind fashion. One week later all joints were removed and replaced by prostheses. The retrieved joints were analyzed for evidence of successful gene transfer and gene expression. In the first three patients reported, the data suggest that transfer of the IL-1Ra gene to the MCP joints was accomplished and that gene expression was achieved[114].

Conclusion

The most promising cytokine-targeted therapies are those in which TNF-α binding proteins are administered parenterally. It is expected that these biologicals will not remain the only tool to achieve decreased TNF-α activity. In the coming years, many data will be generated on therapeutic strategies that inhibit disease mechanisms operating more close to the apex of the pathogenic pyramid. Furthermore, more convenient anti-TNF-α drugs that can be administered orally may become available for use in clinical practice.

Reference

1. Brennan F.M., Gibbons T., Mitchell A.P., Cope R.N., Maini R.N., Feldmann M. Enchance expression of TNF-α receptor mRNA and protein in mononuclear cells isolated from rheumatoid arthritis synovial joints. *Eur J Immunol*, 1992;**22**:1907–12.

2. Feldmann M., Brennan F.M., Maini R.N. Role of cytokines in rheumatoid arthritis. *Ann Rev Immunol*, 1996;**14**:397–440.

3. Brennan F.M., Chantry D., Jackson A., Maini R.N., Feldmann M. Inhibitory effect of TNF alpha antibodies on synovial cell Il1 production in rheumatoid arthritis. *Lancet*, 1989;**2**:244–7.

4. Probert L., Plows D., Kontogeorgos G., Kollias G. The type I interleukin-1 receptor acts in series with tumor necrosis factor (TNF) to induce arthritis in TNF-transgenic mice. *Eur J Immunol*, 1995;**25**:1794–7.

5. Joosten L.A.B., Helsen M.M.A., Vandeloo F.A.J., Vandenberg W.B. Anticytokine treatment of established type II collagen-induced arthritis in DBA/1 mice: A comparative study using anti-TNF alpha, anti-IL-1 alpha/beta, and IL-1Ra. *Arthritis Rheum*, 1996;**39**:797–809.

6. Corti A., Poiesi C., Merli S., Cassani G. Tumor necrosis factor (TNF) alpha quantification by ELISA and bioassay: Effects on TNF alpha-soluble TNF receptor (p55) complex dissociation during assay incubations. *J Immunol Methods*, 1994;**177**:191–8.

7. Hale K.K., Smith C.G., Baker S.L., Vanderslice R.W., Squires C.H., Gleason T.M.,*et al.* Multifunctional regulation of the biological effects of TNF-alpha by the soluble type II TNF receptors. *Cytokine*, 1995;**7**:26–38.

8. Lennard A.C. Interleukin-1 receptor antagonist. *Crit rev Immunol*, 1995;**15**:77-105

9. Arend W.P., Malyak M. Guthridge C.J., Gabay C. Interleukin-1 receptor antagonist: Role in biology. *Annu Rev Immunol*, 1998;**1**627-55

10. Klein B., Brailly H. Cytokine-binding proteins: Stimulating antagonists. *Immunol Today*, 1995;**16**:216–20.

11. Sebbag M., Parry S.L., Brennan F.M., Feldman M. Cytokine stimulation of T lymphocytes regulates their capacity to induce monocyte production of tumor necrosis factor-alpha, but not interleukin-10: Possible relevance to pathophysiology of rheumatoid arthritis. *Eur J Immunol*, 1997;**27**:624–32.

12. Joosten L.A.B., Lubberts E., Durez P., Helsen M.M.A., Jacobs M.J.M., Goldman M., *et al.* Role of interleukin-4 and interleukin-10 in murine collagen-induced arthritis: Protective effect of interleukin-4 and interleukin-10 treatment on cartilage destruction. *Arthritis Rheum*, 1997;**40**:249–60.

13. Dolhain R.J.E.M., Vanderheiden A.N., Terhaar N.T., Breedveld F.C., Miltenburg A.M.M. Shift toward T lymphocytes with a T helper 1 cytokine-secretion profile in joints of patients with rheumatoid arthritis. *Arthritis Rheum*, 1996;**39**:1961–9.

14. Van der Graaff W.L., Prins A.P.A., Dijkmans B.A.C., Van Lier R.A.W. Prognostic value of Th1/Th2 ratio in rheumatoid arthritis. *Lancet*, 1998;**351**:1931.

15. Saklatvala J. Tumor necrosis factor alpha stimulates resorption and inhibits synthesis of proteoglycan in cartilage. *Nature*, 1986;**322**:547–9.

16. Arend W.P., Dayer J.M. Inhibition of the production and effects of interleukin-1 and tumor necrosis factor alpha in rheumatoid arthritis. *Arthritis Rheum*, 1995;**38**:151–60.

17. Feldmann M., Elliot M.J., Woody J.N., Maini R.N. Anti-tumor necrosis factor-alpha therapy of rheumatoid arthritis. *Adv Immunol*, 1997;**64**:310–50.

18. Feldmann M., Brennan F.M., Williams R.O., Elliott M.J., Maini R.N. Cytokine expression and networks in rheumatoid arthritis: Rationale for anti-TNF alpha antibody therapy and its mechanism of action. *J Inflamm*, 1996;**47**:90–6.

19. Keffer J., Probert L., Cazlaris H., Georgopoulos S., Kaslaris E., Kioussis D., *et al.* Transgenic mice expressing human tumor necrosis factor: a predictive model of arthritis. *EMBO*, 1991;**10**:4 025–31.

20. Williams R.O., Feldmann M., Maini R.N. Anti-tumor necrosis factor ameliorates joint disease in murine collagen induced arthritis. *Proc Natl Acad Sci USA*, 1992;**89**:9784–8..

21. Vreugdenhill G., Lowenberg B., Van Eijk HG, Swaak A.J.G. TNF alpha is associated with disease activity and the degree of anemia in patients with rheumatoid arthritis. *Eur J Clin Invest*, 1992;**22**:488–93.

22. Elliott M.J., Maini R.N., Feldmann M., Long-Fox A., Charles P., Katsikis P., *et al.* Treatment of rheumatoid arthritis with chimeric monoclonal antibodies to tumor necrosis factor alpha. *Arthritis Rheum*, 1993;**36**:1681–90.

23. Elliott M.J., Maini R.N., Feldmann M. Kalden J.R., Antoni C., Smolen J.S. *et al.* Randomised double-blind comparison of chimeric monoclonal antibody to tumour necrosis factor alpha (cA2) versus placebo in rheumatoid arthritis. *Lancet*, 1994;**344**:1105–10.

24. Elliott M.J., Maini R.N., Feldmann M., Longfox A., Charles P., Bijl H., *et al.* Repeated therapy with monoclonal antibody to tumour necrosis factor alpha (cA2) in patients with rheumatoid arthritis. *Lancet*, 1994;**344**:1125–7.

25. Camussi G., Lupia E. The future role of anti-tumor necrosis factor products in the treatment of arthritis. *Drugs*, 1998;**55**:613–20.

26. Rankin E.C.C., Choy E.H.S., Kassimos D., Kingsley G.H., Sopwith A.M., Isenberg D.A., *et al.* The therapeutic effect of an engineered anti-TNF antibody (CDP571) in rheumatoid arthritis. *Br J Rheumatol*, 1995;**34**:334–43.

27. Maini R., Breedveld F.C., Kalden J.R., Smolen J.S., Davis D., Macfarlane J.C., *et al.* Sustained therapeutic efficacy of multiple intravenous infusions of anti-TNF-alpha monoclonal antibody combined with low dose weekly methotrexate in rheumatoid arthritis. *Arthritis Rheum*, 1998, in press.

28. Mohler K.M., Torrance D.S., Smith C.A., Goodwin R.G., Shemler K.E., Fung U.P., Madani H., Witmer M.B. Soluble tumor necrosis factor receptors are effective therapeutic agents and lethal endotoxemia and function simultaneously as both TNF carriers and TNF antagonists. *J Immunol*, 1993;**151**:1548–61.

29. Murray K.M., Dahl S.L. Recombinant human tumor necrosis factor receptor (p75) Fc fusion protein (TNFR.Fc) in rheumatoid arthritis. *Ann Pharmacother*, 1997;**31**:1335–8.

30. Moreland L.W., Margolies G., Heck L.W., Saway A., Blosch C., Hanna R., *et al.* Recombinant soluble tumor necrosis factor receptor (p80) fusion protein: Toxicity and dose finding trial in refractory rheumatoid arthritis. *J Rheumatol*, 1996;**23**:1849–55.

31. Moreland L.W., Baumgartner S.W., Schiff M.H., Tindall E.A., Fleischmann R.M., Weaver A.L., *et al.* Treatment of rheumatoid arthritis with a recombinant human tumor necrosis factor receptor (p75)-Fc fusion protein. *N Engl J Med*, 1997;**337**:141–7.

32. Weinblatt M., Moreland L.W., Schiff M.H., Baumgartner S.W., Tindall E., Fleischmann R.M., *et al.* Longterm and phase III treatment of DMARD failing rheumatoid arthritis with TNF receptor P75 FC fusion protein (TNFR:FC;Enbrel™). *Arthritis Rheum*, 1997;**40**(suppl.9):S126.

33. Paleolog E. Target effector role of vascular endothelium in the inflammatory response: insights from the clinical trial of anti-TNF alpha antibody in rheumatoid arthritis. *J Clin Pathol-Mol Pathol*, 1997;**50**:225–33.

34. Tak P.P., Taylor P.C., Breedveld F.C., Smeets T.J.M., Kluin P.M., Meinders A.E., *et al.* Reduction in cellularity and expression of adhesion molecules in rheumatoid synovial tissue after anti-TNFα monoclonal antibody treatment. *Arthritis Rheum*, 1996;**39**:1077–81.

35. Choy E.H.S., Connolly D.J.A., Rapson N., Kingsley G.H., Johnston J.M., Panayi G.S. Effect of a humanised non-depleting anti-CD4 monoclonal antibody (mAb) on synovial fluid (SF) in rheumatoid arthritis (RA). *Arthritis Rheum*, 1997;**40**:S52.

36. Miesel R., Ehrlich W., Wohlert H., Kurpisz M., Kroger H. The effects of interleukin-1 receptor antagonist on oxidant-induced arthritis in mice. *Clin Exp Rheumatol*, 1995;**13**:595–601.

37. Campion G.V., Lesback M.E., Lookabaugh J., Gordon G., Catalano M. and the IL-1ra Arthritis Study Groups. Dose-range

and dose-frequency study o recombinant human interleukin-1 receptor antagonist in patients with rheumatoid arthritis. *Arthritis Rheum*, 1996;**39**:1092–1101.

38. Drevlow B.E., Lovis R., Haag M.A., Sinacore J.M., Jacobs C., Blosche C., *et al*. Recombinant human interleukin-1 receptor type I in the treatment of patients with active rheumatoid arthritis. *Arthritis Rheum*, 1996;**39**:257–65.

39. Bresnihan B., Lookabaugh J., Witt K., Musikic P. Treatment with recombinant human interleukin-1 receptor antagonist (rhIL-1ra) in rheumatoid arthritis (RA): results of a randomized double-blind, placebo-controlled multicenter trial. *Arthritis Rheum*, 1996;**39**(suppl.9):S73.

40. Watt I., Cobby M., Amgen rhIL-1ra Clinical Research Product Team. Recombinant human IL-1 receptor antagonist (rhIL-1a) reduces the rate of joint erosion in rheumatoid arthritis (RA). *Arthritis Rheum*, 1996;**39**(suppl.9):S123.

41. Cunnane G., Madigan A., FitzGerald O, Bresnihan B. Treatment with recombinant human interleukin-1 receptor antagonist (rhIL-1ra) mya reduces synovial infiltration in rheumatoid arthritis (RA). *Arthritis Rheum*, 1996;**39**(suppl.9):S245.

42. Cunnane G., Madigan A., FitzGerald O., Bresnihan B. Treatment with recombinant human interleukin-1 receptor antagonist (rhIL-1Ra) may reduce synovial infiltration in rheumatoid arthritis (RA). *Arthritis Rheum* 1996;**39**:S245.

43. Nietfeld J.J., Wilbrink B., Helle M., van Roy J.L., den Otter R.W., Swaak A.J., Huber-Bruning O. Interleukin-1 induced interleukin-6 is required for the inhibition of proteoglycan synthesis by interleukin-1 in human articular cartilage. *Arthritis Rheum*, 1990;**33**:1695–1701.

44. Ito A., Ithoh Y., Sasaguri Y., Morimatsu M., Mori Y. Effects of interleukin-6 on the metabolism of connective tissue components in rheumatoid fibroblasts. *Arthritis Rheum*, 1992;**35**:1197–1201.

45. Mihara M., Ikuta M., Koshihara Y., Oshugi Y. Interleukin 6 inhibits delayed-type hypersensitivity and the development of adjuvant arthritis. *Eur J Immunol*, 1991;**21**:2327–31.

46. Wendling D., Raderot E., Wydenes J. Treatment of severe rheumatoid arthritis with an anti-IL6 monoclonal antibody. *J Rheumatol* 1993;**20**:259–262.

47. Klareskog L., Ronnelid J., Holm G. Immunopathogenesis and immunotherapy in rheumatoid arthritis: An area in transition. *J Intern Med*, 1995;**238**:191–206.

48. Steinbrink K., Wolfl M., Jonuleit H., Knop J., Enk A.H. Induction of tolerance by IL-10-treated dendritic cells. *J Immunol*, 1997;**159**:4772–80.

49. Chen Y.H., Inobe J., Marks R., Gonnella P., Kuchroo V.K., Weiner H.L. Peripheral deletion of antigen-reactive T cells in oral tolerance. *Nature*, 1995;**376**:177–80.

50. Gonnella P.A., Chen Y.H., Inobe J., Komagata Y., Quartulli M., Weiner H.L. In situ immune response in gut-associated lymphoid tissue (GALT) following oral antigen in TCR-transgenic mice. *J Immunol*, 1998;**160**:4708–18.

51. Khare S.D., Krco C.J., Griffiths M.M., Luthra H.S., David C.S. Oral administration of an immunodominant human collagen peptide modulates collagen-induced arthritis. *J Immunol*, 1995;**155**:3653–9.

52. Sieper J., Kary S., Sorensen H., Alten R., Eggens U., Huge W., *et al*. Oral type II collagen treatment in early rheumatoid arthritis: A double-blind placebo-controlled, randomized trial. *Arthritis Rheum*, 1996;**39**:41–51.

53. Barnett M.L., Kremer J.M., St. Clair E.W., Clegg D.O., Furst D., Weisman M., *et al*. Treatment of rheumatoid arthritis with oral type II collagen: Results of a multicenter, double-blind, placebo-controlled trial. *Arthritis Rheum*, 1998;**41**:290–7.

54. Trentham D.E., Dynesius-Trentham R.A., Orav E.J., Combitchi D., Lorenzo C., Sewell K.L., *et al*. Effects of oral administration of collagen on RA. *Science*, 1993;**261**:1727–30.

55. Seitz M., Loetscher P., Dewald B., Towbin H., Ceska M., Baggiolini M. Production of interleukin-1 receptor antagonist, inflammatory chemotactic proteins, and prostaglandin E by rheumatoid and osteoarthritic synoviocytes—regulation by IFN-gamma and IL-4. *J Immunol*, 1994;**152**:2060–5.

56. Sugiyama E., Kuroda A., Taki H., Ikemoto M., Hori T., Yamashita N., *et al*. Interleukin 10 cooperates with interleukin 4 to suppress inflammatory cytokine production by freshly prepared adherent rheumatoid synovial cells. *J Rheumatol*, 1995;**22**:2020–6.

57. Isomaki P., Luukkainen R., Saario R., Toivanen P., Punnonen J. Interleukin-10 functions as an antiinflammatory cytokine in rheumatoid synovium. *Arthritis Rheum*, 1996;**39**:386–95.

58. Isomaki P., Luukkainen R., Toivanen P., Punnonen J. The presence of interleukin-13 in rheumatoid synovium and its antiinflammatory effects on synovial fluid macrophages from patients with rheumatoid arthritis. *Arthritis Rheum*, 1996;**39**:1693–702.

59. Hart P.H., Ahern M.J., Smith M.D., Finlayjones J.J. Regulatory effects of IL-13 on synovial fluid macrophages and blood monocytes from patients with inflammatory arthritis. *Clin Exp Immunol*, 1995;**99**:331–7.

60. Chomarat P., Vannier E., Dechanet J., Rissoan M.C., Banchereau J., Dinarello C.A., *et al*. Balance of IL-1 receptor antagonist/IL-1 beta in rheumatoid synovium and its regulation by IL-4 and IL-10. *J Immunol*, 1995;**154**:1432–9.

61. Van Roon J.A.G., Van Roy J.L.A.M., Duits A., Lafeber F.P.J.G., Bijlsma J.W. Proinflammatory cytokine production and cartilage damage due to rheumatoid synovial T helper-1 activation is inhibited by interleukin-4. *Ann Rheum Dis*, 1995;**54**:836–40.

62. Van Roon J.A.G., Van Roy J.L.A.M., Gmelig Meyling F.H.J., Lafeber F.P.J.G., Bijlsma J.W.J. Prevention and reversal of cartilage degradation in rheumatoid arthritis by interleukin-10 and interleukin-4. *Arthritis Rheum* 1996;**39**:829–35.

63. Jorgensen C., Apparailly F., Couret I., Canovas F., Jacquet C., Sany J. Interleukin-4 and interleukin-10 are chondroprotective and decrease mononuclear cell recruitment in human rheumatoid synovium in vivo. *Immunology*, 1998;**93**:518–23.

64. Kawakami A., Eguchi K., Matsuoka N., Tsuboi M., Urayama S., Kawabe Y., *et al*. Inhibitory effects of interleukin-10 on synovial cells of rheumatoid arthritis. *Immunology*, 1997;**91**:252–9.

65. Persson S., Mikulowska A., Narula S., Ogarra A., Holmdahl R., Interleukin-10 suppresses the development of collagen type II-induced arthritis and ameliorates sustained arthritis in rats. *Scand J Immunol*, 1996;**44**:607–14.

66. Walmsley M., Katsikis P.D., Abney E., Parry S., Williams R.O., Maini R.N., *et al*. Interleukin-10 inhibition of the progression of established collagen-induced arthritis. *Arthritis Rheum* 1996;**39**: 495–503.

67. Lubberts E., Joosten L.A.B., Helsen M.M.A., Van den Berg W.B. Regulatory role of interleukin 10 in joint inflammation and cartilage destruction in murine streptococcal cell wall (SCW) arthritis. More therapeutic benefit with IL-4/IL-10 combination therapy than with IL-10 treatment alone. *Cytokine* 1998;**10**:361–9.

68. Bessis N., Boissier M.C., Ferrara P., Blankenstein T., Fradelizi D., Fournier C. Attenuation of collagen-induced arthritis in mice by treatment with vector cells engineered to secrete interleukin-13. *Eur J Immunol*, 1996;**26**:2399–403.

69. Bessis N., Chiocchia G., Kollias G., Minty A., Fournier C., Fradelizi D., *et al*. Modulation of proinflammatory cytokine production in tumour necrosis factor-alpha (TNF-alpha)-transgenic mice by treatment with cells engineered to secrete IL-4, IL-10 or IL-13. *Clin Exp Immunol*, 1998;**111**:391–6.

70. Pajkrt D., Camoglio L., Tielvanbuul M.C.M., De Bruin K., Cutler D.L., Affrime M.B., *et al*. Attenuation of proinflammatory response by recombinant human IL-10 in human endotoxemia—Effect of timing of recombinant human IL-10 administration. *J Immunol*, 1997;**158**:3971–7.

71. Maini R., Paulus H., Breedveld F.C., Moreland L.W., St. Clair E.W., Russel A.S., *et al*. rHUIL-10 in subjects with active rheumatoid arthritis (RA): a phase I and cytokine response study. *Arthritis Rheum*, 1997;**40**(suppl.2):S224.

72. Rosengren S., Bong G.W., Firestein G.S. Anti-inflammatory effects of an adenosine kinase inhibitor—Decreased neutrophil accumulation and vascular leakage. *J Immunol*, 1995;**154**:5444–51.

73. Prabhakar U., Brooks D.P., Lipshlitz D., Esser K.M. Inhibition of LPS-induced TNF alpha production in human monocytes by adeno-

sine (A(2)) receptor selective agonists. *Int J Immunopharmacol*, 1995;17:221–4.

74. Cronstein B.N., Naime D., Firestein G. The antiinflammatory effects of an adenosine kinase inhibitor are mediated by adenosine. *Arthritis Rheum* 1995;38:1040–5.

75. Sajjadi F.G., Takabayashi K., Foster A.C., Domingo R.C., Firestein G.S. Inhibition of TNF-alpha expression by adenosine—Role of A3 adenosine receptors. *J Immunol*, 1996;156:3435–42.

76. Boyle D.L., Sajjadi F.G., Firestein G.S. Inhibition of synoviocyte collagenase gene expression by adenosine receptor stimulation. *Arthritis Rheum*, 1996;39:923–30.

77. Boyle D.L., Han Z.N., Rutter J.L. Brinckerhoff C.E., Firestein G.S. Posttranscriptional regulation of collagenase-1 gene expression in synoviocytes by adenosine receptor stimulation. *Arthritis Rheum*, 1997;40:1772–9.

78. Hasko G., Szabo C., Nemeth Z.H., Kvetan V., Pastores S.M., Vizi E.S. Adenosine receptors agonists differentially regulate IL-10, TNF-alpha and nitric oxide production in RAW 264.7 macrophages and in endotoxemic mice. *J Immunol*, 1996;157:4634–40.

79. Meisel C., Vogt K., Platzer C., Randow D., Liebenthal C., Volk H.D. Differential regulation of monocytic tumor necrosis factor-alpha and interleukin-10 expression. *Eur J Immunol*, 1996;26:1580–6.

80. Edwards C.K., Zhou T., Zhang J., Baker T.J., De M., Long R.E., *et al.* Inhibition of superantigen induced proinflammatory cytokine production and inflammatory arthritis in MRL-lpr/lpr mice by a transcriptional inhibitor of TNF-alpha. *J Immunol*, 1996;157:1758–72.

81. Maksymowych W.P., Avinazubieta A., Luong M.H., Russell A.S. An open study of pentoxifylline in the treatment of severe refractory rheumatoid arthritis. *J Rheumatol*, 1995;22:625–9.

82. Huizinga T.W.J., Dijkmans B.A.C., Van der Velde E.A., Kraan M.C., Verweij C.L., Breedveld F.C. An open study of pentoxyfylline and thalidomide as adjuvant therapy in the treatment of rheumatoid arthritis. *Ann Rheum Dis*, 1996;55:833–6.

83. Sampaio E.P., Sarno E.N., Galilly R., Cohn Z.A., Kaplan G. Thalidomide selectively inhibits tumor necrosis factor alpha production by stimulated human monocytes. *J Exp Med*, 1991;173:699–703.

84. Corral L.G., Muller G.W., Moreira A.L., Chen Y.X., Wu M.D., Stirling D., *et al.* Selection of novel analogs of thalidomide with enhanced tumor necrosis factor alpha inhibitory activity. *Mol Med*, 1996;2:506–15.

85. Niwayama S., Turk B.E., Liu J.O. Potent inhibition of tumor necrosis factor-alpha production by tetrafluorothalidomide and tetrafluorophthalimides. *J Med Chem*, 1996;39:3044–5.

86. Miyachi H., Azuma A., Hashimoto Y. Novel biological response modifiers: Phthalimides with TNF-alpha production regulating activity. *Yakugaku Zasshi-J Pharm Soc J*, 1997;117:91–107

87. Jacobson J.M., Greenspan J.S., Spritzler J., Ketter N., Fahey J.L., Jackson J.B., *et al.* Thalidomide for the treatment of oral aphthous ulcers in patients with human immunodeficiency virus infection. *N Engl J Med*, 1997;336:1487–93.

88. Gearing A.J.H., Beckett P., Christodoulou M., Churchill M., Clements J.M., Crimmin M., *et al.* Matrix metalloproteinases and processing of pro-TNF-alpha. *J Leukocyte Biol*, 1995;57:774–7.

89. Nita I., Ghivizzani S.C., Galealauri J., Bandara G., Georgescu H.I., Robbins P.D., *et al.* Direct gene delivery to synovium: An evaluation of potential vectors in vitro and in vivo. *Arthritis Rheum*, 1996;39:820–8.

90. Evans C.H., Robbins P.D. Progress toward the treatment of arthritis by gene therapy. *Ann Med*, 1995;27:543–6.

91. Evans C.H., Robbins P.D. Getting genes into human synovium. *J Rheumatol*, 1997;24:2061–3.

92. Van Lent P.L.E.M., Holthuysen A.E.M., Van den Bersselaar L.A.M., Van Rooijen N., Joosten L.A.B., Van de Loo F.A.J., *et al.* Phagocytic lining cells determine local expression of inflammation in type II collagen-induced arthritis. *Arthritis Rheum*, 1996;39:1545–55.

93. Bignon Y.J., Dincan C., Dincan M., Souteyrand P. Gene therapy: Its present and future in dermatology. *Eur J Dermatol*, 1996;6:159–63.

94. Fisher K.J., Jooss K., Alson J., Yang Y.P. Haecker S.E., High K., *et al.* Recombinant adeno-associated virus for muscle directed gene therapy. *Nature Med*, 1997;3:306–12.

95. Kessler P.D., Podsakoff G.M., Chen X.J., Mcquiston S.A., Colosi P.C., Matelis L.A., *et al.* Gene delivery to skeletal muscle results in sustained expression and systemic delivery of a therapeutic protein. *Proc Natl Acad Sci USA*, 1996;93:14082–7.

96. Ilan Y., Droguett G., Chowdhury N.R., Li Y., Sengupta K., Thrummala N., *et al.* Insertion of adenoviral E3 region into a recombinant viral vector prevents antiviral humoral and cellular immune responses and permits long-term gene expression. *Proc Natl Acad Sci USA*, 1996;93:12063–8.

97. Sawchuk S.J., Boivin G.P., Duwel L.A., Ball W., Bove K., Trapnell B., *et al.* Anti-T cell receptor mAb prolongs transgene expression following adeno-virus-mediated in-vivo transfer to mouse synovium. *Hum Gene Ther*, 1996;7:499–506.

98. Kolls J.K., Lei D.H., Odom G., Nelson S., Summer W.R., Gerber M.A., *et al.* Use of transient CD4 lymphocyte depletion to prolong transgene expression of E1-deleted adenoviral vectors. *Hum Gene Ther*, 1996;7:489–97.

99. Guerette B., Vilquin J.T., Gingras M., Gravel C., Wood K.J., Tremblay J.P. Prevention of immune reactions triggered by first-generation adenoviral vectors by monoclonal antibodies and CTLA4Ig. *Hum Gene Ther*, 1996;7:1455–63.

100. Ilan Y., Sauter B., Chowdhury N.R., Reddy B.V.N., Thummala N.R., Droguett G., *et al.* Oral tolerization to adenoviral proteins permits repeated adenovirus-mediated gene therapy in rats with pre-existing immunity to adenoviruses. *Hepatology*, 1998;27:1368–76.

101. Roessler B.J., Allen E.D., Wilson J.M., Hartman J.W., Davidson B.L. Adenoviral-mediated gene transfer to rabbit synovium in vivo. *J Clin Invest*, 1993;92:1085–92.

102. Sawchuk S.J., Boivin G.P., Duwel L.E., Ball W., Bove F., Trapnell B., *et al.* Anti-T cell receptor monoclonal antibody prolongs transgene expression following adenovirus-mediated in vivo gene transfer to mouse synovium. *Hum Gene Ther*, 1996;7:499–506.

103. Roessler B.J., Hartman J.W., Vallance D.K., Latta J.M., Janich S.L., Davidson B.L. Inhibition of interleukin-1-induced effects in synoviocytes transduced with the human IL-1 receptor antagonist cDNA using an adenoviral vector. *Hum Gene Ther*, 1995;6:307–16.

104. Le C.H., Nicolson A.G., Morales A., Sewell K.L. Suppression of collagen-induced arthritis through adenovirus-mediated transfer of a modified tumor necrosis factor alpha receptor gene. *Arthritis Rheum*, 1997;40:1662–9.

105. Zhang H.D., Yang Y.P., Horton J.L., Samoilova E.B., Judge T.A., Turka L.A., *et al.* Amelioration of collagen-induced arthritis by CD95 (Apo- 1/Fas)-ligand gene transfer. *J Clin Invest*, 1997;100:1951–7.

106. Makarov S.S., Olsen J.C., Johnston W.N., Schwab J.H., Anderle S.K., Brown R.R., *et al.* Retrovirus-mediated in vivo gene transfer to synovium in bacterial cell wall-induced arthritis in rats. *Gene Therapy*, 1995;2:424–8.

107. Boggs S.S., Patrene K.D., Mueller G.M., Evans C.H., Doughty L.A., Robbins P.D. Prolonged systemic expression of human IL-1 receptor antagonist (hIL-1ra) in mice reconstituted with hematopoietic cells transduced with a retrovirus carrying the hIL-1ra cDNA. *Gene Therapy*, 1995;2:632–8.

108. Otani K., Nita I., Macaulay W., Georgescu H.I., Robbins P.D., Evans C.H. Suppression of antigen-induced arthritis in rabbits by ex vivo gene therapy. *J Immunol* 1996;156:3558–62.

109. Bakker A.C., Joosten L.A.B., Arntz O.J., Helsen M.M.A., Bendele A.M., Van de Loo F.A.J., *et al.* Prevention of murine collagen-induced arthritis in the knee and ipsilateral paw by local expression of human interleukin-1 receptor antagonist protein in the knee. *Arthritis Rheum*, 1997;40:893–900.

110. Pelletier J.P., Caron J.P., Evans C., Robbins P.D., Georgescu H.I, Jovanovic D., *et al.* In vivo suppression of early experimental osteoarthritis by interleukin-1 receptor antagonist using gene therapy. *Arthritis Rheum*, 1997;**40**:1012–9.

111. Mullerladner U., Roberts C.R., Frankin B.N., Gay R.E., Robbins P.D., Evans C.H., *et al.* Human IL-1Ra gene transfer into human synovial fibroblasts is chondroprotective. *J Immunol*, 1997;**158**: 492–8.

112. Evans C.H., Mankin H.J., Ferguson A.B., Robbins P.D., Ghivizzani S.C., Herndon J.H., *et al.* Clinical trial to assess the safety, feasibility, and efficacy of transferring a potentially anti-arthritic cytokine gene to human joints with rheumatoid arthritis. *Hum Gene Ther*, 1996;**7**:1261–80.

113. Mccarthy M. Gene therapy for rheumatoid arthritis starts clinical trials. *Lancet*, 1996;**348**:323.

114. Ghivizzani S.C., Kang R., Muzzonigro T., Whalen J., Watkins S.C., Herndon J.H., *et al.* Gene therapy for arthritis—treatment of the first three patients. *Arthritis Rheum*, 1997;**40**(suppl.9):S223.

40 | *The design of clinical trials*

David L. Scott

Introduction

Background

Clinical trials, especially randomized clinical trials, are the cornerstone of effective medical care. This is particularly true in diseases such as rheumatoid arthritis (RA) where natural fluctuations of disease activity can too easily be ascribed as effects of treatment. This chapter summarizes the key components of designing clinical trials in RA. The principal issues are assessing the likely effects of anti-rheumatic drugs, assessing these using standardized outcome measures, and selecting appropriate clinical trial designs.

An ideal anti-rheumatic drug will rapidly reduce the symptoms of RA, stop the associated progression of joint damages and maintain function with little toxicity. Currently no drugs achieve this and almost all patients take combinations of different drugs. These have only limited benefits on symptoms and marginal slowing of damage and their associated toxicity is relatively high. New therapies are needed which improve the control of symptoms and reduce the rate of joint damage while not causing excessive toxicity. For the foreseeable future it is likely that only combinations of anti-rheumatic drugs will achieve these ends.

Steps in designing a clinical trial

There is no perfect trial, but following a small number of simple rules makes it relatively easy to design and perform a good and effective investigation. The key steps in designing a trial are shown in Table 39.1.

Generating a hypothesis

Clinical trials must answer a relevant and important question. The most difficult step is generating a testable hypothesis that is worth evaluating and can be tested in a trial that is practical and can be completed. While generating a hypothesis is the key step in trial design, it is also the most difficult to describe and to summarize. The definable characteristics of a testable hypothesis are simplicity and clarity combined with a single question as opposed to multiple questions. The trial design, primary outcome measure, size, and duration all stem from the hypothesis. Generating hypotheses depend on expecting specific types of drug effects. This is most easily resolved for drugs in pre-existing groups and is more difficult with completely novel agents.

Table 39.1   Steps in designing a clinical trial

Identify problem
Generate hypothesis
Review relevant previous studies
Select target patients
Determine treatments to be compared
Agree trial design
Define duration of treatment
Agree primary outcome measure
Select secondary outcome measures
Select health status and economic measures
Determine timing of assessments
Calculate sample size
Define likely numbers of dropouts
Determine number of centers and cases per center
Select method of randomization
Select method of analysis

It is best to consider one practical example of a testable hypothesis rather than reviewing the issue in abstract terms. Suppose there is a need to determine whether a new anti-rheumatic drug will decrease joint damage in RA. One testable hypothesis is that the drug will reduce the number of patients developing new erosions compared to patients receiving a placebo. An alternative hypothesis is that it will reduce the rate of progression of radiological damage compared to placebo therapy. These two hypotheses are subtly different. The first relates to a change in status of a proportion of patients (that is the development of one or two new erosions). The second relates to the charge in a continuous or linear measure in all patients (the rate of progression of joint damage). In both cases the hypotheses need to give greater specificity by including a definition of the types of cases (e.g. in relation to a specific disease duration) and their current therapy (e.g. taking methotrexate for a defined period of time between specific dose levels).

Antirheumatic drugs

Classification

These drugs are conventionally divided into anti-inflammatory drug, corticosteroids, and slow-acting drugs. As slow-acting drugs are thought to modify the course of RA they are sometimes termed 'disease-modifying' drugs. This conventional classification is summarized in Table 39.2.

The belief that drugs can influence the course of RA is based on their effects on the radiological progression of joint damage.

Table 39.2 Conventional classification of antirheumatic drugs

Class	Examples
Non-steroidal anti-inflammatory drugs (NSAIDs)	Ibuprofen
	Diclofenac
Corticosteroids	Prednisolone
Slow-acting antirheumatic drugs (SAARDs)	Injectable gold
	Sulfasalazine
	Methotrexate

Although there is evidence that some slow-acting drugs may reduce the rate of progression, the data are open to various interpretations and are not straightforward. These concerns have led to the suggestion that the classification of antirheumatic drugs should be changed and the concept of disease control introduced[1]. Disease control implies beneficial effects on inflammatory synovitis, leading to reduced anatomical damage, improved and maintained function, and an amelioration of systemic rheumatoid disease over long periods of time. Disease control relates as much to an overall management strategy as to therapy with a single drug. The revised classification is summarized in Table 39.3.

Anti-inflammatory drugs

Non-steroidal anti-inflammatory drugs (NSAIDs) are the central focus of anti-rheumatic therapy. They reduce pain and decrease the symptoms of joint inflammation such as tenderness, swelling, and morning stiffness. NSAIDs such as diclofenac, ibuprofen, and naproxen are well established agents. New drugs are being developed aimed particularly at reducing side-effects, especially gastrointestinal toxicity.

The use of multiple end-points within a given study and different end-points across studies make comparisons of drugs difficult. Based on a meta-analysis of 130 placebo-controlled trials Gotzsche[2] recommended the key measures were patient's global assessments of efficacy, pain, and morning stiffness. In short-term trials, lasting from 2–8 weeks, NSAIDs give better symptomatic control than placebo. There is a dose-response, and taking into account the most difficult doses used in clinical practice, the effects of most NSAIDs are comparable. However, there is considerable individual variation in patient's responses to different NSAIDs.

The situation with toxicity, in particular gastrointestinal toxicity is broadly similar. Most NSAIDs cause mild gastrointestinal side-effects, such as nausea, with high frequencies (10–30 per cent of exposures). Serious gastrointestinal toxicity, such as bleeding, perforation, or ulceration are less common and are seen in 1–2 per cent of cases or less. There is a dose-effect response, with most NSAIDs having similar levels of serious toxicity. A few drugs, such as azapropazone, have substantially higher gastrointestinal toxicity and others, such as nabumetone, have substantially lower toxicity[3].

Almost all studies of NSAIDs have been short-term, lasting less than 6 months. There have been a small number of observational studies of long-term NSAID therapy, including drug-survival studies. But these have limited value in determining the long-term efficacy and safety of NSAIDs in RA. In general the value of symptom-controlling therapies in RA is usually only tested in the short-term (up to 3–6 months).

Corticosteroids

The efficacy of corticosteroids in RA was demonstrated in early clinical trials, but their long-term adverse effects, particularly osteoporosis, has substantially limited their routine use[4]. Although steroids are often used and are given to 30–50 per cent of RA patients, the evidence for long-term effectiveness is limited.

Intramuscular injections of depot steroids are often used in active disease when commencing therapy with SAARD to achieve early control of symptoms. Pulse therapy with intravenous corticosteroids such as 0.5 to 1.0 mg of methylprednisolone has rapid onset of action but its advantage is often not maintained and its use remains in some doubt.

The more prolonged use of oral corticosteroids has been shown to be advantageous in early disease. In this situation doses of 7.5 mg prednisolone daily, when used in combination with SAARDs, reduces the progression of erosive disease and does not have excessive adverse reactions. Interestingly, except for the initial 3 months, such low-dose therapy does not have a major clinical impact on clinical disease activity. An alternative approach—high dose step-down corticosteroids—is similarly safe and effective. More studies are needed to establish the value and risks and benefits of corticosteroids in this situation[5].

Table 39.3 Revised classification of antirheumatic drugs

Class of drug	Features
Symptom-modifying antirheumatic drugs (SMARDs)	Improve symptoms and clinical features of synovitis: • Non-steroidal anti-inflammatory drugs • Corticosteroids • Slower-acting drugs
Disease-controlling antirheumatic therapy (DCART)	Change the course of rheumatoid arthritis by: • improving and sustaining function in association with decreased inflammatory synovitis • preventing or significantly decreasing the rate of progression of structural joint damage Changes must be sustained for a minimum period of 1 year

Slow-acting antirheumatic drugs

Slow-acing antirheumatic drugs (SAARDs) include methotrexate, sulfasalazine, injectable and oral gold, antimalarials (hydroxychloroquine and chloroquine), and cytotoxic drugs such as azathioprine. The number of SAARDs is gradually increasing with the introduction of new agents such as leflunomide[6].

As a group, these drugs are chemically diverse and probably have quite different modes of action. Aside from being slow-acting, they are only unique in providing symptomatic relief in RA. In particular, confusion arises when the term 'disease modifying antirheumatic drug' is used in the belief that these agents effect the course of RA. Extensive international discussions have led to a reassessment of the situation and the proposed revised classification is shown in Table 39.3. All current SAARDs have the ability to modify the symptoms of RA and thus meet the criteria for classification as SMARDs. Some may also be disease modifying and make the criteria for DCART status, but at present this is unproven and is not a major justification for their clinical use[1].

The evidence favors using SAARDs in three clinical situations: early disease, erosive disease (defined radiologically), and active disease assessed clinically and by laboratory markers of disease activity such as high levels of erythrocyte sedimentation rate (ESR) or C-reactive protein (CRP). The aim in early disease is to control symptoms and to prevent erosions. The aim in erosive disease is to reduce the progression of damage. The aim in active disease is to control symptoms. SAARDs can be used at most stages of RA for symptomatic relief and are equally effective in both early and late RA. In terms of their symptomatic response, SAARDs reduce symptoms of joint pain and swelling. They decrease the elevated acute phase response. They also make patients feel generally better.

Combination therapy

The use of several antirheumatic drugs concurrently is routine clinical practice. NSAIDs, slow-acting drugs, and corticosteroids are often used together. However, the concept of combination therapy with two slow-acting drugs is more controversial. Although some combinations, such as gold and hydroxychloroquine, have a little apparent benefit, it has been shown that several combinations are effective including the combination use of cyclosporin and methotrexate. At present, this is an area where more research is needed, but it could also well be an important focus of future therapy[7].

Table 39.4 OMERACT core data set

Number of swollen joints
Number of tender joints
Pain assessed by the patient
Patient's global assessments of disease activity
Assessor's global assessments of disease activity
Laboratory evaluation (ESR, C-reactive protein, or equivalent)
Self-administered functional assessment (e.g. Health Assessment Questionnaire)
Radiographic assessment for joint damage

Assessing clinical outcomes and response

Core data set

In chronic diseases such as RA no single outcome measure is universally appropriate. The health benefits of treatment are usually derived from a reduction in symptoms or slowing down the progression of the disease rather than achieving a complete cure. Until recently, outcome measures used in clinical trials seemed to be selected at random and there was no agreement on which measures were best. In the last few years a 'core' set of preferred outcome measures to be included in every clinical trial has been agreed by an international working group meeting—the OMERACT core data set (Table 39.4)[8].

Joint swelling and tenderness

Joint swelling is soft tissue swelling detectable along the joint margins. When a synovial effusion is present it invariably means the joint is swollen. Bony swelling or deformities do not constitute joint swelling. Joint tenderness is pain in a joint which is present: at rest with pressure; on movement of the joint; or from questioning about joint pain, for example movement of the hip joints. Pressure to elicit tenderness should be exerted by the examiner's thumb and index finger sufficient to cause 'whitening' of the examiner's nail bed.

There are a number of different joint counts (Table 39.5). The main joint counts are the ACR 66/68 counts for swollen and tender joints, the Ritchie articular index, and the 28 joint count.

The 66/68 joint count evaluates the following joints:
upper limb—temporomandibular, sternoclavicular, acromioclavicular, shoulder, elbow, wrist, metacarpophalangeal, proximal interphalangeal, and distal interphalangeal;

Table 39.5 Different types of joint counts

Index	Source	Number of joints	Grading
ACR tender joint count	ACR[9]	68	0/1
ACR swollen joint count	ACR[9]	66	0/1
Ritchie index	Ritchie *et al.*[10]	53	0–3
Total tender joint count	Fuchs *et al.*[11]	53	0/1
Total swollen joint count	Fuchs *et al.*	44	0/1
Thompson and Kirwan index	Thompson *et al.*[12]	38	3–95
36 joint count	Fuchs *et al.*[14]	36	0/1
28 joint count	Prevoo *et al.*[13]	28	0/1

lower limb—hip, knee, ankle, tarsus, metatarsophalangeal, and interphalangeal.

The Ritchie articular index evaluates the following joints: *upper*—temporomandibular, sternoclavicular, acromioclavicular, shoulder, elbow, wrist, metacarpophalangeal (as a group), proximal interphalangeal (as a group), and cervical spine; *lower*—hip, knee, ankle, subtalar, midtarsal, and metatarsophalangeal (as a group).

The 28 joint count evaluates the following joints: *upper limb*—shoulder, elbow, wrist, metacarpophalangeal, and proximal interphalangeal; *lower limb*—knee.

A longitudinal study by Prevoo et al.[13] compared the validity and reliability of these different joint counts. The validity and reliability of traditional joint indices did not differ substantially. Weighted joint indices seemed less valid and reliable. No joint index was superior for measuring disease activity.

Fuchs and Pincus[14] investigated whether quantitative assessment of a reduced number of joints by the 28 joint count provides information equivalent to that obtained by the traditional 66-joint evaluation. They were most interested in detecting changes in patients participating in clinical trials. Effect sizes, calculated as mean change in joint score/standard deviation of joint score, were similar for 66 joint and 28 joint scores. The reduced joint count scores gave significant changes for clinical trials involving as few as 15 patients. They concluded that 28 joint count scores might be used in clinical trials without decreasing the ability to detect change over time.

Smolen et al.[15] investigated the validity of the 28-joint count in comparison to the 66/68-joint count in 735 prospectively-studied RA patients. The joints included in the 28-joint count were more commonly involved than other joints. The findings from the 28-joint count correlated highly with those from the 66/68-joint count in all analyses. The 28-joint count seemed a reliable and valid measure for joint assessment, that is easier to perform than the 66/68-joint count, and addresses the joints that are critically involved.

Laboratory measures

The acute phase response can be measured indirectly by the ESR or directly using CRP or serum amyloid A (SAA). Many studies have demonstrated a good correlation between clinical measures of disease activity and the acute phase response, measured using ESR, CRP, or SAA. Longitudinal studies in early RA have shown that CRP and ESR mainly correlate with joint swelling but not with joint pain[16]. This was also found in patients with longer-standing disease, in which the highest correlation with CRP appeared with swollen joints, whereas no correlation was found with tender joints.

A persistently elevated acute phase response is associated with an increased rate of radiological progression compared to those with a normal ESR and CRP or *vice versa*[17]. It has been argued that serial measurements of acute phase protein levels should ideally be transformed into time-integrated values (area under the curve) to allow comparison with outcome measures which

Table 39.6 Composite disease activity scores

Year	Authors	Main features
1956	Lansbury[21]	Morning stiffness, fatigue, aspirin consumption, grip strength, ESR, hemoglobin
1956	Lansbury and Haut[20]	As above plus area weighted articular index
1977	Smyth et al.[21]	A pooled index
1981	Mallya and Mace[22]	An index of disease activity
1990	Davis et al.[23]	Stoke index
1990	Van de Heijde et al.[24]	Disease Activity Score
1990	Stewart et al.[25]	The index of disease activity
1993	Jones et al.[26]	Modified Stoke index
1995	Symmons et al.[27]	Overall status in RA (OSRA)
1995	Prevoo et al.[28]	Modified Disease Activity Score (for 28-joint counts)

are cumulative in nature, like radiographic damage. In a study of 110 patients with RA, van Leeuwen et al.[18] reported a significant correlation between the time integrated CRP and the rate of radiological progression in patients with early RA during the first 3 years and used this relationship to predict subsequent radiological progression. This finding has also been found in patients with longer-standing disease during 5–9 years follow-up[19].

Composite disease activity indices

A number of these are available; the main ones are summarized in Table 39.6. The Stoke[28] and the Mallya and Mace indices require more clinical data and are more complicated and less able to discriminate between patients than the Disease Activity Score (DAS). The DAS index has been independently verified. The DAS, now modified to include the reduced 28-joint counts for tenderness and swelling, has been shown to be a valid as disease activity scores that include more comprehensive articular indices. Symmons et al.[29] developed a measure of overall status in RA (OSRA) to be used in clinical practice. It produces an activity and a damage score based on five items scored 0, 1, and 2. They found the OSRA to be valid, reliable, sensitive to change, and feasible.

Composite response indices

In an attempt to move away from multiple changes in single measures, composite response indices have been developed. Those look at whether individual patients improve with treatment and identifies a single primary efficacy measure.

The American College of Rheumatology[29], using a three-stop process devised the best-known response index. First, they performed a survey of rheumatologists, using actual patient cases from trails, to evaluate which definitions best corresponded to rheumatologists' impressions of improvement, eliminating most candidate definitions of improvement. Second, they tested 20 remaining definitions to determine which maximally discriminated effective treatment from placebo treatment and also minimized placebo response rates. With eight candidate definitions

Table 39.7 American College of Rheumatology preliminary definition of improvement of rheumatoid arthritis

Required	≥ 20% Improvement in tender joint count
	≥ 20% improvement in swollen joint count
	≥ 20% improvement in 3 of following 5:
	Patient pain assessment
	Patient global assessment
	Physician global assessment
	Patient self-assessed

of improvement remaining, they tested to see which were easiest to use and were best in accord with rheumatologists' impressions of improvement. The following definition of improvement was selected: 20 per cent improvement in tender and swollen joint counts and 20 per cent improvement in three of the five remaining ACR core set measures: patient and physician global assessment, pain, disability, and acute-phase reactant. Additional validation of this definition is statistically powerful and does not identify a large percentage of placebo-treated patients as being improved. The criteria are summarized in Tables 39.7 and 39.8.

An alternative approach is to use the disease activity score (DAS)[30]. This is summarized in Table 39.9 and Fig. 39.1. The DAS-based response was developed by combining change from baseline and level of disease activity attained during follow-up. A trial comparing hydroxychloroquine and sulfalasine was used to test construct (radiographic progression), criteria (functional capacity), and discriminate validity. The response criteria had good construct. By contrast ACR criteria showed only good criterion validity.

Radiological assessments

Radiological changes in RA include loss of joint space (reflecting cartilage damage), marginal or juxta-articular bony erosions, subchondral cysts, subluxation and malalignment, ankylosis, reactive sclerosis around healing erosions, and osteophytes in severely damaged joints. Several of these changes are not very specific and there is often poor agreement among observers about their presence and extent of the changes.

Once the radiological cascade of damage starts, rapid progression is seen in the early years, with tapering later on. New techniques such as MRI, isotope scanning, bone densitometry, and

Table 39.8 Disease activity measures suggested by the American College of Rheumatology

1. Tender joint count	ACR tender joint count, an assessment of 28 or more joints. The joint count should be done by scoring several different aspects of tenderness, as assessed by pressure and joint manipulation on physical examination. The information on various types of tenderness should then be collapsed into a single tender-versus-no tender dichotomy.
2. Swollen joint count	ACR swollen joint count, an assessment of 28 or more joints. Joints are classified as either swollen or not swollen.
3. Patient's assessment of pain	A horizontal visual analog scale (usually 10 cm) or Likert scale assessment of the patient's current level of pain.
4. Patient's global assessment of disease activity	The patient's overall assessment of how the arthritis is doing. One acceptable method for determining this is the question from AIMS instrument: 'Considering all the ways your arthritis affects you, mark "X" on the scale for how well you are doing.' An anchored, horizontal, visual analog scale (usually 10 cm) should be provided. A Likert scale response is also acceptable.
5. Physician's global assessment of disease activity	A horizontal visual analogue scale (usually 10 cm) or Likert scale measure of the physician's assessment of the patient's current disease activity.
6. Patient's assessment of physical function	Any patient self-assessment instrument which has been validated, has reliability, has been proven in RA trials to be sensitive to change, and which measures physical function in RA patients is acceptable. Instruments which have been demonstrated to be sensitive in RA trials include the AIMS, the HAQ, the quality (or index) of well being, the MHIQ, and the MACTAR.
7. Acute-phase reactant value	A Westergren erythrocyte sedimentation rate or a C-reactive protein level.

ACR = American College of Rheumatology; ESR = erythrocyte sedimentation rate; CRP = C-reactive protein; AIMS = Arthritis Impact measurement Scales; RA = rheumatoid arthritis; HAQ = Health Assessment Questionnaire; MHIQ = McMaster Health Index Questionnaire; MACTAR = McMaster Toronto Arthritis Patient Preference Disability Questionnaire.

Table 39.9   Means (ranges) of the components of the DAS for low, moderate, and high levels of disease activity*

	Ritchie index	Number of swollen joints	ESR (mm/h)	General health
DAS ≤ 2.4	1 (0–5)	4 (0–18)	13 (1–54)	16 (0–53)
2.4 < DAS ≤ 3.7	5 (0–15)	10 (0–25)	29 (3–99)	33 (0–76)
DAS > 3.7	14 (1–37)	18 (7–35)	45 (3–130)	51 (1–99)

* General health was quantified on a 100-mm visual analog scale. DAS = Disease Activity Score; ESR—erythrocyte sedimentation rate.

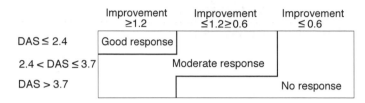

Fig. 39.1   EULAR response criteria based on the DAS. Improvement in the DAS was compared with baseline; categories to the left represent the level of disease activity attained during follow-up.

ultrasound are needed to visualize the earliest stages of the process. All of these techniques are undergoing detailed development and validation. At present radiographs remain the most appropriate approach to evaluate the progression of damage in established RA. In these circumstances serial measurements of radiological progression are better than a single reading. Rapid radiograph progression indicates the need for more aggressive treatment, especially at an early stage where it may be possible to avoid or abort subsequent major joint damage. The progression and increase of radiographic scores correlates significantly with disease duration either in early or late RA.

Methods for scoring radiographs

There are many methods: most restrict the number of joints to those most likely to be involved by RA and least likely to be the site of osteoarthritic or other abnormalities. The main scoring methods are summarized in Table 39.10.

The first approach to standardizing radiographic evaluation was by Steinbroker *et al.* in 1949. They defined four grades of radiographic change: (i) osteoporosis but no erosions; (ii) osteo-

porosis, slight cartilage or subchondral bone destruction; (iii) osteoporosis, cartilage plus bone destruction; (iv) additional ankylosis. Although the ACR adopted their system, the short scale and its bias toward severely affected joints limit its usefulness.

The next step was a semiquantitative method based upon an atlas of standard radiographs of arthritis developed by Kellgren and Lawrence[35]. They also graded damage on a 0–4 scale, with 0 being normal and 4 being the most severely damaged. This method was used in epidemiological studies but is insensitive to change and does not grade individual joints in the hand or feet. Since then many methods have been devised. Two are widely used: (a) the Sharp method[35], which scores a number of joints in the hand and wrist on a graded scale for erosions and narrowing; (b) the Larsen method[38] which scores radiological appearances compared to a set of reference radiographs. The other methods, though usually acceptable, are not widely used.

The Sharp method

This assesses erosions and joint space narrowing (indicating loss of cartilage) in hand and wrist joints. Twenty-seven areas in each hand are read for erosions (up to a maximum of five) and joint narrowing (on a 5-point scale). Subsequent work suggested it was better to reduce the number of joints read. Sharp therefore modified and simplified his method to improve its reproducibility. He suggested scoring 17 joints for erosions and 18 for joint space narrowing in each hand and assigning up to four points for each, bony ankylosis being scored as 4 points. Combining individual scores for multiple joints created an expanded scale, with a range of 0–314. This abbreviated

Table 39.10   Radiological scoring methods in RA

Year	Authors	Main features
1949	Steinbrocker[31]	0–4 grading using standardized ARA criteria
1961	ERC gold study[32]	Separate scores for erosions and joint space narrowing
1963	Kellgren[33]	Standard reference films
1969	Berens and Lin[34]	Global scale from 0 to 5
1971	Sharp *et al.*[35]	Erosion and joint space narrowing scores for hands only
1976	Trentham and Masi[36]	Carpo–metacarpal ratio
1977	Amos *et al.*[37]	Counting new erosions in hands and wrists
1977	Larsen *et al.*[38]	Global scoring using standard reference films for all joints
1983	Genant[39]	Erosion and joint space narrowing scores with standard radiographs
1983	Bluhm *et al.*[40]	Erosion and joint space narrowing scores with standard radiographs
1985	Scott *et al.*[41]	Erosion, joint space narrowing, malalignment, and total scores
1987	Kaye *et al.*[42]	Erosion, joint space narrowing, malalignment, and total scores
1989	Van der Heijde *et al.*[43]	Modified Sharp index including feet

number of joints reduced the time required to read and score a set of films. Kaye *et al.*[44] modified Sharp method to include scores for malalignment. Another modification by van der Heijde *et al.*[45] included the small joints of the feet within the Sharp score.

The Larsen method

Larsen developed this as a semiquantitative evaluation of radiographic changes. Joint damage is scored by comparing the patients' films with standard reference films (the Larsen standard radiographs rheumatoid arthritis were obtained from the Department of Radiology, Oslo Sanitetsforening Rheumatism Hospital, Oslo, Norway) to grade individual joints of the hand and wrist on a scale of 0–5. The grading scale uses a composite evaluation of erosions, cartilage loss, soft tissue swelling, periarticular osteoporosis, joint deformity, and ankylosis. The original method scored metacarpal phalangeal (MCP) joints as one unit, giving one score for all ten joints and similarly for the proximal interphalangeal (PIP) joints, with the wrist being scored as a separate entity. Raunio modified the method and made it more sensitive by using a 12-grade system for each joint. Larsen and his colleagues have since modified the method so MCP and PIP joints are scored individually and the wrist score is multiplied by five. The scores from these joints are added, with weighting for the wrist, to give a scale of 0–150. A modification by Scott *et al.*[44] increases the reliability of scoring 1.

Reproducibility of scoring radiographs

Scoring radiographs using the Sharp, Larsen, or similar indices is reproducible. One study with 13 observers scoring 41 radiographs from 16 RA patients by four different methods found good agreement on scoring across a wide spectrum of disease activity and progression. Other studies have given similar high levels of reproducibility in scoring radiographs[45]. More recently Guth *et al.*[46] evaluated the intraobserver reliability of the Sharp and Larsen methods and the carpo:metacarpal ratio. One observer analysed 71 radiographs from RA patients twice. The intraobserver reliability of each method appeared satisfactory with a good result for the Sharp method (r = 0.97). The correlation was strong (r > 0.80) between the results of Sharp's and Larsen's methods and weaker between these indices and the carpo:metacarpal ratio.

Sensitivity of radiographs to change

There is evidence that the Sharp index is the most sensitive. Cuchacovich *et al.*[47] compared the sensitivity of Sharp's and Larsen's methods in 42 RA patients. They found that the relative sensitivity to change over time was greater for Sharp's method. Similarly Plant *et al.*[48] studied 23 RA patients over 8 years and compared Sharp, Larsen, and carpo:metacarpal ratio methods. Significant changes in scores were detected over the first year using Sharp and Larsen methods but not the carpo:metacarpal ratio. Sharp's method had a greater range and sensitivity of change and better inter and intraobserver reproducibility.

Table 39.11 ACR revized criteria for classification of functional status in RA

Class	Description
Class I	Completely able to perform usual activities of daily living (self-care, vocational, avocational)
Class II	Able to perform usual self-care and vocational activities, but limited in avocational activities
Class III	Able to perform usual self-care activities, but limited in vocational and avocational activities
Class IV	Limited ability to perform usual self-care, vocational, and avocational activities

Assessing health status

Rationale

Measuring health status has concentrated on function as an indicator of disability and latterly on general health status and quality of life. Assessment of function is achieved by 'objective' measures of observed performance and self-completed or interviewer administered questionnaires of the patient's perception of function. Measures range from simple classifications to sophisticated measures of physical, social, and emotional disability and patient preferences.

Simple classification

The oldest, simplest measure is the Steinbrocker functional class[31] revized by Hochberg *et al.*[49] in 1992 (Table 39.11). It classifies groups of RA patients and is useful in broad comparisons between groups of patients but is less useful for monitoring changes over time for individual patients.

Measures of observed functional performance

Observing patients' ability to perform functional tasks such as walking 50 feet, doing up buttons, and standing for periods of time have all been used. Their advantage is that they are 'objective' measures of disability but are limited by the time required to perform them and the fact that they do not place the tasks in a context relevant for patient's everyday life.

The health assessment questionnaire (HAQ)

The HAQ is a self-completed questionnaire that, in its complete form, includes five dimensions of outcome—mortality, disability, discomfort and symptom levels, drug side-effects, and economic impact[50]. In practice, all five dimensions are rarely used; the physical disability scale and the pain visual analogue scale are more commonly used. The physical disability scale assesses upper and lower limb functioning in relation to the degree of difficulty encountered by the patient in performing a range of specified daily living tasks which include walking, dressing, bathing, and shopping. It has been frequently used in research among patients with RA.

There is an extensive literature showing the value of the HAQ in assessing the short-term response to treatment, and as a strong predictor of future disability and premature death it is widely used in clinical research to identify present and potential future health problems[51]. It has been adapted for use in the United Kingdom and has been translated into many other languages. Its popularity is partly based on the fact that it is short and easy to process, reliable, and validated against several other variables. Some studies have demonstrated a significant influence of mood on reported disability. The inherent design of the HAQ creates several 'ceilings' in functional subcategories (such as lower limb function) which may be masked by the overall HAQ score. There are also differences between observed and reported functional ability in RA patients measured using the HAQ; males overestimate their functional ability compared with female patients and patients with early RA tend to underestimate their functional ability.

A modified version of the HAQ—MHAQ—which contains transition questions used at follow-up to assess change was developed by Pincus and colleagues in 1983[52]. Comparisons between the transition questions on the MHAQ and calculated change scores for the original HAQ demonstrated the greater sensitivity of the MHAQ transition questions to changes in clinical status.

The arthritis impact measurement scales (AIMS)

The AIMS was developed by Meenan and coworkers by adapting pre-existing instruments such as the Rand Health Insurance Study Scales[53]. It assesses physical, social, and emotional well being in nine dimensions: mobility, physical activity, ADL, dexterity, household activities, pain, social activity, depression and anxiety. Scale scores are adjusted to fall within a range of 0–10. The original AIMS takes 15–20 min to complete. Both short and longer versions have been developed for use in clinical practice and research that have comparable sensitivity to change. It has been extensively validated and translated into several different languages.

Anderson *et al.*[54] found improvements in AIMS parallel changes in traditional clinical outcome such as tender joint count, morning stiffness, and ESR. The content of the AIMS overlaps with that of the full HAQ by around 65 per cent and both instruments measure three major dimensions of health status: physical disability, psychological disability, and pain.

Generic health status assessment

Generic questionnaires measure multiple aspects of health, including physical function, social function, and pain. They enable comparisons of disease impact to be made across disease groups. They can be divided into two main groups, those which provide a single global score of well being (health indices or utility measures) and those designed to measure a number of dimensions of health status (health profiles).

Single index measures of health status are designed to provide a unitary value of health status, primarily for use in cost-utility analyses. Examples of these include the Quality of Well-being Scale[55] and the European Quality of Life instrument (EuroQol)[56]. The EuroQol assesses perceived health in five dimensions (mobility, self-care, usual activities, pain/discomfort, anxiety/depression) with an overall assessment of health status. Its content is rather too restricted to provide useful information about the impact of RA on the patient and the instrument has been criticized for being crude, highly skewed, unresponsive, and for yielding poor response rates. However, recent work in RA has found EuroQol to be very responsive to self-reported change in RA and better performing than some of disease activity measures[57].

Health profiles provide a measure of the impact of disease on a number of areas of patients' lives, each area being scored and presented separately. Commonly used health profiles include the Nottingham Health Profile[58] and questionnaires from the Rand Health Insurance Study Batteries Experiment, especially the SF-20 and SF-36[59].

The Nottingham health profile (NHP)

This is a two-part, self-completed questionnaire. Since the items of part two are not applicable to all possible respondents, for example work and sex life, the authors have recommended use of part one only. This contains 38 statements designed to measure subjective health status over six dimensions of experience: physical mobility (eight items), pain (eight items), sleep (five items), emotional reaction (nine items), social isolation (five items), and energy (three items). Each section contains a number of statements to which the respondent is required to answer 'yes' or 'no'. Statements are weighted empirically in terms of their perceived severity. The NHP results are analysed in two ways: firstly, whether there are one or more positive responses in a dimension; secondly, the mean scores in each dimension. The number of positive responses in specific categories can be used as an indicator of severity and the total scores in each category presented as a profile. Scores range from zero (no problems or absence of limitations) to 100 (where all problems are present). The NHP has been used to evaluate health status in a variety of arthritides and non-rheumatological conditions. It has been translated into several languages[60].

The SF-36

This questionnaire measures general health status and was developed from the Rand Corporations Health Insurance Experiment and the subsequent Medical Outcomes Study. The SF-36 has become the most widely used general health status measure. It contains 36 items that measure eight dimensions—physical functioning (ten items), role limitations due to physical problems (four items), social functioning (two items), mental health (five items), energy/vitality (four items), pain (two items), and general health perceptions (five items). There is a further single item giving information on change in health over the past year. It is scored to give a profile of health status in eight dimensions on a 0–100 scale. Minor modifications were made to the wording of six items on the SF36 to make it acceptable in the British context[61].

Results from two general population studies in the United Kingdom found high response rates in postal surveys and indicated that respondents found it easy to complete[62]. It contains items that are less severe than those found on the NHP, and as such has been found to be more sensitive to lower levels of disability. Psychometric evaluations have established its criterion and construct validity. Its internal reliability in general population groups is high but there is evidence that some dimensions may be less reliable in seriously ill patients. Tuttleman *et al.*[63] found a significant correlation between SF-36 with HAQ and the physician and patient global assessments. They concluded that SF-36 is a valid instrument for patient with RA. Talamo *et al.*[64] found that SF-36 scores were influenced by comorbidity. Moreover, studies have demonstrated that in contrast to general population studies, elderly and disabled patients find the instrument difficult to complete (due to its relatively complex response formats) and that its content is inappropriate. Consequently, it produces high levels of missing answers with these groups and demonstrates poor reliability and sensitivity. Nevertheless, it has been used extensively in a variety of patient groups and has been translated into a number of different languages. Some disease specific supplementary measures, including one for RA, have been developed in an attempt to overcome these problems.

Defining patients to be studied

Patients

Most patients entered into RA trials are hospital-based cases with established and active disease. It is generally considered suitable to select patients who meet the criteria of the American College of Rheumatology and this provides a relatively homogenous patient population. A disadvantage of the widespread use of these criteria is that we know relatively less about responses of patients with mild or atypical synovitis to antirheumatic drugs as these patients are rarely studied.

Exclusions

It is also conventional to exclude some groups of patients from trials. These include cases with other severe medical problems such as severe cardiac or hepatic disease. Trials with low agents invariably exclude women likely to become pregnant, and this is clearly very important. There is a tendency to exclude patients with very late-stage disease who fall into functional class IV of the Steinbroker classification. Many studies seen to exclude the very elderly, over 80 years or in some cases over 70 to 75 years and finally patients who have been in several previous trials or who have had persisting serious side-effects with antirheumatic drugs. There is a disadvantage in being too selective and excluding too many cases as the trial can then lose its generalizability, and this is a major disadvantage.

'NSAID-like' effects

NSAIDs and drugs with similar effects reduce pain, joint tenderness, and morning stiffness but generally have good effect on the acute phase response, other indicators of systemic inflammation, and radiological progression. Patients for studying these effects should have moderate to high levels of pain, tender joint counts, and morning stiffness. For example they should have moderate to severe pain, over six tender joints and over 30 min morning stiffness.

'SAARD-like' effects

These drugs reduce both local and systemic components of inflammation. Patient should therefore have moderate to high levels of local and systemic features of their RA. For example they should have over six swollen joints, over six tender joints, more than 30 min morning stiffness, and an ESR over 30 mm/h. Usually patients are included if they meet three out of four such criteria If effects on radiographs are to be evaluated patients should not have the majority of their joints already damaged and some upper limit of the extent of damage is needed. An example is a Larsen score of less than 100 (equating to two-thirds of maximum possible damage).

Combination therapy

As most patients with RA receive combinations of different types of antirheumatic drugs this really means combinations of two or more SAARDs or combinations of steroids with SAARDs. There are problems in starting two SAARDs at the same time in a clinical trial: firstly, it is difficult to know whether the effects are due to one or other drug or the combination; secondly, it is often complicated trying to unravel side-effects, especially in blinded studies. The conventional approach is to stabilize patients on one drug and then start the second SAARD after a period of some months. This had led to the concept of studying 'partial' responders and not evaluating patients who have either shown no response to the first drug or have done very well indeed on it. Although this idea is theoretically sound, it is not necessarily simple to agree on what exactly constitutes a 'partial' response. An improvement of 20 per cent is a key measurement as the swollen joint count would be reasonable approximation for a 'partial' response to a SAARD.

Early disease

There is increasing emphasis on treating RA early with aggressive therapy. The variety of this approach is gradually being demonstrated in clinical trials. Most trials use 2 years from diagnosis as an upper limit and 6 weeks or 3 months as a lower limit for defining early disease. Some trials have used 5 years as an upper limit and a few enthusiasts have recommended 1 year or less as an upper limit. There are two main problems with these studies. Firstly, it can be difficult to define the onset of RA, especially in patients whose disease has initially intermittent symptoms. Associated with this is the need to differentiate between the first onset of symptoms and the time at which the diagnosis was first made. Secondly, some patients with RA have a single episode of severe synovitis which does not recur and resolves irrespective of any treatment, such cases would weaken the design of any study as they will improve whether they receive active or placebo therapy.

Numbers of patients

Sample size

The sample size is mainly determined by statistical calculation. This requires considerable experience and it is unwise to proceed without expert statistical advice. An exact description of the statistics lies beyond the scope of this review. In brief, sample size calculations fall into two broad groups. Firstly, they can evaluate continuous variables. Secondly, they can evaluate categorical variables. In both instances investigators must decide on the level of significance sought in the primary outcome measure in the study and the power of the study—that is its ability to exclude a false negative result. These are represented in the alpha and beta values of the power calculation. Most studies use an alpha of 5 per cent and a beta of 90 per cent.

Primary outcome measures are usually continuous variables and will be expressed as means and standard deviations (or 90 per cent confidence intervals). To determine the sample size in these circumstances, investigators need to know the standard deviation of their primary outcome measure in the study population and to have defined the magnitude of difference between treatment and control groups that they consider important. An example is looking at the ability of SAARD to reduce the swollen joint count.

When primary outcome measures are discontinuous variables with two categories, investigators need to know the percentage of patients who fall into one or other category and the effect of change they wish to see. An example is the ability of SAARD to stop the development of new erosions.

Allowing for drop-outs

Patients dropping out of therapy affect all trials. There are many reasons for this, often unrelated to treatment itself. Examples include moving abroad, unrelated severe illness, or even death. It is important to allow for dropouts after calculating the sample size. It is conventional to increase the sample size by 10–20 per cent to take account of such dropouts.

Numbers of centers

Most trials are multicenter studies with between four and 20 or more centers participating. Very few studies in rheumatoid arthritis involve a single center. It is important that each center recruits the adequate number of patients and a minimum number is between six and ten patients per center. In any large study it is important to realize that not all centers will necessarily participate as planned. It is probably important to have too many rather than too few centers agree to take part. It is generally better to have studies arranged with central randomization of patients in any clinical trial. However, as not all centers are comparable and there can be marked difference between patients enrolled and the effects of treatment at individual centers it is important to take this into account.

Rate of enrolment

All clinical trials should have a time frame within which they are completed. This should include planning of the members of patients to be entered in each center and the time allowed for patient entry. At the beginning of any trial there is a period where staff training is needed and the number of patients recruited in the initial weeks is normally small. It is also important that studies invariably take longer to complete than originally envisaged so it is important to take this into account and have a realistic rate of enrolment and involve enough centers. It is conventional for studies in rheumatoid arthritis to enrol patients over periods of 6–12 months. Very large trials, especially those in selected small groups of patients such as early rheumatoid arthritis, may need to enrol patients over longer period of time for up to 2 years. Studies which take longer than this to recruit start to run into a variety of additional problems such as changes in medical staff at the various centers, loss of interest by patients, the withdrawal of patients for other reasons, and the general decline in interest and relevance in the investigation.

Trial design

Types of trial

There are many different types of trial that could be used. But in practice a very small number of approaches are taken. These are summarized in Table 39.12.

The simplest study design randomizes patients into two groups; one receives active therapy and the other placebo. This is a classical parallel group study. When it is important to define the optimal dose for active therapy, a dose-ranging study is needed. There are concerns about the use of placebo controls and many studies therefore use active controls. These can be used to determine whether a new treatment is better than conventional therapy or whether it is equivalent. In general, more patients are usually used to determine equivalence. Factorial designs are needed when the effects of two drugs are to be compared and if there is the possibility that two drugs may interact. Crossover trials and n-of-1 trials have limited roles in

Table 39.12 Types of trial

Common	Uncommon
Parallel groups with placebo controls	Factorial trial with two arms
Dose ranging parallel groups with placebo controls	Cross-over trial
Parallel group with active controls	N of 1 trial

evaluating antirheumatic drugs and should rarely be used. The optimal trial design for combination therapy is contentious and this issue has been considered in detail by Paulus[65].

Controls

The strongest possible trial design compares active therapy with placebo. The disadvantage is that patients given placebo will not receive adequate therapy for their RA. There are major ethical and practical issues involved. In general terms it is possible to use placebo therapy for short periods of time when evaluating new antirheumatic drugs and when patients receive other therapies to control some of their symptoms. It is generally difficult to maintain placebo controls for longer than 4 to 6 months.

The alternative to placebo therapy is to give active treatment with a comparator drug. This is acceptable but does carry some disadvantages. Firstly, it is important to pick an optimal dose of comparative drug. Secondly, the equivalence is less relevant than showing a difference between therapists and the average study comparing two similar types of drugs shows no difference between therapists rather than the new treatment being better than the conventional medication. If a drug is dramatically better than current therapy, showing it in a randomized control trial is a major advantage and demonstrating such an effect should be the major objective in clinical trials.

Randomization

It is important that all clinical trials should be randomized so that patients have an equal chance of receiving any of the treatment options. The number of patients randomized into each group does not necessarily need to be the same, in some circumstances it is possible to have twice as many patients randomized to receive active therapy than to receive control treatment. A personal preference is to have a single randomized schedule held at one site for all patients in the clinical trial. Irrespective of the center in which they were enrolled, it is possible to stratify randomization to take account of one or two major factors likely to contribute towards the results of the study. My personal preference is to avoid this, as it is an unnecessary complication in the majority of instances. It is important that studies remain blinded in the majority of circumstances and when blinding is in place it must continue until the study has finished. It is inappropriate to unblind a study for the individual patient at the end of their period of treatment this has implications for open label extension.

Other treatments

Patients require multiple therapies for their arthritis and it is important that the majority of these continue in the setting of the randomized trial. However, it is also best if changes in treatments could be kept to a minimum in these circumstances. All patients with rheumatoid arthritis use analgesics usually taking the medication when required. It is sensible to continue this in the setting of the trials but to record the dose of analgesics used. If patients are in a trial of a slow-acting drug, NSAIDs should be given with, as far as possible, dose remaining static to those patients who need it. Some studies require patients to be confined to a small number or even one in NSAID but this is not necessarily important. It is also possible when studying a slow-acting drug to look at patients who are receiving steroids provided the dose of steroids is constant. It is often best to exclude patients who are taking very high doses of steroids such as above 7.5 or 10 mg of prednisone daily. If patients are participating in a study of non-steroidal or an equivalent drug then they should be able to take a fixed dose of a slow-acting drug during the course of the study but should not receive additional non-steroidal drugs outside the study treatment regime. When studying a slow-acting drug it is conventional to require a period of 4–6 weeks without a slow-acting drug being used, but with a non-steroidal there is also a concept of washing out period and this is a shorter duration, usually lasting 4–7 days. The evidence that supports these periods of non-steroidal treatment is extremely thin but convention has led to their wide-spread use.

Open label extensions

When patients are enrolled in a trial, especially of a new drug, it is often advantageous to allow them to continue on a fixed dose at the end of the study period. This will give further information about potential adverse effects and will also allow them to see a potentially effective treatment if they believe they have gained advantage from it. The nature of blinding means that it is impossible to identify whether a patient has received active treatment and the dose of that treatment prior to them going into the open label extension. This does create some weakness.

Analysis

It is better to analyse all patients who were enrolled in the study and properly randomized than simply to compare those patients who have completed a course of treatment. The former analysis is called an intention to treat analysis and the latter a valid complaints completed analysis. In practice it is possible, in many circumstances, to gain full information on all patients randomized and an intention to treat analysis invariably has to exclude one or two patients who were randomized but were never followed further. It is important to analyze the primary outcome measure on which the trials design has been based in a single, simple statistical analysis. The active and control groups can be compared at the end of study to define significant differences using appropriate parametric or non-parametric tests. The secondary outcome measures should then be analyzed separately. When multiple statistical analyses have been undertaken, it is important to include some correction for the number of significant tests undertaken.

Ethical issue

All clinical trials should conform to the highest possible ethical standards. The protocol should be reviewed by an ethics committee, patients should be given complete information about the trial and its risks and benefits, and there should be the opportunity to review the results of the trial by external and independent experts assessing efficacy and adverse events.

Other problems

Meta-analysis

There is an increasing number of meta-analyses published. Some give contentious results. For example Gotzsche et al.[66] suggests the benefits of SAARDs are not very marked. Chernoff et al.[67] have proposed that an archive of data from clinical trials should be created to improve methods of meta-analysis. This is sensible but time consuming and expensive. There are secular changes in the reporting of clinical trials[68] and this will create problems in standardization. There is also debate about the best approach for meta-analysis and using multiple outcome models may be better than assessing each outcome individually[69].

Differences between trials and clinical practice

Generalizing is a key issue in trials. Selecting a carefully defined patient group to determine efficacy must be balanced against the problem of generalizing results. A series of papers in the last 4 years have suggested that clinical trial data is often irrelevant in terms of results of clinical practice studies[70,71,72]. This is a relatively unproductive debate as so many different variables effect clinical practice and these variations between results at different centers probably exceed the variations between clinical trial reports and observational studies is clinical practice. Nevertheless, the issue is important and studies should follow on maximizing their generalizability.

Standardization

Medicine is becoming more standardized and clinical trials cannot escape from this pressure. An example of consensus recommendations is the rheumatoid arthritis section of the GREES group[73]. The impact of these standards is as yet unknown. However, it is important to ensure that clinical trial data is made available and especially important that negative studies are not unreported thereby creating positive publication bias. There is evidence that this is a potential problem in NSAID studies[74] and strenuous action is needed to guard against it.

References

1. Edmonds J.P., Scott D.L., Furst D.E., Brooks P.M., Paulus H.E. Anti-rheumatic drugs: a proposed new classification. *Arthritis Rheum*, 1993a;**36**:336–9.
2. Gotzsche P.C. Meta-analysis of NSAIDs: contribution of drugs, doses trial designs and leta-analytic techniques. *Scand J Rheumatol*, 1993;**22**:255–260.
3. Henry D., Lim L.L., Garcia-Rodriguez L.A., Perez-Gutthann S., Carson J.L., Griffin M., Savage R., Logan R., Moride Y., Hawkey C., Hill S., Fries J.T. Variability in risk of gastrointestinal complications with individual non-steroidal anti-inflammatory drugs: results of a collaborative meta-analysis. *BMJ*, 1996;**312**:1563–6.
4. Gotzsche P.C., Johansen H.K. Meta-analysis of short-term low dose prednisolone versus placebo and non-steroidal anti-inflammatory drugs in rheumatoid arthritis. *BMJ*, 1998;**315**:811–818.
5. Cohen M.D., Conn D.L. Benefits of low-dose corticosteroids in rheumatoid arthritis. *Bull Rheum Dis*, 1997;**46**:4–7.
6. Furst D.E. Innovative treatment approaches for rheumatoid arthritis. Cyclosporing, leflunomide and nitrogen mustard. *Baillieres Clin Rheumatol*, 1995;**9**:711-729.
7. Choy E.H., Scott D.L. Drug treatment of rheumatic diseases in the 1990's. Achievements and future developments. *Drugs*, 1997;**53**:337–348.
8. Boers M., Tugwell P., Felson D.T. *et al.*, World Health Organization and International League Against Rheumatism core endpoints for symptom modifying antirheumatic drugs in rheumatoid arthritis clinical trials. *J Rheumatol (Suppl)*, 1994;**41**:86–9.
9. The Co-operating Clinics Committee of the American Rheumatism Association: a seven-day variability study of 499 patients with rheumatoid arthritis. *Arthritis Rheum*, 1965;**8**:302–34.
10. Ritchie D.M., Boyle J.A., McInnes J.M., *et al.*, Clinical studies with an articular index for the assessment of joint tenderness in patients with rheumatoid arthritis. *Q J Med*, 1968;**37**:393–406.
11. Fuchs H.A., Brooks R.H., Callahan L.F., Pincus T. A simplified 28 joint quantitative articular index in rheumatoid arthritis. *Arthritis Rheum*, 1989;**32**:531–7.
12. Thompson P.W., Silman A.J., Kirwan J.R., Currey H.L.F. Articular indices of joint inflammation in rheumatoid arthritis. *Arthritis Rheum*, 1987;**30**:618–23.
13. Prevoo M.L., van Riel P.L., van-'t Hof M.A., van Rijswijk M.H., van Leeuwen M.A., Kuper H.H., van de Putte L.B. Validity and reliability of joint indices. A longitudinal study in patients with recent onset rheumatoid arthritis. *Br J Rheumatol*, 1993;**32**:589–94.
14. Fuchs H.A., Pincus T. Reduced joint counts in controlled clinical trials in rheumatoid arthritis. *Arthritis Rheum*, 1994;**37**:470–5.
15. Smolen J.S., Breedveld F.C., Eberl G., Jones I., Leeming M., Wylie G.L., Kirkpatrick J. Validity and reliability of the twenty-eight-joint count for the assessment of rheumatoid arthritis activity. *Arthritis Rheum*, 1995;**38**:38–43.
16. Otterness I. The value of C-reactive protein measurement in rheumatoid arthritis. *Semin Arthritis Rheum*, 1994;**24**:91–103.
17. Dawes T., Fowler D., Jackson R., *et al.* Prediction of progressive joint damage in patients with rheumatoid arthritis receiving gold or D-penicillamine therapy. *Ann Rheum Dis*, 1986;**45**:945–9.
18. van Leeuwen M.A., van der Heijde D.M., van Riel P.L., *et al.* Interrelationship of outcome measures and process variables in early rheumatoid arthritis: a comparison of radiological damage, physical disability, joint counts, and acute phase reactants. *J Rheumatol*, 1994;**21**:425–9.
19. Hassell A.B., Davis M.J., Fowler P.D., Clarke S., Fisher J., Shadforth M.F., Jones P.W., Dawes P.T. The relationship between serial measures of disease activity and outcome in rheumatoid arthritis. *Q J Med*, 1993;**86**:601–7.
20. Lansbury and Haut 1956.
21. Smythe H.A., Helewa A., Goldsmith C.H. 'Independent assessor' and 'pooled index' as techniques for measuring treatment effects in rheumatoid arthritis. *J Rheumatol*, 1977;**4**:144–52.
22. Mallya R.K., Mace B.E. The assessment of disease activity in rheumatoid arthritis using a multivariate analysis. *Rheumatol Rehabil*, 1981;**20**:14–7.
23. Davis M., Dawes P., Fowler P., *et al.* Comparison and evaluation of a disease activity index for use in patients with rheumatoid arthritis. *Br J Rheumatol*, 1990;**29**:111–5.
24. Van der Heijde D.M., van't Hof M., van Riel P.L., van de Putte L.B. Development of a disease activity score based on judgement in clinical practice by rheumatologists. *J Rheumatol*, 1993;**20**:566–567.
25. Stewart M.W., Palmer D.G., Knight R.G., Highton J. A self-report articular index: relationship to variations in mood and disease activity measures. *Br J Rheumatol*, 1993;**32**:631–2.

26. Jones P.W., Ziade M.F.M., Davis M.J., Dawes P.T. An index of disease activity in rheumatoid arthritis. *Stat Med*, 1993;**12**: 1171–81.

27. Symmons D.P.M., Hassell A.B., Gunatillaka K.A.N., *et al.* Development and preliminary assessment of a simple measure of overall status in rheumatoid arthritis (OSRA) for routine clinical use. *Q J Med*, 1995;**88**:429–37.

28. Prevoo M.L.L., van't Hof M.A., Kuper H.H., van Leeuwen M.A., van de Putte L.D.A., van Riel P.L.C.M. Modified disease activity scores that include twenty eight joint counts. *Arthritis Rheum*, 1995;**38**:44–8.

29. Felson D.T., Anderson J.J., Boers M., *et al.* American College of Rheumatology. Preliminary definition of improvement in rheumatoid arthritis. *Arthritis Rheum*, 1995;**38**:727–735.

30. van Gestel A.M., Prevoo M.L., van't Hof M.A., *et al.* Development and validation of the European League Against Rheumatism response criteria for rheumatoid arthritis. Comparison with the preliminary American College of Rheumatology and the World Health Organization/International League Against Rheumatism Criteria. *Arthritis Rheum*, 1996;**39**:34–40.

31. Steinbroker O., Trager C.H., Batterman R.C. Therapeutic criteria in rheumatoid arthritis. *JAMA*, 1949;**140**:659–65.

32. Research Subcommittee of the Empire Rheumatism Council, 'Gold therapy in rheumatoid arthritis. Final report of a multicentre controlled trial'. *Ann Rheum Dis*, 1961;**20**:315–34.

33. Kellgren J.H., Lawrence J.S. Radiological assessment of rheumatoid arthritis. *Ann Rheum Dis*, 1957;**16**:485–93.

34. Berens D.L., Lin R.K. *Roentgen diagnosis of rheumatoid arthritis*. Springfield Illinois: Charles C. Thomas; 1969.

35. Sharp J.T., Lidsky M.D., Collins L.C., Moreland J. Methods of scoring the progression of radiologic changes in rheumatoid arthritis. Correlation of radiologic, clinical and laboratory abnormalities. *Arthritis Rheum*, 1971;**14**:706–20.

36. Trentham D.E., Masi A.T. Carpo: metacarpal ratio: a new quantitative measure of radiologic progression of wrist involvement in rheumatoid arthritis. *Arthritis Rheum*, 1976;**19**:939–44.

37. Amos R.S., Constable T.J., Crockson R.A., Crockson A.P., McConkey B. Rheumatoid arthritis: relation of serum C-reactive protein and erythrocyte sedimentation rates to radiographic changes. *Br Med J*, 1977;**1**:195–7.

38. Larsen A., Dale K., Eek M. Radiographic evaluation of rheumatoid arthritis and related conditions by standard reference films. *Acta Radiol (Diagn)*, 1977;**18**:481–91.

39. Genant H.K. Methods of assessing radiographic change in rheumatoid arthritis. *Am J Med*, 1983;**75** (**suppl. 6A**):35–47,

40. Bluhm G.B., Smith D.W., Mikulaschek W.M. A radiologic method of assessment of bone and joint destruction in rheumatoid arthritis. *Henry Ford Hosp Med J*, 1983;**31**:152–61.

41. Scott D.L., Houssein D.A., Laassonen L: Proposed modification to larsen's scoring methods for hand and wrist radiographs. *Br J Rheumatol*, 1995;**34**:56.

42. Kaye J.J., Nance E.P., Callahan L.F., *et al.* Observer variation in quantitative assessment of rheumatoid arthritis. II. A simplified scoring system. *Invest Radiol*, 1987;**22**:41–6.

43. van der Heidje D.M., van Riel P.L., Nuver-Zwart I.H., Gribnau F.W., van de Putte L.B. Effects of hydroxychloroquine and sulphasalazine on progression of joint damage in rheumatoid arthritis. *Lancet*, 1989;**I**:1036–8.

44. Scott D.L., Houssein D.A., Laassonen L. Proposed modification to larsen's scoring, methods for hand and wrist radiographs. *Br J Rheumatol*, 1995;**34**:56.

45. Fries J.F., Bloch D.A., Sharp J.T., McShane D.J., Spitz P., Bluhm G.B., Forrester D., Genant H.K., Gofton J.P., Richman S., Weissman B., Wolfe F. Assessment of radiologic progression in rheumatoid arthritis: a randomized controlled trial. *Arthritis Rheum*, 1986;**29**:1–9.

46. Guth A., Coste J., Chagnon S., Lacombe P., Paolaggi J.B. Reliability of three methods of radiologic assessment in patients with rheumatoid arthritis. *Invest Radiol*, 1995;**30**:181–5.

47. Cuchacovich M., Couret M., Peray P., Gatica H., Sany J. Precision of the Larsen and the Sharp methods of assessing radiologic changes in patients with rheumatoid arthritis. *Arthritis Rheum*, 1992;**35**:736–9.

48. Plant M.J., Jones P.W., Dawes P.T. Patterns of radiological progression in rheumatoid arthritis. *Arthritis Rheum*, 1993;**36** (suppl.):S213.

49. Hochberg M.C., Chang R.W., Dwosh l., Lindsey S., Pincus T., Wolfe F. The American College of Rheumatology 1991 revised criteria for the classification of global functional status in rheumatoid arthritis. *Arthritis Rheum*, 1992;**35**:498–502.

50. Fries J.F., Spitz P., Kraincs R.C., Holman H.R. Measurement of patient outcome in arthritis. *Arthritis Rheum*, 1980;**23**:137–45.

51. Ramey D.R., Raynauld J.P., Fries J.F. The Health Assessment Questionnaire 1992: Status and review. *Arthritis Care Res*, 1992;**5**:119–29.

52. Pincus T., Summey J.A., Soraci S.A., Wallston K.A., Rummon N.P. Assessment of patient satisfaction in activities of daily living using a modified Stanford Health Assessment Questionnaire. *Arthritis Rheum*, 1983;**26**:1346–53.

53. Meenan R.F., Gertman P.M., Mason J.H. Measuring health status in arthritis: the Arthritis Impact Measurement Scales. *Arthritis Rheum*, 1980;**23**:146–52.

54. Anderson I.I., Felson D.T., Meenan R.F., Williams H.J. Which traditional measures should be used in rheumatoid arthritis clinical trials? *Arthritis Rheum*, 1989;**32**:1093–99.

55. Kaplan R.M., Anderson J.P. The Quality of Wellbeing Scale: rationale for a single quality of life index. In: Walker S.R. and Rosser R.M., eds. *Quality of Life: assessment and application*. Lancaster: MTP, 1988:51–77.

56. EuroQol Group. EuroQol—a new facility for the measurement of health-related quality of life. *Health Policy*, 1990;**16**:199–208.

57. Hurst, *et al.*, 1996.

58. Hunt S., McEwen P., McKenna S. Measuring health status: a new tool for clinicians and epidemiologists. *J Coll Gen Pract*, 1985;**35**:185–8.

59. Ware J.E., Sherbourne C.D. The MOS 36-item short-form health survey (SF-36): Conceptual framework and item selection. *Med Care*, 1992;**30**:473–83.

60. McKenna S., Hunt S., Tennant A. The development of a patient-completed index of distress from the Nottingham Health Profile: a new measure for use in cost-utility studies. *J Med Econ*, 1993;**6**:13–24.

61. Jenkinson C., Coulter A., Wright L. Short form 36 (SF36) health survey questionnaire: normative data for adults of working age. *Br Med J*, 1993a;**29/306**:1437–40.

62. Brazier J.E., Harper R.A., Jones N.M.B., *et al.* Validating the SF36 health survey questionnaire: new outcome measure for primary care. *Br Med J*, 1992;**305**:160–4.

63. Tuttleman M., Pillemer S.R., Tilley B.C., *et al.* A cross sectional assessment of health status instruments in patients with rheumatoid arthritis participating in a clinical trial. Minocycline in Rheumatoid Arthritis Trial Group. *J Rheumatol*, 1997;**24**: 1910–1915.

64. Talamo J., Frater A., Gallivan S., Young A. Use of the short form 36 (SF36) for health status measurement in rheumatoid arthritis. *Br J Rheumatol*, 1997;**36**:463–9.

65. Paulus H.E. Clinical trial design for evaluating combination therapies. *Br J Rheumatol*, 1995;**34 Suppl 2**:92–95.

66. Gotzche P.C., Podenphant J., Olesen M., Halberg P. Meta-analysis of second-line anti-rheumatic drugs: sample size bias and uncertain benefit. *J Clin Epidemiol*, 1992;**45**:587–594.

67. Chernoff M.C., Wang M., Anderson J.J., Felson D.T. Problems and suggested solutions in creating an archive of clinical trials data to permit later meta-analysis: an example of methotrexate trials in rheumatoid arthritis. *Control Clin Trials*, 1995;**16**:342–355.

68. Anderson J.J., Felson D.T., Meenan R.F. Secular changes in published clinical trials of second-line agents in rheumatoid arthritis. *Arthritis Rheum*, 1991;**34**:1304–1309.

69. Berkey C.S., Anderson J.J., Hoaglin D.C. Multiple-outcome meta-analysis of clinical trials. *Stat Med*, 1996;**15**:537–557.

70. Hawley D.J., Wolfe F. Are the results of controlled clinical trials and observational studies of second-line therapy in rheumatoid arthritis valid and generalisable as measures of rheumatoid arthritis outcome: analysis of 122 studies. *J Rheumatol*, 1991;**18**:1008–1014.

71. Felson D.T. Clinical trials in rheumatoid arthritis under attack: are practice based observational studies the answer? *J Rheumatol*, 1991;**18**:951–953.

72. Pincus T. Limitations of randomised clinical trials to recognize possible advantages of combination therapies in rheumatoid diseases. *Semin Arthritis Rheum*, 1993;**23**:2–10.

73. Anonymous. Recommendations for the registration of drugs used in the treatment of rheumatoid arthritis section. *Br J Rheumatol*, 1998;**37**:211–215.

74. Rochon P.A., Gurwitz J.H., Simm R.W., *et al.* A study of manufacturer-supported trials of non-steroidal anti-inflammatory drugs in the treatment of arthritis. *Arch Intern Med*, 1994;**154**:157–163.

41 | *Anti-T lymphocyte therapies*

Ernest H.S. Choy

Introduction

Rheumatoid arthritis (RA) is an immune-mediated, chronic inflammatory and destructive arthropathy. Current treatment with slow-acting antirheumatic drugs (SAARDs) suppresses inflammation and improves symptoms but does not necessarily improve long-term disease prognosis[1]. The main problem is that SAARDs rarely produce remission[2] and do not halt radiological progression[3]. Furthermore they are toxic, many patients have to terminate treatment after 2 years due to side-effects[4]. New treatments that are more effective are urgently needed. The T cell has been proposed as a therapeutic target in RA. Over the last two decades, numerous anti-T cell strategies have been tested in RA and this is a review of those efforts.

T cells in the pathogenesis of rheumatoid arthritis

Initiation of disease

RA is characterized by a chronic cell-mediated immune response with synovial hypertrophy and pannus formation. The role of T cell in rheumatoid arthritis is reviewed in detail in Chapter 7. The immune response is initiated by presentation of antigenic peptides in the groove of the class II MHC molecule to a CD4+ lymphocyte bearing the appropriate T-cell receptor (TCR). In the presence of other costimulatory signals, such as leukocyte function associated antigen-1 (LFA-1) and CD2 and CD28, this results in activation of the CD4+ lymphocyte. It then produces lymphokines and expresses cell surface molecules that stimulate other immunocytes and mesenchymal cells resulting in amplification of the immune cascade. In a cell-mediated immune response, CD4+ lymphocytes typically produce Th1 lymphokines such as interferon gamma (IFNγ) and interleukin (IL)-2. IFNγ is a powerful stimulant of monocytes/ macrophages[5] while IL-2 stimulates any T cells that express IL-2 receptor (IL-2R). Activated CD4+ lymphocytes also upregulate the expression of many cell surface molecules such as IL-2R, HLA-DR, and CD69. IL-2R leads to an autocrine-positive feedback loop resulting in further expansion of antigen-specific CD4+ lymphocytes. Other cell surface molecules such as CD69, CD40 ligand, and LFA-1, through cell surface contact can stimulate monocytes/macrophages and fibroblasts to release monokines and matrix metalloproteinases (MMP). Monokines, in particular, IL-1[6], and tumor necrosis factor alpha (TNF-α)[7] are potent proinflammatory cytokines with a wide range of actions on mesenchymal and endothelial cells. They increase the expression of adhesion molecules such as intercellular adhesion molecule-1 (ICAM-1) and vascular cellular adhesion molecule-1 (VCAM-1) on endothelial cells. This enhances further recruitment of inflammatory cells into the synovial joints that therefore perpetuates inflammation. Moreover, IL-1 and TNF-α, stimulate the release of MMP by fibroblasts and chondrocytes which degrades connective tissue and leads to joint damage.

Perpetuation of disease in chronic established RA

While there is general consensus on the initiation of RA, the mechanism that perpetuates synovitis remains controversial. The paucity of lymphokines and abundance of monokines in the RA synovium has led some researchers to propose the mesenchymal hypothesis in which established RA is not driven by T cells but is maintained by a positive feedback loop between monokines and mesenchymal cells[8]. However, the protagonists of the T cell hypothesis argue that only a few antigen-specific T cells are needed to sustain a cell-mediated immune response[9]. The frequency of such T cells in other diseases characterized by cell-mediated immune response, such as tuberculosis, leprosy, cutaneous leishamaniasis, and reactive arthritis, varies from 1:500 to 1:3000[10–12]. Thus, the number of RA-specific T cells which would be needed for the continued maintenance of rheumatoid synovitis would be very small and could account for the paucity of Th1 lymphokines. The efficacy of anti-T cell therapy has been regarded by some as the acid test for these conflicting hypotheses.

The rationale of targeting T cells

Scientific basis

The immunogenetic basis of RA is the strongest evidence for the importance of T cells in disease pathogenesis (see Chapter 1). RA is strongly linked to HLA-DR4[13] and DR1[14,15]. The HLA-DR molecule consists of an invariant α and a polymorphic β chain. They form a groove in which an antigenic peptide is presented to the TCR of a CD4+ T cell. This is the only known function of HLA molecules. The third hypervariable region of the β chain is thought to be especially important since it binds to the antigenic peptide. Molecular analysis of this region in HLA-DR4 and DR1 molecules shows that they are identical apart from a conserved substitution. This leads to the proposal of the shared epitode hypothesis[16] in which HLA-DR molecules sharing similar third hypervariable regions are capable of binding to an arthritogenic peptide, rendering individual susceptible to RA. The arthritogenic peptide in RA remains unknown but recently a human chondrocyte antigen, HC-gp39, has been identified as a possible candidate autoantigen[17].

The RA synovial membrane is heavily infiltrated by T cells in a perivascular and diffuse distribution[18]. Monocytes and macrophages infiltrate the subsynovium as well as the synovial lining layer[19]. B cells, which in some synovial membranes may be organized into germinal follicles, are also a feature; they synthesize and secrete immunoglobulins of which only a variable proportion is rheumatoid factor (RF). Macrophages, B lymphocytes, and specialized antigen-presenting cells express HLA molecules and are all capable of presenting antigenic peptides to T cells. T cells in the synovium are activated and express HLA-DR, CD69[20], and the chemokine receptor CCR5[21]; the latter is selectively expressed by Th1 cells. Studies using sensitive immunohistological techniques techniques[22,23] and a semiquantitative polymerase chain reaction have demonstrated the presence of the Th1 lymphokines IL-2 and IFNγ[24,25]. Therefore these activated T cells are potentially capable of sustaining synovitis through the release of lymphokines and direct contact with mesenchymal cells.

Animal models

Compelling evidence for the involvement of T cells in the pathogenesis of destructive inflammatory arthritis comes from animal models. There are three commonly used animal models of RA: adjuvant arthritis in rats, collagen arthritis in mice and rats, and streptococcal cell wall (SCW) arthritis in rats. In all three models, Th1 T cells are central to the pathogenesis. The arthritis cannot be induced in T-cell-deficient animals, it is linked to a particular mouse or rat MHC; it can be transferred by T cells; and the antigenic peptides which stimulates disease-causing T cells are known. Consequently, therapeutic approach based on manipulating T-cell response to antigens have all been tried. These approaches include T-cell vaccination, mucosal tolerance, and monoclonal antibodies (Mabs). Successes of these strategies in ameliorating arthritis lead to their use in human diseases. These will be discussed in detail later in this chapter.

Anti-T cell drug: cyclosporin A

Cyclosporin A (CsA) is a T-cell inhibitor that is widely used in transplantation. It inhibits the release of IL-2 by activated T cells[26]. A number of placebo-controlled trials have shown that it is modestly effective and is now licensed for the treatment of RA[27,28]. Its ability to suppress disease activity in RA argues that T cells remain important in chronic synovitis. However, recently there is evidence suggesting that CsA has an effect on bone and cartilage[29].

Strategies in anti-T cell therapy

One can categorize anti-T-cell therapy into non-specific, semi-specific, and specific. Each category can be further subdivided into those that deplete T cells and those that are imunomodulatory. Clearly, specific therapy is to be preferred to non-specific but it is difficult to implement at the present since the arthritogenic peptide and disease-specific T cells in RA remain unknown.

Non-specific anti-T cell therapies

These treatments target virtually all T cells and can lead to significant immunosuppression. Nevertheless non-specific anti-T-cells drugs such as cyclosporin A can be used effectively in RA. Initially there was a major interest in T-cell depletion but the strategy has largely been abandoned because of prolonged lymphopenia.

Semi-specific anti-T cell therapies

T cells can be divided into many subsets according to the expression of different glycoproteins on their surface. Most of these glycoproteins are cell surface receptors for cytokines or ligands for other cell surface molecules. Specific subsets of T cells can be targeted for depletion using mabs and immunotoxins. Alternatively, blocking or stimulating appropriate surface molecules may be immunomodulatory and able to suppress immune-mediated inflammation.

Specific anti-T cell therapies

Ultimately, only therapy which targets the arthritogenic antigen and/or the specific T cells reacting to it will be disease specific. If exogenous antigen, such as bacteria or viruses, is the cause of RA, antibiotics or antiviral agents may be effective. However, if RA is caused by an autoantigen, mucosal tolerance is probably the only known specific treatment at present. Hitherto, clinical trials of oral tolerance in RA have produced conflicting results. These will be discussed in more detail later.

Tools to target T cells

Monoclonal antibodies

Several mabs have been used in animal models of RA such as collagen type II, SCW, and adjuvant arthritis. The T cell targets have included IL-2R, CD4, CD8, CD5, TCR, and MHC class II. Amongst these, only mabs tageting CD4[30,31], TCR[32,33], and CD5[34] but not CD8[30,34] were effective in preventing arthritis development and reducing the severity of established disease. Interestingly, when anti-CD4 mab was given at the same time as injection of SCW, it rendered the animal resistant to subsequent induction of arthritis with SCW[31]. This resistance to induction of disease may be due to immunological tolerance and will be discussed in more detail later.

Although murine mabs have greatly assisted research in immunology and autoimmune diseases, their therapeutic uses have been restricted since their administration to humans invariably leads to the development of human antimouse antibodies (HAMA). Such HAMA can lead to anaphylaxis or reduced efficacy on retreatment. This is well illustrated by the use of murine anti-ICAM-1 mab in RA[35]. Although initial treatment was clinically efficacious, all the patients developed HAMA, repeated treatment was less effective and anaphylactic reactions occurred in some patients.

Advances in the understanding of the assembly of antibodies from genes to protein and progress in biotechnology have allowed the generation of man-made antibodies by selecting a desired Fc and combining it with any preferred F(ab')$_2$. There are two main types of manmade antibodies: chimeric and humanized. Chimeric antibodies retain the murine F(ab')$_2$ region while the Fc region is replaced by the human isotype. Humanized antibodies retain only the complementarity determining regions of the murine mab while the rest of the molecule is human. It is hoped that with the reduction in the murine component of these antibodies, they would be less immunogenic thus allowing repeated treatments in humans.

Immunotoxin

Immunotoxins are formed by fusion of a toxin with an immunological agent usually a mab or recombinant cytokine. Immunotoxins may be preferred over mabs in therapy because of their superior ability to kill target cells. This is particularly important in diseases in which depletion of target cells is the main objective such as lymphoproliferative diseases[36]. IL-2-DAB and CD5-plus are examples of immunotoxins that have been tested in RA. These agents will be discussed in more detail in this chapter.

Cytokines

Antigenic stimulation of T cells causes them to initiate a program which leads to the secretion of lymphokines, the expression of new markers on their surface, and cell division. The pattern of lymphokines secreted is a property of particular subsets of T cells, Th1, and Th2. Th1 T cells release the classical lymphokines, IL-2 and IFNγ, responsible for cell-mediated immunity. Th2 T cells secrete lymphokines, such as IL-4, IL-6, and IL-10, which are involved in humoral immunity. The products of Th1 and Th2 cells exert mutually antagonistic effects one upon the other. The rheumatoid synovium is characterized by a Th1 response hence treatment with Th2 cytokines such as IL4 and IL-10 may suppress inflammation.

Vaccination

Similar to vaccination in infectious diseases, T cells and their unique cell surface antigens, the TCRs can also be used as vaccines to induce regulatory T cells which suppress the pathogenic T cells in RA. These approaches have been successful in animal models of autoimmune diseases and recently have been used in rheumatoid patients. The major problem with this approach in RA is that the disease-specific T cell has yet to be identified. Although some studies have suggested expansion of certain Vβ T cells, their results are often conflicting. Details of these will be discussed later in this chapter.

Mucosal tolerance

This refers to the ability to suppress an immune response to an antigen delivered through gut or nasal mucosa. The mechanism of action is not fully-defined but appears to involve apoptosis, the release of immunoregulatory cytokines, and the generation of regulatory T cells[37]. Mucosal tolerance is effective in experimental models; for example it prevents the induction of collagen-induced arthritis[38]. Importantly, it is not necessary to feed the disease-inducing antigen but merely an antigen from the target tissue; this effect is called bystander suppression. Since the antigen in RA is unknown, the exploitation of the bystander suppression effect is critical.

Non-specific anti-T cell therapies

Non-specific T cell immunosuppressants

Cyclosporin A

Cyclosporin A is a cyclic endecapeptide isolated from the fungi *Tolypoclasium inflatum* and *Cylindrocarpon lucidium*. It is a potent immunomodulator and initially is thought to inhibit T cells specifically. T-cell inhibition is mediated by the inhibition of IL-2 gene transcription via an effect on the transcription factor NF-AT[26,39]. During T-cell activation, extracellular signals lead to a sharp rise in intracellular calcium. This binds to calmodulin which, in turn, binds to calcineurin; the activated calcineurin dephosforylates the cytoplasmic subunit of the transcription factor NF-AT, resulting in its translocation from the cytoplasm into the nucleus to form a competent transcriptional activator for the production of IL-2. Recent work has shown that CsA binds to cyclophilin (Cyp), which has enzymatic functions and regulates protein folding during proteins synthesis[40]. The Cyp/CsA complex binds to calcineurin and calmodulin, thereby inhibiting its phosphatase activity. This prevents translocation of transcription factor into the nucleus and inhibits gene expression of IL-2[26]. *In vitro* CsA is known to inhibit IL-2 secretion when peripheral blood mononuclear cells are stimulated either by mitogen or antigen[41]. Although CsA is primarily a T cell-directed drug, there is some evidence for effects on other cell types including bone and cartilage[29]. A number of placebo-controlled trials have confirmed its clinical efficacy in RA[27,42]. Interestingly, a recent study suggested it may be more effective than other slow-acting drugs in reducing radiological damage in early RA[28]. However, its therapeutic value in RA has been hampered by renal toxicity particularly when high doses are given.

FK506

FK506 is an immunosuppressant used in transplantation. It has similar immunosuppressive action to CSA but binds to FK506-binding protein instead of cyclophilin. FK506 inhibits the transcription of a group of T-cell cytokine genes including IL-2, IL-3, IL-4, TNF-α, and IFNγ[43]. The blocking of these key cytokines results in the inhibition of T cell activation and inflammation. FK506 has been evaluated in collagen-induced arthritis in rats[44]. FK506 appears to be more potent than CyA in suppressing arthritis. A clinical trial of FK506 in RA is currently being conducted.

Rapamycin

Rapamycin exerts its action primarily by the inhibition of cytokine and growth factor-dependent stimulation of T cells without affecting cytokine production[45]. In addition, rapamycin is capable of inhibiting the growth of T cells[46] and rheumatoid synoviocytes[47]. In preliminary studies, rapamycin has been found to be effective in inhibiting SCW arthritis but only if treatment was initiated at the time of antigen presentation[48]. Initiation of rapamycin treatment during established arthritis was found to have no beneficial effect.

Mycophenolate mofetil

Mycophenolate mofetil is a T and B-cell immunosuppressant that has been used successfully in transplantation. Recently it has been tested in phase II clinical trials in RA[49]. It was well tolerated and produced significant symptomatic improvement. Currently it is being tested in a large phase III multicenter, placebo-controlled trial.

Non-specific T cell depletion

Once T cells were recognized to be pathogenic in RA, a number of strategies aiming to deplete T cells were tested in clinical trials. These included total lymphoid irradiation (TLI), lymphocytapheresis, and thoracic duct drainage (TDD).

Total lymphoid irradiation

TLI has been shown to suppress cell-mediated immune response in patients treated for Hodgkin's lymphoma[50]. It has also been used in collagen arthritis[51]. Subsequent open and double-blind, randomised trials have demonstrated significant clinical improvement in RA patients[52–55]. Benefit lasted 6 months in 80 per cent of the patients and most have benefit lasting up to 1 year. Profound and sustained lymphopenia, especially depletion of CD4+T-cells, was a consistent feature after treatment[56]. Peripheral blood mononuclear cell proliferative responses to phytohemagglutinin and concanavalin A were suppressed[57]. No significant changes in the level of RF, immunoglobulin, immune complexes, and erythrocyte sedimentation rate (ESR) were seen. The main limitation of TLI is the frequency of adverse effects which are often serious[58–60]. These include fatigue, malaise, gastrointestinal symptoms, alopecia, weight loss, opportunistic infections, and a substantial mortality from sepsis. As a result, this treatment is now rarely used in RA.

Lymphocytapheresis

Apheresis means the removal of a component from blood. Trials using plasmapheresis alone were ineffective[61]; this suggested that plasma components, which include RF and immune complexes, were not important in the maintenance of synovitis. In contrast, Karsh et al. in a controlled study using lymphocytapheresis demonstrated a transient improvement in the number of tender and swollen joints in refractory RA patients lasting 5 to 7 weeks[62]. However, clinical response did not correlate with the degree of lymphopenia. The lack of prolonged benefit and practical difficulties prevents its routine use in clinical practice. However, it supports the notion that lymphocytes are important in RA.

Thoracic duct drainage

TDD is another method to remove lymphocytes. Paulus et al. studied nine patients with refractory RA who were treated with TDD over an average of 53 days[63]. A mean of 46×10^{10} lymphocytes were removed. Considerable lymphopenia resulted both in peripheral blood and lymph which returned to normal after 15 weeks. Statistically significant improvement was seen in the TDD treated group when compared to controls. Suppression of cell-mediated immune response was seen after treatment. Interestingly, reinfusion of live lymphocytes led to exacerbation of RA. Side-effects of TDD included sepsis, especially at the wound site, and gastrointestinal hemorrhage[64]. Although TDD seems to be effective in RA, the complicated and difficult technique of continuous drainage, combined with enormous cost and transient clinical benefit, preclude its use in everyday clinical practice.

Semispecific anti-T cell therapies

Depleting T cell subsets

Murine and chimeric anti-CD7 monoclonal antibodies

The exact function of the T lymphocyte specific antigen CD7 remains unknown. Activating CD7+ T cells with anti-CD7 Mab and a suboptimal level of mitogen or antigen led to increased secretion of IL-2 and expression of IL-2R[65]. In vitro, a blocking anti-CD7 mab inhibited mitogen stimulated lymphocyte proliferation[66]. In transplant rejection, anti-CD7 Mab has been shown to be an effective treatment[67]. Both murine and chimeric anti-CD7 Mabs have been used in refractory rheumatoid patient[68,69]. They reduce the number of peripheral blood and synovial CD7+ lymphocytes but did not produce any significant clinical improvement. These results questioned the role of CD7+ lymphocytes in the pathogenesis of RA. Indeed, it was found subsequently that CD7+ lymphocytes did not accumulate preferentially in rheumatoid joints when compared with peripheral blood[70]. Therefore CD7+ lymphocytes are probably unimportant in the pathogenesis of RA and the use of anti-CD7 Mabs has been abandoned.

CD5-plus

CD5-plus is an immunotoxin formed by conjugating a murine anti-CD5 Mab to the A chain of ricin. CD5 is expressed on most thymocytes, all mature T cells, and a subset of B cells. In an open study[71], CD5-plus, led to a 50 and 70 per cent clinical improvement in disease activity according to the Paulus criteria in established and early RA patients respectively. All the patients showed a marked reduction in peripheral blood CD5+ T cells. However, a subsequent double-blind, placebo-controlled trial of CD5-plus failed to show any significant clinical improvement despite inducing significant lymphopenia[72]. The results of the open studies and the placebo-controlled trial are difficult to interpret since different treatment regimens were used. Furthermore, in the randomised control trial, 40 per cent of patients in the placebo group showed significant clinical improvement. This reduces the power of the study but the cause of this high placebo response is unknown. In common with other murine mabs, all but one patient developed a HAMA by day 15 after CD5-plus treatment although no allergic side-effects were reported.

IL-2-DAB

The IL-2R is an early marker of activated T cells suggesting that this molecule could provide a specific therapeutic target. IL2-DAB is an immunotoxin composed of human IL-2 and diphtheria toxin. Once IL2-DAB binds to IL-2R on the surface of the activated lymphocytes, the diphtheria toxin is internalised and kills its target. In a placebo-controlled trial, IL2-DAB was more effective than placebo although only a small number of patient improved (18 versus 0 per cent)[73]. However, its use is limited by its toxicity as many patients developed fever, chills, rigor, and elevated liver transaminases. These side-effects were attributed to transient T cell activation since IL-2R has a cytoplasmic tail which can deliver a intracellular signal after binding to IL-2 before the lymphocyte is killed. Consequently, the development of IL2-DAB has been abandoned.

Campath-1H

Campath-1H is a humanized antibody targeting the surface antigen CDw52 expressed by lymphocytes, monocytes/macrophages, and natural killer cells. Its function is unknown but mabs binding to CDw52 leads to complement-mediated cytolysis[74]. Campath-1H has been used in the treatment of lymphoproliferative diseases[75], vasculitis[76], and RA[77,78]. In vasculitis, combining Campath-1H with non-depleting anti-CD4 mab produced prolonged disease improvement in a patient with refractory systemic vasculitis[76]. An initial open study[77] in nine patients with RA, Campath-1H treatment induced significant symptomatic improvement but the ESR remained unchanged. All patients developed profound lymphopenia which was severe and protracted. It affected both CD4 and CD8 lymphocytes and their numbers never returned to the pretreatment level. Obviously, prolonged lymphopenia is a potential risk for non-specific immunosuppression and a number of opportunistic infections including generalized herpes zoster and *Listeria monocytogene*

septicemia have been reported in patients treated with Campath-1H, particularly for lymphoproliferative diseases[79].

Interestingly, the decreased lymphocyte number showed no correlation with clinical response. Indeed, clinical relapse occurred in the presence of severe peripheral blood lymphopenia. Ruderman *et al.* studied the synovia during arthroplasty from a number of patients who had previously received Campath-1H and subsequently relapsed[80]. Although there was profound peripheral blood lymphopenia, the synovia of these patients showed normal mononuclear cell infiltration including CD4+ T lymphocytes. This suggested that Campath-1H is more effective in depleting peripheral blood lymphocytes than those in the joint.

Side-effects are common in Campath-1H infusions especially during the first dose. Nearly all the patients developed fever (up to 40°C), chills, rigors, hypotension, diarrhea, and dyspnea. These symptoms were similar to those seen after treatment with OKT3 for transplant rejection[81] which was associated with elevated serum levels of IL-2 and TNF-α, the so-called cytokine release syndrome. The intensity of the cytokine release syndrome could be reduced by administering Campath-1H subcutaneously; unfortunately this also reduced its therapeutic efficacy[82]. The severity of cytokine release syndrome and profound lymphopenia limit the clinical usefulness of Campath-1H in RA. Consequently the development of Campath-1H has been terminated.

Depleting anti-CD4 monoclonal antibody

Since CD4+ T cells are thought by many to be pivotal in the pathogenesis of RA, they are obvious targets for immunotherapy. Both murine and chimeric anti-CD4 mabs have been tested in RA clinical trials.

Murine anti-CD4 monoclonal antibodies

Several groups have used different murine anti-CD4 mabs in open clinical trials in refractory RA (Table 41.1)[83–87]. Antibodies were administered intravenously daily for 7 to 10 days. The dosage of Mab varied from 10 to 20 mg/day. Mild cytokine release syndrome was seen in some patients[88]. Significant clinical improvements were seen after treatment in these trials but there was a large variation in clinical response. Changes in acute phase response was only seen in two trials[84,87]. In a few cases clinical improvement persisted beyond 9 months[87]. Interestingly, the frequency of HAMA response was only 50[89], 60[86], and 20 per cent[87] which is less than other murine Mabs. One possible explanation is that treatment with murine anti-CD4 Mabs led to development of tolerance to itself[90].

Chimeric anti-CD4 monoclonal antibody

After the initial, promising results from murine mabs, the chimeric anti-CD4 mab, cM-T412 , was tested in refractory RA patients. It contains the F(ab)$_2$ of the murine anti-CD4 Mab, M-T412, joined to a human IgG1 Fc. It inhibits antigen stimulated lymphocyte proliferation but does not lead to complement-mediated lysis.

Two placebo-controlled trials have shown that cM-T412 was ineffective when administered weekly or monthly despite

Table 41.1 Murine anti-CD4 monoclonal antibodies used in rheumatoid arthritis

Name of antibody	Investigators
M-T151	Herzog C. *et al.*[85]
	Reiter C. *et al.*[86]
VIT4	Herzog C. *et al.*[85]
16H5	Horneff G. *et al.*[84]
BL4	Goldberg D. *et al.*[83]
BF5	Wendling D. *et al.*[87]

dose-related CD4 lymphopenia[91,92]. The clinical efficacy of cM-T412 when it was given daily remains controversial. Open studies suggested cM-T412 was effective[93-95] although clinical response was highly variable. However, a few patients showed sustained disease remission lasting over 2 years. In these studies, cM-T412 was given daily for 5 days and the dose varied between 10 and 100 mg/day. No studies showed a correlation between clinical response and peripheral blood CD4 lymphopenia. Immediately after treatment there was a sustained and profound CD4 lymphopenia which was dose dependent. In most patients, the CD4 lymphocyte numbers returned to the normal range after 6–12 months. However, in some it remained below pretreatment levels. Recovery of CD4 lymphocyte number may be delayed by the concurrent use of steroids[94] and methotrexate[96]. Indeed, one patient treated with oral steroids, methotrexate, and high dose cM-T412 died from *Pneumocytis carinii* infection[96]. However, most patients did not develop infectious complications after cM-T412 treatment despite profound CD4 lymphopenia.

The lack of correlation between CD4 lymphopenia and clinical response might be due to poor antibody penetration into the joint[94]. When paired peripheral blood and synovial fluid samples were analysed before and after treatment on the first and last day of therapy, there was a marked difference between the two compartments. In the peripheral blood, similar to previous studies, there was a rapid and profound CD4 lymphopenia after a single 50 mg dose of cM-T412 while synovial fluid CD4 lymphocyte numbers did not change. Most of the peripheral blood CD4 lymphocytes were coated with cM-T412 but only 11 per cent were coated in the synovial fluid. The percentage of antibody-coated synovial fluid CD4 lymphocytes rose to 49 per cent after five daily doses of cM-T412 although there was a wide range among patients. Interestingly, the percentage of synovial fluid cM-T412 coated CD4 lymphocyte correlated with the degree of clinical improvement[94].

A double-blind, placebo-controlled trial of cM-T412 in early RA patients failed to show any significant clinical response[97]. However, the dose of cM-T412 in this study was limited by the degree of CD4 lymphopenia. Interestingly, synovial histology from patients in this study showed a reduction in the number of inflammatory cells and adhesion molecule expression on endothelial cells although cytokine staining remained unchanged. There was no change in the CD4/CD8 lymphocyte ratio in the joint suggesting that in the synovium, cM-T412 at the dosage used did not deplete CD4 lymphocytes. Although higher doses of cM-T412 may lead to greater clinical efficacy, it

will undoubtedly result in severe and unacceptable CD4 lymphopenia. Hence the strategy of lymphocyte depletion has largely been abandoned in RA. However, recently, some researchers have advocated the use of stem cell rescue as a strategy for aggressive lymphocyte depletion treatment[98].

Semi-specific T cell immunomodulation

Non-depleting anti-CD4 monoclonal antibodies

The rationale for using non-depleting anti-CD4 Mab in RA was developed initially in animal models in which the treatment induced 'immunological tolerance'[31]. In SCW arthritis, a single course of a non-depleting anti-CD4 Mab, given at the time of disease induction, prevented the development of arthritis. Moreover, the treated animals acquired a resistance to further attempts at disease induction because of the induction of immunological tolerance. In non-obese diabetic mice, an animal model of diabetes, anti-CD4 Mab induced tolerance even in established disease[99]. Interestingly, CD4 lymphocyte depletion was not necessary to produce tolerance[100]. On the contrary, established anti-CD4 Mab mediated tolerance could be broken by lymphocyte depletion[101]. If anti-CD4 Mabs could induce tolerance in established human autoimmune diseases such as RA, it could lead to 'reprogramming' of the immune response and result in long-term disease improvement[102].

Three non-depleting anti-CD4 Mabs have been tested in RA. In an open-label, dose-escalating study using a humanized non-depleting anti-CD4 Mab, 4162W94 (Glaxo Wellcome), 24 patients in four cohorts were treated with five daily doses of 10 mg, 30 mg, 100 mg, or 300 mg. Clinical improvement with reduction in ESR and CRP was seen in patients treated with either 100 or 300 mg doses[103]. Interestingly, there were reductions in synovial fluid IL-6 and TNF-α levels. Treatments were well tolerated but half the patients developed a cytokine release syndrome. The concentration of synovial fluid 4162W94 was approximately 30 per cent of the corresponding plasma level[104]. A recent placebo-controlled trial has confirmed the clinical efficacy of the antibody although high-dose treatment was associated with lymphopenia and vasculitic skin rashes[105].

IDEC-CE9.1/SB-210396 is a primatized non-depleting anti-CD4 Mab developed in macaque monkeys. In a randomised, placebo-controlled trial[106], patients with refractory RA were treated either with placebo or three different doses (40, 80, and 140 mg) twice weekly for 4 weeks. In the two high-dose groups, there were statistically significant clinical improvements although some patients in the 140 mg group developed leukocytoclastic vasculitis that necessitated termination of treatment.

The results of a placebo-controlled trial using the humanized non-depleting anti-CD4 Mab, OKT4-cdr4a are not yet available although a preliminary communication suggested that it was efficacious[107].

Although short-term clinical trials suggest that non-depleting anti-CD4 Mabs suppress inflammation, long-term studies are necessary to assess whether they could induce prolonged disease remission in RA. If the latter is possible then they would transform the current treatment strategy for RA.

Immunomodulatory cytokine: IL-10

IL-10 is an immunosuppressive cytokine which inhibits the production of IL-1 and TNF-α *in vitro*[108]. It is found in the rheumatoid joint but the concentration is probably insufficient to abolish inflammation. In a double-blind, placebo-controlled trial, daily subcutaneous injections of IL-10 or placebo were given to 72 RA patients[109]. The doses given were placebo, 0.5, 1, 5, 10, or 20 μg/kg daily for 4 weeks. There was a trend towards clinical improvement in the 5 μg group after treatment for 4 weeks but further studies are necessary to assess its clinical efficacy in RA.

MHC and MHC-peptide vaccines

Since RA is linked with the HLA-DR4 and DR1 in Northern Europeans and North Americans, vaccination using the disease-associated MHC and MHC-peptide may be efficacious. This approach is effective in experimental allergic encephalomyelitis, an animal model of multiple sclerosis. In RA, three doses (1.3 mg, 4 mg, and 13 mg) of HLA-DR4/1-peptide were administered to 52 RA patients who were heterozygous for the shared epitope as an adjunct to methotrexate[110]. Treatment was well tolerated and no significant immunosuppression was seen. However, only 33 and 31 per cent of the patients developed IgG and IgM antibody response to the vaccine, respectively. Currently, there are plans to investigate the use of HLA-DR4/1 conjugated with the putative RA autoantigen HC-gp39 as a vaccine in RA[111].

T-cell vaccination

The concept of T-cell vaccination has arisen from an impressive body of experimental work. In adjuvant arthritis, the arthritogenic T cells can be chemically modified and used as a vaccine to prevent or treat disease[112]. The pathogenic T cell is first identified by showing that it is able to transfer disease from arthritic to naïve animals. Once identified, it is expanded as a cell line or clone and they are then rendered non-pathogenic by chemical or physical treatment. Finally, these T cells are injected into naïve animals as vaccines. Such vaccines then prevent disease induction and, more relevantly, suppress established disease. It is now clear that T-cell vaccination works by stimulating regulatory T cells, primarily directed against the T-cell receptor on the disease-inducing T cells (anti-idiotypic cells) but also against various T-cell activation antigens (antiergotypic cells)[113]. These regulatory cells are probably not generated *de novo* by vaccination but form part of a natural immunoregulatory network which is upregulated by vaccination[113].

The most obvious problem of T-cell vaccination in RA is the impossibility of determining which is the pathogenic T cell. Nonetheless, T-cell vaccination has been attempted using vaccines derived from synovial fluid T cells on the premise that the pathogenic T cells will be found at highest concentration at the site of disease. Three small open trials have been undertaken[114-116]. In the first study, there was no significant clinical or immunological response except slight reduction of RF. In the second study, two patients were treated but neither improved convincingly, although an antivaccine response was demonstrated in both. In the third study, three patients were treated of whom only one showed a clinical response; and interestingly, this was the only patient in whom an immunological response against the vaccine developed. These studies are difficult to analyse since the vaccines and the treatment protocols were different. In addition, it is impossible to detect any effect on the immune responses specific for RA since the causative antigen is not known. Consequently no further studies are planned in RA.

T-cell receptor vaccination

In many autoimmune diseases, an expansion of T cells with particular TCR Vβ chains are found in lesional sites, such as the synovium, compared to blood. It was proposed that such expanded T cells would be pathogenetically relevant. Furthermore, vaccination with peptides from TCR on pathogenic T cells inhibits disease in animal models of autoimmune diseases[117]. In RA, many different Vβ populations were reported to be expanded. A number of investigators have embarked on a clinical trial of a Vβ17-derived peptide in RA[118] based on the finding that there was an expansion of Vβ17 positive CD4 lymphocytes among the recently-activated T cells as defined by the expression of IL-2R[119] within the rheumatoid synovium. The initial uncontrolled, open, dose-finding study noted a reduction in joint scores and Vβ17+IL-2R+T cells in the blood. Approximately 40 per cent of patients developed a T-cell response to the vaccinated peptide. Treatment was well tolerated and no toxicity was observed. Subsequently, these investigators have used a combination of three TCR peptides (Vβ3, Vβ14, Vβ17) in incomplete Freund's adjuvant as a vaccine (IR501, Immune Response Corp) in a placebo-controlled trial of 99 RA patients[120]. The vaccine (90 μg or 300 μg) or placebo was administered as intramuscular injections at week 0, 4, 8, and 20. In only the 90 μg group there was a statistically significant improvement when compared with placebo although only a third of the patients showed a response to the vaccine. Hence, further studies are necessary to assess the efficacy and safety of TCR peptide-vaccines in RA.

Specific T cell immunomodulation: mucosal tolerance

Oral tolerance

Native type II collagen has been used to induce mucosal tolerance in RA. The initial study[121] showed a clinical improvement in patients treated with chicken-derived type II collagen compared to placebo; there was also an increase in the number of patients who went into remission. Disappointingly, a study from a different group, using bovine type II collagen[122], failed to demonstrate any significant effect. Both studies were underpowered and the former had serious trial design faults. The results of a large, placebo-controlled trial of 274 RA patients treated with oral chicken type II collagen has been published recently[123]. In this study, patients were treated with either placebo, 20, 100, 500, or 2500 μg/day of chicken type II collagen for 24 weeks. Three response criteria were used: Paulus, ACR, and ≥30 per cent reduction in both tender and swollen joint counts. Statistically significant improvement was only detected in the 2 µg/day group when compared with placebo (39 per cent versus 19 per cent) using Paulus criteria. Interestingly, presence of serum antibody to CII was associated with clinical improvement.

Current evidence suggests that oral tolerance may be efficacious although the clinical effect is small. New strategies to enhance the immunomodulatory effect of mucosal tolerance, such as administration via the nasal mucosa[124] or conjugation with cholera toxin[125], may lead to more effective treatment.

Nasal tolerance

In experimental allergic encephalomyelitis, attempts to induce oral tolerance with the pathogenic antigen, myelin basic protein, have been difficult. However, inhalation of myelin basic protein or its immunodominant peptides were effective[124]. Nasal tolerance has yet to be tested in RA but may be an important strategy for the future.

Conclusion

Current evidence suggests that CD4+ Th1 T cells are pathogenic in RA so that inhibiting T-cell function can suppress inflammation and reduce disease activity. In animal models of RA, immunomodulation of T cells can produce prolonged disease remission. This has yet to be demonstrated in human disease. Increased understanding of T-cell activation in RA may lead to more specific therapy in the future as most of our current attempts are relatively nonspecific.

References

1. Scott D.L., Symmons D.P., Coulton B.L., Popert A.J. Long-term outcome of treating rheumatoid arthritis: results after 20 years. *Lancet*, 1987;l:1108–11.
2. Wolfe F., Hawley D.J. Remission in rheumatoid arthritis. *J Rheumatol*, 1985;12:245–52.
3. Iannuzzi L., Dawson N., Zein N., Kushner I. Does drug therapy slow radiographic deterioration in rheumatoid arthritis? *N Engl J Med*, 1983;309:1023–8.
4. Wijnands M.J., vant Hof M.A., van Leeuwen M.A., van Rijswijk M.H., van de Putte L.B., van Riel P.L. Long-term second-line treatment: a prospective drug survival study. *Br J Rheumatol*, 1992;31:253–8.
5. Paulnock D.M. Macrophage activation by T cells. *Curr Opin Immunol*, 1992;4:344–9.
6. Kirkham B.W. Interleukin-1, immune activation pathways, and different mechanisms in osteoartbritis and rheumatoid arthritis. *Ann Rheum Dis*, 1991;50:395–400.
7. Brennan F.M., Feldmann M. Cytokines in autoimmunity. *Curr Opin Immunol*, 1992;4:754–9.
8. Firestein G.S., Zvaifler N.J. How important are T cells in chronic rheumatoid synovitis? *Arthritis Rheum*, 1990;33:768–73.
9. Panayi G.S., Lanchbury J.S., Kingsley G.H. The importance of the T cell in initiating and maintaining the chronic synovitis of rheumatoid arthritis. *Arthritis Rheum*, 1992;35:729–35.
10. Conceicao-Silva F., Schubach A.O., Nogueria R.S., Coutinho S.G. Quantitation of T cells which recognize Leishmania braziliensis braziliersis (Lbb) antigens in lesions and periopheral blood of cutaneous or mucosal leishmaniasis patients by limiting dilution analysis. *Mem Inst Oswaldo*, 1978;82:118.
11. Modlin R.L., Melancon-Kaplan J., Young S.M.M., *et al.* Learning from lesions: patterns of tissue inflammation in leprosy. *Proc Natl Acad Sci USA*, 1988;1213:1217.
12. Sieper J., Braun J., Wu P., Kingsley G.H. T cells are responsible for enhancing synovial cellular immune response to triggering antigen in reactive arthritis. *Clin Exp Immunol*, 1993;91:96–102.
13. Lanchbury J.S., Sakkas L.I., Panayi G.S., Smolen J.R. Kalden J.R., Maini R.N., eds. *Rheumatoid arthritis: recent research advances.* Berlin: Springer-Verlag, 1992; Genetic factors in rheumatoid arthritis. p. 17–28.
14. Boki K.A., Panayi G.S., Vaughan R.W., Drosos A.A., Moutsopoulos H.M., Lanchbury J.S. HLA class II sequence polymorphisms and susceptibility to rheumatoid arthritis in Greeks. The HLA-DR beta shared-epitope hypothesis accounts for the disease in only a minority of Greek patients. *Arthritis Rheum*, 1992;35:749–55.
15. Gao X., Gazit E., Livneh A., Stastny P. Rheumatoid arthritis in Israeli Jews: shared sequences in the third hypervariable region of DRB 1 alleles are associated with susceptibility. *J Rheumatol*, 1991;18:801–3.
16. Gregersen P.K., Silver J., Winchester R.J. The shared epitope hypothesis. An approach to understanding the molecular genetics of susceptibility to rheumatoid arthritis. *Arthritis Rheum*, 1987;30:1205–13.
17. Verheijden G.F., Rijnders A.W., Bos E., *et al.* Human cartilage glycoprotein-39 as a candidate autoantigen in rheumatoid arthritis. *Arthritis Rheum*, 1997;40:1115–25.
18. Duke O., Panayi G.S., Janossy G., Poulter L.W. An immunohistological analysis of lymphocyte subpopulations and their microenvironment in the synovial membranes of patients with RA using monoclonal antibodies. *Clin Exp Immunol*, 1982;49:23–30.
19. Duke O., Panayi G.S. The pathogenesis of rheumatoid arthritis. In vivo, 1988;2:95–104.
20. Galeazzi M., Afeltra A., Porzio F., Bonomo L. The activation markers on synovial T cells of rheumatoid arthritis. *Clin Rheumatol*, 1990;9
21. Loetscher P., Uguccioni M., Bordoli L., *et al.* CCR5 is characteristic of Th1 lymphocytes. *Nature*, 1998;391:344–5.
22. Combe B., Pope R.M., Fischbach M., Darnell B., Baron S., Talal N. Interleukin-2 in rheumatoid arthritis: production of and response to interleukin-2 in rheumatoid synovial fluid, synovial tissue and peripheral blood. *Clin Exp Immunol*, 1985;59:520–8.
23. Dolhain R.J., ter Haar N.T., Hoefakker S., *et al.* Increased expression of interferon (IFN)-gamma together with IFN-gamma receptor in the rheumatoid synovial membrane compared with synovium of patients with osteoarthritis. *Br J Rheumatol*, 1996;35:24–32.
24. Buchan G., Barrett K., Fujita T., Taniguchi T., Maini R.N., Feldmann M. Detection of activated T cell products in the rheumatoid joint using cDNA probes to interleukin 2 (1L2), 1L2 receptor and IFNτ. *Clin Exp Immunol*, 1988;71:295–301.
25. Waalen K., Sioud M., Natvig J.B., Fxrre O. Spontaneous in vivo gene transcription of interleukin-2, interleukin-3, interleukin-4, interleukin-6, interferon-gamma, interleukin-2 receptor (CD25) and proto-oncogene c-myc by rheumatoid synovial T cells. *Scand J Immunol*, 1992;36:865–73.
26. Schreiber S.L., Crabtree G.R. The mechanism of action of cyclosporin A and FK506. *Immunol Today*, 1992;13:136–42.
27. Weinblatt M.E., Coblyn J.S., Fraser P.A., *et al.* Cyclosporin A treatment of refractory rheumatoid arthritis. *Arthritis Rheum*, 1987;30:11–7.
28. Pasero G., Priolo F., Marubini E., *et al.* Slow progression of joint damage in early rheumatoid arthritis treated with cyclosporin A. *Arthritis Rheum*, 1996;39:1006–15.

29. Russell R.G.G., Graveley R. Skjodt H. The effects of cyclosporin A on bone and cartilage. *Br J Rheumatol*, 1993;32(suppl 1):42–6.

30. Levitt N.G., Fernandez Madrid F., Wooley P.H. Pristane induced arthritis in mice. IV. Immunotherapy with monoclonal antibodies directed against lymphocyte subsets. *J Rheumatol*, 1992;19:1342–7.

31. Van den Broek M.E., Van de Langerijt L.G., Van Bruggen M.C., Billingham M.E,. Van den Berg W.B. Treatment of rats with monoclonal anti-CD4 induces long-term resistance to streptococcal cell wall-induced arthritis. *Eur J Immunol*, 1992;22:57–61.

32. Yoshino S., Cleland L.G., Mayrhofer G. Treatment of collagen-induced arthritis in rats with a monoclonal antibody against the alpha beta T cell antigen receptor. *Arthritis Rheum*, 1991;34:1039–47.

33. Chiocchia G., Boissier M.C., Fournier C. Therapy against murine collagen-induced arthritis with T cell receptor V beta-specific antibodies. *Eur J Immunol*, 1991;21:2899–905.

34. Larsson P., Holmdahl R. Klareskog L. In vivo treatment with anti-CD8 and anti-CD5 monoclonal antibodies alters induced tolerance to adjuvant arthritis. *J Cell Biochem*, 1989;40:49–56.

35. Kavanaugh A.F., Schulze-Koops H., Davis L.S., Lipsky P.E. Repeat treatment of rheumatoid arthritis patients with a murine anti-intercellular adhesion molecule-I monoclonal antibody. *Arthritis Rheum*, 1997;40:849–53.

36. Waldmann T.A. Monoclonal antibodies in diagnosis and therapy. *Science*, 1991;252:1657–62.

37. Weiner H.L., Friedman A., Miller A., et al. Oral tolerance: immunologic mechanisms and treatment of animal and human organ-specific autoimmune disease by oral administration of autoantigens. *Ann Rev Immunol*, 1994;12:809–37.

38. Staines N.A. Oral tolerance and collagen arthritis. *Br J Rheumatol*, 1991;30:40–3.

39. Kronke M., Leonard W.J., Depper J.M., et al. Cyclosporin A inhibits T-cell growth factor gene expression at the level of mRNA transcription. *Proc Natl Acad Sci USA*, 1984;81:5214–8.

40. Walsh C.T., Zydowsky L.D., McKeon F.D. Cyclosporin A, the cyclophilin class of peptidylprolyl isomerases, and blockade of T cell signal transduction. *J Biol Chem*, 1992;267:13115–8.

41. Yocum D.E. Cyclosporine, FK-506, rapamycin, and other immunomodulators. *Rheum Dis Clin N Am*, 1996;22:133–54.

42. Dougados M., Torley H. Efficacy of cyclosporin A in rheumatoid arthritis: worldwide experience. *Br J Rheumatol*, 1993;32 (suppl l):57–9.

43. Schreiber S.L., Crabtree G.R. The mechanism of action of cyclosporin A and FK506. *Immunol Today*, 1992;13:136–42.

44. Inamura N., Hashimoto M., Nakahara K., Aoki H., Yamaguchi I., Kohsaka M. Immunosuppressive effect of FK506 on collagen-induced arthritis in rats. *Clin Immunol Immunop*, 1988;46:82–90.

45. Dumont F.J., Su Q. Mechanism of action of the immunosuppressant rapamycin. *Life Sciences*, 1996;58:373–95.

46. Flanagan W.M., Crabtree G.R. Rapamycin inhibits p34cdc2 expression and arrests T lymphocyte proliferation at the G1/S transition. *Ann New York Acad Sci* 1993;696:31–7.

47. Migita K., Eguchi K., Aoyagi T., et al. The effects of the immunosuppressant rapamycin on the growth of rheumatoid arthritis (RA) synovial fibroblast. *Clin Exp Immunol*, 1996;104:86–91.

48. Carlson R.P., Baeder W.L., Caccese R.G., Warner L.M., Sehgal S.N. Effects of orally administered rapamycin in animal models of arthritis and other autoimmune diseases. *Ann New York Acad Sci*, 1993;685:86–113.

49. Schiff M., Stein G., Leischman B. Cellcept (Mycophenolate Mofetil—MMF) a new treatment for RA: a 9-month, randomized, double-blind trial comparing 1 g bid and 2 g bid. [Abstract] *Arthritis Rheum*, 1997;40(Suppl):S194.

50. Colonna P., Andrieu J.M., Ghouadni R. et al. Advanced Hodgkin disease (clinical stages IIIB and IV): low relapse rate after brief chemotherapy followed by high-dose total lymphoid irradiation. *Am J Hematol*, 1989;30:121–7.

51. Lindsley H.B., Jamieson T.W., De Smet A.A., Kimler B.F., Cremer M.A., Hassanein K.M. Total lymphoid irradiation retards evolution of articular erosions in collagen induced arthritis. *J Rheumatol*, 1988;15:742–4.

52. Kotzin B.L., Strober S., Engleman E.G., et al. Treatment of intractable rheumatoid arthritis with total lymphoid irradiation. *N Engl J Med*, 1981;305:969–76.

53. Strober S., Tanay A., Field E., et al. Efficacy of total lymphoid irradiation in intractable rheumatoid arthritis. A double-blind, randomized trial. *Ann Intern Med*, 1985;102:441–9.

54. Field E.H., Strober S., Hoppe R.T., et al. Sustained improvement of intractable rheumatoid arthritis after total lymphoid irradiation. *Arthritis Rheum*, 1983;26:937–46.

55. Strober S., Kotzin B.L., Hoppe R.T., et al. The treatment of intractable rheumatoid arthritis with lymphoid irradiation. *Int J Radiat Oncol Biol Phys*, 1981;7:1–7.

56. Kotzin E.L., Kansas G.S., Engleman E.G., Hoppe R.T., Kaplan H.S., Strober S. Changes in T cell subsets in patients with rheumatoid arthritis treated with total lymphoid irradiation. *Clin Immunol Immunopathol*, 1983;27:250–60.

57. Strober S., Field E.M., Kotzin B.L., et al. Treatment of intractable rheumatoid arthritis with total lymphoid irradiation (TLI): immunological and clinical changes. *Radiother Oncol*, 1983; 1:43–52.

58. Sherrer Y., Bloch D., Strober S., Fries J. Comparative toxicity of total lymphoid irradiation and immunosuppressive drug treated patients with intractable rheumatoid arthritis. *J Rheumatol*, 1987;14:46–51.

59. Tanay A., Field E.H., Hoppe R.T., Strober S. Long-term followup of rheumatoid arthritis patients treated with total lymphoid irradiation. *Arthritis Rheum*, 1987;30:1–10.

60. Brahn E., Helfgott S.M., Belli J.A., et al. Total lymphoid irradiation therapy in refractory rheumatoid arthritis. Fifteen- to forty-month followup. *Arthritis Rheum*, 1984;27:481–8.

61. Dwosh I.L., Giles A.R., Ford P.M., Pater J.L., Anastassiades TP. Plasmapheresis therapy in rheumatoid arthritis. A controlled, double-blind, crossover trial. *N Engl J Med*, 1983;308:1124–9.

62. Karsh J., Klippel J.H., Plotz P.H., Decker J.L., Wright D.G., Flye M.W. Lymphapheresis in rheumatoid arthritis. A randomized trial. *Arthritis Rheum*, 1981;24:867–73.

63. Paulus H.E., Machleder H.I., Levine S., Yu D.T., MacDonald N.S. Lymphocyte involvement in rheumatoid arthritis. Studies during thoracic duct drainage. *Arthritis Rheum*, 1977;20:1249–62.

64. Decker J.L. Apheresis and rheumatoid arthritis. *Ann Intern Med*, 1983;98:666–7.

65. Jung L.K., Roy A.K., Chakkalath H.R. CD7 augments T cell proliferation via the interleukin-2 autocrine pathway. *Cell Immunol*, 1992;141:189–99

66. Costantinides Y., Kingsley G.H., Pitzalis C., Panayi G.S. Inhibition of lymphocyte proliferation by a monoclonal antibody (RFT2) against CD7. *Clin Exp Immunol*, 1991;85:164–7.

67. Lazarovits A.I., Rochon J., Banks L. et al. Human mouse chimeric CD7 monoclonal antibody (SDZCHH3 80) for the prophylaxis of kidney transplant rejection. *J Immunol*, 1993;150:5163–74.

68. Kirkham B.W., Pitzalis C., Kingsley G.H., et al. Monoclonal antibody treatment in rheumatoid arthritis: Clinical and immunological effects of a CD7 monoclonal antibody. *Br J Rheumatol*, 1991;30:459–63.

69. Kirkham B.W., Thien F., Pelton B.K., et al. Chimeric CD7 monoclonal antibody therapy in rheumatoid arthritis. *J Rheumatol*, 1992;19:1348–52.

70. Lazarovits A.I., White M.J., Karsh J. CD7- T cells in rheumatoid arthritis. *Arthritis Rheum*, 1992;35:615–24.

71. Strand V., Lipsky P.E., Cannon G.W., et al. Effects of administration of an anti-CD5 plus immunoconjugate in rheumatoid arthritis. Results of two phase II studies. The CD5 Plus Rheumatoid Arthritis Investigators Group. *Arthritis Rheum*, 1993;36:620–30.

72. Olsen N.J., Brooks R.H., Cush J.J., et al. A double-blind, placebo-controlled study of antiCD5 immunoconjugate in patients with rheumatoid arthritis. *Arthritis Rheum*, 1996;39:1102–8.

73. Moreland L.W., Sewell K.L., Trentham D.E., et al. Interleukin-2 diphtheria fusion protein (DAB486IL-2) in refractory rheumatoid arthritis. A double-blind, placebo-controlled trial with open-label extension. *Arthritis Rheum*, 1995;38:1177–86.

74. Greenwood J., Clark M., Waldmann H. Structural motifs involved in human IgG antibody effector functions. *Eur J Immunol*, 1993;23:1098–104.

75. Hale G., Dyer M.J., Clark M.R., *et al.* Remission induction in non-Hodgkin lymphoma with reshaped human monoclonal antibody CAMIPATh-1H. *Lancet*, 1988;2:1394–9.

76. Lockwood C.M., Thiru S., Isaacs J.D., Hale G., Waldmann H. Long-term remission of intractable systemic vasculitis with monoclonal antibody therapy. *Lancet*, 1993;341:1620–2.

77. Isaacs J.D., Watts R.A., Hazelman B.L., *et al.* Humanised monoclonal antibody therapy for rheumatoid arthritis. *Lancet*, 1992;340:748–52.

78. Isaacs J.D., Manna V.K., Rapson N., *et al.* Campath-1H in rheumatoid arthritis—an intravenous dose-ranging study. *Br J Rheumatol*, 1996;35:231–40.

79. Poynton C.H., Mort D., Maughan T.S. Adverse reactions to Campath-1H monoclonal antibody. *Lancet*, 1993;341:1037.

80. Ruderman E.M., Weinblatt M.E., Thurmond L.M., Pinkus G.S., Gravallese E.M. Synovial tissue response to treatment with Campath-1H. *Arthritis Rheum*, 1995;38:254–8.

81. Norman D.J., Chatenoud L., Cohen D., Goldman M., Shield C.F., 3d. Consensus statement regarding OKT3 -induced cytokine-release syndrome and human antimouse antibodies. *Transplantation Proceedings*, 1993;25:89–92.

82. Matteson E.L., Yocum D.E., St Clair E.W., *et al.* Treatment of active refractory rheumatoid arthritis with humanized monoclonal antibody CAMPATh-IH administered by daily subcutaneous injection. *Arthritis Rheum*, 1995;38:1187–93.

83. Goldberg D., Morel P., Chatenoud L., *et al.* Immunological effects of high dose administration of anti-CD4 antibody in rheumatoid arthritis patients. *J Autoimmunity*, 1991;4:617–30.

84. Horneff G., Burmester G.R., Emmrich F., Kalden J.R. Treatment of rheumatoid arthritis with an anti-CD4 monoclonal antibody. *Arthritis Rheum*, 1991;34:129–40.

85. Herzog C., Walker C., Muller W., *et al.* Anti-CD4 antibody treatment of patients with rheumatoid arthritis: I. Effect on clinical course and circulating T cells. *J Autoimmunity*, 1989;2:627–42.

86. Reiter C., Kakavand B., Rieber E.P., Schattenkirchner M., Riethmuller G., Kruger K. Treatment of rheumatoid arthritis with monoclonal CD4 antibody M-T151. Clinical results and immunopharmacologic effects in an open study, including repeated administration. *Arthritis Rheum*, 1991;34:525–36.

87. Wendling D., Racadot E., Morel-Fourrier B., Wijdenes J. Treatment of rheumatoid arthritis with anti-CD4 monoclonal antibody. Open study of 25 patients with the B-F25 clone. *Clin Rheumatol*, 1992;11:542–7.

88. Horneff G., Krause A., Emmrich F., Kalden J.R., Burmester G.R. Elevated levels of circulating tumor necrosis factor-alpha, interferon-gamma, and interleukin-2 in systemic reactions induced by anti-CD4 therapy in patients with rheumatoid arthritis. *Eur Cytokine Netw*, 1991;3:266–7.

89. Horneff G., Winkler T., Kalden J.R., Emmrich F., Burmester G.R. Human anti-mouse antibody response induced by anti-CD4 monoclonal antibody therapy in patients with rheumatoid arthritis. *Clin Immunol Immunopathol*, 1991;59:89–103.

90. Benjamin R.J., Waldmann H. Induction of tolerance by monoclonal antibody therapy. *Nature*, 1986;320:449–51.

91. Choy E.H.S., Chikanza I.C., Kingsley G.H., Corrigall V., Panayi G.S. Treatment of rheumatoid arthritis with single dose or weekly pulses of chimaeric anti-CD4 monoclonal antibody. *Scand J Immunol*, 1992;36:291–8.

92. Moreland L.W., Pratt P.W., Mayes M.D., *et al.* Double-blind, placebo-controlled multicenter trial using chimeric monoclonal anti-CD4 antibody, cM-T4 12, in rheumatoid arthritis patients receiving concomitant methotrexate. *Arthritis Rheum*, 1995;38:1581–8.

93. Moreland L.W., Bucy R.P., Tilden A., *et al.* Use of a chimeric monoclonal anti-CD4 antibody in patients with refractory rheumatoid arthritis. *Arthritis Rheum*, 1993;36:307–18.

94. Choy E.H., Pitzalis C., Cauli A., *et al.* Percentage of anti-CD4 monoclonal antibody-coated lymphocytes in the rheumatoid joint is associated with clinical improvement. Implications for the development of immunotherapeutic dosing regimens. *Arthritis Rheum*, 1996;39:52–6.

95. van der Lubbe P.A., Reiter C., Breedveld F.C., *et al.* Chimeric CD4 monoclonal antibody cMT412 as a therapeutic approach to rheumatoid arthritis. *Arthritis Rheum*, 1993;36:1375–9.

96. Moreland L.W., Pratt P.W., Bucy R.P., Jackson B.S., Feldman J.W., Koopman W.J. Treatment of refractory rheumatoid arthritis with chimaeric anti-CD4 antibody. Long-term follow up of CD4+ T cell counts. *Arthritis Rheum*, 1994;37:834–8.

97. van der Lubbe P.A., Dijkmans B.A., Markusse H.M., Nassander U., Breedveld F.C. A randomized, double-blind, placebo-controlled study of CD4 monoclonal antibody therapy in early rheumatoid arthritis. *Arthritis Rheum*, 1995;38:1097–106.

98. Tyndall A., Gratwohl A. Haepopoietic stem and progenitor cells in the treatment of severe autoimmune disease. *Ann Rheum Dis*, 1996;55:149–51.

99. Hutchings P., O'Reilly L., Parish N.M., Waldmann H., Cooke A. The use of a non-depleting anti-CD4 monoclonal antibody to re-establish tolerance to beta cells in NOD mice. *Eur J Immunol*, 1992;22:1913–8.

100. Carteron N.L., Wofsy D., Seaman W.E. Induction of immune tolerance during administration of monoclonal antibody to L3T4 does not depend on depletion of L3T4+ cells. *J Immunol*, 1988;140:713–6.

101. Parish N.M., Hutchings P.R., Waldmann H., Cooke A. Tolerance to IDDM induced by CD4 antibodies in nonobese diabetic mice is reversed by cyclophosphamide. *Diabetes*, 1993;42:1601–5.

102. Cobbold S.P., Qin S.X., Waldmann H. Reprogramming the immune system for tolerance with monoclonal antibodies. *Semin Immunol*, 1990;2:377–87.

103. Panayi G.S., Choy E.H.S., Connolly D.J.A., *et al.* T cell hypothesis in rheumatoid arthritis (RA) tested by humanised non-depleting anti-CD4 monoclonal antibody (mAb) treatment I suppression of disease activity and acute phase response. [Abstract] *Arthritis Rheum*, 1996;39(Suppl):S244.

104. Choy E.H.S., Connolly D.J.A., Rapson N., Kingsley G.H., Johnston J.M., Panayi G.S. Effect of a humanised non-depleting anti-CD4 monoclonal antibody (mAb) on synovial fluid (SF) in rheumatoid arthritis (RA). [Abstract] *Arthritis Rheum*, 1997;40(Suppl):552.

105. Panayi G.S., Choy E.H.S., Emery P., *et al.* Repeat-cycle study of high-dose intravenous (iv) 4162w94 anti-CD4 monoclonal antibody (mAb) in rheumatoid arthritis (RA). [Abstract] *Arthritis Rheum*, 1998;41:In press.

106. Levy R., Weisman M., Wiesenhutter C., *et al.* Results of a Placebo-Controlled, Multicenter Trial Using a Primatized, Non-Depleting, Anti-CD4 Monoclonal Antibody in the Treatment of Rheumatoid Arthritis. [Abstract] *Arthritis Rheum*, 1996;39(suppl):S122

107. Schulze-Koops H., Davis L.S., Haverty P., Wacholtz M.C., Lipsky P. Reduction of Th1 cell activity in patients with rheumatoid arthritis after treatment with a non-depleting mono-clonal antibody to CD4. [Abstract] *Arthritis Rheum*, 1997;40(Suppl): S191,

108. Katsikis P.D., Chu C.Q., Brennan F.M., Maini R.N., Feldmann M. Immunoregulatory role of interleukin 10 in rheumatoid arthritis. *J Exp Med*, 1994;179:1517–27.

109. Maini R.N., Paulus H., Breedveld F.C., *et al.* rHUIL-10 in subjects with active rheumatoid arthritis (RA): A phase I and cytokine response study. *Arthritis Rheum*, 1997;40(Suppl):S224.

110. St Clair E.W., Cohen S.B., Fleischmann R.M. *et al.* Vaccination of rheumatoid arthritis patients with DR4/1-peptide. [Abstract] *Arthritis Rheum*, 1997;40:S96.

111. Pitzalis C., Choy E. Fourth international symposium on the immunotherapy of the rheumatic diseases. *Ann Rheum Dis*, 1998;57:177–179.

112. Cohen P.L., Naparstek Y., Ben-Nun A., Cohen I.R. Lines of T lymphocytes induce or vaccinate against autoimmune arthritis. *Science*, 1983;219:56–8.

113. Lohse A.W., Cohen I.R. Immunoregulation: studies of physiological and therapeutic autoreactivity by T cell vaccination. *Springer Seminars In Immunopathology*, 1992;14:179–86.

114. van Laar J.M., Miltenburg A.M.M., Verdonk M.J., Daha M.R., de Vries R.R.P., Breedveld F.C. T cell vaccination in rheumatoid arthritis. *Br J Rheumatol*, 1991;**30**:28–9

115. Lohse A.W., Bakker N.P., Hermann E., Poralla T., Jonker M., Meyer zumBuschenfelde K.H. Induction of an anti-vaccine response by T cell vaccination in non-human primates and humans. *Autoimmunity*, 1993;**6**:121–30.

116. Kingsley G., Verwilghen J., Chikanza I., Panayi G.S. T cell vaccination (TCV) in rheumatoid arthritis: a controlled double-blinded pilot study. [Abstract] *Arthritis Rheum*, 1992;**35**:S44.

117. Howell M.D., Winters S.T., Olee T., Powell H.C., Carlo D.J., Brostoff S.W. Vaccination against experimental allergic encephalomyelitis with T cell receptor peptides. *Science*, 1989;**246**:668–70.

118. Moreland L.W., Heck Jr L.W., Koopman W.J., *et al.* Vf317 T cell receptor peptide vaccination in rheumatoid arthritis: results of phase I dose escalation study. *J Rheumatol*, 1996;**23**:1353–62.

119. Howell M.D., Diveley Y.P., Lundeen K.A., *et al.* Limited T-cell receptor β-chain heterogeneity among interleukin 2 receptor-positive synovial T cells suggests a role for superantigen in rheumatoid arthritis. *Proc Natl Acad Sci USA*, 1991;**88**:10921–5.

120. Moreland L., Koopman W.J., Adamson T., *et al.* Results of phase II rheumatoid arthrtis clinical trial using T cell receptor peptides. [Abstract] *Arthritis Rheum*, 1997;**40**:S223.

121. Trentham D.E., Dynesius-Trentham R.A., Orav E.J., *et al.* Effects of oral administration of type II collagen on rheumatoid arthritis. *Science*, 1993;**261**:1727–30.

122. Sieper J., Kary S., Sorensen H., *et al.* Oral type II collagen treatment in early rheumatoid arthritis. A double-blind, placebo-controlled, randomized trial. *Arthritis Rheum*, 1996;**39**:41–51.

123. Barnett M.L., Kremer J.M., St. Clair E.W., Clegg D.O., Furst D., Weisman M., Fletcher M.J.F., Chasan-Taber S., Finger E., Morales A., *et al.* Treatment of rheumatoid arthritis with oral type II collagen: results of a multicenter, double-blind, placebo-controlled trial. *Arthritis Rheum*, 1998;**41**:290–7.

124. Metzler B., Wraith D.C. Mucosal tolerance in a murine model of experimental autoimmune encephalomyelitis. *Ann NY Acad Sci*, 1996;**778**:228–42.

125. Sun J.B., Rask C., Olsson T., Holmgren J., Czerkinsky C. Treatment of experimental autoimmune encephalomyelitis by feeding myelin basic protein conjugated to cholera toxin B subunit. *Proc Natl Acad Sci USA*, 1996;**93**:7196–201.

42 | *Antimacrophage therapies*

Alison M. Badger

Introduction

Rheumatoid arthritis (RA) is a chronic inflammatory disease of unknown etiology that targets the synovial membrane as well as the extra-articular tissues. The disease is characterized by bone and cartilage destruction leading to gross crippling joint deformities, significant levels of pain, and increased mortality. A successful therapy would reduce inflammation and pain as well as retarding or reversing joint destruction. The current first line therapies for RA are non-steroidal anti-inflammatory drugs (NSAIDs) and steroids. These are followed by second line agents which have a slower mechanism of action and are known as slow-acting or disease-modifying drugs (SMARDs or DMARDs). The DMARDs currently in use have mainly been adapted from other specialties for the treatment of RA. Unfortunately, the mechanism of action for these compounds is not always well defined and most of them have side-effects that are not tolerable for long-term therapy and their ability to reverse joint destruction is questionable.

RA is considered to be the result of an autoimmune reaction. However the causative antigen is still unknown. Intense efforts to define an infectious agent have failed, although several pathogens have been proposed as being the culprits in initiation of the disease[1]. However, the concept that RA is infectious in origin continues to be attractive. The lack of knowledge of the etiological agent has hampered the straightforward approach of being able to target a specific antigen, molecule, or infectious agent. Therefore, considerable effort has been invested in targeting the cells, and/or the soluble factors that they produce, generally thought to be responsible for disease pathology. The progress that has been made in recent years in understanding the cellular and molecular events in the disease pathology, and in the immune response in general, has contributed greatly to the current therapeutic approaches under investigation.

Role of macrophages in RA

RA is characterized by a mononuclear infiltration into the synovial tissue of the joints. This occurs during joint inflammation where there is an abnormal proliferation of the lining of the synovium resulting in a considerable increase in thickness. Coupled with this is a huge infiltration of both macrophages and lymphocytes. Examination of cytokine production in the synovial tissue of the inflamed joint reveals an abundance of cytokines and growth factors produced by macrophages compared with the relatively low levels of T cell-

derived mediators[2]. Macrophages release proinflammatory cytokines, chemokines, growth factors, and enzymes, all of which contribute to the disease process. Therefore, in an attempt to develop new therapies for RA, it is a reasonable approach to target either the macrophage itself, or one or more of the factors that this cell produces. This not to say that the macrophage is wholly responsible for the initiating event in RA, although this hypothesis has been proposed[3].

Regardless of whether these cells initiate the disease, or whether they are a secondary phenomenon that exacerbates a T-cell instigated event, it is clear that the inflammatory events in the joint are sustained by these cells and the mediators that they produce. This chapter will describe some of those therapies, both currently in use as well as those in preclinical experimental evaluation, that target the monocyte/macrophage population(s) of cells. This includes compounds that inactivate or interfere with the proinflammatory potential of the cells themselves, as well as compounds that inhibit their ability to produce proinflammatory cytokines such as TNF-α, IL-1, IL-6, IL-8, GM-CSF, and other small molecules such as nitric oxide (NO).

In addition to targeting the production and/or activity of pro-inflammatory cytokines, there are additional cytokines that have been identified as having anti-inflammatory or immunosuppressive activity. Examples of these cytokines are IL-4, IL-10, and IL-13, as well as transforming growth factor-β (TGF-β) all of which have been shown to have anti-inflammatory activity both *in vitro* and *in vivo*. Evaluation of these cytokines as therapeutic agents, or attempts to stimulate their production, is another area with therapeutic potential that is being aggressively pursued. Other strategies, such as induction of apoptosis, modulation of macrophage inhibitory factor (MIF), and inhibition of those chemokines that attract monocyte/macrophages to the sites of inflammation, will be discussed.

Antimacrophage therapy: targeting the macrophage at the cellular level

Leukapheresis

The efficacy of leukapheresis has long been proven in RA and systemic connective tissue diseases and the procedure may now be improved by new equipment allowing peripheral elimination by specific leukocyte filters (reviewed in Ref. 4). In severe RA, it has been demonstrated that repeated leukapheresis can be effective in depleting activated monocytes from the circulation[5,6,7]. Cells of the monocyte/macrophage system are already highly activated in the peripheral blood of RA patients with active disease[8] and cells obtained from a first leukapheresis were shown to constitutively release large amounts of prostaglandin E2 (PGE2), neopterin, IL-1β, and TNF-α. In addition, the IL-1 and neopterin levels produced by these cells could be further enhanced by stimulation with interferon-gamma (IFN-γ) or TNF-α *in vitro*. In a second or third leukapheresis most of the activated monocytes were shown to have been removed and the repopulating cells showed a reduced activation status compared to the cells prior to therapy. Concomitant clinical assessments revealed a significant reduction in the mean Ritchie articular index after the final leukapheresis procedure[8].

Induction of apoptosis

RA is characterized by synovial proliferation and the hyperplasia of synoviocytes resulting in bone and joint destruction. Occasionally, a spontaneous arrest of the synovial hypertrophy is observed in the disease process, strongly suggesting the presence of cell death known as apoptosis (reviewed in Ref. 9). It has been suggested that autoimmune disease, including RA, is a result of defective apoptosis[10]. In fact, apoptotic cells are present in the rheumatoid synovium and the apoptotic process is accelerated by anti-Fas monoclonal antibody (Mab)[11]. In a recent *in vivo* study in SCID mice, anti-Fas monoclonal antibody diminished rheumatoid synovial tissue that had been engrafted into the mice[12]. A search for molecules that could induce apoptosis in activated macrophages could well be a viable strategy for treatment of RA. Further investigation into the role of Fas and Fas-ligand in the rheumatoid synovium and the risks and benefits of manipulating these receptor–ligand interactions will determine the usefulness of this approach. Some compounds, in fact, already being evaluated in the treatment of RA or in preclinical development, have been shown to induce apoptotic events *in vitro*, although not necessarily in monocyte/macrophage cell populations. An example of compounds that appear to be able to modulate apoptotic events are some of the p38 MAP kinase inhibitors. These compounds have been described as both inducing apoptosis[13], enhancing TNF-α mediated apoptosis[14] or inhibiting apoptosis[15]. Another example is the antiarthritic agent bucillamine which has been shown to induce apoptosis in concert with copper[16].

Liposome-encapsulated antimacrophage agents

Synovial lining macrophages are key cells in the onset of RA. When these cells are eliminated from the joint by local injection of toxic liposomes there is a significant improvement in arthritic symptoms. In a mouse model of antigen-induced arthritis, liposome-encapsulated clodronate (dichloromethylene bisphosphonate) injected into the knee joint on day 7 after onset of arthritis, sustained loss of lining cells and at day 21 there was a significant reduction in the cellular infiltrate. The toxic liposomes are taken up by the synovial lining macrophages and the depletion lasts for several weeks. This treatment was shown to be efficacious in a number of animal models of arthritis including immune complex arthritis, antigen-induced arthritis, and

collagen-induced arthritis (reviewed in Ref. 17). Liposomal clodronate is a more potent inactivator of macrophages than liposomal forms of two other bisphosphonate compounds, pamidronate (3-amino-1-hydroxypropylidene bisphosphonate), and etidronate (1-hydroxyethylidene-1,1-bisphosphonate). All three of these bisphosphonates encapsulated in liposomes effectively inhibited the growth of RAW 264 cells while free drugs were 20–1000 times less potent growth inhibitors[18].

One caveat to the approach of deleting monocyte/macrophages is that there may be a population(s) of macrophage in the joint that have more of a protective than a pro-inflammatory function. These cells would be those producing inhibitors such as IL-10 or TGF-β. Selective stimulation of IL-10 producing macrophages or selective elimination of those cells producing IL-1 and TNF has been suggested as an elegant approach[17] and might be achieved by the use of monoclonal antibodies targeted to cell surface markers. In this manner, the overt depletion of macrophages would be avoided, a situation which could compromise the generation of an effective immune response when required.

Antimacrophage therapy: lysosome targeting agents

A number of compounds, already being used to treat RA, have been found to accumulate in macrophage lysosomes. This accumulation could alter the functional activity of these cells and thus reduce or modify their proinflammatory activity. This modulation in functional activity may include changes in antigen presentation, changes in hydrolytic enzyme production and activity, modulation of cytokine and inflammatory mediator production, to name but a few. Different classes of antiarthritic compounds have been shown to accumulate in lysosomes but the functional outcome of this accumulation in macrophages is not identical for the different compounds.

Gold compounds

Gold compounds have been used as DMARDs in RA for many years and their mechanism of action continues to be an area of active research. Administration of gold compounds to RA patients results in the accumulation of gold in the lysosomes of synovial macrophages in RA patients[19,20]. Gold compounds have a number of effects on macrophages which include inhibition of Fc and C3 receptor expression in monocytes[21], reduction in oxygen radical generation[22,23] and inhibition of macrophage accessory cell function as demonstrated by their effects on T cell proliferation to antigen and mitogen[24,25]. They have also been shown to inhibit IL-1, IL-8, and macrophage chemotactic protein-1 (MCP-1) from monocytes and synovial cells[26–29] and to decrease monocyte chemotaxis *in vitro*[21,22]. Intramuscular gold has been shown to decrease cytokine expression and macrophage numbers in biopsies of rheumatoid synovial membrane[30].

It should be noted that the effects of gold compounds on IL-1 and TNF production and activity are actually quite contradictory, and depend on the gold compound being studied, the culture conditions, and the stimulus used[31]. However, several studies have shown that auranofin can inhibit the production of both IL-1 and TNF-α (reviewed in Ref. 31). The effects of gold compounds on macrophage signal transduction pathways and effects on protein kinase C, phospholipases A and C, and 5-lipoxygenase are also very controversial and discussed in the review by Bondeson[31].

Antimalarials—chloroquine, hydroxychloroquine

Antimalarial drugs have been used for many years in the treatment of rheumatoid arthritis[32]. Chloroquine and hydroxychloroquine have become the most frequently used antimalarials in RA because of their relative safety[33]. Their mechanism of action in RA is not entirely clear but the compounds have been shown to accumulate in the lysosomes of various types of cells and to inhibit the degradation of substances that are delivered to these organoids by phagocytosis or endocytosis. This inhibition of lysosomal degradation by chloroquine has been attributed to the increase in intralysosomal pH and is a property of this compound and other weak bases[34]. In the absence of an acidic pH, lysosomal hydrolases do not dissociate from mannose 6-phosphate receptors in the prelysosomal compartment and, as a consequence, these receptors are trapped in a state that cannot transport additional lysosomal hydrolases from the Golgi complex to lysosomes[35]. The neutralization of lysosomal pH could be responsible for the inhibitory effect of antimalarials on neutrophil phagocytosis, locomotion and, hexose monophosphate shunt activity[36]. Chloroquine has been reported to inhibit the production of TNF-α from lipopolysaccharide (LPS)-stimulated macrophages[37,38,39], and in a recent report it was shown that chloroquine inhibited the processing of membrane-bound 26 kD prohormone to the 17-kD native protein rather than inhibiting induction of mRNA or synthesis of protein[40].

Azaspiranes

Atiprimod (SK&F 106615) is an azaspirane being developed as an immunomodulatory macrophage-targeting agent[41,42]. The azaspiranes, examples of which are shown in Fig. 42.1, are novel compounds that display beneficial therapeutic activity in a number of animal models of autoimmune disease[43,44,45] and transplantation[46,47]. The compounds are especially effective in the adjuvant arthritic rat, a model for human RA, where they inhibit the inflammatory response, prevent bone and cartilage degradation[43,48], as well as inhibiting the production of the proinflammatory cytokine IL-6. The compounds are also anti-inflammatory in collagen-induced arthritis in the DBA/1 mouse where they inhibit paw inflammation as well as reducing serum amyloid protein (A. Badger; unpublished data). As cationic amphiphiles, the azaspiranes accumulate in macrophage lysosomes, lowering lysosomal pH, and thereby altering the functional activity of these cells[42,46,49]. The potential effects that this accumulation of compound in the macrophage lysosomes could have on

Fig. 42.1 Structures of immunomodulatory azaspiranes.

macrophage function, and ultimately on the disease process in RA, are depicted in Fig. 42.2 and are summarized as follows:

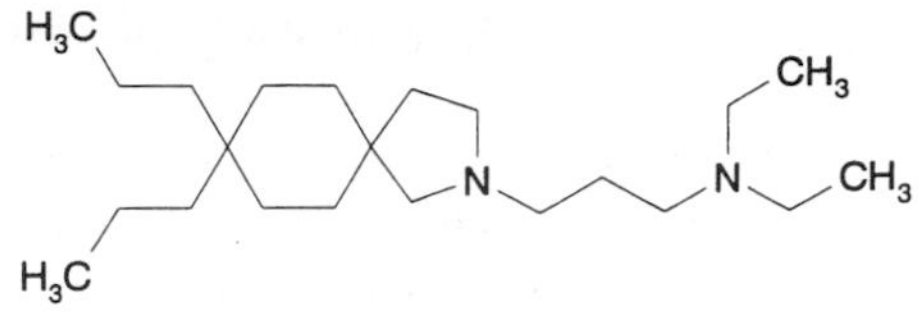

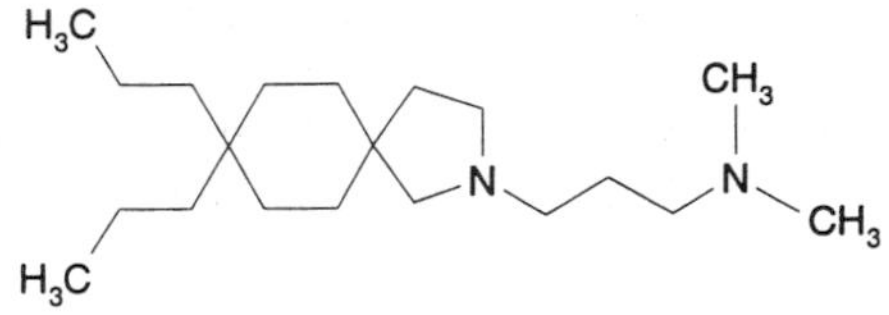

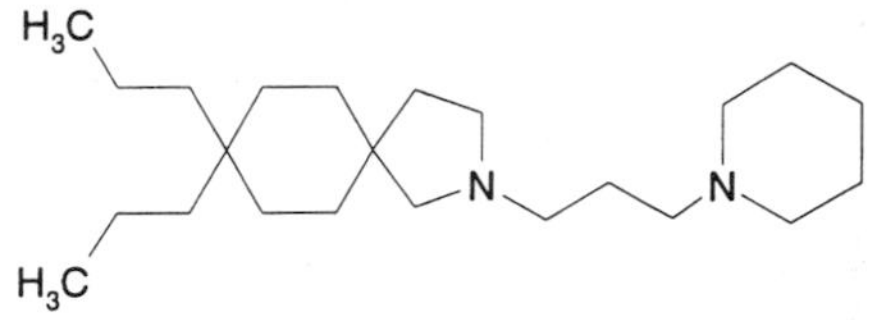

- spleen cells, lymph node cells and macrophages from treated animals are able to suppress T cell responses to mitogen and antigen and this effect is not mediated by the production of prostaglandins or nitric oxide[44,50,51];
- alterations in antigen presentation by macrophages to T cells[52] and D. Olivera (unpublished observations);
- modulation of lysosomal enzymes release (R. Dodds, unpublished observations);
- reduction of superoxide radicals from mouse peritoneal macrophages[23] (and unpublished observations);
- reduction of serum IL-6 in the AA rat[43] and serum TNF-α in mouse models of endotoxin shock (A. Badger, unpublished observation).

Of particular interest is the finding that alveolar macrophages (AM) from rats treated orally with atiprimod, as well as normal AM treated *in vitro* with the compound, have an increased capability to kill *Candida albicans*[49] but the mechanism of this increased capability to inhibit the growth or kill the microorganisms is not known. In addition to the *in vitro* studies, mice infected with *Candida albicans* and treated with azaspiranes are not immunocompromised and have a lifespan equal to or longer than control untreated mice[49,53]. This lack of overt immunosuppression by atiprimod was also observed in mice immunized with ovalbumin, where antibody responses to the antigen were

Mechanisms of Azaspirane-Mediated Anti-Arthritic Activity

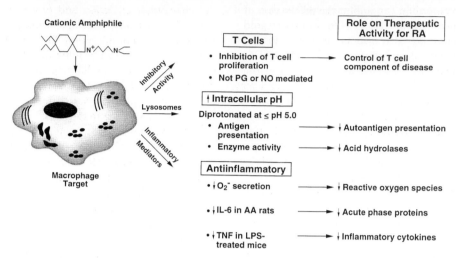

Fig. 42.2 Mechanism(s) of action of the azaspiranes *in vitro* and *in vivo*. PG, prostaglandins; NO, nitric oxide.

normal and cellular responses only minimally affected[54]. Thus, these compounds, with their selectivity for the macrophage, may show beneficial effects in RA.

Targeting the macrophage to inhibit cytokine production—IL-1 and TNF-α

Overproduction of the cytokines IL-1 and TNF-α causes a destructive immune response associated with the inflammation, as well as the cartilage and bone damage, observed in RA. Other cytokines clearly play a role in the disease process but there is no question that these cytokines play a pivotal role and there is now considerable evidence that the inhibition of either IL-1 or TNF-α can have dramatic effects on the progression of RA[55,56,57]. There are several classes of compounds that act directly on macrophages to inhibit the production of cytokines. These compounds may have an advantage over biologicals, such as antibodies and soluble cytokine receptors, as they are usually orally active, have longer half-lives *in vivo* and a reduced potential for antigenicity.

Non-steroidal anti-inflammatory drugs (NSAIDs) and corticosteroids

NSAIDs still provide the cornerstone of symptomatic treatment in RA, effectively reducing the signs and symptoms of acute joint inflammation by inhibiting the enzyme cyclo-oxygenase (COX) and the production of prostaglandins (PGs) and thromboxane. The constitutive enzyme, COX-1, is responsible for PGs that have a gastroprotective role and maintain renal perfusion whereas COX-2, the inducible form of COX, is upregulated at

inflammatory sites. The therapy-limiting side-effects of classical NSAIDs which inhibit both COX-1 and COX-2 are gastric irritation/ulceration and renal damage; this is considered to be the result of inhibiting COX-1[58]. Therefore, the selective inhibition of COX-2 has become a major strategic effort. Macrophages show little or no COX activity unless stimulated with LPS or cytokines and then they become a major source of the enzymes. Although several investigators have suggested that eicosanoids are important factors in the regulation of proinflammatory cytokine induction in macrophages this is a controversial issue[59]. The new COX-2 inhibitors[60] show great promise for the treatment of RA but their use results in inhibition of PG production and will not focus on regulation of the induction of proinflammatory cytokines in mononuclear phagocytes.

Corticosteroids exert potent anti-inflammatory and immunosuppressive effects in RA and reduce the chronic inflammatory infiltrate, which is present in the synovium of diseased patients. They also inhibit inflammation by redirection of lymphocyte traffic, inhibition of cytokine gene expression, inhibition of nitric oxide production, inhibition of expression of adhesion molecules, and increase in the synthesis of lipocortin-1 which inhibits the action phospholipase A2 (reviewed in Ref. 61). The long-term use of steroids is hampered by their side-effects. The recently-described mechanism of action of these drugs by inhibiting NF-κB[62,63] is providing new strategies for developing drugs with steroid-like effects, but with a safer profile of activity.

Methotrexate/adenosine

Methotrexate (MTX) is a folic acid antagonist which is immunosuppressive and/or anti-inflammatory (reviewed in Ref. 64). MTX impairs the chemotaxis of blood monocytes[65] and has been shown by some investigators to inhibit monokine production[66], while at the same time increasing the production of cytokine inhibitors such as soluble TNF-receptor[65,66]. MTX has been shown by others to inhibit certain activities of IL-1 in mononuclear cells without interfering with the production or secretion of the cytokine[67]. However, unlike corticosteroids MTX does not always reduce the chronic inflammatory infiltrate present in the synovium of patients with RA[68] but this may be a dose response effect as other groups have found a decrease in inflammatory infiltrate in synovial biopsies after MTX therapy[69,70].

It has been suggested that the therapeutic effects of MTX may be linked to its ability to inhibit aminoimidazol-4-carboxamide ribonucleoside (AICAR) which, in turn increases adenosine levels[71,72]. Adenosine is an endogenous purine nucleoside which acts as a potent anti-inflammatory agent. Evidence for the anti-inflammatory effect of increased adenosine release at inflamed sites was first shown *in vivo* in the murine air pouch model where the effects of MTX were reversed with an adenosine A2 antagonist[72]. Adenosine has now been shown to inhibit LPS-induced TNF production by mouse macrophages, rat Kupffer cells, and human monocytes[73–76]. In the human monocyte cell line, U937, adenosine inhibits LPS-stimulated TNF-α production and this effect was shown to be mediated through A3 receptors[77]. Of particular interest is the finding that adenosine enhances IL-10 secretion by human monocytes[78] and this phenomenon was not mediated through the occupancy of A1 or A2 receptors. This could well be an additional beneficial effect of increasing adenosine levels as IL-10 has been shown to have anti-inflammatory activity (see below).

Adenosine agonists or adenosine regulating agents could therefore have beneficial therapeutic effects in chronic diseases such as RA. However, adenosine has cardiovascular side-effects when administered systemically so another approach is to regulate adenosine concentrations with an adenosine kinase inhibitor and this concept has been tested with GP-1-515[79,80].

P38 MAP kinase inhibitors

One class of compounds that works directly on the macrophage to inhibit the production of a number of cytokines including IL-1 and TNF-α is the series of inhibitors of the serine/threonine p38 MAP kinase (also known as C5BP, SAPK-2, RK). These compounds block cytokine production from LPS-stimulated monocyte/macrophages at the translational level[81] and they have shown activity in a number of animal models of acute and chronic inflammation[82]. Several orally-active selective p38 inhibitors have been described. Examples shown in Fig. 42.3 are

SB 210313[83], SB 220025[84], and SB 203580[85]. SB 203580 has been used as a model compound to examine the molecular mechanism(s) of action and functional activity of these compounds and many additional consequences have been ascribed to p38 activation/inhibition. SB 203580 is a pyridinyl imidazole that is a highly selective inhibitor of p38 MAP kinase[85], competing with ATP for the binding to p38[86]. X-ray crystallographic studies have elucidated a uniquely shaped binding pocket that offers a potential explanation for the selectivity of this and other inhibitors belonging to this class[87,88].

SB 203580 is a potent inhibitor of inflammatory cytokine production from LPS-stimulated human monocytes and the human monocyte cell line THP-1 *in vitro* with IC$_{50}$s of 50–100 nM[82,89] and *in vivo* in both mice and rats with IC$_{50}$ values of 15 to 25 mg/kg[90]. It has therapeutic activity in collagen-induced arthritis at 50 mg/kg, reducing both paw inflammation as well as serum amyloid protein levels[90]. At 30 and 60 mg/kg the compound inhibits paw inflammation in the adjuvant arthritic rat as well as inhibiting bone loss and improving joint histological parameters[90]. Of particular interest are the findings that these inhibitors are not overtly immunosuppressive either *in vitro* or *in vivo*[90,91]. Recent studies have demonstrated that SB 203580 is capable of inhibiting the release of nitric oxide (NO) from mouse macrophages (RAW 267.4) stimulated with LPS and IFN-γ (F. Barone, unpublished observations). This effect appeared to be a post-transcriptional effect as iNOS gene expression was not affected whereas protein levels were decreased substantially when measured by Western blot analysis. Another consequence of macrophage IL-1 production is the cartilage damage elicited through induction of matrix metalloproteinases (MMPs) and nitric oxide, and SB 203580 has been shown to inhibit NO production from cartilage explants[92].

PDE 4 inhibitors

Inhibitors of cyclic nucleotide phosphodiesterases (PDE) suppress LPS-induced TNF-α production in monocytes and macrophages through the activation of adenylate cyclase[93,94,95]. This indicates that the subsequent increase in intracellular levels of adenosine 3'5'-cyclic monophosphate (cAMP) is a suppressive signal for TNF-α that could be exploited as a potential target. PDE 4 has been shown to be the predominant cAMP-metabolizing enzyme in immune and inflammatory cells[96], and for this reason PDE 4 inhibition has been a major

SB 210313   SB 220025   SB 203580

Fig. 42.3 p38 MAP kinase inhibitors.

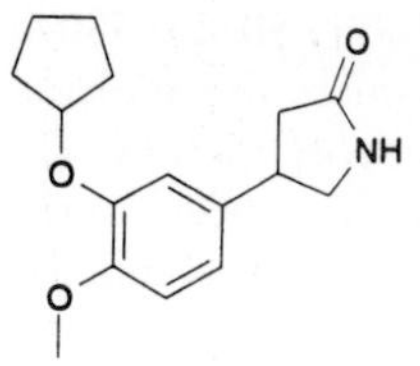

Rolipram 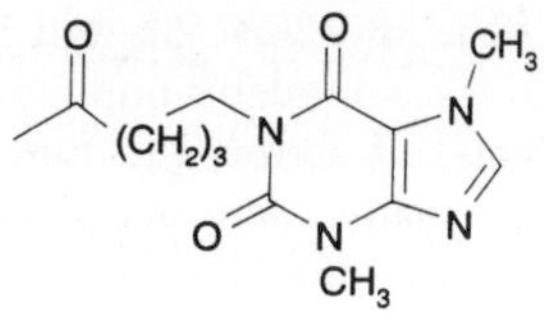　　　　　　　　　　Pentoxiphylline

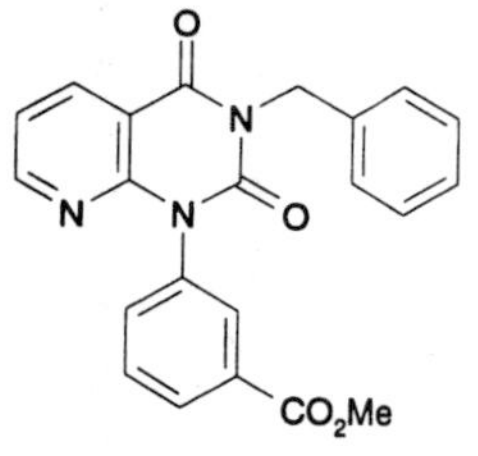

CP-77059 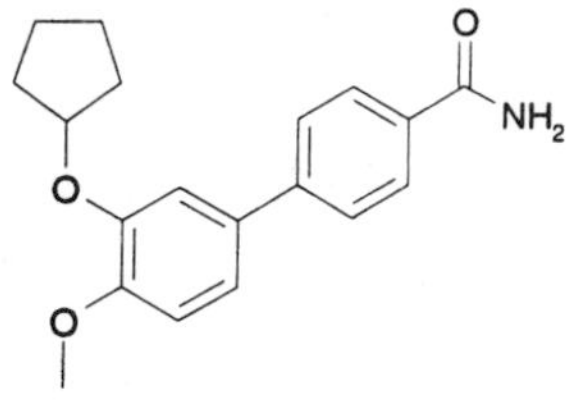　　　　　　　　　　CP-353164

Fig. 42.4　Phosphodiesterase 4 inhibitors.

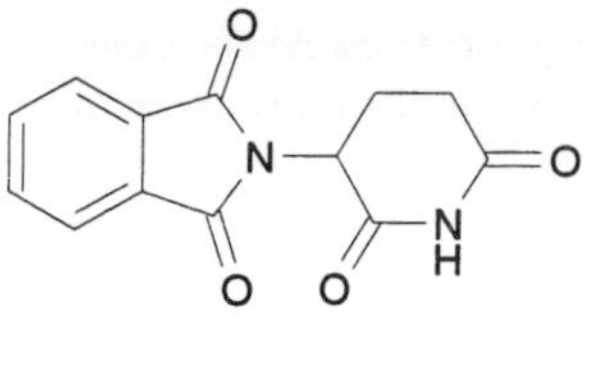

Thalidomide　　　　　　　　　　CC-1069

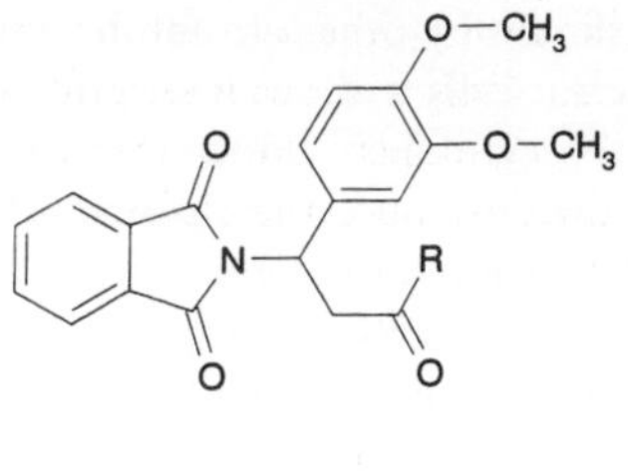

Fig. 42.5　Thalidomide and an analog, CC-1069.

target for the discovery of anti-inflammatory drugs[97]. Both specific inhibitors of this PDE isoform such as rolipram[94,98], as well as non-specific inhibitors such as pentoxifylline (Fig. 42.4) inhibit TNF-α in human monocytes[99] but rolipram is 500-fold more potent than pentoxifylline. These PDE 4 inhibitors reduce serum TNF-α levels and prolong survival in mouse models of endotoxin shock[100]. Rolipram and CP-77059 have been shown to suppress ankle swelling and radiological evidence of joint damage in the AA rat[101]. CP-353164 (Fig. 42.4) has been found to be more effective at blocking the release of TNF-α both *in vitro* in human monocytes and *in vivo* in a murine TNF-α production model than rolipram and may be useful for the treatment of RA[102].

Pentoxifylline has been evaluated in the clinic in RA patients, with significant improvement noted in one study in 50 per cent of the patients[103]. In another study, significant diminution in the number of tender and swollen joints was noted after 3 months although no consistent affects were observed on TNF-α production[104]. However, in a more recent study of patients with severe RA, the therapeutic benefits were too small to warrant the use of this drug in severe RA[105]. Considerable effort has been applied to the synthesis of novel compounds for the treatment of diseases where TNF has been shown to play a significant role such as asthma and AIDS and RA[106].

Thalidomide

Thalidomide was originally introduced in the 1950s as a sedative but was withdrawn following the discovery of its teratogenic effects. It has now been found to have immunomodulatory and anti-inflammatory effects and has been evaluated in a number of animal models of autoimmune disease[107,108]. It is currently being reevaluated in a range of indications[109]. The compound has been shown to inhibit TNF-α production from monocyte/macrophages[110] and is therefore being evaluated in a number of diseases including Crohn's disease, multiple sclerosis, and AIDS as well as RA[111]. Thalidomide is thought to inhibit TNF-α production by enhancing degradation of TNF messenger RNA[112]. Some positive effects have been observed in the clinical trials with thalidomide[113,114] but the side-effect profile may be the limiting factor for its use in RA. A large number of thalidomide analogs have been synthesized in attempts to separate the toxic effects from the TNF inhibitory activity. Some analogs, for example CC-1069 (Fig. 42.5) which lacks the hydrolytically unstable glutarimide ring, are several hundred times more potent as TNF inhibitors and may have more potential for the treatment of RA[115].

Targeting the macrophage to inhibit cytokine production—macrophage inhibitory factor (MIF)

This cytokine has recently generated a great deal of interest. MIF was always considered to be a product of activated T lymphocytes and to exhibit a number of macrophage activating properties[116–118]. However, MIF has now been identified as a protein secreted by the anterior pituitary in response to LPS stimulation[119,120] as well as by macrophages themselves[121]. In addition, MIF has been shown to override the immunosuppresive effects of glucocorticoids on macrophage cytokine production *in vitro*[122]. Monocytes and macrophages synthesize and release MIF following stimulation with LPS, TNF-α, and IFN-γ[121]. Of note is the fact that macrophages can themselves be stimulated with recombinant MIF to produce TNF-α so the macrophage is both an important source and an important target of MIF[121]. These findings would indicate that targeting this macrophage-derived cytokine could be therapeutically beneficial in RA. Experimental evidence that MIF is involved in the pathogenesis of arthritis is provided by animal models of the disease. For example MIF has been shown to be involved in the pathogenesis of collagen type II-induced arthritis in mice as the treatment with neutralizing anti-MIF antibodies prior to immunization with collagen delayed the onset and lowered the frequency of arthritis[123]. In addition, in the rat model of adjuvant arthritis, anti-MIF treatment leads to a profound, dose dependent inhibition of paw swelling and a reduction in synovial lavage leukocyte numbers as well as reduced synovial macrophage and T cell accumulation[124].

Inhibition of the activity of MIF may have utility in the treatment of a broad range of inflammatory and autoimmune disease and ongoing structural and conformational studies[120] will assist in the development of pharmacological agents that can modulate MIF activity.

Macrophage-derived proinflammatory mediators: nitric oxide

Nitric oxide (NO) is produced by a number of cell types which include macrophages, synoviocytes, and endothelial cells. NO is involved in a variety of cellular processes which include platelet aggregation, neurotransmission, and immune activation[125]. Normally there are low constitutive levels of NO, and increases in NO levels produced in inflammatory situations is a result of stimulation of inducible nitric oxide synthase (iNOS). Several inflammatory stimuli including IL-1, TNF, and LPS are responsible for this stimulation but the actual expression of iNOS is regulated by the balance of cytokines. For example the anti-inflammatory cytokines IL-4 and IL-10 (see below) as well as TGFβ inhibit iNOS expression in macrophages[126–129].

Induction of iNOS leads to sustained and abundant NO production which can have a range of activities encompassing both pro- and anti-inflammatory effects[130] and whichever predominates depends on the situation and the disease state. However, numerous studies show an association between inflammation and high NO levels. For example, in the MRL-lpr/lpr mouse, large quantities of NO are produced and the development of joint inflammation coincides with a rise in NO production. Moreover, arthritic disease in these mice can be inhibited with NG-mono-methyl-L-arginine (L-NMMA), a non-specific inhibitor of NOS[131,132]. In the rat adjuvant-induced arthritis model, L-NMMA reduced NO biosynthesis reduced paw swelling and improved histopathological changes in the ankle joints[133].

There is increased expression of blood mononuclear cell iNOS in RA patients[134] and the presence of iNOS in human synovium implies that macrophages, as well as fibroblasts, are major sources of synovial NO[135,136]. As the overproduction of NO has been associated with RA, as well as several other disease states, efforts to identify selective inhibitors of iNOS have been undertaken by several groups and a recent report by Hallinan[137] and coworkers describe a highly selective inhibitor for iNOS which is 700 times more selective for iNOS than for the endothelial NOS (eNOS) isoform. Several antiarthritic compounds, in fact, inhibit NO production. Examples are auranofin, methotrexate, glucocorticoids, and cytokine suppressive p38 inhibitors such as SB 203580[138]. It is important to be aware that, although there is a great deal of support for the concept that NO is dangerous in rheumatic diseases and should be suppressed, this is a controversial issue[130] and there are a number of situations where NO can be protective[138]. In addition, NO is involved in apoptosis and can either increase or decrease apoptotic events depending on the cells and circumstances (reviewed in Ref. 139).

Modulation of anti-inflammatory cytokines that affect functional activity of macrophages

In addition to the cytokines with proinflammatory properties such as IL-1 and TNF-α there are also a number of cytokines produced by T cells that have anti-inflammatory activity. These cytokines, IL-4, IL-10, and IL-13, effectively inhibit a number of macrophage functions and are under investigation as potential therapies for RA.

Interleukin-4 (IL-4)

IL-4 is produced by the CD4$^+$ population of lymphocytes (T cells) which have the characteristics of the Th2 subtype[140]. IL-4 inhibits IL-1 and TNF-α production from human peripheral blood monocytes, human alveolar macrophages, human peritoneal macrophages, and murine macrophages[141,142]. IL-4 does not inhibit all cytokines as it has been shown to increase the levels of IL-1 receptor antagonist (IL-1Ra) released from monocyte/macrophages of RA patients[142]. Mechanistically, IL-4 has been shown to increase cytokine mRNA degradation while IL-10 inhibits NF-kB, thus reducing cytokine gene expression[143]. *In vivo*, in the mouse collagen arthritis model, a combination of IL-4 and IL-10 was shown to be very effective whereas treatment with antibodies to the two cytokines exacerbated disease[143].

Interleukin-10 (IL-10)

IL-10, like IL-4, is an anti-inflammatory cytokine released by Th2 cells (for review see Ref. 144). This cytokine is thought to play a prominent role in the natural suppression of joint inflammation. Of note is the fact that IL-10 decreases class II MHC expression by macrophages and blocks proinflammatory cytokine production by these cells[145]. IL-10 inhibits LPS-induced TNF-α release from human monocytes[146], inhibits LPS-induced TNF-α release *in vivo* in endotoxin shock models[147], inhibits free radical production[148], and adhesion molecule expression[149]. In recent study, IL-10 gene transfer was shown to inhibit the onset of collagen-induced arthritis in DBA/1 mice. Transfer of a replication-defective adenoviral vector expressing viral IL-10, inhibited the arthritis and significant levels of IL-10 were measured in the serum of the treated animals[150]. Therefore, the use of recombinant IL-10 as a therapeutic agent, or stimulation of the production of IL-10 appears to be an attractive therapeutic strategy. As mentioned previously in this chapter, adenosine can increase the production of IL-10 by TNF-stimulated human monocytes[78]. An alternative strategy aimed at maintaining the right 'mix' of regulatory cytokines might be selective inhibition of those cells producing destructive proinflammatory cytokines while sparing an effect on cells producing anti-inflammatory cytokines such as IL-4 and IL-10. This kind of selectivity is difficult to achieve and fraught with the difficulties of multifunctional activities of the cell populations involved and the factors they produce.

Interleukin-13 (IL-13)

As in the case with both IL-4 and IL-10, IL-13 is also a product predominantly of antigen-stimulated Th2-type lymphocytes, although it has also been detected in Th1-like clones. This cytokine shares most investigated biological activity on monocytes and B cells with IL-4[151,152]. IL-13 inhibits LPS-induced TNF-α production by mononuclear cells from peripheral blood but not synovial cells of patients with chronic inflammatory arthritis[153]. IL-13 was able to inhibit IL-1β production from both of these cell populations. IL-13 may be used therapeutically to down regulate monocyte/macrophage activities at the sites of inflammation.

Inhibition of macrophage migration into inflammatory tissues—chemokines

Chemokines released by cells form a concentration gradient which acts as a homing signal for other cells. This directed migration of leukocyte populations from the circulation to sites of inflammation maintains the heightened immune responses observed in these sites[154]. Chemokines are classified into two major groups, CXC and CC, based on the position of the first two of their four invariant cysteines[155]. Each of the chemokines recognizes and induces the chemotaxis of a particular class of cells such as neutrophils, T cells, and/or macrophages. The earliest examples of chemokines released by monocytes that attract other cells such as neutrophils are IL-8 and monocyte chemoattractant protein-1 (MCP-1). There are now around 30 chemokines known, and 14 different seven-transmembrane G-protein-coupled receptors have been identified by cloning[156], making it increasingly difficult to discover selective inhibitors.

MIP-1α and RANTES are ligands for the CCR1 receptor which is located on circulating mononuclear cells and since these ligands appear to play an important role in the pathogenesis of multiple sclerosis and RA this receptor has become a prime therapeutic target. Recently, small molecule functional antagonists of the CCR1 chemokine receptor on monocytes have been identified and characterized[157]. The compounds, 4-hydroxypiperidine analogs, inhibited chemokine binding to CCR1 transfected HEK 293 cells, inhibited calcium mobilization as well as inhibiting MIP-1α and RANTES-induced migration of peripheral blood mononuclear cells. These antagonists may be useful in chronic inflammatory disease involving these chemokines.

Conclusions

One conclusion that can be drawn from this review is that almost all of the therapies currently being used in RA have some kind of effect on macrophages. This can be a direct effect where the compound's primary target is the macrophage or an indirect effect where the primary target is another cell, a T cell population for example. The consequent modification of this T cell's function, or the cytokines it produces, by a DMARD or immunomodulatory agent, could then interfere with its ability to interact with another cell population, in this case macrophages. Macrophage function required for an effective normal, pro- or anti-inflammatory immune response is then impaired.

In targeting macrophages, one must be constantly aware of the fact that too drastic a depletion of a cell type or soluble mediator may not be in the best interest of the patient. Macrophages are needed for antigen presentation in normal immune responses, and for resistance against micro-organisms, and the cytokines they produce are also required for maintenance of a normally active immune response. Selective targeting of those cells which are highly activated, sometimes called 'angry macrophages', which are causing destructive processes in the diseased joint, while sparing those cells required for immune function would be an ideal profile for a macrophage-targeting drug.

Controlling the anti-inflammatory activity of macrophages at the biochemical level will require highly selective targeting of signal transduction pathways by modulating the enzymes and transcription factors involved, hopefully in a cell-specific manner. An example of the kind of selectivity for macrophages that one could envision as a therapeutic has been described recently by Yarovo *et al*[158]. These investigators have discovered an apoptosis-inducing retinoid, MX84, that induces cell death in monocyte/macrophage cells lines but is inactive against more than 30 other cell lines. The compound is a retinoid precursor and is activated by a macrophage-secreted phospholipase to an active retinoid which acts through its specific receptor, activates gene transcription, and induces apoptosis. This is a novel, cell-specific approach to the control of diseases caused by excessive macrophage activity such as RA.

References

1. Kingsley, G., Panayi, G.S. Joint destruction in rheumatoid arthritis: biological bases. *Clin Exptl Rheumatol*, 1997;**15**(Suppl.17): S3–S14.
2. Firestein, G.S., Alvaro-Garcia, J.S., Maki, R. Quantitative analysis of cytokine gene expression in rheumatoid arthritis. *J Immunol*, 1997;**144**:3347–3353.
3. Firestein, G.S., Zvaifler, N.J. How important are T cells in chronic arthritis. *Arthritis Rheum*, 1994;**33**:768–773.
4. Schneider, M. Plasma- and lymphapheresis in autoimmune diseases. *Zeitschrift fur Rheumatologie*, 1994;**55**:90–04.
5. Karsh, J., Wright, D.G., Klippel, J.H., Decker, J.L., Deisseroth, A.B., Flye, M.W. Lymphocyte depletion by continuous flow cell centrifugation in rheumatoid arthritis: clinical effects. *Arthritis Rheum*, 1979;**22**:1055–1059.
6. Tenenbaum, J., Urowitz, M.B., Keystone, E.C., Dwosh, I.L., Curtis, J.E. Leucapheresis in severe rheumatoid arthritis. *Ann Rheum Dis*, 1979;**38**:40–44.
7. Yeadon, C., Karsh, J. Lymphapheresis in rheumatoid arthritis. The Clinical and laboratory effects of a limited course of cell depletion. *Clin Exp Rheumatol*, 1983;**1**:119–124.
8. Hahn, G., Stuhmuller, B., Hain, N., Kalden, J.R., Pfizizenmaier, K., Burmester, G.R. Modulation of monocyte activation in patients with rheumatoid arthritis by leukapheresis therapy. *J Clin Invest*, 1993;**91**:862–870.
9. Nishioka, K., Hasunuma, T., Kato, T., Sumida, T., Kobata, T. Apoptosis in rheumatoid arthritis. *Arthritis Rheum*, 1998; **41**:1–9.

10. Mountz, J.D., Wu, J., Chen, J., Zhou, T. Autoimmune disease: a problem of defective apoptosis. *Arthritis Rheum*, 1994;37:1415–1420.

11. Nakajima, T., Aono, H., Hasunuma, T., Yamamoto, K., Shirai, T., Hirohata, K., Nishioka, K. Apoptosis and functional Fas antigen in rheumatoid arthritis synoviocytes. *Arthritis Rheum*, 1995;38:485–491.

12. Sakai, K., Matsuno, H., Morita, I., Nezuka, T., Tsuji, H., Shirai, T., Yonehara, S., Hasunuma, T., Nishioka, K. Potential withdrawal of rheumatoid synovium by the induction of apoptosis using a novel *in vivo* model of rheumatoid arthritis. *Arhritis Rheum*, 1998;41:1251–1257.

13. Nemoto, S., Xiang, J., Huang, S., Lin, A. Induction of apoptosis by SB 202190 through inhibition of p38β mitogen-activated protein kinase. *J. Biol. Chem*, 1998;273:16415–16420.

14. Roulston, A., Reinhard, C., Amiri, P., Williams, L.T. Early activation of c-jun N-terminal kinase and p38 kinase regulate cell survival in response to tumor necrosis factor α. *J Biol Chem*, 1998;273:10232–10239.

15. Horstmann, S., Kahle, P.J., Borasio, G.D. Inhibitor of p38 mitogen-activated protein kinase promotes nueronal survival in vitro. *J Neuroscience Res*, 1988;52:483–490.

16. Sawada, T., Hashimoto, S., Furukawa, H., Tohma, S., Inoue, T., Ito K. Generation of reactive oxygen species is required for bucillamine, a novel anti-rheumatic drug, to induce apoptosis in concert with copper. *Immunopharmacol*, 1997;35:195–202.

17. van den Berg, W.B., van Lent, P.L.E.M. The role of macrophages in chronic arthritis. *Immunobiology*, 1996;195:614–623.

18. Monkkonen, J., Taskinen, M., Auriola, S.O., Urti, A. Growth inhibition of macrophage-like and other cell types by liposome-encapsulated, calcium-bound, and free bisphophonates in vitro. *J Drug Targeting*, 1994;2:299–308.

19. Norton W.L., Lewis, D.C., Ziff, M. Electron-dense deposits following injection of gold sodium thiomalate and thiomalic acid. *Arthritis Rheum*, 1968;11:436–443.

20. Nakamura, H., Igarashi, M. Localization of gold in synovial membrane of rheumatoid arthritis patients treated with sodium aurothiomalate. Studies by electron microscope and electron probe X-ray microanalysis. *Ann Rheum Dis*, 1977;36:209–215.

21. Scheinberg, M.A., Santos, L.M., Finkelstein, A.A. The effect of auranofin and sodium aurothiomalate on peripheral blood monocytes. *J Rheumatol*, 1982;9:366–369.

22. Harth, M., Keown, P.A., Orange, J.F. Monocyte dependent excited oxygen radical generation in rheumatoid arthritis: inhibition by gold sodium thiomalate. *J Rheumatol*, 1983;10:701–707.

23. Mirabelli, C.K., Sung, C-P., Picker, D.H., Barnard, C., Hydes, P., Badger, A.M. Effect of metal-containing compounds on superoxide release from phorbol myristate acetate stimulated murine peritoneal macrophages: inhibition by auranofin and spirogermanium *J Rheumatol*, 1988;15:1064–1069.

24. Lipsky, P.E., Ziff, M. Inhibition of antigen- and mitogen-induced human lymphocyte proliferation by gold compounds. *J Clin Invest*, 1977;59:455–466.

25. Lee, J.C., Rebar, L., Demuth, S., Hanna, N. Suppressed IL-2 production and response in adjuvant arthritic rats: role of suppressor cells and the effect of auranofin treatment. *J Rheumatol*, 1985;12:885–891.

26. Danis, V.A., Kulesz, A.J., Nelson, D.S., Brooks, P.M. The effect of gold sodium thiomalate and auranofin on lipopolysaccharide-induced interleukin-1 production by blood monocytes in vitro: variation in healthy subjects and patients with arthritis. *Clin Exp Immunol*, 1990;79:335–340.

27. Danis, V.A., Franic, G.M., Brooks, P.M. The effect of slow-acting anti- rheumatic drugs (SAARDs) and combinations of SAARDs on monokine production in vitro. *Drugs Exp Clin Res*, 1991;17:549–554.

28. Seitz, M., Loetscher, P., Dewald, B., Towbin, H., Baggiolini, M. In vitro modulation of cytokine, cytokine inhibitor, and prostaglandin E release from blood mononuclear cells and synovial fibroblasts by antirheumatic drugs. *J Rheumatol*, 1997;24:1471–1476.

29. Loetscher, P., Dewald, B., Baggiolini, M., Seitz, M. Monocyte chemoatractant protein 1 and interleukin 8 production by rheumatoid synoviocytes: effects of anti-rheumatic drugs. *Cytokines* 1994;6:162–170.

30. Yanni, G., Farahat, M.N.M.R., Poston, R.N. *et al.* Instamuscular gold decreases cytokine expression and macrophage numbers in the rheumatoid synovial membrane. *Ann Rheum Dis*, 1994;53: 256–260.

31. Bondeson, J. The mechanisms of action of disease-modifying antirheumatic drugs: a review with emphasis on macrophage signal transduction and the induction of pro-inflammatory cytokines. *Gen Pharmac*, 1997;29:127–150.

32. Mackenzie, A.H. Antimalarial drugs for rheumatoid arthritis. *Am. J. Med*, 1983;30:48–58.

33. Maksymowych, W., Russell, A.S. Antimalarials in rheumatology: efficacy and safety. *Semin. Arthritis Rheum*, 1987;16:206–221.

34. Poole, B., Ohkuma, S. Effect of weak bases on the intralysosomal pH in mouse peritoneal macrophages. *J Cell Biol*, 1981; 90:665–669.

35. Brown, W.J., Constantinescu, E., Farquhar, M.G. Redistribution of mannose-6-phospate receptor-induced by tunicamysin and chloroquine. *J Cell Biol*, 1984;99:320–326.

36. Tsokos, G.C.H. Immunomodulatory treatment in patients with rheumatic diseases: mechanisms of action. *Semin. Arthritis Rheum*, 17:24–38.

37. Ertel, W., Morrison, M.H., Ayalo, A., Chaudry, I.H. Chloroquine attenuates hemorrhagic shock-induced suppression of Kupffer cell antigen presentation and major histocompatibility complex class II antigen expression through blockade of tumor necrosis factor and prostaglandin release. *Blood*, 1991;78:1781–1788.

38. Picot, S., Peyron, F., Donadille, A., Vuillez, J-P., Barbe, G., Ambroise-Thomas, P. Chloroquine-induced inhibition of the production of TNF, but not of IL-6, is affected by disruption of iron metabolism. *Immunology*, 1993;80:127–133.

39. Zhu, X., Ertel, W., Ayala, A., Morrison, M.H., Perrin, M.M., Chaudry, I.H. Chloroquine inhibits macrophage tumor necrosis factor-α mRNA transcription. *Immunology*, 1993;80:122–126.

40. Jeong, J-Y., Jue, D-M. Chloroquine inhibits processing of tumor necrosis factor in lipopolysaccharide-stimulated RAW 264–7 macrophages. *J Immunol*, 1997;158:4901–4907.

41. Badger, A.M., Wright, C.S. SK&F 106615. *Drugs of the Future*, 1995;20:893–896.

42. Badger, A.M. (1995) Discovery and development of the immunomodulatory azaspiranes. In: *The Search for Anti-inflammatory Drugs: Case Histories from Concept to Clinic*, V.J. Merluzzi and J. Adams eds, Birkhauser, pp. 275–305.

43. Bradbeer, J.N., Kapadia, R.D., Sarkar, S.K., Zhao, H., Stroup, G.B., Swift, B.A., Rieman, D.J., Badger, A.M. Disease-modifying activity of SK&F 106615 in rat adjuvant arthritis. *Arthritis Rheum*, 1996;39:504–514.

44. Rabinovitch, A., Suarez, W.L., Qin, H.Y., Power, R.F., Badger, A.M. Prevention of diabetes and induction of non-specific suppressor cell activity in the BB rat by an immunomodulating azaspirane, SK&F 106610. *J Autoimmun*, 1993;1:39–49.

45. Albrightson-Winslow, C.R., Brickson, B.B., King, A., Olivera, D., Short, B., Saunders, C., Badger, A.M. Beneficial effects of long-term treatment with SK&F 105685 in murine lupus nephritis. *J Pharm Exp Ther*, 1990;225:382–387.

46. Hancock, W.W., Schmidbauer, G., Badger, A.M., Kupiec-Weglinski, J.W. SK&F 105685 suppresses allogeneically induced mononuclear and endothelial cell activation and cytokine production and prolongs rat cardiac allograft survival. *Transplant Proc*, 1992;24:231–232.

47. Schmidbauer, G., Hancock, W.W., Badger, A.M., Kupiec-Weglinski, J.W. SK&F 105685, a novel immunoregulatory azaspirane induces non-specific X-irradiation resistant suppressor cell activity *in vivo* and prolongs vascularized allograft survival. *Transplantation*, 1993;55:1236–1234.

48. High, W.B., Bugelski, P.J., Nichols, M.W., Swift, B.A., Solleveld, H.A., Badger, A.M. Effects of a novel azaspirane (SK&F 105685)

on the arthritic lesions in the adjuvant Lewis rat: attenuation of the inflammatory process and preservation of skeletal integrity. *J Rheumatol*, 1994;**21**:476–483.

49. Badger, A.M., Handler, J.A., Genell, C.A., Herzyk, D., Gore, E., Polsky, R., Webb, L., Bugelski, P.J. Atiprimod (SK&F 106615), a novel macrophage targeting agent, enhances alveolar macrophage candidacidal activity and is not immunosuppressive in Candida-infected mice. *Int J Immunopharm*. (In Press).

50. Badger, A.M., DiMartino, M.J., Talmadge, J.E., Picker, D.H., Schwartz, D.A., Dorman, J.W., Mirabelli, C.K., Hanna, N. Inhibition of animal models of autoimmune disease and the induction of non-specific suppressor cells by SK&F 105685 and related azaspiranes. *Int J Immunopharmacol*, 1989;**11**:839–846.

51. Badger, A.M., Schwartz, D.A., Picker, D.H., Dorman, J.W., Bradley, F.C., Cheeseman, E.N., DiMartino, M.J., Hanna, N., Mirabelli, C.K. Antiarthritic and suppressor cell inducing activity of azaspiranes: structure-function relationships of a novel class of immunomodulatory agents. *J Med Chem*, 1990;**33**:2963–2970.

52. Kaplan, J.M., Badger, A.M., Ruggieri, E.V., Swift, B.A., Bugelski, P.J. Effects of SK&F 105685, a novel anti-arthritic agent, on immune function in the dog. *Int J Immunopharm*, 1993;**15**:113–123.

53. Herzyk, D., Ruggieri, E.V., Cunningham, L., Polsky, R., Herold, C., Klinkner, A., Badger, A.M., Kerns, W.D., Bugelski, P.J. Single-organism model of host defense against infection: a novel immunotoxicologic approach to evaluate immunomodulatory drugs. *Toxicol Pathol*, 1997;**25**:351–362.

54. Badger, A.M., Newman-Tarr, T.M., Sattersfield, J.L. Selective immunomodulatory activity of SK&F 106615, a macrophage-targeting antiarthritic compound, on antibody and cellular responses in rats and mice. *Immunopharm*, 1997;**37**:53–61.

55. Feldmann, M., Brennan, F.M., Maini, R.N. Role of cytokines in rheumatoid arthritis. *Annu Rev Immunol*, 1996;**14**:397–440.

56. Brennan, F.M., Chantry, D., Jackson, A., Maini, R.N., Feldmann, M. Inhibitory effect of TNFα antibodies on synovial cell interleukin-1 production in rheumatoid arthritis. *Lancet*, 1989;**2**:244–247.

57. Feldmann, M., Elliott, M.J., Woody, J.N., Maini, R.N. Anti-tumor necrosis factor-alpha therapy of rheumatoid arthritis. *Adv Immunol*, 1997;**64**:283–350.

58. Richardson, C.E., Emery, P. New cyclo-oxygenase and cytokine inhibitors. *Bailliere's Clinical Rheumatol*, 1995;**9**:731–758.

59. Bondeson, J. The mechanisms of action of disease-modifying antirheumatic drugs: a review with emphasis on macrophage signal transduction. *Gen Pharmac*, 1997;**29**:127–150.

60. Parnham, M.J. Selective COX-2 inhibitors. *Drug News and Persp*, 1997;**10**:182–187.

61. Cato, A.C.B., Wade, E. Molecular mechanism of anti-inflammatory action of glucocorticoids. *BioEssays*, 1996;**18**:371–378.

62. Scheinman, R.I., Gogswell, P.C., Lofquist, A.K., Galdwin, A.S. Role of transcriptional activation of IκBα in mediation of immunosuppression by glucocorticoids. *Science*, 1995;**270**:283–286.

63. Auphan, N., DiDonato, J.A., Rosette, C., Helmberg, A., Karin, M. Immunosuppression by glucocorticoids: inhibition of NF-κB activity through induction of IκB synthesis. *Science*, 1995;**270**: 286–290.

64. Markham, A., Faulds, D. Methotrexate. A review of its pharmacodynamic and pharmacokinetic properties, and therapeutic efficacy in rheumatoid arthritis and other immunoregulatory disorders. *Clin Immunother*, 1994;**1**:217–244.

65. Nesher, G., Moore, T.L., Dorner, R.W. *In vitro* effects of methotrexate on peripheral blood monocytes: modulation by folinic acid and S-adenosylmethionine. *Ann Rheum Dis*, 1991;**50**:637–641.

66. Seitz., M., Loetscher, P. Dewald, B., Towbin, H., Rordorf, C., Gallati, H. *et al.* Methotrexate action in rheumatoid arthritis: stimulation of cytokine inhibitor and inhibition of chemokine production by peripheral blood mononuclear cells. *Br J Rheumatol*, 1995;**34**:602–609.

67. Segal, R., Yaron, M., Tartakovsky, B. Methotrexate, mechanism of action in rheumatoid arthritis. *Seminars Arthritis Rheum*, 1990;**20**:190–200.

68. Haraoui, B., Pelletier, J.P., Cloutier, J.M., Faure, M.P., Martel-Pelletier, J. Synovial membrane histology and immunopathology in rheumatoid arthritis and osteoarthritis. *In vivo* effects of antirheumatic drugs. *Arthritis Rheum*, 1991;**34**:153–163.

69. Firestein, G.S., Pain, M.M., Boyle, D.L. Mechanisms of methotrexate action in rheumatoid arthritis: selective decrease in synovial collagenase gene expression. *Arthritis Rheum*, 1994;**37**: 193–200.

70. Balsa, A., Gamallo, C., Martin-Mola, E. *et al.* Histologic changes in rheumatoid synovitis induced by naproxen and methotrexate. *J Rheumatol*, 1993;**30**:1472–1477.

71. Baggott, J.E., Vaughn, W.H., Hudson, B.B. Inhibition of 5-amino-imidazole-4-carboxamide ribotide transformylase, adenosine deaminase and 5′-adenylate deaminase by polyglutamates of methotrexate and oxidized folates and by 5-aminoimidazole-4-carboxamide riboside and ribotide. *Biochem J*, 1986;**236**:193–200.

72. Cronstein, B.N., Naime, D., Ostad, E. The anti-inflammatory mechanism of methotrexate. Increased adenosine release at inflamed sites diminishes leukocyte accumulation in an *in vivo* model of inflammation. *J Clin Invest*, 1993;**92**:2675–2682.

73. Parmely, M.J., Zou, W.W., Edwards, C.K., Borcherding, D.R., Silverstein, R., and Morrison, D.C. Adenosine and a related carbocyclic nucleoside analogue selectively inhibit tumor necrosis factor-α production and protect mice against endotoxin challenge. *J Immunol*, 1993;**151**:389–397.

74. Reinstein, L.J., Lichtman, S.N., Currin, R.T., Wang, J., Thurman, R.G., Lemasters, J.J. Suppression of lipopolysaccharide-stimulated release of tumor necrosis factor by adenosine: evidence for A2 receptors on rat Kupffer cells. *Hepatology*, 1994;**19**:1445–1452.

75. Bouma, M.G., Stad, R.K., van den Wildenberg, F.A.J.M., Buurman, W.A. Differential regulatory effects of adenosine on cytokine release by activated human monocytes. *J Immunol*, 1994;**153**:4159–4168.

76. Prabhakar, U., Brooks, D.P., Lipshutz, D., Esser, K.M. Inhibition of LPS-induced TNF-α production in human monocytes by adenosine (A2) receptor selective agonists. *Int J Immunopharmacol*, 1995;**17**:221–224.

77. Sajjadi, F.G., Takabayashi, K., Foster, A.C., Domingo, R.C., Firestein, G.S. Inhibition of TNF-α expression by adenosine. Role of A3 adenosine receptors. *J Immunol*, 1996;**156**:3435–3442.

78. LeMoine, O., Stordeur, P., Schandere, L., Marchant, A. deGroote, D., Goldman, M., Deviere, J. Adenosine enhances IL-10 secretion by human monocytes. *J Immunol*, 1996;**156**:4408–4414.

79. Rosengren, S., Bong, G.W., Firestein, G.S. Anti-inflammatory effects of an adenosine kinase inhibitor. *J Immunol*, 1995;**154**:5444–5451.

80. Firestein, G.S., Boyle, D., Bullough, D.A., Gruber, H.E., Sajjadi, F.G., Montag, A., Sambol, B., Mullane, K.M. Protective effect of an adenosine kinase inhibitor in septic shock. *J Immunol*, 1994;**152**:5853–5859.

81. Lee, J.C., Laydon, J.T., McDonnell, P.C., Gallagher, T.F., Kumar, S., Green, D., McNulty, D., Blumenthal, M.J., Heys, J.R., Landvatter, S.W., Strickler, J.E., McLaughlin, M.M., Siemens, I.R., Fisher, S.M., Livi, G.P., White, J.R., Adams, J.L., Young, P.R. A protein kinase involved in the regulation of inflammatory cytokine biosynthesis. *Nature*, 1994;**372**:739–746.

82. Lee, J.C., Badger, A.M., Griswold, D.E., Dunnington, D., Truneh, A., Votta, B., White, J.R., Young, P.R., Bender P.E. Bicycle imidazoles as a novel class of cytokine biosynthesis inhibitors. *Ann NY Acad Sci*, 1993;**696**:149–170.

83. Boehm, J.C., Smietana, J.M., Sorenson, M.E., Garigipati, R.S., Gallagher, T.F., Sheldrake, P.L., Bradbeer, J., Badger, A.M., Laydon, J.T., Lee, J.C., Hillegass, L.M., Griswold, D.E., Breton, J.J., Chabot-Fletcher, M.C., Adams, J.L. 1-Substituted 4-aryl-5-pyridinylimidazoles: a new class of cytokine suppressive drugs with low 5-lipoxygenase and cyclooxygenase inhibitory potency. *J Med Chem*, 1996;**39**:3929–3937.

84. Jackson, J.R., Bolognese, B., Hilegass, L., Kassis, S., Adams, J., Griswold, D.E., Winkler, J.D. Effects of SB 220025, a selective inhibitor of p38 mitogen-activated protein kinase, in angiogenesis and chronic inflammatory disease models. *J Pharm Exp Ther*, 1988;284:687–692.

85. Cuenda, A., Rouse, J., Doza, Y.N., Meier, R., Cohen, P., Gallagher, T.F., Young, P.R., Lee, J.C. SB 203580 is a specific inhibitor of a MAP kinase homologue which is stimulated by cellular stresses and interleukin-1. *FEBS Lett*, 1995;364:229–233.

86. Young, P.R., McLaughlin, M.M., Kumar, S., Kassis, S., Doyle, M.L., McNulty, D., Gallagher, T.F., Fisher, S., McDonnell, P.C., Carr, S.A., Huddleston, M.J., Seibel, G., Porter, T.G., Livi, G.P., Adams, J.L., Lee, J.C. Pyridinyl imidazole inhibitors of p38 mitogen-activated protein kinase bind in the ATP site. *J Biol Chem*, 1997;272:12116–12121.

87. Tong, L., Pav, S., White, D.M., Rogers, S., Crane, K.M., Cywin, C.L., Brown, M.L., Pargellis, C.A. A highly specific inhibitor of p38 MAP kinase binds in the ATP pocket. *Nature Structural Biology*, 1997;4:311–316.

88. Wilson, K.P., McCaffrey, P.G., Hsiao, K., Pazhanisamy, S., Galullo, V., Bemis, G.W., Fitzgibbon, M.J., Caron, P.R., Murko, M.A., Su, M. The structural basis for the specificity of pyridinyl-imidazole inhibitors of p38 MAP kinase. *Chem Biol*, 1997;4:423–431.

89. Gallagher, T.F., Fier-Thompson, S.M., Garigipati, R.S., Sorenson, M.E., Smietana, J.M., Lee, D., Bender, P.E., Lee, J.C., Laydon, J.T., Griswold, D.E., Chabot-Fletcher, M.D., Breton, J.J., Adams, J.L. Triarylimidazole inhibitors of IL-1 biosynthesis. *Bioorg Med Chem Lett*, 1995;5:1171–1176.

90. Badger, A.M., Bradbeer, J.N., Botta, B., Lee, J.C., Adams, J.L., Griswold, D.E. Pharmacological profile of SB 203580, a selective inhibitor of cytokine suppressive binding protein/p38 kinase, in animal models of arthritis, bone resorption, endotoxin shock and immune function. *J Pharm Exptl Ther*, 1966;279:1453–1461.

91. Reddy, M.P., Webb, E.F., Cassatt, D., Maley, D., Lee, J.C., Griswold, D.E., Truneh, A. Pyridinyl imidazoles inhibit the inflammatory phase of delayed type hypersensitivity reactions without affecting T-dependent immune responses. *Int J Immunopharmacol*, 1994;16:795–804.

92. Badger, A.M., Cook, M.N., Lark, M.W., Newman-Tarr, T.M., Swift, B.A., Nelson, A.H., Barone, F.C., Kumar, S. SB 203580 inhibits p38 mitogen-activated protein kinase, nitric oxide production, and inducible nitric oxide synthase in bovine cartilage-derived chondrocytes. *J Immunol*, 1998;161:467–473.

93. Molnar Kimber, K.L., Yonno, L., Heaslip, R.J., Weichman, B.M. Differential regulation of TNF-α and IL-1β production from endotoxin stimulated human monocytes by phosphodiesterase inhibitors. *Mediat Inflamm*, 1992;1:411–417.

94. Semmler, J., Wachtel, H., Endres, S. The specific type IV phosphodiesterase inhibitor rolipram suppresses tumor necrosis factor-α production by human mononuclear cells. *Int J Immunopharmacol*, 1993;15:409–413.

95. Endres, S., Sinha, F.B., Stoll, D., Dinarello, C.A., Gerzer, R., Weber, P.C. Cyclic nucleotides differentially regulate the synthesis of tumor necrosis factor-α and interleukin-1β by mononuclear cells. *Immunology*, 1991;72:56–60.

96. Torphy, T.J., Undem, B.J. Phosphodiesterase inhibitors: new opportunities for the treatment of asthma. *Thorax*, 1991;46:512–523.

97. Shire, M.G., Muller, G.W. TNF-α inhibitors and rheumatoid arthritis. *Exp Opin Ther Patents*, 1998;8:531–544.

98. Prabhakar, U., Lipshutz, D., O'Leary Bartus, J., Slivjak, M.J., Smith, E.F., Lee, J.C., Esser, K.M. Characterization of cAMP-dependent inhibition of LPS-induced TNFα production by rolipram, a specific phosphodiesterase IV (PDE IV) inhibitor. *Int J Immunopharm*, 1994;16:805–816.

99. Strieter, R.M., Remick, D.G., Ward, P.A., Spengler, R.N., Lynch III J.P., Larrick, J., Kunkel, S.L. Cellular and molecular regulation of tumor necrosis factor-alpha production by pentoxifyulline. *Biochem Biophys Res Commun*, 1988;155:1230–1236.

100. Badger, A.M., Olivera, D.L., Esser, K.M. Beneficial effects of the phosphodiesterase inhibitors BRL 61063, pentoxifylline, and rolipram in a murine model of endotoxin shock. *Circ Shock*, 1994;44:188–195.

101. Sekut, L., Yarnall, D., Stimpson, S.A., Noel, L.S., Bateman-Fite, R., Clark, R.L., Brackeen, M.F., Menius, L.A., Connolly, K.M. Anti-inflammatory activity of phosphodiesterase (PDE) IV inhibitors in acute and chronic models of inflammation. *Clin Exp Immunol*, 1995;100:126–132.

102. Lloyd, A. Monitor: molecules and profiles. *Drug Discovery Today*, 1997;2:301–305.

103. Chikanza, I.C., Fernandes, L. The current status and future prospects for biological targeted therapies for rheumatoid arthritis. *Exp Opin Invest Drugs*, 1996;5:819–828.

104. Maksymowych, W.P., Avina-Zubieta, A., Luong, M.H., Russell, A.S. An open study of pentoxifylline in the treatment of severe refractory rheumatoid arthritis. *J Rheumatol*, 1995;22:625–629.

105. Dubost, J-J., Soubrier, M., Ristori, M-M., Beaujon, G., Oualid, T., Bussiere, J-L., Sauvezie, B. An open study of the anti-TNF alpha agent pentoxifylline in the treatment of rheumatoid arthritis. *Rev Rheum*, 1997;67:907–911.

106. Hughes, B., Owens, R., Perry, M., Warrellow, G., Allen, R. PDE-4 inhibitors: the use of molecular cloning in the design and development of novel drugs. *Drug Disc Today*, 1997;2:88–101.

107. Zwingenberger, K., Wnendt, S. Immunomodulation by thalidomide: systematic review of the literature and of unpublished observations. *J Inflamm*, 1966;46:177–211.

108. Oliver, S.J., Cheng, T.P., Banquerigo, Brahn, E. The effect of thalidomide and 2 analogs on collagen-induced arthritis. *J Rheumatol*, 1997;25:964–969.

109. Koch, H.P. Thalidomide and congeners as anti-inflammatory agents. *Prog Med Chem*, 1985;22:166–242.

110. Sampaio, E.P., Sarno, E.N., Galilly, R., Cohn, Z.A., Kaplan, G. Thalidomide selectively inhibits tumor necrosis factor α production by stimulated human monocytes. *J Exp Med*, 1991;173:699–703.

111. Gutierrez-Rodriguez, O. Thalidomide: a promising treatment for rheumatoid arthritis. *Arthritis Rheum*, 1984;27:1118–1121.

112. Moreira, A.L., Sampaio, E.P., Zmuidzinas, A., Frindt, P., Smigh, K.A., Kaplan, G. Thalidomide exerts its inhibitory action on tumor necrosis factor alpha by enhancing mRNA degradation. *J Exp Med*, 1993;177:1675–1680.

113. Scoville, C.D. Results of the extension phase of the open trial of thalidomide in the treatment of rheumatoid arthritis. *Arthritis Rheum*, 1996;39(Suppl.):S281.

114. Lee, S., Klausner, S., Oliver, G., Kaplan, E., McCullagh, Abramson, S. Treatment of rheumatoid arthritis (RA) with thalidomide. *Arthritis Rheum*, 1996;39(Suppl.):S282.

115. Corral, L.G., Muller, G.W., Moreira, A.L., Chen, Y., Wu, M., Stirling, D., Kaplan, G. Selection of novel analogs of thalidomide with enhanced tumor necrosis factor α inhibitory activity. *Molecular Med*, 1996;2:506–515.

116. David, J.R. Delayed hypersensitivity *in vitro*: its mediation by cell-free substances formed by lymphoid cell-antigen interaction. *Pathology*, 1966;56:72–77.

117. Nathan, C.F., Karnovsky, M.L., Davie, J.R. Alterations of macrophage functions by mediators from lymphocytes. *J Exp Med*, 1971;133:1356–1376.

118. Bloom B.R., Bennet, B. Mechanism of a reaction *in vitro* associated with delayed type hypersensitivity. *Science*, 1966;153:80–82.

119. Bernhagen, J., Calandra, T., Mitchell, R.A., Martin, S.B., Tracey, K.J., Voelter, W. et al. MIF is a pituitary derived cytokine that potentiates lethal endotoxemia. *Nature*, 1993;365:756–759.

120. Bernhagen, J., Mitchell, R.A., Calandro, T., Voelter, W., Cerami, A., Bucala, R. Purification, bioactivity, and secondary structure analysis of mouse and human macrophage migration inhibitory factor (MIF). *Biochemistry*, 1994;33:1414–14155.

121. Calandro, T., Bernhagen, J., Mitchell, R.A., Bucala, R. The macrophage is an important and previously unrecognized source

of macrophage migration inhibitory factor. *J Exp Med*, 1994;179:1895–1902.

122. Calandra, T., Bernhagen, J., Metz, C.N., Spiegel, L.A., Bacher, M., Donnelly, T., Cerami, A., Bucala, R. MIF as a glucocorticoid-induced modulator of cytokine production. *Nature*, 1995;377:68–71.

123. Mikulowska, A., Metz, C.N., Bucala, R., Holmdahl, R. Macrophage migration inhibitory factor is involved in the pathogenesis of collagen type II-induced arthritis in mice. *J Immunol*, 1997;158:5514–5517.

124. Leech, M., Metz, C., Santos, L., Peng, T., Holdsworth, Bucala, R., Morand, E.F. Involvement of macrophage migration inhibitory factor in the evolution of rat adjuvant arthritis. *Arthritis Rheum*, 1998;41:910–917.

125. Clancy, R.M., Amin, A.R., Abramson, S.B. The role of nitric oxide in inflammation and immunity. *Arthritis Rheum*, 1998;7:1141–1151.

126. Clancy, R.M., Abramson, S.B. Nitric oxide: a novel mediatory of inflammation. *Soc Exp Biol Med*, 1995;210:93–101.

127. Nathan, C. Perspectives series: nitric oxide and nitric oxide synthases. Inducible nitric oxide synthase: what difference does it make? *J Clin Invest*, 1997;100:2417–2423.

128. Billiar, T.R. Nitric oxide: novel biology with clinical relevance. *Ann Surg*, 1995;221:339–349.

129. Gorbunov, N., Esposito, E. Nitric oxide as a mediator of inflammation. *Int J Immunopathol Pharmacol*, 1993;6:67–75.

130. St. Clair, E.W. Nitric oxide—friend or foe in arthritis. *J Rheumatol*, 1998;25:1451–1453.

131. McCartney-Francis, N., Allen, J.B., Mizel, D.E., Albina, J.E., Xie, Q., Nathan, C.F., Wahl, S. Suppression of arthritis by an inhibitor of nitric oxide synthase. *J Exp Med*, 1993;178:749–754.

132. Gilkeson, G.S., Mudgett, J.S., Seldin, M.F., Ruiz, P., Alexander, A.A., Misukonis, M.A., Pisetsky, D.S., Weinberg, J.B. Clinical and serologic manifestations of autoimmune disease in MRL-lpr/lpr mice lacking nitric oxide synthase type 2. *J Exp Med*, 1997;186:365–373.

133. Stefanovic-Racic, M., Stadler, J., Evans, C.H. Nitric oxide and arthritis. *Arthritis Rheum*, 1993;36:1036–1044.

134. St. Clair, E.W., Wilkinson, W.E., Lang, T., Sanders, L., Misukonis, M.A., Gilkeson, G.S., Pisetsky, D.S., Granger, D.I., Weinbert, J.B. Increased expression of blood mononuclear cell nitric oxide synthase type 2 in rheumatoid arthritis patients. *J Exp Med*, 1996;184:1173–1178.

135. Sakurai, H., Kohsaka, H., Liu, M-F., Higashiyama, H., Hirata, Y., Kanno, K., Saito, I., Miyasaki, N. Nitric oxide production and inducible nitric oxide synthase expression in inflammatory arthritides. *J Clin Invest*, 1995;96:2357–2363.

136. McInnes, I.B., Leung, B.P., Field, M., Wei, X.Q., Huang, F-P., Sturrock, R.D., Kinninmouth, A., Weidner, J., Mumford, R., Liew, F.Y. Production of nitric oxide in the synovial membrane of rheumatoid and osteoarthritis patients. *J Exp Med*, 1996;184:1519–1524.

137. Hallinan, E.A., Tsymbalov, S., Finnegan, P.M., Moore, W.M., Jerome, G.M., Currie, M.G., Pitzele, B.S. Acetamidine lysine derivative, N-(5(S)-amino-6,7-dihydroxyheptyl)ethanimidamide dihydrochloride: a highly selective inhibitor of human inducible nitric oxide synthase. *J Med Chem*, 1998;41:775–777.

138. Clancy, R.M., Amin, A.R., Abramson, S.B. The role of nitric oxide in inflammation and immunity. *Arthritis Rheum*, 1998;41:1141–1151.

139. Brune, B., von Knethen, A., Sandau, K.B. Nitric oxide and its role in apoptosis. *Eur J Pharmacol* 1998;351:261–272.

140. Miossec, P., van den Berg, W. Thi/Th2 cytokine balance in arthritis. *Arthritis Rheum*, 1997;40:2105–2115.

141. Sone, S., Yamagawa, H., Nishioka, Y., Orino, E., Bhaska-ran, G., Nii, A., Mizuno, K., Heike, Y., Ogushi, F., Ogura, T. Interleukin-4 as a potent down-regulator for human alveolar macrophages capable of producing tumor necrosis factor-alpha and interleukin-1. *Eur Respir J*, 1992;5:174

142. Hart, P.H., Ahern, M.J., Smith, M.D., Finlay-Jones, J.J. Comparison of the suppressive effects of interleukin-10 and interleukin-4 on synovial fluid macrophages and blood monocytes from patients with inflammatory arthritis. *Immunology*, 1995;84:536–542.

143. Joosten, L.A.B., Lubberts, E., Durez, P., Helsen, M.M.A., Jacobs, M.J.M., Goldman, M., van den Berg, W. Role of interleukin-4 and interleukin-10 in murine collagen-induced arthritis. *Arthritis Rheum*, 1997;40:249–260.

144. Keystone, E., Wherry, J., Grint, P. IL-10 as a therapeutic strategy in the treatment of rheumatoid arthritis. *Rheumatic Dis Clin N Am*, 1998;24:629–639.

145. Weckmann, A.L., Alcocer-Varela, J. Cytokine inhibitors in autoimmune disease. *Semin Arthritis Rheum*, 1996;26:539–557.

146. de Waal Malefyt, R., Abrams, J., Bennett, B., Figdor, C.G., de Vries, J.E. Interleukin-10 (IL-10) inhibits cytokine synthesis by human monocytes: an autoregulatory role of IL-10 produced by monocytes. *J Exp Med*, 1991;174:1209–1219.

147. Marchant, A., Bruyns, C., Vandenabeele, P., Ducarme, M., Gerard, C., Delvaux, A., De Groote, D., Abramowicz, D., Velu, T., Goldman, M. Interleukin-10 reduces the release of tumor necrosis factor and prevents lethality in experimental endotoxemia. *Eur J Immunol*, 1994;24:1167–1171.

148. Bogdan, C., Vodovotz, Y., Nathan, C. Macrophage deactivation by interleukin-10. *J Exp Med*, 1991;174:1549–1555.

149. Willems, F., Marchant, A., Delville, J.P., Gerard, C., Delvaux, A., Velu, T., de Boer, M., Goldman, M. Interleukin-10 inhibits B7 and intercellular adhesion molecule-1 expression on human monocytes. *Eur J Immunol*, 1994;24:1007–1009.

150. Ma, Y., Thornton, S., Duwel, L.E., Boivin, G.P., Giannini, E.H., Leiden, J.M., Bluestone, J.A., Hirsch, R. Inhibition of collagen-induced arthritis in mice by viral IL-10 gene transfer. *J Immunol*, 1998;161:1516–1524.

151. Zurawski, G., de Vries, J.E. Interleukin 13, an interleukin 4-like cytokine that acts on monocytes and B cells, but not on T cells. *Immunol Today*, 1994;15:19–26.

152. Doyle, A.G., Herbein, G., Montaner, L.J., Minty, A.J., Caput, D., Ferrara, P., Gordon, S. Interleukin-13 alters the activation state of murine macrophages *in vitro*: comparison with interleukin-4 and interferon-γ. *Eur J Immunol*, 1994;24:1441–1445.

153. Hart, P.H., Ahern, M.J., Smith, M.D., Finlay-Jones, J.J. Regulatory effects of IL-13 on synovial fluid macrophages and blood monocytes from patients with inflammatory arthritis. *Clin Exp Immunol* 99:331–337.

154. Baggiolini, M., Dewald, B., Moser, B. Interleukin 8 and related chemotactic cytokines—CXC and CC chemokines. *Adv Immunology*, 1994;55:97–179.

155. Schall, T. In: *The Cytokine Handbook* (Thompson, A. ed.) pp. 419–460. Academic Press, San Diego.

156. Mackay, C.R. Chemokine receptors and T cell chemokines. *J Exp Med*, 1966;184:799–802.

157. Hesselgesser, J., Ng, G.P., Liang, M., Zheng, W., May, K., Bauman, J.G., Monahan, S., Islam, I., Wei, G.P., Ghannam, A., Taubb, D.D., Rosser, M., Snider, R.M., Morrissey, M.M., Perez, H.D., Horuk, R. Identification and characterization of small molecule functional antagonists of the CCR1 chemokine receptor. *J Exp Med*, 1988;184:799–802.

158. Yarovoi, S.V., Lu, X-P., Picard, N., Rungta, D., Rideout, D., Pfahl, M. Selective activation of an apoptotic retinoid precursor in macrophage cell lines. *J Biol Chem, 1998;273:*20852–20859.

43 | *Inhibition of matrix metalloproteinases in rheumatoid arthritis*

Tim Shaw

Introduction

Structural joint damage is a characteristic pathology of both rheumatoid (RA) and osteoarthritis (OA) which is accepted by many as a strong predictor for long-term outcome. Given sufficient time this damage contributes to functional decline, disability, and major surgical procedures[1–3]. Indeed, it has been reported that patients with extensive radiographic damage (stages III and IV) have significantly more work disability than those at stages I and II[4]. Similarly, it is also associated with a significant economic impact, with the predicted annual cost of RA related knee replacements alone in the United States reaching over 1 billion dollars[5].

Consequently, protecting bone and articular cartilage from pathological damage has major therapeutic and economic potential. If joint destruction in RA or OA can be prevented or significantly reduced then the long-term functionality of the affected joints could be preserved. It is, therefore, considered that patients whose disease progression is delayed early on in their illness could benefit in terms of improved quality of life throughout their disease course. This may be of particular importance if the later stages of severe disability can be avoided or significantly delayed.

Prevention of structural joint damage is therefore a major goal of antiarthritic therapy, which has been recognized by rheumatologists and health authorities alike[6,7]. Consequently, it is now strongly recommended to investigate the ability of new antirheumatoid drugs to prevent or retard structural joint damage, and this has opened debate as to the potential of new therapies which might be solely targeted towards prevention of damage.

Currently available antirheumatoid therapies are predominantly directed towards the control of pain and joint inflammation associated with synovitis. The effect of these drugs on preventing structural joint damage has been very much a secondary consideration, which was assumed to be related to their ability to reduce inflammation. However, it remains a controversial subject as to how effective these second line, so called disease modifying antirheumatoid drugs (DMARDs), really are in preventing or even slowing joint damage. In a review of six commonly used DMARDs only three (aurothioglucose, sul-fasalazine, and methotrexate) were found to have a statistically significant effect on radiological progression[8]. However, it is also documented that even with what is currently considered the best of these, methotrexate, that progression is only slowed and that erosive damage and joint space narrowing still occur[9–11].

In addition to these DMARDs, there have also been data demonstrating the ability of low dose oral corticosteroids to slow radiological progression[12]. Although still considered controversial, this study was particularly interesting in that slower progression was demonstrated in the corticosteroid group compared to placebo, despite the observation that in both groups the inflammatory component of the disease appeared equally controlled. This, together with other reports, has initiated discussion that radiological progression continues despite relief of clinical symptoms, and therefore suggests the processes causing synovitis and destruction might be separate and independent[13].

More recent additions to the antirheumatiod drug armamentarium include leflunomide, which, like methotrexate, has also demonstrated a favorable slowing of progression[14]. However, based on currently available data the degree of this effect appears similar to that achievable with methotrexate and, therefore, it is reasonable to assume that even with this new therapy structural joint damage is at best slowed and that further progression will still continue. Novel anti-TNF-α antirheumatoid therapies, such as etanercept, have also been reported to produce substantial improvements in relief of clinical symptoms[15], but to date their ability to retard structural joint damage has still to be assessed.

The current situation, therefore, remains that prevention of structural damage is a major therapeutic goal, which is inadequately addressed, even with the most recent therapies. Furthermore, the paradigm that controlled inflammation results in reduced damage may not be the complete story, and it is likely that novel therapies specifically directed towards inhibiting the process of cartilage and bone damage will be required to achieve maximal benefit. As a result there has been a large research effort over many years to understand not only this destructive process, but also what part of this pathway could be influenced by therapeutic intervention to prevent joint damage.

Articular cartilage, its destruction and the role of matrix metalloproteinases (MMPs)

Articular cartilage is a highly specialized tissue that has unique biomechanical properties. First, it permits free articulation of diarthrodial joints, and second it is paramount to the successful weight bearing capacity of the joint by distributing load over a large area of bone. The ability of articular cartilage to resist these forces derives from the organization of its two major structural components, collagen fibers (predominantly type II) and proteoglycan. The collagen network is composed of tightly wound triple helix of amino acid chains, forming fibers that provide cartilage with tensile strength. This provides a dense network of fibers in which is immobilized a high concentration of proteoglycan. The hydrophilic characteristics of these macroproteins create an osmotic pressure within the tissue causing influx of water and a pronounced swelling. This swelling is kept under control by the network of collagen fibers which will compress under weight, spreading load over a larger surface area. It is known that there is physiological variation in the levels of proteoglycan, dependant upon joint use, however, the cartilage will remain undamaged as long as the collagen network remains intact. Articular cartilage is, therefore, a fiber-reinforced composite matrix, the biomechanical properties of which are critically dependent on the integrity of the collagen network[16].

When pathological destruction of cartilage occurs, there is an initial net loss of the proteoglycan matrix, although, providing the supporting collagen network remains intact, this proteoglycan loss can be reversed[17]. However, it is the subsequent cleavage of the collagen network itself which marks the irreversible step in the tissues destruction[18]. Once this fibrillar network is damaged or depleted the cartilage loses its integrity and biomechanical properties, and therefore fails to protect the joint from stress. In conditions such as rheumatoid arthritis, the removal of cartilage then exposes the bone to further damage,

which then produces the characteristic erosions of the disease. In the long term this damage to the structure of the joint can lead to a significant reduction in its functionality and if the damage is severe, to a need for total joint replacement.

The enzymes most frequently implicated in the destruction of articular cartilage are a family of zinc endopeptidases called matrix metalloproteinases (MMPs). This is an ever increasing class of enzymes, which can be broadly classified as collagenases (MMP 1, 8, and 13), stromelysins (MMP 3, 10, and 11), gelatinases (MMP 2 and 9), and membrane-type metalloproteinases or MT-MMP (MMP 14, 15, 16, and 17)[19,20]. All are functional at neutral pH and are produced by a variety of cells including fibroblasts, neutrophils, macrophages, chondrocytes, and osteoblasts in response to inflammatory cytokines, such as interleukin 1 and tumour necrosis factor[21]. Initially synthesized as inactive proenzymes, they are converted to active enzymes by a sequence of events possibly starting with the activation of certain key proenzymes. Many activation mechanisms have been described[22], however, plasmin may be a major contributor in the generation of certain active species, including Stromelysin-1 (MMP-3), which in turn is then capable of activating many of the collagenases enzymes[23]. Collectively, MMPs can degrade all the components of the extracellular matrix[24]; however, at physiological pHs the collagenases are the only mammalian enzymes known which can cleave the triple helix of fibrillar collagen, and therefore induce irreversible destruction of the collagen network of articular cartilage.

Within the arthritic joints of animals and humans the concentrations of most MMPs are known to be raised[25]; as such there is reasonable evidence to implicate the involvement of most of the MMPs in having an active role in the destructive processes in both rheumatoid and osteoarthritis (Table 43.1). However, it is the involvement of the collagenases and stromelysin-1 which has attracted most interest since they appear to be key mediators of cartilage and bone changes in these conditions.

There is good evidence for the involvement of stomelysin-1 (MMP-3) in arthritis with several reports of its elevated levels and localization within arthritic joints[32]. Its activity on minor

Table 43.1   Matrix metalloproteinases and their implication in arthritic diseases

Enzyme group (common nomenclature)	Major substrates	Involvement in arthritis?
Collagenases		
MMP-1 (Fibroblast collagenase)	Collagens, I, II, III, VII, X	Produced by RA synovial fibroblasts,[26] present at the site of erosions[27]
MMP-8 (Neutrophil collagenase)	Collagens I, II, III	Expressed in RA synovial fibroblasts[28] and in OA cartilage[29]
MMP-13 (Collagenase 3)	Collagens I, II, III	Present in rheumatoid synovium[30] and expressed in RA articular cartilage[31]
Stromelysins		
MMP-3 (Stromelysin 1)	Proteoglycan core protein, minor collagens, activates MMPs 1, 8, and 9	Increased in serum and synovial fluid in RA[32] and OA[33] Immunolocalization in RA synovial fibroblasts[34]
MMP-10 (Stromelysin 2)	Aggrecan, gelatin	
MMP-11 (Stromelysin 3)	Weak stromelysin activity	
MMP 7 (Matrilysin)	Aggrecan, gelatins, fibronectin	Expression in OA cartilage[35]
Gelatinases		
MMP-2 (Gelatinase A)	Gelatins, minor collagens, elastin	Present in synovia and destructive regions of femoral heads in coxarthropathy (as is MMP-9)[36]
MMP-9 (Gelatinase B)	Gelatin, minor collagens	Elevated in synovial fluid and sera in RA[37]

collagens and its ability to activate the collagenases has led to much interest in this particular enzyme as being a major cause of the structural joint damage in both rheumatoid and osteoarthritis. However, more recent data from stomelysin-1 deficient mice with collagen-induced arthritis, has shown that loss of articular cartilage and proteoglycan was similar to wild-type mice which possess this MMP[38]. Therefore, it may be reasonable to conclude that sole inhibition of this particular enzyme is unlikely to have a significant effect at preventing structural joint damage in arthritis. Indeed, selective stromelysin inhibitors have been shown to have no protective effects on *in vitro* models of cartilage destruction (internal communication).

In contrast, the collagenases remain heavily implicated as key enzymes in the destructive process and their initial cleavage of the collagen fibril is considered the irreversible step in collagen destruction. Not only do they cleave the collagen most commonly found in articular cartilage (type II), but they have also been shown to be elevated in both synovial joint fluid and serum from arthritic conditions. In addition, early work showing the presence of collagenase-1 (MMP-1) at the site of erosions[27] has now been complimented by the demonstration that this enzyme is expressed early in the RA disease process[39]. This suggests that not only are collagenases an essential element in the destructive processes of arthritis, but that they are present in the cartilage at an extremely early stage of the disease. Consequently, if their effects are to be prevented then therapeutic intervention would need to be initiated as soon after diagnosis as possible.

There is, therefore, substantial evidence to implicate MMPs, and particularly the collagenases, in the destructive process associated with RA and OA. Consequently much attention has been focused on how these enzymes are controlled and in developing novel synthetic inhibitors towards them.

Control of MMPs

Natural inhibitors of matrix metalloproteinases

There are two known natural sources of MMP inhibition. The most prominent of these is α_2 macroglobulin (α_2-M). This is a large protein (~750 kD), produced by the liver, which is found in the serum and synovial fluid from patients with RA and OA. However, while α_2-M may function as an inhibitor in these fluids its large size may exclude its access to other sites of MMP activity in deeper connective tissues, for example layers of cartilage.

The second, and more specific, natural source of inhibition is a family of proteins known as tissue inhibitors of metalloproteinases (TIMPs). All activated MMPs are inhibited by TIMPs, which are synthesized by connective tissue cells and bind to MMPs, forming tight but non-covalent, binding complexes with a 1:1 stoichiometry[40]. Currently, four TIMPs have been identified, all have a relative molecular mass of approximately 21 kD and contain two domains, one responsible for inhibition of MMPs, the other binding to progelatinases and also possessing some growth factor properties.

Much of the structural joint damage associated with arthritic conditions is attributed to an imbalance between the levels of activated MMPs and TIMPs. Should the amount of activated MMPs exceed that of the locally available TIMP, then the outcome is connective tissue turnover. In the arthritic joint this eventually becomes manifest as destruction of cartilage and bone. Indeed, this imbalance between MMP and TIMPs has been demonstrated in cartilage explants from both OA and RA patients. In these patients an increased metalloproteinase activity over TIMP activity was demonstrated in macroscopic lesions compared to normal surrounding tissues[41]. Further work suggests that the level of TIMP gene expression is similar in these diseases, and that the imbalance is due to increased production of MMPs, particularly in RA. Conversely, in areas of osteophyte formation in OA, expression of TIMP mRNA has been shown to be greater than that of MMP mRNA[42].

In vitro studies using bovine nasal cartilage have demonstrated the ability of both TIMP-1 and TIMP-2 to prevent the release of collagen fragments[43]. As TIMPs only inhibit MMPs, and since the system lacked a source of MMP-8, this strongly implicates the role of MMPs 1 and 13 in the breakdown of cartilage. Systemic administration of TIMPs in a type II collagen-induced mouse model has also shown a significant reduction in disease severity compared to controls[44]. However, it is uncertain whether this was due to an increase in TIMPs in the affected joints.

TIMPs are unlikely future therapeutic agents; however, it could be postulated that increasing the local production of TIMPs could lead to readdressing the balance between MMPs and TIMPs and consequently to prevention of cartilage damage. Several substances are known to increase TIMP mRNA and protein, including all trans-retinoic acids and synthetic vitamin A analogues (retinoids)[45], together with several cytokines such as IL-6, IL-1, and possibly TNF-α[46]. TNF-α and IL-6 are of particular interest since their levels are elevated in several inflammatory conditions, including the serum and synovial fluid from RA patients[47]. TNF-α is also heavily implicated in the inflammatory process and indeed much success has been achieved by inhibiting this cytokine in RA. Consequently, the more general actions of these cytokines may restrict their usefulness in being used to elevate TIMP levels. Furthermore, if endogenous substances already elevate the production of TIMPs, then the potential to increase further their production by using an additional exogenous agent may be limited. For this reason, modification of the actions of MMPs has predominantly focused on the development of synthetic low molecular weight inhibitors.

Synthetic MMP inhibitors

Interest in novel synthetic inhibitors has been extremely high over the past decade and the production of different inhibitors with differing inhibitory activities has been prolific[48,49]. Some of these compounds have been developed with the intent of primary use in oncology where MMPs are thought to play a significant role in the spread and growth of cancer cells, and in the process of angiogenesis which further promotes their growth. However, others have targeted arthritic diseases and have produced encouraging animal data supporting the concept

Table 43.2 MMP inhibitors in clinical development

Compound (Company)	Inhibitory profile	Indication	Status
Arthritic indications			
Trocade™ (Ro 32-3555) (Roche)	Collagenases 1, 2, and 3	Rheumatoid arthritis	Phase III
Ro 113, 0830 (Roche)	Gelatinases A and B Collagenases 2 and 3	Osteoarthritis	Phase II
BAY 12-9566* (Bayer)	Gelatinases A and B Stromelysin-1	Osteoarthritis and oncology	Phase III
Other indications			
Marimastat (BB-2576) (British Biotechnology)	Collagenases 1, 2 and 3 Gelatinases A and B Stromelysin-1	Oncology	Phase III
AG3340 (Agouron)	Collagenase 3 Gelatinase A Stromelysin-1	Oncology	Phase II
CGS 27023A* (Novartis)	Gelatinase A and B Collagenase 2 Stromelysin	Oncology (OA also?)	Phase I
D5410 (Chiroscience)	?	Inflammatory bowel disease	Phase I

* no longer in clinical development

that MMP inhibitors have a great potential to reduce the structural damage associated with these indications. Unfortunately, few have progressed into clinical studies and even fewer have remained in development long enough to know if this potential can be realized (Table 43.2).

One of the first synthetic MMP inhibitors to show promise was Ro 31-9790. This compound showed good *in vivo* activity in animal models of arthritis, and was considered to have significant potential to prevent structural damage in RA (internal communication). Unfortunately, while it entered early clinical trials further development was halted due to preclinical evidence of an undesirable drug-related histopathology in certain joints.

Ro 31-9790 belongs to series of compound that utilize a hydroxamic acid as the zinc binding ligand. This class has also lead to a number of other potent, broad spectrum inhibitors, which include batimastat (BB94), marimastat (BB2516), and CGS 27023A. Of these, data in animal models of arthritis appears to be available only for Ro 31-9790 and CGS 27023A, while batimastat and marimastat have been pursued for oncology indications.

Early development work was, however, hampered due to the lack of sufficient oral bioavailability and batimastat had to be administered by intraperitoneal injection due to its poor aqueous solubility[49]. Subsequently, its development was stopped and replaced with an alternative compound, marimastat, that has improved bioavailability. This compound again has broad spectrum activity although there is some selectivity for collagenases and gelatinase over stromelysin. Marimastat is currently in phase III trials for oncology, and whilst no data in either arthritis animal models or RA patients has been published it does

provide extremely useful information on the safety profile of this type of MMP inhibitor in the clinic.

CGS 27023A has demonstrated protective effects in several preclinical models of cartilage degradation. These include the inhibition of glycosaminoglycan and hydroxyproline release from IL-1 stimulated bovine nasal cartilage cultures[50] and the protection of cartilage proteoglycan in a rabbit partial minisectomy osteoarthritis model[51]. In both this model and a spontaneous OA model in the guinea pig, CGS 27023A was also shown to preserve chondrocyte viability compared to controls, thereby further suggesting the potential for MMP inhibitors to prevent cartilage damage in this condition. However, the clinical development of CGS 27023A has been terminated due to an unfavorable safety profile.

As well as the search for novel inhibitors, attention has also focused on readily available drugs that might possess MMP inhibitory activity, the most reported of which are the tetracyclines. The discovery that minocycline inhibited bone loss in diabetic rats, as well as collagenase activity in both gingiva of humans with peridontal disease and the gingiva and skin of rats with experimental diabetes[52], promoted a significant amount of interest in the non-antimicrobial actions of this family of drugs. Since then many other tetracyclines (including minocycline and doxycycline) together with other chemically modified tetracyclines have been reported to have anticollagenase activity[53,54]. In addition to this anticollagenase activity, these compounds also inhibit other MMPs including gelatinases and stromelysins. Further work has also provided evidence that these inhibitory effects may be due to a combination of both a weak direct inhibitory activity together with inhibition of the conversion of the pro-MMP to its active enzyme[54].

Although initially promising, the results from animal and clinical studies on the ability of these compounds to reduce joint damage are somewhat disappointing. In the rat adjuvant-induced arthritis, neither minocycline nor doxycycline significantly reduced the amount of radiological damage, although there was evidence suggesting a reduction in collagenase levels, particularly if combined with a non-steroidal anti-inflammatory such as flurbiprofen[55]. The exact mechanism of this interaction is not known, but may involve improved uptake of the tetraycline. Clinical studies with tetracyclines have also been disappointing in their ability to prevent structural damage. The largest study conducted to date failed to show any statistical difference between placebo and minocycline on the progression of structural damage in patients with RA[56]. Several assessments of damage, including erosion progression rate, joint space narrowing, and newly eroded joints, were analyzed and although there were some positive trends, a significant effect could not be found. Unfortunately, the study was somewhat under powered for these particular endpoints so that a larger study conducted in a suitable population of RA patients for a sufficient duration of time is still required to provide a definitive answer. A smaller study of doxy-cycline in RA did, however, show reduced activity of collaganase-2 (MMP-8) from saliva after 12 weeks of dosing[57].

If collagenases have a role in joint damage, then these clinical results initially seem somewhat surprising. However, it should be remembered that all the tetracyclines are relatively weak inhibitors of collagenase, and that reduction of collagenase activity in the saliva may bear little relationship to collagenase activity in the rheumatoid joint. In addition, tetracyclines do not inhibit all three collagenase enzymes, with collagenase-3 (MMP-13) showing resistance[58]. This could be significant since there is good evidence to promote collagenase-3 as a key enzyme in the cleavage of type II collagen, and therefore its inhibition could be considered essential for any protective effect. This would appear supported by recent data suggesting that inhibition of all the collagenases may be desirable to produce maximal effect[59] although this remains controversial. However, three extremely interesting novel MMP inhibitors, have demonstrated effective joint protection in animal models and have progressed to arthritis clinical trials.

BAY 12-9566 is a broad spectrum inhibitor having activity against stromelysin and gelatinase, with less potency against the collagenases. In dog and guinea pig menisectomy models of osteoarthritis, BAY 12-9566 significantly reduced cartilage lesions and was also suggested to increase function of the affected limb[60]. Good oral bioavailability of over 80 per cent has been reported, and following multiple oral doses of 10 or 25 mg daily there was good penetration into synovial fluid[61]. Consequently, BAY 12-9566 had progressed to Phase III trials in osteoarthritis, as well as being investigated for oncology indications. One such indication was small cell lung cancer, known to be one of the more aggressive neoplasms. Recently released data, however, indicated that tumor growth and survival were significantly worse in the active arms compared with placebo. As a result, this compound has been withdrawn from all indications including OA. The nature of this finding has, understandably, caused much concern over the safety of other MMP inhibitors in clinical development. However, as discussed later it is not neces-

sarily valid to characterize a safety concern from one inhibitor as a class effect and to assume that is applies to all others.

Ro 113,0830 (also referred to in the literature as RS-130830) has a different profile of inhibitory properties with potent activity against several MMPs including collagenase-2 and 3 (MMPs 8 and 13). This compound has been shown to be orally active in a rabbit menisectomy model of OA in which it reduced the incidence of several features of cartilage damage[62]. These included reduced ulceration, pitting, and erosion of cartilage on the femur or tibia. Clinical development of Ro 1130,830 proceeds in phase II trials in osteoarthritis.

The third promising orally active MMP inhibitor being developed for arthritis is Trocade™ (Ro 32-3555). This is also a hydroxamic acid, and has a unique spectrum of inhibitory activity in that it is selective for the collagenases. Specifically, *in vitro* studies have shown that Trocade™ has potent inhibitory activity against human collagenases-1, 2, and 3 (Ki of 3.0 nM, 4.4 nM, and 3.4 nM respectively) while having less activity against stromelysin (Ki of 527 nM) and gelatinases A and B (Ki 154 nM and 59 nM respectively)[63]. Hence, it is distinguished from more broad spectrum inhibitors by being a Collagenase Selective Inhibitor (CSI).

Preclinical data with Trocade™ has been extremely encouraging. *In vitro* experiments have demonstrated protection against IL-1 induced degradation of bovine cartilage, while *in vivo* studies have confirmed the compounds oral activity[63]. In addition to these, Trocade™ has also been shown to preserve articular cartilage in the *P. acnes* induced arthritis model in both the rat and the rabbit. In this assessment rats treated orally with Trocade™ had a significantly greater area of cartilage compared to controls. In the rabbit model, a clear protective effect of Trocade™ was particularly visible when using advanced MRI techniques to image the joint and the cartilage (Fig 43.1). What is evident from these images is that the erosive damage to both the bone and cartilage is markedly reduced despite the presence of active joint inflammation. This is not unexpected since there is currently no evidence to suggest MMP inhibitors can directly reduce the inflammation associated with arthritis. However, it does provide compelling evidence that joint protection is possible with Trocade™ even in the presence of an active inflammatory process. In addition, it provides a strong indication as to how MMP inhibitors should be considered for use in the clinic.

Further to models of rheumatoid arthritis, Trocade™ has also demonstrated efficacy in models of osteoarthrits[64]. The SRT/ORT mouse model of osteoarthritis is a robust reflection of this indications, which produces bone and cartilage changes similar to those observed in the human condition. When administered orally, Trocade™ was effective in reducing joint damage as determined both by radiographic techniques and by histological evaluation. This again provides excellent data to support the critical role of collagenases in the destructive process of the joint, and that the damage characteristic of arthritic conditions can be significantly reduced by their inhibition.

On the basis of these preclinical data Trocade™ is currently under going evaluation in humans. Early clinical experience in healthy volunteers provided evidence of good oral bioavailability and also showed Trocade™ to be well tolerated[65]. Small-

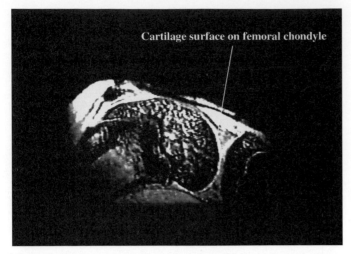

(a)

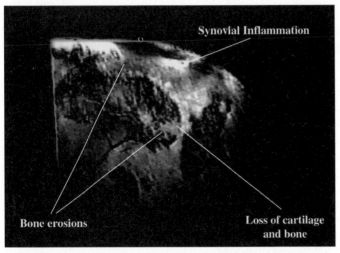

(b)

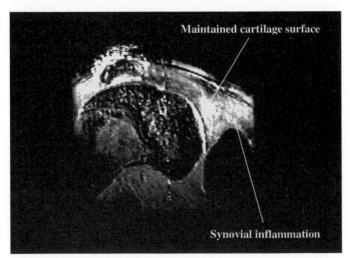

(c)

Fig. 43.1 Effect of Trocade™ in prevention of structural joint damage: representative MRI images from *P. acnes* in rabbit. (a) Normal rabbit knee. (b) Arthritic rabbit knee. (c) Arthritic knee with subcutaneously dosed Trocade™ (50 mg/kg) once daily.

scale investigations in patients with RA have confirmed these findings and consequently large-scale trials are now ongoing in RA to determines if the potential to reduce joint damage seen in the animal models can be realized in the target indication.

Safety of MMP inhibitors

As with all new therapeutic interventions there is always a concern about the potential safety issues that might arise. This is particularly true of MMP inhibition since these enzymes are involved in many homeostatic mechanisms, particularly those associated with tissue turnover. It is also true that our knowledge of the function of these enzymes is still relatively poor and that they may have many other roles that are yet to be elucidated.

Many of the predicted safety issues arise from the pivotal role of MMPs in tissue turnover and remodeling, and of particular concern has been the potential impact of MMP inhibitors on wound healing. The repair process is thought to involve heavily MMPs and, although there are currently no data available on any inhibitor with respect to a detrimental effect on this process, it is probably prudent to consider this a potential concern until further evaluation has been done.

For a similar reason it is expected that any MMP inhibitor is likely to have a significant effect on fetal growth and therefore to be a teratogen. Although this has the potential to be a significant issue it should be remembered that many of the current therapies in RA are also teratogenic in nature. Indeed, even recently-approved antirheumatic drugs carry significant warnings of teratogenic effects. As MMP inhibitors are likely to be given in addition to such drugs, the fact that they too are teratogenic is probably of less concern. In osteoarthritis, however, these potential effects could be considered more of an issue since concomitant medications are unlikely to be teratogenic. Fortunately, in this indication the majority of female patients are postmenopausal and therefore teratogenic drugs may again be of less concern. In either indication, however, this property should not preclude the use of MMP inhibitors in women of childbearing potential who are taking adequate contraceptive therapies.

The effect of MMP inhibition on tissue remodeling is also a critical issue when considering their use in juvenile RA (JRA). Clearly this disease can be extremely erosive and damaging to the joints, and should a MMP inhibitor be successful in preventing damage in adult RA it would be tempting to apply it in JRA. However, until the real benefit of MMP inhibitors in RA is fully established and there is more clarity concerning the effects of these drugs on the growth and development of the skeleton, then their use in JRA can not be recommended.

Given the lack of success in getting many MMP inhibitors to the clinic, there is relatively little data available to judge whether the above are real concerns, or to determine any other safety issues. The most advanced MMP inhibitor for which clinical data has been published is marimastat, which is now in phase III for various cancer indications.

A summary of the safety profile from the phase II trials with this inhibitor found that the most common drug-related toxicity was a characteristic syndrome consisting of musculoskeletal pain and stiffness[66,67]. These effects reportedly commence in the small joints of the hand, spreading to the arms, shoulder, and other joints if drug treatment is continued. The events arose in a dose and time dependant fashion, but were, however, reversible on drug withdrawal. This toxicity was clearly dose limiting and even with patients taking 1–3-week drug holidays and recommencing on reduced doses, a significant number of patients still experienced these effects.

These symptoms are reported to be similar to those seen during toxicological evaluation of marimastal, where a tendonitis was observed[66]. Since the toxicological data on marimastat and Ro 31-9790 have not been published, it is difficult to make a direct comparison of the two compounds, or establish a relationship between the clinical and toxicology finding for marimastat. However, it is interesting to note that the joint lesions in the toxicology studies with Ro 31-9790 led to the decision to stop its development in arthritis.

The cause of these musculoskeletal effects has received much attention and is clearly a great concern for any MMP inhibitor being investigated in any arthritic condition. Many groups have attributed this effect to specific MMPs, for example collagenase-1 (MMP-1). This appeared to be supported by the fact that the available data on BAY-129566 suggests this inhibitor of stromelysin and gelatinases is not associated with such events. However, the association between inhibition of collagenase-1 and these events now seems unlikely given that Trocade™, which is a potent inhibitor or all three collagenases, continues to progress in arthritis trials without any apparent reports of similar musculoskeletal syndromes. Further to this Trocade™, which is equipotent with Ro 31-9790 against collagenase-1, has a superior toxicology profile, despite achieving plasma concentrations several fold higher than those achieved with Ro 31-9790. Therefore, these data strongly dismiss the inhibition of collagenase-1 as being the cause of these musculoskeletal syndromes.

Other theories have proposed the involvement of sheddases, which are involved in the cleavage of TNF-α and its receptor from cell membranes. The resulting increase in free TNF-α being attributed to the inflammation observed. However, why this should lead to specific, localized effects in the tendons and joint remains to be explained, and consequently, the true cause of the musculoskeletal events remains to be identified.

Finally, the recent findings with BAY 12-9566 and its subsequent withdrawal from clinical development have raised the issue that MMP inhibitors may be associated with increased tumor growth and poor survival times in small cell lung, cancer. Clearly any such relationship has to be fully explored. However, there are substantial differences between most of the available MMP inhibitors such that it would be invalid to assume an effect seen with one will automatically be seen with another. These differences relate not only to the compound chemical structure, but also to their metabolism and the inihibitor profile that they exert. For example, BAY 12-9566 is a carboxylic acid and has a chemical structure that is very different from the hydroxamic acids like Trocade™. This difference is likely to result in variable metabolic pathways and ultimately different metabolites. Further, BAY 12-9566 had inhibitory activity predominantly against gelatinases and stromelysins, which is again

different from certain other MMP inhibitors. In addition to this, recent data with marimastat in aggressive pancreatic cancer, while not positive, did not indicate that his MMP inhibitor had an adverse effect on the neoplasm. It should be noted that differing safety profiles between various MMP inhibitors are already emerging. Therefore, while it is prudent to consider this finding as a signal for detailed pharmacovigilance within any clinical evaluation of an MMP inhibitor, it should not immediately be considered a class effect.

Given this, it is likely to be extremely difficult to define categorically a characteristic safety profile for MMP inhibitors in general. It has to be remembered that MMPs are a family of related enzymes and all the inhibitors discussed above inhibit different members of this family to various degrees. Each inhibitor has the potential to have a unique safety profile which, in part, is related to which specific MMPs it affects. Likewise, inhibitors can come from distinct chemical classes, which themselves may have a distinct toxicology.

Clinical evaluation of MMP inhibitors in arthritic indications

Clinical studies with these drugs are probably the most challenging aspect of their development, and there are a number of critical issues in designing and conducting clinical studies of any MMP inhibitor in RA or OA which need to be addressed in order to produce reliable results.

Not the least of these issues is how to measure structural damage as the primary endpoint. Radiographic evaluation is clearly the gold standard with the Larsen or modified Sharp scores being acceptable methods of scoring. Magnetic resonance imaging (MRI) may also be an option to consider given that it may be more sensitive to change over time than plain film radiographs [68]. However, caution should be used with either of these methods with respect to a number of areas, including consistent image acquisition across all participating centers, validation between all readers scoring the images, and finally the validation of MRI as a suitable tool for assessing damage. It should be remembered that this promising technique is still not validated in determining disease progression over time and that a recognized scoring system for MRI images of RA and OA has yet to be developed. This aside, MRI holds many advantages over plain film radiography including 3-D reconstruction and determinations of cartilage volume, both of which could be valuable endpoints, particularly in OA. The necessary validation work needed for MRI to be accepted as a primary imaging tool will undoubtedly become available in the future, however until the plain film radiographic evaluation remains the gold standard for proving efficacy.

Once the assessment of endpoints has been decided, the other issues concerning the duration of study, the specific patient population, the number of patients needed, and the use of background medications can be addressed. The duration of therapy will depend on both the disease (RA or OA) and also the method chosen to determine structural damage. As a guide, using well-controlled radiographic techniques and a suitably progressing patient population, 1 or 2-year trials are recommended as a minimum for RA and OA, respectively. The specific patient population within the chosen disease indication also has some bearing on this time frame since selecting patients with characteristics associated with high rates of disease progression will increase the chances that the control group will progress sufficiently to enable a treatment effect to be seen in the active groups. In knee OA, for example, a high risk population that could be considered is postmenopausal women with a high body mass index.

Determining the number of such patients needed is a relatively easy calculation to make once certain parameters are known. Unfortunately these parameters are difficult to determine for structural damage endpoints since they include (i) the expected amount of progression in the study population over the time of the trial, (ii) the variability of this progression, and (iii) the degree of effect one wants to be able to detect, which itself should be based on detecting a clinically relevant difference. This final point is of particular importance since at present there remains no definitive answer to what is a clinically meaningful retardation of structural joint damage. Unfortunately, this is likely to remain so until an absolute relationship between structural joint damage and long-term functional outcome has been established.

The overall outcome of these requirements is that given the large amount of variability, even in a carefully chosen population, together with the relatively short period of study, it is likely that a suitably powered trial could require several hundred patients per arm to reach statistically significant conclusions. The consequence of requiring large numbers inevitably requires many centers probably from different countries, all of which compound the above issues concerning consistent image acquisition, assessment, and quality control.

Finally, some consideration should be given to the control group and the background medications to be permitted. As discussed above, there is no evidence to suggest any MMP inhibitor will reduce inflammation in the short term and therefore patients, particularly in RA, will require additional anti-inflammatory therapy. Most likely this will include analgesics, DMARDs, NSAIDs, and possibly even corticosteroids. The potential effect of these on the chosen endpoints has to be considered in some depth and should a confounding effect be expected then it should be suitably controlled for within the study design. This does, however, have the advantage of making placebo a suitable control group. If patients are permitted adequate therapy for relief of their symptoms then the addition of an MMP inhibitor or placebo becomes an ethically acceptable design, even if the trial is for several years. Although significant, these hurdles are not insurmountable and there are at least three MMP inhibitors that are in trials designed to establish their efficacy in arthritic conditions.

Future role of MMP inhibitors

The goal of being able to prevent the structural damage associated with both RA and OA has a realistic chance of being achieved with a MMP inhibitor. There is clearly good evidence supporting a role of MMPs in the destructive process, and several inhibitors have demonstrated remarkable protective effects in animal models of both these diseases. However, this is a novel approach to the management of these diseases and the challenge will be to change the current treatment paradigm.

Perhaps one of the major areas still requiring clarification is which of the MMPs is the most relevant, or if one collagenase is more important than the others[69]. It is also possible that different MMPs may be more heavily implicated in different diseases and that a suitable inhibitor profile for one indication may not be optimal for another. Collagenases and possibly stromelysins are likely candidates, but will selective inhibitors of these enzymes be effective, or is broad spectrum inhibition of MMPs needed to obtain maximal effect? Conversely, will broad spectrum inhibitors be associated with a poorer safety profile by inhibiting unnecessary enzymes? Indeed, is inhibition of a specific MMP related to a particular pattern of adverse events?

The situation has also now been expanded with the understanding that certain other closely related enzymes could be important in the disease process. Particular attention has been focused on enzymes involved in the activation or release of membrane-bound cytokines and their soluble receptors. The role of TNF-α in the inflammatory process is well documented and there are now substantial data on the effectiveness of anti-TNF therapy in RA[15,70]. It therefore stimulated a great deal of interest to find that various MMPs were involved in the activation of pro-TNF-α[71], and it is now known that TNF-α converting enzyme (TACE) is a distinct metalloproteinase, belonging to another growing family of enzymes known as ADAMs (a disintegrin and metalloproteinase)[72]. The close relationship of TACE with those MMPs implicated in structural damage has also led to the possibility of synthesizing compounds which inhibit TACE, as well as the important MMPs in the destructive process. Not only would such a compound be a potent anti-inflammatory but it could also have a real protective effect on joint damage. Animal studies have supported this possibility with two broad spectrum MMP inhibitors (BB-1101 and BB-1433) reducing inflammation and radiological damage in adjuvant induce arthritis[73], and at least part of this activity was attributed to the compounds' ability to reduce TNF-α production. In addition to these, there are now a number of selective TACE inhibitors and more broad spectrum inhibitors in preclinical evaluation.

As well as the challenging clinical development, MMP inhibitors for arthritis also face a tough regulatory hurdle to become approved licensed drugs. Although prevention or retardation of structural damage is a recognized goal of new antirheumatoid therapies, there are still questions concerning what this means clinically for the patient. The logical and expected outcome is to maintain joint function, however, assessment of this is dominated initially by the level of inflammation and pain rather than the degree of structural damage. Assessments distinguishing between the loss of function due to joint damage from that due to inflammation have, as yet, not been established, although it has recently been estimated that approximately 25 per cent of disability in RA can be explained by progressive joint damage after the first 5–10 years[74]. Therefore, radiological progression is at most a surrogate for long-term function and studies confirming this relationship are still short of true validation. Consequently, it is likely that regulatory approval of any MMP inhibitor based only on the prevention of structural joint damage will require extensive follow-up investigation to determine its impact on functional outcome.

However, assuming a positive outcome to the ongoing clinical trials and subsequent approval by the regulators then the availability of effective drugs to prevent damage could have a major effect on the way RA patients are treated. Clearly, the best way to prevent damage is to initiate therapy as early after diagnosis as possible, and ideally before any damage has occurred. This would place MMP inhibitors as first line, baseline therapies for RA on top of which anti-inflammatory drugs can then be used to control synovitis. While these therapies can be changed and modified to suit the individual patient, the underlying therapy with the MMP inhibitor should remain constant to maintain protection to the joints. This therapeutic management would require a change in approach to existing treatment regimens and also raises additional issues.

Not least of these is which patients would benefit most from receiving a MMP inhibitor? Given that approximately 20 per cent of patients have little or no structural damage it may be desirable to identify which patients are most likely to progress, and many surrogate markers of future structural joint damage have been proposed. These include markers characteristic of RA, such as rheumatoid factors and genetic susceptibility, as well as elevated acute phase response and possible biochemical markers of cartilage and bone destruction such as fragments of collagen or aggracan[75]. All these still remain as exploratory markers and no definitive relationships between these and radiographic outcome has been established. Until a time where there is available technology to assess certain surrogate markers, together with a therapeutic agent that successfully reduces joint damage, this is likely to remain the case. However, once established it is feasible that in a managed health-care environment, these may be used to target therapy to high-risk patients.

The other issue is that of patient compliance in that patients may have no immediate, perceivable benefits from taking an MMP inhibitor. For instance, it will not address their immediate needs of reduced pain and inflammation. Unless a suitable surrogate marker of structural joint damage becomes not only validated but also widely available, then the only evidence of efficacy will be the lack of radiologically detectable damage. This may be difficult for some patients to accept and therefore patient education will become a critical aspect of the acceptance of these drugs.

Undoubtedly there are still a number of issues and concerns around the development and potential use of MMP inhibitors in arthritic conditions. These are slowly being addressed and the next few years will provide answers or clarifications to many of these. However, until then MMP inhibitors remain one of the most novel of approaches to the treatment of RA and OA which, if successful, has the potential to improve significantly the long-term outcome of these disabling diseases.

References

1. Paulus, H.E., van der Heijde, D.M.F.M., Bulpitt, K.J., and Gold, R.H., Monitoring radiographic changes in early rheumatoid arthritis. *Journal of Rheumatology*, 1996;**23**:801–805.

2. Pincus, T., Long-term outcome in rheumatoid arthritis. *British Journal of Rheumatology*, 1995;**34** (suppl. 2) 59–73.

3. Scott. D.L., Adebajo, A.O., El-Badaway, S., Kirwan, J.R., van de Putte, L.B.A., and van Riel, P.L.C.M. Disease controlling anti-rheumatic therapy: Preventing or significantly decreasing the rate of progression of structural damage. *Journal of Rheumatology,* 1994;Suppl **44**,36–40.

4. Pugner, K.M., Holmes, J.W., Hieke, K., and Scott, D.L., (in preparation). The costs of rheumatoid arthritis: A long-term view.

5. Quam, J.P., Michet, C.J., Wilson, M.G., Ilstrup, D.M., Melton, L.J., and Walrichs, S.L., Total knee arthroplasty: A population-based study. Mayo clinical proceedings, 1991;**66**,589–595.

6. GREES report, Recommendations for the registration of drugs used in the treatment of rheumatiod arthritis. *British Journal of Rheumatology*, 1998;**37**,211–215.

7. Food and Drug Administration, (1998) *Guidance for industry: clinical development programs for drugs, devices and biological products for the treatment of rheumatoid arthritis.* (Draft guidance). FDA, Rockville.

8. van Riel, P.L.C.M., van der Heijde, D.M.F.M., Nuver-Zwart, I.H., and van de Putte, L.B.A. Radiological progression in rheumatoid arthritis: results of 3 comparative trials. *Journal of Rheumatology,* 1995;**22**,1797–1799.

9. Weinblatt, M.E., Trentham, D.E., Fraser, P.A., Holdsworth, D.E., Falchuk, K.R., Weissman, B.N., and Coblyn, J.S. Long-term prospective trial of low dose methotrexate in rheumatoid arthritis. *Arthritis & Rheumatism*, 1998;**31**,167–175.

10. Kremer, J.M., and Lee, J.K. A long-term prospective study of the use of methotrexate in rheumatoid arthritis. *Arthritis & Rheumatism*, 1988;**31**,577–584.

11. Jeurissen, M.E.C., Boerbooms, A.M., van de Putte, L.B.A., Doesburg, W.H., and Lemmens, A.M. Influence of methotrexate and azothiaprine on radiologic progression in rheumatoid arthritis. *Annals of Internal Medicine*, 1991;**114**,999–1004.

12. Kirwan, J.R., The effect of glucocorticoids on joint destruction in rheumatoid arthritis. *New England Journal of Medicine*, 1995;**133**,142–146.

13. Mulherin, D., Fitzgerald, O., and Bresnihan, B., Clinical improvement and radiological deterioration in rheumatoid arthritis: evidence that the pathogenesis of synovial inflammation and articular erosion may differ. *British Journal of Rheumatology*, 1996;**35**,1263–1268.

14. Schiff, M., Kaine, J., Sharp, J., and Strand, V., 1998. X-ray analysis of 12 months treatment of active rheumatoid arthritis with leflunomide compared to placebo or methotrexate. *Arthritis & Rheumatism*, 41,S155(736).

15. Moreland, L.W., Baumgartner, S.W., Schiff, M.H., Tindall, E.A., Fleischmann, R.M., Weaver, A.L., Bulpitt, K.J., Weinblatt, M.E., Keystone, E.C., Ettlinger, R.E., Furst, D., Mease, P., Gruber, B.L., Katz, R.S., Skosey, J.L., Arkfield, D.G., Lies, R.B., Lange, M., Blosch, C.M., and Garrison, L. Optimal dose of the TNF reception p75 fusion protein (TNFR-FC, Enbrel™). *Arthritis & Rheumatism*, 1998;**41**,S59(157).

16. Hardingham, T.E. Biosynthesis, assembly and turnover of cartilage proteoglycans. In:*Research monographs in cell and tissue physiology* (ed. A.M. Glavert) 1998, pp. 41–52.

17. Pettipher, E.R., Higgs, G.A., and Henderson, B., Interleukin-1 induces leukocyte infiltration and cartilage degradation in the synovial joint. *Proceedings of the National Academy of Science*, 1986;**83**,8749–8753.

18. Fell, H.B., Barratt, M.E.J., Welland, H., and Green, R. The capacity of pig articular cartilage in organ culture to regenerate after breakdown induced by complement-sufficient antiserum of pig erthrocytes. *Calcification Tissue Research*, 1976;**20**,3–21.

19. Brikendal-Hansen, H., Moore, W.G.I., Boden, M.K., Windsor, L.J., Birkendal-Hansen, B., Decarlo, A., and Engler, J.A.,Matrix metalloproteinases: a review. *Critical Review of Oral Biology*, 1993;**4**:197–250.

20. Sato, H., Takino, T., and Okada. Y., A matrix metalloprotoenase expressed on the surface of invasive tumour cells. *Nature*, 1994;370,61–65.

21. Krane, S.M., Amento, E.P., Goldring, M.B., Goldring, S.R., and Stephenson, M.L. In: *Research monographs in cell and tissue physiology* (ed A.M. Galvert) 1998, pp.179–195.

22. Nagase, H., Activation mechanisms of matrix metalloproteinases. *Biological Chemistry*, 1997;378,151–160.

23. Murphy, G. Matrix metalloproteinases and their inhibitors. *Acto Orthopedica Scandavia* 1995;(suppl 266), 66:55–60.

24. Woessner, J.F. Jr. Matrix metalloproteinases and their inhibitors in connextive tissue. *FASEB J*, 1991;5:2145–2154.

25. Brinckerhoff, C.E. Joint destruction in arthritis: metalloproteinase in the sportlight. *Arthritis & Rheumatism*, 1991;34,1073–1075.

26. Hiraoka, K., Sasaguri, Y., Komiya, S., Inoue, A., and Morimatsu, M., Cell proliferation-related production of matrix metalloproteinases 1 (Tissue collagenase) and 3 (Stromelysin) by cultured human rheumatoid synovial fibroblasts. *Biochemistry International*, 1992;27,1083–1091.

27. Wooley, D.E., Crossley, M.J., and Evanson, J.M. Collagenase at sites of cartilage erosion in the rheumatoid joint. *Arthritis & Rheumatism*, 1977;20,5625–5628.

28. Hanemaaijer, R., Sorsa, T., Konttinen, Y.T., Ding, Y., Sutinen, M., Visser, H., Van Hinsberg, V.W.M., Helaakoski, T. Kainulainen, T., Ronka, H., Tschesche, H., and Salo, T., Matrix metalloproteinase-8 is expressed in rheumatoid synovial fibroblasts and endothelial cells: Regulation by tumor necrosis factor and doxycycline. *Journal of Biological Chemistry*, 1997;272, 31504–31509.

29. Chubinskaya, S., Huch, K., Mikecz, K., Cs-Szabo, G., Hasty, K.A., Kuettner, K.E., and Cole, A.A. Chondrocyte matrix metalloprotienase-8: up regulation of neutrophil collagenase by interlukin-1 beta in human cartilage from knee and ankle joints. *Laboratory Investigations*, 1996;74, 232–240.

30. Lindy, O., Kottinen, Y.T., Sorsa, T., Ding, Y., Santavirta, S., Ceponis, A., and Lopez-Otin, C. Matrix metalloproteinase 13 (collagenase 3) in human rheumatoid synovium. *Arthritis & Rheumatism*, 1997;40,1391–1399.

31. Stahle-Backdahl, M., Sandstedt, B., Bruce, K., Lindahl, A., Jimenez, M.G., Vega, J.A., and Lopez-Otin, C. Collagenase 3 (MMP-13) is expressed during human fetal ossification and re-expressed in postnatal bone remodelling and in rheumatoid arthritis. *Laboratory Investigations*,1997;76,717–728.

32. Manicourt, D.H., Fujimoto, N., Obata, K., and Thonar, E.J.M. Levels of circulating collagenase, stomelysin-1 and tissue inhibitor of matrix metalloproteinases 1 in patients with rheumatoid arthritis. *Arthritis & Rheumatism*, 995;38,1031–1039.

33. Yoshihara, Y., Obata, K., Fujimoto, N., Yamashita, K., Hayakawa, T., and Shimmei, M. Increased levels of stromelysin-1 and tissue inhibitor of metalloproteinase-1 in sera from patients with rheumatoid arthritis. *Arthritis & Rheumatism*, 1995;38,969–975.

34. Okada, Y., Takeuchi, N., Tomita, K., Nakanishi, I., and Nagase, H. Immunolocalisation of matrix metalloproteinase 3 (stromelysin) in rheumatoid synvioblasts (B cells): correlation with rheumatoid arthritis. *Annals of Rheumatic Diseases*, 1989;48,645–653.

35. Ohta, S., Imai, K., Yamashita, K., Matsumoto, T., Azumano, I., and Okada, Y. Expression of matrix metalloproteinase 7 (matrilysin) in human osteoarthritic cartilage. *Laboratory Investigations*, 1998;78,79–87.

36. Matsumoto, F., Uzuki, M., Kaneko, C., Rikimura, A., Kokubun, S., and Sawai, T. Expression of matrix metalloproteinases (MMPs) and tissue inhibitor of metalloproteinases (TIMPs) in joint tissues of rapidly destructive coxarthropathy (RDC), analyzed by immunohistochemical study. *Ryumachi*, 1997;37,688–95.

37. Gruber, B.L., Sorbi, D., French, D.L., Marchese, M.J., Nuovo, G.J., Kew, R.R., and Arbeit, L.A. Markedly elevated serum MMP-9 (Gelatinase B) levels in rheumatoid arthritis: A potentially useful laboratory marker. *Clinically Immunology and Immunopathology*, 1996;78,161–171.

38. Mudgett, J.S., Hutchinson, N.I., Chartrain, N.A., Forsyth, A.J., McDonnell, J., Singer, I.I., Bayne, E.K., Flanagan, J., Kawaka, D., Shen, C.F., Stevens, K., Chen, H., Trumbauer, M., and Visco, D.M. Susceptibility of stromelysin 1-deficient mice to collagen-induced arthritis and cartilage destruction. *Arthritis & Rheumatism*, 1998;41,110–121.

39. Cunnane, G., Fitzgerald, O., Hummel, K.M., Gay, R.E., Gay, S., and Breshnihan, B. Collagenase, cathepsin B and cathepsin L gene expression in the synovial membrane of patients with early inflammatory arthritis. *Rheumatology*, 1999;38,38–34.

40. Gomis-Ruth, F-X., Maskos, K., Betz, M., Bergner, A., Huber, R., Suzuki, K., Yoshida, N., Nagase, H., Brew, K., Bourenkov, G.P., Bartunik, H., and Bode, W. Mechanism of inhibition of the human matrix metalloproteinase stromelysin-1 by TIMP-1. *Nature*, 1997;389,77–80.

41. Martel-Pelletier, J., Fujimoto, N., Obata, K., Cloutier, J-M., and Pelletier, J-P. The imbalance between the synthesis level of metalloproteinases and TIMPs in osteoarthritic and rheumatoid arthritis cartilage can be enhanced by interlukin-1. *Arthritis & Rheumatism*, 1993;36:S191.

42. Kikuchi, H., Shimade, W., Nonaka, T., Ueshima, S., and Tanaka, S., Significance of serine proteinase and matrix metalloproteinase systems in the destruction of human articular cartilage. *Clinical and Experimental Pharmacology and Physiology*, 1996;23,885–889.

43. Ellis, A.J., Curry, V.A., Powell, E.K., and Cawston, T.E. The prevention of collagen breakdown in bovine nasal cartilage by TIMP, TIMP-2 and a low weight molecular synthetic inhibitor. *Biochemical and Biophysical Research Communications*, 1994;201,94–101.

44. Carmichael, D.F., Stricklin, G.P., and Stuart, J.M. Systemic administration of TIMP in the treatment of collagen-induced arthritis in Mice. *Agents and Actions*, 1989;27,378–9.

45. Wright, J.K., Clark, I.M., Cawston, T.E., and Hazelman, B.L. The secretion of the tissue inhibitor metalloproteinases (TIMP) by human synovial fibroblasts is modulated by all trans-retinoic acid. *Biochemica et Biophysica Acta*, 1991;1133,25–30.

46. Ries, C., and Petrides, P.E. Cytokine regulations of matrix metalloproteinase activity and its regulatory dysfunction in disease. *Biological Chemistry*, 1995;376,345–355.

47. Houssiau, F.A., Devogelaer, J-P., van Damme, J., Nagant de Deuxchaisnes, C., and van Snick, J. Interleukin-6 in synovial fluid and serum of patients with rheumatoid arthritis and other inflammatory arthritis. *Arthritis & Rheumatism*, 1988;31: 784–788.

48. Bottomley, K.M., Johnson, W.H., and Walter, D.S. Matrix metalloproteinase inhibitors in arthritis. *Journal of Enzyme Inhibition*, 1998;13,79–101.

49. Morphy, J.R., Millican, T.A., Porter, J.R. Matrix metalloproteinase inhibitors: current status. *Current Medicinal Chemistry*, 1995;2,743–762.

50. Spitito, S., Doughty, J., O'Byrne, E., Ganu, V., and Goldberg, R.L. Metalloproteinase inhibitors halt collagen breakdown in IL-1 induced bovine nasal cartilage cultures. *Inflammation Research*, 1995;44(Suppl 2),S131–S132.

51. O-Bryne, E.M., Parker, D.T., Roberts, E.D., Goldberg, R.L., MacPherson, L.J., Blancuzzi, V. Wilson, D., Singh, H.N., Ludewig, R., and Ganu, V.S., Oral administration of a matrix metalloproteinase inhibitor, CGS 27023A, protects the cartilage proteoglycan matrix in a partial menisectomy model of osteoarthritis in rabbits. *Inflammation Research*, 1998;44,Suppl 2,S117–S118.

52. Golub, L.M., Lee, H.M., Lehrer, G., Nemiroff, A., McNamara, T.F., Kaplan, R., and Ramamurty, N.S., Minocycline reduces gingival collagenolytic activity during diabetes: preliminary observations and a proposed new mechanism of action. *Journal of Peridontal Research*, 1983;18,516.

53. Golub, L.M., Ramamurthy, N.S., McNamara, T.F., Geenwald, R.A., and Rifkin, B.R. Tetracyclines inhibit connective tissue breakdown: New therapeutic implications for an old family of drugs. *Critical Review of Oral Biological Medicine*, 1991;2,297–322.

54. Ryan, M.E., Greenwald, R.A., and Golub, L.M. Potential of tetracyclines to modify cartilage breakdown in osteoarthritis. *Current Opinion in Rheumatology*, 1995;**8**,238–247.

55. Greenwald, R., Moak, S.A., Ramamurthy, N.S., and Goloub, L.M. Tetracyclines supress matrix metalloproteinase activity in adjuvant arthritis and in combination with fluriprofen, ameliorate bone damage. *Journal of Rheumatology*, 1992;**19**,927–938.

56. Bluhm, G.B., Sharp, J.T., Tilley, B.C., Alarcon, G.S., Cooper, S.M., Pillermer, S.R., Clegg, D.O., Heyse, S.P., Trentham, D.E., Neuner, R., Kaplan, D.A., Leisen, J.C.C., Bukley, L., Duncan, H., Tuttleman, M., Li, S., and Fowler, S.E. Radiographic results from the minocycline in rheumatoid arthritis (MIRA) trial. *Journal of Rheumatology*, 1997;**24**,1295–1302.

57. Nordstorm, D., Lindy, O., Lauhio, A., Sorsa, T., Santavirta, S., and Konttinen, Y.T. Anti-collagenolytic mechanism of aciton of doxycycline treatment in rheumatoid arthritis. *Rheumatology International*, 1998;**17**,175–180.

58. Lindy, O., Kottinen, Y.T., Sorsa, T., Ding, Y., Santavirta, S., Ceponis, A., and Lopez-Otin, C. Matrix metalloproteinase 13 (collagenase 3) in human rheumatoid synovium. *Arthritis & Rheumatism*, 1997;**40**,1391–1399.

59. Rediske, J., Koehne, C., Melton, R., and Ganu, V. OA-affected human cartilage slices spontaneously secrete stromelysin–1 (MMPs), collagenase I (MMP1) and collagenase 3 (MMP13). *Arthritis & Rheumatism*, 1998;**41**,S300 (1604).

60. Chau, T., Jolly, G., Plym, M-J., McHugh, M., Bortolon, E., Wakefield, J., Gianpaolo-Ostravage, C., and Maniglia C. Inhibition of articular cartilage degradation in dog and guinea-pig models of osteoarthritis by the stromelysin inhibitor, BAY 12-9566. *Arthritis & Rheumatism*, 1998;**41**,S300 (1605).

61. Sunndaresan, P.R., Shah, A., and Heller, A.H. Penetration of Bay-12-9566 in synovial fluid and effect of age and gender on the pharmacokinetics of Bay-12-9566. *Annual Meeting of the American Society of Clinical Pharmacology*, 1998I–129.

62. Lollini, L., Haller, J., Eugui, E.M., Womble, S.W., Martin, R., Campbell, J., Hendricks, T., Broka, C., Moskowitz, R., van Wart, H., and Caulfield, J., Disease modification by RS-130830, a collagenase-3 selective inhibitor, in experimental osteoarthritis (OA). *Arthritis & Rheumatism*, 1997;**40**, S87 (341).

63. Lewis, E.J., Bishop, J., Bottomley, K.M.K., Bradshaw, D., Brewster, M., Broadhurst, M.J., Brown, P.A., Budd, J.M., Elliot, L., Greenham, A.K., Johnson, W.H., Nixon, J.S., Rose, F., Sutton, B., and Wilson, K., Ro 32-3555, on orally active collagenase inhibitor, prevents cartilage breakdown in vitro and in vivo. *British Journal of Pharmacology*, 1997;**121**,540–546.

64. Brewster, M., Lewis, E.J., Wilson, K.L., Greenham, A.K., and Bottomley, K.M.K. Ro-32-3555, an orally active collagenase selective inhibitor, prevents structural damage in te4h STR/ORT mouse model of osteoarthritis. *Arthritis & Rheumatism*, 1998;**41**, 1639–1644.

65. Wood, N.D., Aitken, M., Harris, S., Kitchener, S., McClelland, G.R., and Sharp, S., The tolerability and pharmacokinetics of the cartilage protective agent (Ro32-3555) in healthy make volunteers. *British Journal of Clinical Pharmacology*, 1996;**42**, 676–77.

66. Rasmussen, H.S., and McCann, P.P. Matrix metalloproteinase inhibition as a novel anticancer strategy: a review with special focus on batimastat and marimastat. *Pharmacology and Therapeutics*, 1997;**75**,69–75.

67. Nemunaitis, J., Poole, C., Primrose, J., Rosemurgy, A., Malfetano, J., Brown, P., Berrington. A., Cornish, A., Lynch, K., Rasmussen, H., Kerr, D., Cox, D., and Millar, A. Combined analysis of studies of the effects of the matrix metalloproteinase inhibitor marimastat on serum tumor markers in advanced cancer: selection of a biologically active and tolerable dose for longer-term studies. *Clinical Cancer Research*, 1998;**4**,1101–1109.

68. Peterfy, C.G., Dion, E., Miaux, Y., White, D., Jiang, Y., Lu, Y., Zaim, S., Sack, K., Stevens, M., Fye, K., Stevens, R., van der Auwera, P., and Genant, H. Comparison of MRI and X-ray for monitoring erosive changes in rheumatoid arthritis. *Arthritis & Rheumatism*, 1998;**41**,S51 (109).

69. Martel-Pelletier, J., and Pelletier J-P. Wanted-The collagenase responsible for the destruction of the collagen network in human cartilage. *British Journal of Rheumatology*, 1996;**35**, 818–819.

70. Baumgartner, S., Moreland, L.W., Schiff, M.H., Tindall, E., Fleischmann, R.M., Weaver, A., Ettinger, R.E., Gruber, B.L., Kaltz, R.S., Skosey, J.L., Lies, R.B., Robison, A., and Biosch, C.M. Double-blind placebo controlled trial of tumor necrosis factor receptor (p80) fusion protein (TNFR-Fc) in active arthritis. *Arthritis & Rheumatism*, 1996;**39**,S74 (283).

71. Gearing, A.J.H., Beckett, P., Christodoulou, M., Churchill, M., Clements, J., Crimmin, M., Davidson, A.H., Drummond, A.H., Galloway, W.A., Gilbert, R., Gordon, J.L., Leber, T.M., Mangan, M., Miller, K., Nayee, P., Owen, K. Patel, S., Thomas, W., Wells, G., Wood, L.M., and Woolley, K., Processing of tumour necrosis factor-α precursor by metalloproteinases. *Nature*, 1994;**370**,555–561.

72. Moss, M.L., Jin, S.L., Milla, M.E., Burkhart, W., Carter, H.L., Chen, W.J., Clay, W.C., Didsbury, J.R., Hassler, D., Hoffman, C.R., Kost, T.A., Lambert, M.H., Leesnitzer, M.A., McCauley, P., McGeehan, G., Mitchell, J., Moyer, M., Pahel, G., Rocque, W., Overton, L.K., Schoenen, F., Seaton, T., Su, J.L., Warner, J., and Becherer, J.D. Cloning of a disintegrin metalloproteinase that processes precursor tumour-necrosis factor-α. *Nature*, 1997;**385**,733–736.

73. DiMartino, M., Wolff, C., High, W., Stroup, G., Hoffman, S., Laydon, J., Lee, J.C., Bertolini, D., Galloway, W.A., Crimmin, M.J., Davis, M., and Davies, S. Anti-arthritic activity of hydroxamic acid based pseudopeptide inhibitors of matrix metalloproteinases and TNFα processing. *Inflammatory Research*, 1997;**46**, 211–215.

74. Scott, D.L., Pugner, K., Kaarela, K., Holmes, J., and Hieke, K., (in press). The link between joint damage and the long-term consequences of rheumatoid arthritis.

75. Wollheim, F.A. Predictors of joint damage in rheumatoid arthritis. *APMIS*, 1996;**104**,81–93.

44 | *Small molecule inhibitors of signal transduction*

Anthony M. Manning

Inflamed tissues invariably contain many activated cells, including T and B cells, monocyte/macrophages, fibroblasts, and endothelium[1]. These activated cells are characterized by elevated expression of many genes encoding inflammatory molecules, including cytokines, growth factors, cell adhesion molecules, and degradative enzymes. Indeed, altered expression of a variety of proinflammatory genes appears fundamental to the etiology of inflammatory disease. Over-expression of inflammatory cytokines is thought to be consequential to most inflammatory disease. In rheumatoid arthritis (RA), for example, elevated mRNAs for IL-1α, IL-1β, IL-6, IL-8, IL-10, GM-CSF, G-CSF, M-CSF, TNF-α, EGF, PDGF, and TGF-β are detected in synovial cells or fluid from RA patients[2]. TNF-α and IL-1, in particular, appear to play a key role in RA disease progression, and in other inflammatory conditions[3]. In the RA joint, both cytokines stimulate leukocyte recruitment, osteoclast activation, cartilage degradation, synovial cell and fibroblast proliferation, and the enhanced production of inflammatory mediators from a large number of difference cell types. Antagonism of these cytokines using either antibodies, soluble receptors or receptor antagonists results in clinical improvement[4,5], providing further validation for their pivotal role in joint inflammation.

In response to tissue injury or infection, resident tissue cells such as mast cells or tissue macrophages release cytokines capable of activating the transcription of genes encoding endothelial cell adhesion molecules, including P-selectin, E-selectin, vascular cell adhesion molecule-1 (VCAM-1), and intercellular adhesion molecule-1 (ICAM-1)[6]. Endothelial cell adhesion molecules play a key role in inflammation through their ability to enhance recruitment of blood leukocytes to inflamed tissues. In the RA joint, there is elevated expression of E-selectin, VCAM-1, and ICAM-1[7], correlating with enhanced recruitment of blood leukocytes and the perpetuation of chronic joint inflammation[8]. Antagonism of ICAM-1 function using monoclonal antibodies results in clinical improvement in RA[9]. In Crohn's disease, a form of inflammatory bowel disease, antisense inhibitor of ICAM-1 production results in clinical improvement and a reduction in the need for glucocorticoid therapy[10], again confirming the critical role of adhesion molecules in inflammation. In RA joints, treatment with monoclonal antibody to TNF-α decreased adhesion molecule expression, T cell infiltration, and joint inflammation, thus demonstrating a link between this proinflammatory cytokine, adhesion molecule expression, and RA[11]. Such findings reinforce the integrated nature of inflammatory processes, and suggest the possibility for

development of disease-modifying agents which act at points critical to inflammatory gene expression.

Leukotriene synthetic enzymes and other metabolic enzymes, including cyclooxygenase 2 (COX2) and inducible nitric oxide synthase (iNOS), are responsible for the enhanced production of inflammatory mediators at sites of inflammation (reviewed in Ref. 12). Transcriptional activity of the genes encoding these enzymes is also elevated in inflamed tissues[13]. In many inflammatory diseases, specific matrix degrading enzymes, such as stromelysin or collagenase, or protein-degrading enzymes such as tryptase, are also over-expressed and contribute to irreversible joint and tissue destruction[14].

New technologies for the large-scale analysis of gene expression in cultured cells and tissue samples have highlighted the dramatic changes in gene transcription which occur during the initiation and progression of inflammatory disease. Using cDNA microarray analysis[15] the relative expression of 96 genes, including cytokines, chemokines, growth factors, cell adhesion molecules, matrix degrading enzymes, and transcription factors, was determined in cultured macrophages, synoviocytes, and chondrocytes, and in biopsies from rheumatoid arthritis and inflammatory bowel disease patients[16]. Enhanced transcription of many of these genes was revealed, and differences between RA and inflammatory bowel disease samples were noted. Such analyses support and extend earlier reports of up-regulation of inflammatory gene transcription at sites of inflammation.

Because the products of multiple genes contribute to tissue destruction indicative of inflammatory disease, altered gene transcription must be considered as a fundamental process promoting the etiology of these diseases. Several classes of agents with well-established clinical utility, including corticosteroids, cyclosporin A and gold, are known to mediate their anti-inflammatory effects through modulating gene transcription. These agents, discovered through serendipity, exhibit a number of undesirable side-effects primarily due to the cellular processes they inhibit, Molecular definition of the mechanisms by which specific genes are turned on or off offers the opportunity for the discovery of novel agents with enhanced efficacy and reduced side-effects.

A rational approach to the discovery of gene-regulating drugs has resulted from an enhanced understanding of specific mechanism regulating inflammatory gene transcription (Fig. 44.1)[17]. In particular, four transcription factor families — AP-1/ATF2, NF-κB, NFAT and STAT—are likely to be critical regulators of inflammatory gene expression. The activity of at least three of

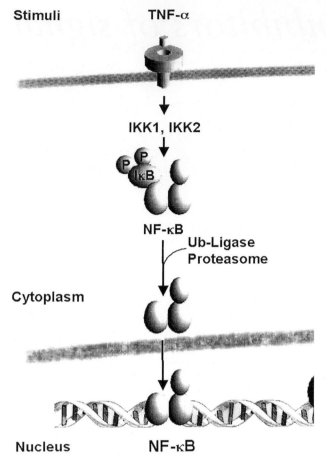

Fig. 44.1 Diversity of signal transduction pathways regulating inflammatory gene expression.

these transcription factors is regulated, directly or indirectly, by mitogen-activated protein kinase (MAP kinase) pathways, which are discussed below. The following sections discuss the relevant pathways and novel inhibitors that have merged as a consequence of using these transcription factors and their upstream activators as targets for the discovery of novel anti-inflammatory drugs. Glucocorticoids (GCs), cyclosporin A (CsA), and FK506 serve as key examples of established therapeutics which act to inhibit signal transduction and gene transcription in inflammatory cells. These mechanism of action of these compounds is described below.

Glucocorticoids

Glucocorticoids (GCs) have and continue to be the most effective therapeutics available for the clinical suppression of the immune response and the process of inflammation[18]. The molecular mechanisms which underlie the clinical efficacy of GCs have, until recently, been poorly understood. Many hormones, including corticosteroids, estrogen, androgen, vitamin D and progesterone, modulate gene expression through direct binding to a large family of specific intracellular receptors belonging to the steroid hormone receptor supergene family[19]. These receptors act as transcription factors (TFs), binding specific steroid

response elements (SREs) within the promoters of a wide range of genes. Over a hundred members of the steroid/thyroid hormone receptor family have been cloned, comprising the largest family of TFs known[20]. Ligand binding of these receptors induces nuclear translocation, DNA binding, and the transcription of a range of hormone-responsive genes. GCs bind to an intracellular GC receptor GR), promoting nuclear translocation and binding to GC-response elements (GRE) in the promoters of genes. However, in some settings, these TFs can actually repress gene expression. GCs suppress inflammation through their ability to repress the expression of multiple inflammatory genes, including cytokines and cell adhesion molecules, and genes responsible for the generation of inflammatory mediators such as prostaglandin H2, thromboxanes, and leukotrienes. Cell adhesion molecule and cytokine gene expression is repressed by GCs even though these genes lack GREs. The suppression of expression of these genes by GCs is now known to function through interference of the GR with the activity of key transcription factors such as NF-κB, AP-1, NFATp, and C/EBP[21].

NF-κB represents a key regulator of genes central to the inflammatory response[22–24]. GCs inhibit activation of NF-κB both *in vitro* and *in vivo* through transcriptional activation of the IκB-α gene[25,26]. GC inhibition of NF-κB activation could account for many of its anti-inflammatory properties. AP-1 is another TF required for transcription of inflammatory cytokines, matrix metalloproteinases, and genes associated with abnormal cell proliferation[27]. GCs inhibit AP-1 activity through physical interference of the GR with the Fos and Jun subunits of AP-1 (reviewed in Ref. 22). These actions of GCs have revealed the key role of NF-κB and AP-1 in the inflammatory and immune response. Key components of the NF-κB and AP-1 signal transduction pathways have been identified and cloned, and represent attractive targets for the development of a new class of anti-inflammatory agents with the efficacy of steriods, but without the hormonal properties associated with the GR. These components include receptor-associated adaptor proteins, protein kinases, and members of the MAPK family of signal transduction enzymes[28,29].

The pharmaceutical industry has focused significant attention over the past two decades on the empirical discovery of synthetic glucocorticoids that retain their anti-inflammatory properties but not their hormonal side-effects, most notably enhanced bone loss. With the definition of the AP-1 and NF-κB-inhibitory activities associated with GC efficacy, efforts have been renewed to identity synthetic GCs with AP-1 and NF-κB transrepression activity but without activity in classical GRE-mediated transcription assays. Studies of GR structure and function are providing insights for the design sequences of improved GCs[30]. Recognition of GRE sequences in gene promoters is determined by discrete sequences present in the zinc finger region of the GR and by homodimer formation of the receptor. The exact nature of the dimers formed determines the specificity of promoter element binding. Binding of specific ligands to the GR and other members of the nuclear hormone receptor superfamily determines dimerization by recruiting specific regions in the ligand binding domains of each receptor type. In the case of the GR, transcriptional activation is mediated by homodimers, and chiefly requires a region in the second zinc finger of the receptor

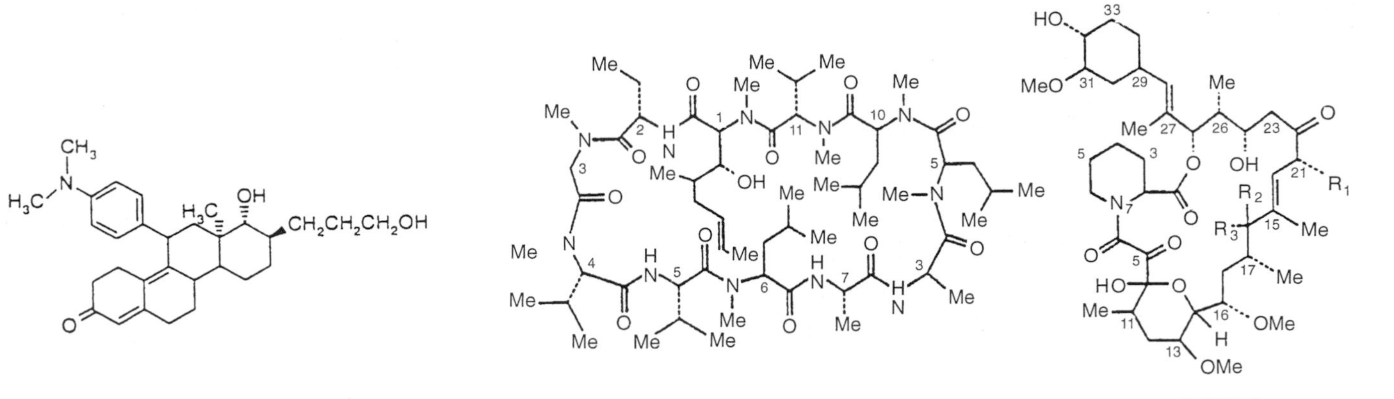

Fig. 44.2 Compound structures for ZD26489, an AP-1 selective glucocorticoid, CsA, and FK506.

known as the D-loop. The domains of the GR required for transrepression of AP-1 have not been completely mapped; however, deletion mutants of the GR have allowed the assignment of the N-terminal amino acid sequence between positions 272 and 400, the DNA and ligand binding domains as essential components for the repression. In the case of AP-1, sequences comprising the bZip region appear critical for interaction with the GR. Of note, transrepression of AP-1 activity occurs at lower hormone concentrations than that required to activate transcription from the GRE, which may indicate that AP-1 repression is mediated by GR monomers in contrast to an absolute requirement for dimers. Mutations in the dimerization interaction loop, which inhibit dimer formation, prevent the activation of the GRE, but still retain the ability to fully repress AP-1 activity. Several examples of ligands (Fig. 44.2) which can selectively repress AP-1 activity without activating the GRE have been reported[31], and these and other agents may show promise as therapeutic agents with improved side-effect profiles.

CsA and FK506

The immunosuppressive agents cyclosporin A (CsA) and FK506 (Fig. 44.2) have established organ transplantation as a viable medical alternative for patients facing imminent organ failure. These agents effectively inhibit T cell activation and proliferation, a process central to immune function. The identification of the intracellular targets of these drugs in T cells revealed that these agents modulate T-cell receptor signal transduction and immune gene expression. An early and critical step in T cell activation is the induction of expression of the cytokine interleukin-2 (IL-2) gene. Engagement of the T cell receptor by antigen-MHC complex activates a signal transduction cascade involving early CA^{2+} influx. Increase in intracellular Ca^{2+} leads to the activation of calcineurin, a Ca^{2+}/calmodulin-dependent Ser/Thr phosphatase. Activated calcineurin dephosphorylates a subunit (NFATp) of the nuclear factor in activated T cells, NFAT[32,33]. Dephosphorylation of NFATp results in its translocation to the nucleus, where it forms a transcriptional activation complex

with the AP-1 subunits Fos and Jun, and thereby activating IL-2 transcription. Activated NFAT has also implicated in the inducible expression of a growing number of inflammatory genese, inlcuding IL-2, IL-3, IL-4, IL-5, IL-8, IL-13, GM-CSF, interferon γ, and TNF-α[34]. CsA and FK506 inhibit IL-2 production in activated T cells by inactivating calcineurin[35]. Their immediate target proteins, termed immunophilins, are cyclophilins A and B[36,37]. The immunophilins display cis-trans peptidyl-isomerase activities, and binding of CsA or FK506 results in the interaction of these complexes with calcineurin and inhibition of its activity. In patients with early RA, low-dose CsA is as effective as traditional DMARDs in controlling clinical symptoms, decreasing the rate of further joint damage in previously involved joints as well as the rate of new joint involvement[38]. However, the toxicity of CsA and FK506, which arises from their ability to inhibit calcineurin in cells outside the immune system, has limited their clinical utility[39]. Pharmacologic agents that target NFAT independent of calcineurin might lack the toxicity of CsA and FK506 whilst retaining their antirheumatic activity. In this regard, T cell receptor (TCR) crosslinking leads to the activation of tyrosine kinases, including Lck and ZAP-70, and the tyrosine phosphorylation of multiple intracellular substrates including Vav[40]. These kinases appear to be components of the NFAT activation pathway emanating from TCR activation, and as such represent potential targets for novel NFAT inhibitors. Drugs discovery efforts targeting these kinases have been initiated, but no reports of selective inhibitors have appeared to date. Additional downstream kinases involved in regulating NFAT activity have been identified[41], however, their molecular identity is as yet unknown.

MAP kinase inhibitors

Activator protein-1 (AP-1) is a pivotal transcription factor which regulates T-cell activation, cytokine production, and production of matrix metalloproteinases[42]. AP-1 includes members of Jun and Fos families of transcription factors, which are characterized by basic region-leucine zipper (bZIP) DNA-binding

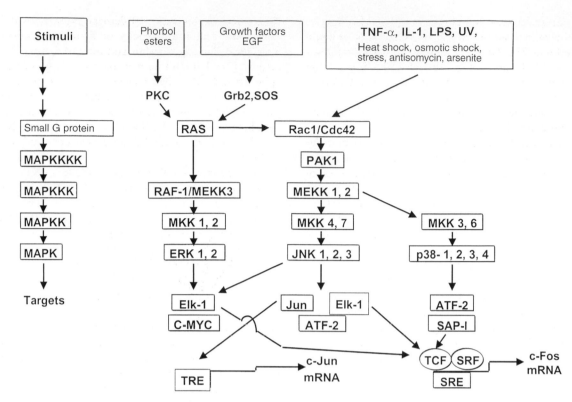

Fig. 44.3   MAP kinase regulation of AP-1. Extracellular stimuli activate the ERK, JNK, and p38 MAPK pathways through Ras and Rac-mediated processes. The ERK, JNK, and p38 MAPKs phosphorylate the Elk-1 and SAP-1a transcription factors, resulting in enhanced c-Jun and c-Fos transcription and protein production. In addition, JNK 1, 2, and 3 phosphorylate the Jun subunit of AP-1 and directly enhance AP-1 transactivating potential.

domains. AP-1 proteins bind to DNA and activate transcription as Jun homodimers, Jun–Jun heterodimers, or Jun–Fos heterodimers. There are multiple Jun and Fos family members (c-Jun, JunB, JunD and c-Fos, FosB, Fra-1, Fra-2) which are expressed in different cell types and mediate the transcription of both unique and overlapping genes. AP-1 is also a component of the nuclear factor of activated T cells (NFAT) complex responsible for the transcription of the IL-2 gene and other cytokine genes in activated t Cells[43].

MAP Kinase (MAPK) pathways regulate the transcriptional activity of AP-1, both at the level of *de novo* synthesis of AP-1 family proteins and by controlling their transactivation function (Fig. 44.3)[44,45]. MAPK cascades consists of three- or four-tiered signaling modules in which the MAPK is activated by a MAP kinase kinase (MAPKK), which in turn is activated by a MAP kinase kinase kinase (MAPKKK) (Fig. 44.1). The MAPKKK is itself activated by a small G protein such as Ras, either directly or via another upstream kinase[46]. Three such MAPK signaling cascades, culminating in activation of the ERK, JNK and, p38 MAP families of MAPK have been investigated in detail. The JNKs and p38 kinases area activated in response to the proinflammatory cytokines TNF-α and IL-1, and by cellular stress (e.g. heat shock, osmotic shock, reactive oxygen metabolites, protein synthesis inhibitors, UV irradiation). The MAPKs are proline-directed serine/threonine kinases, which are activated by phosphorylation on closely-spaced threonine and tyrosine residues within the activation loop; the activation sequences characteristic of the ERK, JNK, and p38 MAP kinase families

are TEY, TPY, and TGY, respectively. These sequences are targets for phosphyrolation by specific MAPKKs, dual specificity threonine/tyrosine kinases which are themselves activated by MAPKKK-mediated phosphorylation at a pair of serine residues in the activation loop.

While there is some crosstalk between the major MAPK pathways, cells maintain exquisite specificity with extracellular signals only activating their proper targets. This is a result of several factors that include preferred interactions between kinases within a module and between MAPKs and their substrates[47]. Recently, scaffold proteins that bind multiple components of the signaling cascade have been described. For example, JIP-1 (JNK-interacting protein-1) first characterized as a cytoplasmic inhibitor of the JNK pathway has been shown to selectively bind the MAPK module, MLK*arMKK7*arJNK[48]. It has no binding affinity for a variety of other MAPK cascade enzymes. Different scaffold proteins are likely to exist for other MAPK signaling cascades to preserve substrate specificity. Many of the studies that have reported cross-talks between the different pathways have employed over-expression of members of the signaling cascades. This often leads to the erroneous conclusion that no fidelity exists between the cascades.

All three MAPK pathways are involved in the transcription regulation of Fos- and Jun- family genes. The ERKs, JNKs, and p38 MAPKs each contribute to upregulation of c-Fos gene transcription, by phosphorylating and activating the Ets-family transcription factors Elk-1 and SAP-1[49]. A major component of AP-1 regulation is a consequence of post-translational modification; for example, c-Jun is regulated by phosphorylation at two N-terminal serines in the transactivation domain (amino acids 63 and 73). This is accomplished by the c-Jun N-terminal kinases JNK1 and JNK2, although JNK2 binds c-Jun with 10-fold higher affinity than JNK1 and may be the physiologically relevant activator of AP-1[47].

The JNKs are encoded by three genes: *JNK1, JNK2,* and *JNK3*. JNK1 and 2 are ubiquitously expressed whereas *JNK3* is selectively expressed in the brain, heart, and testis. Gene transcripts are alternatively spliced to produce four-JNK1 isoforms, four-JNK2 isoforms, and two-JNK3 isoforms. Inhibitors of JNK-mediated AP-1 activation may prove to be novel anti-inflammatory/immunosuppressive agents that will inhibit inducible expression of inflammatory genes, without affecting AP-1 mediated housekeeping functions. In T cells JNK activation by costimulation through the antigen and CD28 receptors correlates with IL-2 induction[50]. Recently, the examination of JNK-deficient mice revealed that the JNK pathway is induced in Th1 cells (producers of IFN-γ and TNF-β) but not in Th2 effector cells (producers of IL-4, IL-5, IL-6, IL-10, and IL-13) upon antigen stimulation[51]. Deletion of either *JNK1* or *JNK2* in mice resulted in a selective defect in the ability of Th1 effector cells to express IFNγ. This suggests that JNK1 and JNK2 do not have redundant functions in T cells and that they play different roles in the control of cell growth, differentiation, and death. Mice with homozygous disruption of the *JNK3* gene are viable[52]. However, they are resistant to the excitotoxic stress response elicited by kainic acid, a glutamate receptor agonist.

Kainic acid causes neuronal damage especially within the hippocampus. The neurotoxicity of kainic acid possibly results from the induction of c-Jun and increased AP-1 DNA binding activity. JNK3 inhibitors may be potentially useful in treating epilepsy and other neurodegenerative disease such as stoke. Recently, the X-ray crystal structure of the unphosphorylated form of JNK3 was reported and should provide assistance in designing selective JNK3 inhibitors[53]. JNK3 reveals similarities to the structure of cAMP-dependent protein kinase and ERK2 and p38.

PD98059 (Fig. 44.4) was discovered in a biochemical screen of inhibitors of the ERK cascade[54]. PD98059 binds to the inactive form of MEK1, a primary MAPKK in the ERK cascade and blocks the phosphorylation required for MEK activation. Specificity of action was indicated by the inability of PD098059 to inhibit phosphorylation mediated by c-Raf, JNK, p38, PKA, PKC, v-Src, active MEK1, and several other serine/threonine and protein tyrosine kinases (including receptor tyrosin kinases). U0126 is another MEK inhibitor that was discovered in a cell-based screen for compounds which inhibited the activity of an AP-1 driven luciferase promoter–reporter construct[55]. U0126 has potent *in vitro* activity and blocks T cell activation and proliferation in response to Con A or CD3 stimulation. In addition, this inhibitor demonstrated potent *in vivo* efficacy in models of inflammation and delayed type hypersensitivity. Of note, competition studies with radiolabelled compounds demonstrated that PD98059 and U0126 compete for a similar site on MEK that is distinct from the ATP or peptide substrate binding sites. Ro

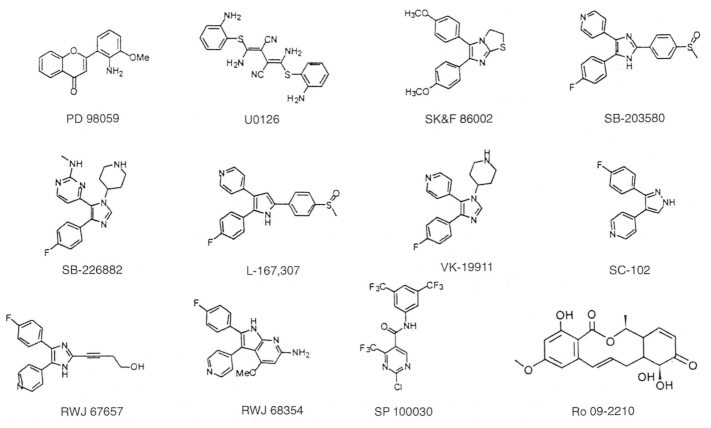

Fig. 44.4 Selected inhibitors of MAP kinases affecting AP-1.

09-2210, another inhibitor of MEK1, was reported recently[56]. This compound was identified during high throughput screening of microbial broths for inhibitors of anti-CD3 induced T cell proliferation. Ro 09-2210 is a potent inhibitor of MEK1 (IC50 = 59 nM) and appears to function through a mechanism distinct from that of PD98059 and U0126.

While no specific JNK inhibitors have been described, isoform-specific inhibitors are being sought. The greatest attention and most progress has been made in the discovery of p38 MAPK inhibitors[57]. The important role of the p38 pathway in inflammatory processes resulted from studies using a series of pyridinyl imidazoles, exemplified by SK&F 86002 and SB203580[58]. These potent inhibitors of p38 activity block IL-1 and TNF production in lipopolysacharide-stimulated human monocytes. SB203580 competes with ATP for binding to p38 and is remarkably selective[59]. It does inhibit JNK2 but with a 10–20 fold lower potency than p38. SB 203580 binds p38 by inserting into the ATP-binding pocket. While the 4-fluorophenyl ring of the compound does not make contact with residues in the ATP-binding pocket it is in near proximity to the Thr 106 of the enzyme. Mutation of this amino acid to Met 106 makes p38 insensitive to SB 203580[60]. Thr 106 is conserved in p38β, another isoform of p38, that is sensitive to SB 203580, but is replaced by methionine in p38γ, p38δ, JNK1, and JNK2 (all

much less sensitive to SB 203580). Mutation of p38β Thr106 to Met 106 rendered p38β almost resistant to SB 203580 and the reverse mutation of Met 106 to Thr106 in p38γ and p38δ resulted in SB 203580 sensitivity.

Some of the earlier p38 inhibitors, including SB 203580, are inhibitory towards several cytochrome p450 isoforms (1A2, 2C9, 2C19, 3A4, 2D6). This is due to the high-affinity binding of the 4-pyridyl group of heme iron. As a consequence, replacements for the 4-pyridyl ring were sought and the pyrimidine analog as represented by SB 226882 has equivalent p38 inhibitory potency *in vitro* and is effective in *in vivo* mouse models measuring circulating TNF levels. Several other p38 inhibitors have been reported including L-167,307[61], VK 19911[62], and SC-102 RWJ 67657 and RWJ 68354[63].

NF-κB pathways

Nuclear factor-κB (NF-κB) was first described as a B-cell-specific factor which bound to a short DNA sequence motif located in the immunoglobulin κ light chain enhancer, but it is now clear that NF-κB is expressed in all cell types and plays a broader role in gene transcription[64–66]. NF-κB plays a key role in the expres-

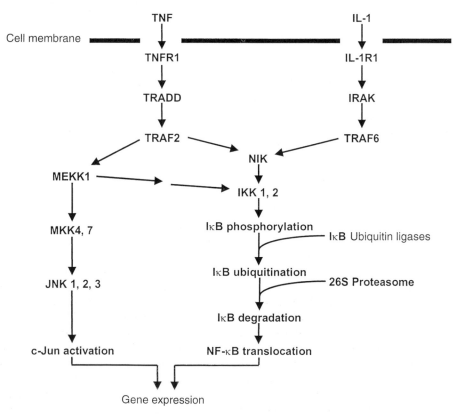

Fig. 44.5 Signal transduction pathway regulating NF-κB activation by TNF-a and IL-1. Activation of the TNF receptor type 1 (TNFR1) leads to recruitment of the TNF-receptor-associated proteins TRADD and TRAF2, resulting in activation of the MAPK kinase kinases MEKK1 and NIK. Both these kinases have been implicated in the activation of the IκB kinases IKK1 and IKK2. NIK is also activated by IL-1 through the IL-1 receptor-associated kinase IRAK and TRAF6. Phosphorylation of the cytoplasmic inhibitor of NF-κB, IκB, leads to its ubiquitination and protelytic degradation by components of the ubiquitin-proteasome system. Free NF-κB within the cytoplasm is rapidly translocated to the nucleus where it modulates gene transcription.

sion of an many as 70 genes central to the inflammatory response and has been detected in a variety of inflammatory settings *in vivo* including in atherosclerotic and restenotic lesions, in septicemia in humans, in rheumatoid synovium, and in UV-damaged skin. NF-κB exists in the cytoplasm in an inactive form associated with inhibitory proteins termed IκB, of which the most important may be IκBα, IκBβ, and IκB*ye. Activation is achieved through the signal-induced proteolytic degradation of IκB in the cytoplasm (Fig. 44.5).

Extracellular stimuli initiate a signaling cascade leading to activation of two IκB kinases, IKK-1 (IKKα) and IKK-2 (IKKβ), which phosphorylate IκB as specific N-terminal serine residues (S32 and S36 for IκBα, S19 and S23 for IκBβ) (Fig. 44.4)[67–71]. Phosphorylated IκB is then selectively ubiquinated, by an E3 ubiquitin ligase, the terminal member of a cascade of ubiquitin-conjugating enzymes. In the last step of this signaling cascade, phosphorylated and ubiquinated IκB, which is still associated with NK-κB in the cytoplasm, is selectively degraded by the 26S proteasome[72]. This process exposes the nuclear localization sequence (NLS), thereby freeing NF-κB to interact with the nuclear import machinery and translocate the nucleus, where it binds its target to initiate transcription.

The IκB kinases IKK-1 and IKK-2 are related members of a new family of intracellular signal transduction enzymes, containing an amino-terminal kinase domain and a C-terminal region with two protein interaction motifs, a leucine zipper and a helix–loop motif. There is strong evidence that IKK-1 and IKK-2 are themselves phosphorylated and activated by one or more upstream activating kinases, which are likely to be members of the MAPKKK family of enzymes. NF-κB inducing kinase (NIK) was identified by its ability to bind directly to TRAF2, an adapter protein thought to couple both TNF-α and IL-1 receptors to NF-κB[73]. A second MAPKKK, MEKK-1, was shown to be present in the IKK signalsome complex[70,74].

Recently, the pIκBα-ubiquitin ligase was isolated from HeLa cells, through its specific association with the pIκBα/NF-κB complex[75]. The small polypeptide ubiquitin is transferred to specific proteins via a cascade of ligases that catalyze covalent attachment of ubiquitin to proteins. It appears there are only a small number of E1 ubiquitin ligases, and that specificity of ubiquitin transfer is mediated, in large part, by specific combinations of E2 and E3 ubiquitin ligases. In some cases, the E3 ligase does not directly transfer ubiquitin, but simply acts to mediate interaction of a specific protein substrate with an E2 ligase charged with ubiquitin. We initially purified an activity capable of specifically phosphorylating IκB in the presence of purified E1 and partially-purified E3 ligases from HeLa cells. This protein was identified as Ubc5c, an E2 ubiquitin ligase. The exquisite specificity of this system was demonstrated by the inability of Ubc5b, a related family member with approximately 90 per cent sequence identity to Ubc5c, to reconstitute IκB ubiquitination *in vitro*. Using recombinant NF-κB:IκB complexes, we purified two proteins which specifically bound when IκB was phosphorylated by IKK2. Nanoelectrospray mass spectrometry identified these polypeptides as two versions of the same protein and belonging to the recently-identified β-TrCP/Slimb family. These proteins contain F box and WD domains, known to be involved in protein:protein interactions.

The IκB-specific F box/WD protein bound specifically to pIκBα and promoted its ubiquitination in the presence of an E1 and Ubc5c, the IκB-specific E2 ubiquitin ligase. We therefore designated this IκB E3 ligase the E3 receptor subunit specific for IκBα, or E3RS^{I}κB. A truncated version of this protein, containing only the F box IκB recognition motif, acted as a dominant negative molecule, inhibiting IκBα degradation and NF-κB activation in HeLa cells.

In addition to the IKKs and IαB ubiquitin ligase, there are additional kinase targets associated with the upstream activation of NF-κB[76]. Receptor–interacting protein (RIP) is a part of the TNF-receptor (TNF-R1) associated signaling complex along with TRADD and TRAF2. RIP is serine/threonine kinase and the only component of the TNF-R1 signaling complex with enzymatic activity. However, no substrates have been identified for RIP. Analogous signaling components exist for the IL-1 receptor, they include IRAK, which is also a serine/threonine kinase that is autophosphorylated upon receptor activation. IRAK associates with TRAF6 to activate NF-κB; however, recombinant IRAK has not kinase activity. IKK-1 and IKK-2, their upstream activating kinases MEKK, and NIK, and their downstream effector, the E3 ligase, all represent attractive targets for the discovery of drugs which selectively regulate NF-κB function.

NF-κB inhibitors

There are multiple targets that are amenable to small molecular blockade within the NF-κB activation pathway. No specific inhibitors of the enzymes mentioned above have been described. Two excellent reviews have summarized the effects and (where known) the mechanism of action of many compounds reported to inhibit the activation or function of NF-κB[77,78]. Here we focus on three classes of NF-κB inhibitory compounds: proteasome inhibitors, antioxidants, and dual NF-κB-AP-1 inhibitors with specificity for T cells.

As detailed in the previous section, IκB degradation is mediated by the 26S proteasome, the organelle thought to be responsible foro the degradation of abnormal and denatured proteins in the cytoplasm. The 20S proteasome is a large multi-catalytic protease complex that forms the core of the 26S proteasome. The 20S proteasome was identified as the specific cellular target of lactacystin, a steptomyces metabolite that inhibits cell cycle progression and promotes neurite outgrowth in a murine neuroblastoma cell line[79,80]. Proteasome inhibitors such as lactacystin, MG132, and MG341 (Fig. 44.6) have been shown to inhibit NF-κB activation[81,82], and a subset of these (lactacystin, MG341) have been shown to inhibit the transcriptional activation of endothelial cell adhesion molecules as well as leukocyte adhesion[83]. Proteasome inhibitors also induce cell cycle arrest and apoptosis[84], making them potentially useful agents in the treatment of proliferative diseases. Note, however, that tyrosine phosphorylation of IκB at Tyr-42 has been reported to induce IκB dissociation and NF-κB activation by a mechanism not involving the proteolytic degradation of IκB[85], and inhibitors of IκB degradation would not be expected to block NF-κB activation via this mechanism.

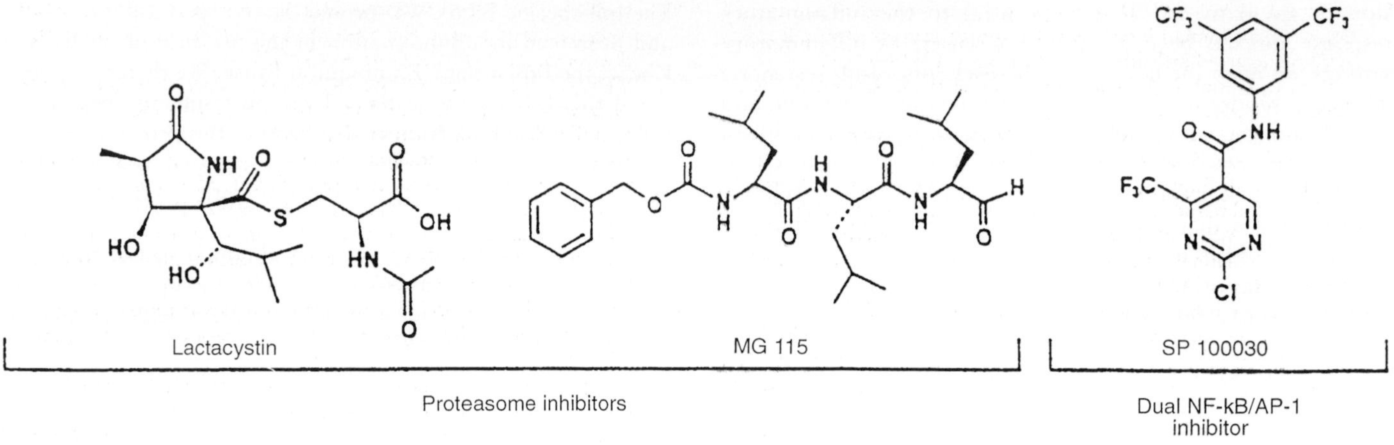

Fig. 44.6 Representative inhibitors of NF-κB.

Inflammatory reactions are generally accompanied by the local production of reactive oxygen metabolites, including hydroxy and nitroxy radicals, hydrogen peroxide, and superoxide. Although the exact role of these metabolites in the pathogenesis of inflammatory disease is controversial, there is extensive evidence for their role as second messengers regulating NF-κB expression[86] and Ras-mediated mitogenesis[87]. Reactive oxygen activates NF-κB in cultured cells, and antioxidants such as pyrrolidone dithiocarbamate (PDTC) can inhibit NF-κB activation by a range of stimuli[88]. Several antioxidants have been tested *in vivo* and found to modulate NF-κB activation and endothelial cell adhesion molecule gene transcription[89]. It should be noted, however, that antioxidants exert a plethora of effects on cells, inlcuding activation of MAP kinases and other transcription factors such as AP-1[90-92]. It is unlikely that antioxidants could be developed as specific inhibitors of NF-κB activation, although their potential as anti-inflammatory agents may be realized because of their pleotropic effects on inflammatory gene expression.

Dual NF-κB and AP-1 inhibitors

A novel class of T cell-specific inhibitors of NF-κB and AP-1 activity was recently identified in a cell-based screening effort to identify modulators of inflammatory gene expression[77,93]. The most potent inhibitor in this series, SP100030, inhibits NF-@κB- and AP-1- dependent reporter gene expression in stably-transfected Jurkat T cells with an IC50 of 30 nM. In stimulated Jurkat T Cells, SP100030 inhibited the induced transcription of the IL-2, IL-8, TNF-α, and GM-CSF genes with a similar IC50. The effects of SP100030 were specific for human T cells, demonstrating activity in four separate T cell lines and in primary T cells isolated from whole human blood. SP100030 displayed no activity in non-T cell lines, including monocytes, epithelial cells, fibroblasts, synoviocytes, osteoblasts, and endothelial cells. SP100030 demonstrated efficacy in preclinical models of autoimmune disease, including adjuvant-induced arthritis, delayed type hypersensitivity, inflammatory bowel disease, and

allograft rejection[94]. SP100030 represents a new class of T cell specific dual inhibitors of NF-κB and AP-1 mediated inflammatory gene expression, and suggests that cell-specific inhibitors of inflammatory gene expression can indeed be identified. An interesting implication, possibly related to the cross-regulation of NF-κB and AP-1 activity by MAP kinase pathways, is that T cells possess a common target protein that controls the functions of both NF-κB and AP-1.

Future prospects

Insights into the molecular mechanism underlying inflammatory disease have highlighted the role so signal transduction and gene expression in joint inflammation and erosion. A multitude of signal transduction pathways and transcription factors have been identified, and many of them represent attractive drug discovery targets. The small molecules discussed herein are likely to represent only the first of many inhibitors to be identified from drug discovery efforts. Key challenges for the future will include the successful transition of these early stage compounds into viable drugs. Issues such as safety and tolerability will be of paramount importance if such agents are to be useful additions to the rheumatologist's therapeutic armament. Virtually every major pharmaceutical company is pursuing these agents, and it is anticipated that these concerted efforts will eventually bear fruit.

References

1. Fieldmann M. *et al*. Rheumatoid arthritis. *Cell* 1996;**85**:307.
2. Firestein G.S. Cytokine networks in rheumatoid arthritis: implications for therapy. *Agents Actions* 1995;**S47**:37.
3. Arend W.P., Dayer J. Inhibition of the production and effects of interleukin-1 and tumor necrosis factor a in rheumatoid arthritis. *Arthritis Rheum* 1995;**38**:151.
4. Elliott M.J. *et al*. Treatment of rheumatoid arthritis with chimeric monoclonal antibodies to tumor necrosis factor alpha. *Arthritis Rheum* 1993;**12**:1681.

5. Campion G.V. *et al.* Dose-range and dose-frequency study of recombinant human interleukin-1 receptor antagonist in patients with rheumatoid arthritis. *Arthritis Rheum* 1996;**39**:1092.

6. Carlos T., Harlan J.M. Leukocyte-endothelial adhesion molecules. *Blood* 1994;**84**:2068.

7. Johnson B.A. *et al.* Adhesion molecule expression in human synovial tissue. *Arthritis Rheum* 1993;**36**:137

8. Tak P.P. et al. Expression of adhesion nolecules in early rheumatoid synovial tissue. *Clin Immunol Immunopathol* 1995;**77**:236.

9. Kavanaugh A.F. *et al.* Treatment of refractory rheumatoid arthritis with a monoclonal antibody to intercellular adhesion molecule 1. *Arthritis Rheum* 37:992

10. Isis positive Crohn' s disease trial. *SCRIP* 1997;**2212**:23

11. Tak P.P. *et al.* Decrease in cellularity and expression of adhesion molecules by anti-tumor necrosis factor a monoclonal antibody treatment in patients with rheumatoid arthritis. *Arthritis Rheum* **39**:1077.

12. Lewis A.J., Keft A.F. A review on the strategies for the development and application of new anti-arthritic agents. *Immunopharm Immunotoxicol* 1995;**17**:607.

13. Seibert K. *et al.* Pharmacological and biochemcial demonstration of the role of cyclooxygenase 2 in inflammation and pain. *Proc Nat Acad Sci USA* 1994;**91**:12013.

14. Firestein G.S. *et al.* Gene expression (collagenase, tissue inhibitor of metalloproteinases, complement, and HLA-DR) in rheumatoid arthritis and osteoarthritis synovium: Quantitative analysis and effect of intraarticular corticosteroids. *Arthritis Rheum* 1994;**34**:1094.

15. Schena M. *et al.* Parallel human genome analysis: microarray-based expression monitoring of 1000 genes. *Proc Nat Acad Sci USA* 1996;**93**:10614.

16. Heller R.A. *et al.* Discovery and analysis of inflammatory disease-related genes using cDNA microarrays. *Proc Nat Acad Sci USA* 1997;**94**:2150.

17. Karin M., Hunter T. Transcriptional control by protein phosphorylation: signal transmission from the cell surface to the nucleus. *Curr Biol.* 1995;**5**:747.

18. Mobley J.L. *et al.* Glucocorticosteroids, old and new: biological function and use in the treatment of asthma. *Exp Opn Invest Drugs* 1996;**5**:871.

19. Rosen J. *et al.* Intracellular receptors and signal transducers of transcription superfamilies: novel targets for small molecule drug discovery. *J Med Chem* 1995;**38**:4855.

20. Mangelsdorf D.J. *et al.* The nuclear receptor superfamily: the second decade. *Cell* 1995;**83**:835.

21. Cato A.C.B., Wade E. Molecular mechanisms of anti-inflammatory action of glucocorticoids. *BioEssays* 1996;**18**:371.

22. Lenardo M.J., Baltimore D. NF-κB:A pleiotropic mediator of inducible and tissue-specific gene control. *Cell* 1989;**58**:227.

23. Baeuerle P.A., Henkel T. Function and activation of NF-κB in the immune system. *Annu Rev Immunol*, 1994;**12**:141.

24. Manning A.M., Anderson D.C. Transcription factor NF-κB: an emerging regulator of inflammation. *Annu Rep Med Chem* 1994;**29**:235.

25. Auphan N. *et al.* Immunosuppression by glucocorticoids: inhibition of NF-κB activity through induction of IκB-α synthesis. *Science* 1995;**270**:286.

26. Scheinman R.I. *et al.* Role of transcriptional activation of IκB-α in mediation of the immunosuppression by glucocorticoids. *Science* 1995;**270**:283.

27. Angel P., Karin M. The role of Jun, Fos and the AP-1 complex in cell proliferation and transformation. *Biochim Biophys Acta* 1991;**1072**:129.

28. Manning A.M., Lewis A.J. Transcription factors, rheumatoid arthritis and the search for improved antirheumatic agents. *Rheum Arth* 1997;**1**:65.

29. Stein B, Andersen D. The MAP kinase family: new "MAPs" for signal transduction pathways and novel targets for drug discovery. *Ann Rep Med Chem* 1996;**31**:289.

30. Heck S. *et al.* A distinct modulating domain in glucocorticoid receptor monomers in the repression of activity of the transcription factor AP-1. *EMBO J* 1994;**13**:4087.

31. Webster, N.J.G. *et al.* The hormone-binding domains of the estrogen and glucocorticoid receptors contain an inducible transcription activation function. *Cell* 1988;**54**:199.

32. Shaw K.T. *et al.* Immunosuppressive drugs prevent a rapid dephosphorylation of transcription factor NFAT1 in stimulated immune cells, *Proc Nat Acad Sci USA* 1995;**92**:11205.

33. Luo C. *et al.* Interaction of calcineurin with a domain of the transcription factor NFAT, that controls nuclear import. *Proc Nat Acad Sci USA* 1996;**93**:8907.

34. Rao A. (1994) NF-ATp: a transcription factor required for the coordinate induction of several cytokine genes. *Immunol Today* 15:274.

35. Liu J. *et al.* Calcineurin is a common target for cyclophilin-cyclosporin A and FKBP-FK506 complex. *Cell* 1991;**66**:807.

36. Sewell T.J. *et al.* Inhibition of calcineurin by a novel FK506-binding protein. *J Biol Chem* 1994;**269**:21094.

37. Bram J. *et al.* Identification of the immunophilins capable of mediating inhibition of signal transduction by cyclosporin A and FK506: role of calcineurin binding and cellular location. *Mol Cell Biol* 1993;**13**:4760.

38. Pasero G. *et al.* Slow progression of joint damage in early onset rheumatoid arthritis treated with cyclosporin A. *Arth Rheum* 1996;**39**:1006.

39. Dumont F.J. *et al.* The immunosuppressive and toxic effects of FK-506 are mechanistically related: pharmacology of a novel antagonist of FK-506 and rapamycin. *J Exp Med* 1992;**176**:751.

40. Howe LR, Weiss A. Multiple kinase mediate T cell receptor signaling. *Trends Biochem Sci* 1995;**20**:59.

41. Shibasaki F. *et al.* Role of kinases nd the phosphatase calcineurin in the nuclear shuttling of transcription factor NFAT4. *Nature* 1996;**382**:370.

42. Foletta V.C. *et al.* Transcriptional regulation in the immune system: all roads leads to AP-1 *J Leukoc Biol* 1998;**63**:139.

43. Rao A. *et al.* Transcriptional factors of the NFAT family: regulation and function. *Ann Rev Immunol* 1997;**15**:707.

44. Su B., Karin M. Mitogen-activated protein kinase cascades and the regulation of gene expression. *Curr Opin Immunol* 1996;**8**:402.

45. Whitmarsh A.J., Davis R.J. Transcription factor AP-1 regulation by mitogen-activated protein kinase signal transduction pathways. *J Molec Med* 1996;**74**:589.

46. Fanger G.R. *et al.* MEKKs, GCKs, MLKs, PAKs, TAKs, and Tpls: upstream regulators of the c-Jun amino-terminal kinases? *Curr Opin Genet Devel* 1997;**7**:67.

47. Kallunki T. *et al.* JNK2 contains a specificity-determining region responsible for efficient c-Jun binding and phosphorylation. *Genes Dev* 1994;**8**:2996.

48. Dickens M. *et al.* A cytoplasmic inhibitor of the JNK signal transduction pathway. *Science* 1997;**277**:693.

49. Whtimarsh A.J. Integration of MAP kinase signal transduction pathways at the serum response element. *Science* 1995;**269**:403.

50. Su B. *et al.* JNK is involved in signal integration during co-stimulation of T lymphocytes. *Cell* 1994;**77**:727.

51. Yang D.D. *et al.* Differentiation of CD4+ T cells of Th1 cells requires MAP kinase JNK2. *Immunity* 1998;**9**:575.

52. Yang D. *et al.* Absence of excitotoxicity-induced apoptosis in the hippocampus of mice lacking the JNK3 gene. *Nature* 1997;**389**:865.

53. Xie X. *et al. Structure* 1998;**6**:983.

54. Dudley D.T. *et al.* A synthetic inhibitor of the mitogen-activated protein kinase cascade. *Proc Nat Acad Sci USA* 1995;**95**:7686.

55. Favata M.F. *et al.* Identification of a novel inhibitor of MAP kinase kinase. *J Biol Chem* 1998;**273**:18:623.

56. Williams D.H. *et al.* Ro 09-2210 exhibits potent anti-proliferative effects on activated T cells by selectively blocking MKK activity. *Biochem* 1998;**37**:9579.

57. Lee J.C. *et al*. A protein kinase involved in the regulation of inflammatory cytokine biosynthesis. *Nature* 1994;**372**:39.

58. Badger A.M. *et al*. Pharmacological profile of SB203590, a selective inhibitor of cytokine suppressive binding protein/p38 kinase, in animal models of arthritis, bone resorption, endotoxin shock and immune function. *J Pharmacol Exp Ther* 1996;**279**:1453.

59. Tong L. *et al*. A highly specific inhibitor of human p38 MAP kinase binds in the ATP packet. *Nature Struct Biol* 1997;**4**:311.

60. Eyers P.A. *et al*. Conversion of SB203580 insensitive MAP kinase family members to drug-sensitive forms by a single amino acid substitution. *Chem Biol* 1998;**5**:321.

61. De Losazlo E. *et al*. Pyrroles and other heterocycles as inhibitors of p38 kinase. *J Bioinorg Med Chem* 1998;**8**:2689.

62. Wilson K.P. *et al*. Structural basis for specificity of pyridinylimidazole inhibitors of p38 MAP kinases. *Chem Biol* 1997;**4**:423.

63. Henry J. R. *et al*. 6-amino-2-(4-fluorphenyl)-4-methoxy-3-(4-pyridyl)-1H-pyrrolo[2,3-b]pyridine (RWJ 68354): a potent and selective p38 kinase inhibitor. *J Med Chem* 1998;**4**:4196.

64. Baeuerle P.A., Baichwal V.R. Activation and function of NF-κB in the immune system. *Adv Immunol* 1997;**65**:111.

65. Manning A.M. NF-κB as a drug discovery target. *Curr Opin Drug Disc Dev* 1998;**1**:147.

66. Manning A.M., Anderson D.C. NF-κB: An emerging regulator of inflammation. *Ann Rep Med Chem* 1994;**29**:235.

67. Regnier C.H. *et al*. Identification and characterization of an IκB Kinase. *Cell* 1997;**90**:373.

68. DiDonato J.A. *et al*. A cytokine-responsive IκB kinase that activates the transcription factor NF-κB. *Nature* 1997;**388**:853.

69. Zandi E. *et al*. The IκB kinase complex (IKK) contains two kinase subunits, IKKα and IKKβ, necessary for IκB phosphorylation and NF-κB activation. *Cell* 1997;**91**:243.

70. Mercurio F. *et al*. IKK-1 and IKK-2: Cytokine-activated IκB kinases essential for NF-κB activation. *Science* 1997;**278**:860.

71. Woronicz J.D. *et al*. IκB kinase-β: NF-κB activation and complex formation with IκB kinase-α and NIK. *Science* 1997;**278**:866.

72. Chen Z. *et al*. Signal-induced site-specific phosphorylation targets IκB-α to the ubiquitin-proteasome pathway. *Genes Dev* 1995;**9**:1586.

73. Malini N.L. *et al*. MAP3K-related kinase involved in NF-κB induction by TNF, CD95 and IL-1. *Nature* 1997;**385**:540.

74. Lee F.S. *et al*. Activation of the IκBα complex by MEKK1, a kinase of the JNK pathway. *Cell* 1997;**88**:1586.

75. Yaron A. *et al*. Identification of the receptor component of the IκB-α ubiquitin ligase. *Nature* 1998;**396**:590.

76. Baichwal V.J., Baeuerle P.A. TNF signal transduction cascades. *Ann Rep Med Chem* 1998;**33**:233.

77. Manning, A.M., Mercurio F. Transcription inhibitors in inflammation. *Exp Opin Invest Drugs* 1997;**6**:555.

78. Baeuerle PA, Baichwal VR. NF-κB as a frequent target for immunosuppressive and anti-inflammatory molecules. *Adv Immunol* 1997;**65**:111.

79. Fenteany G.F. *et al*. Inhibition of proteasome activities and subunit-specific amino-terminal threonine modification by lactacystin. *Science* 1995;**268**:726.

80. Omura S. *et al*. Lactacystin, a novel microbial metabolite, induces neuritogenesis of neuroblastoma cells. @2J Antibiot 1991;**44**:113.

81. Palomella V.J., Rando O.L., Goldberg A.L., Maniatis T. The ubiquitin-proteasome pathway is required for processing the NF-κB1 precursor protein and the activation of NF-κB. *Cell* 1994;**78**:773.

82. Traenckner B-M.E., Wilk S., Baeuerle P.A. A proteasome inhibitor prevents NF-κB activation and stabilizes a newly phosphorylated form of Iκ-Bα that is still bound to NF-κB. *EMBO J* 1995;**13**:5433.

83. Read M.A., *et al*. The proteasome pathway is required for cytokine-induced endothelial leukocyte adhesion molecule expression. *Immunity* 1995;**2**:493.

84. Maki C.G., Huibregtse J.M., Howley P.M. In vivo ubiquitination and proteasome-mediated degradation of p53. *Cancer Res* 1996;**6**:2649.

85. Imbert V. *et al*. Tyrosine phosphorylation of IκB-α activates NF-κB without proteolytic degradation of IκB-α. *Cell* 1996;**86**:787.

86. Schreck R., Rieber P., Baeuerle P.A. Reactive oxyen intermediates as apparently widely used messengers in the activation of the NF-κB transcription factor and HIV-1. *EMBO J* 1991;**10**:2247.

87. Irani K., Xia Y., Zweier J.L. *et al*. Mitogenic signaling mediated by oxidants in Ras-transformed fibroblasts. *Science* 1997;**275**:1649.

88. Ziegler-Heitbrock H.W.L. *et al*. Pyrrolidine dithiocarbamate inhibits NF-κB mobilization and TNF production in human monocytes. *J Immunol* 1993;**151**:6986.

89. Gerritsen M.E. *et al*. Flavonoids inhibit cytokine-induced endothelial cell adhesion protein gene expression. *Am J Pathol* 1995;**147**:278.

90. Coso O.A., Chiariello M., Yu J.C. *et al*. The small GTP-binding proteins Rac1 and Cdc42 regulate the activity of the JNK/SAPK signaling pathway. *Cell* 1995;**81**:1137.

91. Meyer M., Schreck R., Baeuerle P.A. H2O2 and antioxidants have opposite effects on activation of NF-kappa B and AP-1 in intact cells: AP-1 as secondary antioxidant-responsive factor. *EMBO J* 1993;**12**:2005.

92. Gomez del Arco P. *et al*. JNK is a target for antioxidants in T lymphocytes. *J Biol Vhem* 1996;**271**:26335.

93. Sullivan R.W. *et al*. 2-chloro-4-trifluoromethyl-pyridine-5-N-carboxamide: a potent inhibitor of NF-κB and AP-1-mediated gene expression identified using solution phase combinatorial chemistry. *J Med Chem* 1998;**4**:413.

94. Goldman M.E. *et al*. SP100030 is a novel T-cell-specific transcription factor inhibitor that possesses immunosuppressive activity in vivo. *Trans Proc* 1996;**28**:3106.

Index

Page numbers in **bold** indicate main discussion, those in *italic* refer to figures and tables.